BNF 39

MARCH 2000

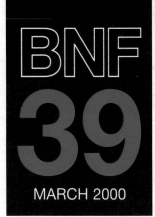

BRITISH NATIONAL FORMULARY

British Medical Association

Royal Pharmaceutical Society of Great Britain

Published by the British Medical Association
Tavistock Square, London WC1H 9JP, UK
and the **Royal Pharmaceutical Society of Great Britain**
1 Lambeth High Street, London, SE1 7JN, UK

© 2000 British Medical Association and the Royal Pharmaceutical Society of Great Britain

ISBN: 0 85369 462 1

ISSN: 0260-535X

Printed in Great Britain by Bemrose Security Printing, Derby

Copies may be obtained through any bookseller or direct from the publishers:

BMJ Books
PO Box 295
London WC1H 9TE
UK
Tel: +44 (0) 20 7383 6185/6245
Fax: +44 (0) 20 7383 6662
E-mail: orders@bmjbookshop.com
www.bmjbookshop.com

Pharmaceutical Press
PO Box 151
Wallingford
Oxon OX10 8QU
UK
Tel: +44 (0) 1491 829272
Fax:+44 (0) 1491 829292
E-mail: rpsgb@cabi.org
www.pharmpress.com

For a list of name changes required by Directive 92/27/EEC, see p. x

Contents

Preface

The BNF is a joint publication of the British Medical Association and the Royal Pharmaceutical Society of Great Britain. It is published under the authority of a Joint Formulary Committee which comprises representatives of the two professional bodies and of the Department of Health. The BNF aims to provide doctors, pharmacists and other healthcare professionals with sound up-to-date information about the use of medicines.

The BNF presents, in a readily accessible way, key information on the prescribing, dispensing and administration of medicines. It is designed to provide clear guidance on the selection of medicines. All drugs that are generally prescribed in the UK are included and those that are considered less suitable for prescribing are clearly identified. Little or no information is included on medicines that are promoted for purchase by the public.

Basic information about drugs is drawn from the manufacturers' product literature, from medical and pharmaceutical literature, from regulatory and professional authorities, and from the data used for pricing prescriptions. Advice on the therapeutic use of medicines and on the choice of drugs is constructed from clinical literature and reflects, wherever possible, an evaluation of the evidence. In addition, the Joint Formulary Committee receives expert clinical advice on all therapeutic areas, particularly those that are not yet supported by good evidence; this ensures that the BNF's recommendations are relevant to practice. Many individuals and organisations contribute towards the preparation of each edition of the BNF.

The BNF is designed as a digest for rapid reference and it may not always include all the information necessary for prescribing and dispensing. Also, less detail is given in the BNF on areas such as obstetrics, malignant disease, and anaesthesia since it is expected that those undertaking treatment will have specialist knowledge and access to specialist literature. The BNF should therefore be supplemented as necessary by specialised publications and by reference to the manufacturers' product literature. Information is also available from local drug information services (see inside front cover).

Biannual publication allows the BNF to reflect promptly changes in product availability as well as emerging safety concerns and shifts in clinical practice. The more important changes for this edition are listed on p. viii.

Electronic versions of the BNF—including intranet versions—are produced in parallel with the paper version. An internet version is being developed.

> The BNF welcomes comments from healthcare professionals; such comments help to ensure that the BNF remains relevant to practice. Comments and constructive criticism should be sent to:
>
> Executive Editor, British National Formulary,
> c/o Royal Pharmaceutical Society of Great Britain,
> 1 Lambeth High Street, London SE1 7JN.
> Email: editor@bnf.rpsgb.org.uk

Acknowledgements

The Joint Formulary Committee is grateful to individuals and organisations that have provided advice and information to the BNF.

The principal contributors for this edition were:

J.M. Aitken, S.P. Allison, F.H. Anderson,
D.G. Arkell, T.P. Baglin, R.H. Behrens,
D.T. Beswick, D. Bowsher, R.J. Buckley, I. Burgess,
A.J. Camm, D.A. Chamberlain, C. Cooper,
W.A.M. Cutting, C. Diamond, R. Dinwiddie,
G.H. Elder, T.S.J. Elliott, B.G. Gazzard,
A.M. Geddes, A.H. Ghodse, P.W. Golightly,
E.C. Gordon-Smith, M.W. Greaves, I.A. Greer,
J. Guillebaud, C.H. Hawkes, C.J. Hawkey,
D.F. Hawkins, A.A. Jackson, S.H. Jackson,
R.M. Jones, J.A. Kanis, J.R. Kirwan,
P.G. Kopelman, M. Lader, M.J.S. Langman,
T.H. Lee, J. Leese, P.N. Leigh, L. Luzzatto,
G.M. Mead, J.M. Neuberger, A.J. Nunn, D.J. Oliver,
L.P. Ormerod, P.A. Poole-Wilson, R.E. Pounder,
L.E. Ramsay, F. Reynolds, P.A. Routledge,
P.C. Rubin, D.M. Salisbury, R.S. Sawers,
M.C. Sheppard, S.D. Shorvon, T. Sizer, P. Sleight,
I. Stockley, M. Summerhayes, A.E. Tattersfield,
R.N. Thin, H. Thomas, S. Thomas, G.R. Thompson,
J.H. Tripp, D.G. Waller, D.A. Warrell, P.J. Watkins,
G.B. Wyatt.

Members of the British Association of Dermatologists Therapy Guidelines and Audit Subcommittee, C.E.M. Griffiths (chairman), A.V. Anstey, C.B. Bunker, N.H. Cox, K.L. Dalziel, M.R. Judge, H.C. Williams and E.J.M. Rehm (Secretariat) have provided valuable advice.

Correspondents in the pharmaceutical industry have provided information on new products and commented on products in the BNF. The Prescription Pricing Authority has provided the prices of drugs in the BNF.

Numerous doctors, pharmacists, nurses and others have sent comments and suggestions.

The BNF has valuable access to the *Martindale* data banks by courtesy of the *Martindale* staff. A.B. Prasad has once again provided valuable comments.

S.M. Townsend-Smith has assisted with the processing of data on interactions. E.J. Laughton and L.J. Whitley have also provided considerable assistance during the production of this edition of the BNF.

E.I. Connor has assisted with the development of the electronic BNF. P.D. Johnson and B. Thomas of Quartet Software have provided technical assistance and have continued to support the production of the electronic BNF. M. Bagley and C. Elmes have assisted with the production of illustrations in the BNF.

Joint Formulary Committee 1999–2000

Chairman
Sir Charles George
BSc, MD, FRCP, FFPM

Deputy Chairman
Nicholas L. Wood
BPharm, FRPharmS

Committee Members
Alison Blenkinsopp
PhD, BPharm, MRPharmS

Peter Clappison
MB, ChB, MRCGP

Doreen Hepburn
BSc, FRPharmS, MCPP

Frank P. Marsh
MA, MB, BChir, FRCP

Helen St.C. Remington
MPharm, BSc, DMS, MRPharmS

Jane Richards
*OBE, MB BS, MRCS, LRCP, FRCGP,
D(Obst)RCOG, DCH*

James Smith
BPharm, PhD, FRPharmS, MCPP, MIInfSc

Robert M. Weatherstone
MA, MB, BChir, FRCP

Joint Secretaries
José L. García de Ancos
LMS, MSc(Econ)

James E. F. Reynolds
PhD, FRPharmS

Executive Secretary
Susan M. Thomas
BSc(Econ), MA

Editorial Staff

Executive Editor
Dinesh K. Mehta
BPharm, MSc, MRPharmS

Senior Assistant Editor
John Martin
BPharm, PhD, MRPharmS

Staff Editors
Harriet K. L. Blackley
BPharm, MRPharmS

Stephen G. Coleman
BPharm, MRPharmS

Parastou Donyai
BPharm, PhD, MRPharmS

Bryony Jordan
BSc, DipPharmPract, MRPharmS

Rachel S. M. Ryan
BPharm, MRPharmS

Shama M. S. Wagle
BPharm, DipPharmPract, MRPharmS

Editorial Assistants
Gerard P. Gallagher

Louise M. E. Wykes
BSc

How to use the BNF

Notes on conditions, drugs and preparations

The main text consists of classified notes on clinical conditions, drugs and preparations. These notes are divided into 15 chapters, each of which is related to a particular system of the body or to an aspect of medical care. Each chapter is then divided into sections which begin with appropriate *notes for prescribers*. These notes are intended to provide information to doctors, pharmacists, nurses, and other healthcare professionals to facilitate the selection of suitable treatment. The notes are followed by details of relevant drugs and preparations.

Guidance on prescribing

This part includes information on prescription writing, controlled drugs and dependence, prescribing for children and the elderly, and prescribing in palliative care. Advice is given on the reporting of adverse reactions.

Emergency treatment of poisoning

This chapter provides information on the management of acute poisoning when first seen in the home, although aspects of hospital-based treatment are mentioned.

Appendixes and indexes

The appendixes include information on interactions, liver disease, renal impairment, pregnancy, breast-feeding, intravenous additives, borderline substances, appliances, wound management products, and cautionary and advisory labels for dispensed medicines. They are designed for use in association with the main body of the text.

The Dental Practitioners' List and the Nurse Prescribers' List are also included in this section. The indexes consist of the Index of Manufacturers and the Main Index.

DRUG NAME ◤ ●

Indications: details of uses and indications

Cautions: details of precautions required (with cross-references to appropriate Appendixes) and also any monitoring required

COUNSELLING. Verbal explanation to the patient of specific details of the drug treatment (e.g. posture when taking a medicine)

Contra-indications: details of any contra-indications to use of drug

Side-effects: details of common and more serious side-effects

Dose: dose and frequency of administration (max. dose). CHILD and ELDERLY details of dose for specific age group

By alternative route, dose and frequency

*Approved Name (Non-proprietary) PoM ●
Pharmaceutical form, colour, coating, active ingredient and amount in dosage form, net price, pack size = basic NHS price. Label: (as in Appendix 9)

Proprietary Name® (Manufacturer) PoM NHS ●
Pharmaceutical form, sugar-free, active ingredient mg/mL, net price, pack size = basic NHS price. Label: (as in Appendix 9)
Excipients: includes clinically important excipients or electrolytes
* exceptions to the prescribing status indicated by a footnote.
Note. Specific notes about the product e.g. handling

Drugs

Drugs appear under pharmacopoeial or other non-proprietary titles. When there is an *appropriate current monograph* (Medicines Act 1968, Section 65) preference is given to a name at the head of that monograph; otherwise a British Approved Name (BAN), if available, is used (see also p. x).

The symbol ◤ is used to denote those preparations that are considered by the Joint Formulary Committee to be less suitable for prescribing. Although such preparations may not be considered as drugs of first choice, their use may be justifiable in certain circumstances.

Prescription-only medicines PoM

This symbol has been placed against those preparations that are available only on medical or dental prescription. For more detailed information see *Medicines, Ethics and Practice*, No. 23, London, Pharmaceutical Press, 2000 (and subsequent editions as available).

The symbol CD indicates that the preparation is subject to the prescription requirements of the Misuse of Drugs Act. For regulations governing prescriptions for such preparations see pages 7-9.

Preparations not available for NHS prescription NHS

This symbol has been placed against those preparations included in the BNF that are not prescribable under the NHS. Those prescribable only for specific disorders have a footnote specifying the condition(s) for which the preparation remains available. Some preparations which are not *prescribable* by brand name under the NHS may nevertheless be *dispensed* using the brand name providing that the prescription shows an appropriate non-proprietary name.

Preparations

Preparations usually follow immediately after the drug which is their main ingredient.

Preparations are included under a non-proprietary title, if they are marketed under such a title, or if they are not otherwise prescribable under the NHS, or if they may be prepared extemporaneously.

If proprietary preparations are of a distinctive colour this is stated.

In the case of compound preparations the indications, cautions, contra-indications, side-effects, and interactions of all constituents should be taken into account for prescribing.

Prices

Prices have been calculated from the basic cost used in pricing NHS prescriptions dispensed in October 1999 or later, see p. vii for further details.

Patient Packs

On January 1 1994, Directive 92/27/EEC came into force, outlining requirements for the labelling of medicines and for the format and content of patient information leaflets to be supplied with each medicine.

All medicines now have approved labelling and patient information leaflets; anyone who supplies a medicine is responsible for providing the relevant information to the patient.

Many medicines are available in manufacturers' original packs complete with patient information leaflets. Where patient packs are available, the BNF shows the number of dose units in the packs. In particular clinical circumstances, where patient packs need to be split or medicines are provided in bulk dispensing packs, manufacturers will provide additional supplies of patient information leaflets on request.

During the revision of each edition of the BNF careful note is taken of the information that appears on the patient information leaflets. Where it is considered appropriate to alert a prescriber to some specific limitation appearing on the patient information leaflet (for example, in relation to pregnancy) this advice now appears in the BNF.

The patient information leaflet also includes details of all inactive ingredients in the medicine. A list of common E numbers and the inactive ingredients to which they correspond is now therefore included in the BNF (see inside back cover).

PACT and SPA

PACT (Prescribing Analyses and Cost) and SPA (Scottish Prescribing Analysis) automatically provide general practitioners with information about their prescribing. The information is sent on a quarterly basis direct from the Prescription Pricing Authority (and may be obtained for individual months on request). It is now available as a 'standard report' which replaces the previous *level 1* and *level 2 reports*. The previous *level 3 report* is replaced by a 'catalogue' which provides the data in a more helpful manner and is available on request for periods of one or more months.

Prices in the BNF

Basic **net prices** are given in the BNF to provide an indication of relative cost. Where there is a choice of suitable preparations for a particular disease or condition the relative cost may be used in making a selection. Cost-effective prescribing must, however, take into account other factors (such as dose frequency and duration of treatment) that affect the total cost. The use of more expensive drugs is justified if it will result in better treatment of the patient or a reduction of the length of an illness or the time spent in hospital.

Prices have generally been calculated from the net cost used in pricing NHS prescriptions dispensed in October 1999, but where available later prices have been included; unless an original pack is available these prices are based on the largest pack size of the preparation in use in community pharmacies. The price for an extemporaneously prepared preparation has been omitted where the net cost of the ingredients used to make it would give a misleadingly low impression of the final price.

The unit of 20 is still sometimes used as a basis for comparison, but where suitable original packs or patient packs are available these are priced instead.

Gross prices vary as follows:
1. Costs to the NHS are greater than the net prices quoted and include professional fees and overhead allowances;
2. Private prescription charges are calculated on a separate basis;
3. Over-the-counter sales are at retail price, as opposed to basic net price, and include VAT.

BNF prices are NOT, therefore, suitable for quoting to patients seeking private prescriptions or contemplating over-the-counter purchases.

A fuller explanation of costs to the NHS may be obtained from the Drug Tariff.

It should be noted that separate Drug Tariffs are applicable to England and Wales, Scotland, and Northern Ireland. Prices in the different tariffs may vary.

Changes

The BNF is revised twice yearly and numerous changes are made between issues. All copies of BNF No. 38 (September 1999) should therefore be withdrawn and replaced by BNF No. 39 (March 2000). Significant changes have been made in the following sections for BNF No. 39:

Taking medicines to best effect [new text], Guidance on prescribing
Antihypertensive therapy [revised text], section 2.5
Advice on antibacterial therapy for sexually transmitted infections [revised text], table 1, section 5.1
Influenza [new text], section 5.3
Viral hepatitis [new text], section 5.3
Osteoporosis [new text], section 6.6
Emergency contraception [revised text], section 7.3.1
Cytotoxic drugs [reorganisation], section 8.1
Vitamin K [revised text], section 9.6.6
Corticosteroids for the eye [revised text], section 11.4.1
Anogenital warts [revised text], section 13.7
Preparations for warts and calluses [revised text], section 13.7

Dose changes

Changes in dose statements introduced into BNF No. 39:

Begrivac®, p. 549
Camcolit®, p. 184
Cefotaxime, p. 259
Dihydroergotamine mesilate, p. 219
Doxycycline, p. 264
Fluvirin®, p. 549
Fucidin®, p. 270
Glipizide, p. 320
Inactivated influenza vaccine (split viron), p. 549
Metronidazole [rectal], p. 279
Premique® Cycle, p. 335
Procaine benzylpenicillin/Procaine penicillin, p. 253
Vigabatrin, p. 229

Classification Changes

Classification changes have been made in the following sections for BNF No. 39:

Section 5.1.1.5 Mecillinams [section re-introduced]
Section 5.3 Amantadine [moved from herpes section to influenza section]
Section 7.5 [title no longer exists]
Section 8.1 Calcium folinate and calcium levofolinate [moved from section 8.1.3]
Section 8.1 Mesna [moved from section 8.1.1]
Section 8.1 Amifostine [moved from section 9.1.6]
Section 13.7 Anogenital warts [title change]
Section 13.11.7 Preparations for promotion of wound healing [title change]

New names

Name changes introduced into BNF No. 39 (see also p. x):

Spasmonal Fibre® [formerly *Alvercol*®], p. 35
Duraphat® [formerly *Fluorigard*® weekly dental rinse], p. 436
Co-cyprindiol [new British Approved Name for cyproterone acetate with ethinylestradiol], p. 522

Discontinued preparations

Preparations discontinued during the compilation of BNF No. 39:

Atromid-S®
Blocadren®
Cobadex®
Dalacin C® paediatric suspension
Decadron Shock-Pak®
Double Check®
Dyspamet Chewtab®
Edecrin®
Femeron®
Fleet® *Micro-enema*
Fluzone®
Gyne T 380®
Innovace Melt®
Metosyn® scalp lotion
Migravess®
Mysoline® oral suspension
Nizoral® suspension
Ophthaine®
Pendramine®
Prepidil®
Prostin F2 alpha®
Raxar®
Robaxin® injection
Ronicol®
Saluric®
Securopen®
Soframycin® ointment
Spiroctan-M®
Sulfadimidine
Timecef®
Triludan®
Trobicin®
Tryptizol®
Ukidan®
Urokinase®
Vancocin® 250 mg vials
Ventolin® aerosol inhalation [replaced by *Ventolin Evohaler*®]
Wellferon®
Z Span®

Late additions

Ammonaps® (Orphan Europe) ▼ PoM

Granules, sodium phenylbutyrate 940 mg/g, net price 266-g pack = £860.00.

Tablets, sodium phenylbutyrate 500 mg, net price 250-tab pack = £493.00. BNF section 9.8.1

For the treatment of urea cycle disorders (under specialist supervision)

Aromasin® (Pharmacia & Upjohn) ▼ PoM

Tablets, s/c, exemestane 25 mg, net price 15-tab pack = £51.43, 30-tab pack = £102.86, 90-tab pack = £308.58. BNF section 8.3.4.1

For the treatment of advanced breast cancer in post-menopausal women whose disease has progressed despite anti-oestrogen therapy

Cardicor® (Merck) ▼ PoM

Tablets, f/c, bisoprolol fumarate 1.25 mg, net price 28-tab pack = £8.56; 2.5 mg (scored), 28-tab pack = £8.56; 3.75 mg (scored, white-yellow), 28-tab pack = £8.56; 5 mg (scored, light yellow), 28-tab pack = £8.56; 7.5 mg (scored, yellow), 28-tab pack = £9.09; 10 mg (scored, orange), 28-tab pack = £9.61. BNF section 2.4

For stable moderate to severe heart failure, as an adjunct to treatment with an ACE inhibitor, a diuretic and possibly a cardiac glycoside (under specialist supervision)

GyneFix® (Contrel) PoM

GyneFix® IN, intra-uterine device, 6 copper sleeves with surface area of 330 mm² on polypropylene thread, net price = £24.75. BNF section 7.3.4

For use as an intra-uterine contraceptive

GyneFix® PT, intra-uterine device, 6 copper sleeves with surface area of 330 mm² on polypropylene thread, net price = £24.75. BNF section 7.3.4

For use as an intra-uterine contraceptive; to be inserted after abortion of less than 10 weeks' gestation

Infanrix-Hib® (SmithKline Beecham) ▼ PoM

Injection, powder for reconstitution, capsular polysaccharide of *Haemophilus influenzae* type b (conjugated to a protein carrier), with diluent containing diphtheria toxoid, tetanus toxoid, and acellular pertussis vaccine components adsorbed on a mineral carrier, net price 0.5-mL prefilled syringe = £12.40. BNF Section 14.4

For primary immunisation against diphtheria, tetanus, pertussis and *Haemophilus influenzae* type b infection

OxyContin® (Napp) ▼ CD

Tablets, f/c, m/r, oxycodone hydrochloride 10 mg (white), net price 56-tab pack = £21.43; 20 mg (pink), 56-tab pack = £42.86; 40 mg (yellow), 56-tab pack = £85.73; 80 mg (green), 56-tab pack = £171.46. Label: 2, 25. BNF section 4.7.2

For moderate to severe pain in patients with cancer or postoperative pain

OxyNorm® (Napp) ▼ CD

Capsules, oxycodone hydrochloride 5 mg (orange/beige), net price 56-cap pack = £10.56; 10 mg (white/beige), 56-cap pack = £21.12; 20 mg (pink/beige), 56-cap pack = £42.24. Label: 2

Liquid (= oral solution), oxycodone hydrochloride 5 mg/5 mL, net price 250 mL = £9.43. Label: 2

Concentrate (= concentrated oral solution), oxycodone hydrochloride 10 mg/mL, net price 120 mL = £45.25. Label: 2. BNF section 4.7.2

For moderate to severe pain in patients with cancer or postoperative pain

Renagel® (Genzyme) ▼ PoM

Capsules, sevelamer 403 mg, net price 200-cap pack = £73.00. Label: 21, 25. BNF section 9.5.2.2

For the treatment of hyperphosphataemia in haemodialysis patients

Teveten® (Solvay) ▼ PoM

Tablets, f/c, eprosartan (as mesilate) 300 mg, net price 28-tab pack = £12.50; 400 mg (pink), 56-tab pack = £16.96; 600 mg, 28-tab pack = £14.75. BNF section 2.5.5.2

For hypertension

Tobi® (PathoGenesis) ▼ PoM

Nebuliser solution, tobramycin 60 mg/mL, net price 56 × 5-mL (300-mg) unit = £1540.00. BNF section 5.1.4

For chronic pulmonary *Pseudomonas aeruginosa* infection in cystic fibrosis patients aged over 6 years

Zyomet® (Goldshield) PoM

Gel, metronidazole 0.75%, net price 30 g = £12.00. Label: 10 patient information leaflet. BNF section 13.10.1.2

Excipients: include benzyl alcohol, disodium edetate, propylene glycol

For the treatment of acute inflammatory exacerbations of acne rosacea

---

New preparations included in this edition

Preparations included in the relevant sections of BNF No. 39:

Name changes

Directive 92/27/EEC requires use of the Recommended International Non-proprietary Name (rINN) for medicinal substances. In most cases the British Approved Name (BAN) and rINN were identical. Where the two differed, the BAN has been modified to accord with the rINN.

List 1 includes those substances where a change of name was considered to pose the highest potential risk to public health—it is anticipated that the MCA will announce arrangements that require both the rINN and the former BAN to appear on manufacturers' labels and leaflets (giving precedence to the rINN) for at least 5 years. The BNF shows both names in the main drug entries.

List 2 includes those substances for which the former BAN has been modified to accord with the rINN; the new BAN is required to appear on manufacturers' labels and leaflets. Former BANs have been retained as synonyms in the BNF.

List 1—Both names to appear

UK name	rINN
[1]adrenaline	epinephrine
amethocaine	tetracaine
bendrofluazide	bendroflumethiazide
benzhexol	trihexyphenidyl
chlorpheniramine	chlorphenamine
dicyclomine	dicycloverine
dothiepin	dosulepin
eformoterol	formoterol
flurandrenolone	fludroxycortide
frusemide	furosemide
hydroxyurea	hydroxycarbamide
lignocaine	lidocaine
methotrimeprazine	levomepromazine
methylene blue	methylthioninium chloride
mitozantrone	mitoxantrone
mustine	chlormethine
nicoumalone	acenocoumarol
[1]noradrenaline	norepinephrine
oxpentifylline	pentoxifylline
procaine penicillin	procaine benzylpenicillin
salcatonin	calcitonin (salmon)
thymoxamine	moxisylyte
thyroxine sodium	levothyroxine sodium
trimeprazine	alimemazine

1. In common with the BP, precedence will continue to be given to the terms adrenaline and noradrenaline

List 2—rINN/new BAN to appear exclusively

former BAN	rINN/new BAN
aminacrine	aminoacridine
amoxycillin	amoxicillin
amphetamine	amfetamine
amylobarbitone	amobarbital
amylobarbitone sodium	amobarbital sodium
beclomethasone	beclometasone
benorylate	benorilate
benzphetamine	benzfetamine
benztropine	benzatropine
busulphan	busulfan
butobarbitone	butobarbital
carticaine	articane
cephalexin	cefalexin
cephamandole nafate	cefamandole nafate
cephazolin	cefazolin
cephradine	cefradine
chloral betaine	cloral betaine

List 2 (*continued*)

former BAN	rINN/new BAN
chlorbutol	chlorobutanol
chlormethiazole	clomethiazole
chlorthalidone	chlortalidone
cholecalciferol	colecalciferol
cholestyramine	colestyramine
clomiphene	clomifene
colistin sulphomethate sodium	colistimethate sodium
corticotrophin	corticotropin
cyclosporin	ciclosporin
cysteamine	mercaptamine
danthron	dantron
desoxymethasone	desoximetasone
dexamphetamine	dexamfetamine
dibromopropamidine	dibrompropamidine
dienoestrol	dienestrol
dimethicone(s)	dimeticone
dimethyl sulphoxide	dimethyl sulfoxide
doxycycline hydrochloride (hemihydrate hemiethanolate)	doxycycline hyclate
ethacrynic acid	etacrynic acid
ethamsylate	etamsylate
ethinyloestradiol	ethinylestradiol
ethynodiol	etynodiol
flumethasone	flumetasone
flupenthixol	flupentixol
gestronol	gestonorone
guaiphenesin	guaifenesin
hexachlorophane	hexachlorophene
hexamine hippurate	methenamine hippurate
hydroxyprogesterone hexanoate	hydroxyprogesterone caproate
indomethacin	indometacin
lysuride	lisuride
methyl cysteine	mecysteine
methylphenobarbitone	methylphenobarbital
monosulfiram	sulfiram
oestradiol	estradiol
oestriol	estriol
oestrone	estrone
oxethazaine	oxetacaine
pentaerythritol tetranitrate	pentaerithrityl tetranitrate
phenobarbitone	phenobarbital
pipothiazine	pipotiazine
polyhexanide	polihexanide
potassium clorazepate	dipotassium clorazepate
pramoxine	pramocaine
prothionamide	protionamide
quinalbarbitone	secobarbital
riboflavine	riboflavin
sodium calciumedetate	sodium calcium edetate
sodium cromoglycate	sodium cromoglicate
sodium ironedetate	sodium feredetate
sodium picosulphate	sodium picosulfate
sorbitan monostearate	sorbitan stearate
stibocaptate	sodium stibocaptate
stilboestrol	diethylstilbestrol
sulphacetamide	sulfacetamide
sulphadiazine	sulfadiazine
sulphadimidine	sulfadimidine
sulphaguanidine	sulfaguanidine
sulphamethoxazole	sulfamethoxazole
sulphapyridine	sulfapyridine
sulphasalazine	sulfasalazine
sulphathiazole	sulfathiazole
sulphinpyrazone	sulfinpyrazone
tetracosactrin	tetracosactide
thiabendazole	tiabendazole
thioguanine	tioguanine
thiopentone	thiopental
urofollitrophin	urofollitropin

Guidance on prescribing

General guidance

Medicines should be prescribed only when they are necessary, and in all cases the benefit of administering the medicine should be considered in relation to the risk involved. This is particularly important during pregnancy where the risk to both mother and fetus must be considered (for further details see Prescribing in Pregnancy, Appendix 4).

TAKING MEDICINES TO BEST EFFECT. Difficulties in compliance with drug treatment occur regardless of age. Factors contributing to poor compliance with prescribed medicines include:

- Prescription not collected or not dispensed
- Purpose of medicine not clear
- Perceived lack of efficacy
- Real or perceived side-effects
- Instructions for administration not clear
- Physical difficulty in taking medicines (e.g. with handling small tablets or opening medicine containers)
- Unattractive formulation (e.g. unpleasant taste)
- Complicated regimen

The prescriber and the patient should agree on the health outcomes that the patient desires and on the strategy for achieving them ('concordance'). Further information on concordance is available on the Internet (http://www.concordance.org).

Taking the time to explain to the patient (and relatives) the rationale and the potential adverse effects of treatment may improve compliance. Advising the patient of the possibility of alternative treatments may encourage the patient to seek advice rather than merely abandon unacceptable treatment.

Simplifying the drug regimen may help; the need for frequent administration may reduce compliance although there appears to be little difference in compliance between once-daily and twice-daily administration. Combination products reduce the number of drugs taken but this may be at the expense of the ability to titrate individual doses.

ABBREVIATION OF TITLES. In general, titles of drugs and preparations should be written *in full*. Unofficial abbreviations should not be used as they may be misinterpreted; obsolete titles, such as Mist. Expect. should not be used.

NON-PROPRIETARY TITLES. Where non-proprietary ('generic') titles are given, they should be used in prescribing. This will enable any suitable product to be dispensed, thereby saving delay to the patient and sometimes expense to the health service. The only exception is where bioavailability problems are so important that the patient should always receive the same brand; in such cases, the brand name or the manufacturer should be stated. Non-proprietary titles should **not** be invented for the purposes of prescribing generically since this can lead to confusion, particularly in the case of compound and modified-release preparations.

Titles used as headings for monographs may be used freely in Great Britain and Northern Ireland but in other countries may be subject to restriction.

Many of the non-proprietary titles used in this book are titles of monographs in the European Pharmacopoeia, British Pharmacopoeia or British Pharmaceutical Codex 1973. In such cases the preparations must comply with the standard (if any) in the appropriate publication, as required by the Medicines Act (Section 65).

PROPRIETARY TITLES. Names followed by the symbol ® are or have been used as proprietary names in the United Kingdom. These names may in general be applied only to products supplied by the owners of the trade marks.

DOSES. The doses stated in the BNF are intended for general guidance and represent, unless otherwise stated, the usual range of doses that are generally regarded as being suitable for adults. In general the *doses, indications, cautions, contra-indications and side-effects* in the BNF reflect those in the manufacturers' data sheets or Summaries of Product Characteristics (SPCs) which, in turn, reflect those in the corresponding Marketing Authorisations (formerly known as Product Licences). On the few occasions that an unlicensed drug is included in the BNF, this is now indicated in brackets after the entry. Where a use (or route) is recommended outside the licensed indication of an available product this too is indicated.

> It has been noted (*Drug and Therapeutics Bulletin* 1992; **30:** 97–9) that prescribing of licensed medicines outside the recommendations of the Marketing Authorisation alters (and probably increases) the doctor's professional responsibility.

ORAL SYRINGES. An **oral syringe** is supplied when oral liquid medicines are prescribed in doses other than multiples of 5 mL. The oral syringe is marked in 0.5-mL divisions from 1 to 5 mL to measure doses of less than 5 mL. It is provided with an adaptor and an instruction leaflet. The *5-mL spoon* is used for doses of 5 mL (or multiples thereof).

STRENGTHS AND QUANTITIES. The strength or quantity to be contained in capsules, lozenges, tablets, etc. should be stated by the prescriber.

If a pharmacist receives an incomplete prescription for a systemically administered preparation other than a prescription for a controlled drug and considers it would not be appropriate for the patient to return to the doctor, the following procedures will apply:

(a) an attempt must always be made to contact the prescriber to ascertain the intention;

(b) if the attempt is successful the pharmacist must, where practicable, subsequently arrange for details of quantity, strength where applicable, and dosage to be inserted by the prescriber on the incomplete form;

(c) where, although the prescriber has been contacted, it has not proved possible to obtain the written intention regarding an incomplete prescription, the pharmacist may endorse the form 'p.c.' (prescriber contacted) and add details of the quantity and strength where applicable of the preparation supplied, and of the dose indicated. The endorsement should be initialled and dated by the pharmacist;

(d) where the prescriber cannot be contacted and the pharmacist has sufficient information to make a professional judgment the preparation may be dispensed. If the quantity is missing the pharmacist may supply sufficient to complete up to 5 days' treatment; except that where a combination pack (i.e. a proprietary pack containing more than one medicinal product) or oral contraceptive is prescribed by name only, the smallest pack shall be dispensed. In all cases the prescription must be endorsed 'p.n.c.' (prescriber not contacted) the quantity, the dose, and the strength (where applicable) of the preparation supplied must be indicated, and the endorsement must be initialled and dated;

(e) if the pharmacist has any doubt about exercising discretion, an incomplete prescription must be referred back to the prescriber.

EXCIPIENTS. Oral liquid preparations that do not contain *fructose, glucose* or *sucrose* are described as 'sugar-free' in the BNF. Preparations containing hydrogenated glucose syrup, mannitol, sorbitol or xylitol are also marked 'sugar-free' since there is evidence that they do not cause dental caries. Patients receiving medicines containing cariogenic sugars should be advised of appropriate dental hygiene measures to prevent caries.

Where information on the presence of *aspartame, gluten, tartrazine, arachis (peanut) oil* or *sesame oil* is available, this is indicated in the BNF against the relevant preparation; the manufacturer should be contacted in the absence of information on excipients in the BNF and in the product literature, if it is essential to check details.

Information is provided on *preservatives* in eye-drops and on *selected excipients* in skin preparations (see section 13.1.3). Pressurised metered aerosols containing *chlorofluorocarbons* (CFCs) have also been identified throughout the BNF (see section 3.1.1.1)

EXTEMPORANEOUS PREPARATION. The BP direction that a preparation must be *freshly prepared* indicates that it must be made not more than 24 hours before it is issued for use. The direction that a preparation should be *recently prepared* indicates that deterioration is likely if the preparation is stored for longer than about 4 weeks at 15–25° C.

DRUGS AND DRIVING. Prescribers should advise patients if treatment is likely to affect their ability to drive motor vehicles. This applies particularly to drugs with sedative effects and patients should be warned that these effects are increased by alcohol. See also Appendix 9.

PATENTS. In the BNF certain drugs have been included notwithstanding the existence of actual or potential patent rights. In so far as such substances are protected by Letters Patent, their inclusion in this Formulary neither conveys, nor implies, licence to manufacture.

HEALTH AND SAFETY. When handling chemical or biological materials particular attention should be given to the possibility of allergy, fire, explosion, radiation, or poisoning. Some substances, including corticosteroids, antibiotics, phenothiazines, and many cytotoxics, are irritant or very potent and should be handled with caution. Contact with the skin and inhalation of dust should be avoided.

SAFETY IN THE HOME. Patients must be warned to keep all medicines out of the reach of children. All solid dose and all oral and external liquid preparations must be dispensed in a reclosable *child-resistant container* unless:

- the medicine is in an original pack or patient pack such as to make this inadvisable;
- the patient will have difficulty in opening a child-resistant container;
- a specific request is made that the product shall not be dispensed in a child-resistant container;
- no suitable child-resistant container exists for a particular liquid preparation.

All patients should be advised to dispose of *unwanted medicines* by returning them to a supplier for destruction.

NAME OF MEDICINE. The name of the medicine should appear on the label unless the prescriber indicates otherwise.

1. Subject to the conditions of paragraphs 4 and 6 below, the name of the prescribed medicine is stated on the label unless the prescriber deletes the letters 'NP' which appear on NHS prescription forms.

2. The strength is also stated on the label in the case of tablets, capsules, and similar preparations that are available in different strengths.

3. If it is the wish of the prescriber that a description such as 'The Sedative Tablets' should appear on the label, the prescriber should write the desired description on the prescription form.

4. The arrangement will extend to approved names, proprietary names or titles given in the BP, BPC, BNF, or DPF. The arrangement does not apply when a prescription is written so that several ingredients are given.

5. The name written on the label is that used by the prescriber on the prescription.

6. If more than one item is prescribed on one form and the prescriber does not delete the letters 'NP', each dispensed medicine is named on the label, subject to the conditions given above in paragraph 4. If the prescriber wants only selected items on such a prescription to be so labelled this should be indicated by deleting the letters 'NP' on the form and writing 'NP' alongside the medicines to be labelled.

7. When a prescription is written other than on an NHS prescription form the name of the prescribed preparation will be stated on the label of the dispensed medicine unless the prescriber indicates otherwise.

8. The Council of the Royal Pharmaceutical Society advises that the labels of dispensed medicines should indicate the total quantity of the product dispensed in the container to which the label refers. This requirement applies equally to solid, liquid, internal, and

external preparations. If a product is dispensed in more than one container, the reference should be to the amount in each container.

Generic names of **compound preparations** which appear in the BNF are those approved by the British Pharmacopoeia Commission; whenever possible they reflect the names of the active ingredients.

Prescribers should avoid creating their own compound names for the purposes of generic prescribing; such names do not have an approved definition and can be misinterpreted.

Special care should be taken to avoid errors when prescribing compound preparations; in particular the hyphen in the prefix 'co-' should be retained.

Special care should also be taken to avoid creating generic names for **modified-release** preparations where the use of these names could lead to confusion between formulations with different lengths of action.

SECURITY AND VALIDITY OF PRESCRIPTIONS. The Councils of the British Medical Association and the Royal Pharmaceutical Society have issued a joint statement on the security and validity of prescriptions.

In particular, prescription forms should:

- not be left unattended at reception desks;
- not be left in a car where they may be visible; and
- when not in use, be kept in a locked drawer within the surgery and at home.

Where there is any doubt about the authenticity of a prescription, the pharmacist should contact the prescriber. If this is done by telephone, the number should be obtained from the directory rather than relying on the information on the prescription form, which may be false.

Prescription writing

Prescriptions[1] should be written legibly in ink or otherwise so as to be indelible[2], should be dated, should state the full name and address of the patient, and should be signed in ink by the prescriber[3]. The age and the date of birth of the patient should preferably be stated, and it is a legal requirement in the case of prescription-only medicines to state the age for children under 12 years.

The following should be noted:

(a) The unnecessary use of decimal points should be avoided, e.g. 3 mg, not 3.0 mg.

Quantities of 1 gram or more should be written as 1 g etc.

Quantities less than 1 gram should be written in milligrams, e.g. 500 mg, not 0.5 g.

Quantities less than 1 mg should be written in micrograms, e.g. 100 micrograms, not 0.1 mg.

When decimals are unavoidable a zero should be written in front of the decimal point where there is no other figure, e.g. 0.5 mL, not .5 mL.

Use of the decimal point is acceptable to express a range, e.g. 0.5 to 1 g.

(b) 'Micrograms' and 'nanograms' should **not** be abbreviated. Similarly 'units' should **not** be abbreviated.

(c) The term 'millilitre' (ml or mL)[4] is used in medicine and pharmacy, and cubic centimetre, c.c., or cm^3 should not be used.

(d) Dose and dose frequency should be stated; in the case of preparations to be taken 'as required' a **minimum dose interval** should be specified.

When doses other than multiples of 5 mL are prescribed for *oral liquid preparations* the dose-volume will be provided by means of an **oral syringe**, see p. 1 (except for preparations intended to be measured with a pipette).

Suitable quantities:

Elixirs, Linctuses, and Paediatric Mixtures (5-mL dose), 50, 100, or 150 mL

Adult Mixtures (10-mL dose), 200 or 300 mL

Ear Drops, Eye-drops, and Nasal Drops, 10 mL (or the manufacturer's pack)

Eye Lotions, Gargles, and Mouth-washes, 200 mL

(e) For suitable quantities of dermatological preparations, see section 13.1.2.

(f) The names of drugs and preparations should be written clearly and **not** abbreviated, using approved titles **only** (see also advice in box on p. 3 to **avoid** creating generic titles for modified-release preparations).

(g) The symbol 'NP' on NHS forms should be deleted if it is required that the name of the preparation should not appear on the label. For full details see p. 2.

(h) The quantity to be supplied may be stated by indicating the number of days of treatment required in the box provided on NHS forms. In most cases the exact amount will be supplied. This does not apply to items directed to be used as required—if the dose and frequency are not given the quantity to be supplied needs to be stated.

When several items are ordered on one form the box can be marked with the number of days of treatment providing the quantity is added for any item for which the amount cannot be calculated.

(i) Although directions should preferably be in **English without abbreviation**, it is recognised that some Latin abbreviations are used (for details see Inside Back Cover).

(j) A prescription for a preparation that has been withdrawn or needs to be specially imported for a named patient should be handwritten. The name of the preparation should be endorsed with the prescriber's signature and the letters 'WD' (withdrawn or specially-imported drug); there may be considerable delay in obtaining a withdrawn medicine.

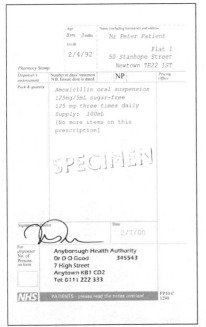

---

1. The above recommendations are acceptable for **prescription-only medicines** (PoM). For items marked CD see also Controlled Drugs and Drug Dependence p. 7.

2. It is permissible to issue carbon copies of NHS prescriptions as long as they are signed in ink.

3. Computer-generated facsimile signatures do not meet the legal requirement.

4. The use of capital 'L' in mL is a printing convention throughout the BNF; both 'mL' and 'ml' are recognised SI abbreviations.

Computer-issued prescriptions

For computer-issued prescriptions the following recommendations of the Joint Computing Group of the General Practitioners Committee and the Royal College of General Practitioners should also be noted:

1. The computer must print out the date,[1] the patient's surname, one forename, other initials, and address, and may also print out the patient's title and date of birth. The age of children under 12 years and of adults over 60 years must be printed in the box available; the age of children under 5 years should be printed in years and months. A facility may also exist to print out the age of patients between 12 and 60 years.

2. The doctor's name must be printed at the bottom of the prescription form; this will be the name of the doctor responsible for the prescription (who will normally sign it). The doctor's surgery address, reference number, and Health Authority (HA)[2] are also necessary. In addition, the surgery telephone number should be printed.

3. When prescriptions are to be signed by general practitioner registrars, assistants, locums, or deputising doctors, the name of the doctor printed at the bottom of the form must still be that of the responsible principal.

4. Names of medicines must come from a dictionary held in the computer memory, to provide a check on the spelling and to ensure that the name is written in full. The computer can be programmed to recognise both the non-proprietary and the proprietary name of a particular drug and to print out the preferred choice, but must not print out both names. For medicines not in the dictionary, separate checks are required—the user must be warned that no check was possible and the entire prescription must be entered in the lexicon.

5. The dictionary may contain information on the usual doses, formulations, and pack sizes to produce standard predetermined prescriptions for common preparations, and to provide a check on the validity of an individual prescription on entry.

6. The prescription must be printed in English without abbreviation; information may be entered or stored in abbreviated form. The dose must be in numbers, the frequency in words, and the quantity in numbers in brackets, thus: 40 mg four times daily (112). It must also be possible to prescribe by indicating the length of treatment required, see (h) above.

7. The BNF recommendations should be followed as in (a), (b), (c), (d), and (e) above.

8. Checks may be incorporated to ensure that all the information required for dispensing a particular drug has been filled in. For instructions such as 'as directed' and 'when required', the maximum daily dose should normally be specified.

9. Numbers and codes used in the system for organising and retrieving data must never appear on the form.

10. Supplementary warnings or advice should be written in full, should not interfere with the clarity of the prescription itself, and should be in line with any warnings or advice in the BNF; numerical codes should not be used.

11. A mechanism (such as printing a series of non-specific characters) should be incorporated to cancel out unused space, or wording such as 'no more items on this prescription' may be added after the last item. Otherwise the doctor should delete the space manually.

12. To avoid forgery the computer may print on the form the number of items to be dispensed (somewhere separate from the box for the pharmacist). The number of items per form need be limited only by the ability of the printer to produce clear and well-demarcated instructions with sufficient space for each item and a spacer line before each fresh item.

13. Handwritten alterations should only be made in exceptional circumstances—it is preferable to print out a new prescription. Any alterations must be made in the doctor's own handwriting and counter-signed; computer records should be updated to fully reflect any alteration. Prescriptions for drugs used for contraceptive purposes (but which are not promoted as contraceptives) may need to be marked in handwriting with the symbol (or endorsed in another way to indicate that the item is prescribed for contraceptive purposes).

14. Prescriptions for controlled drugs must not be printed from the computer. Blank forms may be computer-printed with the doctor's name, surgery address and telephone number, reference number and Health Authority (HA)[2]; the remaining details must be handwritten.[3]

15. The strip of paper on the side of the FP10[4](Comp) may be used for various purposes but care should be taken to avoid including confidential information. It may be advisable for the patient's name to appear at the top, but this should be preceded by 'confidential'.

16. In rural dispensing practices prescription requests (or details of medicines dispensed) will normally be entered in one surgery. The prescriptions (or dispensed medicines) may then need to be delivered to another surgery or location; if possible the computer should hold up to 10 alternatives.

17. Prescription forms that are reprinted or issued as a duplicate should be labelled clearly as such.

---

1. The exemption for own handwriting regulations for phenobarbital does not apply to the date; a computer-generated date need not be deleted but the date must also be added by the prescriber.

2. Health Board in Scotland.

3. Except in the case of phenobarbital (but see also footnote 1) or where the prescriber has been exempted from handwriting requirements, for details see Controlled Drugs and Drug Dependence p. 7.

4. GP10 in Scotland.

Emergency supply of medicines

For details of emergency supply at the request of a doctor, see *Medicines, Ethics and Practice*, No. 23, London, Pharmaceutical Press, 2000 (and subsequent editions).

The Medicines (Products Other Than Veterinary Drugs) (Prescription Only) Order 1983, as amended, allows exemptions from the Prescription Only requirements for emergency supply to be made by a person lawfully conducting a retail pharmacy business provided:

(a) that the pharmacist has interviewed the person requesting the prescription-only medicine and is satisfied:

    (i) that there is immediate need for the prescription-only medicine and that it is impracticable in the circumstances to obtain a prescription without undue delay;

    (ii) that treatment with the prescription-only medicine has on a previous occasion been prescribed by a doctor[1] for the person requesting it;

    (iii) as to the dose which it would be appropriate for the person to take;

(b) that no greater quantity shall be supplied than will provide five days' treatment except when the prescription-only medicine is:

    (i) an ointment, cream, or preparation for the relief of asthma in an aerosol dispenser when the smallest pack can be supplied;

    (ii) an oral contraceptive when a full cycle may be supplied;

    (iii) an antibiotic in liquid form for oral administration when the smallest quantity that will provide a full course of treatment can be supplied;

(c) that an entry shall be made in the prescription book stating:

    (i) the date of supply;

    (ii) the name, quantity and, where appropriate, the pharmaceutical form and strength;

    (iii) the name and address of the patient;

    (iv) the nature of the emergency;

(d) that the container or package must be labelled to show:

    (i) the date of supply;

    (ii) the name, quantity and, where appropriate, the pharmaceutical form and strength;

    (iii) the name of the patient;

    (iv) the name and address of the pharmacy;

    (v) the words 'Emergency supply'.

(e) that the prescription-only medicine is not a substance specifically excluded from the emergency supply provision, and does not contain a Controlled Drug specified in schedules 1, 2, or 3 to the Misuse of Drugs Regulations 1985 except for phenobarbital or phenobarbital sodium for the treatment of epilepsy: for details see *Medicines, Ethics and Practice*, No. 23, London, Pharmaceutical Press, 2000 (and subsequent editions as available).

Royal Pharmaceutical Society's Guidelines

(1) The pharmacist should consider the medical consequences of *not* supplying.

(2) If the patient is not known to the pharmacist, the patient's identity should be established by way of appropriate documentation.

(3) It may occasionally be desirable to contact the prescriber, e.g. when the medicine requested has a potential for misuse or the prescriber is not known to the pharmacist.

(4) Care should be taken to ask whether the patient's doctor has stopped the treatment, or whether the patient is taking any other medication.

(5) Except for conditions which occur infrequently (e.g. hay fever, asthma attack or migraine), a supply should not be made if the item requested was last prescribed more than 6 months ago.

(6) Consideration should be given to supplying less than 5 days' quantity if this is justified.

(7) Where a prescription is to be provided later, a record of emergency supply as required by law must still be made. It is good practice to add to the record the date on which the prescription is received. Payment for the medicine supplied is not a legal requirement, but may help to minimise the abuse of the emergency supply exemption. If an NHS prescription is to be provided, a refundable charge may be made.

---

1. The doctor must be a UK-registered doctor.

Controlled drugs and drug dependence

PRESCRIPTIONS. Preparations which are subject to the prescription requirements of the Misuse of Drugs Regulations 1985, i.e. preparations specified in schedules 2 and 3, are distinguished throughout the BNF by the symbol CD (Controlled Drugs). The principal legal requirements relating to medical prescriptions are listed below.

Prescriptions ordering Controlled Drugs subject to prescription requirements must be *signed* and *dated*[1] by the prescriber and specify the prescriber's *address*. The prescription must always state *in the prescriber's own handwriting*[2] in ink or otherwise so as to be indelible:

1. The name and address of the patient;

2. In the case of a preparation, the form[3] and where appropriate the strength[4] of the preparation;

3. The total quantity of the preparation, or the number of dose units, *in both words and figures;*[5]

4. The dose.[6]

A prescription may order a Controlled Drug to be dispensed by instalments; the amount of the instalments and the intervals to be observed must be specified.[7] Prescriptions ordering 'repeats' on the same form are **not** permitted.

It is an offence for a doctor to issue an incomplete prescription and a pharmacist is **not** allowed to dispense a Controlled Drug unless all the information required by law is given on the prescription. Failure to comply with the regulations concerning the writing of prescriptions will result in inconvenience to patients and delay in supplying the necessary medicine.

DEPENDENCE AND MISUSE. The most serious drugs of addiction are **cocaine, diamorphine** (heroin), **morphine**, and the **synthetic opioids**. For arrangements for prescribing of diamorphine, dipipanone or cocaine for addicts, see p. 9.

Despite marked reduction in the prescribing of **amphetamines** there is concern that abuse of illicit amfetamine and related compounds is widespread.

Owing to problems of abuse, **flunitrazepam** and **temazepam** are subject to additional controlled drug requirements (but temazepam remains exempt from the additional prescribing requirements).

The principal **barbiturates** are now Controlled Drugs, but phenobarbital (phenobarbitone) and phenobarbital sodium (phenobarbitone sodium) or a preparation containing either of these are exempt from the handwriting requirement but must fulfil all other controlled drug prescription requirements (**important:** the own handwriting exemption does **not** apply to the date; a computer-generated date need not be deleted but the date must also be added by the prescriber). Moreover, for the treatment of epilepsy phenobarbital and phenobarbital sodium are available under the emergency supply regulations (p. 6).

Cannabis (Indian hemp) has no approved medicinal use and cannot be prescribed by doctors. Its use is illegal but has become widespread. Cannabis is a mild hallucinogen seldom accompanied by a desire to increase the dose; withdrawal symptoms are unusual. **Lysergide** (lysergic acid diethylamide, LSD) is a much more potent hallucinogen; its use can lead to severe psychotic states in which life may be at risk.

---

1. A prescription is valid for 13 weeks from the date stated thereon.

2. Does not apply to prescriptions for temazepam. Otherwise applies unless the prescriber has been specifically exempted from this requirement or unless the prescription contains no controlled drug other than phenobarbital or phenobarbital sodium or a preparation containing either of these; the exemption does **not** apply to the date—a computer-generated date need not be deleted but the date must also be added by the prescriber.

3. The dosage form (e.g. tablets) must be included on a Controlled Drugs prescription irrespective of whether it is implicit in the proprietary name (e.g. *MST Continus*) or of whether only one form is available.

4. When more than one strength of a preparation exists the strength required must be specified.

5. Does not apply to prescriptions for temazepam.

6. The instruction 'one as directed' constitutes a dose but 'as directed' does not.

7. A total of 14 days' treatment by instalment of any drug listed in Schedule 2 of the Misuse of Drugs Regulations may be prescribed. In *England and Wales*, form FP10HP(AD) (pink—mainly used by hospital-based treatment units) or form FP10(MDA) (blue—mainly used by general practitioners) should be used; in *Scotland*, forms HBP(A) (hospital-based prescribers) or GP10 (general practitioners) should be used.

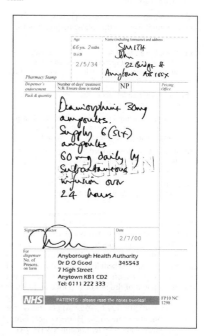

PRESCRIBING DRUGS LIKELY TO CAUSE DEPENDENCE OR MISUSE. The prescriber has three main responsibilities:

1. To avoid creating dependence by introducing drugs to patients without sufficient reason. In this context, the proper use of the morphine-like drugs is well understood. The dangers of other controlled drugs are less clear because recognition of dependence is not easy and its effects, and those of withdrawal, are less obvious. Perhaps the most notable result of uninhibited prescribing is that a very large number of patients in the country take tablets which do them neither much good nor much harm, but are committed to them indefinitely because they cannot readily be stopped.

2. To see that the patient does not gradually increase the dose of a drug, given for good medical reasons, to the point where dependence becomes more likely. This tendency is seen especially with hypnotics and anxiolytics (for CSM advice see section 4.1). The prescriber should keep a close eye on the amount prescribed to prevent patients from accumulating stocks that would enable them to arrange their own dosage or even that of their families and friends. A minimal amount should be prescribed in the first instance, or when seeing a new patient for the first time.

3. To avoid being used as an unwitting source of supply for addicts. Methods include visiting more than one doctor, fabricating stories, and forging prescriptions.

Patients under temporary care should be given only small supplies of drugs unless they present an unequivocal letter from their own doctors. Doctors should also remember that their own patients may be doing a collecting round with other doctors, especially in hospitals. It is sensible to decrease dosages steadily or to issue weekly or even daily prescriptions for small amounts if it is apparent that dependence is occurring.

The stealing and misuse of prescription forms could be minimised by the following precautions:

(a) do not leave unattended if called away from the consulting room or at reception desks; do not leave in a car where they may be visible; when not in use, keep in a locked drawer within the surgery and at home;

(b) draw a diagonal line across the blank part of the form under the prescription;

(c) write the quantity in words and figures when prescribing drugs prone to abuse; this is obligatory for controlled drugs (see Prescriptions, above);

(d) alterations are best avoided but if any are made they should be clear and unambiguous; add initials against altered items;

(e) if prescriptions are left for collection they should be left in a safe place in a sealed envelope.

TRAVELLING ABROAD. Prescribed drugs listed in schedules 4 and 5 to the Misuse of Drugs Regulations 1985 are not subject to import or export licensing but doctors are advised that patients intending to carry Schedule 2 and 3 drugs abroad may require an export licence. This is dependent upon the amount of drug to be exported and further details may be obtained from the Home Office by telephoning (020) 7273 3806. Applications for licences should be sent to the Home Office, Drugs Branch, Queen Anne's Gate, London SW1H 9AT.

There is no standard application form but applications must be supported by a letter from a doctor giving details of:

- the patient's name and current address;
- the quantities of drugs to be carried;
- the strength and form in which the drugs will be dispensed;
- the dates of travel to and from the United Kingdom.

Ten days should be allowed for processing the application.

Individual doctors who wish to take Controlled Drugs abroad while accompanying patients, may similarly be issued with licences. Licences are not normally issued to doctors who wish to take Controlled Drugs abroad solely in case a family emergency should arise.

These import/export licences for named individuals do not have any legal status outside the UK and are only issued to comply with the Misuse of Drugs Act and facilitate passage through UK Customs and Excise control. For clearance in the country to be visited it would be necessary to approach that country's consulate in the UK.

Misuse of Drugs Act

The Misuse of Drugs Act, 1971 prohibits certain activities in relation to 'Controlled Drugs', in particular their manufacture, supply, and possession. The penalties applicable to offences involving the different drugs are graded broadly according to the *harmfulness attributable to a drug when it is misused* and for this purpose the drugs are defined in the following three classes:

Class A includes: alfentanil, cocaine, dextromoramide, diamorphine (heroin), dipipanone, lysergide (LSD), methadone, morphine, opium, pethidine, phencyclidine, and class B substances when prepared for injection

Class B includes: oral amphetamines, barbiturates, cannabis, cannabis resin, codeine, ethylmorphine, glutethimide, pentazocine, phenmetrazine, and pholcodine

Class C includes: certain drugs related to the amphetamines such as benzfetamine and chlorphentermine, buprenorphine, diethylpropion, mazindol, meprobamate, pemoline, pipradrol, most benzodiazepines, androgenic and anabolic steroids, clenbuterol, chorionic gonadotrophin (HCG), non-human chorionic gonadotrophin, somatotropin, somatrem, and somatropin

The Misuse of Drugs Regulations 1985 define the classes of person who are authorised to supply and possess controlled drugs while acting in their professional capacities and lay down the conditions under which these activities may be carried out. In the regulations drugs are divided into five schedules each specifying the requirements governing such activities as import, export, production, supply, possession, prescribing, and record keeping which apply to them.

Schedule 1 includes drugs such as cannabis and lysergide which are not used medicinally. Possession and supply are prohibited except in accordance with Home Office authority.

Schedule 2 includes drugs such as diamorphine (heroin), morphine, pethidine, secobarbital, gluteth-imide, amfetamine, and cocaine and are subject to the full controlled drug requirements relating to pre-scriptions, safe custody (except for secobarbital), the need to keep registers, etc. (unless exempted in schedule 5).

Schedule 3 includes the barbiturates (except secobarbi-tal, now schedule 2), buprenorphine, diethylpropion, flunitrazepam, mazindol, meprobamate, pentazocine, phentermine, and temazepam. They are subject to the special prescription requirements (except for pheno-barbital and temazepam, see p. 7) but not to the safe custody requirements (except for buprenorphine, diethylpropion, flunitrazepam, and temazepam) nor to the need to keep registers (although there are requirements for the retention of invoices for 2 years).

Schedule 4 includes in Part II 33 benzodiazepines (flunitrazepam and temazepam are now in schedule 3) and pemoline which are subject to minimal con-trol. Part I includes androgenic and anabolic steroids, clenbuterol, chorionic gonadotrophin (HCG), non-human chorionic gonadotrophin, somatotropin, somatrem, and somatropin. Controlled drug prescrip-tion requirements do not apply and Schedule 4 Con-trolled Drugs are not subject to safe custody requirements.

Schedule 5 includes those preparations which, because of their strength, are exempt from virtually all Con-trolled Drug requirements other than retention of invoices for two years.

Notification of drug misusers

In May 1997, the Misuse of Drugs (Supply to Addicts) Regulations 1997 revoked the requirement for doctors to send to the Home Office particulars of drug addicts. However, doctors are expected to report on a standard form cases of drug misuse to their local Drug Misuse Database (DMD)—see below for contact telephone numbers.

A report (notification) to the Drug Misuse Data-base should be made when a patient first presents with a drug problem or re-presents after a gap of six months or more. All types of problem drug misuse should be reported including opioid, benzodi-azepine, and CNS stimulant.

The Drug Misuse Databases are now the only national and local source of epidemiological data on people presenting with problem drug misuse and as such provide valuable information to those work-ing with, and those planning services for drug mis-users. The databases cannot however be used as a check on multiple prescribing for drug addicts because the data are anonymised.

Enquiries about the regional and national Drug Misuse Databases (including requests for supplies of notification forms) can be made by contacting one of the centres listed below:

ENGLAND

Anglia and Oxford
Telephone (01865) 226734; fax (01865) 226652
North Thames
Telephone (020) 8846 6563; fax (020) 8846 6555
North West
Merseyside and Cheshire: telephone (0151) 231 4294; fax (0151) 231 4320
North Western: telephone (0161) 772 3782; fax (0161) 772 3445
Northern and Yorkshire
Telephone (0113) 295 1337; fax (0113) 295 1310

South and West (including Wessex)
Telephone (0117) 958 4384; fax (0117) 958 6569
South Thames
Telephone (020) 8846 6563; fax (020) 8846 6555
Trent
Telephone (0116) 225 6360; fax (0116) 225 6370
West Midlands
Telephone (0121) 580 4331; fax (0121) 525 7980

SCOTLAND
Telephone (0131) 551 8715; fax (0131) 551 1392

WALES
Telephone (029) 2066 7766; fax (029) 2066 5940

In **Northern Ireland**, the Misuse of Drugs (Notifi-cation of and Supply to Addicts) (Northern Ireland) Regulations 1973 require doctors to send particu-lars of persons whom they consider to be addicted to certain controlled drugs to Chief Medical Officer of the Department of Health and Social Services. The Northern Ireland contacts are:

Medical contact:
Dr Ian McMaster
C3 Castle Buildings
Belfast BT4 3PP
Telephone (028) 9052 2421
Fax (028) 9052 0781

Administrative contact:
Health Promotion Branch
C4.22 Castle Buildings
Belfast BT4 3PP
Telephone (028) 9052 0532

Prescribing of diamorphine (heroin), dipipanone, and cocaine for addicts

The Misuse of Drugs (Supply to Addicts) Regula-tions 1997 require that only medical practitioners who hold a special licence issued by the Home Sec-retary may prescribe, administer or supply diamor-phine, dipipanone[1] (*Diconal®*) or cocaine in the treatment of drug addiction; other practitioners must refer any addict who requires these drugs to a treatment centre. Whenever possible the addict will be introduced by a member of staff from the treat-ment centre to a pharmacist whose agreement has been obtained and whose pharmacy is conveniently sited for the patient. Prescriptions for weekly sup-plies will be sent to the pharmacy by post and will be dispensed on a daily basis as indicated by the doctor. If any alterations of the arrangements are requested by the addict, the portion of the prescrip-tion affected must be represcribed and not merely altered. *General practitioners and other doctors may still prescribe diamorphine, dipipanone, and cocaine for patients (including addicts) for relief of pain due to organic disease or injury without a spe-cial licence.*

For prescription-writing guidelines, see p. 7.

1. Dipipanone in *Diconal®* tablets has been much mis-used by opioid addicts in recent years. Doctors and others should be suspicious of people who ask for the tablets, especially if temporary residents.

Adverse reactions to drugs

Any drug may produce unwanted or unexpected adverse reactions. Detection and recording of these is of vital importance. Doctors and pharmacists are urged to help by reporting adverse reactions to:

Medicines Control Agency
CSM Freepost
London SW8 5BR
(0800 731 6789)

Prepaid Yellow Cards for reporting are available from the above address and are also bound in this book (inside back cover).

A 24-hour Freefone service is available to all parts of the UK for advice and information on suspected adverse drug reactions; contact the National Yellow Card Information Service at the MCA on 0800 731 6789. Outside office hours a telephone-answering machine will take messages.

The following regional centres also collect data:

CSM Mersey
Freepost
Liverpool L3 3AB
(0151) 794 8113

CSM Wales
Freepost
Cardiff CF4 1ZZ
(029) 2074 4181
(Direct Line)

CSM Northern
Freepost 1085
Newcastle upon Tyne
NE1 1BR
(0191) 232 1525 (Direct Line)

CSM West Midlands
Freepost SW2991
Birmingham B18 7BR
[No telephone number]

The CSM's Adverse Drug Reactions On-line Information Tracking (ADROIT) facilitates the monitoring of adverse drug reactions.

Suspected adverse reactions to *any* therapeutic agent should be reported, including drugs (*self-medication* as well as *prescribed* ones), blood products, vaccines, X-ray contrast media, dental or surgical materials, intra-uterine devices, herbal products, and contact lens fluids.

NEWER DRUGS. These are indicated by the symbol ▼. Doctors and pharmacists are asked to report *all* suspected reactions (i.e. any adverse or any unexpected event, however minor, which could conceivably be attributed to the drug). Reports should be made despite uncertainty about a causal relationship, irrespective of whether the reaction is well recognized, and even if other drugs have been given concurrently.

ESTABLISHED DRUGS AND VACCINES. Doctors and pharmacists are asked to report *all* serious suspected reactions, including those that are fatal, life-threatening, disabling, incapacitating, or which result in or prolong hospitalisation; they should be reported even if the effect is well recognised.

Examples include anaphylaxis, blood disorders, endocrine disturbances, effects on fertility, haemorrhage from any site, renal impairment, jaundice, ophthalmic disorders, severe CNS effects, severe skin reactions, reactions in pregnant women, and any drug interactions. Reports of serious adverse reactions are required to enable comparison with other drugs of a similar class. For established drugs doctors and pharmacists are asked not to report well-known, relatively minor side-effects, such as dry mouth with tricyclic antidepressants, constipation with opioids, or nausea with digoxin.

Special problems

Delayed drug effects. Some reactions (e.g. cancers, chloroquine retinopathy, and retroperitoneal fibrosis) may become manifest months or years after exposure. Any suspicion of such an association should be reported.

The elderly. Particular vigilance is required to identify adverse reactions in the elderly.

Congenital abnormalities. When an infant is born with a congenital abnormality or there is a malformed aborted fetus doctors are asked to consider whether this might be an adverse reaction to a drug and to report all drugs (including self-medication) taken during pregnancy.

Children. Particular vigilance is required to identify adverse reactions in children, including those due to the unlicensed use of medicines; all suspected reactions should be reported.

Prevention of adverse reactions

Adverse reactions may be prevented as follows:

1. Never use any drug unless there is a good indication. If the patient is pregnant do not use a drug unless the need for it is imperative.
2. Allergy and idiosyncrasy are important causes of adverse drug reactions. Ask if the patient had previous reactions.
3. Ask if the patient is already taking other drugs *including self-medication drugs*; interactions may occur.
4. Age and hepatic or renal disease may alter the metabolism or excretion of drugs, so that much smaller doses may be needed. Genetic factors may also be responsible for variations in metabolism, notably of isoniazid and the tricyclic antidepressants.
5. Prescribe as few drugs as possible and give very clear instructions to the elderly or any patient likely to misunderstand complicated instructions.
6. When possible use a familiar drug. With a new drug be particularly alert for adverse reactions or unexpected events.
7. If serious adverse reactions are liable to occur warn the patient.

Defective Medicines

During the manufacture or distribution of a medicine an error or accident may occur whereby the finished product does not conform to its specification. While such a defect may impair the therapeutic effect of the product and could adversely affect the health of a patient, it should **not** be confused with an Adverse Drug Reaction where the product conforms to its specification.

The Defective Medicines Report Centre assists with the investigation of problems arising from licensed medicinal products thought to be defective and co-ordinates any necessary protective action. Reports on suspect defective medicinal products should include the brand or the non-proprietary name, the name of the manufacturer or supplier, the strength and dosage form of the product, the product licence number, the batch number or numbers of the product, the nature of the defect, and an account of any action already taken in consequence. The Centre can be contacted at:

The Defective Medicines Report Centre
Medicines Control Agency
Room 1801, Market Towers
1 Nine Elms Lane
London SW8 5NQ
(020) 7273 0574 (weekdays 9.00 am–5.00 pm)
or (020) 7210 3000 or 5371 (any other time)

Prescribing for children

Children, and particularly neonates, differ from adults in their response to drugs. Special care is needed in the neonatal period (first 30 days of life) and doses should always be calculated with care. At this age, the risk of toxicity is increased by inefficient renal filtration, relative enzyme deficiencies, differing target organ sensitivity, and inadequate detoxifying systems causing delayed excretion.

Whenever possible painful intramuscular injections should be **avoided** in children.

PRESCRIPTION WRITING. Prescriptions should be written according to the guidelines in Prescription Writing (p. 4). Inclusion of age is a legal requirement in the case of prescription-only medicines for children under 12 years of age, but it is preferable to state the age for **all** prescriptions for children.

It is particularly important to state the strengths of capsules or tablets. Although liquid preparations are particularly suitable for children, they may contain sugar which encourages dental decay. Sugar-free medicines are preferred for long-term treatment.

When a prescription for a liquid oral preparation is written and the dose ordered is smaller than 5 mL an **oral syringe** will be supplied (for details, see p. 1). Parents should be advised not to add any medicines to the infant's feed, since the drug may interact with the milk or other liquid in it; moreover the ingested dosage may be reduced if the child does not drink all the contents.

Parents must be warned to keep **all** medicines out of the reach of children, see Safety in the Home, p. 2.

Rare paediatric conditions

Information on substances such as *biotin* and *sodium benzoate* used in rare metabolic conditions can be obtained from:

Drug Information Centre, Alder Hey Children's Hospital, Liverpool L12 2AP. Telephone (0151) 252 5381;
Pharmacy, Great Ormond Street Hospital for Children, Great Ormond St, London, WC1N 3JH. Telephone (020) 7405 9200

Dosage in Children

Children's doses in the BNF are stated in the individual drug entries as far as possible, except where paediatric use is not recommended, information is not available, or there are special hazards.

Doses are generally based on body-weight (in kilograms) or the following age ranges:

first month (neonate)
up to 1 year (infant)
1–5 years
6–12 years

Unless the age is specified, the term 'child' in the BNF includes persons aged 12 years and younger.

DOSE CALCULATION. Children's doses may be calculated from adult doses by using age, body-weight, or body-surface area, or by a combination of these factors. The most reliable methods are those based on body-surface area.

Body-weight may be used to calculate doses expressed in mg/kg. Young children may require a higher dose per kilogram than adults because of their higher metabolic rates. Other problems need to be considered. For example, calculation by body-weight in the obese child may result in much higher doses being administered than necessary; in such cases, dose should be calculated from an ideal weight, related to height and age.

Body-surface area (BSA) estimates are more accurate for calculation of paediatric doses than body-weight since many physiological phenomena correlate better to body-surface area. The average body-surface area of a 70-kilogram human is about 1.8 m². Thus, to calculate the dose for a child the following formula may be used:

Approximate dose for patient =

$$\frac{\text{surface area of patient } (m^2) \times \text{adult dose}}{1.8}$$

The **percentage method** below may be used to calculate paediatric doses of drugs that have a wide margin between the therapeutic and the toxic dose.

Age	Ideal body-weight		Height		Body-surface	Percentage of adult dose
	kg	lb	cm	inch	m²	
Newborn*	3.5	7.7	50	20	0.23	12.5
1 month*	4.2	9	55	22	0.26	14.5
3 months*	5.6	12	59	23	0.32	18
6 months	7.7	17	67	26	0.40	22
1 year	10	22	76	30	0.47	25
3 years	15	33	94	37	0.62	33
5 years	18	40	108	42	0.73	40
7 years	23	51	120	47	0.88	50
12 years	39	86	148	58	1.25	75
Adult						
Male	68	150	173	68	1.80	100
Female	56	123	163	64	1.60	100

* The figures relate to full term and not preterm infants who may need reduced dosage according to their clinical condition.

More precise body-surface values may be calculated from height and weight by means of a nomogram (e.g. J. Insley, *A Paediatric Vade-Mecum*, 13th Edition, London, Arnold, 1996).

DOSE FREQUENCY. Doses for antibiotics are usually stated as every 6 hours. Some flexibility should be allowed in children to avoid waking them during the night. For example, the night-time dose may be given at the parent's bedtime.

Where new or potentially toxic drugs are used, the manufacturers' recommended doses should be carefully followed.

Prescribing in palliative care

Palliative care is the active total care of patients whose disease is not responsive to curative treatment. Control of pain, of other symptoms, and of psychological, social and spiritual problems, is paramount to provide the best quality of life for patients and their families. Careful assessment of symptoms and needs of the patient should be undertaken by a multidisciplinary team.

Specialist palliative care is available in most areas as day hospice care, home care teams (often known as Macmillan teams), in-patient hospice care, and hospital teams. Many acute hospitals and teaching centres now have consultative, hospital-based teams.

Hospice care of terminally ill patients has shown the importance of symptom control and psychosocial support of the patient and family. Families should be included in the care of the patient if they wish.

Many patients wish to remain at home with their families. Although some families may at first be afraid of caring for the patient at home, support can be provided by community nursing services, social services, voluntary agencies and hospices together with the general practitioner. The family may be reassured by the knowledge that the patient will be admitted to a hospital or hospice if the family cannot cope.

DRUG TREATMENT. The number of drugs should be as few as possible, for even the taking of medicine may be an effort. Oral medication is usually satisfactory unless there is severe nausea and vomiting, dysphagia, weakness, or coma, in which case parenteral medication may be necessary.

Pain

Analgesics are more effective in preventing pain than in the relief of established pain; it is important that they are given regularly.

The non-opioid analgesics **aspirin** or **paracetamol** given regularly will often make the use of opioids unnecessary. Aspirin (or other NSAIDs if preferred) may also control the pain of *bone secondaries*; naproxen, flurbiprofen, and indometacin (section 10.1.1) are valuable and if necessary can be given rectally. Radiotherapy, bisphosphonates (section 6.6.2) and radioactive isotopes of **strontium** (*Metastron®* available from Amersham) may also be useful for pain due to bone metastases.

An opioid such as **codeine** or **dextropropoxyphene**, alone or in combination with a non-opioid analgesic at adequate dosage, may be helpful in the control of moderate pain if non-opioids alone are not sufficient. If these preparations are not controlling the pain, **morphine** is the most useful opioid analgesic. Alternatives to morphine are **hydromorphone** (section 4.7.2) and transdermal **fentanyl** (see below and section 4.7.2).

ORAL ROUTE. Morphine is given *by mouth* as an oral solution or as standard ('immediate release') tablets regularly every 4 hours, the initial dose depending largely on the patient's previous treatment. A dose of 5–10 mg is enough to replace a weaker analgesic (such as paracetamol or co-proxamol), but 10–20 mg or more is required to replace a strong one (comparable to morphine itself). If the first dose of morphine is no more effective than the previous analgesic it should be increased by 50%, the aim being to choose the lowest dose which prevents pain. The dose should be adjusted with careful assessment of the pain and the use of other drugs (such as NSAIDs) should also be considered. Although morphine in a dose of 5–20 mg is usually adequate there should be no hesitation in increasing it stepwise according to response to 100 mg or occasionally up to 500 mg or higher if necessary. If pain occurs between doses the next dose due is increased; in the interim an additional dose is given.

Modified-release preparations of morphine are an alternative to the oral solution or standard formulation tablets. Depending on the formulation of the modified-release preparation, the total daily morphine requirement may be given in two equal doses or as a single dose.

Preparations suitable for twice daily administration include *MST Continus®* tablets or suspension, *Oramorph® SR* tablets, and *Zomorph®* capsules. Preparations that allow administration of the total daily morphine requirement as a single dose include *MXL®* capsules. *Morcap SR®* capsules may be given either twice daily or as a single daily dose.

The starting dose of modified-release preparations designed for twice daily administration is usually 10–20 mg every 12 hours if no other analgesic (or only paracetamol) has been taken previously, but to replace a weaker opioid analgesic (such as co-proxamol) the starting dose is usually 20–30 mg every 12 hours. Increments should be made to the dose, not to the frequency of administration, which should remain at every 12 hours.

The effective dose of modified-release preparations can alternatively be determined by giving the oral solution of morphine every 4 hours in increasing doses until the pain has been controlled, and then transferring the patient to the same total 24-hour dose of morphine given as the modified-release preparation (divided into two portions for 12-hourly administration). The first dose of the modified-release preparation is given 4 hours after the last dose of the oral solution.[1]

Morphine, as oral solution or standard formulation tablets, should be prescribed for breakthrough pain.

PARENTERAL ROUTE. If the patient becomes unable to swallow, the equivalent intramuscular dose of morphine is half the oral solution dose; in the case of the modified-release tablets it is half the total 24-hour dose (which is then divided into 6 portions to be given every 4 hours). **Diamorphine** is preferred for injection because, being more soluble, it can be given in a smaller volume. The equivalent intramuscular (or subcutaneous) dose of diamorphine is approximately a third of the oral dose of morphine. *Subcutaneous infusion* of diamorphine via syringe driver can be useful (for details, see p. 14).

---

1. Studies have indicated that administration of the last dose of the *oral solution* with the first dose of the *modified-release tablets* is not necessary.

RECTAL ROUTE. Morphine is also available for *rectal administration* as suppositories; alternatively **oxycodone** suppositories can be obtained on special order.

TRANSDERMAL ROUTE. Transdermal preparations of fentanyl are available (section 4.7.2). Careful conversion from oral morphine to transdermal fentanyl is necessary; a 25 micrograms/hour patch is equivalent to a total dose of morphine up to 135 mg/24 hours

GASTRO-INTESTINAL PAIN. The pain of *bowel colic* may be reduced by loperamide 2–4 mg 4 times daily. Hyoscine hydrobromide may also be helpful, given sublingually at a dose of 300 micrograms 3 times daily as *Kwells®* (Roche Consumer Health) tablets. For the dose by subcutaneous infusion using a syringe driver, see p.14.

Gastric distension pain due to pressure on the stomach may be helped by a preparation incorporating an antacid with an antiflatulent (section 1.1.1) and by domperidone 10 mg 3 times daily before meals.

MUSCLE SPASM. The pain of muscle spasm can be helped by a muscle relaxant such as diazepam 5–10 mg daily or baclofen 5–10 mg 3 times daily.

NEUROPATHIC PAIN. Tricyclic antidepressants can be useful; amitriptyline may be given initially at a dose of 10–25 mg each night and the dose increased gradually. If pain persists, an anticonvulsant such as *either* sodium valproate initially 200 mg twice daily increased to 1.6 g daily in divided doses *or* carbamazepine initially 200 mg at night increased to 400 mg twice daily, may be added or substituted.

Pain due to nerve compression may be reduced by a corticosteroid such as dexamethasone 8 mg daily, which reduces oedema around the tumour, thus reducing compression.

Nerve blocks may be considered when pain is localised to a specific area. **Transcutaneous electrical nerve stimulation** (TENS) may also help.

Miscellaneous conditions

Non-licensed indications or routes

Several recommendations in this section involve non-licensed indications or routes.

RAISED INTRACRANIAL PRESSURE. Headache due to raised intracranial pressure often responds to a high dose of a corticosteroid, such as dexamethasone 16 mg daily for 4 to 5 days, subsequently reduced to 4–6 mg daily if possible; dexamethasone should be given before 6 p.m. to reduce the risk of insomnia.

INTRACTABLE COUGH. Intractable cough may be relieved by moist inhalations or by regular administration of oral morphine hydrochloride (or sulphate) in an initial dose of 5 mg every 4 hours. Methadone linctus should be avoided because it has a long duration of action and tends to accumulate.

DYSPNOEA. Dyspnoea may be relieved by regular oral morphine hydrochloride (or sulphate) in carefully titrated doses, starting at 5 mg every 4 hours. Diazepam 5–10 mg daily may be helpful; a corticosteroid, such as dexamethasone 4–8 mg daily, may also be helpful if there is bronchospasm or partial obstruction.

EXCESSIVE RESPIRATORY SECRETION. Excessive respiratory secretion (death rattle) may be reduced by subcutaneous injection of hyoscine hydrobromide 400–600 micrograms every 4 to 8 hours; care must however be taken to avoid the discomfort of dry mouth. For the dose by subcutaneous infusion using a syringe driver, see next page.

RESTLESSNESS AND CONFUSION. Restlessness and confusion may require treatment with haloperidol 1–3 mg by mouth every 8 hours. Chlorpromazine 25–50 mg by mouth every 8 hours is an alternative, but causes more sedation. Levomepromazine (methotrimeprazine) is also used occasionally for restlessness. For the dose by subcutaneous infusion using a syringe driver, see next page

HICCUP. Hiccup due to gastric distension may be helped by a preparation incorporating an antacid with an antiflatulent (section 1.1). If this fails, metoclopramide 10 mg every 6 to 8 hours by mouth or by intramuscular injection can be added; if this also fails, chlorpromazine 10–25 mg every 6 to 8 hours can be tried.

ANOREXIA. Anorexia may be helped by prednisolone 15–30 mg daily or dexamethasone 2–4 mg daily.

CONSTIPATION. Constipation is a very common cause of distress and is almost invariable after administration of an opioid. It should be prevented if possible by the regular administration of laxatives; a faecal softener with a peristaltic stimulant (e.g. co-danthramer), or lactulose solution with a senna preparation should be used (section 1.6.2 and section 1.6.3).

FUNGATING GROWTH. Fungating growth may be treated by cleansing with a mixture of 1 part of 4% povidone–iodine skin cleanser solution and 4 parts of liquid paraffin. Oral administration of metronidazole (section 5.1.11) may eradicate the anaerobic bacteria responsible for the odour of fungating tumours; topical application (section 13.10.1.2) is also used.

CAPILLARY BLEEDING. Capillary bleeding may be reduced by applying gauze soaked in adrenaline (epinephrine) solution 1 mg/mL (1 in 1000).

DRY MOUTH. Dry mouth may be relieved by good mouth care and measures such as the sucking of ice or pineapple chunks or the use of artificial saliva (section 12.3.5); dry mouth associated with candidiasis can be treated by oral preparations of nystatin or miconazole (section 12.3.2); alternatively, fluconazole can be given by mouth (section 5.2). Dry mouth may be caused by certain medication including opioids, antimuscarinic drugs (e.g. hyoscine), antidepressants and some anti-emetics; if possible, an alternative preparation should be considered.

PRURITUS. Pruritus, even when associated with obstructive jaundice, often responds to simple measures such as application of emollients (section 13.2.1). In the case of obstructive jaundice, further measures include administration of colestyramine or an anabolic steroid, such as stanozolol 5–10 mg daily; antihistamines can be helpful (section 3.4.1).

CONVULSIONS. Patients with cerebral tumours or uraemia may be susceptible to convulsions. Prophylactic treatment with phenytoin or carbamazepine (section 4.8.1) should be considered. When oral medication is no longer possible, diazepam as suppositories 10–20 mg every 4 to 8 hours, or phenobarbital by injection 50–200 mg twice daily is continued as prophylaxis. For the use of midazolam by subcutaneous infusion using a syringe driver, see below.

DYSPHAGIA. A corticosteroid such as dexamethasone 8 mg daily may help, temporarily, if there is an obstruction due to tumour. See also under Dry Mouth.

NAUSEA AND VOMITING. Nausea and vomiting are common in patients with advanced cancer. Ideally, the cause should be determined before treatment with anti-emetics (section 4.6) is started.

Nausea and vomiting may occur with opioid therapy particularly in the initial stages but can be prevented by giving an anti-emetic such as haloperidol or metoclopramide. An anti-emetic is usually necessary only for the first 4 or 5 days and therefore combined preparations containing an opioid with an anti-emetic are not recommended because they lead to unnecessary anti-emetic therapy (and associated side-effects when used long-term).

Metoclopramide has a prokinetic action and is used in a dose of 10 mg 3 times daily by mouth for nausea and vomiting associated with gastritis, gastric stasis, and functional bowel obstruction. Alternatively, cisapride 20 mg twice daily by mouth may produce a stronger prokinetic action. Drugs with antimuscarinic effects antagonise prokinetic drugs and, where possible, should not therefore be used concurrently.

Haloperidol is used in a dose of 1.5 mg daily (or twice daily if nausea continues) by mouth for most chemical causes of vomiting (e.g. hypercalcaemia, renal failure).

Cyclizine is given in a dose of 50 mg up to 3 times daily by mouth. It is used for nausea and vomiting due to mechanical bowel obstruction, raised intracranial pressure, and motion sickness.

Anti-emetic therapy should be reviewed every 24 hours; it may be necessary to substitute the anti-emetic or to add another one.

Levomepromazine (methotrimeprazine) 12.5–25 mg daily by mouth may be used if first-line anti-emetics are inadequate. Dexamethasone 8–16 mg daily by mouth may be used as an adjunct.

For the administration of anti-emetics by subcutaneous infusion using a syringe driver, see below.

For the treatment of nausea and vomiting associated with cancer chemotherapy, see section 8.1.

INSOMNIA. Patients with advanced cancer may not sleep because of discomfort, cramps, night sweats, joint stiffness, or fear. There should be appropriate treatment of these problems before hypnotics are used. Benzodiazepines, such as temazepam, may be useful (section 4.1.1).

HYPERCALCAEMIA. See section 9.5.1.2.

Syringe drivers

Although drugs can usually be administered *by mouth* to control the symptoms of advanced cancer, the parenteral route may sometimes be necessary. If the parenteral route is necessary, repeated administration of *intramuscular injections* can be difficult in a cachectic patient. This has led to the use of a portable syringe driver to give a *continuous subcutaneous infusion*, which can provide good control of symptoms with little discomfort or inconvenience to the patient.

Syringe driver rate settings. Staff using syringe drivers should be **adequately trained** and different rate settings should be **clearly identified** and **differentiated**; incorrect use of syringe drivers is a common cause of drug errors.

Indications for the **parenteral route** are:
- the patient is unable to take medicines by mouth owing to *nausea and vomiting, dysphagia, severe weakness*, or *coma;*
- there is *malignant bowel obstruction* in patients for whom further surgery is inappropriate (avoiding the need for an intravenous infusion or for insertion of a nasogastric tube);
- occasionally when the patient *does not wish* to take regular medication by mouth.

NAUSEA AND VOMITING. Haloperidol is given in a *subcutaneous infusion* dose of 2.5–10 mg/24 hours.

Levomepromazine (methotrimeprazine) causes sedation in about 50% of patients; it is given in a *subcutaneous infusion dose* of 25–200 mg/24 hours, although lower doses of 5–25 mg/24 hours may be effective with less sedation.

Cyclizine is particularly liable to precipitate if mixed with diamorphine or other drugs (see under Mixing and Compatibility, below); it is given in a *subcutaneous infusion dose* of 150 mg/24 hours.

Metoclopramide may cause skin reactions; it is given in a *subcutaneous infusion dose* of 30–100 mg/24 hours.

Octreotide (section 8.3.4.3), which stimulates water and electrolyte absorption and inhibits water secretion in the small bowel, can be used by subcutaneous infusion, in a dose of 300–600 micrograms/24 hours to reduce intestinal secretions and vomiting.

BOWEL COLIC AND EXCESSIVE RESPIRATORY SECRETIONS. Hyoscine hydrobromide effectively reduces respiratory secretions and is sedative (but occasionally causes paradoxical agitation); it is given in a *subcutaneous infusion dose* of 0.6–2.4 mg/24 hours.

Hyoscine butylbromide is effective in bowel colic, is less sedative than hyoscine hydrobromide, but is not always adequate for the control of respiratory secretions; it is given in a *subcutaneous infusion dose* of 20–60 mg/24 hours (**important:** this dose of *hyoscine butylbromide* must not be confused with the much lower dose of *hyoscine hydrobromide*, above).

Glycopyrronium 0.6–1.2 mg/24 hours may also be used.

RESTLESSNESS AND CONFUSION. Haloperidol has little sedative effect; it is given in a *subcutaneous infusion dose* of 5–15 mg/24 hours.

Levomepromazine (methotrimeprazine) has a sedative effect; it is given in a *subcutaneous infusion dose* of 50–200 mg/24 hours.

Midazolam is a sedative and an antiepileptic, and is therefore suitable for a very restless patient; it is given in a *subcutaneous infusion dose* of 20–100 mg/24 hours.

CONVULSIONS. If a patient has previously been receiving an antiepileptic *or* has a primary or secondary cerebral tumour *or* is at risk of convulsion (e.g. owing to uraemia) antiepileptic medication should not be stopped. Midazolam is the benzodiazepine antiepileptic of choice for *continuous subcutaneous infusion*, and is given in a dose of 20–40 mg/24 hours.

PAIN CONTROL. Diamorphine is the preferred opioid since its high solubility permits a large dose to be given in a small volume (see under Mixing and Compatibility, below). The table below gives the approximate doses of *morphine by mouth* (as oral solution or standard formulation tablets or as modified-release tablets) equivalent to *diamorphine by injection* (intramuscularly or by subcutaneous infusion).

MIXING AND COMPATIBILITY. The general principle that injections should be given into separate sites (and should not be mixed) does not apply to the use of syringe drivers in palliative care. Provided that there is evidence of compatibility, selected medication can be mixed in syringe drivers. Not all types of medication can be used in a subcutaneous infusion. In particular, chlorpromazine, prochlorperazine and diazepam are **contra-indicated** as they cause skin reactions at the injection site; to a lesser extent cyclizine and levomepromazine (methotrimeprazine) may also sometimes cause local irritation.

In theory injections dissolved in water for injections are more likely to be associated with pain (possibly owing to their hypotonicity). The use of physiological saline (sodium chloride 0.9%) however increases the likelihood of precipitation when more than one drug is used; moreover subcutaneous infusion rates are so slow (0.1–0.3 mL/hour) that pain is not usually a problem when water is used as a diluent.

Diamorphine can be given by subcutaneous infusion in a strength of up to 250 mg/mL; up to a strength of 40 mg/mL either *water for injections* or *physiological saline* (sodium chloride 0.9%) is a suitable diluent—above that strength only *water for injections* is used (to avoid precipitation).

The following can be mixed with *diamorphine:*

Cyclizine[1]	Hyoscine hydrobromide
Dexamethasone[2]	Levomepromazine
Haloperidol[3]	Metoclopramide[4]
Hyoscine butylbromide	Midazolam

Subcutaneous infusion solution should be monitored regularly both to check for precipitation (and discoloration) and to ensure that the infusion is running at the correct rate.

PROBLEMS ENCOUNTERED WITH SYRINGE DRIVERS. The following are problems that may be encountered with syringe drivers and the action that should be taken:

- if the subcutaneous infusion runs *too quickly* check the rate setting and the calculation;
- if the subcutaneous infusion runs *too slowly* check the start button, the battery, the syringe driver, the cannula, and make sure that the injection site is not inflamed;
- if there is an *injection site reaction* make sure that the site does not need to be changed—firmness or swelling at the site of injection is not in itself an indication for change, but pain or obvious inflammation is.

1. Cyclizine may precipitate at concentrations above 10 mg/mL *or* in the presence of physiological saline *or* as the concentration of diamorphine relative to cyclizine increases; mixtures of diamorphine and cyclizine are also liable to precipitate after 24 hours.

2. Special care is needed to avoid precipitation of dexamethasone when preparing.

3. Mixtures of haloperidol and diamorphine are liable to precipitate after 24 hours if haloperidol concentration is above 2 mg/mL.

4. Under some conditions metoclopramide may become discoloured; such solutions should be discarded.

Equivalent doses of morphine sulphate by mouth (as oral solution or standard tablets *or* as modified-release tablets) *or* of diamorphine hydrochloride by intramuscular injection *or by* subcutaneous infusion

These equivalences are approximate only and may need to be adjusted according to response

ORAL MORPHINE		PARENTERAL DIAMORPHINE	
Morphine sulphate oral solution or standard tablets	Morphine sulphate modified-release tablets	Diamorphine hydrochloride by intramuscular injection	Diamorphine hydrochloride by subcutaneous infusion
every 4 hours	every 12 hours	every 4 hours	every 24 hours
5 mg	20 mg	2.5 mg	15 mg
10 mg	30 mg	5 mg	20 mg
15 mg	50 mg	5 mg	30 mg
20 mg	60 mg	7.5 mg	45 mg
30 mg	90 mg	10 mg	60 mg
40 mg	120 mg	15 mg	90 mg
60 mg	180 mg	20 mg	120 mg
80 mg	240 mg	30 mg	180 mg
100 mg	300 mg	40 mg	240 mg
130 mg	400 mg	50 mg	300 mg
160 mg	500 mg	60 mg	360 mg
200 mg	600 mg	70 mg	400 mg

If breakthrough pain occurs give a subcutaneous (preferable) or intramuscular injection of diamorphine equivalent to one-sixth of the total 24-hour subcutaneous infusion dose. It is kinder to give an intermittent bolus injection *subcutaneously*—absorption is smoother so that the risk of adverse effects at peak absorption is avoided (an even better method is to use a subcutaneous butterfly needle).

To minimise the risk of infection no individual subcutaneous infusion solution should be used for longer than 24 hours.

Prescribing for the elderly

Old people, especially the very old, require special care and consideration from prescribers.

POLYPHARMACY. Elderly patients often receive multiple drugs for their multiple diseases. This greatly increases the risk of drug interactions as well as adverse reactions. Moreover, symptoms such as headache, sleeplessness, and lightheadedness which may be associated with social stress, as in widowhood, loneliness, and family dispersal can lead to further prescribing, especially of psychotropics. The use of drugs in such cases can at best be a poor substitute for effective social measures and at worst pose a serious threat from adverse reactions. Whilst unnecessary medication should be avoided, elderly patients should not be denied effective treatments such as those for stroke prophylaxis in atrial fibrillation or for osteoporosis.

FORM OF MEDICINE. Frail elderly patients may have difficulty swallowing tablets; if left in the mouth, ulceration may develop. They should always be encouraged to take their tablets or capsules with enough fluid, and in some cases it may be helpful to discuss with the patient the possibility of prescribing the drug as a liquid if available.

MANIFESTATIONS OF AGEING. In very old subjects, manifestations of normal ageing may be mistaken for disease and lead to inappropriate prescribing. For example, drugs such as prochlorperazine are commonly misprescribed for giddiness due to age-related loss of postural stability. Not only is such treatment ineffective but the patient may experience serious side-effects such as parkinsonism, postural hypotension, and confusion.

SELF-MEDICATION. Self-medication with over-the-counter products or with drugs prescribed for a previous illness (or even for another person) may be an added complication. Discussion with both the patient and relatives as well as a home visit may be needed to establish exactly what is being taken.

SENSITIVITY. The ageing nervous system shows increased *susceptibility* to many commonly used drugs, such as opioid analgesics, benzodiazepines, antipsychotics, and antiparkinsonian drugs, all of which must be used with caution.

Pharmacokinetics

The most important effect of age is reduction in renal clearance. Many aged patients thus *excrete drugs slowly*, and are *highly susceptible to nephrotoxic drugs*. Acute illness may lead to rapid reduction in renal clearance, especially if accompanied by dehydration. Hence, a patient stabilised on a drug with a narrow margin between the therapeutic and the toxic dose (e.g. digoxin) may rapidly develop adverse effects in the aftermath of a myocardial infarction or a respiratory-tract infection. Metabolism of drugs in the liver may be reduced in the elderly.

The net result of pharmacokinetic changes is that the tissue concentration of a drug is commonly increased by over 50%, and debilitated patients may show even larger changes.

Adverse reactions

Adverse reactions often present in the elderly in a vague and non-specific fashion. *Confusion* is often the presenting symptom (caused by almost any of the commonly used drugs). Other common manifestations are *constipation* (with antimuscarinics and many tranquillisers) and postural *hypotension* and *falls* (with diuretics and many psychotropics).

HYPNOTICS. Many hypnotics with long half-lives have serious hangover effects of drowsiness, unsteady gait, and even slurred speech and confusion. Those with short half-lives should be used but they too can present problems (section 4.1.1). Short courses of hypnotics are occasionally useful for helping a patient through an acute illness or some other crisis but every effort must be made to avoid dependence. Benzodiazepines impair balance, which may result in falls.

DIURETICS. Diuretics are overprescribed in old age and should **not** be used on a long-term basis to treat simple gravitational oedema which will usually respond to increased movement, raising the legs, and support stockings. A few days of diuretic treatment may speed the clearing of the oedema but it should rarely need continued drug therapy.

NSAIDs. Bleeding associated with *aspirin* and *other NSAIDs* is more common in the elderly who are more likely to have a fatal or serious outcome. NSAIDs are also a special hazard in patients with cardiac disease or renal impairment which may again place older patients at particular risk.

Owing to the *increased susceptibilty of the elderly* to the *side-effects of NSAIDs* the following recommendations are made:

- for *osteoarthritis, soft-tissue lesions* and *back pain* first try measures such as weight reduction (if obese), warmth, exercise and use of a walking stick;
- for *osteoarthritis, soft-tissue lesions, back pain* and *pain in rheumatoid arthritis*, paracetamol should be used first and can often provide adequate pain relief;
- alternatively, a low-dose NSAID (e.g. ibuprofen up to 1.2 g daily may be given;
- for pain relief when either drug is inadequate, paracetamol in a full dose plus a low-dose NSAID may be given;
- if necessary, the NSAID dose can be increased or a low-dose opioid analgesic given with paracetamol (e.g. co-codamol 8/500 or co-dydramol 10/500);
- do not give two NSAIDs at the same time.

For advice on prophylaxis of NSAID-induced peptic ulcers if continued NSAID treatment is necessary, see section 1.3.

OTHER DRUGS. Other drugs which commonly cause adverse reactions are *antiparkinsonian drugs, antihypertensives, psychotropics*, and *digoxin*. The usual maintenance dose of digoxin in very old patients is 125 micrograms daily (62.5 micrograms in those with renal disease); lower doses are often inadequate but toxicity is common in those given 250 micrograms daily.

Drug-induced blood disorders are much more common in the elderly. Therefore drugs with a tendency to cause bone marrow depression (e.g. *co-trimoxazole, mianserin*) should be avoided unless there is no acceptable alternative.

The elderly generally require a lower maintenance dose of *warfarin* than younger adults; once again, the outcome of bleeding tends to be more serious.

Guidelines

First always question whether a drug is indicated at all.

LIMIT RANGE. It is a sensible policy to prescribe from a limited range of drugs and to be thoroughly familiar with their effects in the elderly.

REDUCE DOSE. Dosage should generally be substantially lower than for younger patients and it is common to start with about 50% of the adult dose. Some drugs (e.g. long-acting antidiabetic drugs such as glibenclamide and chlorpropamide) should be avoided altogether.

REVIEW REGULARLY. Review repeat prescriptions regularly. It may be possible to stop the drug (e.g. digoxin can often be withdrawn) or it may be necessary to reduce the dose to match diminishing renal function.

SIMPLIFY REGIMENS. Elderly patients benefit from simple treatment regimens. Only drugs with a clear indication should be prescribed and whenever possible given once or twice daily. In particular, regimens which call for a confusing array of dosage intervals should be avoided.

EXPLAIN CLEARLY. Write full instructions on every prescription (*including* repeat prescriptions) so that containers can be properly labelled with full directions. Avoid imprecisions like 'as directed'. Child-resistant containers may be unsuitable.

REPEATS AND DISPOSAL. Instruct patients what to do when drugs run out, and also how to dispose of any that are no longer necessary. Try to prescribe matching quantities.

If these guidelines are followed most elderly people will cope adequately with their own medicines. If not then it is essential to enrol the help of a third party, usually a relative or a friend.

Drugs and sport

Doping Classes and Methods of the International Olympic Committee Medical Commission 1999

The following are examples of classes and methods prohibited in sport:

Classes	**Stimulants** eg. amphetamine, bromantan, caffeine (above 12mcg/mL), carphedon, cocaine, ephedrine, certain beta$_2$ agonists*. **Narcotics** eg. diamorphine (heroin), morphine, methadone, pethidine. **Anabolic Agents** eg. methandienone, nandrolone, stanozolol, testosterone, clenbuterol, DHEA, androstenedione, 19-norandrostenadiol, certain beta$_2$ agonists*. **Diuretics** eg. acetazolamide, frusemide, hydrochlorothiazide, triamterene, mannitol. **Peptide Hormones, Mimetics & Analogues** eg. growth hormone, corticotrophin, chorionic gonadotrophin, erythropoietin, insulin*, and all respective releasing factors and their analogues.
Methods	**Blood Doping** **Pharmacological, Chemical & Physical Manipulation** eg. substances and methods that alter the integrity and validity of the urine; eg. diuretics, probenecid, catheterisation, sample substitution or tampering.
Classes of drugs subject to certain restrictions	**Alcohol & Cannabinoids** Restricted in certain sports. Refer to regulations of national or international sports federations. **Local Anaesthetics** Route of administration restricted to local or intra-articular injection, when medically justified*. **Corticosteroids** Route of administration restricted to anal, aural, dermatological, inhalational, nasal and opthalmological (but not rectal), local or intra-articular injection*. **Beta-blockers** Restricted in certain sports. Refer to regulations of national or international sports federations.

*Written notification of administration to the relevant medical authority may be required, eg. governing body medical officer. Check with your governing body.

Treatment Guidelines
Examples of permitted & prohibited substances

	ALLOWED	BANNED
ASTHMA	sodium cromoglycate, theophylline, salbutamol*, terbutaline*, salmeterol*, beclomethasone**, fluticasone**, (*by inhalation only and written notification of administration should be given to relevant medical authority) (** by inhalation only).	products containing sympathomimetics eg. ephedrine, isoprenaline, fenoterol, rimiterol, orciprenaline.
COLD/ COUGH	all antibiotics, steam & menthol inhalations, permitted antihistamines, terfenadine, astemizole, pholcodine, guaiphenesin, dextromethorphan, paracetamol.	products containing sympathomimetics eg. ephedrine, pseudoephedrine, phenylpropanolamine.
DIARRHOEA	diphenoxylate, loperamide, products containing electrolytes (eg. Dioralyte, Rehidrat).	products containing opioids eg. morphine.
HAYFEVER	antihistamines, nasal sprays containing a corticosteroid or xylometazoline, eyedrops containing sodium cromoglycate.	products containing ephedrine, pseudoephedrine.
PAIN	aspirin, codeine, dihydrocodeine, ibuprofen, paracetamol, all non-steroidal anti-inflammatories, dextropropoxyphene.	products containing opioids, caffeine.
VOMITING	domperidone, metoclopramide.	

WARNING. Prescribed medicines may contain prohibited substances. Some vitamin, herbal and nutritional substances may contain prohibited substances, such as Guarana, Ma Huang, Chinese Ephedra.

The substances listed are only examples of substances permitted or prohibited by the IOC. Not all sports adopt the IOC Medical Code. If in doubt check with the relevant governing body or with the UK Sport Drug Information Line (020) 7380 8030.

Supplies of this card are available from: UK Sport, Ethics & Anti-Doping, Walkden House, 10 Melton Street, London NW1 2EB.

Similar cards detailing classes of drugs and doping methods prohibited by the Football Association and the Lawn Tennis Association are also available from the respective governing bodies.

General information about drugs and sports together with more comprehensive lists of permitted medications in sport is published in *Competitors and Officials Guide to Drugs and Sport* which may be purchased from UK Sport.

Emergency treatment of poisoning

These notes are only guidelines and it is strongly recommended that **poisons information centres** (see below) be consulted in cases where there is doubt about the degree of risk or about appropriate management.

HOSPITAL ADMISSION. All patients who show features of poisoning should generally be admitted to hospital. Patients who have taken poisons with delayed actions should also be admitted, even if they appear well; delayed-action poisons include aspirin, iron, paracetamol, tricyclic antidepressants, co-phenotrope (diphenoxylate with atropine, *Lomotil*®), and paraquat; this also applies to modified-release preparations. A note should be sent of what is known and what treatment has been given.

It is often impossible to establish with certainty the identity of the poison and the size of the dose. Fortunately this is not usually important because only a few poisons (such as opioids, paracetamol, and iron) have specific antidotes and few patients require active removal of the poison. Most patients must be treated symptomatically. Nevertheless, knowledge of the type of poisoning does help in anticipating the course of events. Patients' reports may be of little help, because they may be confused or may only be able to say that they have taken an undefined amount, possibly of mixed drugs. Parents may think a child has taken something which could be poisonous and may exaggerate or underplay the risks out of anxiety or guilt. Sometimes symptoms are due to an illness such as appendicitis. Accidents can arise from a number of domestic and industrial products (the contents of which are not generally known).

TOXBASE

TOXBASE, the primary clinical toxicology database of the National Poisons Information Service, has recently become available on the Internet (http://www.spib.axl.co.uk/). It provides information about routine diagnosis, treatment and management of patients exposed to drugs, household products, and industrial and agricultural chemicals. For further information contact 0131-536 2298. **Important:** for specialised information telephone the Poisons Information Centres.

TICTAC

TICTAC is a computer-aided tablet and capsule identification system. It is available to authorised users including Regional Drug Information Centres (see inside front cover) and Poisons Information Centres.

> The **poisons information centres** (see below) will provide advice on all aspects of poisoning day and night

Poisons information centres (consult day and night)

Belfast	(028) 9024 0503
Birmingham	0121-507 5588
or	0121-507 5589
Cardiff	(029) 2070 9901
Dublin	Dublin 837 9964
Edinburgh	0131-536 2300
London	(020) 7635 9191
Newcastle	0191-282 0300

Note. Some of these centres also advise on laboratory analytical services which may be of help in the diagnosis and management of a small number of cases

General care

Respiration

Respiration is often impaired in unconscious patients. An obstructed airway requires immediate attention. Pull the tongue forward, remove dentures and oral secretions, hold the jaw forward, insert an oropharyngeal airway if one is available, and turn the patient semiprone. The risk of inhaling vomit is minimised with the patient positioned semiprone and head down.

Most poisons that impair consciousness also depress respiration. Assisted ventilation by mouth-to-mouth or *Ambu-bag* inflation may be needed. Oxygen is not a substitute for adequate ventilation, though it should be given in the highest concentration possible in poisoning with carbon monoxide and irritant gases.

Respiratory stimulants do not help and are **potentially dangerous**.

Blood pressure

Hypotension is common in severe poisoning with central nervous system depressants. A systolic blood pressure of less than 70 mmHg may lead to irreversible brain damage or renal tubular necrosis. The patient should be carried head downwards on a stretcher and nursed in this position in the ambulance. Oxygen should be given to correct hypoxia and an intravenous infusion set up if practicable. Vasopressor drugs should **not** be used.

Fluid depletion without hypotension is common after prolonged coma and after aspirin poisoning due to vomiting, sweating, and hyperpnoea.

Hypertension, often transient, occurs less frequently than hypotension in poisoning; it may be associated with sympathomimetic drugs such as amphetamines, phencyclidine, and cocaine.

Heart

Cardiac conduction defects and arrhythmias may occur in acute poisoning, notably with tricyclic antidepressants. Arrhythmias often respond to correction of underlying hypoxia or acidosis. Ventricular arrhythmias that have been confirmed by emergency ECG and which are causing serious hypotension may require treatment with lidocaine (lignocaine) (section 2.3.2). Supraventricular arrhythmias are seldom life-threatening and drug treatment is best withheld until the patient reaches hospital.

Body temperature

Hypothermia may develop in patients of any age who have been deeply unconscious for some hours particularly following overdose with barbiturates or phenothiazines. It may be missed unless core temperature is measured using a low-reading rectal thermometer or by some other means. It is best treated by wrapping the patient (e.g. in a 'space blanket') to conserve body heat. A *mild* source of heat (such as water bottles heated to 42°C) may be used and care must be taken to avoid causing burns.

Hyperthermia can develop in patients taking CNS stimulants; children and the elderly are also at risk when taking drugs with antimuscarinic properties at therapeutic doses. It is initially managed by removing all unnecessary clothing. Active cooling with water will promote evaporation; iced water should **not** be used.

Both hypothermia and hyperthermia require urgent hospitalisation for assessment and supportive treatment.

Convulsions

Single short-lived convulsions do not require treatment. Diazepam, up to 10 mg by slow intravenous injection, preferably in emulsion form, should be given if convulsions are protracted or recur frequently; it should not be given intramuscularly.

Removal and elimination

Removal from the stomach

The dangers of attempting to empty the stomach have to be balanced against the toxicity of the ingested poison, as assessed by the quantity ingested, the inherent toxicity of the poison, and the time since ingestion. Gastric emptying is clearly unnecessary if the risk of toxicity is small or if the patient presents too late.

Emptying the stomach by **gastric lavage** is of doubtful value if attempted more than 1 hour after ingestion. The chief danger of gastric aspiration and lavage is inhalation of stomach contents, and it should **not** be attempted in drowsy or comatose patients unless there is a good enough cough reflex or the airway can be protected by a cuffed endotracheal tube. Stomach tubes should **not** be passed after corrosive poisoning.

Petroleum products are more dangerous in the lungs than in the stomach and therefore removal from the stomach is **not** advised because of the risk of inhalation.

On balance gastric lavage is seldom practicable or desirable before the patient reaches hospital.

Emesis induced by **ipecacuanha** (Paediatric Ipecacuanha Emetic Mixture BP) has been used in adults and children, but is of very limited value. There is no evidence that it prevents clinically sig-

nificant absorption (even if used within 1–2 hours) and its adverse effects may often complicate diagnosis particularly in iron poisoning. It should only be considered if the patient is fully conscious, if the poison ingested is neither corrosive nor a petroleum distillate, if it is not adsorbed by activated charcoal, or if gastric lavage is inadvisable or refused (for advice call a poisons information centre).

Salt solutions, copper sulphate, apomorphine, and mustard are dangerous and should **not** be used.

IPECACUANHA

Indications: induction of emesis in selected patients, see notes above

Cautions: avoid in poisoning with corrosive or petroleum products owing to risk of aspiration (see notes above); also avoid if risk of aspiration, in shock, or if risk of convulsions; cardiovascular disease

Side-effects: excessive vomiting and mucosal damage; cardiac effects if absorbed

Dose: see under preparation below

Ipecacuanha Emetic Mixture, Paediatric, BP
Paediatric Ipecacuanha Emetic
> *Note.* Paediatric Ipecacuanha Emetic Mixture is equivalent in strength to Ipecac Syrup USP
> *Mixture,* ipecacuanha liquid extract 0.7 mL, hydrochloric acid 0.025 mL, glycerol 1 mL, syrup to 10 mL
> *Dose:* ADULT 30 mL; CHILD 6–18 months 10 mL, older children 15 mL; the dose is followed by a tumblerful of water and repeated after 20 minutes if necessary

Prevention of absorption

Given by mouth, **activated charcoal** can bind many poisons in the stomach, thereby *reducing their absorption.* The **sooner** it is given the **more effective** it is, but it may still be effective up to 1 hour after ingestion of the poison—longer in the case of modified-release preparations or of drugs with antimuscarinic (anticholinergic) properties. It is relatively safe and is particularly useful for the prevention of absorption of poisons which are toxic in small amounts, e.g. antidepressants.

For the use of charcoal in active elimination techniques, see below.

Actidose-Aqua® (Cambridge)
Oral suspension, activated charcoal, net price 50-g pack (240 mL) = £12.50
> *Dose:* reduction of absorption, 50–100 g; INFANT under 1 year 1 g/kg (approx. 5 mL/kg), CHILD 1–12 years 25–50 g
> Active elimination (see below), 25–50 g every 4–6 hours; INFANT under 1 year, 1 g/kg (approx. 5 mL/kg) every 4–6 hours; CHILD 1–12 years, 25–50 g every 4–6 hours

Carbomix® (Penn)
Powder, activated charcoal, net price 25-g pack = £8.50, 50-g pack = £11.90
> *Dose:* reduction of absorption, 50 g; CHILD under 12 years 25 g (50 g in severe poisoning)
> Active elimination, see below

Charcodote® (Dominion)
Oral suspension, activated charcoal, net price 50-g pack = £12.50
> *Dose:* reduction of absorption, 50 g; CHILD under 12 years 25 g (50 g in severe poisoning)
> Active elimination, see below

Liqui-Char® (Oxford)

Oral suspension, activated charcoal, net price 25-g pack = £7.50, 50-g pack = £12.50

Dose: reduction of absorption, 50 g; CHILD under 12 years 25 g (50 g in severe poisoning)

Active elimination, see below

Medicoal® (Concord)

Granules, effervescent, activated charcoal 5 g/sachet. Contains Na⁺ 17.9 mmol/sachet. Net price 5-sachet pack = £6.52, 30-sachet pack = £30.16

Dose: reduction of absorption, initially 2 sachets repeated every 15–20 minutes until dose of charcoal given is 10 times that of poison ingested (if amount known) or until max. 10 sachets/24 hours have been given; each sachet suspended in approx. 100 mL water (may be administered in divided doses for children)

Active elimination techniques

Repeated doses of **activated charcoal** by mouth *enhance the elimination* of some drugs after they have been absorbed; repeated doses are given after overdosage with:

Carbamazepine	Quinine
Dapsone	Theophylline
Phenobarbital	

The usual adult dose of activated charcoal is 50 g initially then 50 g every 4 hours. Vomiting should be treated (e.g. with an anti-emetic drug) since it may reduce the efficacy of charcoal treatment. In cases of intolerance, the dose may be reduced and the frequency increased (e.g. 25 g every 2 hours *or* 12.5 g every hour) but this may compromise efficacy.

Other techniques intended to enhance the elimination of poisons after absorption are only practicable in hospital and are only suitable for a small number of severely poisoned patients. Moreover, they only apply to a limited number of poisons. Examples include:

Haemodialysis for salicylates, phenobarbital, methyl alcohol (methanol), ethylene glycol, and lithium

Haemoperfusion for medium- and short-acting barbiturates, chloral hydrate, meprobamate, and theophylline.

Alkalinisation of the urine increases elimination of salicylates, but forced alkaline diuresis is no longer recommended.

Specific drugs

Alcohol

Acute intoxication with alcohol (ethanol) is common in adults but also occurs in children. The features include ataxia, dysarthria, nystagmus, and drowsiness, which may progress to coma, with hypotension and acidosis. Aspiration of vomit is a special hazard and hypoglycaemia may occur in children and some adults. Patients are managed supportively with particular attention to maintaining a clear airway and measures to reduce the risk of aspiration of gastric contents. The blood glucose is measured and glucose given if indicated.

Analgesics (non-opioid)

ASPIRIN. The chief features of salicylate poisoning are hyperventilation, tinnitus, deafness, vasodilatation, and sweating. Coma is uncommon but indicates very severe poisoning. The associated acid-base disturbances are complex.

Treatment must be in hospital where plasma salicylate, pH, and electrolytes can be measured. Fluid losses are replaced and sodium bicarbonate (1.26%) given to enhance urinary salicylate excretion when the plasma-salicylate concentration is greater than

500 mg/litre (3.6 mmol/litre) in adults *or*
350 mg/litre (2.5 mmol/litre) in children.

Haemodialysis is the treatment of choice for severe salicylate poisoning and should be given serious consideration when the plasma-salicylate concentration is greater than 700 mg/litre (5.1 mmol/litre) or in the presence of severe metabolic acidosis.

NSAIDs. Mefenamic acid is an important member of this group encountered in overdosage. Convulsions are the most important feature of toxicity and are treated with diazepam.

Ibuprofen may cause nausea, vomiting, and tinnitus, but more serious toxicity is very uncommon. Gastric emptying is indicated if more than 400 mg/kg has been ingested within the preceding hour, followed by symptomatic measures.

PARACETAMOL. As little as 10–15 g (20–30 tablets) of paracetamol may cause severe hepatocellular necrosis and, less frequently, renal tubular necrosis. Nausea and vomiting, the only early features of poisoning, usually settle within 24 hours. Persistence beyond this time, often associated with the onset of right subcostal pain and tenderness, usually indicates development of hepatic necrosis. Liver damage is maximal 3–4 days after ingestion and may lead to encephalopathy, haemorrhage, hypoglycaemia, cerebral oedema, and death.

Therefore, despite a lack of significant early symptoms, patients who have taken an overdose of paracetamol should be transferred to hospital urgently.

Administration of activated charcoal should be considered if paracetamol 150 mg/kg or more is thought to have been ingested within the previous hour.

Antidotes such as **acetylcysteine** and **methionine** protect the liver if given within 10–12 hours of ingestion; acetylcysteine is effective up to and possibly beyond 24 hours.

Patients at risk of liver damage and therefore requiring treatment can be identified from a single measurement of the plasma-paracetamol concentration, related to the time from ingestion, provided this time interval is not less than 4 hours; earlier samples may be misleading. The concentration is plotted on a paracetamol treatment graph of a reference line ('normal treatment line') joining plots of 200 mg/litre (1.32 mmol/litre) at 4 hours and 6.25 mg/litre (0.04 mmol/litre) at 24 hours (see below). Those whose plasma-paracetamol concentrations are above the *normal treatment line* are treated with acetylcysteine by intravenous infusion (or with methionine by mouth, provided the overdose has been taken **within 10–12 hours** *and* the patient is not vomiting). Patients on enzyme-inducing drugs (e.g. carbamazepine, phenobarbital, phenytoin, rifampicin, and alcohol) or who are malnourished (e.g. in anorexia, in alcoholism, or those who are HIV-positive) may develop toxicity at **lower** plasma-paracetamol concentrations and should be treated if concentrations are above the *high-risk treatment line* (which joins plots that are at 50% of the plasma-paracetamol concentrations of the normal treatment line).

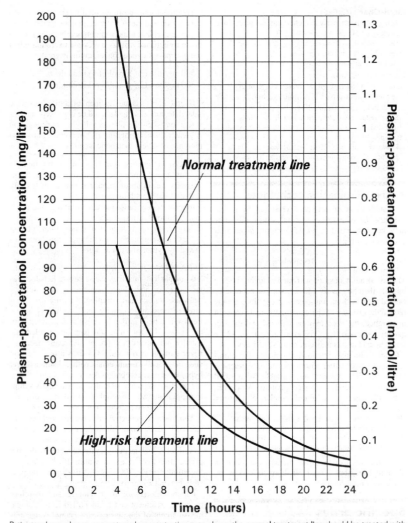

Normal treatment line

High-risk treatment line

Time (hours)

Patients whose plasma-paracetamol concentrations are above the **normal treatment line** should be treated with acetylcysteine by intravenous infusion (or with methionine by mouth, provided the overdose has been taken **within 10–12 hours** *and* the patient is not vomiting). Patients on enzyme-inducing drugs (e.g. carbamazepine, phenobarbital, phenytoin, rifampicin, and alcohol) or who are malnourished (e.g. in anorexia, in alcoholism, or those who are HIV-positive) should be treated if their plasma-paracetamol concentrations are above the **high-risk treatment line**.
Graph reproduced courtesy of University of Wales College of Medicine Therapeutics and Toxicology Centre

Plasma-paracetamol concentration may be difficult to interpret when paracetamol has been ingested over several hours. If there is doubt about timing or the need for treatment then the patient should be treated with an antidote.

In remote areas methionine (2.5 g) should be given by mouth since it is seldom practicable to give acetylcysteine outside hospital. Once the patient reaches hospital the need to continue treatment with the antidote will be assessed from the plasma-paracetamol concentration (related to the time from ingestion).

See also Co-proxamol, under Analgesics (opioid).

ACETYLCYSTEINE

Indications: paracetamol overdosage (see notes above)

Cautions: asthma

Side-effects: rashes, anaphylaxis

Dose: *by intravenous infusion,* in glucose intravenous infusion 5%, initially 150 mg/kg in 200 mL over 15 minutes, followed by 50 mg/kg in 500 mL over 4 hours, then 100 mg/kg in 1000 mL over 16 hours

Parvolex® (Medeva) [PoM]
Injection, acetylcysteine 200 mg/mL. Net price 10-mL amp = £2.65

METHIONINE

Indications: paracetamol overdosage, see notes above
Dose: by mouth, 2.5 g initially, followed by 3 further doses of 2.5 g every 4 hours

Methionine (Non-proprietary)
Tablets, DL-methionine 250 mg. Net price course of 40 tabs = £13.22
Available from Norton

Analgesics (opioid)

Opioids (narcotic analgesics) cause varying degrees of coma, respiratory depression, and pinpoint pupils. The specific antidote **naloxone** is indicated if there is coma or bradypnoea. Since naloxone has a shorter duration of action than many opioids, close monitoring and repeated injections are necessary according to the respiratory rate and depth of coma. Alternatively, it may be given by continuous intravenous infusion, the rate of administration being adjusted according to response. The effects of some opioids, such as buprenorphine, are only partially reversed by naloxone.

CO-PROXAMOL. Combinations of dextropropoxyphene and paracetamol (co-proxamol) are frequently taken in overdosage. The initial features are those of acute opioid overdosage with coma, respiratory depression, and pinpoint pupils. Patients may die of acute cardiovascular collapse before reaching hospital (particularly if alcohol has also been consumed) unless adequately resuscitated or given **naloxone** as antidote to the dextropropoxyphene. Paracetamol hepatotoxicity may develop later and should be anticipated and treated as indicated above.

NALOXONE HYDROCHLORIDE

Indications: overdosage with opioids; postoperative respiratory depression (section 15.1.7)
Cautions: physical dependence on opioids; cardiac irritability; naloxone is short-acting, see notes above
Dose: *by intravenous injection*, 0.8–2 mg repeated at intervals of 2–3 minutes to a max. of 10 mg if respiratory function does not improve (then question diagnosis); CHILD 10 micrograms/kg; subsequent dose of 100 micrograms/kg if no response
By subcutaneous or intramuscular injection, as intravenous injection but only if intravenous route not feasible (onset of action slower)
By continuous intravenous infusion, 2 mg diluted in 500 mL intravenous infusion solution at a rate adjusted according to the response
IMPORTANT. Doses used in acute opioid overdosage may not be appropriate for the management of opioid-induced respiratory depression and sedation in those receiving palliative care and in chronic opioid use, see also section 15.1.7 for management of postoperative respiratory depression

Naloxone (Non-proprietary) [PoM]
Injection, naloxone hydrochloride
400 micrograms/mL. Net price 1-mL amp = £4.10
Available from Antigen, Faulding DBL

Min-I-Jet® Naloxone (IMS) [PoM]
Injection, naloxone hydrochloride
400 micrograms/mL. Net price 1-mL disposable syringe = £5.23; 2-mL disposable syringe = £9.74
Narcan® (Du Pont) [PoM]
Injection, naloxone hydrochloride
400 micrograms/mL, net price 1-mL amp = £4.54
Neonatal preparations —section 15.1.7

Antidepressants

Tricyclic and related antidepressants cause dry mouth, coma of varying degree, hypotension, hypothermia, hyperreflexia, extensor plantar responses, convulsions, respiratory failure, cardiac conduction defects, and arrhythmias. Dilated pupils and urinary retention also occur. Metabolic acidosis may complicate severe poisoning; delirium with confusion, agitation, and visual and auditory hallucinations, is common during recovery.

Symptomatic treatment and activated charcoal by mouth may reasonably be given in the home before transfer but hospital admission is strongly advised, and supportive measures to ensure a patent airway and adequate ventilation during transfer are mandatory. Intravenous diazepam may be required for control of convulsions (preferably in emulsion form). Although arrhythmias are worrying, some will respond to correction of hypoxia and acidosis; the use of anti-arrhythmic drugs is best avoided. Diazepam given by mouth is usually adequate to sedate delirious patients but large doses may be required.

Antimalarials

Overdosage with chloroquine and hydroxychloroquine is extremely hazardous and difficult to treat. Urgent advice from a poisons information centre is essential. Life-threatening features include arrhythmias (which can have a very rapid onset) and convulsions (which can be intractable). Quinine overdosage is also a severe hazard and calls for urgent advice from a poisons information centre.

Beta-blockers

Therapeutic overdosages with beta-blockers may cause lightheadedness, dizziness, and possibly syncope due to impaired circulation secondary to bradycardia and hypotension; heart failure may be precipitated or exacerbated. These complications are most likely in patients with pre-existing conduction system disorders or impaired myocardial function. Bradycardia is the most common arrhythmia caused by beta-blockers, but sotalol occasionally induces ventricular tachyarrhythmias (sometimes of the torsades de pointes type). The effects of massive overdosage may vary from one beta-blocker to another; propranolol overdosage in particular may cause coma and convulsions.

Acute massive overdosage must be managed in hospital and expert advice should be obtained. Maintenance of a clear airway and adequate ventilation is mandatory. An intravenous injection of atropine is required to treat bradycardia and hypotension (3 mg for an adult, 40 micrograms/kg for a child). Cardiogenic shock unresponsive to atropine is probably best treated with an intravenous injection of glucagon 50–150 micrograms/kg [unlicensed indication and dose] in glucose 5% (with precautions to protect the airway in case of vomiting). A further dose of glucagon (or an intravenous infusion) may be required if the response is not maintained. If glucagon is not available, intravenous isoprenaline or intravenous prenalterol [not on UK market] are alternatives to glucagon.

Hypnotics and anxiolytics

BARBITURATES. These cause drowsiness, coma, respiratory depression, hypotension, and hypothermia. The duration and depth of cerebral depression vary greatly with the drug, the dose, and the tolerance of the patient. The severity of poisoning is often greater with a large dose of barbiturate hypnotics than with the longer-acting phenobarbital. The majority of patients survive with supportive measures alone. Repeated doses of activated charcoal (see Active Elimination Techniques, above) may be used for phenobarbital poisoning. Charcoal haemoperfusion is the treatment of choice for the small minority of patients with very severe barbiturate poisoning who fail to improve, or who deteriorate despite good supportive care.

BENZODIAZEPINES. Benzodiazepines taken alone cause drowsiness, ataxia, dysarthria, and occasionally minor and short-lived depression of consciousness. They potentiate the effects of other central nervous system depressants taken concomitantly. Flumazenil, a benzodiazepine antagonist, may be used in the *differential diagnosis* of unclear cases of multiple drug overdose but expert advice is **essential** since adverse effects may occur (e.g. convulsions in patients dependent on benzodiazepines).

Iron salts

Iron poisoning is commonest in childhood and is usually accidental. The symptoms are nausea, vomiting, abdominal pain, diarrhoea, haematemesis, and rectal bleeding. Hypotension, coma, and hepatocellular necrosis occur later. Mortality is reduced with intensive and specific therapy with **desferrioxamine**, which chelates iron. The stomach should be emptied at once by gastric lavage. The serum-iron concentration is measured as an emergency and intravenous desferrioxamine given to chelate absorbed iron in excess of the expected iron binding capacity. In **severe toxicity** intravenous desferrioxamine should be given *immediately* without waiting for the result of the serum-iron measurement (contact a poisons information centre for advice).

DESFERRIOXAMINE MESILATE
(Deferoxamine Mesilate)
Indications: iron poisoning; chronic iron overload (section 9.1.3)
Cautions: section 9.1.3
Side-effects: section 9.1.3
Dose: *by continuous intravenous infusion*, up to 15 mg/kg/hour; max. 80 mg/kg in 24 hours

Preparations
Section 9.1.3

Lithium

Most cases of lithium intoxication occur as a complication of long-term therapy and are caused by reduced excretion of the drug due to a variety of factors including dehydration, deterioration of renal function, infections, and co-administration of diuretics or NSAIDs (or other drugs that interact). Acute deliberate overdoses may also occur with delayed onset of symptoms (12 hours or more) due to slow entry of lithium into the tissues and continuing absorption from modified-release formulations.

The early clinical features are non-specific and may include apathy and restlessness which could be confused with mental changes due to the patient's depressive illness. Vomiting, diarrhoea, ataxia, weakness, dysarthria, muscle twitching, and tremor may follow. Severe poisoning is associated with convulsions, coma, renal failure, electrolyte imbalance, dehydration, and hypotension.

Therapeutic lithium concentrations are within the range of 0.4–1.0 mmol/litre; concentrations in excess of 2.0 mmol/litre are usually associated with serious toxicity and such cases may need treatment with haemodialysis (if there is renal failure). In acute overdosage much higher serum concentrations may be present without features of toxicity and all that is usually necessary is to take measures to increase urine production (e.g. by ensuring adequate fluid intake; but avoid diuretics). Otherwise treatment is supportive with special regard to electrolyte balance, renal function, and control of convulsions.

Phenothiazines and related drugs

Phenothiazines cause less depression of consciousness and respiration than other sedatives. Hypotension, hypothermia, sinus tachycardia, and arrhythmias (particularly with thioridazine) may complicate poisoning. Dystonic reactions can occur with therapeutic doses, (particularly with prochlorperazine and trifluoperazine) and convulsions may occur in severe cases. Arrhythmias may respond to correction of hypoxia and acidosis but anti-arrhythmic drugs may also be needed. Dystonic reactions are rapidly abolished by injection of drugs such as benzatropine or procyclidine (section 4.9.2).

Stimulants

AMPHETAMINES. These cause wakefulness, excessive activity, paranoia, hallucinations, and hypertension followed by exhaustion, convulsions, hyperthermia, and coma. The early stages can be controlled by chlorpromazine and, if necessary, beta-blockers. Later, tepid sponging, anticonvulsants, and artificial respiration may be needed. Amfetamine excretion can be increased by forced acid diuresis but this is seldom necessary.

COCAINE. Cocaine can be smoked, sniffed, or injected. It stimulates the central nervous system causing agitation, dilated pupils, tachycardia, hypertension, hallucinations, hypertonia, and hyperreflexia. Convulsions, coma and metabolic acidosis may develop in the worst cases. Sedation, with intravenous diazepam, may be all that is necessary (and will also control convulsions); intravenous propranolol may be indicated for severe arrhythmias (labetalol may be preferred if there is associated hypertension).

ECSTASY. Ecstasy (methylenedioxymethamphetamine) may cause severe reactions, even at doses that were previously tolerated. The most serious effects are delirium, coma, convulsions, ventricular arrhythmias, hyperpyrexia, rhabdomyolysis, acute renal failure, acute hepatitis, disseminated intravascular coagulation, adult respiratory distress syndrome, hyperreflexia, hypotension and intracerebral haemorrhage; hyponatraemia has also been associated with ecstasy use.

Treatment is supportive, with diazepam to control severe agitation or persistent convulsions and close monitoring including ECG. Self-induced water intoxication should be considered in patients with ecstasy poisoning.

Theophylline

Theophylline and related drugs are often prescribed as modified-release formulations and toxicity may therefore be delayed. They cause vomiting (which may be severe and intractable), agitation, restlessness, dilated pupils, sinus tachycardia, and hyperglycaemia. More serious effects are haematemesis, convulsions, and supraventricular and ventricular arrhythmias. Profound **hypokalaemia** may develop rapidly.

The stomach should be emptied if the patient presents within 2 hours. Elimination of theophylline may be enhanced by repeated doses of activated charcoal by mouth (see also under Active Elimination Techniques). Hypokalaemia is corrected by intravenous infusion of potassium chloride and may be so severe as to require 60 mmol/hour (high doses under ECG monitoring). Convulsions should be controlled by intravenous administration of diazepam (emulsion preferred). Sedation with diazepam may be necessary in agitated patients.

Providing the patient is **not** an asthmatic, extreme tachycardia, hypokalaemia, and hyperglycaemia may be reversed by intravenous administration of propranolol (section 2.4).

Other poisons

Consult poisons information services day and night—p. 19.

Cyanides

Cyanide antidotes include dicobalt edetate, given alone, and sodium nitrite followed by sodium thiosulphate. These antidotes are held for emergency use in hospitals as well as in centres where cyanide poisoning is a risk such as factories and laboratories.

DICOBALT EDETATE

Indications: acute poisoning with cyanides
Cautions: owing to toxicity to be used only when patient tending to lose, or has lost, consciousness; not to be used as a precautionary measure
Side-effects: hypotension, tachycardia, and vomiting

Dose: *by intravenous injection,* 300 mg (20 mL) over 1 minute (5 minutes if condition less serious) followed immediately by 50 mL of glucose intravenous infusion 50%; if response inadequate a second dose of both may be given; if no response after further 5 minutes a third dose of both may be given

Dicobalt Edetate (Cambridge) [PoM]
Injection, dicobalt edetate 15 mg/mL. Net price 20-mL (300-mg) amp = £9.08

SODIUM NITRITE

Indications: poisoning with cyanides (used in conjunction with sodium thiosulphate)
Side-effects: flushing and headache due to vasodilatation
Dose: see under preparation below

Sodium Nitrite Injection [PoM]
Injection, sodium nitrite 3% (30 mg/mL) in water for injections
Dose: 10 mL by intravenous injection over 3 minutes, followed by 25 mL of sodium thiosulphate injection 50%, by intravenous injection over 10 minutes
'Special-order' [unlicensed] product: contact Martindale, Oxford, or regional hospital manufacturing unit

SODIUM THIOSULPHATE

Indications: poisoning with cyanides (used in conjunction with sodium nitrite)

Sodium Thiosulphate Injection [PoM]
Injection, sodium thiosulphate 50% (500 mg/mL) in water for injections
Dose: see above under Sodium Nitrite Injection
'Special-order' [unlicensed] product: contact Martindale, Oxford, or regional hospital manufacturing unit

Ethylene glycol

Fomepizole is licensed for the treatment of ethylene glycol poisoning. Ethanol (by mouth or by intravenous infusion) has also been used for the treatment of ethylene glycol poisoning. Advice from Poisons Information Centres should be obtained for the treatment of ethylene glycol poisoning.

FOMEPIZOLE

Indications: poisoning by ethylene glycol
Side-effects: abdominal pain, vomiting, hypotension, vertigo, headache, seizures, eosinophilia, rash, pain and inflammation at injection site
Dose: *by intravenous infusion* over 30 minutes, initially 15 mg/kg followed by 10 mg/kg every 12 hours for 4 doses, then 15 mg/kg every 12 hours until plasma ethylene glycol concentration is below 200 mg/litre (3.2 millimol/litre)
Patients requiring haemodialysis, consult product literature

Antizol® (Cambridge) ▼ [PoM]
Concentrate for intravenous infusion, fomepizole 1 g/mL, net price 1.5-mL vial = £606.00

Heavy metals

Heavy metal antidotes include dimercaprol, penicillamine, and sodium calcium edetate.

DIMERCAPROL
(BAL)

Indications: poisoning by antimony, arsenic, bismuth, gold, mercury, possibly thallium; adjunct (with sodium calcium edetate) in lead poisoning

Cautions: hypertension, renal impairment (discontinue or use with extreme caution if impairment develops during treatment), elderly, pregnancy and breast-feeding

Contra-indications: not indicated for iron, cadmium, or selenium poisoning; severe hepatic impairment (unless due to arsenic poisoning)

Side-effects: hypertension, tachycardia, malaise, nausea, vomiting, salivation, lacrimation, sweating, burning sensation (mouth, throat, and eyes), feeling of constriction of throat and chest, headache, muscle spasm, abdominal pain, tingling of extremities; pyrexia in children; local pain and abscess at injection site

Dose: *by intramuscular injection,* 2.5–3 mg/kg every 4 hours for 2 days, 2–4 times on the third day, then 1–2 times daily for 10 days or until recovery

Dimercaprol (Sovereign) PoM
Injection, dimercaprol 50 mg/mL. Net price 2-mL amp = £38.84
Note. Contains arachis (peanut) oil as solvent

PENICILLAMINE

Indications: poisoning by certain toxic metal ions, particularly by copper and lead

Cautions: see section 10.1.3

Contra-indications: see section 10.1.3

Side-effects: see section 10.1.3

Dose: 1–2 g daily in divided doses before food until urinary lead is stabilised at less than 500 micrograms/day; CHILD 20 mg/kg daily

Preparations
Section 10.1.3

SODIUM CALCIUM EDETATE
(Sodium Calciumedetate)

Indications: poisoning by heavy metals, especially lead

Cautions: renal impairment

Side-effects: nausea, diarrhoea, abdominal pain, pain at site of injection, thrombophlebitis if given too rapidly, renal damage particularly in overdosage; hypotension, lacrimation, myalgia, nasal congestion, sneezing, malaise, thirst, fever, chills, headache also reported

Dose: *by intravenous infusion,* adults and children, up to 40 mg/kg twice daily in sodium chloride intravenous infusion 0.9% or glucose intravenous infusion 5% for up to 5 days, repeated if necessary after 48 hours

Ledclair® (Sinclair) PoM
Injection, sodium calcium edetate 200 mg/mL. Net price 5-mL amp = £4.38

Noxious gases

CARBON MONOXIDE. Carbon monoxide poisoning is now usually due to inhalation of smoke, car exhaust, or fumes caused by blocked flues or incomplete combustion of fuel gases in confined spaces. Its toxic effects are entirely due to hypoxia.

Immediate treatment is essential. The person should be removed into the fresh air, the airway cleared, and **oxygen** 100% administered as soon as available. Artificial respiration should be given as necessary and continued until adequate spontaneous breathing starts, or stopped only after persistent and efficient treatment of cardiac arrest has failed. Admission to hospital is desirable because complications may arise after a delay of hours or days. Cerebral oedema should be anticipated in severe poisoning and is treated with an intravenous infusion of mannitol (section 2.2.5). Referral for hyperbaric oxygen treatment should be discussed with the poisons information services if the victim is or has been unconscious, or has a blood carboxyhaemoglobin concentration of more than 20%, or is pregnant.

CS GAS. CS gas, which has been used for riot control, causes irritation of the eyes and respiratory tract which normally settles spontaneously within 15 minutes. If symptoms persist, the patient should be removed to a well-ventilated area, and the exposed skin washed with soap and water after removal of contaminated clothing. Contact lenses should be removed and hard ones washed (soft ones should be discarded). Persistent eye symptoms should be treated by irrigating the eyes with water or physiological saline and the patient referred to an ophthalmologist. Patients with features of severe poisoning, particularly respiratory complications, should be admitted to hospital for symptomatic treatment.

SULPHUR DIOXIDE, CHLORINE, PHOSGENE, AMMONIA. All of these gases can cause upper respiratory tract and conjunctival irritation. Pulmonary oedema, with severe breathlessness and cyanosis may develop suddenly up to 36 hours after exposure. Death may occur. Patients are kept under observation and those who develop pulmonary oedema are given corticosteroids and oxygen. Assisted ventilation may be necessary in the most serious cases.

Pesticides

PARAQUAT. Concentrated liquid paraquat preparations (e.g. *Gramoxone®*), available to farmers and horticulturalists, contain 10–20% paraquat and are extremely toxic. Granular preparations, for garden use, contain only 2.5% paraquat and have caused few deaths.

Paraquat has local and systemic effects. Splashes in the eyes irritate and ulcerate the cornea and conjunctiva. Copious washing of the eye and instillation of antibacterial eye-drops, should aid healing but it may be a long process. Skin irritation, blistering, and ulceration can occur from prolonged contact both with the concentrated and dilute forms. Inhalation of spray, mist, or dust containing paraquat may cause nose bleeding and sore throat but not systemic toxicity.

Ingestion of concentrated paraquat solutions is followed by nausea, vomiting, and diarrhoea. Painful ulceration of the tongue, lips, and fauces may appear after 36 to 48 hours together with renal failure. Some days later there may be dyspnoea with pulmonary fibrosis due to proliferative alveolitis and bronchiolitis.

Treatment should be started immediately. The single most useful measure is oral administration of repeat-dose **activated charcoal**[1]; the first dose of 100 g is given with a laxative (e.g. magnesium sulphate), followed by activated charcoal 50 g every 4 hours (or more frequently if tolerated) until the charcoal is seen in the stool. Vomiting may preclude the use of activated charcoal and an anti-emetic may be required. Gastric lavage is of doubtful value. Intravenous fluids and analgesics are given as necessary. Oxygen therapy should be avoided in the early stages of management since this may exacerbate damage to the lungs, but oxygen may be required in the late stages to palliate symptoms. Measures to enhance elimination of absorbed paraquat are probably valueless but should be discussed with the poisons information services who will also give guidance on predicting the likely outcome from plasma concentrations. Paraquat absorption can be confirmed by a simple qualitative urine test.

ORGANOPHOSPHORUS INSECTICIDES. Organophosphorus insecticides are usually supplied as powders or dissolved in organic solvents. All are absorbed through the bronchi and intact skin as well as through the gut and inhibit cholinesterase activity thereby prolonging and intensifying the effects of acetylcholine. Toxicity between different compounds varies considerably, and onset may be delayed after skin exposure.

Anxiety, restlessness, dizziness, headache, miosis, nausea, hypersalivation, vomiting, abdominal colic, diarrhoea, bradycardia, and sweating are common. Muscle weakness and fasciculation may develop and progress to generalised flaccid paralysis including the ocular and respiratory muscles. Convulsions, coma, pulmonary oedema with copious bronchial secretions, hypoxia, and arrhythmias occur in severe cases. Hyperglycaemia and glycosuria without ketonuria may also be present.

Further absorption should be prevented by emptying the stomach, removing the patient to fresh air, or removing soiled clothing and washing contaminated skin. In severe poisoning it is vital to ensure a clear airway, frequent removal of bronchial secretions, and adequate ventilation and oxygenation. **Atropine** will reverse the muscarinic effects of acetylcholine and is given in a dose of 2 mg as atropine sulphate (intramuscularly or intravenously according to the severity of poisoning) every 20 to 30 minutes until the skin becomes flushed and dry, the pupils dilate, and tachycardia develops.

---

1. **Fuller's earth** and **bentonite** given by mouth have also been used as adsorbents. A suspension of Fuller's earth 30% was used in three doses of 200–500 mL given at two-hour intervals; magnesium sulphate or mannitol were given with Fuller's earth to promote diarrhoea and empty the gut.

Pralidoxime mesilate (P2S), a cholinesterase reactivator, is indicated, as an adjunct to atropine, in moderate or severe poisoning but is only effective if given within 24 hours. It may be obtained from designated centres, the names of which are held by the poisons information centres (see p. 19). A dose of 30 mg/kg (diluted with 10–15 mL water for injections) by slow intravenous injection should produce improvement in muscle power within 30 minutes but repeated doses or, in severe cases, an intravenous infusion of up to 500 mg/hour may be required.

PRALIDOXIME MESILATE

(P2S)

Indications: adjunct to atropine in the treatment of organophosphorus poisoning

Cautions: renal impairment, myasthenia gravis

Contra-indications: poisoning due to carbamates and to organophosphorus compounds without anticholinesterase activity

Side-effects: drowsiness, dizziness, disturbances of vision, nausea, tachycardia, headache, hyperventilation, and muscular weakness

Dose: *by slow intravenous injection* (diluted to 10–15 mL with water for injections and given over 5–10 minutes), 30 mg/kg initially followed by 1–2 further doses if necessary; usual max. 12 g in 24 hours

CHILD 20–60 mg/kg as required depending on severity of poisoning and response

Note. Pralidoxime mesilate doses in BNF may differ from those in product literature

Pralidoxime Mesilate PoM

Injection, pralidoxime mesilate 200 mg/mL

Available as 5-mL amps (from designated centres)

Snake bites and insect stings

SNAKE BITE. Acute envenoming from snake bite is rare in the UK. Many exotic snakes are kept, some illegally, but the only indigenous venomous snake is the adder (*Vipera berus*). The bite may cause local and systemic effects. Local effects include pain, swelling, bruising, and tender enlargement of regional lymph nodes. Systemic effects include early transient hypotension with syncope, angioedema, abdominal colic, diarrhoea, and vomiting, with later persistent or recurrent hypotension, ECG abnormalities, spontaneous systemic bleeding, coagulopathy, adult respiratory distress syndrome, and acute renal failure. There is a small risk of fatal envenoming especially in children and the elderly.

Indications for antivenom treatment include systemic envenoming, especially hypotension (see above), ECG abnormalities, vomiting, haemostatic abnormalities, polymorphonuclear leucocytosis, elevated serum creatine kinase and local envenoming if, after bites on the hand or foot, swelling extends beyond the wrist or ankle within 4 hours of the bite. For both **adults** and **children**, the contents of one vial (10 mL) of **European viper venom antiserum** (available from Farillon) is given *by intravenous injection* over 10–15 minutes or *by intravenous infusion* over 30 minutes after diluting in sodium chloride intravenous infusion 0.9% (use 5 mL diluent/kg body-weight). The **same dose**

should be used for **adults** and **children**. The dose
can be repeated in 1–2 hours if symptoms of **systemic envenoming** persist. Adrenaline (epinephrine) injection must be immediately to hand for
treatment of anaphylactic reactions to the antivenom (for full details see section 3.4.3).

Antivenom is available for certain foreign snakes,
spiders and scorpions. For information on identification, management, and supply, telephone:

Oxford	(01865) 220968
or	(01865) 221332
or	(01865) 741166
Liverpool	(0151) 708 9393
Liverpool (Fazakerley Hospital Pharmacy)	
(supply only)	(0151) 525 5980
London	(020) 7635 9191

INSECT STINGS. Stings from ants, wasps, hornets,
and bees cause local pain and swelling but seldom
cause severe direct toxicity unless many stings are
inflicted at the same time. If the sting is in the
mouth or on the tongue marked swelling may cause
respiratory distress. The stings from these insects
are usually treated by cleaning the area, applying a
cooling lotion (such as a calamine preparation), and
giving an antihistamine by mouth. Bee stings
should be removed as quickly as possible. Anaphylactic reactions require treatment with intramuscular **adrenaline** (**epinephrine**); self-administered
intramuscular adrenaline (e.g. *EpiPen*®) is the best
first-aid treatment for patients with severe hypersensitivity. For full details of the management of
anaphylaxis, see section 3.4.3.

1: Gastro-intestinal system

1.1 Antacids and other drugs for dyspepsia

1.1.1 Aluminium- and magnesium-containing antacids
1.1.2 Sodium bicarbonate
1.1.3 Other drugs for dyspepsia and gastro-oesophageal reflux disease

Dyspepsia

Dyspepsia, typically as heartburn or food-related discomfort (indigestion), occurs with gastro-oesophageal reflux disease (section 1.1.3), gastric and duodenal ulceration (section 1.3) and gastric cancer. Most commonly dyspepsia is of uncertain origin. *Helicobacter pylori* infection may be present in some patients with non-ulcer dyspepsia but there is little evidence that *H. pylori* eradication provides symptomatic relief in these patients; for reference to the benefit of eradication treatment in duodenal and gastric ulcer, see section 1.3.

Antacids

Antacids (usually containing aluminium or magnesium compounds) can often relieve symptoms in *ulcer dyspepsia* and in *gastro-oesophageal reflux disease* (reflux oesophagitis); they are also sometimes used in non-ulcer dyspepsia but the evidence of benefit is uncertain. Antacids are best given when symptoms occur or are expected, usually between meals and at bedtime, 4 or more times daily; additional doses may be required up to once an hour. Conventional doses e.g. 10 mL 3 or 4 times daily of liquid magnesium–aluminium antacids promote ulcer healing, but less well than antisecretory drugs (section 1.3); proof of a relationship between healing and neutralising capacity is lacking. Liquid preparations are more effective than solids.

Bismuth-containing antacids (unless chelates) are best avoided because absorbed bismuth can be neurotoxic, causing encephalopathy; they tend to be constipating. Calcium-containing antacids can induce rebound acid secretion: with modest doses the clinical significance is doubtful, but prolonged high doses also cause hypercalcaemia and alkalosis, and can precipitate the milk alkali syndrome. For **preparations** on sale to the public (not prescribable on the NHS), see p. 33

See also section 1.3 for drugs used in the treatment of peptic ulcer.

INTERACTIONS. Antacids should preferably not be taken at the same time as other drugs since they may impair absorption. Antacids may also damage enteric coatings designed to prevent dissolution in the stomach. See also **Appendix 1** (antacids).

1.1.1 Aluminium- and magnesium-containing antacids

Aluminium- and **magnesium-containing** antacids, such as magnesium carbonate, hydroxide and trisilicate, and aluminium glycinate and hydroxide, being relatively insoluble in water, are long-acting if retained in the stomach. They are suitable for most antacid purposes. Magnesium-containing antacids tend to be laxative whereas aluminium-containing antacids may be constipating. Aluminium accumulation does not appear to be a risk if renal function is normal (see also Appendix 3).

Compound preparations have no clear advantages over simpler preparations: neutralising capacity may be the same. Complexes such as **hydrotalcite** confer no special advantage.

Activated **dimeticone** (simethicone) is added to an antacid as an antifoaming agent to relieve flatulence. These preparations may be useful for the relief of hiccup in palliative care. **Alginates** added as protectants against gastro-oesophageal reflux disease (section 1.1.3) may be useful, but surface anaesthetics (e.g. oxetacaine) added to improve symptom relief are of doubtful efficacy. The amount of additional ingredient or antacid in individual preparations varies widely, as does their sodium content, so that preparations may not be freely interchangeable.

ALUMINIUM HYDROXIDE

Indications: dyspepsia; hyperphosphataemia (section 9.5.2.2)

Cautions: see notes above; **interactions:** Appendix 1 (antacids)

Contra-indications: hypophosphataemia; porphyria (section 9.8.2)

Side-effects: see notes above

■ Aluminium-only preparations

Aluminium Hydroxide (Non-proprietary)
Tablets, dried aluminium hydroxide 500 mg. Net price 20 = 28p
Dose: 1–2 tablets chewed 4 times daily and at bedtime or as required
Mixture (gel), about 4% w/w Al_2O_3 in water, with a peppermint flavour. Net price 200 mL = 41p
Dose: antacid, 5–10 mL 4 times daily between meals and at bedtime or as required; CHILD 6–12 years, up to 5 mL 3 times daily
Note. The brand name *Aludrox®* [NHS] (Pfizer Consumer) is used for aluminium hydroxide mixture; net price 200 mL = £1.34. *Aludrox®* [NHS] tablets also contain magnesium.

Alu-Cap® (3M)
Capsules, green/red, dried aluminium hydroxide 475 mg (low Na⁺). Net price 120-cap pack = £4.03
Dose: antacid, 1 capsule 4 times daily and at bedtime; CHILD not recommended for antacid therapy

■ Co-magaldrox

Co-magaldrox is a mixture of aluminium hydroxide and magnesium hydroxide; the proportions are expressed in the form x/y where x and y are the strengths in milligrams per unit dose of magnesium hydroxide and aluminium hydroxide respectively

Maalox® (Rhône-Poulenc Rorer)
Suspension, sugar-free, co-magaldrox 195/220 (magnesium hydroxide 195 mg, dried aluminium hydroxide 220 mg/5 mL (low Na⁺)). Net price 500 mL = £2.16
Dose: 10–20 mL 20 minutes–1 hour after meals and at bedtime or when required; CHILD under 14 years not recommended

Maalox TC® (Rhône-Poulenc Rorer)
Tablets, co-magaldrox 300/600 (magnesium hydroxide 300 mg, dried aluminium hydroxide 600 mg (low Na⁺)). Net price 100 = £4.25
Suspension, sugar-free, co-magaldrox 300/600 (magnesium hydroxide 300 mg, dried aluminium hydroxide 600 mg/5 mL (low Na⁺)). Net price 500 mL = £4.25
Dose: antacid, 1–2 tablets chewed or 5–10 mL suspension 4 times daily 20 minutes–1 hour after meals and at bedtime; duodenal ulcer, 3 tablets or 15 mL suspension 4 times daily (treatment) *or* twice daily (prevention of recurrence)

Mucogel® (Pharmax)
Suspension, sugar-free, co-magaldrox 195/220 (magnesium hydroxide 195 mg, dried aluminium hydroxide 220 mg/5 mL (low Na⁺)). Net price 500 mL = £1.82
Dose: 10–20 mL 3 times daily, 20 minutes–1 hour after meals, and at bedtime or when required; CHILD under 12 years not recommended

---

Low Na⁺
The words low Na⁺ added after some preparations indicate a sodium content of less than 1 mmol per tablet or 10-mL dose.

MAGNESIUM CARBONATE

Indications: dyspepsia

Cautions: renal impairment; see also notes above; **interactions:** Appendix 1 (antacids)

Contra-indications: hypophosphataemia

Side-effects: diarrhoea; belching due to liberated carbon dioxide

Aromatic Magnesium Carbonate Mixture, BP (Aromatic Magnesium Carbonate Oral Suspension)
Oral suspension, light magnesium carbonate 3%, sodium bicarbonate 5%, in a suitable vehicle containing aromatic cardamom tincture. Contains about 6 mmol Na⁺/10 mL. Net price 200 mL = 60p
Dose: 10 mL 3 times daily in water
For **preparations** also containing aluminium, see above and section 1.1.3.

MAGNESIUM TRISILICATE

Indications: dyspepsia

Cautions: see under Magnesium Carbonate

Contra-indications: see under Magnesium Carbonate

Side-effects: diarrhoea

Magnesium Trisilicate Tablets, Compound, BP
Tablets, magnesium trisilicate 250 mg, dried aluminium hydroxide 120 mg
Dose: 1–2 tablets chewed when required

Magnesium Trisilicate Mixture, BP
(Magnesium Trisilicate Oral Suspension)
Oral suspension, 5% each of magnesium trisilicate, light magnesium carbonate, and sodium bicarbonate in a suitable vehicle with a peppermint flavour. Contains about 6 mmol Na⁺/10 mL
Dose: 10 mL 3 times daily in water

Magnesium Trisilicate Oral Powder, Compound, BP

Oral powder, magnesium trisilicate 250 mg, chalk 250 mg, heavy magnesium carbonate 250 mg, sodium bicarbonate 250 mg/g. Contains about 3 mmol Na+/g. Label: 13

Dose: 1–5 g in liquid when required

For **preparations** also containing aluminium, see above and section 1.1.3.

Aluminium-magnesium complexes

HYDROTALCITE

Aluminium magnesium carbonate hydroxide hydrate

Indications: dyspepsia

Cautions: see notes above; **interactions:** Appendix 1 (antacids)

Side-effects: see notes above

Hydrotalcite (Peckforton)

Suspension, hydrotalcite 500 mg/5 mL (low Na+). Net price 500-mL pack = £1.96

Dose: 10 mL between meals and at bedtime; CHILD under 6 years not recommended, 6–12 years 5 mL

Note. The brand name *Altacite®* DHS is used for hydrotalcite suspension; for *Altacite Plus®* suspension, see below.

Other compound antacid preparations

Altacite Plus® (Peckforton)

Suspension, sugar-free, co-simalcite 125/500 (activated dimeticone 125 mg, hydrotalcite 500 mg)/5 mL (low Na+). Net price 500 mL = £1.96

Dose: 10 mL between meals and at bedtime when required; CHILD 8–12 years 5 mL

Tablets DHS, see p. 33

Asilone® (SSL)

Suspension, sugar-free, dried aluminium hydroxide 420 mg, activated dimeticone 135 mg, light magnesium oxide 70 mg/5 mL (low Na+). Net price 500 mL = £1.95

Dose: 5–10 mL after meals and at bedtime or when required up to 4 times daily; CHILD under 12 years not recommended

Tablets DHS, see p. 33

Liquid DHS, see p. 33

Diovol® (Pharmax)

Suspension, sugar-free, aluminium hydroxide 200 mg, activated dimeticone 25 mg, magnesium hydroxide 200 mg/5 mL (low Na+). Net price 300 mL = £1.08

Dose: 5–10 mL 3 times daily between meals and at bedtime or when required

Maalox Plus® (Rhône-Poulenc Rorer)

Suspension, sugar-free, dried aluminium hydroxide 220 mg, activated dimeticone 25 mg, magnesium hydroxide 195 mg/5 mL (low Na+). Net price 500 mL = £2.16

Dose: 5–10 mL 4 times daily (after meals and at bedtime or when required); CHILD under 5 years 5 mL 3 times daily, over 5 years appropriate proportion of adult dose

Tablets DHS, see p. 33

Mucaine® (Wyeth) PoM

Suspension, sugar-free, aluminium hydroxide mixture 4.75 mL, magnesium hydroxide 100 mg, oxetacaine 10 mg/5 mL. Net price 200-mL pack = 76p

Dose: 5–10 mL (without fluid) 3–4 times daily (15 minutes before meals and at bedtime or when required), but evidence of value of local anaesthetic uncertain; CHILD not recommended

For **preparations** containing aluminium and magnesium on sale to the public and not prescribable on the NHS, see p. 33

1.1.2   Sodium bicarbonate

Sodium bicarbonate dissolved in water, used occasionally in doses of 1–5 g when required, acts rapidly in the relief of dyspepsia, but absorbed bicarbonate can cause alkalosis in excessive doses. Sodium bicarbonate should be avoided in patients on salt-restricted diets (in heart failure and in hepatic and renal impairment).

SODIUM BICARBONATE

Indications: rapid relief of dyspepsia; urinary tract (section 7.4.3); acidosis (section 9.2.1.3 and section 9.2.2)

Cautions: hepatic and renal impairment, cardiac disease, pregnancy; patients on sodium-restricted diet; elderly; avoid prolonged use; **interactions:** Appendix 1 (antacids)

Side-effects: belching, alkalosis on prolonged use

Dose: see notes above and under preparation below

Sodium Bicarbonate Tablets, Compound, BP (Soda Mint Tablets) sodium bicarbonate 300 mg. Contains about 4 mmol Na+/tab

Dose: 2–6 tablets sucked when required

denotes preparations that are considered to be less suitable for prescribing (see p. vi)

1.1.3   Other drugs for dyspepsia and gastro-oesophageal reflux disease

Gastro-oesophageal reflux disease (reflux oesophagitis) results from reflux of gastric or duodenal contents into the oesophagus and causes symptoms, which include heartburn, acid regurgitation, and difficulty in swallowing (dysphagia); oesophageal inflammation, ulceration, and stricture formation may occur and there may be an association with asthma.

Initial management of mild gastro-oesophageal reflux disease includes lifestyle changes (raising the head of the bed, weight reduction, avoidance of alcohol, cessation of smoking, and avoidance of aggravating foods such as fats—but evidence of benefit with all these measures not established) and treatment with **antacids** and **alginates**. Alginate-containing antacids form a 'raft' that floats on the surface of the stomach contents to reduce reflux and protect the oesophageal mucosa.

For those with gastro-oesophageal reflux disease who do not respond to these measures, and those with more severe symptoms, suppression of gastric acid secretion with a **histamine H₂-antagonist** (section 1.3.1) may relieve symptoms and reduce antacid consumption. Alternatively, a prokinetic drug such as **metoclopramide** (section 4.6) or **cisapride** (section 1.2) may improve gastro-oesophageal sphincter function and accelerate gastric emptying. The extent of oesophageal healing depends on the severity of the disease and duration of therapy. Endoscopically confirmed erosive, ulcerative, or stricturing disease responds best to treatment with a proton pump inhibitor (section 1.3.5) which usually needs to be maintained.

CHILDREN. Gastro-oesophageal reflux disease is common in infancy but most symptoms resolve between 12 and 18 months of age. Mild or moderate reflux without complications can be managed initially by changes in posture and thickening of liquid feeds (see Appendix 7 for suitable products) followed if necessary by treatment with an alginate product (low sodium and aluminium content for use in infants). For older children, life-style changes similar to those for adults (see above) may be helpful followed if necessary by treatment with an alginate.

Children who do not respond to these measures or who have complications such as respiratory disorders or suspected oesophagitis should be referred to hospital; an H₂-receptor antagonist such as cimetidine (section 1.3.1) may be needed to reduce acid secretion. If the oesophagitis is resistant to H₂-receptor blockade, the proton pump inhibitor omeprazole (section 1.3.5) can be tried.

Compound alginic acid preparations

Algicon® (Rhône-Poulenc Rorer)
Tablets, aluminium hydroxide-magnesium carbonate co-gel 360 mg, magnesium alginate 500 mg, heavy magnesium carbonate 320 mg, potassium bicarbonate 100 mg, sucrose 1.5 g (low Na⁺). Net price 60-tab pack = £2.64
Caution: diabetes mellitus (high sugar content)
Dose: 1–2 tablets 4 times daily (chewed after meals and at bedtime); CHILD under 12 years not recommended
Suspension, yellow, aluminium hydroxide-magnesium carbonate co-gel 140 mg, magnesium alginate 250 mg, magnesium carbonate 175 mg, potassium bicarbonate 50 mg/5 mL (low Na⁺). Net price 500 mL (lemon and mint-flavoured) = £3.07
Dose: 10–20 mL 4 times daily (after meals and at bedtime); CHILD under 12 years not recommended

Gastrocote® (SSL)
Tablets, alginic acid 200 mg, dried aluminium hydroxide 80 mg, magnesium trisilicate 40 mg, sodium bicarbonate 70 mg. Contains about 1 mmol Na⁺/tablet. Net price 100-tab pack = £3.51
Caution: diabetes mellitus (high sugar content)
Dose: 1–2 tablets chewed 4 times daily (after meals and at bedtime); CHILD under 6 years not recommended
Liquid, sugar-free, peach-coloured, dried aluminium hydroxide 80 mg, magnesium trisilicate 40 mg, sodium alginate 220 mg, sodium bicarbonate 70 mg/5 mL. Contains 1.8 mmol Na⁺/5 mL. Net price 500 mL = £2.67
Dose: 5–15 mL 4 times daily (after meals and at bedtime)

Gaviscon® (R&C)
Tablets, sugar-free, alginic acid 500 mg, dried aluminium hydroxide 100 mg, magnesium trisilicate 25 mg, sodium bicarbonate 170 mg. Contains 2 mmol Na⁺/tablet. Net price 60-tab pack (peppermint or lemon flavour) = £2.25
Dose: 1–2 tablets chewed after meals and at bedtime, followed by water; CHILD 2–6 years 1 tablet (on doctor's advice only) and 6–12 years 1 tablet
Liquid, sugar-free, sodium alginate 250 mg, sodium bicarbonate 133.5 mg, calcium carbonate 80 mg/5 mL. Contains about 3 mmol Na⁺/5 mL. Net price 500 mL (aniseed- or peppermint-flavour) = £2.70
Dose: 10–20 mL after meals and at bedtime; CHILD 2–6 years (on doctor's advice only) and 6–12 years 5–10 mL
Gaviscon 250® [NHS], *Gaviscon 500® Tablets*, and *Gaviscon® Liquid Sachets*, see p. 33

Gaviscon® Advance (R&C)
Suspension, sugar-free, sodium alginate 500 mg, potassium bicarbonate 100 mg/5 mL. Contains 2.3 mmol Na⁺, 1 mmol K⁺/5 mL. Net price 500 mL = £5.40
Dose: ADULT and CHILD over 12 years, 5–10 mL after meals and at bedtime

Gaviscon® Infant (R&C)
Oral powder, sugar-free, sodium alginate 225 mg, magnesium alginate 87.5 mg, with colloidal silica and mannitol/dose (half dual-sachet). Contains 0.92 mmol Na⁺/dose. Net price 15 dual-sachets (30 doses) = £2.46
Dose: INFANT under 4.5 kg 1 dose (half dual-sachet) mixed with feeds (or water in breast-fed infants) when required; over 4.5 kg 2 doses (1 dual-sachet); CHILD 2 doses (1 dual-sachet) in water after each meal
Note. Not to be used in premature infants, or where excessive water loss likely (e.g. fever, diarrhoea, vomiting, high room temperature), or if intestinal obstruction. Not to be used with other preparations containing thickening agents
IMPORTANT. Each half of the dual-sachet is identified as 'one dose'. To avoid errors prescribe as 'dual-sachet' with directions in terms of 'dose'

Peptac® (Norton)
Suspension, sugar-free, sodium bicarbonate 133.5 mg, sodium alginate 250 mg, calcium carbonate 80 mg/5 mL. Contains 3.1 mmol Na⁺/5mL. Net price 500 mL (aniseed flavour) = £2.16
Dose: 10–20 mL after meals and at bedtime; CHILD 6–12 years 5–10 mL

Topal® (Ceuta)
Tablets, alginic acid 200 mg, dried aluminium hydroxide 30 mg, light magnesium carbonate 40 mg with lactose 220 mg, sucrose 880 mg, sodium bicarbonate 40 mg (low Na⁺). Net price 42-tab pack = £1.67
Caution: diabetes mellitus (high sugar content)
Dose: 1–3 tablets chewed 4 times daily (after meals and at bedtime); CHILD half adult dose

Indigestion **preparations** on sale to the public (not prescribable on the NHS) include:

Actal® (alexitol = aluminium), **Actonorm Gel**® (aluminium, magnesium, activated dimeticone, peppermint oil), **Actonorm Powder**® (section 1.2), **Altacite**® (hydrotalcite = aluminium, magnesium), **Aludrox Liquid**® (aluminium), **Aludrox Tablets**® (aluminium, magnesium), **Andrews Antacid**® (calcium, magnesium), **APP**® (section 1.2), **Asilone Antacid Liquid**® (aluminium, activated dimeticone, magnesium; suspension is prescribable), **Asilone Antacid Tablets**® (aluminium, activated dimeticone)

Barum Antacid® (calcium), **Birley**® (aluminium, magnesium), **Bismag**® (magnesium, sodium bicarbonate), **Bisma-Rex**® (bismuth, calcium, magnesium, peppermint oil), **Bisodol Heartburn Relief Tablets**® (alginic acid, magaldrate, sodium bicarbonate), **Bisodol Indigestion Relief Powder**® (magnesium, sodium bicarbonate), **Bisodol Indigestion Relief Tablets**® and **Bisodol Extra Strong Mint Tablets**® (calcium, magnesium, sodium bicarbonate), **Bisodol Wind Relief Tablets**® (calcium, magnesium, sodium bicarbonate, activated dimeticone), **Boots Heartburn Relief**® (alginic acid, calcium, sodium bicarbonate), **Boots Indigestion Relief Tablets**® (aluminium, magnesium, activated dimeticone), **Boots Indigestion Tablets**® (calcium, magnesium, sodium bicarbonate), **Boots Children's 1 month Plus Gripe Mixture**® (sodium bicarbonate)

Carbellon® (magnesium, charcoal, peppermint oil)

De Witt's Antacid Powder® (calcium, magnesium, sodium bicarbonate, light kaolin, peppermint oil), **De Witt's Antacid Tablets**® (calcium, magnesium, peppermint oil), **Dijex**® (aluminium, magnesium), **Dynese**® (magaldrate = aluminium, magnesium)

Entrotabs® (aluminium, attapulgite, pectin)

Gaviscon 250® **Tablets** (alginic acid, aluminium, magnesium, sodium bicarbonate; **Gaviscon**® and **Gaviscon 500**® **Tablets** are prescribable), **Gaviscon**® **Liquid Sachets** (sodium alginate, calcium, sodium bicarbonate), **Gelusil**® (aluminium, magnesium)

Maalox Plus Tablets® (aluminium, magnesium, activated dimeticone; suspension is prescribable), **Maclean**® (aluminium, calcium, magnesium), **Magnatol**® (alexitol, magnesium, potassium bicarbonate, xanthan gum), **Moorland**® (aluminium, bismuth, calcium, magnesium, light kaolin)

Nulacin® (calcium, magnesium, peppermint oil; *contains* gluten)

Opas® (calcium, magnesium, sodium bicarbonate)

Pepto-Bismol® (bismuth), **Phillips' Milk of Magnesia**® (magnesium), **Premiums**® (aluminium, calcium, magnesium, peppermint oil)

Rap-eze® (calcium), **Remegel**® (calcium), **Rennie**® (calcium, magnesium), **Rennie Deflatine**® (calcium, magnesium, activated dimeticone), **Roter**® (bismuth, magnesium, sodium bicarbonate, frangula)

Setlers Antacid® (calcium), **Setlers Heartburn and Indigestion Liquid**® (calcium, sodium alginate, sodium bicarbonate), **Setlers Wind-eze**® (activated dimeticone), **Simeco**® (aluminium, magnesium, activated dimeticone), **Sovol**® (aluminium, magnesium, activated dimeticone)

Tums® (calcium)

Unigest® (aluminium, activated dimeticone)

Windcheaters® (activated dimeticone)

Activated dimeticone alone

Activated dimeticone (also known as simethicone) is an antifoaming agent. It is licensed for infantile colic but evidence of benefit is uncertain.

Dentinox® (DDD) ◼︎
Colic drops (= emulsion), activated dimeticone 21 mg/2.5-mL dose. Net price 100 mL = £1.36
Dose: gripes, colic or wind pains, INFANT 2.5 mL with or after each feed (max. 6 doses in 24 hours); may be added to bottle feed
Note. The brand name *Dentinox*® is also used for other preparations including teething gel

Infacol® (Pharmax) ◼︎
Liquid, sugar-free, activated dimeticone 40 mg/mL (low Na⁺). Net price 50 mL = £1.82. Counselling, use of dropper
Dose: gripes, colic or wind pains, INFANT 0.5–1 mL before feeds

Woodward's Colic Drops® (SSL) ◼︎
Oral drops, activated dimeticone 20 mg/0.3-mL dose, net price 30 mL = £1.57
Dose: gripes, colic or wind pains, CHILD under 2 years 0.3–0.6 mL 4 times daily before feeds

---

1.2   Antispasmodics and other drugs altering gut motility

The smooth muscle relaxant properties of antimuscarinic and other antispasmodic drugs may be useful as adjunctive treatment in *non-ulcer dyspepsia*, in *irritable bowel syndrome*, and in *diverticular disease*. The gastric antisecretory effects of conventional antimuscarinic drugs are of little practical significance since dosage is limited by atropine-like side-effects. Moreover, they have been superseded by more powerful and specific antisecretory drugs, including the histamine H₂-receptor antagonists.

The dopamine-receptor antagonists metoclopramide and domperidone, and the acetylcholine-release promoter cisapride all tend to stimulate transit in the gut.

Antimuscarinics

Antimuscarinics (formerly termed 'anticholinergics') reduce intestinal motility and gastric secretion and may be useful in some forms of dyspepsia, in irritable bowel syndrome and in diverticular disease. Other indications of antimuscarinic drugs include arrhythmias (section 2.3.1), asthma and airways disease (section 3.1.2), motion sickness (section 4.6), parkinsonism (section 4.9.2), urinary incontinence (section 7.4.2), mydriasis and cycloplegia (section 11.5), premedication (section 15.1.3) and as an antidote to organophosphorus poisoning (p. 27).

Antimuscarinics that are used for gastro-intestinal smooth muscle spasm include the tertiary amines **atropine sulphate** and **dicycloverine hydrochloride (dicyclomine hydrochloride)** and the quaternary ammonium compounds **propantheline bromide** and **hyoscine butylbromide**. The quaternary ammonium compounds are less lipid soluble than atropine and so may be less likely to cross the blood-brain barrier; they are also less well absorbed. Although central atropine-like side-effects, such as confusion, are thereby reduced, peripheral side-effects are common with quaternary ammonium compounds.

Propantheline bromide is indicated as an adjunct in the treatment of gastro-intestinal disorders characterised by smooth muscle spasm (including non-ulcer dyspepsia and irritable bowel syndrome); atropine sulphate is also licensed for these indications. Dicycloverine hydrochloride (dicyclomine hydrochloride) has a much less marked antimuscarinic action than atropine and may also have some direct action on smooth muscle. Hyoscine butylbromide is advocated as a gastro-intestinal antispasmodic, but it is poorly absorbed; the injection is useful in endoscopy and radiology. Non-selective antimuscarinics (e.g. belladonna alkaloids, included in preparations on sale to the public) are outmoded as ulcer treatments, any clinical virtues being outweighed by atropinic side-effects.

CAUTIONS. Antimuscarinics should be used with caution (due to increased risk of side-effects) in Down's syndrome, in children and in the elderly; they should also be used with caution in reflux oesophagitis, diarrhoea, ulcerative colitis, acute myocardial infarction, hypertension, conditions characterised by tachycardia (including hyperthyroidism, cardiac insufficiency, cardiac surgery), pyrexia, pregnancy and breast-feeding. **Interactions:** Appendix 1 (antimuscarinics).

CONTRA-INDICATIONS. Antimuscarinics are contra-indicated in angle-closure glaucoma, myasthenia gravis (but may be used to decrease muscarinic side-effects of anticholinesterases—section 10.2.1), paralytic ileus, pyloric stenosis and prostatic enlargement.

SIDE-EFFECTS. Side-effects of antimuscarinics include constipation, transient bradycardia (followed by tachycardia, palpitations and arrhythmias), reduced bronchial secretions, urinary urgency and retention, dilatation of the pupils with loss of accommodation, photophobia, dry mouth, flushing and dryness of the skin. Side-effects that occur occasionally include confusion (particularly in the elderly), nausea, vomiting and giddiness.

ATROPINE SULPHATE

Indications: symptomatic relief of gastro-intestinal disorders characterised by smooth muscle spasm; mydriasis and cycloplegia (section 11.5); pre-medication (section 15.1.3); see also notes above

Cautions: see notes above

Contra-indications: see notes above

Side-effects: see notes above

Atropine (Non-proprietary) PoM
Tablets, atropine sulphate 600 micrograms. Net price 28-tab pack = £5.90
Available from CP
Dose: 0.6–1.2 mg at night

Preparations on sale to the public (not prescribable on the NHS) containing atropine or related alkaloids include:

Actonorm Powder® (atropine, aluminium, calcium, magnesium, sodium bicarbonate, peppermint oil),
APP® (homatropine, aluminium, bismuth, calcium, magnesium)

denotes preparations that are considered to be less suitable for prescribing (see p. vi)

DICYCLOVERINE HYDROCHLORIDE/ DICYCLOMINE HYDROCHLORIDE

Indications: symptomatic relief of gastro-intestinal disorders characterised by smooth muscle spasm

Cautions: see notes above

Contra-indications: see notes above; infants under 6 months

Side-effects: see notes above

Dose: 10–20 mg 3 times daily; CHILD 6–24 months 5–10 mg up to 3–4 times daily, 15 minutes before feeds, 2–12 years 10 mg 3 times daily

¹ **Merbentyl®** (Florizel) PoM
Tablets, dicycloverine hydrochloride 10 mg, net price 20 = £1.08
Syrup, dicycloverine hydrochloride 10 mg/5 mL, net price 500 mL = £8.23
1. Dicycloverine hydrochloride can be sold to the public provided that max. single dose is 10 mg and max. daily dose is 60 mg

Merbentyl 20® (Florizel) PoM
Tablets, dicycloverine hydrochloride 20 mg, net price 84-tab pack = £9.11

■ Compound preparations

Kolanticon® (Peckforton)
Gel, sugar-free, dicycloverine hydrochloride 2.5 mg, dried aluminium hydroxide 200 mg, light magnesium oxide 100 mg, activated dimeticone (simethicone USP) 20 mg/5 mL, net price 200 mL = £1.52, 500 mL = £1.85
Dose: 10–20 mL every 4 hours when required

HYOSCINE BUTYLBROMIDE

Indications: symptomatic relief of gastro-intestinal or genito-urinary disorders characterised by smooth muscle spasm; dysmenorrhoea (but see section 4.7.1)

Cautions: see notes above

Contra-indications: see notes above; avoid in porphyria (section 9.8.2)

Side-effects: see notes above

Dose: *by mouth,* 20 mg 4 times daily; CHILD 6–12 years, 10 mg 3 times daily
Irritable bowel syndrome, 10 mg 3 times daily, increased if required up to 20 mg 4 times daily

By intramuscular or intravenous injection, acute spasm and spasm in diagnostic procedures, 20 mg repeated after 30 minutes if necessary (may be repeated more frequently in endoscopy); CHILD not recommended

¹ **Buscopan®** (Boehringer Ingelheim) PoM
Tablets, coated, hyoscine butylbromide 10 mg. Net price 56-tab pack = £2.59
1. Hyoscine butylbromide can be sold to the public provided single dose does not exceed 20 mg, daily dose does not exceed 80 mg, and pack does not contain a total of more than 240 mg.
Injection, hyoscine butylbromide 20 mg/mL. Net price 1-mL amp = 20p

PROPANTHELINE BROMIDE

Indications: symptomatic relief of gastro-intestinal disorders characterised by smooth muscle spasm; urinary frequency (section 7.4.2); gustatory sweating (section 6.1.5)

Cautions: see notes above

Contra-indications: see notes above

Side-effects: see notes above

Dose: 15 mg 3 times daily at least 1 hour before meals and 30 mg at night, max. 120 mg daily; CHILD not recommended

Pro-Banthine® (Hansam) P̲o̲M̲
Tablets, pink, s/c, propantheline bromide 15 mg. Net price 100-tab pack = £13.68. Label: 23

Other antispasmodics

Alverine, **mebeverine**, and **peppermint oil** are believed to be direct relaxants of intestinal smooth muscle and may relieve pain in *irritable bowel syndrome* and *diverticular disease*. They have no serious adverse effects but, like all antispasmodics, should be avoided in paralytic ileus. Peppermint oil occasionally causes heartburn.

ALVERINE CITRATE

Indications: adjunct in gastro-intestinal disorders characterised by smooth muscle spasm; dysmenorrhoea

Cautions: pregnancy and breast-feeding

Contra-indications: paralytic ileus; when combined with sterculia, intestinal obstruction, faecal impaction, colonic atony

Side-effects: nausea, headache, pruritus, rash and dizziness reported

Dose: 60–120 mg 1–3 times daily; CHILD under 12 years not recommended

Spasmonal® (Norgine)
Capsules, alverine citrate 60 mg (blue/grey), net price 100-cap pack = £10.92; 120 mg (*Spasmonal® Forte*, blue/grey), 60-cap pack = £13.10
Note. A proprietary brand of alverine citrate 60 mg (*Relaxyl®*) is on sale to the public for irritable bowel syndrome

■ Compound preparations

Spasmonal Fibre® (Norgine)
Granules, beige, coated, sterculia 62%, alverine citrate 0.5%. Net price 500 g = £12.19. Label: 25, 27, counselling, see below
Dose: irritable bowel syndrome, 1–2 heaped 5-mL spoonfuls swallowed without chewing with water once or twice daily after meals; CHILD not recommended
COUNSELLING. Preparations that swell in contact with liquid should always be carefully swallowed with water and should not be taken immediately before going to bed

MEBEVERINE HYDROCHLORIDE

Indications: adjunct in gastro-intestinal disorders characterised by smooth muscle spasm

Cautions: paralytic ileus; pregnancy and breast-feeding; avoid in porphyria (section 9.8.2.)

Dose: ADULT and CHILD over 10 years 135–150 mg 3 times daily preferably 20 minutes before meals

¹ **Mebeverine Hydrochloride** (Non-proprietary) P̲o̲M̲
Tablets, mebeverine hydrochloride 135 mg, net price 20 = £1.51
Available from APS, Berk (*Fomac®*), Cox, Generics, Hillcross, Norton

1. Mebeverine hydrochloride can be sold to the public for symptomatic relief of irritable bowel syndrome provided that max. single dose is 135 mg and max. daily dose is 405 mg; for uses other than symptomatic relief of irritable bowel syndrome provided that max. single dose is 100 mg and max. daily dose is 300 mg; proprietary brands on sale to the public include *Colofac 100®*, *Colofac IBS®* (135 mg), *Equilon®* (135 mg), *IBS Relief®*

Colofac® (Solvay) P̲o̲M̲
Tablets, s/c, mebeverine hydrochloride 135 mg. Net price 20 = £1.67
Liquid, yellow, sugar-free, mebeverine hydrochloride 50 mg (as embonate)/5 mL. Net price 300 mL = £3.50

■ Modified release

Colofac® MR (Solvay) P̲o̲M̲
Capsules, m/r, mebeverine hydrochloride 200 mg, net price 60-cap pack = £7.41. Label: 25
Dose : irritable bowel syndrome, 1 capsule twice daily preferably 20 minutes before meals; CHILD not recommended

■ Compound preparations

¹ **Fybogel® Mebeverine** (R&C) P̲o̲M̲
Granules, buff, effervescent, ispaghula husk 3.5 g, mebeverine hydrochloride 135 mg/sachet. Contains 7 mmol K⁺/sachet (caution in renal impairment). Net price 60 sachets = £15.00. Label: 13, 22, counselling, see below
Dose: irritable bowel syndrome, ADULT, 1 sachet in water, morning and evening 30 minutes before food; an additional sachet may also be taken before the midday meal if necessary; CHILD not recommended
COUNSELLING. Preparations that swell in contact with liquid should always be carefully swallowed with water and should not be taken immediately before going to bed
1. 10-sachet pack can be sold to the public

PEPPERMINT OIL

Indications: relief of abdominal colic and distension, particularly in irritable bowel syndrome

Cautions: rarely sensitivity to menthol

Side-effects: heartburn, perianal irritation; rarely, allergic reactions (including rash, headache, bradycardia, muscle tremor, ataxia)
LOCAL IRRITATION. Capsules should not be broken or chewed because peppermint oil may irritate mouth or oesophagus

Colpermin® (Pharmacia & Upjohn)
Capsules, m/r, e/c, light blue/dark blue, blue band, peppermint oil 0.2 mL. Net price 100-cap pack = £10.96. Label: 5, 25
Excipients: include arachis (peanut) oil
Dose: 1–2 capsules, swallowed whole with water, 3 times daily for up to 2–3 months if necessary; CHILD under 15 years not recommended

Mintec® (Monmouth)
Capsules, e/c, green/ivory, peppermint oil 0.2 mL. Net price 100-cap pack = £12.80. Label: 5, 22, 25
Dose: 1–2 capsules swallowed whole with water, 3 times daily before meals for up to 2–3 months if necessary; CHILD not recommended

Motility stimulants

Metoclopramide and **domperidone** (section 4.6) are dopamine antagonists which stimulate gastric emptying and small intestinal transit, and enhance the strength of oesophageal sphincter contraction. They are used in some patients with *non-ulcer dyspepsia*. Metoclopramide is also used to speed the transit of barium during intestinal follow-through examination, and as accessory treatment for *gastro-oesophageal reflux disease*. Metoclopramide and domperidone are useful in non-specific and in cytotoxic-induced nausea and vomiting. Metoclopramide and occasionally domperidone may induce an acute dystonic reaction, particularly in young women and children—for further details of this and other side-effects, see section 4.6.

Cisapride is a motility stimulant believed to promote release of acetylcholine in the gut wall; it does not have dopamine-antagonist properties. It is of use in *gastro-oesophageal reflux disease* and *gastric stasis* and in the short-term management of *non-ulcer dyspepsia*. Concomitant administration with drugs which inhibit the metabolism of cisapride can lead to disturbances of cardiac rhythm (see under Cisapride).

CISAPRIDE

Indications: see under dose

Cautions: hepatic and renal impairment (Appendixes 2 and 3); pregnancy (Appendix 4); elderly; perform ECG to exclude prolonged QT interval before treating at-risk patients (see also Arrhythmias below); **interactions:** Appendix 1 (cisapride)

Contra-indications: where gastro-intestinal stimulation dangerous; breast-feeding (Appendix 5); **important:** see also Arrhythmias, below

ARRHYTHMIAS. Serious cardiac arrhythmias and cases of sudden death have been reported. Recommendations include:

- avoid concomitant administration of drugs known to prolong the QT interval; for details, see **interactions:** Appendix 1 (cisapride)
- avoid concomitant administration of oral or parenteral drugs which inhibit metabolism of cisapride and can raise plasma-cisapride concentration; avoid concomitant administration of grapefruit juice (increases plasma-cisapride concentration); for details, see **interactions:** Appendix 1 (cisapride)
- avoid if personal or family history of QT interval prolongation, or if history of ventricular arrhythmias or torsades de pointes
- avoid in bradycardia, clinically significant heart disease, and in those with second- or third- degree AV block
- avoid in premature infants for up to 3 months after birth (risk of QT interval prolongation)
- avoid in uncorrected electrolyte disturbances, particularly potassium or magnesium
- avoid in renal or respiratory failure

Side-effects: abdominal cramps and diarrhoea, occasional hypersensitivity (including rash, pruritus, urticaria, bronchospasm), headaches and lightheadedness; convulsions, extrapyramidal effects and increased urinary frequency; liver function abnormalities (and possibly cholestasis) also reported; **important:** ventricular arrhythmias (including torsades de pointes) have been reported (see Arrhythmias above)

Dose: ADULT and CHILD over 12 years

Symptoms and mucosal lesions associated with gastro-oesophageal reflux disease, 10 mg 3–4 times daily *or* 20 mg twice daily (12-week course recommended); maintenance treatment, 20 mg at bedtime *or* 10 mg twice daily (20 mg twice daily if initial lesions very severe) (halve 20-mg dose and double frequency of administration if severe abdominal cramps)

Symptoms of impaired gastric motility secondary to disturbed and delayed gastric emptying associated with diabetes, systemic sclerosis and autonomic neuropathy, 10 mg 3–4 times daily initially for 6 weeks (longer if necessary)

Symptoms of dyspepsia (peptic ulcer or other lesions excluded), 10 mg 3 times daily (usually for 4 weeks)

COUNSELLING. Advise patient to take 15–30 minutes before meals and at bedtime (for night symptoms)

Prepulsid® (Janssen-Cilag) PoM

Tablets, scored, cisapride (as monohydrate) 10 mg, net price 120-tab pack = £28.20. Counselling, administration, see above

Suspension, cisapride (as monohydrate) 5 mg/5 mL. Net price 500 mL = £15.60. Counselling, administration, see above

Quicklet® tablets, cisapride (as monohydrate) 20 mg, net price 56-tab pack = £35.09. Counselling, see below

COUNSELLING. *Quicklet®* tablets should be placed on the tongue and allowed to dissolve. Advise patient to take 15–30 minutes before meals and at bedtime (for night symptoms)

Excipients: include aspartame (section 9.4.1)

1.3   Ulcer-healing drugs

1.3.1	H_2-receptor antagonists
1.3.2	Selective antimuscarinics
1.3.3	Chelates and complexes
1.3.4	Prostaglandin analogues
1.3.5	Proton pump inhibitors
1.3.6	Other ulcer-healing drugs

Peptic ulceration commonly involves the stomach, duodenum, and lower oesophagus; after gastric surgery it involves the gastro-enterostomy stoma.

Healing can be promoted by general measures, stopping smoking and taking antacids and by antisecretory drug treatment, but relapse is common when treatment ceases. Nearly all duodenal ulcers and most gastric ulcers not associated with NSAIDs are caused by *Helicobacter pylori*.

The management of *H. pylori* infection and of NSAID-associated ulcers is discussed below.

Helicobacter pylori infection

Long-term healing of duodenal and gastric ulcers can be achieved by eradicating *Helicobacter pylori*; it is recommended that the presence of *H. pylori* is confirmed before starting eradication treatment. Acid inhibition combined with antibiotic treatment is highly effective in the eradication of *H. pylori*; reinfection with *H. pylori* is rare.

Studies have demonstrated the efficacy of one-week eradication regimens that include a proton pump inhibitor and clarithromycin with either metronidazole or amoxicillin; these regimens produce *H. pylori* eradication in 90% or more of patients. Treatment failure may reflect poor compliance, metronidazole resistance or, less commonly, clarithromycin resistance. If clarithromycin cannot be used, both amoxicillin and metronidazole need to be used instead. Ranitidine bismuth citrate may be substituted for a proton pump inhibitor if necessary.

Two-week triple therapy regimens are associated with high eradication rates, but adverse effects are common and compliance is a problem.

Two-week dual therapy regimens using a proton pump inhibitor and a single antibiotic are licensed, but produce low rates of *H. pylori* eradication and are **not** recommended.

A two-week regimen using tripotassium dicitrato-bismuthate *plus* a proton pump inhibitor *plus* two antibiotics may have a role in the treatment of resistant cases after confirmation of the presence of *H. pylori*.

Other drugs used for *H. pylori* eradication include tinidazole (section 5.1.11) and tetracycline; they should be used in combination with antisecretory drugs and other antibiotics.

Antibiotic-induced colitis is a possible (but uncommon) risk.

Test for *Helicobacter pylori*

^{13}C-Urea breath test kits are available for the diagnosis of gastro-duodenal infection with *Helicobacter pylori*. The test involves collection of breath samples before and after ingestion of an oral solution of ^{13}C-urea; the samples are sent for analysis by an appropriate laboratory. The test should not be performed within 4 weeks of treatment with an antibiotic or an antisecretory drug.

Helicobacter Test INFAI® (Infai) PoM
Oral powder, ^{13}C-urea 75 mg for dissolving in water. Net price 1 kit (including 4 breath sample containers, straws) = £21.01 (analysis included)

Pylobactell® (BSIA) PoM
Soluble tablets, ^{13}C-urea 100 mg. Net price 1 kit (including 6 breath sample containers, 30-mL mixing and administration vial, straws) = £21.75 (analysis included)

NSAID-associated ulcers

Gastro-intestinal bleeding and ulceration may occur with NSAID use (section 10.1.1).

Omeprazole or misoprostol may be used to prevent NSAID-associated gastric and duodenal ulcers; colic and diarrhoea may limit the dose of misoprostol. H$_2$-receptor antagonists may be effective in preventing NSAID-associated duodenal ulcers.

In patients who need to continue NSAID treatment, NSAID-associated ulcers may be treated with H$_2$-receptor antagonists, proton pump inhibitors or misoprostol; omeprazole may produce more rapid healing since the rate of healing probably correlates with the intensity of acid suppression.

Recommended regimens for *Helicobacter pylori* eradication

Regimens that include clarithromycin

Omeprazole 20 mg twice daily
Clarithromycin 500 mg twice daily
Amoxicillin 1 g twice daily
Total net price for 7-day course = £40.65

Lansoprazole 30 mg twice daily
Clarithromycin 500 mg twice daily
Amoxicillin 1 g twice daily
Total net price for 7-day course = £40.44

Pantoprazole 40 mg twice daily
Clarithromycin 500 mg twice daily
Amoxicillin 1 g twice daily
Total net price for 7-day course = £40.47

Omeprazole 20 mg twice daily
Clarithromycin 500 mg twice daily
Metronidazole 400 mg twice daily
Total net price for 7-day course = £40.88

Lansoprazole 30 mg twice daily
Clarithromycin 500 mg twice daily
Metronidazole 400 mg twice daily
Total net price for 7-day course = £40.67

Pantoprazole 40 mg twice daily
Clarithromycin 500 mg twice daily
Metronidazole 400 mg twice daily
Total net price for 7-day course = £40.70

Ranitidine bismuth citrate 400 mg twice daily
Clarithromycin 500 mg twice daily
Amoxicillin 1 g twice daily
Total net price for 7-day course = £38.59

Ranitidine bismuth citrate 400 mg twice daily
Clarithromycin 500 mg twice daily
Metronidazole 400 mg twice daily
Total net price for 7-day course = £38.82

Regimens that do not include clarithromycin

Omeprazole 20 mg twice daily
Amoxicillin 500 mg 3 times daily
Metronidazole 400 mg 3 times daily
Total net price for 7-day course = £22.38

Lansoprazole 30 mg twice daily
Amoxicillin 1 g twice daily
Metronidazole 400 mg twice daily
Total net price for 7-day course = £21.27

Ranitidine bismuth citrate 400 mg twice daily
Amoxicillin 1 g twice daily
Metronidazole 400 mg twice daily
Total net price for 7-day course = £19.42

Antisecretory treatment (with a proton pump inhibitor or H$_2$-receptor antagonist) may need to be continued for 4–8 weeks to promote ulcer healing (particularly after ulcer haemorrhage or perforation)

H$_2$-receptor antagonists

All H$_2$-receptor antagonists heal *gastric and duodenal ulcers* by reducing gastric acid output as a result of histamine H$_2$-receptor blockade; they can also be expected to relieve *gastro-oesophageal reflux disease*. High doses of H$_2$-receptor antagonists have been used in the *Zollinger–Ellison syndrome*, but omeprazole may now be preferred.

Maintenance treatment with low doses has largely been replaced in *Helicobacter pylori* positive patients by eradication regimens (section 1.3). Maintenance treatment may occasionally be used for those with frequent severe recurrences and for the elderly who suffer ulcer complications.

Treatment of *undiagnosed dyspepsia* with H$_2$-receptor antagonists may be acceptable in younger patients but is undesirable in older people because the diagnosis of gastric cancer may be delayed.

Therapy can promote healing of *NSAID-associated ulcers* (particularly duodenal) (section 1.3).

Treatment has not been shown to be beneficial in haematemesis and melaena, but prophylactic use reduces the frequency of bleeding from gastroduodenal erosions in hepatic coma, and possibly in other conditions requiring intensive care. Treatment also reduces the frequency of acid aspiration in obstetric patients at delivery (Mendelson's syndrome).

CAUTIONS. H$_2$-receptor antagonists should be used with caution in hepatic impairment (Appendix 2), in renal impairment (Appendix 3), pregnancy (Appendix 4), and in breast-feeding (Appendix 5). H$_2$-receptor antagonists may mask symptoms of gastric cancer; particular care is required in those whose symptoms change and in those who are middle-aged or over.

SIDE-EFFECTS. Side-effects of the H$_2$-receptor antagonists include diarrhoea and other gastro-intestinal disturbances, altered liver function tests (rarely liver damage), headache, dizziness, rash, and tiredness. Rare side-effects include acute pancreatitis, bradycardia, AV block, confusion, depression, and hallucinations particularly in the elderly or the very ill, hypersensitivity reactions (including fever, arthralgia, myalgia, anaphylaxis), and blood disorders (including agranulocytosis, leucopenia, pancytopenia, thrombocytopenia). There have been occasional reports of gynaecomastia and impotence.

INTERACTIONS. Cimetidine retards oxidative hepatic drug metabolism by binding to microsomal cytochrome P450. It should be avoided in patients stabilised on warfarin, phenytoin, and theophylline (or aminophylline), but other interactions (see **Appendix 1**) may be of less clinical relevance. Famotidine, nizatidine, and ranitidine do not share the drug metabolism inhibitory properties of cimetidine.

CIMETIDINE

Indications: benign gastric and duodenal ulceration, stomal ulcer, reflux oesophagitis, Zollinger-Ellison syndrome, other conditions where gastric acid reduction is beneficial (see notes above and section 1.9.4)

Cautions: see notes above; preferably avoid intravenous injection (use intravenous infusion) particularly in high dosage and in cardiovascular impairment (risk of arrhythmias); **interactions:** Appendix 1 (histamine H$_2$-antagonists) and notes above

Side-effects: see notes above; alopecia; rarely tachycardia, interstitial nephritis

Dose: *by mouth*, 400 mg twice daily (with breakfast and at night) *or* 800 mg at night (benign gastric and duodenal ulceration) for at least 4 weeks (6 weeks in gastric ulceration, 8 weeks in ulcer associated with continued NSAID); when necessary the dose may be increased to 400 mg 4 times daily or rarely (e.g. as in stress ulceration) to a max. of 2.4 g daily in divided doses; INFANT under 1 year, 20 mg/kg daily in divided doses has been used; CHILD over 1 year, 25–30 mg/kg daily in divided doses

Maintenance, 400 mg at night *or* 400 mg morning and night

Reflux oesophagitis, 400 mg 4 times daily for 4–8 weeks

Zollinger–Ellison syndrome (but see notes above), 400 mg 4 times daily or occasionally more

Gastric acid reduction (prophylaxis of acid aspiration; do not use syrup), obstetrics 400 mg at start of labour, then up to 400 mg every 4 hours if required (max. of 2.4 g daily); surgical procedures 400 mg 90–120 minutes before induction of general anaesthesia

Short-bowel syndrome, 400 mg twice daily (with breakfast and at bedtime) adjusted according to response

To reduce degradation of pancreatic enzyme supplements, 0.8–1.6 g daily in 4 divided doses according to response 1–1½ hours before meals

By intramuscular injection, 200 mg every 4–6 hours; max. 2.4 g daily

By slow intravenous injection, 200 mg given over at least 5 minutes; may be repeated every 4–6 hours; if a larger dose is needed or there is cardiovascular impairment, the dose should be diluted and given over at least 10 minutes (infusion is preferable); max. 2.4 g daily

By intravenous infusion, 400 mg in 100 mL of sodium chloride 0.9% intravenous infusion infused over ½–1 hour (may be repeated every 4–6 hours) *or* by continuous infusion at an average rate of 50–100 mg/hour over 24 hours, max. 2.4 g daily; INFANT under 1 year, *by intramuscular injection or slow intravenous injection or infusion*, 20 mg/kg daily in divided doses has been used; CHILD over 1 year, 25–30 mg/kg daily in divided doses

¹ **Cimetidine** (Non-proprietary) ▢PoM

Tablets, cimetidine 200 mg, net price 120-tab pack = £14.59; 400 mg, 60-tab pack = £17.35; 800 mg, 30-tab pack = £16.83

Available from APS, Ashbourne (*Peptimax®*), Berk (*Ultec®*), BHR (*Phimetin®*), Bioglan, Cox, CP, Dexcel Pharma, Eastern (*Zita®*), Galen (*Galenamet®*), Hillcross, Norton, Opus (*Acitak®*)

1. Cimetidine can be sold to the public for adults and children over 16 years (provided packs do not contain more than 2 weeks' supply) for the short-term symptomatic relief of heartburn, dyspepsia, and hyperacidity (max. single dose 200 mg, max. daily dose 800 mg), and for the prophylactic management of nocturnal heartburn (single night-time dose 100 mg); a proprietary brand (*Tagamet 100®* containing cimetidine 100 mg) is on sale to the public

Dyspamet® (SmithKline Beecham) [PoM]
Suspension, sugar-free, cimetidine 200 mg/5 mL. Contains sorbitol 2.79 g/5 mL. Net price 600 mL = £24.08

Tagamet® (SmithKline Beecham) [PoM]
Tablets, all green, f/c, cimetidine 200 mg, net price 120-tab pack = £19.58; 400 mg, 60-tab pack = £22.62; 800 mg, 30-tab pack = £22.62
Effervescent tablets, sugar-free, cimetidine 400 mg. Contains 17.6 mmol Na+/tablet. Net price 60-tab pack = £20.56. Label: 13
Excipients: include aspartame 70 mg/tablet (section 9.4.1)
Syrup, orange, cimetidine 200 mg/5 mL. Net price 600 mL = £28.49
Injection, cimetidine 100 mg/mL. Net price 2-mL amp = 36p

FAMOTIDINE

Indications: see under Dose
Cautions: see notes above; **interactions:** Appendix 1 (histamine H$_2$-antagonists) and notes above
Side-effects: see notes above; rarely anxiety, toxic epidermal necrolysis, urticaria, anorexia, dry mouth
Dose: benign gastric and duodenal ulceration, treatment, 40 mg at night for 4–8 weeks; maintenance (duodenal ulceration), 20 mg at night; CHILD not recommended
Reflux oesophagitis, 20–40 mg twice daily for 6–12 weeks; maintenance, 20 mg twice daily
Zollinger–Ellison syndrome (but see notes above), 20 mg every 6 hours (higher dose in those who have previously been receiving another H$_2$-antagonist); doses up to 800 mg daily in divided doses have been used

[1] **Pepcid®** (MSD) [PoM]
Tablets, f/c, famotidine 20 mg (beige), net price 28-tab pack = £14.00; 40 mg (brown), 28-tab pack = £26.60
1. Famotidine can be sold to the public for adults and children over 16 years (provided packs do not contain more than 2 weeks' supply) for the short-term symptomatic relief of heartburn, dyspepsia, and hyperacidity, and for the prevention of these symptoms when associated with consumption of food or drink including when they cause sleep disturbance (max. single dose 10 mg, max. daily dose 20 mg); proprietary brands (*Boots Excess Acid Control®*, *Pepcid® AC*, *Pepcid® AC Chewable* all containing famotidine 10 mg) are on sale to the public

NIZATIDINE

Indications: see under Dose
Cautions: see notes above; hepatic impairment; avoid rapid intravenous injection (risk of arrhythmias and postural hypotension); **interactions:** Appendix 1 (histamine H$_2$-antagonists) and notes above
Side-effects: see notes above; sweating; rarely vasculitis, hyperuricaemia, exfoliative dermatitis
Dose: *by mouth*, benign gastric, duodenal or NSAID-associated ulceration, treatment, 300 mg in the evening *or* 150 mg twice daily for 4–8 weeks; maintenance, 150 mg at night; CHILD not recommended
Gastro-oesophageal reflux disease, 150–300 mg twice daily for up to 12 weeks
By intravenous infusion, for short-term use in peptic ulcer hospital inpatients as alternative to oral route, *by intermittent intravenous infusion* over 15 minutes, 100 mg 3 times daily, *or by continuous intravenous infusion*, 10 mg/hour; max. 480 mg daily; CHILD not recommended

[1] **Nizatidine** (Non-proprietary) [PoM]
Capsules, nizatidine 150 mg, net price 60-cap pack = £22.68; 300 mg, 30-cap pack = £21.74
Available from Ashbourne (*Zinga®*)
1. Nizatidine can be sold to the public for the prevention and treatment of symptoms of food-related heartburn and meal-induced indigestion in adults and children over 16 years; max. single dose 75 mg, max. daily dose 150 mg for max. 14 days

Axid® (Lilly) [PoM]
Capsules, nizatidine 150 mg (pale yellow/dark yellow), net price 28-cap pack = £7.72, 30-cap pack = £8.27; 300 mg (pale yellow/brown), 30-cap pack = £16.40
Injection, nizatidine 25 mg/mL. For dilution and use as an intravenous infusion. Net price 4-mL amp = £1.14

RANITIDINE

Indications: see under Dose, other conditions where reduction of gastric acidity is beneficial (see notes above and section 1.9.4)
Cautions: see notes above; avoid in porphyria (section 9.8.2); **interactions:** Appendix 1 (histamine H$_2$-antagonists) and notes above
Side-effects: see notes above; rarely tachycardia, agitation, visual disturbances, erythema multiforme, alopecia
Dose: *by mouth*, 150 mg twice daily *or* 300 mg at night (benign gastric and duodenal ulceration) for 4 to 8 weeks, up to 6 weeks in chronic episodic dyspepsia, and up to 8 weeks in NSAID-associated ulceration (in duodenal ulcer 300 mg can be given twice daily for 4 weeks to achieve a higher healing rate); maintenance, 150 mg at night; CHILD (peptic ulcer) 2–4 mg/kg twice daily, max. 300 mg daily
Duodenal ulcer associated with *H. pylori* (but see p. 37 for recommended regimens), ranitidine 300 mg daily in 1–2 divided doses (plus amoxicillin 750 mg 3 times daily and metronidazole 500 mg 3 times daily) for 2 weeks; ranitidine treatment continued for a further 2 weeks
Prophylaxis of NSAID-induced duodenal ulcer, 150 mg twice daily
Reflux oesophagitis, 150 mg twice daily *or* 300 mg at night for up to 8 weeks, or if necessary 12 weeks (moderate to severe, 150 mg 4 times daily for up to 12 weeks); long-term treatment of healed oesophagitis, 150 mg twice daily
Zollinger–Ellison syndrome (but see notes above), 150 mg 3 times daily; doses up to 6 g daily in divided doses have been used
Gastric acid reduction (prophylaxis of acid aspiration) in obstetrics, *by mouth*, 150 mg at onset of labour, then every 6 hours; surgical procedures, *by intramuscular or slow intravenous injection*, 50 mg 45–60 minutes before induction of anaesthesia (intravenous injection diluted to 20 mL and given over at least 2 minutes), or *by mouth*, 150 mg 2 hours before induction of anaesthesia, and also, when possible on the preceding evening
By intramuscular injection, 50 mg every 6–8 hours
By slow intravenous injection, 50 mg diluted to 20 mL and given over at least 2 minutes; may be repeated every 6–8 hours
By intravenous infusion, 25 mg/hour for 2 hours; may be repeated every 6–8 hours
Prophylaxis of stress ulceration, initial slow intravenous injection of 50 mg (as above) then *continuous infusion*, 125–250 micrograms/kg per hour (may be followed by 150 mg twice daily *by mouth* when oral feeding commences)

¹**Ranitidine** (Non-proprietary) PoM
Tablets, ranitidine (as hydrochloride) 150 mg, net price 60-tab pack = £19.46; 300 mg, 30-tab pack = £19.28

Available from APS, Ashbourne (*Zaedoc®*), Berk (*Rantec®*), Cox, CP, Dominion, Galen, Generics, Genus, Goldshield, Hillcross, Norton, Ranbaxy, Sovereign, Sterwin, Tillomed (*Ranitic®*)

1. Ranitidine can be sold to the public for adults and children over 16 years (provided packs do not contain more than 2 weeks' supply) for the short-term symptomatic relief of heartburn, dyspepsia, and hyperacidity, and for the prevention of these symptoms when associated with consumption of food or drink (max. single dose 75 mg, max. daily dose 300 mg); a proprietary brand (*Zantac® 75* containing ranitidine (as hydrochloride) 75 mg) is on sale to the public

Zantac® (GlaxoWellcome) PoM
Tablets, f/c, ranitidine (as hydrochloride) 150 mg, net price 60-tab pack = £19.52; 300 mg, 30-tab pack = £19.20
Effervescent tablets, pale yellow, ranitidine (as hydrochloride) 150 mg (contains 14.3 mmol Na⁺/ tablet), net price 60-tab pack = £27.88; 300 mg (contains 20.8 mmol Na⁺/tablet), 30-tab pack = £27.42. Label: 13

Note. The effervescent tablets contain aspartame (section 9.4.1)

Syrup, sugar-free, ranitidine (as hydrochloride) 75 mg/5 mL. Net price 300 mL = £22.32
Injection, ranitidine (as hydrochloride) 25 mg/mL. Net price 2-mL amp = 64p

---

RANITIDINE BISMUTH CITRATE
(Ranitidine Bismutrex)
Indications: see under Dose
Cautions: see notes above; see also under Tripotassium Dicitratobismuthate; **interactions:** Appendix 1 (histamine H₂-antagonists) and notes above
Contra-indications: moderate to severe renal impairment; pregnancy (Appendix 4); breast-feeding (Appendix 5); porphyria (section 9.8.2)
Side-effects: see notes above; may darken tongue or blacken faeces; rarely tachycardia, agitation, visual disturbances, erythema multiforme, alopecia
Dose: 400 mg twice daily, preferably with food, for 8 weeks in benign gastric ulceration or 4–8 weeks in duodenal ulceration; CHILD not recommended
Eradication of *Helicobacter pylori*, see eradication regimens on p. 37; ranitidine bismuth citrate treatment may be continued for a total of 4 weeks; long-term (maintenance) treatment not recommended (max. total of 16 weeks treatment in any 1 year); CHILD not recommended
COUNSELLING. May darken tongue and blacken faeces

Pylorid® (GlaxoWellcome) PoM
Tablets, blue, f/c, ranitidine bismuth citrate 400 mg. Net price 14-tab pack = £13.00; Counselling (discoloration of tongue and faeces)

1.3.2 ## Selective antimuscarinics

Pirenzepine is a selective antimuscarinic drug which was used for the treatment of gastric and duodenal ulcers. It has now been discontinued.

1.3.3 # Chelates and complexes

Tripotassium dicitratobismuthate is a bismuth chelate effective in healing gastric and duodenal ulcers, but not on its own in maintaining remission. For the role of tripotassium dicitratobismuthate in a *Helicobacter pylori* eradication regimen for those who have not responded to first-line regimens, see section 1.3.

The bismuth content of tripotassium dicitratobismuthate is low but absorption has been reported; encephalopathy (described with older high-dose bismuth preparations) has not been reported.

Ranitidine bismuth citrate (section 1.3.1) is used in the management of peptic ulcer, and in combination with two antibiotics for the eradication of *H. pylori* (section 1.3).

Sucralfate may act by protecting the mucosa from acid-pepsin attack in gastric and duodenal ulcers. It is a complex of aluminium hydroxide and sulphated sucrose but has minimal antacid properties. It should be used with caution in patients under intensive care (**important**: reports of bezoar formation, see CSM advice below)

TRIPOTASSIUM DICITRATOBISMUTHATE
(Bismuth Chelate)
Indications: benign gastric and duodenal ulceration; see also *Helicobacter pylori* infection, section 1.3
Cautions: see notes above; **interactions:** Appendix 1 (tripotassium dicitratobismuthate)
Contra-indications: renal impairment, pregnancy
Side-effects: may darken tongue and blacken faeces; nausea and vomiting reported

De-Noltab® (Yamanouchi)
Tablets, f/c, tripotassium dicitratobismuthate 120 mg. Net price 112-tab pack = £29.40. Counselling, see below
Dose: 2 tablets twice daily *or* 1 tablet 4 times daily; taken for 28 days followed by further 28 days if necessary; maintenance not indicated but course may be repeated after interval of 1 month; CHILD, not recommended
COUNSELLING. Each dose to be swallowed with half a tumblerful of water; twice daily dosage to be taken 30 minutes before breakfast and main evening meal; four times daily dosage to be taken as follows: one dose 30 minutes before breakfast, midday meal and main evening meal, and one dose 2 hours after main evening meal; milk should not be drunk by itself during treatment but small quantities may be taken in tea or coffee or on cereal; antacids should not be taken half an hour before or after a dose; may darken tongue and blacken faeces

SUCRALFATE
Indications: see under dose
Cautions: renal impairment (avoid if severe, see Appendix 3); pregnancy and breast-feeding; administration of sucralfate and enteral feeds should be separated by 1 hour; **interactions:** Appendix 1 (sucralfate)
BEZOAR FORMATION. Following reports of bezoar formation associated with sucralfate, the **CSM** has advised caution in seriously ill patients, especially those receiving concomitant enteral feeds or those with predisposing conditions such as delayed gastric emptying

Side-effects: constipation; diarrhoea, nausea, indigestion, gastric discomfort, dry mouth, rash, hypersensitivity reactions, back pain, dizziness, headache, vertigo and drowsiness, bezoar formation (see above)

Dose: benign gastric and duodenal ulceration and chronic gastritis, 2 g twice daily (on rising and at bedtime) *or* 1 g 4 times daily 1 hour before meals and at bedtime, taken for 4–6 weeks or in resistant cases up to 12 weeks; max. 8 g daily
Prophylaxis of stress ulceration (suspension), 1 g 6 times daily (max. 8 g daily)
CHILD not recommended

Sucralfate (Non-proprietary) [PoM]
Tablets, sucralfate 1 g. Net price 112-tab pack = £10.59. Label: 5
Available from Hillcross

Antepsin® (Chugai) [PoM]
Tablets, scored, sucralfate 1 g. Net price 112-tab pack = £9.80. Label: 5
COUNSELLING. Tablets may be dispersed in water
Suspension, sucralfate, 1 g/5 mL. Net price 560 mL = £9.80. Label: 5

1.3.4   Prostaglandin analogues

Misoprostol, a synthetic prostaglandin analogue has antisecretory and protective properties, promoting *gastric and duodenal ulcer* healing. It can prevent NSAID-associated ulcers, its use being most appropriate for the frail or very elderly from whom NSAIDs cannot be withdrawn.

MISOPROSTOL

Indications: see notes above and under Dose

Cautions: conditions where hypotension might precipitate severe complications (e.g. cerebrovascular disease, cardiovascular disease); **interactions:** Appendix 1 (misoprostol)

Contra-indications: pregnancy or planning pregnancy (increases uterine tone)—**important:** women of childbearing age, see also below, and breast-feeding
WOMEN OF CHILDBEARING AGE. Manufacturer advises that misoprostol should not be used in women of childbearing age unless the patient requires non-steroidal anti-inflammatory (NSAID) therapy and is at high risk of complications from NSAID-induced ulceration. In such patients it is advised that misoprostol should only be used if the patient takes *effective contraceptive measures* and has been advised of the *risks of taking misoprostol if pregnant.*

Side-effects: diarrhoea (may occasionally be severe and require withdrawal, reduced by giving single doses not exceeding 200 micrograms and by avoiding magnesium-containing antacids); also reported: abdominal pain, dyspepsia, flatulence, nausea and vomiting, abnormal vaginal bleeding (including intermenstrual bleeding, menorrhagia, and postmenopausal bleeding), rashes, dizziness

Dose: benign gastric and duodenal ulceration and NSAID-associated ulceration, 800 micrograms daily (in 2–4 divided doses) with breakfast (or main meals) and at bedtime; treatment should be

continued for at least 4 weeks and may be continued for up to 8 weeks if required
Prophylaxis of NSAID-induced gastric and duodenal ulcer, 200 micrograms 2–4 times daily taken with the NSAID
CHILD not recommended

Cytotec® (Searle) [PoM]
Tablets, scored, misoprostol 200 micrograms, net price 60-tab pack = £11.14. Label: 21

■ With diclofenac or naproxen
Section 10.1.1

1.3.5   Proton pump inhibitors

The proton pump inhibitors **omeprazole, lansoprazole, pantoprazole** and **rabeprazole** inhibit gastric acid by blocking the hydrogen-potassium adenosine triphosphatase enzyme system (the 'proton pump') of the gastric parietal cell. Proton pump inhibitors are effective short-term treatments for *gastric and duodenal ulcers*; they are also used in combination with antibiotics for the eradication of *Helicobacter pylori* (see p. 37 for specific regimens). Proton pump inhibitors are the treatment of choice for severe symptoms in gastro-oesophageal reflux disease (section 1.1.3). Omeprazole is effective in the treatment of the *Zollinger-Ellison syndrome* (including cases resistant to other treatment); lansoprazole is also indicated for this condition.

CAUTIONS. Proton pump inhibitors should be used with caution in patients with liver disease (Appendix 2), in pregnancy (Appendix 4) and in breast-feeding. Proton pump inhibitors may mask symptoms of gastric cancer; particular care is required in those whose symptoms change and in those over 45 years of age; before treatment the presence of gastric malignancy should be excluded.

SIDE-EFFECTS. Side-effects of the proton pump inhibitors include gastro-intestinal disturbances (including diarrhoea, nausea and vomiting, constipation, flatulence, abdominal pain), headache, hypersensitivity reactions (including rash, urticaria, angioedema, bronchospasm), pruritus, dizziness, peripheral oedema, muscle and joint pain, malaise, blurred vision, depression and dry mouth. Proton pump inhibitors decrease gastric acidity and may increase the risk of gastro-intestinal infections.

OMEPRAZOLE

Indications: see under Dose

Cautions: see notes above; **interactions:** Appendix 1 (proton pump inhibitors)

Side-effects: see notes above; also reported, bullous eruption, Stevens-Johnson syndrome, toxic epidermal necrolysis, anaphylaxis, fever, photosensitivity, paraesthesia, vertigo, interstitial nephritis, alopecia, somnolence, insomnia, sweating, gynaecomastia, rarely impotence, taste disturbance, stomatitis, liver enzyme changes and liver dysfunction, encephalopathy in severe liver disease; haematological changes (including agranulocytosis, leucopenia, pancytopenia, thrombocytopenia), hyponatraemia; reversible confusion, agitation, and hallucinations in the severely ill; visual impairment reported with high-dose injection

Dose: *by mouth*, benign gastric and duodenal ulcers, 20 mg once daily for 4 weeks in duodenal ulceration or 8 weeks in gastric ulceration; in severe or recurrent cases increase to 40 mg daily; maintenance for recurrent duodenal ulcer, 20 mg once daily; prevention of relapse in duodenal ulcer, 10 mg daily increasing to 20 mg once daily if symptoms return

NSAID-associated duodenal or gastric ulcer and gastroduodenal erosions, 20 mg once daily for 4 weeks, followed by a further 4 weeks if not fully healed; prophylaxis in patients with a history of NSAID-associated duodenal or gastric ulcers, gastroduodenal lesions, or dyspeptic symptoms who require continued NSAID treatment, 20 mg once daily

Duodenal ulcer associated with *Helicobacter pylori*, see eradication regimens on p. 37

Benign gastric ulcer associated with *H. pylori*, omeprazole 40 mg daily in 1–2 divided doses (plus amoxicillin 0.75–1 g twice daily) for 2 weeks

Zollinger–Ellison syndrome, initially 60 mg once daily; usual range 20–120 mg daily (above 80 mg in 2 divided doses)

Gastric acid reduction during general anaesthesia (prophylaxis of acid aspiration), 40 mg on the preceding evening then 40 mg 2–6 hours before surgery

Gastro-oesophageal reflux disease, 20 mg once daily for 4 weeks, followed by a further 4–8 weeks if not fully healed; 40 mg once daily has been given for 8 weeks in gastro-oesophageal reflux disease refractory to other treatment; may be continued at 20 mg once daily

Acid reflux disease (long-term management), 10 mg daily increasing to 20 mg once daily if symptoms return

Acid-related dyspepsia, 10–20 mg once daily for 2–4 weeks according to response

CHILD over 2 years, severe ulcerating reflux oesophagitis, 0.7–1.4 mg/kg daily for 4–12 weeks; max. 40 mg daily (to be initiated by hospital paediatrician)

By intravenous infusion, gastric acid reduction during anaesthesia (prophylaxis of acid aspiration), 40 mg completed 1 hour before surgery

Benign gastric ulcer, duodenal ulcer and gastro-oesophageal reflux, 40 mg once daily until oral administration possible

CHILD not recommended

COUNSELLING. Swallow whole, *or* disperse tablets in water, *or* mix capsule contents or tablets with fruit juice or yoghurt

Losec® (Astra) PoM

MUPS® (= dispersible tablets), f/c, omeprazole 10 mg (light pink), net price 28-tab pack = £18.91 (also 7-tab pack, hosp. only); 20 mg (pink), 28-tab pack = £28.56 (also 7-tab pack, hosp. only); 40 mg (red-brown), 7-tab pack = £14.28. Counselling, administration

Capsules, enclosing e/c granules, omeprazole 10 mg (pink), net price 28-cap pack = £18.91 (also 7-cap pack, hosp. only); 20 mg (pink/brown), 28-cap pack = £28.56 (also 7-cap pack, hosp. only); 40 mg (brown), 7-cap pack = £14.28. Counselling, administration

▼ *Intravenous infusion*, powder for reconstitution, omeprazole (as sodium salt), net price 40-mg vial = £5.21

LANSOPRAZOLE

Indications: see under Dose

Cautions: see notes above; **interactions:** Appendix 1 (proton pump inhibitors)

Side-effects: see notes above; also reported, bullous eruption, erythema multiforme, alopecia, photosensitivity, paraesthesia, interstitial nephritis, anaphylaxis, liver enzyme changes and liver dysfunction, haematological changes (including eosinophilia, leucopenia, pancytopenia, thrombocytopenia), bruising, purpura, petechiae, fatigue, taste disturbance, vertigo, hallucinations, confusion, rarely gynaecomastia, impotence

Dose: benign gastric ulcer, 30 mg daily in the morning for 8 weeks

Duodenal ulcer, 30 mg daily in the morning for 4 weeks; maintenance 15 mg daily

NSAID-associated duodenal or gastric ulcer, 15–30 mg once daily for 4 weeks, followed by a further 4 weeks if not fully healed

Duodenal ulcer associated with *Helicobacter pylori*, see eradication regimens on p. 37

Zollinger-Ellison syndrome (and other hypersecretory conditions), initially 60 mg once daily adjusted according to response; daily doses of 120 mg or more given in two divided doses

Gastro-oesophageal reflux disease, 30 mg daily in the morning for 4 weeks, followed by a further 4 weeks if not fully healed; maintenance 15–30 mg daily

Acid-related dyspepsia, 15–30 mg daily in the morning for 2–4 weeks

CHILD not recommended

Zoton® (Lederle) PoM

Capsules, enclosing e/c granules, lansoprazole 15 mg (yellow), net price 28-cap pack = £14.21, 56-cap pack = £28.42; 30 mg (lilac/purple), 14-cap pack = £14.08, 28-cap pack = £28.15, 56-cap pack = £56.29 (also 7-cap pack, hosp. only). Label: 5, 25

Suspension, pink, powder for reconstitution, lansoprazole 30 mg/sachet (strawberry flavour), net price 28-sachet pack = £34.14. Label: 5, 13

■ With antibiotics

For additional cautions, contra-indications and side-effects see Amoxicillin (section 5.1.1) and Clarithromycin (section 5.1.5)

HeliClear® (Wyeth) PoM

Triple pack, lansoprazole capsules 30 mg (*Zoton®*), amoxicillin (as trihydrate) capsules 500 mg, clarithromycin tablets 500 mg (*Klaricid®*). Net price 7-day pack (14 × lansoprazole caps, 28 × amoxicillin caps, 14 × clarithromycin tabs) = £34.14. Label: 5, 9, 25

Dose: eradication of *Helicobacter pylori* in patients with duodenal ulcer, lansoprazole 30 mg twice daily, clarithromycin 500 mg twice daily, and amoxicillin 1 g twice daily for 7–14 days; CHILD not recommended

PANTOPRAZOLE

Indications: see under Dose
Cautions: see notes above; renal impairment (Appendix 3); **interactions:** Appendix 1 (proton pump inhibitors)
Side-effects: see notes above; also reported fever, liver enzyme changes, raised triglycerides
Dose: *By mouth,* benign gastric ulcer, 40 mg in the morning for 4 weeks, continued for further 4 weeks if not fully healed
Gastro-oesophageal reflux disease, 40 mg daily in the morning for 4 weeks, continued for further 4 weeks if not fully healed; may be continued at 20 mg daily (long-term management), increased to 40 mg daily if symptoms return
Duodenal ulcer, 40 mg daily in the morning for 2 weeks, continued for further 2 weeks if not fully healed
Duodenal ulcer associated with *Helicobacter pylori*, see eradication regimens on p. 37
CHILD not recommended
By intravenous injection, over 2–15 minutes, duodenal ulcer, gastric ulcer, and gastro-oesophageal reflux, 40 mg daily until oral administration can be resumed
CHILD not recommended

Protium® (Knoll) [PoM]
Tablets, e/c, pantoprazole (as sodium sesquihydrate) 20 mg, net price 28-tab pack = £14.21; 40 mg 28-tab pack = £26.50. Label: 25
▼ *Injection,* powder for reconstitution, pantoprazole (as sodium sesquihydrate), net price 40-mg vial = £5.71

RABEPRAZOLE SODIUM

Indications: see under Dose
Cautions: see notes above; **interactions:** Appendix 1 (proton pump inhibitors)
Side-effects: see notes above; also reported, stomatitis, chest pain, cough, rhinitis, sinusitis, leucocytosis, insomnia, nervousness, drowsiness, asthenia, taste disturbance, pharyngitis, anorexia, influenza-like syndrome, sweating, weight gain
Dose: benign gastric ulcer, 20 mg daily in the morning for 6 weeks, followed by a further 6 weeks if not fully healed
Duodenal ulcer, 20 mg daily in the morning for 4 weeks, followed by a further 4 weeks if not fully healed
Gastro-oesophageal reflux disease, 20 mg daily in the morning for 4–8 weeks; may be continued at 10–20 mg daily
CHILD not recommended

Pariet® (Eisai, Janssen-Cilag) ▼ [PoM]
Tablets, e/c, rabeprazole sodium 10 mg (pink), net price 28-tab pack = £12.98; 20 mg (yellow), 28-tab pack = £23.75. Label: 25

1.3.6   Other ulcer-healing drugs

Carbenoxolone is a synthetic derivative of glycyrrhizinic acid (a constituent of liquorice).
The only oral preparation of carbenoxolone remaining on the UK market is in the form of a combination with antacids for *oesophageal ulceration and inflammation.*
Side-effects of carbenoxolone (commonly sodium and water retention and occasionally hypokalaemia) may cause or exacerbate hypertension, oedema, cardiac failure, and muscle weakness. For these reasons other drugs are preferred; if used, regular monitoring of weight, blood pressure, and electrolytes is advisable during treatment. Carbenoxolone may act by protecting the mucosal barrier from acid–pepsin attack and increasing mucosal mucin production.

CARBENOXOLONE SODIUM [▨]

Indications: oesophageal inflammation and ulceration
Cautions: cardiac disease, hypertension, hepatic and renal disease (see contra-indications); elderly (see under preparation); not recommended in children; see also notes above; **interactions:** Appendix 1 (carbenoxolone)
Contra-indications: hypokalaemia, cardiac failure and in those receiving cardiac glycosides (unless electrolyte levels monitored weekly and measures taken to avoid hypokalaemia); hepatic and renal impairment (see Appendixes 2 and 3); pregnancy
Side-effects: sodium and water retention (provoking hypertension and cardiac failure), hypokalaemia (leading to impaired neuromuscular function and muscle damage and to renal damage if prolonged)
Dose: see under preparations

■ Compound preparation
Pyrogastrone® (Sanofi-Synthelabo) [PoM] [▨]
Tablets, chewable, carbenoxolone sodium 20 mg, alginic acid 600 mg, dried aluminium hydroxide 240 mg, magnesium trisilicate 60 mg, sodium bicarbonate 210 mg (Na+ 3 mmol/tablet). Net price 100-tab pack = £24.85. Label: 21, 24
Liquid, carbenoxolone sodium 10 mg, dried aluminium hydroxide 150 mg (Na+ 0.85 mmol, K+ 1.5 mmol)/5 mL when reconstituted with water. Net price 500 mL = £12.39. Label: 21
Dose: for oesophageal inflammation and ulceration, 1 tablet, chewed, 3 times daily after meals, and 2 at night, for 6–12 weeks or 10 mL liquid 3 times daily after meals and 20 mL at night, for 6–12 weeks; not recommended for children or for adults over 75 years

1.4   Antidiarrhoeal drugs

1.4.1   Adsorbents and bulk-forming drugs
1.4.2   Antimotility drugs

The **first line** of treatment in acute diarrhoea, as in gastro-enteritis, is prevention or treatment of fluid and electrolyte depletion. This is particularly important in infants and in frail and elderly patients. For details of **oral rehydration preparations**, see section 9.2.1.2. Severe dehydration requires immediate admission to hospital and urgent replacement of fluid and electrolytes.
Antimotility drugs (section 1.4.2) are used for short-term symptomatic relief of acute diarrhoea in adults.

Antispasmodics (section 1.2) are occasionally of value in treating abdominal cramp associated with diarrhoea but they should **not** be used for primary treatment. Antispasmodics and antiemetics should be **avoided** in young children with gastro-enteritis since they are rarely effective and have troublesome side-effects.

Antibacterial drugs are generally unnecessary in simple gastro-enteritis, even when a bacterial cause is suspected, because the complaint will usually resolve quickly without such treatment, and infective diarrhoeas in the UK are often caused by viral infections. Systemic bacterial infection does, however, need appropriate systemic treatment. **Erythromycin** (section 5.1.5) or **ciprofloxacin** (section 5.1.12) can be used for treating Campylobacter enteritis. For drugs for shigellosis and salmonellosis, see section 5.1, table 1. Ciprofloxacin is occasionally used for prophylaxis against travellers' diarrhoea, but this is not recommended. Poorly absorbed drugs such as neomycin should be **avoided** altogether in gastro-intestinal infection. They prolong rather than shorten the time taken to control diarrhoea by causing masked bacterial diarrhoea, carrier states, or antibiotic-associated colitis (pseudomembranous colitis). Clioquinol should also be **avoided** as it is neurotoxic; both it and lactobacillus preparations are valueless.

Colestyramine (cholestyramine, section 1.5) and **aluminium hydroxide mixture** (section 1.1.1), bind unabsorbed bile salts and provide symptomatic relief of diarrhoea following ileal disease or resection, in bacterial colonisation of the small bowel, and in post-vagotomy diarrhoea.

1.4.1 Adsorbents and bulk-forming drugs

Adsorbents such as kaolin are **not** recommended for *acute diarrhoeas*. Bulk-forming drugs, such as ispaghula, methylcellulose, and sterculia (section 1.6.1) are useful in controlling faecal consistency in ileostomy and colostomy, and in controlling diarrhoea associated with diverticular disease.

KAOLIN, LIGHT ◢

Indications: diarrhoea but see notes above
Cautions: interactions: Appendix 1 (kaolin)

Kaolin Mixture, BP ◢
(Kaolin Oral Suspension)
Oral suspension, light kaolin or light kaolin (natural) 20%, light magnesium carbonate 5%, sodium bicarbonate 5% in a suitable vehicle with a peppermint flavour.
Dose: 10–20 mL every 4 hours
Note. Kaolin-containing preparations on sale to the public include *KLN®*

1.4.2 Antimotility drugs

In *acute diarrhoeas* antimotility drugs have a limited role as adjuncts to fluid and electrolyte replacement (section 9.2.1.2); they are **not** recommended for acute diarrhoeas in young children.

For comments on their role in *chronic diarrhoeas* see section 1.5.

CODEINE PHOSPHATE

Indications: see notes above; cough suppression (section 3.9.1); pain (section 4.7.2)
Cautions: see section 4.7.2; not recommended for children; tolerance and dependence may occur with prolonged use; **interactions:** Appendix 1 (opioid analgesics)
Contra-indications: see section 4.7.2; conditions where inhibition of peristalsis should be avoided, where abdominal distension develops, or in acute diarrhoeal conditions such as acute ulcerative colitis or antibiotic-associated colitis
Side-effects: see section 4.7.2
Dose: see under Preparations

Codeine Phosphate (Non-proprietary) PoM
Tablets, codeine phosphate 15 mg, net price 20 = 52p; 30 mg, 20 = £1.57; 60 mg, 20 = £1.35. Label: 2
Dose: 30 mg 3–4 times daily (range 15–60 mg); CHILD not recommended
Note. Travellers needing to take codeine phosphate tablets abroad may require a doctor's letter explaining why they are necessary.

Diarrest® (Galen) PoM ◢
Liquid, yellow, codeine phosphate 5 mg, dicycloverine hydrochloride (dicyclomine hydrochloride) 2.5 mg, potassium chloride 40 mg, sodium chloride 50 mg, sodium citrate 50 mg/5 mL. Net price 200 mL = £3.34
Dose: for diarrhoea, vomiting, and cramp, 20 mL 4 times daily with water; CHILD 4–5 years 5 mL, 6–9 years 10 mL, 10–13 years 15 mL but see cautions and notes above

Kaodene® (Sovereign) NHS ◢
Suspension, codeine phosphate 5 mg, light kaolin 1.5 g/5 mL. Net price 250 mL = £2.16
Dose: 20 mL 3–4 times daily; CHILD under 5 years not recommended, over 5 years 10 mL but see cautions and notes above

CO-PHENOTROPE

A mixture of diphenoxylate hydrochloride and atropine sulphate in the mass proportions 100 parts to 1 part respectively
Indications: adjunct to rehydration in acute diarrhoea (but see notes above); chronic mild ulcerative colitis
Cautions: see under Codeine Phosphate; young children are particularly susceptible to **overdosage** and symptoms may be delayed and observation is needed for at least 48 hours after ingestion; presence of subclinical doses of atropine may give rise to atropine side-effects in susceptible individuals or in overdosage; **interactions:** Appendix 1 (opioid analgesics)
Contra-indications: see under Codeine Phosphate
Side-effects: see under Codeine Phosphate, section 4.7.2

Lomotil® (Searle) PoM
Tablets, co-phenotrope 2.5/0.025 (diphenoxylate hydrochloride 2.5 mg, atropine sulphate 25 micrograms). Net price 20 = £1.57
Dose: initially 4 tablets, followed by 2 tablets every 6 hours until diarrhoea controlled; CHILD under 4 years not recommended, 4–8 years 1 tablet 3 times daily, 9–12 years 1 tablet 4 times daily, 13–16 years 2 tablets 3 times daily, but see also notes above
Note. Co-phenotrope 2.5/0.025 tablets are also available from Mepra-pharm (*Diarphen®*) and Norgine (*Tropergen®*)

LOPERAMIDE HYDROCHLORIDE

Indications: adjunct to rehydration in acute diarrhoea in adults and children over 4 years (but see notes above); chronic diarrhoea in adults only

Cautions: see notes above; liver disease; pregnancy (Appendix 4)

Contra-indications: conditions where inhibition of peristalsis should be avoided, where abdominal distension develops, or in acute diarrhoeal conditions such as ulcerative colitis or antibiotic-associated colitis

Side-effects: abdominal cramps, dizziness, drowsiness, and skin reactions, including urticaria reported; paralytic ileus and abdominal bloating also reported

Dose: acute diarrhoea, 4 mg initially followed by 2 mg after each loose stool for up to 5 days; usual dose 6–8 mg daily; max. 16 mg daily; CHILD under 4 years not recommended, 4–8 years 1 mg 3–4 times daily for up to *3 days only*, 9–12 years 2 mg 4 times daily for up to 5 days

Chronic diarrhoea in adults, initially, 4–8 mg daily in divided doses, subsequently adjusted according to response and given in 2 divided doses for maintenance; max. 16 mg daily

¹ **Loperamide** (Non-proprietary) PoM

Capsules, loperamide hydrochloride 2 mg. Net price 30-cap pack = £1.41

Available from Ashbourne (*Lodiar*®), Berk (*Diocaps*®), Cox, Generics, Hillcross, Norgine (*LoperaGen*®), Norton, Tillomed (*Norimode*®), Unichem

1. Loperamide can be sold to the public, for adults and children over 12 years, provided it is licensed and labelled for the treatment of acute diarrhoea; proprietary brands including *Arret*® capsules NHS, *Boots Diareze*® capsules, *Diasorb*® capsules, *Diocalm Ultra*® capsules NHS and *Imodium*® NHS (8- and 12-cap packs), *Imodium*® liquid and *Normaloe*® tablets are on sale to the public

Imodium® (Janssen-Cilag) PoM

Capsules, green/grey, loperamide hydrochloride 2 mg. Net price 30 = £1.22

Syrup, red, sugar-free, loperamide hydrochloride 1 mg/5 mL. Net price 100 mL = £1.05

■ Compound preparations

Imodium®**Plus** (Janssen-Cilag)

Tablets (chewable), scored, loperamide hydrochloride 2 mg, activated dimeticone 125 mg, net price 6-tab pack = £1.97, 18-tab pack = £4.54. Label: 24.

Dose: acute diarrhoea with abdominal colic, initially 2 tablets (ADOLESCENT 12–18 years 1 tablet) then 1 tablet after each loose stool; max. 4 tablets daily for up to 2 days; CHILD not recommended

MORPHINE

Indications: see notes above

Cautions: see notes above and under Codeine Phosphate (section 4.7.2)

Contra-indications: see notes above and under Codeine Phosphate

Side-effects: see notes above and under Codeine Phosphate (section 4.7.2); sedation and the risk of dependence are greater

Kaolin and Morphine Mixture, BP ◢

(Kaolin and Morphine Oral Suspension)

Oral suspension, light kaolin or light kaolin (natural) 20%, sodium bicarbonate 5%, and chloroform and morphine tincture 4% in a suitable vehicle. Contains anhydrous morphine 550–800 micrograms/10 mL.

Dose: 10 mL every 4 hours in water

Preparations on sale to the public containing morphine include:

Diocalm® (attapulgite, morphine)
Enterosan® (belladonna, morphine, kaolin)
Opazimes® (belladonna, morphine, aluminium, kaolin)

> ◢ denotes preparations that are considered to be less suitable for prescribing (see p. vi)

1.5 Treatment of chronic diarrhoeas

Once tumours are ruled out individual complaints need specific treatment including dietary manipulation as well as drug treatment and the maintenance of a liberal fluid intake.

Irritable bowel syndrome

Irritable bowel syndrome can present with pain, constipation, or diarrhoea, all of which may benefit from a high-fibre diet, with bran or with other agents which increase stool bulk (section 1.6.1). In some patients there may be important psychological aggravating factors which respond to reassurance. Antimotility drugs such as loperamide (section 1.4.2) may relieve diarrhoea and antispasmodic drugs (section 1.2) may relieve pain. Opioids with a central action such as codeine are better avoided because of the risk of dependence.

Malabsorption syndromes

Individual conditions need specific management and also general nutritional consideration. Thus coeliac disease (gluten enteropathy) usually needs a gluten-free diet (Appendix 7) and pancreatic insufficiency needs pancreatin supplements (section 1.9.4).

Ulcerative colitis

For *acute attacks* of ulcerative colitis local **corticosteroid** treatment such as budesonide or prednisolone enemas or prednisolone suppositories for localised rectal disease will induce remission; foam preparations are especially useful where patients have difficulty retaining liquid enemas. More extensive disease requires oral corticosteroid treatment and severe extensive or fulminant disease needs hospital admission and intravenous corticosteroid administration.

The **aminosalicylates**, sulfasalazine (sulphasalazine), mesalazine, balsalazide and olsalazine are useful in the treatment of symptomatic disease. The aminosalicylates also have value in maintenance of remission in ulcerative colitis. Corticosteroids are unsuitable for *maintenance treatment* because of side-effects. In resistant cases **azathioprine** (section 8.2.1), 2 mg/kg daily, given under close supervision may be helpful [unlicensed indication].

Laxatives are required to facilitate bowel movement when proctitis is present but a high-fibre diet and bulk-forming drugs such as **methylcellulose** are more useful in adjusting faecal consistency (section 1.6.1).

Antimotility drugs such as codeine and loperamide should not be used in severe colitis as they can precipitate paralytic ileus and megacolon. They have limited value in mild disease, but treatment of the inflammation is more logical. For similar reasons antispasmodics should **not** be used in ulcerative colitis.

General nutritional care and appropriate supplements are essential.

Crohn's disease

Treatment of Crohn's disease (particularly of colonic disease) is similar to that for ulcerative colitis. In small bowel disease the **aminosalicylates** may have marginal value. Symptoms and inflammation associated with disease exacerbation are suppressed by **oral corticosteroids** such as prednisolone; modified-release budesonide is also effective and causes fewer systemic side-effects. **Metronidazole** may be beneficial possibly through its antibacterial activity. Other antibacterials should be given if specifically indicated and for managing bacterial overgrowth in the small bowel.

Infliximab (*Remicade*®, Schering-Plough) is a monoclonal antibody which inhibits the pro-inflammatory cytokine, tumour necrosis factor α. It has been introduced recently for the treatment of severe active Crohn's disease refractory to corticosteroid or immunosuppressant therapy and for the treatment of refractory fistulas of Crohn's disease; infliximab should be used by specialists in the presence of adequate resuscitation facilities.

General nutritional care and appropriate supplements are essential.

Antibiotic-associated colitis

Antibiotic-associated colitis (pseudomembranous colitis) is caused by colonisation of the colon with *Clostridium difficile* which may follow antibiotic therapy. It is usually of acute onset, but may run a chronic course; it is a particular hazard of clindamycin but few antibiotics are free of this side-effect. Oral **vancomycin** (see section 5.1.7) or **metronidazole** (see section 5.1.11) are used as specific treatment; vancomycin may be preferred for very sick patients.

Diverticular disease

Diverticular disease is treated with a high-fibre diet, **bran supplements**, and **bulk-forming drugs**. **Antispasmodics** may provide symptomatic relief when colic is a problem (section 1.2). **Antibiotics** are used only when the diverticula in the intestinal wall become infected (specialist referral). **Antimotility** drugs which slow intestinal motility, e.g. codeine, diphenoxylate, and loperamide could possibly exacerbate the symptoms of diverticular disease and are **contra-indicated**.

Aminosalicylates

Sulfasalazine is a combination of 5-aminosalicylic acid ('5-ASA') and sulfapyridine; sulfapyridine acts only as a carrier to the colonic site of action but still causes side-effects. In the newer aminosalicylates, **mesalazine** (5-aminosalicylic acid), **balsalazide** (a prodrug of 5-aminosalicylic acid) and **olsalazine** (a dimer of 5-aminosalicylic acid which cleaves in the lower bowel), the sulphonamide-related side-effects of sulfasalazine are avoided, but 5-aminosalicylic acid alone can still cause side-effects including blood disorders (see recommendation below) and lupoid phenomenon also seen with sulfasalazine. Olsalazine may also be particularly prone to cause watery diarrhoea. Some manufacturers of sulfasalazine and mesalazine recommend renal function tests, but evidence of practical value is unsatisfactory.

CAUTIONS. Aminosalicylates should be used with caution during pregnancy (Appendix 4) and breastfeeding (Appendix 5); blood disorders can occur (see recommendation below).

> **Blood disorders**
> It is recommended that patients receiving aminosalicylates should be advised to report any unexplained bleeding, bruising, purpura, sore throat, fever or malaise that occurs during treatment. A blood count should be performed and the drug stopped immediately if there is suspicion of a blood dyscrasia.

CONTRA-INDICATIONS. Aminosalicylates should be avoided in salicylate hypersensitivity and in moderate or severe renal impairment.

SIDE-EFFECTS. Side-effects of the aminosalicylates include diarrhoea, nausea, headache, exacerbation of symptoms of colitis, hypersensitivity reactions (including rash, urticaria, interstitial nephritis and lupus erythematosus-like syndrome); side-effects that occur rarely include acute pancreatitis, hepatitis, nephrotic syndrome, blood disorders (including agranulocytosis, aplastic anaemia, leucopenia, neutropenia, thrombocytopenia—see also recommendation above)

BALSALAZIDE SODIUM

Indications: treatment of mild to moderate ulcerative colitis and maintenance of remission

Cautions: see notes above; history of asthma

Contra-indications: see notes above; severe hepatic impairment
BLOOD DISORDERS. See recommendation above

Side-effects: see notes above; abdominal pain, vomiting, cholelithiasis

Dose: acute attack, 2.25 g 3 times daily until remission occurs or for up to max. 12 weeks
Maintenance, 1.5 g twice daily, adjusted according to response (max. 6 g daily)
CHILD not recommended

Colazide® (Astra) ▼ PoM
Capsules, beige, balsalazide sodium 750 mg. Net price 130-cap pack = £39.00. Label: 21, 25, counselling, blood disorder symptoms (see recommendation above)

MESALAZINE

Indications: treatment of mild to moderate ulcerative colitis and maintenance of remission; see also under preparations

Cautions: see notes above; elderly

Contra-indications: see notes above; severe hepatic impairment; blood clotting abnormalities BLOOD DISORDERS. See recommendation above

Side-effects: see notes above; abdominal pain; rarely allergic lung reactions, allergic myocarditis, methaemoglobinaemia

Dose: see under preparations, below

Note. The delivery characteristics of enteric-coated mesalazine preparations may vary; these preparations should not be considered interchangable

Asacol® (SmithKline Beecham) PoM
Tablets, red, e/c, mesalazine 400 mg, net price 90-tab pack = £32.69, 120-tab pack = £43.58. Label: 5, 25, counselling, blood disorder symptoms (see recommendation above)

Dose: ulcerative colitis, acute attack, 6 tablets daily in divided doses; maintenance of remission of ulcerative colitis and Crohn's ileo-colitis, 3–6 tablets daily in divided doses; CHILD not recommended

Note. Preparations that lower stool pH (e.g. lactulose) may prevent release of mesalazine

Foam enema, mesalazine 1 g/metered application. Net price 14 g (14 applications) with disposable applicators and plastic bags = £39.60. Counselling, blood disorder symptoms (see recommendation above)

Dose: acute attack affecting the rectosigmoid region, 1 metered application (mesalazine 1 g) into the rectum daily for 4–6 weeks; acute attack affecting the descending colon, 2 metered applications (mesalazine 2 g) once daily for 4–6 weeks; CHILD not recommended

Suppositories, mesalazine 250 mg, net price 20-suppos pack = £7.15; 500 mg, 10 = £7.15. Counselling, blood disorder symptoms (see recommendation above)

Dose: 3–6 suppositories of 250 mg (max. 3 suppositories of 500 mg) daily in divided doses, with last dose at bedtime; CHILD not recommended

Pentasa® (Ferring) PoM
Slow Release tablets, m/r, both scored, mesalazine 250 mg (grey), net price 200-tab pack = £25.82; 500 mg (grey), 100-tab pack = £32.28. Counselling, administration, see dose, blood disorder symptoms (see recommendation above)

Dose: acute attack, up to 4 g daily in 2–3 divided doses; maintenance, 1.5 g daily in 2–3 divided doses; tablets may be dispersed in water, but should not be chewed; CHILD under 15 years not recommended

Granules, m/r, pale brown, mesalazine 1 g/sachet, net price 50-sachet pack = £31.60. Counselling, administration, see dose, blood disorder symptoms (see recommendation above)

Dose: acute attack, up to 4 g daily in 2–4 divided doses; maintenance, 2 g daily in 2 divided doses; granules should be placed on tongue and washed down with water or orange juice without chewing; CHILD under 12 years not recommended

Retention enema, mesalazine 1 g in 100-mL pack. Net price 7 enemas = £19.45. Counselling, blood disorder symptoms (see recommendation above)

Dose: 1 enema at bedtime; CHILD not recommended

Suppositories, mesalazine 1 g. Net price 28-suppos pack = £44.68. Counselling, blood disorder symptoms (see recommendation above)

Dose: ulcerative proctitis, acute attack, 1 suppository daily for 2–4 weeks; maintenance, 1 suppository daily; CHILD under 15 years not recommended

Salofalk® (Cortecs) PoM
Tablets, e/c, yellow, mesalazine 250 mg. Net price 100-tab pack = £18.41. Label: 5, 25, counselling, blood disorder symptoms (see recommendation above)

Dose: acute attack, 6 tablets daily in 3 divided doses; maintenance 3–6 tablets daily in divided doses; CHILD not recommended

Suppositories, mesalazine 500 mg. Net price 30-suppos pack = £16.75. Counselling, blood disorder symptoms (see recommendation above)

Dose: acute attack, 1–2 suppositories 2–3 times daily adjusted according to response; CHILD not recommended

Enema, mesalazine 2 g in 59-mL pack. Net price 7 enemas = £32.95. Counselling, blood disorder symptoms (see recommendations above)

Dose: acute attack *or* maintenance, 1 enema daily at bedtime; CHILD not recommended

OLSALAZINE SODIUM

Indications: treatment of mild ulcerative colitis and maintenance of remission

Cautions: see notes above

Contra-indications: see notes above
BLOOD DISORDERS. See recommendation above

Side-effects: see notes above; watery diarrhoea, arthralgia

Dose: acute attack, 1 g daily in divided doses after meals increased if necessary over 1 week to max. 3 g daily (max. single dose 1 g)
Maintenance, 500 mg twice daily after meals

Dipentum® (Pharmacia & Upjohn) PoM
Capsules, brown, olsalazine sodium 250 mg. Net price 112-cap pack = £27.42. Label: 21, counselling, blood disorder symptoms (see recommendation above)

Tablets, yellow, scored, olsalazine sodium 500 mg. Net price 60-tab pack = £29.38. Label: 21, counselling, blood disorder symptoms (see recommendation above)

SULFASALAZINE

(Sulphasalazine)

Indications: treatment of mild to moderate and severe ulcerative colitis and maintenance of remission; active Crohn's disease; rheumatoid arthritis (section 10.1.3)

Cautions: see notes above; history of allergy; hepatic and renal impairment; G6PD deficiency (section 9.1.5); slow acetylator status; risk of haematological and hepatic toxicity (differential white cell, red cell and platelet counts initially and at monthly intervals for first 3 months; liver function tests at monthly intervals for first 3 months); kidney function tests at regular intervals; upper gastro-intestinal side-effects common over 4 g daily; porphyria (section 9.8.2); **interactions:** Appendix 1 (sulfasalazine)

Contra-indications: see notes above; sulphonamide hypersensitivity; CHILD under 2 years of age

BLOOD DISORDERS. See recommendation above

Side-effects: see notes above; loss of appetite; fever; blood disorders (including Heinz body anaemia, megaloblastic anaemia); hypersensitivity reactions (including Stevens-Johnson syndrome, exfoliative dermatitis, epidermal necrolysis, pruritus, photosensitisation, anaphylaxis, serum sickness); lung complications (including eosinophilia, fibrosing alveolitis); ocular complications (including periorbital oedema); stomatitis, parotitis; ataxia, aseptic meningitis, vertigo, tinnitus, alopecia, peripheral neuropathy, insomnia, depression, hallucinations; kidney reactions (including proteinuria, crystalluria, haematuria); oligospermia; urine may be coloured orange; some soft contact lenses may be stained

Dose: *by mouth*, acute attack 1–2 g 4 times daily (but see **cautions**) until remission occurs (if necessary corticosteroids may also be given), reducing to a maintenance dose of 500 mg 4 times daily; CHILD over 2 years, acute attack 40–60 mg/kg daily, maintenance dose 20–30 mg/kg daily

By rectum, in suppositories, alone or in conjunction with oral treatment 0.5–1 g morning and night after a bowel movement. As an enema, 3 g at night, retained for at least 1 hour

Sulfasalazine (Non-proprietary) PoM

Tablets, sulfasalazine 500 mg. Net price 100 = £6.86. Label: 14, counselling, blood disorder symptoms (see recommendation above), contact lenses may be stained

Available from Ashbourne (*Ucine*®), Berk, Cox, Hillcross

Tablets, e/c, sulfasalazine 500 mg. Net price 112-tab pack = £12.11. Label: 5, 14, 25, counselling, blood disorder symptoms (see recommendation above), contact lenses may be stained

Available from Cox (*Sulazine EC*®)

Salazopyrin® (Pharmacia & Upjohn) PoM

Tablets, yellow, scored, sulfasalazine 500 mg. Net price 112-tab pack = £7.74. Label: 14, counselling, blood disorder symptoms (see recommendation above), contact lenses may be stained

EN-Tabs® (= tablets e/c), yellow, f/c, sulfasalazine 500 mg. Net price 112-tab pack = £9.69. Label: 5, 14, 21, 25, counselling, blood disorder symptoms (see recommendation above), contact lenses may be stained

Suspension, yellow, sulfasalazine 250 mg/5 mL. Net price 500 mL = £15.70. Label: 14, counselling, blood disorder symptoms (see recommendation above), contact lenses may be stained

Suppositories, yellow, sulfasalazine 500 mg. Net price 10 = £2.75. Label: 14, counselling, blood disorder symptoms (see recommendation above), contact lenses may be stained

Retention enema, sulfasalazine 3 g in 100-mL single-dose disposable packs fitted with a nozzle. Net price 7 × 100 mL = £11.87. Label: 14, counselling, blood disorder symptoms (see recommendation above), contact lenses may be stained

Anion-exchange resins

COLESTYRAMINE
(Cholestyramine)

Indications: diarrhoea associated with Crohn's disease, ileal resection, vagotomy, diabetic vagal neuropathy, and radiation; pruritus in liver disease, and hypercholesterolaemia, see section 2.12

Cautions: see section 2.12

Contra-indications: see section 2.12

Side-effects: see section 2.12

Dose: diarrhoea, after initial introduction over 3–4 week period, 12–24 g daily mixed with water (or other suitable liquid), in single or up to 4 divided doses, subsequently adjusted as required; max. 36 g daily

CHILD 6–12 years, consult product literature

COUNSELLING. Other drugs should be taken at least 1 hour before or 4–6 hours after colestyramine to reduce possible interference with absorption

Preparations
Section 2.12

Corticosteroids

BUDESONIDE

Indications: see under preparations

Cautions: see section 6.3.2

Contra-indications: see section 6.3.2

Side-effects: see section 6.3.2

Dose: see under preparations

Budenofalk® (Cortecs) PoM

Capsules, e/c, pink, budesonide 3 mg, net price 100-cap pack = £81.20. Label: 5, 10 steroid card, 22, 25

Dose: mild to moderate Crohn's disease affecting the ileum or ascending colon, 3 mg 3 times daily for up to 8 weeks; reduce dose for the last 2 weeks of treatment. See also section 6.3.2

CHILD not recommended

Entocort® (Astra) PoM

CR Capsules, e/c, m/r, grey/pink, budesonide 3 mg. Net price 100-cap pack = £90.00. Label: 5, 10 steroid card, 22, 25

Note. Dispense in original container (contains desiccant)

Dose: mild to moderate Crohn's disease affecting the ileum or ascending colon, 9 mg once daily in the morning before breakfast for up to 8 weeks; reduce dose for the last 2–4 weeks of treatment. See also section 6.3.2

CHILD not recommended

Enema, budesonide 2 mg/100 mL when dispersible tablet reconstituted in isotonic saline vehicle. Net price pack of 7 dispersible tablets and bottles of vehicle = £30.00

Dose: ulcerative colitis involving rectal and recto-sigmoid disease, 1 enema at bedtime for 4 weeks; CHILD not recommended

HYDROCORTISONE

Indications: ulcerative colitis, proctitis, proctosigmoiditis

Cautions: see section 6.3.2; systemic absorption may occur; prolonged use should be avoided

Contra-indications: use of enemas and rectal foams in obstruction, bowel perforation, and extensive fistulas; untreated infection

Side-effects: see section 6.3.2; local irritation

Dose: rectal, see under Preparations

Colifoam® (Stafford-Miller) PoM
Foam in aerosol pack, hydrocortisone acetate 10%. Net price 20.8 g (14 applications) with applicator = £6.80

Dose: initially 1 metered application (125 mg hydro-cortisone acetate) inserted into the rectum once or twice daily for 2–3 weeks, then once on alternate days

PREDNISOLONE

Indications: ulcerative colitis, and Crohn's disease; other indications, see section 6.3.2, see also preparations

Cautions: see under Hydrocortisone and section 6.3.2

Contra-indications: see under Hydrocortisone and section 6.3.2

Side-effects: see under Hydrocortisone and section 6.3.2

Dose: *by mouth,* initially 20–40 mg daily, in single or divided doses, until remission occurs, followed by reducing doses

By rectum, see under preparations

■ Oral preparations, section 6.3.2

■ Rectal preparations

Predenema® (Pharmax) PoM
Retention enema, prednisolone 20 mg (as sodium metasulphobenzoate) in 100-mL single-dose disposable pack. Net price 1 (standard tube) = 76p, 1 (long tube) = £1.29

Dose: ulcerative colitis, initially 1 enema at bedtime for 2–4 weeks, continued if good response; CHILD not recommended

Predfoam® (Pharmax) PoM
Foam in aerosol pack, prednisolone 20 mg (as metasulphobenzoate sodium)/metered application. Net price 25 g (14 applications) with disposable applicators = £6.74

Dose: proctitis and distal ulcerative colitis, 1 metered application (containing 20 mg prednisolone) inserted into the rectum once or twice daily for 2 weeks, continued for further 2 weeks if good response; CHILD not recommended

Predsol® (Medeva) PoM
Retention enema, prednisolone 20 mg (as sodium phosphate) in 100-mL single-dose disposable packs fitted with a nozzle. Net price 7 = £5.24

Dose: rectal and rectosigmoidal ulcerative colitis and Crohn's disease, initially 1 enema at bedtime for 2–4 weeks, continued if good response; CHILD not recommended

Suppositories, prednisolone 5 mg (as sodium phosphate). Net price 10 = £1.00

Dose: ADULT and CHILD proctitis and rectal complications of Crohn's disease, 1 suppository inserted night and morning after a bowel movement

Cromoglicate

Allergy with classical symptoms of vomiting, colic and diarrhoea caused by specific foods such as shellfish should be managed by strict avoidance. The condition should be distinguished from symptoms of occasional food intolerance in those with irritable bowel syndrome. **Sodium cromoglicate** (sodium cromoglycate) may be helpful as an adjunct to dietary avoidance.

SODIUM CROMOGLICATE
(Sodium cromoglycate)

Indications: food allergy (in conjunction with dietary restriction); asthma, section 3.3; allergic conjunctivitis, section 11.4.2; allergic rhinitis, section 12.2.1

Side-effects: occasional nausea, rashes, and joint pain

Dose: 200 mg 4 times daily before meals; CHILD 2–14 years 100 mg; capsules may be swallowed whole or the contents dissolved in hot water and diluted with cold water before taking. May be increased if necessary after 2–3 weeks to a max. of 40 mg/kg daily and then reduced according to the response

Nalcrom® (Pantheon) PoM
Capsules, sodium cromoglicate 100 mg. Net price 100-cap pack = £66.85. Label: 22, counselling, see dose above

1.6   Laxatives

1.6.1	Bulk-forming laxatives
1.6.2	Stimulant laxatives
1.6.3	Faecal softeners
1.6.4	Osmotic laxatives
1.6.5	Bowel cleansing solutions

Before prescribing laxatives it is important to be sure that the patient *is* constipated and that the constipation is *not* secondary to an underlying undiagnosed complaint.

It is also important for those who complain of constipation to understand that bowel habit can vary considerably in frequency without doing harm. Some people tend to consider themselves constipated if they do not have a bowel movement each day. A useful definition of constipation is the passage of hard stools less frequently than the patient's own normal pattern and this can be explained to the patient.

Misconceptions about bowel habits have led to excessive laxative use. Abuse may lead to hypokalaemia and an atonic non-functioning colon.

Thus, laxatives should generally be **avoided** except where straining will exacerbate a condition (such as angina) or increase the risk of rectal bleeding as in haemorrhoids. Laxatives are also of value in *drug-induced constipation,* for the expulsion of *parasites* after anthelmintic treatment, and to clear the alimentary tract before *surgery and radiological procedures.* Prolonged treatment of constipation is seldom necessary except occasionally in the elderly.

CHILDREN. The use of laxatives in children should be discouraged unless prescribed by a doctor. Infrequent defaecation may be normal in breast-fed babies or in response to poor intake of fluid or fibre. Delays of greater than 3 days between stools may increase the likelihood of pain on passing hard stools leading to anal fissure, anal spasm and eventually to a learned response to avoid defaecation.

If increased fluid and fibre intake is insufficient, an osmotic laxative such as lactulose or a bulk-forming laxative such as methylcellulose may be effective; methylcellulose is given in a dose of 0.5–1 g twice daily for a child over 7 years [unlicensed use]—an appropriate formulation for a younger child is not readily available. If there is evidence of minor faecal retention, the addition of a stimulant laxative such as senna may overcome withholding but may lead to colic or, in the presence of faecal impaction in the rectum, an increase of faecal overflow. Referral to hospital may be needed unless the child evacuates the impacted mass spontaneously. In hospital, enemas or suppositories may clear the mass but their use is frequently distressing for the child and may lead to a persistence of withholding. Enemas may be administered under heavy sedation in hospital or alternatively a bowel cleansing solution (section 1.6.5) may be tried. In severe cases or where the child is afraid, a manual evacuation under anaesthetic may be appropriate.

Long-term use of stimulant laxatives such as senna or sodium picosulfate (sodium picosulphate, section 1.6.2) is essential to prevent recurrence of the faecal impaction. Parents should be encouraged to use them regularly for many months; intermittent use may provoke a series of relapses.

> The laxatives that follow have been divided into 5 main groups (sections 1.6.1–1.6.5). This simple classification disguises the fact that some laxatives have a complex action.

1.6.1   Bulk-forming laxatives

Bulk-forming laxatives relieve constipation by increasing faecal mass which stimulates peristalsis; the full effect may take some days to develop and patients should be told this.

Bulk-forming laxatives are of particular value in those with small hard stools, but should not be required unless fibre cannot be increased in the diet. A balanced diet, including adequate fluid intake and fibre is of value in preventing constipation.

Bulk-forming laxatives are useful in the management of patients with *colostomy, ileostomy, haemorrhoids, anal fissure, chronic diarrhoea associated with diverticular disease, irritable bowel syndrome*, and as adjuncts in *ulcerative colitis* (section 1.5). Adequate fluid intake must be maintained to avoid intestinal obstruction. Unprocessed wheat **bran**, taken with food or fruit juice, is a most effective bulk-forming preparation. Finely ground bran, though more palatable, has poorer water-retaining properties, but can be taken as bran bread or biscuits in appropriately increased quantities. Oat bran is also used.

Methylcellulose, ispaghula, and **sterculia** are useful in patients who cannot tolerate bran. Methylcellulose also acts as a faecal softener.

BRAN

Indications: see notes above
Cautions: see under Ispaghula Husk
Contra-indications: see under Ispaghula Husk; gluten enteropathies and coeliac disease
Side-effects: see under Ispaghula Husk
Dose: see preparation below

COUNSELLING. Preparations that swell in contact with liquid should always be carefully swallowed with water and should not be taken immediately before going to bed

Trifyba® (Sanofi-Synthelabo)
Powder, brown, wheat fibre 80%. Net price 56 sachets containing 3.5 g = £3.28. Counselling, see below
Note. Contains gluten
Dose: 1 sachet 2–3 times daily added to food; CHILD (but see section 1.6) half to one sachet 1–2 times daily added to food

COUNSELLING. At least one glass of water or other liquid should be drunk with the meal

ISPAGHULA HUSK

Indications: see notes above; hypercholesterolaemia (section 2.12)
Cautions: adequate fluid intake should be maintained to avoid intestinal obstruction—it may be necessary to supervise elderly or debilitated patients or those with intestinal narrowing or decreased motility
Contra-indications: difficulty in swallowing, intestinal obstruction, colonic atony, faecal impaction
Side-effects: flatulence, abdominal distension, gastro-intestinal obstruction or impaction; hypersensitivity reported
Dose: see preparations below

COUNSELLING. Preparations that swell in contact with liquid should always be carefully swallowed with water and should not be taken immediately before going to bed

Fybogel® (R&C)
Granules, buff, effervescent, sugar- and gluten-free, ispaghula husk 3.5 g/sachet (low Na⁺). Net price 60 sachets (plain, lemon, or orange flavoured) = £4.24. Label: 13, counselling, see above
Note. Contains aspartame 50 mg/sachet (see section 9.4.1)
Dose: 1 sachet in water twice daily preferably after meals; CHILD (but see section 1.6) 6–12 years ½–1 level 5-mL spoonful (children under 6 years on doctor's advice only)

Konsyl® (Eastern)
Powder, gluten-free, ispaghula husk (micronised), *Konsyl Sugar Free* (6 g/sachet); net price 30-sachet pack = £3.99; *Konsyl Orange* (3.4 g/sachet), 60-sachet pack = £3.99. Label 13, counselling, see above
Dose: 1 sachet in water 1–3 times daily before or after meals; CHILD (but see section 1.6) over 6 years, ½ adult dose or less (children under 6 years on doctor's advice only)
Diarrhoea (section 1.4.1), 1 sachet in water 3 times daily
Important. Each sachet of *Konsyl Sugar Free* contains almost twice as much ispaghula husk as *Konsyl Orange*

Isogel® (Pfizer Consumer)

Granules, brown, sugar- and gluten-free, ispaghula husk 90%. Net price 300 g = £3.53. Label: 13, counselling, see above

Dose: constipation, 2 teaspoonfuls in water once or twice daily, preferably at mealtimes; CHILD (but see section 1.6) 1 teaspoonful

Diarrhoea (section 1.4.1), 1 teaspoonful 3 times daily

Regulan® (Procter & Gamble)

Powder, beige, sugar- and gluten-free, ispaghula husk 3.4 g/5.85-g sachet (orange or lemon/lime flavour). Net price 30 sachets = £1.57. Label: 13, counselling, see above

Excipients: include aspartame (section 9.4.1)

Dose: 1 sachet in 150 mL water 1–3 times daily; CHILD (but see section 1.6) 6–12 years 2.5–5 mL

METHYLCELLULOSE

Indications: see notes above; obesity (section 4.5.1)

Cautions: see under Ispaghula Husk

Contra-indications: see under Ispaghula Husk

Side-effects: see under Ispaghula Husk

Dose: see preparations below

COUNSELLING. Preparations that swell in contact with liquid should always be carefully swallowed with water and should not be taken immediately before going to bed

Celevac® (Monmouth)

Tablets, pink, scored, methylcellulose '450' 500 mg. Net price 112-tab pack = £2.69. Counselling, see above and dose

Dose: 3–6 tablets twice daily. In constipation the dose should be taken with at least 300 mL of water. In diarrhoea, ileostomy, and colostomy control, minimise liquid intake for 30 minutes before and after the dose

---

STERCULIA

Indications: see notes above

Cautions: see under Ispaghula Husk

Contra-indications: see under Ispaghula Husk

Side-effects: see under Ispaghula Husk

Dose: see under preparations below

COUNSELLING. Preparations that swell in contact with liquid should always be carefully swallowed with water and should not be taken immediately before going to bed

Normacol® (Norgine)

Granules, coated, gluten-free, sterculia 62%. Net price 500 g = £5.53; 60 × 7-g sachets = £4.65. Label: 25, 27, counselling, see above

Dose: 1–2 heaped 5-mL spoonfuls, or the contents of 1–2 sachets, washed down without chewing with plenty of liquid once or twice daily after meals; CHILD (but see section 1.6) 6–12 years half adult dose

Normacol Plus® (Norgine)

Granules, brown, coated, gluten-free, sterculia 62%, frangula (standardised) 8%. Net price 500 g = £5.92; 60 × 7 g sachets = £4.98. Label: 25, 27, counselling, see above

Dose: constipation and after haemorrhoidectomy, 1–2 heaped 5-mL spoonfuls or the contents of 1–2 sachets washed down without chewing with plenty of liquid once or twice daily after meals

---

1.6.2 Stimulant laxatives

The recognised stimulant laxatives include **bisacodyl** and members of the **anthraquinone** group, e.g. senna. **Docusate** sodium probably acts both as a stimulant and as a softening agent. **Dantron** (danthron) has limited indications (see below) because *rodent* studies indicate potential carcinogenic risk. Powerful stimulants such as **cascara** and **castor oil** are obsolete.

Stimulant laxatives increase intestinal motility and often cause abdominal cramp; they should be avoided in intestinal obstruction. Prolonged use of stimulant laxatives can precipitate the onset of an atonic non-functioning colon and hypokalaemia; however, prolonged use may be justifiable in some circumstances (see section 1.6 for the use of stimulant laxatives in children).

Glycerol suppositories act as a rectal stimulant by virtue of the mildly irritant action of glycerol.

Soft soap is a more severe irritant; the use of soft soap enema should be **avoided**, especially in pregnancy, as it may inflame the colonic mucosa.

The **parasympathomimetics** bethanechol, distigmine, neostigmine, and pyridostigmine (see section 7.4.1 and section 10.2.1) enhance parasympathetic activity in the gut and increase intestinal motility. They are rarely used for their gastro-intestinal effects. Organic obstruction of the gut must first be excluded and they should not be used shortly after bowel anastomosis.

BISACODYL

Indications: see under Dose; tablets act in 10–12 hours; suppositories act in 20–60 minutes

Cautions: see notes above

Contra-indications: see notes above

Side-effects: see notes above; tablets, griping; suppositories, local irritation

Dose: *by mouth* for constipation, 5–10 mg at night; occasionally necessary to increase to 15–20 mg; CHILD (but see section 1.6) under 10 years 5 mg

By rectum in suppositories for constipation, 10 mg in the morning; CHILD (but see section 1.6) under 10 years 5 mg

Before radiological procedures and surgery, 10 mg by mouth at bedtime for 2 days before examination and, if necessary, a 10-mg suppository 1 hour before examination; CHILD half adult dose

Bisacodyl (Non-proprietary)

Tablets, e/c, bisacodyl 5 mg. Net price 20 = 62p. Label: 5, 25

Suppositories, bisacodyl 10 mg. Net price 12 = £1.49

Paediatric suppositories, bisacodyl 5 mg. Net price 5 = 89p

Note. The brand name *Dulco-lax®* NHS (Windsor) is used for bisacodyl tablets, net price 10-tab pack = 59p; suppositories (10 mg), 10 = £1.48; paediatric suppositories (5 mg), 5 = 89p

The brand name *Dulco-lax® Liquid* is used for sodium picosulfate elixir

---

DANTRON

(Danthron)

Indications: only for: prophylaxis and treatment of analgesic-induced constipation in terminally ill patients of all ages; constipation in cardiac failure and coronary thrombosis (conditions in which bowel movement must be free of strain); acts within 6–12 hours

Cautions: see notes above; avoid prolonged contact with skin (as in incontinent patients)—risk of irritation and excoriation; avoid in pregnancy and

breast-feeding; *rodent* studies indicate potential carcinogenic risk
Contra-indications: see notes above
Side-effects: see notes above; urine may be coloured red
Dose: see under preparations

■ With poloxamer '188' (as co-danthramer)
Note. Co-danthramer suspension 5 mL = one co-danthramer capsule, **but** strong co-danthramer suspension 5 mL = two strong co-danthramer capsules
Co-danthramer (Non-proprietary) [PoM]
Capsules, co-danthramer 25/200 (dantron 25 mg, poloxamer '188' 200 mg). Net price 60-cap pack = £13.82. Label: 14 (urine red)
  Dose: 1–2 capsules at bedtime; CHILD 1 capsule at bedtime (restricted indications, see notes above)
Available from Napp
Strong capsules, co-danthramer 37.5/500 (dantron 37.5 mg, poloxamer '188' 500 mg). Net price 60-cap pack = £16.72. Label: 14 (urine red)
  Dose: 1–2 capsules at bedtime (restricted indications, see notes above); CHILD under 12 years not recommended
Available from Napp
Suspension, co-danthramer 25/200 in 5 mL (dantron 25 mg, poloxamer '188' 200 mg/5 mL). Net price 300 mL = £11.28, 1 litre = £37.53. Label: 14 (urine red)
  Dose: 5–10 mL at night; CHILD 2.5–5 mL (restricted indications, see notes above)
Available from Galen (*Ailax®*), Hillcross, Napp (*Codalax®* [NHS]), Sovereign (*Danlax®*)
Strong suspension, co-danthramer 75/1000 in 5 mL (dantron 75 mg, poloxamer '188' 1 g/5 mL). Net price 300 mL = £30.15. Label: 14 (urine red)
  Dose: 5 mL at night (restricted indications, see notes above); CHILD under 12 years not recommended
Available from Cox, Galen (*Ailax® Forte*), Hillcross, Napp (*Codalax Forte®* [NHS])

■ With docusate sodium (as co-danthrusate)
Co-danthrusate (Non-proprietary) [PoM]
Capsules, co-danthrusate 50/60 (dantron 50 mg, docusate sodium 60 mg). Net price 63-cap pack = £13.46. Label: 14 (urine red)
  Dose: 1–3 capsules, usually at night; CHILD 6–12 years 1 capsule (restricted indications, see notes above)
Available from Cox, Galen (*Capsuvac®*), Hillcross, Medeva (*Normax®* [NHS]), Norton, Sterwin
Suspension, yellow, co-danthrusate 50/60 (dantron 50 mg, docusate sodium 60 mg/5 mL). Net price 200 mL = £6.40. Label: 14 (urine red)
  Dose: 5–15 mL at night; CHILD 6–12 years 5 mL at night (restricted indications, see notes above)
Available from Medeva (*Normax®*)

DOCUSATE SODIUM
(Dioctyl Sodium Sulphosuccinate)
Indications: constipation (oral preparations act within 1–2 days); adjunct in abdominal radiological procedures
Cautions: see notes above; do not give with liquid paraffin; rectal preparations not indicated if haemorrhoids or anal fissure
Contra-indications: see notes above
Side-effects: see notes above
Dose: *by mouth*, chronic constipation, up to 500 mg daily in divided doses; CHILD (but see section 1.6) over 6 months 12.5 mg 3 times daily, 2–12 years 12.5–25 mg 3 times daily (use paediatric oral solution only)
With barium meal, 400 mg

Dioctyl® (Schwarz)
Capsules, yellow/white, docusate sodium 100 mg, net price 30-cap pack = £1.67, 100-cap pack = £4.44
Docusol® (Typharm)
Adult oral solution, sugar-free, docusate sodium 50 mg/5 mL, net price 300 mL = £2.48
Paediatric oral solution, sugar-free, docusate sodium 12.5 mg/5 mL, net price 300 mL = £1.63

■ Rectal preparations
Fletchers' Enemette® (Pharmax)
Enema, docusate sodium 90 mg, glycerol 3.78 g/5 mL with macrogol and sorbic acid. Net price 5-mL unit = 31p
  Dose: ADULT and CHILD (but see section 1.6) over 3 years, 5-mL unit when required
Norgalax Micro-enema® (Norgine)
Enema, docusate sodium 120 mg in 10-g single-dose disposable packs. Net price 10-g unit = 64p
  Dose: ADULT and CHILD (but see section 1.6) over 12 years, 10-g unit

GLYCEROL
(Glycerin)
Indications: constipation
Dose: see below

Glycerol Suppositories, BP
(Glycerin Suppositories)
Suppositories, gelatin 140 mg, glycerol 700 mg, purified water to 1 g. Net price 12 = 78p (infant), 79p (child), 67p (adult)
  Dose: 1 suppository moistened with water before use. The usual sizes are for *infants* small (1-g mould), *children* medium (2-g mould), *adults* large (4-g mould)

SENNA
Indications: constipation; acts in 8–12 hours
Cautions: see notes above
Contra-indications: see notes above
Side-effects: see notes above
Dose: see under preparations

Senna (Non-proprietary)
Tablets, total sennosides (calculated as sennoside B) 7.5 mg. Net price 20 = 30p
  Dose: 2–4 tablets, usually at night; initial dose should be low then gradually increased; CHILD (but see section 1.6) over 6 years, half adult dose in the morning (on doctor's advice only)
  Note. Lower dose on packs on sale to the public
Available from Cox, R&C (*Senokot®* [NHS])
Manevac® (Galen)
Granules, coated, senna fruit 12.4%, ispaghula 54.2%. Net price 400 g = £5.76, 56 × 4-g sachets = £3.80. Label: 25, 27, counselling, see Ispaghula Husk
  Dose: 1–2 level 5-mL spoonfuls (or sachets) with water or warm drink after supper and, if necessary, before breakfast *or* every 6 hours in resistant cases for 1–3 days; CHILD (but see section 1.6) 5–12 years 1 level 5-mL spoonful (or sachet) daily
  Note. One level 5-mL spoonful is equivalent to one 4-g sachet
  COUNSELLING. Preparations that swell in contact with liquid should always be carefully swallowed with water and should not be taken immediately before going to bed

Senokot® (R&C)

Tablets NHS, see above

Granules, brown, total sennosides (calculated as sennoside B) 15 mg/5 mL or 5.5 mg/g (one 5-mL spoonful = 2.7 g). Net price 100 g = £2.92

Dose: 5–10 mL, usually at bedtime; CHILD (but see section 1.6) over 6 years 2.5–5 mL in the morning

Note. Lower dose on sale to the public

Syrup, brown, total sennosides (calculated as sennoside B) 7.5 mg/5 mL. Net price 100 mL pack = £1.98

Dose: 10–20 mL, usually at bedtime; CHILD (but see section 1.6) 2–6 years 2.5–5 mL in the morning (doctor's advice only), over 6 years 5–10 mL

Note. Lower dose on packs on sale to the public

SODIUM PICOSULFATE

(Sodium Picosulphate)

Indications: constipation; bowel evacuation before abdominal radiological procedures, endoscopy, and surgery (section 1.6.5)

Cautions: see notes above

Contra-indications: see notes above

Side-effects: see notes above

Dose: see below

Sodium Picosulfate Elixir, sodium picosulfate 5 mg/5 mL. Acts within 10–14 hours. Net price 100 mL = £1.85

Dose: 5–15 mL at night; CHILD (but see section 1.6) 2–5 years 2.5 mL, 5–10 years 2.5–5 mL

Note. The brand names *Laxoberal®* NHS and *Dulcolax® Liquid* (both Windsor) are used for sodium picosulfate elixir 5 mg/5 mL

The brand name *Dulco-lax®* is also used for bisacodyl tablets and suppositories

■ Bowel cleansing solutions
Section 1.6.5

Other stimulant laxatives

Unstandardised preparations of cascara, frangula, rhubarb, and senna should be **avoided** as their laxative action is unpredictable. Aloes, colocynth, and jalap should be **avoided** as they have a drastic purgative action.

Phenolphthalein can cause rashes. It may colour alkaline urine pink.

Stimulant laxative preparations on sale to the public (not prescribable on the NHS) together with their significant ingredients:

Boots Compound Laxative Syrup of Figs® (fig, senna), **Boots Senna Tablets®** (senna)

Califig® (fig, senna), **Calsalettes®** (aloin)

Ex-lax Senna® (senna)

Fam-Lax Senna® (Irish moss, rhubarb, senna)

Juno Junipah Salts® (juniper berry oil, sodium bicarbonate, sodium phosphate, sodium sulphate)

Nylax with Senna® (senna)

Potter's Cleansing Herb® (aloes, cascara, senna)

Rhuaka® (cascara, rhubarb, senna)

Faecal softeners

Liquid paraffin, the classical lubricant, has disadvantages (see below). Bulk laxatives (section 1.6.1) and non-ionic surfactant 'wetting' agents e.g. docusate sodium (section 1.6.2) also have softening properties. Such drugs are useful for oral adminis-

tration in the management of haemorrhoids and anal fissure; glycerol suppositories (section 1.6.2) are useful for rectal use.

Enemas containing **arachis oil** (ground-nut oil, peanut oil) lubricate and soften impacted faeces and promote a bowel movement.

ARACHIS OIL

Indications: see notes above

Dose: see below

Fletchers' Arachis Oil Retention Enema® (Pharmax)

Enema, arachis (peanut) oil in 130-mL single-dose disposable packs. Net price 130 mL = £1.02

Dose: to soften impacted faeces, 130 mL; the enema should be warmed before use; CHILD (but see section 1.6) under 3 years not recommended; over 3 years reduce adult dose in proportion to body-weight (medical supervision only)

LIQUID PARAFFIN ◢

Indications: constipation

Cautions: CSM recommends avoid prolonged use, and has contra-indicated in children less than 3 years of age

Side-effects: anal seepage of paraffin and consequent anal irritation after prolonged use, granulomatous reactions caused by absorption of small quantities of liquid paraffin (especially from the emulsion), lipoid pneumonia, and interference with the absorption of fat-soluble vitamins

Dose: see under preparation

Liquid Paraffin Oral Emulsion, BP ◢

Oral emulsion, liquid paraffin 5 mL, vanillin 5 mg, chloroform 0.025 mL, benzoic acid solution 0.2 mL, methylcellulose-20 200 mg, saccharin sodium 500 micrograms, water to 10 mL

Dose: 10–30 mL at night when required

COUNSELLING. Should not be taken immediately before going to bed

> ◢ denotes preparations that are considered to be less suitable for prescribing (see p. vi)

Osmotic laxatives

These act by retaining fluid in the bowel by osmosis or by changing the pattern of water distribution in the faeces.

Saline purgatives such as **magnesium hydroxide** are commonly abused but are satisfactory for occasional use; adequate fluid intake should be maintained. **Magnesium salts** are useful where rapid bowel evacuation is required. **Sodium salts** should be avoided as they may give rise to sodium and water retention in susceptible individuals. **Phosphate enemas** are useful in bowel clearance before radiology, endoscopy, and surgery.

Lactulose is a semi-synthetic disaccharide which is not absorbed from the gastro-intestinal tract. It produces an osmotic diarrhoea of low faecal pH, and discourages the proliferation of ammonia-producing organisms. It is therefore useful in the treatment of *hepatic encephalopathy*. **Lactitol** is a similar disaccharide.

LACTITOL

Indications: see under Lactulose
Contra-indications: see under Lactulose
Side-effects: see under Lactulose
Dose: constipation, initially 20 g daily in a single dose with morning or evening meal, subsequently adjusted to produce one stool daily (dose of 10 g daily may be sufficient); CHILD (but see section 1.6) 1–6 years 2.5–5 g, 6–12 years 5–10 g, 12–16 years 10–20 g daily, subsequently adjusted to produce one stool daily
Hepatic encephalopathy, 500–700 mg/kg daily in 3 divided doses with meals, subsequently adjusted to produce 2 soft stools daily
By nasogastric administration, as a 40% solution (200 g/500 mL), 1–2 mL/kg body-weight daily
COUNSELLING. Powder should be mixed with food or liquid and one to two glasses of liquid should be drunk with the meal

Lactitol (Non-proprietary)
Powder, lactitol 10 g/sachet. Net price 10-sachet pack = £1.00. Counselling, see above
Available from Novartis Consumer Health

LACTULOSE

Indications: constipation (may take up to 48 hours to act), hepatic encephalopathy (portal systemic encephalopathy)
Cautions: lactose intolerance
Contra-indications: galactosaemia, intestinal obstruction
Side-effects: flatulence, cramps, and abdominal discomfort
Dose: see under preparations below
COUNSELLING. Powder can be placed on tongue and washed down with water or other liquid *or* sprinkled on food *or* mixed with water or other liquid before swallowing

Lactulose (Non-proprietary)
Solution, lactulose 3.1–3.7 g/5 mL with other ketoses. Net price 500-mL pack = £2.75
Dose: constipation, initially 15 mL twice daily, adjusted according to patient's needs; CHILD (but see section 1.6) under 1 year 2.5 mL twice daily, 1–5 years 5 mL twice daily, 5–10 years 10 mL twice daily
Hepatic encephalopathy, 30–50 mL 3 times daily, subsequently adjusted to produce 2–3 soft stools daily
Available from APS, Ashbourne (*Osmolax®*), Berk (*Laxose®*), Cox, CP, Hillcross, Intrapharm (*Lactugal®*), Lagap, Norton, Novartis (*Regulose®*), Solvay (*Duphalac®* [NHS])
Note. A proprietary brand of lactulose 3.3 g/5 mL (*Regulose®*) is on sale to the public
Powder, lactulose 10 g/sachet, with other ketoses. Net price 30-sachet pack = £3.00. Counselling, see above
Dose: constipation, 10 g twice daily, adjusted according to patient's needs; CHILD (but see section 1.6) 5–10 years 5 g twice daily, under 5 years lactulose solution recommended
Hepatic encephalopathy, 20–30 g 3 times daily, subsequently adjusted to produce 2–3 soft stools daily
Available from Solvay (*Lactulose Dry, Duphalac Dry®*)

MACROGOLS

(Polyethylene glycols)
Indications: see preparation below
Cautions: pregnancy and breast-feeding; discontinue if symptoms of fluid and electrolyte disturbance
Contra-indications: intestinal perforation or obstruction, paralytic ileus, severe inflammatory conditions of the intestinal tract (such as Crohn's disease, ulcerative colitis, and toxic megacolon)
Side-effects: abdominal distension and pain, nausea
Dose: see preparation below

Movicol® (Norgine)
Oral powder, macrogol '3350' (polyethylene glycol '3350') 13.125 g, sodium bicarbonate 178.5 mg, sodium chloride 350.7 mg, potassium chloride 46.6 mg/sachet. Net price 20-sachet pack (lime and lemon flavour) = £8.70, 30-sachet pack = £13.05. Label: 13
Dose: chronic constipation, 2–3 sachets daily in divided doses; each sachet dissolved in 125 mL water and drunk immediately usually for up to 2 weeks, course repeated if required; ELDERLY initially 1 sachet daily; CHILD not recommended
Faecal impaction, 8 sachets daily dissolved in 1 litre water; the solution should be drunk within 6 hours, usually for max. 3 days; CHILD not recommended.
After reconstitution the solution should be kept in a refrigerator and discarded if unused after 6 hours
Caution: patients with impaired cardiovascular function should not take more than 2 sachets in any 1 hour

MAGNESIUM SALTS

Indications; Dose: see under preparations
Cautions: renal impairment (risk of magnesium accumulation); hepatic impairment (see Appendix 2); elderly and debilitated; see also notes above; **interactions:** Appendix 1 (magnesium salts)
Contra-indications: acute gastro-intestinal conditions
Side-effects: colic

■ Magnesium hydroxide

Magnesium Hydroxide Mixture, BP
(Cream of Magnesia)
Aqueous suspension containing about 8% hydrated magnesium oxide. Do not store in cold place
Dose: constipation, 25–50 mL when required

■ Magnesium hydroxide with liquid paraffin

Liquid Paraffin and Magnesium Hydroxide Oral Emulsion, BP ◤
Oral emulsion, 25% liquid paraffin in aqueous suspension containing 6% hydrated magnesium oxide
Dose: constipation, 5–20 mL when required
Note. Liquid paraffin and magnesium hydroxide preparations on sale to the public include: *Milpar®* [NHS]

◤ denotes preparations that are considered to be less suitable for prescribing (see p. vi)

■ Magnesium sulphate
Magnesium Sulphate. Label: 13, 23
Dose: rapid bowel evacuation (acts in 2–4 hours) 5–
10 g in a tumblerful of water preferably before breakfast
Note. Magnesium sulphate is on sale to the public as
Epsom Salts; *Andrews Liver Salts*® [NHS] (citric acid,
magnesium sulphate, sodium bicarbonate) is also on sale
to the public

■ Bowel cleansing solutions
Section 1.6.5

PHOSPHATES (RECTAL)

Indications: rectal use in constipation; bowel
evacuation before abdominal radiological procedures, endoscopy, and surgery
Cautions: elderly and debilitated; see also notes
above
Contra-indications: acute gastro-intestinal conditions
Side-effects: local irritation
Dose: see below

Carbalax® (Pharmax)
Suppositories, sodium acid phosphate (anhydrous)
1.3 g, sodium bicarbonate 1.08 g, net price 12 =
£2.14
Dose: constipation, 1 suppository, inserted 30 minutes
before evacuation required; moisten with water before
use; CHILD under 12 years not recommended

Fleet® **Ready-to-use Enema** (De Witt)
Enema, sodium acid phosphate 21.4 g, sodium
phosphate 9.4 g/118 mL. Net price single-dose
pack (standard tube) = 46p
Dose: ADULT and CHILD (but see section 1.6) over 12
years, 118 mL; CHILD 3–12 years, on doctor's advice
only (under 3 years not recommended)

Fletchers' Phosphate Enema® (Pharmax)
Enema, sodium acid phosphate 12.8 g, sodium
phosphate 10.24 g, purified water, freshly boiled
and cooled, to 128 mL (corresponds to Phosphates Enema Formula B). Net price 128 mL with
standard tube = 44p, with long rectal tube = 61p
Dose: 128 mL; CHILD (but see section 1.6) over 3 years,
reduced according to body weight (under 3 years not
recommended)

SODIUM CITRATE (RECTAL)

Indications: rectal use in constipation
Cautions: elderly and debilitated; see also notes
above
Contra-indications: acute gastro-intestinal con-
ditions
Dose: see below

Micolette Micro-enema® (Dexcel)
Enema, sodium citrate 450 mg, sodium lauryl sul-
phoacetate 45 mg, glycerol 625 mg, together with
citric acid, potassium sorbate, and sorbitol in a
viscous solution, in 5-mL single-dose disposable
packs with nozzle. Net price 5 mL = 32p
Dose: ADULT and CHILD over 3 years, 5–10 mL (but see
section 1.6)

Micralax Micro-enema® (Medeva)
Enema, sodium citrate 450 mg, sodium alkylsul-
phoacetate 45 mg, sorbic acid 5 mg, together with
glycerol and sorbitol in a viscous solution in 5-
mL single-dose disposable packs with nozzle. Net
price 5 mL = 33p
Dose: ADULT and CHILD over 3 years, 5 mL (but see section 1.6)

Relaxit Micro-enema® (Crawford)
Enema, sodium citrate 450 mg, sodium lauryl sulphate 75 mg, sorbic acid 5 mg, together with
glycerol and sorbitol in a viscous solution in 5-
mL single-dose disposable packs with nozzle. Net
price 5 mL = 31p
Dose: ADULT and CHILD (but see section 1.6) 5 mL
(insert only half nozzle length in child under 3 years)

1.6.5 Bowel cleansing solutions

Bowel cleansing solutions are used before colonic
surgery, colonoscopy, or radiological examination
to ensure the bowel is free of solid contents. They
are **not** treatments for constipation.

BOWEL CLEANSING SOLUTIONS

Indications: see above
Cautions: pregnancy; renal impairment; heart disease; ulcerative colitis; diabetes mellitus; reflux
oesophagitis; impaired gag reflex; unconscious or
semiconscious or possibility of regurgitation or
aspiration
Contra-indications: gastro-intestinal obstruction, gastric retention, gastro-intestinal ulceration,
perforated bowel, congestive cardiac failure;
toxic colitis, toxic megacolon or ileus
Side-effects: nausea and bloating; less frequently
abdominal cramps (usually transient—reduced by
taking more slowly); vomiting
Dose: see under preparations

Citramag® (Bioglan)
Powder, effervescent, magnesium carbonate
11.57 g, anhydrous citric acid 17.79 g/sachet, net
price 10-sachet pack (lemon and lime flavour) =
£11.92. Label 10, patient information leaflet, 13,
counselling, see below
Dose: bowel evacuation for radiological examination or
surgery, on day before procedure, 1 sachet at 8 a.m. and
1 sachet between 2 and 4 p.m.; CHILD 5–9 years one-
third adult dose; over 10 years and frail ELDERLY one-
half adult dose
COUNSELLING. The patient information leaflet advises
that hot water (200 mL) is needed to make the solution
and provides guidance on the timing and procedure for
reconstitution; it also mentions need for high fluid, low
residue diet beforehand (according to hospital advice),
and explains that only clear fluids can be taken after *Citramag*® until procedure completed

Fleet Phospho-soda® (De Witt)
Oral solution, sugar-free, sodium dihydrogen
phosphate dihydrate 24.4 g, disodium phosphate
dodecahydrate 10.8 g/45 mL. Net price 2 × 45-mL
bottles = £4.79. Label: 10 patient information
leaflet, counselling
Dose: 45 mL diluted with half a glass (120 mL) of cool
water, followed by one full glass (240 mL) of cool water
Timing of doses is dependent on the time of the procedure
For morning procedure, first dose should be taken at
7 a.m. and second at 7 p.m. on day before the procedure
For afternoon procedure, first dose should be taken at
7 p.m. on day before and second dose at 7 a.m. on day of
the procedure
Solid food must not be taken during dosing period; clear
liquids or water should be substituted for meals
CHILD not recommended

Klean-Prep® (Norgine)
Oral powder, macrogol '3350' (polyethylene glycol '3350') 59 g, anhydrous sodium sulphate 5.685 g, sodium bicarbonate 1.685 g, sodium chloride 1.465 g, potassium chloride 743 mg/sachet. Contains aspartame (see section 9.4.1). Net price 4 sachets = £8.39. Label: 10 patient information leaflet, counselling
Four sachets when reconstituted with water to 4 litres provides an iso-osmotic solution for bowel cleansing before surgery, colonoscopy or radiological procedures
Dose: 250 mL (1 tumblerful) of reconstituted solution every 10–15 minutes, or by nasogastric tube 20–30 mL/minute, until 4 litres have been consumed or watery stools are free of solid matter; CHILD not recommended
The solution from all 4 sachets should be drunk within 4–6 hours (250 mL drunk rapidly every 10–15 minutes); flavouring such as clear fruit cordials may be added if required; to facilitate gastric emptying domperidone or metoclopramide may be given 30 minutes before starting.
Alternatively the administration may be divided into two, e.g. taking the solutions from 2 sachets on the evening before examination and the remaining 2 on the morning of the examination
After reconstitution the solution should be kept in a refrigerator and discarded if unused after 24 hours
Note. Contra-indicated in patients under 20 kg body-weight; allergic reactions reported

Picolax® (Nordic)
Oral powder, sugar-free, sodium picosulfate 10 mg/sachet, with magnesium citrate (for bowel evacuation before radiological procedure, endoscopy, and surgery). Net price 2 sachets = 59p. Label: 10, patient information leaflet, 13, counselling, see below
Dose: ADULT and CHILD over 9 years, 1 sachet in water in morning (before 8 a.m.) and a second in afternoon (between 2 and 4 p.m.) of day preceding procedure; CHILD 1–2 years quarter sachet morning and afternoon, 2–4 years half sachet morning and afternoon, 4–9 years 1 sachet morning and half sachet afternoon
Acts within 3 hours of first dose
Note. Low residue diet recommended for 2 days before procedure and copious intake of water or other clear fluids recommended during treatment
COUNSELLING. Patients should be warned that heat is generated on addition to water; for this reason the powder should be added initially to 30 mL (2 tablespoonfuls) of water; after 5 minutes (when reaction complete) the solution should be further diluted to 150 mL (about a tumblerful)

1.7 Local preparations for anal and rectal disorders

1.7.1	Soothing haemorrhoidal preparations
1.7.2	Compound haemorrhoidal preparations with corticosteroids
1.7.3	Rectal sclerosants

Anal and perianal pruritus, soreness, and excoriation are best treated by application of bland ointments and suppositories (section 1.7.1). These conditions occur commonly in patients suffering from haemorrhoids, fistulas, and proctitis. Careful local toilet with attention to any minor faecal soiling, adjustment of the diet to avoid hard stools, the use of bulk-forming materials such as bran (section

1.6.1) and a high residue diet are helpful. In proctitis these measures may supplement treatment with corticosteroids or sulfasalazine (see section 1.5).

When necessary topical preparations containing **local anaesthetics** (section 1.7.1) or **corticosteroids** (section 1.7.2) are used provided perianal thrush has been excluded. Perianal thrush is best treated with **nystatin** by mouth and by local application (see sections 5.2, 7.2.2, and 13.10.2).

The management of *anal fissures* requires stool softening by increasing dietary fibre in the form of bran or by using a bulk-forming laxative. Short-term use of local anaesthetic preparations may help (section 1.7.1). If these measures are inadequate, the patient should be referred for specialist treatment in hospital; surgery or the use of a topical nitrate (e.g. glyceryl trinitrate 0.2–0.3% ointment) may be considered [unlicensed indication].

1.7.1 Soothing haemorrhoidal preparations

Soothing preparations containing mild astringents such as bismuth subgallate, zinc oxide, and hamamelis may give symptomatic relief in haemorrhoids. Many proprietary preparations also contain lubricants, vasoconstrictors, or mild antiseptics.

Local anaesthetics are used to relieve pain associated with *haemorrhoids,* and *pruritus ani* but good evidence is lacking. Lidocaine (lignocaine) ointment (section 15.2) is used before emptying the bowel to relieve pain associated with *anal fissure.* Alternative local anaesthetics include tetracaine (amethocaine), cinchocaine, and pramocaine (pramoxine), but they are more irritant. Local anaesthetic ointments can be absorbed through the rectal mucosa therefore excessive application should be **avoided,** particularly in infants and children. They should be used for short periods only (no longer than a few days) since they may cause sensitisation of the anal skin.

Soothing haemorrhoidal preparations on sale to the public together with their significant ingredients include:

Anacal® (heparinoid, laureth '9'), **Anodesyn®** (allantoin, lidocaine (lignocaine)), **Anusol® cream** (bismuth oxide, Peru balsam, zinc oxide), **Anusol® ointment and suppositories** (bismuth oxide, bismuth subgallate, Peru balsam, zinc oxide)

Boots Haemorrhoid Ointment® (lidocaine (lignocaine), zinc oxide), **Boots Suppositories for Haemorrhoids®** (benzyl alcohol, glycol monosalicylate, methyl salicylate, zinc oxide)

Germoloids® (lidocaine (lignocaine), zinc oxide)

Hemocane® (benzoic acid, bismuth oxide, cinnamic acid, lidocaine (lignocaine), zinc oxide)

Lanacane® cream (benzocaine, chlorothymol)

Nupercainal® (cinchocaine)

Preparation H® gel (hamamelis water), **Preparation H® ointment and suppositories** (shark liver oil, yeast cell extract)

1.7.2 Compound haemorrhoidal preparations with corticosteroids

Corticosteroids are often combined with local anaesthetics and soothing agents in preparations for haemorrhoids. They are suitable for occasional short-term use after exclusion of infections, such as herpes simplex; prolonged use can cause atrophy of the anal skin. See section 13.4 for general comments on topical corticosteroids and section 1.7.1 for comment on local anaesthetics.

Haemorrhoids in children are rare. Treatment is usually symptomatic and the use of a locally applied cream is appropriate for short periods; however, local anaesthetics can cause stinging initially and this may aggravate the child's fear of defaecation.

Anugesic-HC® (Parke-Davis) [PoM]

Cream, benzyl benzoate 1.2%, bismuth oxide 0.875%, hydrocortisone acetate 0.5%, Peru balsam 1.85%, pramocaine hydrochloride 1%, zinc oxide 12.35%. Net price 30 g (with rectal nozzle) = £3.09

Apply night and morning and after a bowel movement; do not use for longer than 7 days; CHILD not recommended

Suppositories, buff, benzyl benzoate 33 mg, bismuth oxide 24 mg, bismuth subgallate 59 mg, hydrocortisone acetate 5 mg, Peru balsam 49 mg, pramocaine hydrochloride 27 mg, zinc oxide 296 mg. Net price 12 = £2.24

Insert 1 suppository night and morning and after a bowel movement; do not use for longer than 7 days; CHILD not recommended

Anusol-HC® (Kestrel) [PoM]

Ointment, benzyl benzoate 1.25%, bismuth oxide 0.875%, bismuth subgallate 2.25%, hydrocortisone acetate 0.25%, Peru balsam 1.875%, zinc oxide 10.75%. Net price 30 g (with rectal nozzle) = £3.04

Apply night and morning and after a bowel movement; do not use for longer than 7 days; CHILD not recommended

Note. A proprietary brand (*Anusol Plus HC®* ointment) is on sale to the public

Suppositories, benzyl benzoate 33 mg, bismuth oxide 24 mg, bismuth subgallate 59 mg, hydrocortisone acetate 10 mg, Peru balsam 49 mg, zinc oxide 296 mg. Net price 12 = £2.14

Insert 1 suppository night and morning and after a bowel movement; do not use for longer than 7 days; CHILD not recommended

Note. A proprietary brand (*Anusol Plus HC®* suppositories) is on sale to the public

Betnovate® (GlaxoWellcome) [PoM]

Rectal ointment, betamethasone valerate 0.05%, lidocaine hydrochloride (lignocaine hydrochloride) 2.5%, phenylephrine hydrochloride 0.1%. Net price 30 g (with applicator) = £1.50

Apply 2–3 times daily until inflammation subsides then once daily, externally or by rectum; do not use for longer than 7 days; CHILD under 1 year not recommended

Perinal® (Dermal)

Spray application, hydrocortisone 0.2%, lidocaine hydrochloride (lignocaine hydrochloride) 1%. Net price 30-mL pack = £6.87

Spray twice over the affected area up to 3 times daily; do not use for longer than 1–2 weeks; CHILD under 14 years not recommended

Proctocream HC® (Stafford-Miller)

Cream, hydrocortisone acetate 1%, pramocaine hydrochloride 1%. Net price 15 g (with applicator) = £2.29

ADULT over 18 years, apply morning and night after a bowel movement up to 4 times daily, externally or by rectum; do not use for longer than 7 days

Proctofoam HC® (Stafford-Miller) [PoM]

Foam in aerosol pack, hydrocortisone acetate 1%, pramocaine hydrochloride 1%. Net price 21.2-g pack (approx. 40 applications) with applicator = £4.71

Dose: haemorrhoids and proctitis, 1 applicatorful (4–6 mg hydrocortisone acetate, 4–6 mg pramocaine hydrochloride) by rectum 2–3 times daily and after a bowel movement (max. 4 times daily); do not use for longer than 7 days; CHILD not recommended

Proctosedyl® (Hoechst Marion Roussel) [PoM]

Ointment, cinchocaine (dibucaine) hydrochloride 0.5%, hydrocortisone 0.5%. Net price 30 g = £6.48 (with cannula)

Apply morning and night and after a bowel movement, externally or by rectum; do not use for longer than 7 days

Suppositories, cinchocaine (dibucaine) hydrochloride 5 mg, hydrocortisone 5 mg. Net price 12 = £2.93

Insert 1 suppository night and morning and after a bowel movement; do not use for longer than 7 days

Scheriproct® (Schering Health) [PoM]

Ointment, cinchocaine (dibucaine) hydrochloride 0.5%, prednisolone hexanoate 0.19%. Net price 30 g = £4.41

Apply twice daily for 5–7 days (3–4 times daily on 1st day if necessary), then once daily for a few days after symptoms have cleared

Suppositories, cinchocaine (dibucaine) hydrochloride 1 mg, prednisolone hexanoate 1.3 mg. Net price 12 = £2.08

Insert 1 suppository daily after a bowel movement, for 5–7 days (in severe cases initially 2–3 times daily)

Ultraproct® (Schering Health) [PoM]

Ointment, cinchocaine (dibucaine) hydrochloride 0.5%, fluocortolone hexanoate 0.095%, fluocortolone pivalate 0.092%. Net price 30 g (with rectal nozzle) = £4.57

Apply twice daily for 5–7 days (3–4 times daily on 1st day if necessary), then once daily for a few days after symptoms have cleared

Suppositories, cinchocaine (dibucaine) hydrochloride 1 mg, fluocortolone hexanoate 630 micrograms, fluocortolone pivalate 610 micrograms. Net price 12 = £2.15

Insert 1 suppository daily after a bowel movement, for 5–7 days (in severe cases initially 2–3 times daily) then 1 suppository every other day for 1 week

Uniroid-HC® (Unigreg) [PoM]

Ointment, cinchocaine (dibucaine) hydrochloride 0.5%, hydrocortisone 0.5%. Net price 30 g (with applicator) = £4.43

Apply twice daily and after a bowel movement, externally or by rectum; do not use for longer than 7 days; CHILD under 12 years not recommended

Suppositories, cinchocaine (dibucaine) hydro-chloride 5 mg, hydrocortisone 5 mg. Net price 12 = £2.00

Insert 1 suppository twice daily and after a bowel movement; do not use for longer than 7 days; CHILD under 12 years not recommended

Xyloproct® (Astra) PoM
Ointment (water-miscible), aluminium acetate 3.5%, hydrocortisone acetate 0.275%, lidocaine (lignocaine) 5%, zinc oxide 18%. Net price 30 g (with applicator) = £3.39

Apply several times daily; short-term use only

Suppositories, aluminium acetate 50 mg, hydro-cortisone acetate 5 mg, lidocaine (lignocaine) 60 mg, zinc oxide 400 mg. Net price 10 = £1.59

Insert 1 suppository at night and after a bowel movement; short-term use only

1.7.3   Rectal sclerosants

Oily phenol injection is used to inject haemorrhoids particularly when unprolapsed.

PHENOL

Indications: see notes above
Side-effects: irritation, tissue necrosis

Oily Phenol Injection, BP, PoM phenol 5% in a suitable fixed oil. Net price 5-mL amp = £4.14

Dose: 2–3 mL into the submucosal layer at the base of the pile; several injections may be given at different sites, max. total injected 10 mL at any one time
Available from Medeva

1.8   Stoma care

Prescribing for patients with stoma calls for special care. The following is a brief account of some of the main points to be borne in mind.

Enteric-coated and *modified-release* preparations are **unsuitable**, particularly in patients with ileosto-mies, as there may not be sufficient release of the active ingredient.

Laxatives. Enemas and washouts should **not** be prescribed for patients with ileostomies as they may cause rapid and severe dehydration.

Colostomy patients may suffer from constipation and whenever possible should be treated by increasing fluid intake or dietary fibre. **Bulk-forming drugs** (section 1.6.1) should be tried. If they are insufficient, as small a dose as possible of senna (section 1.6.2) should be used.

Antidiarrhoeals. Drugs such as **loperamide, codeine phosphate**, or **co-phenotrope** (diphenoxylate with atropine) are effective. Bulk-forming drugs (section 1.6.1) may be tried but it is often difficult to adjust the dose appropriately.

Antibiotics should **not** be given for an episode of acute diarrhoea.

Antacids. The tendency to diarrhoea from magnesium salts or constipation from aluminium salts may be increased in these patients.

Diuretics should be used with caution in patients with ileostomies as they may become excessively dehydrated and potassium depletion may easily occur. It is usually advisable to use a **potassium-sparing** diuretic (see section 2.2.3).

Digoxin. Patients with a stoma are particularly susceptible to hypokalaemia if on digoxin therapy and potassium supplements or a potassium-sparing diuretic may be advisable (for comment see section 9.2.1.1).

Potassium supplements. Liquid formulations are preferred to modified-release formulations (see above).

Analgesics. Opioid analgesics (see section 4.7.2) may cause troublesome constipation in colostomy patients. When a non-opioid analgesic is required **paracetamol** is usually suitable but anti-inflamm-atory analgesics may cause gastric irritation and bleeding.

Iron preparations may cause loose stools and sore skin in these patients. If this is troublesome and if iron is definitely indicated an intramuscular iron preparation (see section 9.1.1.2) should be used. Modified-release preparations should be **avoided** for the reasons given above.

Patients are usually given advice about the use of *cleansing agents, protective creams, lotions, deo-dorants*, or *sealants* whilst in hospital, either by the surgeon or by the health authority stoma care nurses. Voluntary organisations offer help and support to patients with stoma.

1.9   Drugs affecting intestinal secretions

1.9.1   Drugs acting on the gall bladder
1.9.2   Drugs which increase gastric acidity
1.9.3   Aprotinin
1.9.4   Pancreatin

1.9.1   Drugs acting on the gall bladder

The use of laparoscopic cholecystectomy and of endoscopic biliary techniques has limited the place of the bile acid **ursodeoxycholic acid** in gallstone disease. Ursodeoxycholic acid is suitable for patients not treatable by other means who have mild symptoms, unimpaired gall bladder function, and small or medium-sized radiolucent stones; it is not suitable for radio-opaque stones, which are unlikely to dissolve. Patients should be given appropriate dietary advice (including avoidance of excessive cholesterol and calories) and should preferably be supervised in hospital because radiological moni-toring is required. Long-term prophylaxis may be needed after complete dissolution of the gallstones has been confirmed (preferably with cholecysto-grams and ultrasound on two separate occasions) because gallstones may recur in up to 25% of patients within one year of stopping treatment.

Ursodeoxycholic acid is also used in primary biliary cirrhosis; liver tests improve in most patients but an overall increase in survival has not been demonstrated. Ursodeoxycholic acid has also been tried in primary sclerosing cholangitis [unlicensed indication].

URSODEOXYCHOLIC ACID

Indications: see under Dose and under prepara-tions
Cautions: see notes above
Contra-indications: radio-opaque stones, pregnancy (see Appendix 4; non-hormonal con-

traceptive measures should be taken in women of childbearing age), non-functioning gall bladder, chronic liver disease, peptic ulceration, inflammatory diseases and other conditions of the small intestine and colon which interfere with entero-hepatic circulation of bile salts

Side-effects: nausea, vomiting, diarrhoea; gallstone calcification; pruritis

Dose: dissolution of gallstones, 8–12 mg/kg daily as a single dose at bedtime *or* in two divided doses, for up to 2 years; treatment is continued for 3–4 months after stones dissolve

Primary biliary cirrhosis, see under *Ursofalk*®

Ursodeoxycholic Acid (Non-proprietary) [PoM]

Tablets, ursodeoxycholic acid 150 mg, net price 60-tab pack = £18.87; 250 mg, 60-tab pack = £36.13. Label: 21

Available from Hillcross

Destolit® (Norgine) [PoM]

Tablets, scored, ursodeoxycholic acid 150 mg, net price 60-tab pack = £18.07. Label: 21

Urdox® (CP) [PoM]

Tablets, f/c, ursodeoxycholic acid 300 mg, net price 60-tab pack = £30.24. Label: 21

Ursofalk® (Cortecs) [PoM]

Capsules, ursodeoxycholic acid 250 mg. Net price 60 = £32.95. Label: 21

Suspension, sugar-free, ursodeoxycholic acid 250 mg/5 mL, net price 250 mL = £30.20. Label: 21

Dose: primary biliary cirrhosis, 10–15 mg/kg daily in 2–4 divided doses
Dissolution of gallstones, see Dose, above

Ursogal® (Galen) [PoM]

Tablets, scored, ursodeoxycholic acid 150 mg, net price 60-tab pack = £17.05. Label: 21

Capsules, ursodeoxycholic acid 250 mg, net price 60-cap pack = £30.50. Label: 21

Other preparations for biliary disorders

A **terpene** mixture (Rowachol®) raises biliary cholesterol solubility. It is not considered to be a useful adjunct.

Rowachol® (Rowa) [PoM] [▬]

Capsules, green, e/c, borneol 5 mg, camphene 5 mg, cineole 2 mg, menthol 32 mg, menthone 6 mg, pinene 17 mg in olive oil. Net price 50-cap pack = £7.35. Label: 22

Dose: 1–2 capsules 3 times daily before food (but see notes above)

Interactions: Appendix 1 (*Rowachol*®)

[▬] denotes preparations that are considered to be less suitable for prescribing (see p. vi)

1.9.2   Drugs which increase gastric acidity

Muripsin®, which contained glutamic acid hydrochloride, was formerly used in achlorhydria and hypochlorhydria but was of uncertain value. It has now been discontinued.

1.9.3   Aprotinin

Section 2.11.

1.9.4   Pancreatin

Supplements of pancreatin are given by mouth to compensate for reduced or absent exocrine secretion in cystic fibrosis, and following pancreatectomy, total gastrectomy, or chronic pancreatitis. They assist the digestion of starch, fat, and protein.

Pancreatin is inactivated by gastric acid therefore pancreatin preparations are best taken with food (or immediately before or after food). Gastric acid secretion may be reduced by giving cimetidine or ranitidine an hour beforehand (section 1.3). Concurrent use of antacids also reduces gastric acidity. The newer enteric-coated preparations such as *Creon*®, *Nutrizym GR*®, and *Pancrease*® deliver a higher enzyme concentration in the duodenum (provided the granules are swallowed whole without chewing). Higher-strength versions are now also available (**important:** see CSM advice below).

Since pancreatin is also inactivated by heat, excessive heat should be avoided if preparations are mixed with liquids or food; the resulting mixtures should not be kept for more than one hour.

Dosage is adjusted according to size, number, and consistency of stools, so that the patient thrives; extra allowance may be needed if snacks are taken between meals.

Pancreatin can irritate the perioral skin and buccal mucosa if retained in the mouth, and excessive doses can cause perianal irritation. The most frequent side-effects are gastro-intestinal including nausea, vomiting, and abdominal discomfort; hyperuricaemia and hyperuricosuria have been associated with very high doses. Hypersensitivity reactions occur occasionally and may affect those handling the powder.

PANCREATIN

Note. The pancreatin preparations which follow are all of porcine origin

Indications: see above

Cautions: see above and (for higher-strength preparations) see below

Side-effects: see above and (for higher-strength preparations) see below

Creon® (Solvay)

Granules, brown, e/c, pancreatin, providing: protease 1 125 units, lipase 20 000 units, amylase 22 500 units/sachet. Net price 40-sachet pack = £13.33. Counselling, see dose

Dose: ADULT and CHILD initially 1 sachet with meals either washed down or sprinkled on soft food (then swallowed immediately without chewing); higher doses may be required according to response

Creon® 10 000 (Solvay)
Capsules, brown/clear, enclosing buff-coloured e/c granules of pancreatin, providing: protease 600 units, lipase 10 000 units, amylase 8000 units. Net price 100-cap pack = £16.66. Counselling, see dose
Dose: ADULT and CHILD initially 1–2 capsules with meals either taken whole or contents mixed with fluid or soft food (then swallowed immediately without chewing)

Nutrizym GR® (Merck)
Capsules, green/orange, enclosing e/c pellets of pancreatin, providing minimum of: protease 650 units, lipase 10 000 units, amylase 10 000 units. Net price 100 = £13.15. Counselling, see dose
Dose: ADULT and CHILD 1–2 capsules with meals swallowed whole or contents sprinkled on soft food (then swallowed immediately without chewing); higher doses may be required according to response

Nutrizym 10® (Merck)
Capsules, red/yellow, enclosing e/c minitablets of pancreatin providing minimum of: protease 500 units, lipase 10 000 units, amylase 9000 units. Net price 100 = £13.15. Counselling, see dose
Dose: ADULT and CHILD 1–2 capsules with meals and 1 capsule with snacks, swallowed whole or contents taken with water or sprinkled on soft food (then swallowed immediately without chewing); higher doses may be required according to response

Pancrease® (Janssen-Cilag)
Capsules, enclosing e/c beads of pancrelipase USP, providing minimum of: protease 330 units, lipase 5000 units, amylase 2900 units. Net price 100 = £17.07. Counselling, see dose
Dose: ADULT and CHILD 1–2 (occasionally 3) capsules during each meal and 1 capsule with snacks swallowed whole or contents sprinkled on liquid or soft food (then swallowed immediately without chewing); higher doses may be required according to response

Pancrex® (Paines & Byrne)
Granules, pancreatin, providing minimum of: protease 300 units, lipase 5000 units, amylase 4000 units/g. Net price 300 g = £20.39. Label: 25, counselling, see dose
Dose: ADULT and CHILD 5–10 g just before meals washed down or mixed with liquid

Pancrex V® (Paines & Byrne)
Capsules, pancreatin, providing minimum of: protease 430 units, lipase 8000 units, amylase 9000 units. Net price 300-cap pack = £15.80. Counselling, see dose
Dose: ADULT and CHILD over 1 year 2–6 capsules with meals, swallowed whole or sprinkled on food; CHILD up to 1 year 1–2 capsules mixed with feeds
Capsules '125', pancreatin, providing minimum of: protease 160 units, lipase 2950 units, amylase 3300 units. Net price 300-cap pack = £9.72. Counselling, see dose
Dose: NEONATE 1–2 capsules with feeds
Tablets, e/c, s/c, pancreatin, providing minimum of: protease 110 units, lipase 1900 units, amylase 1700 units. Net price 300-tab pack = £4.51. Label: 5, 25, counselling, see dose
Dose: ADULT and CHILD 5–15 tablets before meals
Tablets forte, e/c, s/c, pancreatin, providing minimum of: protease 330 units, lipase 5600 units, amylase 5000 units. Net price 300-tab pack = £13.74. Label: 5, 25, counselling, see dose
Dose: ADULT and CHILD 6–10 tablets before meals

Powder, pancreatin, providing minimum of: protease 1400 units, lipase 25 000 units, amylase 30 000 units/ g. Net price 300 g = £24.28. Counselling, see dose
Dose: ADULT and CHILD 0.5–2 g with meals washed down or mixed with liquid; NEONATE 250–500 mg with each feed

■ Higher-strength preparations

The **CSM** has advised of data associating the high-strength pancreatin preparations *Nutrizym 22®* and *Pancreatin HL®* with the development of large bowel strictures (fibrosing colonopathy) in children with cystic fibrosis aged between 2 and 13 years. No association was found with *Creon® 25 000*. The following was recommended:
* *Pancrease HL®, Nutrizym 22®, Panzytrat® 25 000* [now discontinued] should not be used in children aged 15 years or less with cystic fibrosis;
* the total dose of pancreatic enzyme supplements used in patients with cystic fibrosis should not usually exceed 10 000 units of lipase per kg body-weight daily;
* if a patient on any pancreatin preparation develops new abdominal symptoms (or any change in existing abdominal symptoms) the patient should be reviewed to exclude the possibility of colonic damage.

Possible risk factors are gender (boys at greater risk than girls), more severe cystic fibrosis, and concomitant use of laxatives. The peak age for developing fibrosing colonopathy is between 2 and 8 years.
COUNSELLING. It is important to ensure adequate hydration at all times in patients receiving higher-strength pancreatin preparations.

Creon® 25 000 (Solvay) ▼ [PoM]
Capsules, orange/clear, enclosing brown-coloured e/c pellets of pancreatin, providing: protease (total) 1000 units, lipase 25 000 units, amylase 18 000 units. Net price 100-cap pack = £39.00. Counselling, see above and under dose
Dose: ADULT and CHILD initially 1 capsule with meals either taken whole or contents mixed with fluid or soft food (then swallowed immediately without chewing)

Nutrizym 22® (Merck) ▼ [PoM]
Capsules, red/yellow, enclosing e/c minitablets of pancreatin, providing minimum of: protease 1100 units, lipase 22 000 units, amylase 19 800 units. Net price 100-cap pack = £30.30. Counselling, see above and under dose
Dose: 1–2 capsules with meals and 1 capsule with snacks, swallowed whole or contents taken with water or sprinkled on soft food (then swallowed immediately without chewing)
CHILD under 15 years not recommended

Pancrease HL® (Janssen-Cilag) ▼ [PoM]
Capsules, enclosing light brown e/c minitablets of pancreatin, providing minimum of: protease 1250 units, lipase 25 000 units, amylase 22 500 units. Net price 100 = £36.18. Counselling, see above and under dose
Dose: 1–2 capsules during each meal and 1 capsule with snacks swallowed whole or contents sprinkled on liquid or soft food (then swallowed immediately without chewing)
CHILD under 15 years not recommended

2: Cardiovascular system

2.1 Positive inotropic drugs

2.1.1 Cardiac glycosides
2.1.2 Phosphodiesterase inhibitors

Positive inotropic drugs increase the force of contraction of the myocardium; for sympathomimetics with inotropic activity see section 2.7.1.

2.1.1 Cardiac glycosides

Cardiac glycosides increase the force of myocardial contraction and reduce conductivity within the atrioventricular (AV) node. Digoxin is the most commonly used cardiac glycoside.

Cardiac glycosides are most useful in the treatment of supraventricular tachycardias, especially for controlling ventricular response in atrial fibrillation (section 2.3). For reference to the role of digoxin in heart failure, see section 2.5.5.

For management of atrial fibrillation the maintenance dose of the cardiac glycoside can usually be determined by the ventricular rate at rest which should not be allowed to fall below 60 beats per minute except in special circumstances, e.g. with the concomitant administration of beta-blockers.

When rapid control is needed, **digoxin** may be given intravenously in a digitalising dose of 0.75 to 1 mg, preferably as an intravenous infusion (suggested volume 50 mL) over at least 2 hours (too rapid a rate of administration is associated with nausea and risk of arrhythmias); this is followed by normal maintenance therapy. The intramuscular route is **not** recommended.

In patients with mild heart failure a loading dose is not required, and a satisfactory plasma-digoxin concentration can be achieved over a period of about a week, using a dose of digoxin 125 to 250 micrograms twice a day which is then reduced.

Digoxin has a long half-life and maintenance doses need to be given only once daily (although higher doses may be divided to avoid nausea). **Digitoxin** also has a long half-life and maintenance doses need to be given only once daily or on alternate days. Renal function is the most important determinant of digoxin dosage, whereas elimination of digitoxin depends on metabolism by the liver.

Unwanted effects depend both on the plasma concentration of the drug and on the sensitivity of the conducting system or of the myocardium, which is often increased in heart disease. Thus plasma concentration alone cannot indicate toxicity reliably but the likelihood of toxicity increases progressively through the range 1.5 to 3 micrograms/litre for digoxin. Cardiac glycosides should be used with special care in the elderly who may be particularly susceptible to digitalis toxicity.

Regular monitoring of plasma-digoxin concentration during maintenance treatment is not necessary unless problems occur. Hypokalaemia predisposes to toxicity; therefore when diuretics are used with a cardiac glycoside the plasma-potassium concentration should be determined and potassium-sparing diuretics or, if necessary, potassium supplements (or foods rich in potassium) should be given.

Toxicity can often be managed by discontinuing digoxin and correcting hypokalaemia if appropriate; serious manifestations require urgent specialist management. **Digoxin-specific antibody fragments** are available for reversal of life-threatening overdosage (see below).

CHILDREN. The dose is based on body-weight; they require a relatively larger dose of digoxin than adults.

DIGOXIN

Indications: heart failure, supraventricular arrhythmias (particularly atrial fibrillation)

Cautions: recent infarction; sick sinus syndrome; thyroid disease; reduce dose in the elderly and in renal impairment; avoid hypokalaemia; avoid rapid intravenous administration (nausea and risk of arrhythmias); pregnancy (see also Appendix 4); **interactions:** Appendix 1 (cardiac glycosides)

Contra-indications: intermittent complete heart block, second degree AV block; supraventricular arrhythmias caused by Wolff-Parkinson-White syndrome; hypertrophic obstructive cardiomyopathy (unless concomitant atrial fibrillation and heart failure — but with caution)

Side-effects: usually associated with excessive dosage, include: anorexia, nausea, vomiting, diarrhoea, abdominal pain; visual disturbances, headache, fatigue, drowsiness, confusion, delirium, hallucinations; arrhythmias, heart block; see also notes above

Dose: *by mouth*, rapid digitalisation, 1–1.5 mg in divided doses over 24 hours; less rapid digitalisation, 250–500 micrograms daily (higher dose may be divided)

Maintenance, 62.5–500 micrograms daily (higher dose may be divided) according to renal function and, in atrial fibrillation, on heart-rate response; usual range, 125–250 micrograms daily (lower dose may be appropriate in elderly)

Emergency loading dose *by intravenous infusion*, total dose of 0.5–1 mg given in divided doses with approx. half of the total dose given over 10–20 minutes (see also Cautions), followed by further fractions of the total dose (also given over 10–20 minutes) at intervals of 4–8 hours according to response (see notes above for an alternative regimen)

Note. The above doses may need to be reduced if digoxin (or another cardiac glycoside) has been given in the preceding 2 weeks. For plasma concentration monitoring blood should ideally be taken at least 6 hours after a dose

Digoxin (Non-proprietary) PoM
Tablets, digoxin 62.5 micrograms, net price 20 = 31p; 125 micrograms, 20 = 32p; 250 micrograms, 20 = 33p
Paediatric injection, digoxin 100 micrograms/mL (hosp. only, available from BCM Specials)

Lanoxin® (GlaxoWellcome) PoM
Tablets, digoxin 125 micrograms, net price 20 = 32p; 250 micrograms (scored), 20 = 32p
Injection, digoxin 250 micrograms/mL. Net price 2-mL amp = 65p

Lanoxin-PG® (GlaxoWellcome) PoM
Tablets, blue, digoxin 62.5 micrograms. Net price 20 = 32p
Elixir, yellow, digoxin 50 micrograms/mL. Do not dilute, measure with pipette. Net price 60 mL = £5.23. Counselling, use of pipette

DIGITOXIN

Indications: heart failure, supraventricular arrhythmias (particularly atrial fibrillation)

Cautions: see under Digoxin but not necessary to reduce dose in renal impairment

Contra-indications: see under Digoxin

Side-effects: see under Digoxin

Dose: maintenance, 100 micrograms daily *or* on alternate days; may be increased to 200 micrograms daily if necessary

Digitoxin (Non-proprietary) PoM
Tablets, digitoxin 100 micrograms, net price 20 = £2.92

Digoxin-specific antibody

Digoxin-specific antibody fragments are indicated for the treatment of known or strongly suspected digoxin or digitoxin overdosage, where measures beyond the withdrawal of the cardiac glycoside and correction of any electrolyte abnormality are felt to be necessary (see also notes above).

Digibind® (GlaxoWellcome) PoM
Injection, powder for preparation of infusion, digoxin-specific antibody fragments (F(ab)) 38 mg. Net price per vial = £87.44 (hosp. and poisons centres only)
Dose: consult product literature

2.1.2   Phosphodiesterase inhibitors

Enoximone and **milrinone** are selective phosphodiesterase inhibitors which exert most of their effect on the myocardium. Sustained haemodynamic benefit has been observed after administration, but there is no evidence of any beneficial effect on survival.

ENOXIMONE

Indications: congestive heart failure where cardiac output reduced and filling pressures increased

Cautions: heart failure associated with hypertrophic cardiomyopathy, stenotic or obstructive valvular disease or other outlet obstruction; monitor blood pressure, heart rate, ECG, central venous pressure, fluid and electrolyte status, platelet count, hepatic enzymes; reduce dose in renal impairment; avoid extravasation; pregnancy and breast-feeding

Side-effects: ectopic beats; less frequently ventricular tachycardia or supraventricular arrhythmias (more likely in patients with pre-existing arrhythmias); hypotension; also headache, insomnia, nausea and vomiting, diarrhoea; occasionally, chills, oliguria, fever, urinary retention; upper and lower limb pain

Dose: *by slow intravenous injection* (rate not exceeding 12.5 mg/minute), diluted before use, initially 0.5–1 mg/kg, then 500 micrograms/kg every 30 minutes until satisfactory response or total of 3 mg/kg given; maintenance, initial dose of up to 3 mg/kg may be repeated every 3–6 hours as required

By intravenous infusion, initially 90 micrograms/kg/minute over 10–30 minutes, followed by continuous or intermittent infusion of 5–20 micrograms/kg/minute

Total dose over 24 hours should not usually exceed 24 mg/kg

Perfan® (Hoechst Marion Roussel) PoM
Injection, enoximone 5 mg/mL. For dilution before use. Net price 20-mL amp = £15.02
Note. Plastic apparatus should be used; crystal formation if glass used

MILRINONE

Indications: short-term treatment of severe congestive heart failure unresponsive to conventional maintenance therapy (not immediately after myocardial infarction); acute heart failure, including low output states, following heart surgery
Cautions: see under Enoximone; also correct hypokalaemia, monitor renal function
Side-effects: see under Enoximone; also chest pain reported
Dose: *by intravenous injection* over 10 minutes, diluted before use, 50 micrograms/kg followed by *intravenous infusion* at a rate of 375–750 nanograms/kg/minute, usually for up to 12 hours following surgery or for 48–72 hours in congestive heart failure; max. daily dose 1.13 mg/kg

Primacor® (Sanofi-Synthelabo) PoM
Injection, milrinone (as lactate) 1 mg/mL. For dilution before use. Net price 10-mL amp = £17.39

2.2	**Diuretics**
2.2.1	Thiazides and related diuretics
2.2.2	Loop diuretics
2.2.3	Potassium-sparing diuretics
2.2.4	Potassium-sparing diuretics with other diuretics
2.2.5	Osmotic diuretics
2.2.6	Mercurial diuretics
2.2.7	Carbonic anhydrase inhibitors
2.2.8	Diuretics with potassium

Thiazides (section 2.2.1) are used to relieve oedema due to chronic heart failure (section 2.5.5) and, in lower doses, to reduce blood pressure.

Loop diuretics (section 2.2.2) are used in pulmonary oedema due to left ventricular failure and in patients with chronic heart failure (section 2.5.5).

Combination diuretic therapy may be effective in patients with oedema resistant to treatment with one diuretic. Vigorous diuresis, particularly with loop diuretics, may induce acute hypotension; rapid reduction of plasma volume should be avoided.

ELDERLY. Lower initial doses of diuretics should be used in the elderly because they are particularly susceptible to the side-effects. The dose should then be adjusted according to renal function. Diuretics should not be used continuously on a long-term basis to treat simple gravitational oedema (which will usually respond to increased movement, raising the legs, and support stockings).

POTASSIUM LOSS. Hypokalaemia may occur with both thiazide and loop diuretics. The risk of hypokalaemia depends on the duration of action as well as the potency and is thus greater with thiazides than with an equipotent dose of a loop diuretic.

Hypokalaemia is dangerous in severe coronary artery disease and in patients also being treated with cardiac glycosides. Often the use of potassium-sparing diuretics (section 2.2.3) avoids the need to take potassium supplements.

In hepatic failure hypokalaemia caused by diuretics can precipitate encephalopathy, particularly in alcoholic cirrhosis; diuretics may also increase the risk of hypomagnesaemia in alcoholic cirrhosis, leading to arrhythmias.

Potassium supplements are seldom necessary when thiazides are used in the routine treatment of hypertension (see also section 9.2.1.1).

2.2.1 Thiazides and related diuretics

Thiazides and related compounds are moderately potent diuretics; they inhibit sodium reabsorption at the beginning of the distal convoluted tubule. They act within 1 to 2 hours of oral administration and most have a duration of action of 12 to 24 hours; they are usually administered early in the day so that the diuresis does not interfere with sleep.

In the management of *hypertension* a low dose of a thiazide, e.g. bendroflumethiazide (bendrofluazide) 2.5 mg daily, produces a maximal or near-maximal blood pressure lowering effect, with very little biochemical disturbance. Higher doses cause more marked changes in plasma potassium, uric acid, glucose, and lipids, with no advantage in blood pressure control, and should not be used. For reference to the use of thiazides in chronic heart failure see section 2.5.5.

Bendroflumethiazide (**bendrofluazide**) is widely used for mild or moderate heart failure and for hypertension—alone in the treatment of mild hypertension or with other drugs in more severe hypertension.

Chlortalidone (chlorthalidone), a thiazide-related compound, has a longer duration of action than the thiazides and may be given on alternate days to control oedema. It is also useful if acute retention is liable to be precipitated by a more rapid diuresis or if patients dislike the altered pattern of micturition promoted by other diuretics.

Other thiazides and related diuretics (including benzthiazide, clopamide, cyclopenthiazide, hydrochlorothiazide, hydroflumethiazide, mefruside and polythiazide) do not offer any significant advantage over those mentioned above, and newer ones are more expensive than the longer-established thiazides.

Metolazone is particularly effective when combined with a loop diuretic (even in renal failure); profound diuresis may occur and the patient should therefore be monitored carefully.

Xipamide resembles chlortalidone structurally, and is more potent than the other thiazides.

Indapamide is also chemically related to chlortalidone. It is claimed to lower blood pressure with less metabolic disturbance, particularly less aggravation of diabetes mellitus.

BENDROFLUMETHIAZIDE/ BENDROFLUAZIDE

Indications: oedema, hypertension (see also notes above)

Cautions: may cause hypokalaemia, aggravates diabetes and gout; may exacerbate systemic lupus erythematosus; elderly (see notes above); pregnancy (see also Appendix 4) and breast-feeding; hepatic and renal impairment (avoid if severe, see Appendixes 2 and 3); see also notes above; porphyria (see section 9.8.2); **interactions:** Appendix 1 (diuretics)

Contra-indications: refractory hypokalaemia, hyponatraemia, hypercalcaemia; severe renal and hepatic impairment; symptomatic hyperuricaemia; Addison's disease

Side-effects: postural hypotension and mild gastrointestinal effects; impotence (reversible on withdrawal of treatment); hypokalaemia (see also notes above), hypomagnesaemia, hyponatraemia, hypercalcaemia, hypochloraemic alkalosis, hyperuricaemia, gout, hyperglycaemia, and altered plasma lipid concentration; less commonly rashes, photosensitivity; blood disorders (including neutropenia and thrombocytopenia—when given in late pregnancy neonatal thrombocytopenia has been reported); pancreatitis, intrahepatic cholestasis, and hypersensitivity reactions (including pneumonitis, pulmonary oedema, severe skin reactions) also reported

Dose: oedema, initially 5–10 mg in the morning, daily *or* on alternate days; maintenance 5–10 mg 1–3 times weekly

Hypertension, 2.5 mg in the morning; higher doses rarely necessary (see notes above)

Bendroflumethiazide/Bendrofluazide (Non-proprietary) PoM
Tablets, bendroflumethiazide 2.5 mg, net price 20 = 61p; 5 mg, 20 = 72p
Available from APS, Ashbourne (*Neo-Bendromax®*), Berk (*Berkozide®*), Cox, Goldshield (*Neo-NaClex®*, 5 mg only), Hillcross, Norton, Sovereign (*Aprinox®*)

CHLORTALIDONE

(Chlorthalidone)

Indications: ascites due to cirrhosis in stable patients (under close supervision), oedema due to nephrotic syndrome, hypertension (see also notes above), mild to moderate chronic heart failure; diabetes insipidus (see section 6.5.2)

Cautions: see under Bendroflumethiazide

Contra-indications: see under Bendroflumethiazide

Side-effects: see under Bendroflumethiazide

Dose: oedema, up to 50 mg daily for limited period

Hypertension, 25 mg in the morning, increased to 50 mg if necessary (see also notes above)

Heart failure, 25–50 mg in the morning, increased if necessary to 100–200 mg daily

Hygroton® (Alliance) PoM
Tablets, yellow, scored, chlortalidone 50 mg, net price 28-tab pack = £1.68

CYCLOPENTHIAZIDE

Indications: oedema, hypertension (see also notes above)

Cautions: see under Bendroflumethiazide

Contra-indications: see under Bendroflumethiazide

Side-effects: see under Bendroflumethiazide

Dose: oedema, 250–500 micrograms daily in the morning; in heart failure may be increased to 1 mg daily (reduce to lowest effective dose for maintenance)

Hypertension, initially 250 micrograms daily in the morning, increased if necessary to 500 micrograms daily (see also notes above)

Navidrex® (Alliance) PoM
Tablets, scored, cyclopenthiazide 500 micrograms. Net price 28-tab pack = £1.25
Excipients: include gluten

HYDROCHLOROTHIAZIDE

Indications: oedema, hypertension (see also notes above)

Cautions: see under Bendroflumethiazide

Contra-indications: see under Bendroflumethiazide

Side-effects: see under Bendroflumethiazide

Dose: oedema, initially 25–50 mg daily, reduced for maintenance if possible; severe oedema in patients unable to tolerate loop diuretics, initially 75 mg daily

Hypertension, 25 mg daily, increased to 50 mg daily if necessary (see also notes above)

ELDERLY. In some patients (especially the elderly) an initial dose of 12.5 mg daily may be sufficient

HydroSaluric® (MSD) PoM
Tablets, both scored, hydrochlorothiazide 25 mg, net price 30-tab pack = 44p; 50 mg, 30-tab pack = 81p

INDAPAMIDE

Indications: essential hypertension

Cautions: renal impairment (stop if deterioration); monitor plasma potassium and urate concentrations in elderly, hyperaldosteronism, gout, or with concomitant cardiac glycosides; hyperparathyroidism (discontinue if hypercalcaemia); pregnancy and breast-feeding; **interactions:** Appendix 1 (diuretics)

Contra-indications: recent cerebrovascular accident, severe hepatic impairment

Side-effects: hypokalaemia, headache, dizziness, fatigue, muscular cramps, nausea, anorexia, diarrhoea, constipation, dyspepsia, rashes (erythema multiforme, epidermal necrolysis reported); rarely postural hypotension, palpitations, increase in liver enzymes, blood disorders (including thrombocytopenia), hyponatraemia, metabolic alkalosis, hyperglycaemia, increased plasma urate concentrations, paraesthesia, photosensitivity, impotence, renal impairment, reversible acute myopia; diuresis with doses above 2.5 mg daily

Dose: 2.5 mg in the morning

Indapamide (Non-proprietary) [PoM]
Tablets, s/c, indapamide 2.5 mg. Net price 60-tab
pack = £3.76
Available from APS, Ashbourne (*Nindaxa 2.5®*), Bar-
tholomew Rhodes, Cox, Hillcross, Norton, Opus
(*Opumide®*), Trinity (*Natramid®*)
Natrilix® (Servier) [PoM]
Tablets, f/c, indapamide 2.5 mg. Net price 30-tab
pack = £3.89, 60-tab pack = £7.63

■ Modified release
Natrilix SR® (Servier) [PoM]
Tablets, m/r, indapamide 1.5 mg. Net price 30-tab
pack = £4.47. Label: 25
Dose: hypertension, 1 tablet daily, preferably in the morning

MEFRUSIDE

Indications: oedema, hypertension (see also notes
above)
Cautions: see under Bendroflumethiazide
Contra-indications: see under Bendroflumethiazide
Side-effects: see under Bendroflumethiazide
Dose: initially 25–50 mg in the morning, increased
to 75–100 mg for oedema; maintenance 25 mg
daily *or* on alternate days (see also notes above)

Baycaron® (Bayer) [PoM]
Tablets, scored, mefruside 25 mg. Net price 20 = £1.41

METOLAZONE

Indications: oedema, hypertension (see also notes
above)
Cautions: see under Bendroflumethiazide; also
profound diuresis on concomitant administration
with furosemide (monitor patient carefully)
Contra-indications: see under Bendroflumethiazide
Side-effects: see under Bendroflumethiazide
Dose: oedema, 5–10 mg in the morning, increased
if necessary to 20 mg daily in resistant oedema,
max. 80 mg daily
Hypertension, initially 5 mg in the morning;
maintenance 5 mg on alternate days

Metenix 5® (Borg) [PoM]
Tablets, blue, metolazone 5 mg. Net price 100-tab
pack = £20.37

POLYTHIAZIDE

Indications: oedema, hypertension (see also notes
above)
Cautions: see under Bendroflumethiazide
Contra-indications: see under Bendroflumethi-
azide
Side-effects: see under Bendroflumethiazide
Dose: usually 1–4 mg daily; in hypertension
500 micrograms daily may be adequate

Nephril® (Pfizer) [PoM]
Tablets, scored, polythiazide 1 mg. Net price 28-
tab pack = 79p

XIPAMIDE

Indications: oedema, hypertension (see also notes
above)
Cautions: see under Bendroflumethiazide
Contra-indications: see under Bendroflumethiazide

Side-effects: gastro-intestinal disturbances; mild
dizziness; hypokalaemia, more rarely other
electrolyte disturbances such as hyponatraemia
Dose: oedema, initially 40 mg in the morning,
increased to 80 mg in resistant cases; maintenance
20 mg in the morning
Hypertension, 20 mg in the morning

Diurexan® (ASTA Medica) [PoM]
Tablets, scored, xipamide 20 mg. Net price 14-tab
pack = £2.09

2.2.2 Loop diuretics

Loop diuretics are used in pulmonary oedema due to
left ventricular failure; intravenous administration
produces relief of breathlessness and reduces pre-
load sooner than would be expected from the time
of onset of diuresis. Loop diuretics are also used in
patients with longstanding heart failure. Diuretic-
resistant oedema (except oedema due to peripheral
venous stasis or calcium-channel blockers) can be
treated with a loop diuretic combined with a thiazide or related diuretic (e.g. bendroflumethiazide
5–10 mg daily or metolazone 5–20 mg daily).

Loop diuretics inhibit reabsorption from the
ascending limb of the loop of Henlé in the renal
tubule and are powerful diuretics. Hypokalaemia
may develop, and care is needed to avoid hypotension. If there is an enlarged prostate, urinary
retention may occur; this is less likely if small doses
and less potent diuretics are used initially.

Furosemide (frusemide) and **bumetanide** are
similar in activity; both act within 1 hour of oral
administration and diuresis is complete within 6
hours so that, if necessary, they can be given twice
in one day without interfering with sleep. Following
intravenous administration they have a peak effect
within 30 minutes. The diuresis associated with
these drugs is dose related. In patients with
impaired renal function very large doses may occasionally be needed; in such doses both drugs can
cause deafness and bumetanide can cause myalgia.

Torasemide has properties similar to those of
furosemide and bumetanide, and is indicated for
oedema and for hypertension.

FUROSEMIDE/FRUSEMIDE

Indications: oedema, oliguria due to renal failure
Cautions: pregnancy and breast-feeding; may
cause hypokalaemia and hyponatraemia; correct
hypovolaemia before using in oliguria; aggravates
diabetes mellitus and gout; liver failure, prostatic
enlargement; porphyria (section 9.8.2); although
manufacturer advises that rate of intravenous
administration should not exceed 4 mg/minute,
single doses of up to 50 mg may be administered
more rapidly; **interactions:** Appendix 1 (diuretics)
Contra-indications: precomatose states associated with liver cirrhosis; renal failure with anuria
Side-effects: hyponatraemia, hypokalaemia, and
hypomagnesaemia (see also section 2.2),
hypochloraemic alkalosis, increased calcium
excretion, hypotension; less commonly nausea,
gastro-intestinal disturbances, hyperuricaemia
and gout; hyperglycaemia (less common than
with thiazides); temporary increase in plasma
cholesterol and triglyceride concentrations; rarely

rashes, photosensitivity and bone marrow depression (withdraw treatment), pancreatitis (with large parenteral doses), tinnitus and deafness (usually with large parenteral doses and rapid administration and in renal impairment)

Dose: *by mouth,* oedema, initially 40 mg in the morning; maintenance 20 mg daily *or* 40 mg on alternate days, increased in resistant oedema to 80 mg daily or more; CHILD 1–3 mg/kg daily, max. 40 mg daily

Oliguria, initially 250 mg daily; if necessary larger doses, increasing in steps of 250 mg, may be given every 4–6 hours to a max. of a single dose of 2 g (rarely used)

By intramuscular injection or slow intravenous injection (see Cautions, above), initially 20–50 mg; CHILD 0.5–1.5 mg/kg to a max. daily dose of 20 mg

By intravenous infusion (by syringe pump if necessary), in oliguria, initially 250 mg over 1 hour (rate not exceeding 4 mg/minute), if satisfactory urine output not obtained in the subsequent hour further 500 mg over 2 hours, then if no satisfactory response within subsequent hour, further 1 g over 4 hours, if no response obtained dialysis probably required; effective dose (up to 1 g) can be repeated every 24 hours

Furosemide/Frusemide (Non-proprietary) [PoM]
Tablets, furosemide 20 mg, net price 20 = 74p; 40 mg, 28-tab pack = £2.25; 500 mg, 20 = £7.16
Various strengths available from APS, Ashbourne (*Froop®*), Berk (*Dryptal®*), Cox, CP (including *Rusyde®*), Hillcross, Norton, Sovereign
Oral solution, sugar-free, furosemide, net price 4 mg/mL, 150 mL = £13.43; 8 mg/mL, 150 mL = £17.33; 10 mg/mL, 150 mL = £18.75
Available from Rosemont (*Frusol®*)
Injection, furosemide 10 mg/mL, net price 2-mL amp = 24p
Available from Antigen, Medeva, Phoenix (all also 5-mL amp)

Lasix® (Borg) [PoM]
Tablets, all scored, furosemide 20 mg, net price 28-tab pack = £1.57; 40 mg, 28-tab pack = £2.27; 500 mg (yellow), 20 = £21.74
Paediatric liquid, sugar-free, furosemide 1 mg/mL when reconstituted with purified water, freshly boiled and cooled, net price 150 mL = £3.68
Injection, furosemide 10 mg/mL, net price 2-mL amp = 84p
Note. Large volume furosemide injections available from Antigen, Medeva (*Min-I-Jet®*)

BUMETANIDE

Indications: oedema, oliguria due to renal failure
Cautions: see under Furosemide (but has been used in porphyria, see section 9.8.2)
Contra-indications: see under Furosemide
Side-effects: see under Furosemide; also myalgia
Dose: *by mouth,* 1 mg in the morning, repeated after 6–8 hours if necessary; severe cases, increased up to 5 mg or more daily
ELDERLY, 500 micrograms daily may be sufficient
By intravenous injection, 1–2 mg, repeated after 20 minutes; when *intramuscular injection* considered necessary, 1 mg initially then adjusted according to response
By intravenous infusion, 2–5 mg over 30–60 minutes

Bumetanide (Non-proprietary) [PoM]
Tablets, bumetanide 1 mg, net price 28-tab pack = £1.80; 5 mg, 28-tab pack = £11.19
Available from APS, Berk (*Betinex®*), Bioglan, Cox, CP, Hillcross, Norton

Burinex® (Leo) [PoM]
Tablets, both scored, bumetanide 1 mg, net price 28-tab pack = £1.64; 5 mg, 28 = £10.45
Liquid, green, sugar-free, bumetanide 1 mg/5 mL. Net price 150 mL = £3.17
Injection, bumetanide 500 micrograms/mL. Net price 2-mL amp = 38p; 4-mL amp = 66p; 10-mL amp = £1.39

TORASEMIDE

Indications: oedema, hypertension
Cautions: see under Furosemide
Contra-indications: see under Furosemide; pregnancy and breast-feeding
Side-effects: see under Furosemide
Dose: oedema, 5 mg once daily, preferably in the morning, increased if required to 20 mg once daily; usual max. 40 mg daily
Hypertension, 2.5 mg daily, increased if necessary to 5 mg once daily

Torem® (Roche) [PoM]
Tablets, torasemide 2.5 mg, net price 28-tab pack = £4.06; 5 mg (scored), 28-tab pack = £5.95; 10 mg (scored), 28-tab pack = £8.75

2.2.3   Potassium-sparing diuretics

Amiloride and **triamterene** on their own are weak diuretics. They cause retention of potassium and are therefore used as a more effective alternative to giving potassium supplements with thiazide or loop diuretics. (See section 2.2.4 for compound preparations with thiazides or loop diuretics.)

Spironolactone is also a potassium-sparing diuretic, and potentiates thiazide or loop diuretics by antagonising aldosterone. It is of value in the treatment of the oedema of cirrhosis of the liver. Low doses of spironolactone may be beneficial in severe heart failure, see section 2.5.5.

Spironolactone is also used in primary hyperaldosteronism (Conn's syndrome).

Potassium supplements must **not** be given with potassium-sparing diuretics. It is also important to bear in mind that administration of a potassium-sparing diuretic to a patient receiving an ACE inhibitor can cause severe hyperkalaemia.

AMILORIDE HYDROCHLORIDE

Indications: oedema, potassium conservation with thiazide and loop diuretics
Cautions: pregnancy and breast-feeding; monitor in renal impairment (avoid if moderate to severe, see also Appendix 3); diabetes mellitus; elderly; **interactions:** Appendix 1 (diuretics)
Contra-indications: hyperkalaemia, renal failure
Side-effects: include gastro-intestinal disturbances, dry mouth, rashes, confusion, postural hypotension, hyperkalaemia, hyponatraemia

Dose: used alone, initially 10 mg daily *or* 5 mg twice daily, adjusted according to response; max. 20 mg daily

With other diuretics, congestive heart failure and hypertension, initially 5–10 mg daily; cirrhosis with ascites, initially 5 mg daily

Amiloride (Non-proprietary) PoM
Tablets, amiloride hydrochloride 5 mg, net price 20 = 37p
Available from APS, Ashbourne (*Amilospare®*), Cox, CP, Hillcross, Norton
Oral solution, sugar-free, amiloride hydrochloride 5 mg/5 mL, net price 150 mL = £41.58
Available from Rosemont (*Amilamont®*)

■ Compound preparations with thiazide or loop diuretics, see section 2.2.4

TRIAMTERENE

Indications: oedema, potassium conservation with thiazide and loop diuretics
Cautions; Contra-indications: see under Amiloride Hydrochloride; may cause blue fluorescence of urine
Side-effects: include gastro-intestinal disturbances, dry mouth, rashes; slight decrease in blood pressure, hyperkalaemia, hyponatraemia; photosensitivity and blood disorders also reported; triamterene found in kidney stones
Dose: initially 150–250 mg daily, reducing to alternate days after 1 week; taken in divided doses after breakfast and lunch; lower initial dose when given with other diuretics
COUNSELLING. Urine may look slightly blue in some lights

Dytac® (Pharmark) PoM
Capsules, maroon, triamterene 50 mg. Net price 30-cap pack = £16.90. Label: 14 (see above), 21

■ Compound preparations with thiazides or loop diuretics, see section 2.2.4

Aldosterone antagonists

SPIRONOLACTONE

Indications: oedema and ascites in cirrhosis of the liver, malignant ascites, nephrotic syndrome, congestive heart failure (section 2.5.5); primary hyperaldosteronism
Cautions: potential metabolic products carcinogenic in *rodents*; elderly; hepatic impairment; renal impairment (avoid if moderate to severe); monitor electrolytes (discontinue if hyperkalaemia); porphyria (section 9.8.2); **interactions:** Appendix 1 (diuretics)
Contra-indications: hyperkalaemia, hyponatraemia, severe renal impairment; pregnancy and breast-feeding; Addison's disease
Side-effects: gastro-intestinal disturbances; impotence, gynaecomastia; menstrual irregularities; lethargy, headache, confusion; rashes; hyperkalaemia (discontinue); hyponatraemia; hepatotoxicity, osteomalacia, and blood disorders reported
Dose: 100–200 mg daily, increased to 400 mg if required; CHILD initially 3 mg/kg daily in divided doses
Heart failure, see section 2.5.5

Spironolactone (Non-proprietary) PoM
Tablets, spironolactone 25 mg, net price 20 = £1.00; 50 mg, 20 = £2.40; 100 mg, 20 = £3.50
Available from APS, Ashbourne (*Spirospare®*), Berk (*Spirolone®*), Cox, Hillcross, Norton
Oral suspensions, sugar-free, spironolactone 5 mg/5 ml, 10 mg/5 ml, 25 mg/5 ml, 50 mg/5 ml and 100 mg/5 ml available from Rosemont (special order)
Aldactone® (Searle) PoM
Tablets, all f/c, spironolactone 25 mg (buff), net price 100-tab pack = £9.88; 50 mg (off-white), 100-tab pack = £19.76; 100 mg (buff), 28-tab pack = £11.07

■ With thiazides or loop diuretics, see section 2.2.4

Potassium-sparing diuretics with other diuretics

Although it is preferable to prescribe thiazides (section 2.2.1) and potassium-sparing diuretics (section 2.2.3) separately, the use of fixed combinations may be justified if compliance is a problem. Potassium-sparing diuretics are not usually necessary in the routine treatment of hypertension, unless hypokalaemia develops. For **interactions**, see Appendix 1 (diuretics).

■ Amiloride with thiazides

Co-amilozide (Non-proprietary) PoM
Tablets, co-amilozide 2.5/25 (amiloride hydrochloride 2.5 mg, hydrochlorothiazide 25 mg). Net price 28-tab pack = £1.94
Available from CP, Du Pont (*Moduret 25®*)
Dose: hypertension, oedema, 1–4 tablets, increased if necessary to max. 8 daily
Tablets, co-amilozide 5/50 (amiloride hydrochloride 5 mg, hydrochlorothiazide 50 mg). Net price 28 = £1.85
Available from APS, Ashbourne (*Amilmaxco 5/50®*), Baker Norton (*Amil-Co®*), Berk (*Delvas®*), Cox, CP, Du Pont (*Moduretic®*), Hillcross, Norton, Opus (*Zida-Co®*)
Dose: hypertension, oedema, 1–2 tablets, increased if necessary to max. 4 daily

Navispare® (Novartis) PoM
Tablets, f/c, orange, amiloride hydrochloride 2.5 mg, cyclopenthiazide 250 micrograms. Net price 28-tab pack = £2.06
Excipients: include gluten
Dose: hypertension, 1–2 tablets in the morning

■ Amiloride with loop diuretics

Co-amilofruse (Non-proprietary) PoM
Tablets, co-amilofruse 2.5/20 (amiloride hydrochloride 2.5 mg, furosemide 20 mg). Net price 28-tab pack = £4.10, 56-tab pack = £9.49
Available from CP, Helios (*Frumil LS®*), Hillcross
Dose: oedema, 1 tablet in the morning
Tablets, co-amilofruse 5/40 (amiloride hydrochloride 5 mg, furosemide 40 mg). Net price 28-tab pack = £4.09
Available from Ashbourne (*Froop-Co®*), Baker Norton (*Fru-Co®*), Borg (*Lasoride®*), Cox, CP, Helios (*Frumil®*), Hillcross, Lagap
Dose: oedema, 1–2 tablets in the morning
Tablets, co-amilofruse 10/80 (amiloride hydrochloride 10 mg, furosemide 80 mg). Net price 28-tab pack = £11.50, 56-tab pack = £14.20
Available from CP (*Aridil®*), Helios (*Frumil Forte®*)
Dose: oedema, 1 tablet in the morning

Burinex A® (Leo) PoM
Tablets, ivory, scored, amiloride hydrochloride 5 mg,
bumetanide 1 mg. Net price 28-tab pack = £3.06
Dose: oedema, 1–2 tablets daily

■ Triamterene with thiazides
COUNSELLING. Urine may look slightly blue in some lights
Dyazide® (SK&F) PoM
Tablets, peach, scored, co-triamterzide 50/25
(triamterene 50 mg, hydrochlorothiazide 25 mg).
Net price 30-tab pack = £2.41. Label: 14 (see
above), 21
Dose: hypertension, 1 tablet daily after breakfast;
oedema, 2 tablets daily (1 after breakfast and 1 after
midday meal) increased to 3 daily if necessary (2 after
breakfast and 1 after midday meal); usual maintenance,
1 daily or 2 on alternate days; max. 4 daily
Note. Tablets containing co-triamterzide 50/25 (triamterene 50 mg and hydrochlorothiazide 25 mg) are also
available from Ashbourne (TriamaxCo®), Baker Norton
(Triam-Co®)

Dytide® (Goldshield) PoM
Capsules, clear/maroon, triamterene 50 mg, benzthiazide 25 mg. Net price 30-cap pack = £16.90.
Label: 14 (see above), 21
Dose: oedema, initially 3 capsules daily (2 after breakfast and 1 after midday meal) for 1 week then 1 or 2 on
alternate days

Kalspare® (Dominion) PoM
Tablets, orange, f/c, scored, triamterene 50 mg,
chlortalidone 50 mg. Net price 28-tab pack =
£3.05. Label: 14 (see above), 21
Dose: hypertension, oedema, 1–2 tablets in the morning

■ Triamterene with loop diuretics
COUNSELLING. Urine may look slightly blue in some lights
Frusene® (Orion) PoM
Tablets, yellow, scored, triamterene 50 mg, furo-
semide 40 mg. Net price 56-tab pack = £5.67.
Label: 14 (see above), 21
Dose: oedema, ½–2 tablets daily in the morning

■ Spironolactone with thiazides
Co-flumactone (Non-proprietary) PoM
Tablets, co-flumactone 25/25 (hydroflumethiazide
25 mg, spironolactone 25 mg). Net price 100-tab
pack = £22.83
Available from Searle (*Aldactide 25*®)
Dose: congestive heart failure, initially 4 tablets daily;
range 1–8 daily
Tablets, co-flumactone 50/50 (hydroflumethiazide
50 mg, spironolactone 50 mg). Net price 28-tab
pack = £8.92
Available from Searle (*Aldactide 50*®)
Dose: congestive heart failure, initially 2 tablets daily;
range 1–4 daily

■ Spironolactone with loop diuretics
Lasilactone® (Borg) PoM
Capsules, blue/white, spironolactone 50 mg, furo-
semide 20 mg. Net price 28-cap pack = £8.91
Dose: resistant oedema, 1–4 capsules daily

2.2.5   Osmotic diuretics

Osmotic diuretics are rarely used in heart failure as
they may acutely expand the blood volume. **Mannitol** is used in cerebral oedema—a typical dose is
1 g/kg as a 20% solution given by rapid intravenous
infusion.

MANNITOL

Indications: see notes above; glaucoma (section 11.6)
Cautions: extravasation causes inflammation and
thrombophlebitis
Contra-indications: congestive cardiac failure,
pulmonary oedema
Side-effects: chills, fever
Dose: *by intravenous infusion,* diuresis, 50–200 g
over 24 hours, preceded by a test dose of 200 mg/
kg by slow intravenous injection
Cerebral oedema, see notes above

Mannitol (Non-proprietary) PoM
Intravenous infusion, mannitol 10% and 20%
Available from Baxter

2.2.6   Mercurial diuretics

Mercurial diuretics are effective but are now almost
never used because of their nephrotoxicity.

2.2.7   Carbonic anhydrase inhibitors

The carbonic anhydrase inhibitor **acetazolamide** is
a weak diuretic and is little used for its diuretic
effect. It is used for prophylaxis against mountain
sickness [unlicensed indication] but is not a substitute for acclimatisation.
    Acetazolamide and eye drops of dorzolamide
inhibit the formation of aqueous humour and are
used in glaucoma (section 11.6)

2.2.8   Diuretics with potassium

Many patients on diuretics do not need potassium
supplements (section 9.2.1.1). For many of those
who do, the amount of potassium in combined preparations may not be enough, and for this reason
their use is to be discouraged.
    Diuretics with potassium and potassium-sparing
diuretics should **not** usually be given together.

COUNSELLING. Modified-release potassium tablets
should be swallowed whole with plenty of fluid during
meals while sitting or standing
Burinex K® (Leo) PoM ▱
Tablets, bumetanide 500 micrograms, potassium
7.7 mmol for modified release. Net price 20 =
85p. Label: 25, 27, counselling, see above
Diumide-K Continus® (ASTA Medica) PoM
▱
Tablets, f/c, white/orange, furosemide 40 mg, potassium 8 mmol for modified release. Net price 30-tab
pack = £2.99. Label: 25, 27, counselling, see above
Lasikal® (Borg) PoM ▱
Tablets, white/yellow, f/c, furosemide 20 mg,
potassium 10 mmol for modified release. Net
price 100-tab pack = £15.21. Label: 25, 27, counselling, see above
Neo-NaClex-K® (Goldshield) PoM ▱
Tablets, pink/white, f/c, bendroflumethiazide 2.5 mg,
potassium 8.4 mmol for modified release. Net price
20 = £1.59. Label: 25, 27, counselling, see above

┌───┐
│ ▱ denotes preparations that are considered to │
│ be less suitable for prescribing (see p. vi) │
└───┘

2.3 Anti-arrhythmic drugs

2.3.1   Management of arrhythmias
2.3.2   Drugs for arrhythmias

2.3.1 Management of arrhythmias

Management of an arrhythmia, apart from the treatment of associated heart failure, requires precise diagnosis of the type of arrhythmia, and electrocardiography is essential.

ECTOPIC BEATS. If spontaneous with a normal heart, these rarely require treatment beyond reassurance. If they are particularly troublesome, beta-blockers are sometimes effective and may be safer than other suppressant drugs.

ATRIAL FIBRILLATION. The ventricular rate at rest can usually be controlled with digoxin. If adequate control at rest or during exercise cannot be achieved readily, a beta-blocker or verapamil may be added if ventricular function is adequate. In some cases other classes of drugs may be appropriate. Anticoagulants are indicated especially in valvular or myocardial disease, and in the elderly; younger patients with lone atrial fibrillation in the absence of heart disease probably do not require anticoagulation. Aspirin is less effective than warfarin at preventing emboli but may be appropriate if there are no other risk factors for stroke. Doses of aspirin within the range 75–300 mg daily are used.

ATRIAL FLUTTER. The ventricular rate at rest can often be controlled with digoxin. Reversion to sinus rhythm (if indicated) may be achieved by appropriately synchronised d.c. shock. Alternatively, amiodarone may be used to restore, and amiodarone or sotalol to maintain sinus rhythm. If the arrhythmia is long-standing a period of treatment with anticoagulants should be considered before cardioversion to avoid the complication of emboli.

PAROXYSMAL SUPRAVENTRICULAR TACHYCARDIA. In most patients this remits spontaneously or can be returned to sinus rhythm by reflex vagal stimulation with respiratory manoeuvres, prompt squatting, or pressure over one carotid sinus (**important:** pressure over carotid sinus should be restricted to monitored patients—it can be dangerous in recent ischaemia, digitalis toxicity, or the elderly).

If vagal stimulation fails, intravenous administration of adenosine is usually the treatment of choice. Intravenous administration of verapamil is useful for patients without myocardial or valvular disease (**important:** never in patients recently treated with beta-blockers, see p. 105). For arrhythmias that are poorly tolerated, synchronised d.c. shock usually provides rapid relief.

In cases of paroxysmal supraventricular tachycardia with block, digitalis toxicity should be suspected. In addition to stopping administration of the cardiac glycoside and giving potassium supplements, intravenous administration of a beta-blocker may be useful. Specific digoxin antibody is available if the toxicity is considered life-threatening (section 2.1.1).

ARRHYTHMIAS AFTER MYOCARDIAL INFARCTION. In patients with a paroxysmal tachycardia or rapid irregularity of the pulse it is best not to administer an antiarrhythmic until an ECG record has been obtained. If the condition of the patient is such that death due to the arrhythmia seems possible lidocaine (lignocaine) should be given intravenously (see p. 74). Bradycardia, particularly if complicated by hypotension, should be treated with atropine sulphate, given intravenously in a dose of 0.3 to 1 mg. If the initial dose is effective it may be repeated if necessary.

VENTRICULAR TACHYCARDIA. Drug treatment is used both for the treatment of ventricular tachycardia and for prophylaxis of recurrent attacks that merit suppression. Ventricular tachycardia requires treatment most commonly in the acute stage of myocardial infarction, but the likelihood of this and other life-threatening arrhythmias diminishes sharply over the first 24 hours after the attack, especially in patients without heart failure or shock. Lidocaine (lignocaine) is the preferred drug for emergency use. Other drugs are best administered under specialist supervision. Very rapid ventricular tachycardia causes profound circulatory collapse and should be treated urgently with d.c. shock.

Torsades de pointes is a special form of ventricular tachycardia which tends to occur in the presence of a long QT interval (usually drug induced, but other factors including hypokalaemia, severe bradycardia, and genetic predisposition may also be implicated). The episodes are usually self-limiting, but are frequently recurrent and may cause impairment (or loss) of consciousness. If not controlled, the arrhythmia may progress to ventricular fibrillation. Intravenous infusion of magnesium sulphate (section 9.5.1.3) is usually effective. A beta-blocker (but not sotalol) and atrial (or ventricular) pacing may be considered. Antiarrhythmics (including lidocaine) may further prolong the QT interval, thus worsening the condition.

2.3.2 Drugs for arrhythmias

Anti-arrhythmic drugs can be classified clinically into those that act on supraventricular arrhythmias (e.g. verapamil), those that act on both supraventricular and ventricular arrhythmias (e.g. disopyramide), and those that act on ventricular arrhythmias (e.g. lidocaine (lignocaine)).

They can also be classified according to their effects on the electrical behaviour of myocardial cells during activity:

Class Ia, b, c: membrane stabilising drugs (e.g. quinidine, lidocaine, flecainide respectively)
Class II: beta-blockers
Class III: amiodarone, bretylium, and sotalol (also Class II)
Class IV: calcium-channel blockers (includes verapamil but not dihydropyridines)

This latter classification (the Vaughan Williams classification) is of less clinical significance.

CAUTIONS. The negative inotropic effects of anti-arrhythmic drugs tend to be additive therefore special care should be taken if two or more are used, especially in impaired myocardial function. Most or all drugs that are effective in countering arrhythmias can also provoke them in some circumstances; moreover, hypokalaemia enhances the arrhythmogenic (pro-arrhythmic) effect of many drugs.

Supraventricular arrhythmias

Adenosine is usually the treatment of choice for terminating paroxysmal supraventricular tachycardia. As it has a very short duration of action (half-life only about 8 to 10 seconds, but prolonged in those taking dipyridamole), most side-effects are short lived. Unlike verapamil, adenosine may be used after a beta-blocker. Verapamil may be preferable to adenosine in asthma.

Oral administration of a **cardiac glycoside** (such as digoxin, section 2.1.1) is the treatment of choice in slowing ventricular response in cases of atrial fibrillation and atrial flutter. Intravenous digoxin, preferably infused slowly, is occasionally required if the ventricular rate needs rapid control.

Verapamil (section 2.6.2) is usually effective for supraventricular tachycardias. An initial intravenous dose (**important**: serious beta-blocker interaction hazard, see p. 105) may be followed by oral treatment; hypotension may occur with larger doses. It should not be used for tachyarrhythmias where the QRS complex is wide (i.e. broad complex) unless a supraventricular origin has been established beyond reasonable doubt. It is also contra-indicated in atrial fibrillation with pre-excitation (e.g.Wolff-Parkinson-White syndrome). It should not be used in children with arrhythmias without specialist advice; some supraventricular arrhythmias in childhood can be accelerated by verapamil with dangerous consequences.

Intravenous administration of a **beta-blocker** (section 2.4) such as esmolol or propranolol, can achieve rapid control of the ventricular rate.

Drugs for both supraventricular and ventricular arrhythmias include **amiodarone**, **beta-blockers**, **disopyramide**, **flecainide**, **procainamide**, **propafenone** and **quinidine**, see below under Supraventricular and Ventricular Arrhythmias.

ADENOSINE

Indications: rapid reversion to sinus rhythm of paroxysmal supraventricular tachycardias, including those associated with accessory pathways (e.g. Wolff-Parkinson-White syndrome); aid to diagnosis of broad or narrow complex supraventricular tachycardias

Cautions: atrial fibrillation or flutter with accessory pathway (conduction down anomalous pathway may increase); heart transplant (see below); **interactions:** Appendix 1 (adenosine)

Contra-indications: second- or third-degree AV block and sick sinus syndrome (unless pacemaker fitted); asthma

Side-effects: include transient facial flush, chest pain, dyspnoea, bronchospasm, choking sensation, nausea, light-headedness; severe bradycardia reported (requiring temporary pacing); ECG may show transient rhythm disturbances

Dose: *by rapid intravenous injection* into central or large peripheral vein, 3 mg over 2 seconds with cardiac monitoring; if necessary followed by 6 mg after 1–2 minutes, and then by 12 mg after a further 1–2 minutes; increments should not be given if high level AV block develops at any particular dose
Note. 3-mg dose ineffective in a number of patients, therefore higher initial dose sometimes used but patients with *heart transplant* are **very sensitive** to effects of adenosine, and should **not** receive higher initial dose. Also if essential to give with dipyridamole reduce initial dose to 0.5–1 mg

Adenocor® (Sanofi-Synthelabo) [PoM]
Injection, adenosine 3 mg/mL in physiological saline. Net price 2-mL vial = £4.05 (hosp. only)
Note. Intravenous infusion of adenosine (*Adenoscan®*, Sanofi Winthrop) may be used in conjunction with radionuclide myocardial perfusion imaging in patients who cannot exercise adequately or for whom exercise is inappropriate—consult product literature

Supraventricular and ventricular arrhythmias

Amiodarone is used in the treatment of arrhythmias particularly when other drugs are ineffective or contra-indicated. It may be used for paroxysmal supraventricular, nodal and ventricular tachycardias, atrial fibrillation and flutter, and ventricular fibrillation. It should be initiated only under hospital or specialist supervision. Amiodarone may be given by intravenous infusion as well as by mouth, and has the advantage of causing little or no myocardial depression. Unlike oral amiodarone, intravenous amiodarone may act relatively rapidly.

Amiodarone has a very long half-life (extending to several weeks) and only needs to be given once daily (but high doses may cause nausea unless divided). Many weeks or months may be required to achieve steady-state plasma concentrations; this is particularly important when interactions with amiodarone are considered (see also Appendix 1).

Most patients taking amiodarone develop corneal microdeposits (reversible on withdrawal of treatment); these rarely interfere with vision, but drivers may be dazzled by headlights at night. Because of the possibility of phototoxic reactions, patients should be advised to shield the skin from light and to use a wide-spectrum sunscreen (section 13.8.1) to protect against both long ultraviolet and visible light.

Amiodarone contains iodine and can cause disorders of thyroid function; both hypothyroidism and hyperthyroidism may occur. Clinical assessment is unreliable, and laboratory tests should be performed every 6 months. Thyroxine (T4) may be raised in the absence of hyperthyroidism; therefore tri-iodothyronine (T3), T4, and thyroid-stimulating hormone (thyrotrophin, TSH) should all be measured. A raised T3 and T4 with a very low or undetectable TSH concentration suggests the development of thyrotoxicosis. The thyrotoxicosis may be very refractory, and amiodarone should usually be withdrawn at least temporarily to help achieve control; treatment with carbimazole may be required. Hypothyroidism can be treated with replacement therapy without withdrawing amiodarone if it is essential.

Pneumonitis should always be suspected if new or progressive shortness of breath or cough develops in a patient taking amiodarone. Fresh neurological symptoms should raise the possibility of peripheral neuropathy.

Amiodarone is also associated with hepatotoxicity and treatment should be discontinued if severe liver function abnormalities or clinical signs of liver disease develop.

Beta-blockers act as anti-arrhythmic drugs principally by attenuating the effects of the sympathetic system on automaticity and conductivity within the heart, for details see section 2.4. For special reference to the role of **sotalol** in ventricular arrhythmias, see also p. 76.

Disopyramide may be given by intravenous injection to control arrhythmias after myocardial infarction (including those not responding to lidocaine (lignocaine)), but it impairs cardiac contractility. Oral administration of disopyramide is useful but it has an antimuscarinic effect which limits its use in patients with glaucoma or prostatic hypertrophy.

Flecainide belongs to the same general class as lidocaine. It may be of value in serious symptomatic ventricular arrhythmias. It may also be indicated for junctional re-entry tachycardias and for paroxysmal atrial fibrillation. As with quinidine it may precipitate serious arrhythmias in a small minority of patients (including those with otherwise normal hearts).

Procainamide can be given by intravenous injection to control ventricular arrhythmias, but prolonged oral use can cause a syndrome resembling systemic lupus erythematosus.

Propafenone is used for the prophylaxis and treatment of ventricular arrhythmias and also for some supraventricular arrhythmias. It has complex mechanisms of action, including weak beta-blocking activity (therefore caution is needed in obstructive airways disease—contra-indicated if severe).

Quinidine may be effective in suppressing supraventricular and ventricular arrhythmias. It may itself precipitate rhythm disorders, and is best used on specialist advice; it can cause hypersensitivity reactions and gastro-intestinal upsets.

Drugs for supraventricular arrhythmias include **adenosine, cardiac glycosides** and **verapamil**, see above under Supraventricular Arrhythmias. Drugs for ventricular arrhythmias include **bretylium, lidocaine, mexiletine, moracizine** and **phenytoin**, see below under Ventricular Arrhythmias.

AMIODARONE HYDROCHLORIDE

Indications: see notes above (should be initiated in hospital or under specialist supervision)

Cautions: liver-function and thyroid-function tests required before treatment and then every 6 months (see notes above for tests of thyroid function); chest x-ray required before treatment; heart failure; renal impairment; elderly; severe bradycardia and conduction disturbances in excessive dosage; intravenous use may cause moderate and transient fall in blood pressure (circulatory collapse precipitated by rapid administration or overdosage); porphyria (section 9.8.2); **interactions:** Appendix 1 (amiodarone)

Contra-indications: sinus bradycardia, sino-atrial heart block; unless pacemaker fitted avoid in severe conduction disturbances or sinus node disease; history of thyroid dysfunction; pregnancy and breast-feeding (see also Appendixes 4 and 5); iodine sensitivity; avoid *intravenous use* in severe respiratory failure, circulatory collapse, severe arterial hypotension

Side-effects: reversible corneal microdeposits (sometimes with night glare), rarely impaired vision due to optic neuritis; peripheral neuropathy and myopathy (usually reversible on withdrawal); bradycardia and conduction disturbances (see Cautions); phototoxicity and rarely persistent slate-grey skin discoloration (see also notes); hypothyroidism, hyperthyroidism, diffuse pulm-

onary alveolitis, pneumonitis, and fibrosis; raised serum transaminases (may require dose reduction or withdrawal if accompanied by acute liver disorders); jaundice, hepatitis and cirrhosis reported; rarely nausea, vomiting, metallic taste, tremor, nightmares, vertigo, headache, sleeplessness, fatigue, alopecia, paraesthesia, benign raised intracranial pressure, impotence, epididymoorchitis; ataxia, rashes (including exfoliative dermatitis), hypersensitivity including vasculitis, renal involvement and thrombocytopenia; haemolytic or aplastic anaemia; anaphylaxis on rapid injection, also bronchospasm or apnoea in respiratory failure

Dose: *by mouth*, 200 mg 3 times daily for 1 week reduced to 200 mg twice daily for a further week; maintenance, usually 200 mg daily or the minimum required to control the arrhythmia

By intravenous infusion via caval catheter, 5 mg/kg over 20–120 minutes with ECG monitoring; max. 1.2 g in 24 hours

Amiodarone (Non-proprietary) PoM
Tablets, amiodarone hydrochloride 100 mg, net price 28-tab pack = £4.49; 200 mg, 28-tab pack = £6.87. Label: 11
Available from APS, Berk (*Amidox®*), Cox, Generics, Hillcross, Norton, Sterwin

Cordarone X® (Sanofi-Synthelabo) PoM
Tablets, both scored, amiodarone hydrochloride 100 mg, net price 28-tab pack = £5.00; 200 mg, 28-tab pack = £8.19. Label: 11
Injection, amiodarone hydrochloride 50 mg/mL. Net price 3-mL amp = £1.50. For dilution and use as an infusion

DISOPYRAMIDE

Indications: ventricular arrhythmias, especially after myocardial infarction; supraventricular arrhythmias

Cautions: discontinue if hypotension, hypoglycaemia, ventricular, tachycardia, ventricular fibrillation or torsades de pointes develop; atrial flutter or tachycardia with partial block, bundle branch block, heart failure (avoid if severe); prostatic enlargement; glaucoma; hepatic and renal impairment (see Appendixes 2 and 3); pregnancy and breast-feeding (see Appendixes 4 and 5); **interactions:** Appendix 1 (disopyramide)

Contra-indications: second- and third-degree heart block and sinus node dysfunction (unless pacemaker fitted); cardiogenic shock; severe uncompensated heart failure

Side-effects: ventricular tachycardia, ventricular fibrillation or torsades de pointes (usually associated with prolongation of QRS complex or QT interval—see Cautions above), myocardial depression, hypotension, AV block; antimuscarinic effects include dry mouth, blurred vision, urinary retention; gastro-intestinal irritation; psychosis, cholestatic jaundice, hypoglycaemia also reported (see Cautions above)

Dose: *by mouth*, 300–800 mg daily in divided doses
By slow intravenous injection, 2 mg/kg over at least 5 minutes to a max. of 150 mg, with ECG monitoring, followed immediately *either* by 200 mg *by mouth*, then 200 mg every 8 hours for 24 hours *or* 400 micrograms/kg/hour *by intravenous infusion*; max. 300 mg in first hour and 800 mg daily

Disopyramide (Non-proprietary) [PoM]
Capsules, disopyramide (as phosphate) 100 mg,
net price 20 = £3.95; 150 mg, 20 = £3.33
Available from Hillcross, Norton (100 mg)

Rythmodan® (Borg) [PoM]
Capsules, disopyramide 100 mg (green/beige), net
price 84-cap pack = £15.82; 150 mg, 84-cap pack
= £20.99
Injection, disopyramide (as phosphate) 10 mg/mL,
net price 5-mL amp = £2.92

■ Modified release

Dirythmin SA® (Astra) [PoM]
Durules® (= tablets, m/r), f/c, disopyramide (as
phosphate) 150 mg. Net price 20 = £2.47. Label:
25
Dose: 300 mg every 12 hours; max. 750 mg daily

Rythmodan Retard® (Borg) [PoM]
Tablets, m/r, scored, f/c, disopyramide (as phos-
phate) 250 mg. Net price 56-tab pack = £31.02.
Label: 25
Dose: 250–375 mg every 12 hours

FLECAINIDE ACETATE

Indications: (should be initiated in hospital)
Tablets and injection: AV nodal reciprocating
tachycardia, arrhythmias associated with Wolff-
Parkinson-White syndrome and similar conditions with accessory pathways, paroxysmal atrial
fibrillation in patients with disabling symptoms
(arrhythmias of recent onset will respond more
readily)
Tablets only: symptomatic sustained ventricular
tachycardia, premature ventricular contractions
and/or non-sustained ventricular tachycardia
causing disabling symptoms in patients resistant
to or intolerant of other therapy
Injection only: ventricular tachyarrhythmias
resistant to other treatment
Cautions: patients with pacemakers (especially
those who may be pacemaker dependent because
stimulation threshold may rise appreciably);
avoid in sinus node dysfunction, atrial conduction
defects, second-degree or greater AV block, bundle branch block or distal block unless pacing rescue available; atrial fibrillation following heart
surgery; elderly (see Dose); hepatic and renal
impairment (see Appendixes 2 and 3); pregnancy
(toxicity in *animal* studies) and breast-feeding;
interactions: Appendix 1 (flecainide)
Contra-indications: heart failure; history of myocardial infarction and either asymptomatic ventricular ectopics or asymptomatic non-sustained
ventricular tachycardia; long-standing atrial
fibrillation where no attempt has been made to
convert to sinus rhythm; haemodynamically significant valvular heart disease
Side-effects: dizziness, visual disturbances
(corneal deposits reported); arrhythmogenic (pro-
arrhythmic) effect; rarely nausea and vomiting,
urticaria, hallucinations, amnesia, confusion,
depression, dyskinesia, convulsions; reversible
increases in liver enzymes, jaundice; ataxia,
peripheral neuropathy, paraesthesia, photosensitivity, pulmonary fibrosis, pneumonitis also
reported

Dose: *by mouth*, ventricular arrhythmias, 100 mg
twice daily; max. 400 mg daily (usually reserved
for rapid control or in heavily built patients),
reduced after 3–5 days if possible
Supraventricular arrhythmias, 50 mg twice daily,
increased if required to max. 300 mg daily
ELDERLY. Rate of elimination may be reduced—care on
dose adjustment
By slow intravenous injection, 2 mg/kg over 10–30
minutes, max. 150 mg, with ECG monitoring; followed if required by *infusion* at a rate of 1.5 mg/
kg/hour for 1 hour, subsequently reduced to 100–
250 micrograms/kg/hour for up to 24 hours; max.
cumulative dose in first 24 hours, 600 mg; transfer to *oral* treatment, as above

Tambocor® (3M) [PoM]
Tablets, flecainide acetate 50 mg, net price 60-tab
pack = £15.55; 100 mg (scored), 60-tab pack =
£22.21
Injection, flecainide acetate 10 mg/mL. Net price
15-mL amp = £4.73

PROCAINAMIDE HYDROCHLORIDE

Indications: ventricular arrhythmias, especially
after myocardial infarction; atrial tachycardia
Cautions: elderly; hepatic and renal impairment,
asthma, myasthenia gravis; pregnancy; **interactions:** Appendix 1 (procainamide)
Contra-indications: heart block, heart failure,
hypotension; systemic lupus erythematosus; not
indicated for torsades de pointes (can exacerbate);
breast-feeding
Side-effects: nausea, diarrhoea, rashes, fever,
myocardial depression, heart failure, lupus
erythematosus-like syndrome, agranulocytosis
after prolonged treatment; psychosis and angioedema also reported
Dose: *by mouth*, ventricular arrhythmias, up to
50 mg/kg daily in divided doses, preferably controlled by monitoring serum-procainamide concentration (dosage intervals can range from 3–6
hours); atrial arrhythmias, higher doses may be
required
By slow intravenous injection, rate not exceeding
50 mg/minute, 100 mg with ECG monitoring,
repeated at 5-minute intervals until arrhythmia
controlled; max. 1 g
By intravenous infusion, 500–600 mg over 25–30
minutes with ECG monitoring, followed by maintenance at rate of 2–6 mg/minute, then if necessary oral treatment as above, starting 3–4 hours
after infusion
Note. Serum procainamide concentration for optimum
response 3–10 mg/litre

Pronestyl® (Squibb) [PoM]
Tablets, scored, procainamide hydrochloride
250 mg. Net price 100-tab pack = £4.70
Injection, procainamide hydrochloride 100 mg/
mL. Net price 10-mL vial = £1.90

PROPAFENONE HYDROCHLORIDE

Indications: ventricular arrhythmias; paroxysmal
supraventricular tachyarrhythmias which include
paroxysmal atrial flutter or fibrillation and paroxysmal re-entrant tachycardias involving the AV
node or accessory pathway, where standard therapy ineffective or contra-indicated

Cautions: heart failure; hepatic and renal impairment; elderly; pacemaker patients; pregnancy and breast-feeding (see Appendixes 4 and 5); great caution in obstructive airways disease owing to beta-blocking activity (contra-indicated if severe); **interactions:** Appendix 1 (propafenone)

Contra-indications: uncontrolled congestive heart failure, cardiogenic shock (except arrhythmia induced), severe bradycardia, uncontrolled electrolyte disturbances, severe obstructive pulmonary disease, marked hypotension; myasthenia gravis; unless adequately paced avoid in sinus node dysfunction, atrial conduction defects, second degree or greater AV block, bundle branch block or distal block

Side-effects: constipation, blurred vision, dry mouth (due to antimuscarinic action); dizziness, nausea and vomiting, fatigue, bitter taste, diarrhoea, headache, and allergic skin reactions reported; postural hypotension, particularly in elderly; bradycardia, sino-atrial, atrioventricular, or intraventricular blocks; arrhythmogenic (pro-arrhythmic) effect; rarely hypersensitivity reactions (cholestasis, blood disorders, lupus syndrome), seizures; myoclonus also reported

Dose: 70 kg and over, initially 150 mg 3 times daily after food under direct hospital supervision with ECG monitoring and blood pressure control (if QRS interval prolonged by more than 20%, reduce dose or discontinue until ECG returns to normal limits); may be increased at intervals of at least 3 days to 300 mg twice daily and, if necessary, to max. 300 mg 3 times daily; under 70 kg, reduce dose

ELDERLY may respond to lower doses

Arythmol® (Knoll) [PoM]
Tablets, both f/c, propafenone hydrochloride 150 mg, net price 90-tab pack = £21.43; 300 mg (scored), 60-tab pack = £21.43. Label: 21, 25

QUINIDINE

Indications: suppression of supraventricular tachycardias and ventricular arrhythmias (see notes above)

Cautions: 200-mg test dose to detect hypersensitivity reactions; **interactions:** Appendix 1 (quinidine)

Contra-indications: heart block

Side-effects: see under Procainamide Hydrochloride; also ventricular arrhythmias, thrombocytopenia, haemolytic anaemia; rarely granulomatous hepatitis; also cinchonism (see Quinine, section 5.4.1)

Dose: *by mouth*, quinidine sulphate 200–400 mg 3–4 times daily

Note. Quinidine sulphate 200 mg ≡ quinidine bisulphate 250 mg

Quinidine Sulphate (Non-proprietary) [PoM]
Tablets, quinidine sulphate 200 mg, net price 100-tab pack = £21.45
Available from Regent

■ Modified release
Kinidin Durules® (Astra) [PoM]
Tablets, m/r, f/c, quinidine bisulphate 250 mg. Net price 100-tab pack = £11.05. Label: 25
Dose: 500 mg every 12 hours, adjusted as required

Ventricular arrhythmias

Bretylium is only used as an anti-arrhythmic drug in resuscitation. It is given both intramuscularly and intravenously but can cause severe hypotension, particularly after intravenous administration; nausea and vomiting can occur with either route. The intravenous route should only be used in emergency when there is doubt about absorption because of inadequate circulation.

Lidocaine (lignocaine) is relatively safe when used by slow intravenous injection and should be considered first for emergency use. Though effective in suppressing ventricular tachycardia and reducing the risk of ventricular fibrillation following myocardial infarction, it has not been shown to reduce mortality when used prophylactically in this condition. In patients with cardiac or hepatic failure doses may need to be reduced to avoid convulsions, depression of the central nervous system, or depression of the cardiovascular system.

Mexiletine may be given as a slow intravenous injection if lidocaine is ineffective; it has a similar action. Adverse cardiovascular and central nervous system effects may limit the dose tolerated; nausea and vomiting may prevent an effective dose being given by mouth.

Moracizine is available on a named-patient basis for the prophylaxis and treatment of serious and life-threatening ventricular arrhythmias for patients already stabilised on moracizine.

Phenytoin (section 4.8.2) by slow intravenous injection was formerly used in ventricular arrhythmias particularly those caused by cardiac glycosides, but this use is now obsolete.

Tocainide has been re-introduced recently. It has been associated with pulmonary infiltrates and with a high incidence of blood disorders; it is restricted for use in circumstances where other treatment has failed or is inappropriate (see Tocainide Hydrochloride, below).

Drugs for both supraventricular and ventricular arrhythmias include **amiodarone, beta-blockers, disopyramide, flecainide, procainamide, propafenone** and **quinidine**, see above under Supraventricular and Ventricular Arrhythmias.

BRETYLIUM TOSILATE

Indications: ventricular arrhythmias resistant to other treatment

Cautions: do not give noradrenaline (norepinephrine) or other sympathomimetic amines; may exacerbate ventricular arrhythmias due to cardiac glycosides; **interactions:** Appendix 1 (adrenergic neurone blockers)

Contra-indications: phaeochromocytoma

Side-effects: hypotension, nausea and vomiting; tissue necrosis reported after intramuscular injection (rotate sites)

Dose: *by slow intravenous injection*, 5–10 mg/kg over 8–10 minutes (preferably 15–30 minutes) with blood pressure and ECG monitoring; may be repeated after 1–2 hours to a total dosage of 30 mg/kg (intravenous dose being diluted to 10 mg/mL in glucose 5% or sodium chloride intravenous infusion) Maintenance 5–10 mg/kg *by intramuscular injection, by intravenous infusion* (over 15–30 minutes) every 6–8 hours, *or* 1–2 mg/minute *by continuous intravenous infusion*

Bretylate® (GlaxoWellcome) PoM
Injection, bretylium tosilate 50 mg/mL, net price 10-mL amp = £18.92

Min-I-Jet® Bretylium Tosylate (Medeva) PoM
Injection, bretylium tosilate 50 mg/mL, net price 10-mL disposable syringe = £19.75

LIDOCAINE HYDROCHLORIDE/ LIGNOCAINE HYDROCHLORIDE

Indications: ventricular arrhythmias, especially after myocardial infarction

Cautions: lower doses in congestive cardiac failure, in hepatic failure, and following cardiac surgery; elderly; **interactions:** Appendix 1 (lidocaine)

Contra-indications: sino-atrial disorders, all grades of atrioventricular block, severe myocardial depression; porphyria (see section 9.8.2)

Side-effects: dizziness, paraesthesia, or drowsiness (particularly if injection too rapid); other CNS effects include confusion, respiratory depression and convulsions; hypotension and bradycardia (may lead to cardiac arrest); hypersensitivity reported

Dose: *by intravenous injection*, in patients without gross circulatory impairment, 100 mg as a bolus over a few minutes (50 mg in lighter patients or those whose circulation is severely impaired), followed immediately by *infusion* of 4 mg/minute for 30 minutes, 2 mg/minute for 2 hours, then 1 mg/minute; reduce concentration further if infusion continued beyond 24 hours (ECG monitoring and specialist advice for infusion)

IMPORTANT. Following intravenous injection lidocaine has a short duration of action (lasting for 15–20 minutes). If an *intravenous infusion* is not immediately available the initial *intravenous injection* of 50–100 mg can be repeated if necessary once or twice at intervals of not less than 10 minutes

Lidocaine/Lignocaine (Non-proprietary) PoM
Injection 2%, lidocaine hydrochloride 20 mg/mL, net price 2-mL amp = 27p; 5-mL amp = 23p; 10-mL amp = 60p; 20-mL amp = 61p
Available from Braun
Infusion, lidocaine hydrochloride 0.1% (1 mg/mL) and 0.2% (2 mg/mL) in glucose intravenous infusion 5%. 500-mL containers
Available from Baxter

Min-I-Jet® Lignocaine (Medeva) PoM
Injection, lidocaine hydrochloride 1% (10 mg/mL), net price 10-mL disposable syringe = £3.39; 2% (20 mg/mL), 5-mL disposable syringe = £3.07

Xylocard® (Astra) PoM
Injection 100 mg, lidocaine hydrochloride (anhydrous) 20 mg/mL. Net price 5-mL syringe = £1.61

MEXILETINE HYDROCHLORIDE

Indications: ventricular arrhythmias, especially after myocardial infarction

Cautions: hepatic impairment; close monitoring on initiation of therapy (including ECG, blood pressure, etc.); **interactions:** Appendix 1 (mexiletine)

Contra-indications: bradycardia, cardiogenic shock; high degree AV block (unless pacemaker fitted)

Side-effects: nausea, vomiting, constipation; bradycardia, hypotension, atrial fibrillation, palpitations, conduction defects, exacerbation of arrhythmias, torsades de pointes; drowsiness, confusion, convulsions, psychiatric disorders, dysarthria, ataxia, paraesthesia, nystagmus, tremor; jaundice, hepatitis, and blood disorders reported; see also notes above

Dose: *by mouth*, initial dose 400 mg (may be increased to 600 mg if opioid analgesics also given), followed after 2 hours by 200–250 mg 3–4 times daily
By intravenous injection, 100–250 mg at a rate of 25 mg/minute with ECG monitoring followed by *infusion* of 250 mg as a 0.1% solution over 1 hour, 125 mg/hour for 2 hours, then 500 micrograms/minute

Mexitil® (Boehringer Ingelheim) PoM
Capsules, mexiletine hydrochloride 50 mg (purple/red), net price 100-cap pack = £4.95; 200 mg (red), 100-cap pack = £11.87
Injection, mexiletine hydrochloride 25 mg/mL. Net price 10-mL amp = £1.49

■ Modified release
Mexitil PL® (Boehringer Ingelheim) PoM
Perlongets® (= capsules, m/r, each enclosing 5 miniature tablets), turquoise/scarlet, mexiletine hydrochloride 360 mg. Net price 60-cap pack = £12.82. Label: 25
Dose: 1 capsule twice daily

MORACIZINE HYDROCHLORIDE

Indications: ventricular arrhythmias[1]

Cautions: sick sinus syndrome; pre-existing conduction abnormalities; congestive heart failure; hepatic and renal impairment; pregnancy and breast-feeding; **interactions:** Appendix 1 (moracizine)

Contra-indications: second-degree or greater AV block (unless paced); cardiogenic shock

Side-effects: include gastro-intestinal disturbances; dizziness, headache, fatigue, palpitations, dyspnoea; arrhythmogenic (pro-arrhythmic effect); chest pain; congestive heart failure; reversible increases in liver enzymes, jaundice; thrombocytopenia

Dose: (initiated in hospital[1]) usually 600–900 mg daily in 3 divided doses, adjusted by steps of 150 mg daily at intervals of 3 days; max. recommended daily dose 900 mg; rapid control, initially 400–500 mg, then 200 mg every 8 hours
Note. Patients well controlled on 3 divided doses daily may be given same total daily dosage in 2 divided doses (every 12 hours)

Ethmozine® (Monmouth) ▼ PoM
[1]*Tablets*, all f/c, moracizine hydrochloride 200 mg, 250 mg and 300 mg
1. *Ethmozine®* tablets available only on named-patient basis for patients already stabilised on moracizine

TOCAINIDE HYDROCHLORIDE

Indications: life-threatening symptomatic ventricular tachyarrhythmias associated with severely compromised left-ventricular function when other therapy has failed or is contra-indicated

Cautions: weekly blood counts essential for first 12 weeks, then monthly; correct hypokalaemia; severe hepatic impairment (Appendix 2), renal impairment (Appendix 3); elderly; uncompensated heart failure, bradycardia and hypotension; pregnancy (Appendix 4); breast-feeding (Appendix 5); **interactions:** Appendix 1 (tocainide)
BLOOD OR PULMONARY DISORDERS. Patients or their carers should be told how to recognise signs of blood or pulmonary disorders, and advised to seek immediate medical attention if symptoms develop

Contra-indications: second- or third-degree AV block (unless paced)

Side-effects: CNS effects including tremor, dizziness, confusion, convulsions, paraesthesia, rarely psychosis, hallucinations; nausea and vomiting; abnormal liver-function tests (hepatitis and jaundice reported); fever, rash (including Stevens-Johnson syndrome and exfoliative dermatitis), vasculitis; lupus erythematosus-like syndrome; pulmonary fibrosis, interstitial pneumonitis, fibrosing alveolitis; agranulocytosis, aplastic anaemia, and thrombocytopenia; arrhythmias, bradycardia, hypotension; blurred vision, tinnitus, taste disturbance

Dose: 1.2 g daily in 3 divided doses; max. 2.4 g daily

Tonocard® (Astra) PoM
Tablets, yellow, f/c, tocainide hydrochloride 400 mg, net price 100-tab pack = £16.35

2.4 Beta-adrenoceptor blocking drugs

Beta-adrenoceptor blocking drugs (beta-blockers) block the beta-adrenoreceptors in the heart, peripheral vasculature, bronchi, pancreas, and liver.

Many beta-blockers are now available and in general they are all equally effective. There are, however, differences between them which may affect choice in treating particular diseases or individual patients; esmolol and sotalol are used for the management of arrhythmia only (see below).

Intrinsic sympathomimetic activity (ISA, partial agonist activity) represents the capacity of beta-blockers to stimulate as well as to block adrenergic receptors. **Oxprenolol, pindolol, acebutolol** and **celiprolol** have intrinsic sympathomimetic activity; they tend to cause less bradycardia than the other beta-blockers and may also cause less coldness of the extremities.

Some beta-blockers are lipid soluble and some are water soluble. **Atenolol, celiprolol, nadolol,** and **sotalol** are the most water-soluble; they are less likely to enter the brain, and may therefore cause less sleep disturbance and nightmares. Water-soluble beta-blockers are excreted by the kidneys; they accumulate in renal impairment and dosage reduction is therefore often necessary.

Beta-blockers with a relatively short duration of action have to be given two or three times daily. Many of these are, however, available in modified-release formulations so that administration once daily is adequate for hypertension. For angina twice-daily treatment may sometimes be needed even with a modified-release formulation. Some beta-blockers such as atenolol, betaxolol, bisoprolol, carvedilol, celiprolol, and nadolol have

an intrinsically longer duration of action and need to be given only once daily.

All beta-blockers slow the heart and may induce myocardial depression. They should therefore not be given to patients with second- or third-degree heart block. Beta-blockers may precipitate or worsen heart failure. However, **carvedilol** (which also has vasodilating properties), may be used cautiously for the treatment of moderate heart failure under the supervision of a hospital specialist. **Sotalol** may prolong the QT interval, and has occasionally caused life-threatening ventricular arrhythmias (**important**: particular care should be taken to avoid hypokalaemia in patients taking sotalol).

Labetalol, celiprolol, carvedilol and **nebivolol** are beta-blockers which have, in addition, an arteriolar vasodilating action, by diverse mechanisms, and thus lower peripheral resistance. There is no evidence that these drugs have important advantages over other beta-blockers in the treatment of hypertension.

Beta-blockers may precipitate asthma and this effect can be dangerous. Beta-blockers should be **avoided** in patients with a history of asthma or chronic obstructive airways disease; if there is no alternative, a cardioselective beta-blocker may be used with extreme caution under specialist supervision. **Atenolol, betaxolol, bisoprolol, metoprolol, nebivolol** and (to a lesser extent) **acebutolol**, have less effect on the beta$_2$ (bronchial) receptors and are, therefore, relatively *cardioselective*, but they are **not** *cardiospecific*. They have a lesser effect on airways resistance but are **not** free of this side-effect.

Beta-blockers are also associated with fatigue, coldness of the extremities (may be less common with those with ISA, see above), and sleep disturbances with nightmares (may be less common with the water-soluble ones, see above).

Beta-blockers are not contra-indicated in diabetes; however they can lead to a small deterioration of glucose tolerance and interfere with metabolic and autonomic responses to hypoglycaemia. Cardioselective beta-blockers (see above) may be preferable and beta-blockers should be avoided altogether in those with frequent episodes of hypoglycaemia.

HYPERTENSION. Beta-blockers are effective antihypertensives but their mode of action is not understood; they reduce cardiac output, alter baroceptor reflex sensitivity, and block peripheral adrenoceptors. Some beta-blockers depress plasma renin secretion. It is possible that a central effect may also explain their mode of action. Blood pressure can usually be controlled with relatively few side-effects. In general the dose of beta-blocker does not have to be high; for example **atenolol** is given in a dose of 50 mg daily and it is not necessary to increase the dose to 100 mg.

Combined thiazide and beta-blocker preparations may help compliance but combined preparations should only be used when blood pressure is not adequately controlled by a thiazide or a beta-blocker alone. Beta-blockers reduce, but do not abolish, the tendency for diuretics to cause hypokalaemia.

Beta-blockers can be used to control the pulse rate in patients with *phaeochromocytoma*. However, they should never be used alone as beta-blockade without concurrent alpha-blockade may lead to a hypertensive crisis. For this reason phenoxybenzamine should always be used together with the beta-blocker.

ANGINA. By reducing cardiac work beta-blockers improve exercise tolerance and relieve symptoms in patients with *angina* (for further details on the management of stable and unstable angina see section 2.6). As with hypertension there is no good evidence of the superiority of any one drug, although occasionally a patient will respond better to one beta-blocker than to another. There is some evidence that sudden withdrawal may cause an exacerbation of angina and therefore gradual reduction of dose is preferable when beta-blockers are to be stopped. There is a risk of precipitating heart failure when beta-blockers and verapamil are used together in established ischaemic heart disease (**important**: see p. 105).

MYOCARDIAL INFARCTION. For advice on the management of myocardial infarction see section 2.10.1.

Several studies have shown that some beta-blockers can reduce the recurrence rate of *myocardial infarction*. However, uncontrolled heart failure, hypotension, bradyarrhythmias, and obstructive airways disease render beta-blockers unsuitable in some patients following a myocardial infarction. **Atenolol** and **metoprolol** may reduce early mortality after intravenous and subsequent oral administration in the acute phase, while **acebutolol**, **metoprolol**, **propranolol**, and **timolol** have protective value when started in the early convalescent phase. The evidence relating to other beta-blockers is less convincing; some have not been tested in trials of secondary protection. It is also not known whether the protective effect of beta-blockers continues after 2–3 years; it is possible that sudden cessation may cause a rebound worsening of myocardial ischaemia.

ARRHYTHMIAS. Beta-blockers act as *anti-arrhythmic drugs* principally by attenuating the effects of the sympathetic system on automaticity and conductivity within the heart. They may be used in conjunction with digoxin to control the ventricular response in atrial fibrillation, especially in patients with thyrotoxicosis. Beta-blockers are also useful in the management' of supraventricular tachycardias, and are used to control those following myocardial infarction, see above.

Esmolol is a relatively cardioselective beta-blocker with a very short duration of action, used intravenously for the short-term treatment of supraventricular arrhythmias, sinus tachycardia, or hypertension, particularly in the peri-operative period. It may also be used in other situations, such as acute myocardial infarction, where sustained beta blockade might be hazardous.

Sotalol, a non-cardioselective beta-blocker with additional class III anti-arrhythmic activity, is used for prophylaxis in paroxysmal supraventricular arrhythmias. It also suppresses ventricular ectopic beats and non-sustained ventricular tachycardia. It has been shown to be more effective than lidocaine (lignocaine) in the termination of spontaneous sustained ventricular tachycardia due to coronary disease or cardiomyopathy. However, it may induce torsades de pointes in susceptible patients.

THYROTOXICOSIS. Beta-blockers are used in pre-operative preparation for thyroidectomy. Administration of propranolol can reverse clinical symptoms of *thyrotoxicosis* within 4 days. Routine tests of increased thyroid function remain unaltered. The thyroid gland is rendered less vascular thus making surgery easier (section 6.2.2).

OTHER USES. Beta-blockers have been used to alleviate some symptoms of *anxiety*; probably patients with palpitations, tremor, and tachycardia respond best (see also section 4.1.2 and section 4.9.3). Beta-blockers are also used in the *prophylaxis of migraine* (section 4.7.4.2). Betaxolol, carteolol, levobunolol, metipranolol and timolol are used topically in *glaucoma* (section 11.6).

PROPRANOLOL HYDROCHLORIDE

Indications: see under Dose

Cautions: pregnancy and breast-feeding (see also Appendixes 4 and 5); avoid abrupt withdrawal in angina; first-degree AV block; reduce oral dose of propranolol in liver disease; liver function deteriorates in portal hypertension; reduce initial dose in renal impairment; diabetes; myasthenia gravis; history of hypersensitivity—may increase sensitivity to allergens and result in more serious hypersensitivity response, also may reduce response to adrenaline (epinephrine) (see also section 3.4.3); see also notes above; **interactions:** Appendix 1 (beta-blockers), **important:** verapamil interaction, see also p. 105

Contra-indications: asthma or history of obstructive airways disease (**important: see Bronchospasm** below); uncontrolled heart failure, Prinzmetal's angina, marked bradycardia, hypotension, sick sinus syndrome, second- or third-degree AV block, cardiogenic shock, metabolic acidosis, severe peripheral arterial disease; phaeochromocytoma (apart from specific use with alpha-blockers, see also notes above)

BRONCHOSPASM. The CSM has advised that beta-blockers, including those considered to be cardioselective, should not be given to patients with a history of asthma or bronchospasm. However, in these patients there are very rare situations where there is no alternative to the use of a beta-blocker, when a cardioselective one is given with extreme caution and under specialist supervision

Side-effects: bradycardia, heart failure, hypotension, conduction disorders, bronchospasm, peripheral vasoconstriction (including exacerbation of intermittent claudication and Raynaud's phenomenon), gastro-intestinal disturbances, fatigue, sleep disturbances; rare reports of rashes and dry eyes (reversible on withdrawal), exacerbation of psoriasis; see also notes above; **overdosage:** see Emergency Treatment of Poisoning, p. 23

Dose: *by mouth*, hypertension, initially 80 mg twice daily, increased at weekly intervals as required; maintenance 160–320 mg daily

Portal hypertension, initially 40 mg twice daily, increased to 80 mg twice daily according to heart-rate; max. 160 mg twice daily

Phaeochromocytoma (only with an alpha-blocker), 60 mg daily for 3 days before surgery *or* 30 mg daily in patients unsuitable for surgery

Angina, initially 40 mg 2–3 times daily; maintenance 120–240 mg daily

Arrhythmias, hypertrophic obstructive cardiomyopathy, anxiety tachycardia, and thyrotoxicosis (adjunct), 10–40 mg 3–4 times daily

Anxiety with symptoms such as palpitations, sweating, tremor, 40 mg once daily, increased to 40 mg 3 times daily if necessary

Prophylaxis after myocardial infarction, 40 mg 4

times daily for 2–3 days, then 80 mg twice daily, beginning 5 to 21 days after infarction

Migraine prophylaxis and essential tremor, initially 40 mg 2–3 times daily; maintenance 80–160 mg daily

By intravenous injection, arrhythmias and thyrotoxic crisis, 1 mg over 1 minute; if necessary repeat at 2-minute intervals; max. 10 mg (5 mg in anaesthesia)

Note. Excessive bradycardia can be countered with intravenous injection of atropine sulphate 0.6–2.4 mg in divided doses of 600 micrograms; for **overdosage** see Emergency Treatment of Poisoning, p. 23

Propranolol (Non-proprietary) PoM

Tablets, propranolol hydrochloride 10 mg, net price 20 = 8p; 40 mg, 20 = 10p; 80 mg, 20 = 23p 160 mg, 20 = 43p. Label: 8

Available from APS (*Apsolol®*), Ashbourne (*Propanix®*), Berk (*Berkolol®*), Cox, CP (*Cardinol®*), DDSA (*Angilol®*), Hillcross

Oral solution (syrup), propranolol hydrochloride 5 mg/5 mL, 10 mg/5 mL, 40 mg/5 ml, 50 mg/5 ml and 80 mg/5 mL available from Rosemont (special order)

Inderal® (Zeneca) PoM

Tablets, all pink, f/c, propranolol hydrochloride 10 mg, net price 100-tab pack = 89p; 40 mg, 100-tab pack = £2.40; 80 mg, 60-tab pack = £2.35. Label: 8

Injection, propranolol hydrochloride 1 mg/mL, net price 1-mL amp = 21p

■ Modified release

Half-Inderal LA® (Zeneca) PoM

Capsules, m/r, lavender/pink, propranolol hydrochloride 80 mg. Net price 28-cap pack = £5.40. Label: 8, 25

Note. Modified-release capsules containing propranolol hydrochloride 80 mg also available from APS, Tillomed (*Half Beta Prograne®*)

Inderal-LA® (Zeneca) PoM

Capsules, m/r, lavender/pink, propranolol hydrochloride 160 mg. Net price 28-cap pack = £6.67. Label: 8, 25

Note. Modified-release capsules containing propranolol hydrochloride 160 mg also available from APS, Ashbourne (*Propanix SR®*), Hillcross, Lagap (*Bedranol SR®*), Opus (*Lopranol LA®*), Tillomed (*Beta Prograne®*), Trinity (*Probeta LA®*)

■ With diuretic

Inderetic® (Zeneca) PoM

Capsules, propranolol hydrochloride 80 mg, bendroflumethiazide 2.5 mg. Net price 60-cap pack = £5.85. Label: 8

Dose: hypertension, 1 capsule twice daily

Inderex® (Zeneca) PoM

Capsules, pink/grey, propranolol hydrochloride 160 mg (m/r), bendroflumethiazide 5 mg. Net price 28-cap pack = £7.45. Label: 8, 25

Dose: hypertension, 1 capsule daily

ACEBUTOLOL

Indications: see under Dose

Cautions: see under Propranolol Hydrochloride

Contra-indications: see under Propranolol Hydrochloride

Side-effects: see under Propranolol Hydrochloride

Dose: hypertension, initially 400 mg once daily *or* 200 mg twice daily, increased after 2 weeks to 400 mg twice daily if necessary

Angina, initially 400 mg once daily *or* 200 mg twice daily; 300 mg 3 times daily in severe angina; up to 1.2 g daily has been used

Arrhythmias, 0.4–1.2 g daily in 2–3 divided doses

Sectral® (Akita) PoM

Capsules, acebutolol (as hydrochloride) 100 mg (buff/white), net price 84-cap pack = £16.10; 200 mg (buff/pink), 56-cap pack = £20.63. Label: 8

Tablets, f/c, acebutolol 400 mg (as hydrochloride). Net price 28-tab pack = £20.02. Label: 8

■ With diuretic

Secadrex® (Akita) PoM

Tablets, f/c, acebutolol 200 mg (as hydrochloride), hydrochlorothiazide 12.5 mg. Net price 28-tab pack = £18.91. Label: 8

Dose: hypertension, 1 tablet daily, increased to 2 daily as a single dose if necessary

ATENOLOL

Indications: see under Dose

Cautions: see under Propranolol Hydrochloride; reduce dose in renal impairment

Contra-indications: see under Propranolol Hydrochloride

Side-effects: see under Propranolol Hydrochloride

Dose: *by mouth,*

Hypertension, 50 mg daily (higher doses rarely necessary)

Angina, 100 mg daily in 1 or 2 doses

Arrhythmias, 50–100 mg daily

By intravenous injection, arrhythmias, 2.5 mg at a rate of 1 mg/minute, repeated at 5-minute intervals to a max. of 10 mg

Note. Excessive bradycardia can be countered with intravenous injection of atropine sulphate 0.6–2.4 mg in divided doses of 600 micrograms; for **overdosage** see Emergency Treatment of Poisoning, p. 23

By intravenous infusion, arrhythmias, 150 micrograms/kg over 20 minutes, repeated every 12 hours if required

Early intervention within 12 hours of myocardial infarction (section 2.10.1), *by intravenous injection* over 5 minutes, 5 mg, then *by mouth*, 50 mg after 15 minutes, 50 mg after 12 hours, then 100 mg daily

Atenolol (Non-proprietary) PoM

Tablets, atenolol 25 mg, net price 28-tab pack = £2.24; 50 mg, 28-tab pack = £1.59; 100 mg, 28-tab pack = £2.10. Label: 8

Various strengths available from Antigen, APS, Ashbourne (*Atenix®*), Berk (*Antipressan®*), Cox, CP, Hillcross, Norton, Tillomed

Tenormin® (Stuart) PoM

'25' tablets, f/c, atenolol 25 mg. Net price 28-tab pack = £4.41. Label: 8

LS tablets, orange, f/c, scored, atenolol 50 mg. Net price 28-tab pack = £5.11. Label: 8

Tablets, orange, f/c, scored, atenolol 100 mg. Net price 28-tab pack = £6.50. Label: 8

Syrup, sugar-free, atenolol 25 mg/5mL. Net price 300 mL = £7.77. Label: 8

Injection, atenolol 500 micrograms/mL. Net price 10-mL amp = 96p (hosp. only)

■ With diuretic

Co-tenidone (Non-proprietary) PoM
Tablets, co-tenidone 50/12.5 (atenolol 50 mg, chlortalidone 12.5 mg), net price 28-tab pack = £6.01; co-tenidone 100/25 (atenolol 100 mg, chlortalidone 25 mg), 28-tab pack = £7.72. Label: 8
Available from APS, Ashbourne (*AtenixCo*®), Berk (*Tenchlor*®), Bioglan, Cox, CP (*Totaretic*®), Hillcross, Norton
Dose: hypertension, 1 tablet daily (but see also under Dose above)

Kalten® (Stuart) PoM
Capsules, red/ivory, atenolol 50 mg, co-amilozide 2.5/25 (anhydrous amiloride hydrochloride 2.5 mg, hydrochlorothiazide 25 mg). Net price 28-cap pack = £8.39. Label: 8
Dose: hypertension, 1 capsule daily

Tenben® (Galen) PoM
Capsules, pink/red, atenolol 25 mg, bendroflumethiazide 1.25 mg, net price 56-cap pack = £4.95. Label: 8
Dose: hypertension, 1–2 capsules daily

Tenoret 50® (Stuart) PoM
Tablets, brown, f/c, co-tenidone 50/12.5 (atenolol 50 mg, chlortalidone 12.5 mg). Net price 28-tab pack = £5.70. Label: 8
Dose: hypertension, 1 tablet daily

Tenoretic® (Stuart) PoM
Tablets, brown, f/c, co-tenidone 100/25 (atenolol 100 mg, chlortalidone 25 mg). Net price 28-tab pack = £8.12. Label: 8
Dose: hypertension, 1 tablet daily (but see also under Dose above)

■ With calcium-channel blocker
Note. Only indicated when calcium-channel blocker or beta-blocker alone proves inadequate

Beta-Adalat® (Bayer) PoM
Capsules, reddish-brown, atenolol 50 mg, nifedipine 20 mg (m/r). Net price 28-cap pack = £10.41. Label: 8, 25
Dose: hypertension, 1 capsule daily, increased if necessary to twice daily; elderly, 1 daily
Angina, 1 capsule twice daily

Tenif® (Stuart) PoM
Capsules, reddish-brown, atenolol 50 mg, nifedipine 20 mg (m/r). Net price 28-cap pack = £10.63. Label: 8, 25
Dose: hypertension, 1 capsule daily, increased if necessary to twice daily; elderly, 1 daily
Angina, 1 capsule twice daily

BETAXOLOL HYDROCHLORIDE

Indications: hypertension; glaucoma (section 11.6)
Cautions: see under Propranolol Hydrochloride
Contra-indications: see under Propranolol Hydrochloride
Side-effects: see under Propranolol Hydrochloride
Dose: 20 mg daily (elderly patients 10 mg), increased to 40 mg if required

Kerlone® (Sanofi-Synthelabo) PoM
Tablets, f/c, scored, betaxolol hydrochloride 20 mg. Net price 28-tab pack = £7.51. Label: 8

BISOPROLOL FUMARATE

Indications: hypertension, angina
Cautions: see under Propranolol Hydrochloride; reduce dose in hepatic and renal impairment
Contra-indications: see under Propranolol Hydrochloride
Side-effects: see under Propranolol Hydrochloride
Dose: usual dose 10 mg daily (5 mg may be adequate in some patients); max. recommended dose 20 mg daily

Emcor® (Merck) PoM
LS Tablets, yellow, f/c, scored, bisoprolol fumarate 5 mg. Net price 28-tab pack = £8.56. Label: 8
Tablets, orange, f/c, scored, bisoprolol fumarate 10 mg. Net price 28-tab pack = £9.61. Label: 8

Monocor® (Lederle) PoM
Tablets, both f/c, bisoprolol fumarate 5 mg (pink), net price 28-tab pack = £8.56; 10 mg, 28-tab pack £9.61. Label: 8

■ With diuretic
Monozide 10® (Lederle) PoM
Tablets, f/c, bisoprolol fumarate 10 mg, hydrochlorothiazide 6.25 mg. Net price 28-tab pack = £11.20. Label: 8
Dose: hypertension, 1 tablet daily

CARVEDILOL

Indications: hypertension; angina; adjunct to diuretics, digoxin, or ACE inhibitors in symptomatic chronic heart failure (under hospital supervision)
Cautions: see under Propranolol Hydrochloride; hepatic impairment (Appendix 2); in heart failure monitor clinical status for 2–3 hours after initiation and after each dose increase; before increasing dose ensure renal function and heart failure not deteriorating; not to be initiated in severe heart failure
Contra-indications: see under Propranolol Hydrochloride
Side-effects: postural hypotension, dizziness, headache, fatigue, gastro-intestinal disturbances, bradycardia; occasionally diminished peripheral circulation, peripheral oedema and painful extremities, dry mouth, dry eyes, eye irritation or disturbed vision, impotence, disturbances of micturition, influenza-like symptoms; rarely angina, AV block, exacerbation of intermittent claudication or Raynaud's phenomenon; allergic skin reactions, exacerbation of psoriasis, nasal stuffiness, wheezing, depressed mood, sleep disturbances, paraesthesia, heart failure, changes in liver enzymes, thrombocytopenia, leucopenia also reported
Dose: hypertension, initially 12.5 mg once daily, increased after 2 days to usual dose of 25 mg once daily; if necessary may be further increased at intervals of at least 2 weeks to max. 50 mg daily in single or divided doses; ELDERLY initial dose of 12.5 mg daily may provide satisfactory control
Angina, initially 12.5 mg twice daily, increased after 2 days to 25 mg twice daily
Heart failure, initially 3.125 mg twice daily (with food), dose increased at intervals of at least 2 weeks to 6.25 mg twice daily, then to 12.5 mg twice daily, then to 25 mg twice daily; increase to highest dose tolerated, max. 25 mg twice daily in patients less than 85 kg body-weight and 50 mg twice daily in patients over 85 kg

Eucardic® (Roche) ▼ PoM
Tablets, all scored, carvedilol 3.125 mg (pink), net price 28-tab pack = £8.14; 6.25 mg (yellow), 28-tab pack = £9.04; 12.5 mg (peach), 28-tab pack = £10.05; 25 mg, 28-tab pack = £12.56. Label: 8

CELIPROLOL HYDROCHLORIDE

Indications: mild to moderate hypertension
Cautions: see under Propranolol Hydrochloride
Contra-indications: see under Propranolol Hydrochloride; also avoid in severe renal impairment
Side-effects: headache, dizziness, fatigue, nausea and somnolence; also bradycardia, bronchospasm; depression and pneumonitis reported rarely
Dose: 200 mg once daily in the morning, increased to 400 mg once daily if necessary

Celiprolol (Non-proprietary) PoM
Tablets, celiprolol hydrochloride 200 mg, net price 28-tab pack = £17.19; 400 mg, 28-tab pack = £34.38. Label 8, 22
Available from Generics, Norton

Celectol® (Pantheon) PoM
Tablets, both f/c, scored, celiprolol hydrochloride 200 mg (yellow), net price 28-tab pack = £17.19; 400 mg, 28-tab pack = £34.38. Label: 8, 22

ESMOLOL HYDROCHLORIDE

Indications: short-term treatment of supraventricular arrhythmias (including atrial fibrillation, atrial flutter, sinus tachycardia); tachycardia and hypertension in peri-operative period
Cautions: see under Propranolol Hydrochloride; renal impairment
Contra-indications: see under Propranolol Hydrochloride
Side-effects: see under Propranolol Hydrochloride
Dose: *by intravenous infusion*, usually within range 50–200 micrograms/kg/minute (consult product literature for details of dose titration and doses during peri-operative period)

Brevibloc® (Baxter) PoM
Injection, esmolol hydrochloride 10 mg/mL, net price 10-mL vial = £5.90
Injection concentrate, esmolol hydrochloride 250 mg/mL (for dilution before infusion), 10-mL amp = £65.90

LABETALOL HYDROCHLORIDE

Indications: hypertension (including hypertension in pregnancy, hypertension with angina, and hypertension following acute myocardial infarction); hypertensive crisis (but see section 2.5); controlled hypotension in anaesthesia
Cautions: see under Propranolol Hydrochloride; interferes with laboratory tests for catecholamines; liver damage (see below)
LIVER DAMAGE. Severe hepatocellular damage reported after both short-term and long-term treatment. Appropriate laboratory testing needed at first symptom of liver dysfunction and if laboratory evidence of damage (or if jaundice) labetalol should be stopped and not restarted
Contra-indications: see under Propranolol Hydrochloride
Side-effects: postural hypotension (avoid upright position during and for 3 hours after intravenous administration), tiredness, weakness, headache,

rashes, scalp tingling, difficulty in micturition, epigastric pain, nausea, vomiting; liver damage (see above); rarely lichenoid rash
Dose: *by mouth*, initially 100 mg (50 mg in elderly) twice daily with food, increased at intervals of 14 days to usual dose of 200 mg twice daily; up to 800 mg daily in 2 divided doses (3–4 divided doses if higher); max. 2.4 g daily
By intravenous injection, 50 mg over at least 1 minute, repeated after 5 minutes if necessary; max. 200 mg
Note. Excessive bradycardia can be countered with intravenous injection of atropine sulphate 0.6–2.4 mg in divided doses of 600 micrograms; for **overdosage** see Emergency Treatment of Poisoning, p. 23
By intravenous infusion, 2 mg/minute until satisfactory response then discontinue; usual total dose 50–200 mg, higher doses in phaeochromocytoma
Hypertension of pregnancy, 20 mg/hour, doubled every 30 minutes; usual max. 160 mg/hour
Hypertension following infarction, 15 mg/hour, gradually increased to max. 120 mg/hour

Labetalol Hydrochloride (Non-proprietary) PoM
Tablets, all f/c, labetalol hydrochloride 100 mg, net price 20 = £1.81; 200 mg, 20 = £2.39; 400 mg, 20 = £3.98. Label: 8, 21
Available from Cox, Hillcross, Norton

Trandate® (Medeva) PoM
Tablets, all orange, f/c, labetalol hydrochloride 50 mg, net price 56-tab pack. £5.05; 100 mg, 56-tab pack = £5.56; 200 mg, 56-tab pack = £9.02; 400 mg, 56-tab pack = £12.56. Label: 8, 21
Injection, labetalol hydrochloride 5 mg/mL. Net price 20-mL amp = £2.83

METOPROLOL TARTRATE

Indications: see under Dose
Cautions: see under Propranolol Hydrochloride; reduce dose in hepatic impairment
Contra-indications: see under Propranolol Hydrochloride
Side-effects: see under Propranolol Hydrochloride
Dose: *by mouth*, hypertension, initially 100 mg daily, maintenance 100–200 mg daily in 1–2 doses
Angina, 50–100 mg 2–3 times daily
Arrhythmias, usually 50 mg 2–3 times daily; up to 300 mg daily in divided doses if necessary
Migraine prophylaxis, 100–200 mg daily in divided doses
Thyrotoxicosis (adjunct), 50 mg 4 times daily
By intravenous injection, arrhythmias, up to 5 mg at rate 1–2 mg/minute, repeated after 5 minutes if necessary, total dose 10–15 mg
Note. Excessive bradycardia can be countered with intravenous injection of atropine sulphate 0.6–2.4 mg in divided doses of 600 micrograms; for **overdosage** see Emergency Treatment of Poisoning, p. 23
In surgery, 2–4 mg *by slow intravenous injection* at induction or to control arrhythmias developing during anaesthesia; 2-mg doses may be repeated to a max. of 10 mg
Early intervention within 12 hours of infarction, 5 mg *by intravenous injection* every 2 minutes to a max. of 15 mg, followed after 15 minutes by 50 mg *by mouth* every 6 hours for 48 hours; maintenance 200 mg daily in divided doses

Metoprolol Tartrate (Non-proprietary) PoM
Tablets, metoprolol tartrate 50 mg, net price 20 = 67p; 100 mg, 20 = £1.23. Label: 8
Available from APS, Ashbourne (*Mepranix*®), Cox, Hill-cross, Norton

Betaloc® (Astra) PoM
Tablets, both scored, metoprolol tartrate 50 mg, net price 100-tab pack = £3.30; 100 mg, 100-tab pack = £6.13. Label: 8
Injection, metoprolol tartrate 1 mg/mL. Net price 5-mL amp = 42p

Lopresor® (Novartis) PoM
Tablets, both f/c, scored, metoprolol tartrate 50 mg (pink), net price 56-tab pack = £2.57; 100 mg (blue), 56-tab pack = £6.68. Label: 8

■ Modified release

Betaloc-SA® (Astra) PoM
Durules® (= tablets, m/r), metoprolol tartrate 200 mg. Net price 28-tab pack = £4.56. Label: 8, 25
Dose: hypertension, angina, 200–400 mg daily; migraine prophylaxis, 200 mg daily

Lopresor SR® (Novartis) PoM
Tablets, m/r, yellow, f/c, metoprolol tartrate 200 mg. Net price 28-tab pack = £8.98. Label: 8, 25
Dose: hypertension, 200 mg daily; angina, 200–400 mg daily; migraine prophylaxis, 200 mg daily

■ With diuretic

Co-Betaloc® (Astra) PoM
Tablets, scored, metoprolol tartrate 100 mg, hydrochlorothiazide 12.5 mg. Net price 28-tab pack = £4.66. Label: 8
Dose: hypertension, 1–3 tablets daily in single or divided doses

Co-Betaloc SA® (Astra) PoM
Tablets, yellow, f/c, metoprolol tartrate (m/r) 200 mg, hydrochlorothiazide 25 mg. Net price 28-tab pack = £5.74. Label: 8, 25
Dose: hypertension, 1 tablet daily

NADOLOL

Indications: see under Dose
Cautions: see under Propranolol Hydrochloride; reduce dose in renal impairment
Contra-indications: see under Propranolol Hydrochloride
Side-effects: see under Propranolol Hydrochloride
Dose: hypertension, 80 mg daily, increased at weekly intervals if required; max. 240 mg daily
Angina, 40 mg daily, increased at weekly intervals if required; usual max. 160 mg daily
Arrhythmias, initially 40 mg daily, increased to 160 mg if required; reduce to 40 mg if brady-cardia occurs
Migraine prophylaxis, initially 40 mg daily, increased by 40 mg at weekly intervals; usual maintenance dose 80–160 mg daily
Thyrotoxicosis (adjunct), 80–160 mg daily

Corgard® (Sanofi-Synthelabo) PoM
Tablets, both blue, nadolol 40 mg, net price 28-tab pack = £3.76; 80 mg, 28-tab pack = £5.45. Label: 8

■ With diuretic

Corgaretic 40® (Sanofi-Synthelabo) PoM
Tablets, scored, nadolol 40 mg, bendroflumethi-azide 5 mg. Net price 28-tab pack = £5.92. Label: 8
Dose: hypertension, 1–2 tablets daily

Corgaretic 80® (Sanofi-Synthelabo) PoM
Tablets, scored, nadolol 80 mg, bendroflumethi-azide 5 mg. Net price 28-tab pack = £8.47. Label: 8
Dose: hypertension, 1–2 tablets daily

NEBIVOLOL

Indications: essential hypertension
Cautions: see under Propranolol Hydrochloride; reduce dose in renal impairment (Appendix 3); elderly
Contra-indications: see under Propranolol Hydrochloride; hepatic impairment
Side-effects: see under Propranolol Hydro-chloride; oedema, headache, depression, visual disturbances, paraesthesia, impotence
Dose: 5 mg daily; ELDERLY initially 2.5 mg daily, increased if necessary to 5 mg daily

Nebilet® (Menarini) ▼ PoM
Tablets, scored, nebivolol (as hydrochloride) 5 mg, net price 28-tab pack = £9.80

OXPRENOLOL HYDROCHLORIDE

Indications: see under Dose
Cautions: see under Propranolol Hydrochloride
Contra-indications: see under Propranolol Hydrochloride
Side-effects: see under Propranolol Hydrochloride
Dose: hypertension, 80–160 mg daily in 2–3 divided doses, increased as required; max. 320 mg daily
Angina, 80–160 mg daily in 2–3 divided doses; max. 320 mg daily
Arrhythmias, 40–240 mg daily in 2–3 divided doses; max. 240 mg daily
Anxiety symptoms (short-term use), 40–80 mg daily in 1–2 divided doses

Oxprenolol (Non-proprietary) PoM
Tablets, all coated, oxprenolol hydrochloride 20 mg, net price 20 = 46p; 40 mg, 20 = £1.25; 80 mg, 20 = £2.05; 160 mg, 20 = £2.36. Label: 8
Available from Hillcross, Norton

Trasicor® (Novartis) PoM
Tablets, all f/c, oxprenolol hydrochloride 20 mg (contain gluten), net price 56-tab pack = £1.29; 40 mg (contain gluten), 56-tab pack = £2.59; 80 mg (yellow), 56-tab pack = £5.17. Label: 8

■ Modified release

Slow-Trasicor® (Novartis) PoM
Tablets, m/r, f/c, oxprenolol hydrochloride 160 mg. Net price 28-tab pack = £6.08. Label: 8, 25
Dose: hypertension, angina, initially 160 mg once daily; if necessary may be increased to max. 320 mg daily
Note. Modified-release tablets containing oxprenolol hydrochloride 160 mg also available from Norton

■ With diuretic

Trasidrex® (Novartis) PoM
Tablets, red, s/c, co-prenozide 160/0.25 (oxprenolol hydrochloride 160 mg (m/r), cyclopenthiazide 250 micrograms). Net price 28-tab pack = £7.40. Label: 8, 25
Dose: hypertension, 1 tablet daily, increased if necessary to 2 daily as a single dose

PINDOLOL

Indications: see under Dose
Cautions: see under Propranolol Hydrochloride; reduce dose in renal impairment
Contra-indications: see under Propranolol Hydrochloride
Side-effects: see under Propranolol Hydrochloride
Dose: hypertension, initially 5 mg 2–3 times daily *or* 15 mg once daily, increased as required at weekly intervals; usual maintenance 15–30 mg daily; max. 45 mg daily
Angina, 2.5–5 mg up to 3 times daily

Visken® (Novartis) PoM
Tablets, both scored, pindolol 5 mg, net price 56-tab pack = £4.07; 15 mg, 28-tab pack = £6.10. Label: 8

■ With diuretic

Viskaldix® (Novartis) PoM
Tablets, scored, pindolol 10 mg, clopamide 5 mg. Net price 28-tab pack = £5.58. Label: 8
Dose: hypertension, 1 tablet daily in the morning, increased if necessary to 2 daily; max. 3 daily

SOTALOL HYDROCHLORIDE

Indications: *Tablets and injection:* life-threatening arrhythmias including ventricular tachyarrhythmias, symptomatic non-sustained ventricular tachyarrhythmias
Tablets only: prophylaxis of paroxysmal atrial tachycardia or fibrillation, paroxysmal AV re-entrant tachycardias (both nodal and involving accessory pathways), paroxysmal supraventricular tachycardia after cardiac surgery, maintenance of sinus rhythm following cardioversion of atrial fibrillation or flutter
Injection only: electrophysiological study of inducible ventricular and supraventricular arrhythmias; temporary substitution for tablets
CSM advice. The use of sotalol should be limited to the treatment of ventricular arrhythmias or prophylaxis of supraventricular arrhythmias (see above). It should no longer be used for angina, hypertension, thyrotoxicosis or for secondary prevention after myocardial infarction; when stopping sotalol for these indications, the dose should be reduced gradually
Cautions: see under Propranolol Hydrochloride; reduce dose in renal impairment (avoid if severe); correct hypokalaemia, hypomagnesaemia, or other electrolyte disturbances; severe or prolonged diarrhoea; **interactions:** Appendix 1 (beta-blockers), **important:** verapamil interaction see also p. 105
Contra-indications: see under Propranolol Hydrochloride; congenital or acquired long QT syndrome; torsades de pointes; renal failure
Side-effects: see under Propranolol Hydrochloride; arrhythmogenic (pro-arrhythmic) effect (torsades de pointes—increased risk in women)

Dose: *by mouth* with ECG monitoring and measurement of corrected QT interval, arrhythmias, initially 80 mg daily in 1–2 divided doses increased gradually at intervals of 2–3 days to usual dose of 160–320 mg daily in 2 divided doses; higher doses of 480–640 mg daily for life-threatening ventricular arrhythmias under specialist supervision
By intravenous injection over 10 minutes, acute arrhythmias, 20–120 mg with ECG monitoring, repeated if necessary with 6-hour intervals between injections
Diagnostic use, see product literature
Note. Excessive bradycardia can be countered with intravenous injection of atropine sulphate 0.6–2.4 mg in divided doses of 600 micrograms; for **overdosage** see Emergency Treatment of Poisoning, p. 23

Sotalol (Non-proprietary) PoM
Tablets, both scored, sotalol hydrochloride 80 mg, net price 28-tab pack = £1.64; 160 mg, 28-tab pack = £6.37. Label: 8
Available from Generics, Hillcross
Beta-Cardone® (Medeva) PoM
Tablets, all scored, sotalol hydrochloride 40 mg (green), net price 100-tab pack = £3.96; 80 mg (pink), 100-tab pack = £5.87; 200 mg, 30-tab pack = £4.15. Label: 8
Sotacor® (Bristol-Myers) PoM
Tablets, sotalol hydrochloride 80 mg, net price 28-tab pack = £3.49; 160 mg, 28-tab pack = £6.89. Label: 8
Injection, sotalol hydrochloride 10 mg/mL. Net price 4-mL amp = £1.76

TIMOLOL MALEATE

Indications: see under Dose; glaucoma (section 11.6)
Cautions: see under Propranolol Hydrochloride
Contra-indications: see under Propranolol Hydrochloride
Side-effects: see under Propranolol Hydrochloride
Dose: hypertension, initially 5 mg twice daily *or* 10 mg once daily; gradually increased if necessary to max. 60 mg daily (given in divided doses above 20 mg daily)
Angina, initially 5 mg 2–3 times daily, usual maintenance 35–45 mg daily (range 15–45 mg daily)
Prophylaxis after myocardial infarction, initially 5 mg twice daily, increased after 2 days to 10 mg twice daily, starting 7 to 28 days after infarction
Migraine prophylaxis, 10–20 mg once daily

Betim® (Leo) PoM
Tablets, scored, timolol maleate 10 mg. Net price 30-tab pack = £2.45. Label: 8

■ With diuretic

Moducren® (MSD) PoM
Tablets, blue, scored, timolol maleate 10 mg, co-amilozide 2.5/25 (amiloride hydrochloride 2.5 mg, hydrochlorothiazide 25 mg). Net price 28-tab pack = £8.00. Label: 8
Dose: hypertension, 1–2 tablets daily as a single dose
Prestim® (Leo) PoM
Tablets, scored, timolol maleate 10 mg, bendroflumethiazide 2.5 mg. Net price 30-tab pack = £4.11. Label: 8
Dose: hypertension, 1–2 tablets daily; max. 4 daily

2.5 Drugs affecting the renin-angiotensin system and some other antihypertensive drugs

Lowering raised blood pressure decreases the frequency of stroke, coronary events, heart failure, and renal failure. Advice on antihypertensive therapy in this section reflects the recommendations of the British Hypertension Society (Guidelines for management of hypertension: report of the third working party of the British Hypertension Society. *J Hum Hypertens* 1999; **13**: 569–92).

Possible causes of hypertension (e.g. renal disease, endocrine causes), contributory factors, risk factors, and the presence of any complications of hypertension, such as left ventricular hypertrophy, should be established. Patients should be given advice on lifestyle changes to reduce blood pressure or cardiovascular risk; these include smoking cessation, weight reduction, reduction of alcohol intake, reduction of dietary sodium, reduction of total and saturated fat, increasing exercise, and increasing fruit and vegetable intake.

THRESHOLDS AND TARGETS FOR TREATMENT. The following thresholds for treatment are recommended:

- Accelerated (malignant) hypertension (with papilloedema or fundal haemorrhages and exudates) *or* impending cardiovascular complications, admit for **immediate treatment**;
- Where the initial blood pressure is systolic ≥ 220 mmHg *or* diastolic ≥ 120 mmHg, **treat immediately**;
- Where the initial blood pressure is systolic 200–219 mmHg *or* diastolic 110–119 mmHg, confirm over 1–2 weeks then **treat** if these values are sustained;
- Where the initial blood pressure is systolic 160–199 mmHg *or* diastolic 100–109 mmHg, *and* the patient has cardiovascular complications, end-organ damage (e.g. left ventricular hypertrophy, renal impairment) or diabetes mellitus (type 1 or 2), confirm over 3–4 weeks then **treat** if these values are sustained;
- Where the initial blood pressure is systolic 160–199 mmHg *or* diastolic 100–109 mmHg, but *no* cardiovascular complications, end-organ damage or diabetes, advise lifestyle changes, reassess weekly initially and **treat** if these values are sustained on repeat measurements over 4–12 weeks;
- Where the initial blood pressure is systolic 140–159 mmHg *or* diastolic 90–99 mmHg *and* the patient has cardiovascular complications, end-organ damage or diabetes, confirm within 4–12 weeks and **treat** if these values are sustained;

- Where the initial blood pressure is systolic 140–159 mmHg *or* diastolic 90–99 mmHg and *no* cardiovascular complications, end-organ damage or diabetes, advise lifestyle changes and **reassess** monthly; if mild hypertension persists, **treat** if coronary heart disease risk[1] is ≥ 15% over 10 years.

An optimal target systolic blood pressure < 140 mmHg *and* diastolic blood pressure < 85 mmHg is suggested; the target in diabetes and in renal disease is lower—see below.

DRUG TREATMENT OF HYPERTENSION. Low-dose *thiazides* (section 2.2.1) reduce coronary events, cardiovascular mortality and all-cause mortality. A thiazide is first-line treatment for hypertension unless there is a contra-indication or a compelling indication for another drug (see below). A low dose is adequate and higher doses (e.g. more than 2.5 mg bendroflumethiazide (bendrofluazide) or 25 mg hydrochlorthiazide) have no additional antihypertensive effect and increase metabolic side-effects.

In the majority of people with hypertension, a low-dose thiazide or a beta-blocker is preferred as first-line therapy; however, in some individuals there may be contra-indications to these drugs or compelling indications for other antihypertensive drugs. No consistent or important differences have been found between the major classes of antihypertensive drugs in terms of antihypertensive efficacy, side-effects or changes to quality of life (although there have been differences in average response related to age and ethnic group). The choice of antihypertensive drug will depend on the relevant indications or contra-indications for the individual patient; where there are no special considerations, the least expensive drug should be selected. *Some* compelling indications and contra-indications for various antihypertensive drugs are shown below (see also under individual drug entries for details):

- **Thiazides** (section 2.2.1)—a compelling *indication* is hypertension in the elderly (see below); a compelling *contra-indication* is gout;
- **Beta-blockers** (section 2.4)—compelling *indications* include myocardial infarction, angina; compelling *contra-indications* include asthma, chronic obstructive pulmonary disease, heart block;
- **ACE inhibitors** (section 2.5.5.1)—compelling *indications* include heart failure, left ventricular dysfunction and diabetic nephropathy; compelling *contra-indications* include renovascular disease (but see section 2.5.5.1) and pregnancy;
- **Calcium-channel blockers**. There are important differences between calcium-channel blockers (section 2.6.2). For **dihydropyridine calcium-channel blockers** a compelling *indication* is isolated systolic hypertension in the elderly when a low-dose thiazide is contra-indicated or not tolerated (see below). For **'rate-limiting' calcium-channel blockers** (e.g. diltiazem, verapamil) a compelling *indication* is angina; compelling *contra-indications* include heart failure and heart block;
- **Alpha-blockers** (section 2.5.4)—a compelling *indication* is prostatism; a compelling *contra-indication* is urinary incontinence;
- **Angiotensin-II receptor antagonists** (section 2.5.5.2) are alternatives for those who cannot tolerate ACE inhibitors because of persistent dry cough, but they have the same compelling *contra-indications* as ACE inhibitors.

---

1. Coronary heart disease risk may be formally estimated using the Joint British Societies' 'Cardiac Risk Assessor' computer program or chart (British Cardiac Society, British Hyperlipidaemia Association, British Hypertension Society. *Heart* 1998; **80**(suppl 2): S1–29)

A single antihypertensive drug is often not adequate and other antihypertensive drugs are usually added in a step-wise manner until control is achieved. Unless it is necessary to lower the blood pressure urgently, an interval of at least 4 weeks should be allowed to determine response. In uncomplicated mild hypertension (systolic blood pressure < 160 mmHg and diastolic < 100 mmHg), drugs may be substituted rather than added.

Response to drug treatment for hypertension may be affected by the patient's ethnic background; in Afro-Caribbean subjects the response to beta-blockers and to ACE inhibitors may be reduced.

OTHER MEASURES TO REDUCE CARDIOVAS-CULAR RISK. **Aspirin** (section 2.9) in a dose of 75 mg daily prevents cardiovascular events and myocardial infarction; however, concerns about an increased risk of bleeding need to be considered. Unless it is contra-indicated, aspirin is recommended for *secondary prevention* in patients with cardiovascular complications (myocardial infarction, angina, non-haemorrhagic cerebrovascular disease, peripheral vascular disease, or atherosclerotic renovascular disease), and for *primary prevention* in patients aged over 50 years with controlled blood pressure (systolic pressure < 150 mmHg and diastolic pressure < 90 mmHg) who have end-organ damage, type 2 diabetes, or a coronary heart disease risk ≥ 15% over 10 years.

A **statin** (section 2.12) is indicated when serum total cholesterol concentration is ≥ 5 mmol/litre, for *secondary prevention* (in patients with a history of myocardial infarction, coronary artery bypass graft, angioplasty, non-haemorrhagic cerebrovascular disease, peripheral vascular disease or atherosclerotic renovascular disease), for *primary prevention* in patients who have a coronary heart disease risk of ≥ 30% over 10 years, and for *familial hypercholesterolaemia*.

HYPERTENSION IN THE ELDERLY. Benefit from antihypertensive therapy is evident up to at least 85 years of age, but it is probably inappropriate to apply a strict age limit when deciding on drug therapy. Elderly subjects who have a good outlook for longevity should have their blood pressure lowered if they are hypertensive. The thresholds for treatment are diastolic pressure averaging ≥ 90 mmHg *or* systolic pressure averaging ≥ 160 mmHg over 3 to 6 months' observation (despite appropriate non-drug treatment). A low dose of a thiazide is the clear drug of first choice, with addition of a beta-blocker when necessary.

ISOLATED SYSTOLIC HYPERTENSION. Isolated systolic hypertension (systolic pressure ≥ 160 mmHg, diastolic pressure < 90 mmHg) is associated with an increased risk of stroke and coronary events, particularly in those aged over 60 years. Systolic blood pressure averaging 160 mmHg or higher over 3 to 6 months (despite appropriate non-drug treatment) should be lowered in those over 60 years, even if diastolic hypertension is absent. Treatment with a low dose of a thiazide, with addition of a beta-blocker when necessary is effective; a long-acting dihydropyridine calcium-channel blocker is recommended when a thiazide is contra-indicated or not tolerated. Patients with severe postural hypotension should not receive blood pressure lowering drugs.

Isolated systolic hypertension in younger patients is uncommon but treatment may be indicated in those with a threshold systolic pressure of 160 mmHg (or less if at increased risk of coronary heart disease, see above).

HYPERTENSION IN DIABETES. Hypertension is common in type 2 (non-insulin-dependent) diabetes and treatment prevents both macrovascular and microvascular complications. Systolic blood pressure ≥ 140 mmHg *or* diastolic pressure ≥ 90 mmHg should be lowered to a target systolic blood pressure < 140 mmHg and a diastolic pressure < 80 mmHg. Low-dose thiazides, beta-blockers, ACE inhibitors and dihydropyridine calcium-channel blockers have all shown benefit in type 2 diabetes.

In type 1 (insulin-dependent) diabetes, hypertension usually indicates the presence of diabetic nephropathy and ACE inhibitors have a specific role in this condition (section 6.1.5). The threshold for treatment of hypertension in type 1 diabetes is the same as that for type 2 diabetes, and the target for patients without nephropathy is a systolic blood pressure < 140 mmHg and a diastolic pressure < 80 mmHg; if nephropathy is present the target is a systolic blood pressure < 130 mmHg and a diastolic pressure < 80 mmHg, or even lower if proteinuria exceeds 1 g in 24 hours.

HYPERTENSION IN RENAL DISEASE. The threshold for antihypertensive treatment in patients with renal impairment or persistent proteinuria is a systolic blood pressure ≥ 140 mmHg *or* a diastolic blood pressure ≥ 90 mmHg. Optimal blood pressure is a systolic blood pressure < 130 mmHg and a diastolic pressure < 85 mmHg, or lower if proteinuria exceeds 1 g in 24 hours. Thiazides may be ineffective and high doses of loop diuretics may be required. Specific cautions apply to the use of ACE inhibitors in renal impairment, see section 2.5.5.1.

HYPERTENSION IN PREGNANCY. High blood pressure in pregnancy may be due to pre-existing essential hypertension or to pre-eclampsia. Oral methyldopa is safe in pregnancy. Beta-blockers are effective and safe in the third trimester but may cause intra-uterine growth restriction when used earlier. Modified-release preparations of nifedipine are also used for hypertension in pregnancy. Intravenous administration of hydralazine or of labetalol can be used to control hypertensive crises. For use of magnesium sulphate in eclampsia, see section 9.5.1.3.

ACCELERATED OR VERY SEVERE HYPERTENSION. Accelerated (or malignant) hypertension or very severe hypertension (e.g. diastolic blood pressure > 140 mmHg) requires urgent treatment in hospital but it is not an indication for parenteral antihypertensive therapy. Normally treatment should be by mouth with a beta-blocker (atenolol or labetalol) or a long-acting calcium-channel blocker (e.g. amlodipine or modified-release nifedipine). Within the first 24 hours the diastolic blood pressure should be reduced to 100–110 mmHg. Over the next 2 or 3 days blood pressure should be normalised by using beta-blockers, calcium-channel blockers, diuretics, vasodilators, or ACE inhibitors. Very rapid reduction in blood pressure can reduce organ perfusion leading to cerebral infarction and blindness, deterioration in renal function, and myocardial ischaemia. Parenteral antihypertensive drugs are rarely necessary; sodium nitroprusside by infusion is the drug of choice on the rare occasions when parenteral treatment is necessary.

2.5.1   Vasodilator antihypertensive drugs

These are potent drugs, especially when used in combination with a beta-blocker and a thiazide. **Important:** for a warning on the hazards of a very rapid fall in blood pressure, see section 2.5.

Diazoxide has been used by intravenous injection in hypertensive emergencies.

Hydralazine given by mouth is a useful adjunct to other treatment, but when used alone causes tachycardia and fluid retention. Side-effects can be few if the dose is kept below 100 mg daily, but systemic lupus erythematosus should be suspected if there is unexplained weight loss, arthritis, or any other unexplained ill health.

Sodium nitroprusside is given by intravenous infusion to control severe hypertensive crises on the rare occasions when parenteral treatment is necessary.

Minoxidil should be reserved for the treatment of severe hypertension resistant to other drugs. Vasodilatation is accompanied by increased cardiac output and tachycardia and the patients develop fluid retention. For this reason a beta-blocker and a diuretic (usually furosemide, in high dosage) are mandatory. Hypertrichosis is troublesome and renders this drug unsuitable for women.

Prazosin, doxazosin, and terazosin (section 2.5.4) have alpha-blocking and vasodilator properties.

DIAZOXIDE

Indications: severe hypertension associated with renal disease (but see section 2.5); hypoglycaemia (section 6.1.4)

Cautions: ischaemic heart disease, pregnancy, labour, impaired renal function; **interactions:** Appendix 1 (diazoxide)

Side-effects: tachycardia, hyperglycaemia, sodium and water retention

Dose: *by rapid intravenous injection* (less than 30 seconds), 1–3 mg/kg to max. single dose of 150 mg (see below); may be repeated after 5–15 minutes if required

Note. Single doses of 300 mg have been associated with angina and with myocardial and cerebral infarction

Eudemine® (Goldshield) [PoM]
Injection, diazoxide 15 mg/mL. Net price 20-mL amp = £30.00

 denotes preparations that are considered to be less suitable for prescribing (see p. vi)

HYDRALAZINE HYDROCHLORIDE

Indications: moderate to severe hypertension (adjunct); heart failure (with long-acting nitrate, but see section 2.5.5); hypertensive crisis (but see section 2.5)

Cautions: hepatic impairment (Appendix 2), renal impairment (Appendix 3); coronary artery disease (may provoke angina, avoid after myocardial infarction until stabilised), cerebrovascular disease; check acetylator status before increasing dose above 100 mg daily (consult product literature); occasionally over-rapid blood pressure reduction even with low parenteral doses; pregnancy (Appendix 4), breast-feeding; **interactions:** Appendix 1 (hydralazine)

Contra-indications: idiopathic systemic lupus erythematosus, severe tachycardia, high output heart failure, myocardial insufficiency due to mechanical obstruction, cor pulmonale, dissecting aortic aneurysm; porphyria (section 9.8.2)

Side-effects: tachycardia, palpitations, flushing, hypotension, fluid retention, gastro-intestinal disturbances; headache, dizziness; systemic lupus erythematosus-like syndrome after long-term therapy with over 100 mg daily (or less in women and in slow acetylator individuals) (see also notes above); rarely rashes, fever, peripheral neuritis, polyneuritis, paraesthesia, arthralgia, myalgia, increased lacrimation, nasal congestion, dyspnoea, agitation, anxiety, anorexia; blood disorders (including leucopenia, thrombocytopenia, haemolytic anaemia), abnormal liver function, jaundice, raised plasma creatinine, proteinuria and haematuria reported

Dose: *by mouth,* hypertension, 25 mg twice daily, increased to usual max. 50 mg twice daily (see notes above)

Heart failure (initiated in hospital) 25 mg 3–4 times daily, increased every 2 days if necessary; usual maintenance dose 50–75 mg 4 times daily

By slow intravenous injection, hypertension with renal complications and hypertensive crisis, 5–10 mg diluted with 10 mL sodium chloride 0.9%; may be repeated after 20–30 minutes (see Cautions)

By intravenous infusion, hypertension with renal complications and hypertensive crisis, initially 200–300 micrograms/minute; maintenance usually 50–150 micrograms/minute

Hydralazine (Non-proprietary) [PoM]
Tablets, hydralazine hydrochloride 25 mg, net price 20 = 48p; 50 mg, 20 = 76p

Apresoline® (Alliance) [PoM]
Tablets, yellow, s/c, hydralazine hydrochloride 25 mg, net price 84-tab pack = £2.35
Excipients: include gluten
Injection, powder for reconstitution, hydralazine hydrochloride. Net price 20-mg amp = £1.54

MINOXIDIL

Indications: severe hypertension, in addition to a diuretic and a beta-blocker

Cautions: see notes above; angina; after myocardial infarction (until stabilised); lower doses in dialysis patients; pregnancy; porphyria (section 9.8.2); **interactions:** Appendix 1 (minoxidil)

Contra-indications: phaeochromocytoma

Side-effects: sodium and water retention; weight gain, peripheral oedema, tachycardia, hypertrichosis; reversible rise in creatinine and blood urea nitrogen; occasionally, gastro-intestinal disturbances, breast tenderness, rashes

Dose: initially 5 mg (elderly, 2.5 mg) daily, in 1–2 doses, increased by 5–10 mg every 3 or more days; max. usually 50 mg daily

Loniten® (Pharmacia & Upjohn) PoM
Tablets, all scored, minoxidil 2.5 mg, net price 100-tab pack = £11.78; 5 mg, 100-tab pack = £20.99; 10 mg, 100-tab pack = £40.70

SODIUM NITROPRUSSIDE

Indications: hypertensive crisis (but see section 2.5); controlled hypotension in anaesthesia; acute or chronic heart failure

Cautions: hypothyroidism, renal impairment, hyponatraemia, ischaemic heart disease, impaired cerebral circulation, elderly; hypothermia; monitor blood pressure and blood-cyanide concentration and if treatment exceeds 3 days, also blood-thiocyanate concentration; avoid sudden withdrawal—terminate infusion over 15–30 minutes; pregnancy and breast-feeding; **interactions:** Appendix 1 (nitroprusside)

Contra-indications: severe hepatic impairment; severe vitamin B$_{12}$ deficiency; Leber's optic atrophy; compensatory hypertension

Side-effects: associated with over rapid reduction in blood pressure (reduce infusion rate): headache, dizziness, nausea, retching, abdominal pain, perspiration, palpitations, apprehension, retrosternal discomfort; occasionally reduced platelet count, acute transient phlebitis

CYANIDE. Side-effects caused by excessive plasma concentration of the cyanide metabolite include tachycardia, sweating, hyperventilation, arrhythmias, marked metabolic acidosis (discontinue and give antidote, see p. 25)

Dose: hypertensive crisis, *by intravenous infusion*, initially 0.5–1.5 micrograms/kg/minute, then adjusted by increments of 0.5 micrograms/kg/minute every 5 minutes within range 0.5–8 micrograms/kg/minute (lower doses in patients already receiving other antihypertensives); stop if marked response not obtained with max. dose in 10 minutes

Note. Lower initial dose of 0.3 micrograms/kg/minute has been used

Maintenance of blood pressure at 30–40% lower than pretreatment diastolic blood pressure, 20–400 micrograms/minute (lower doses for patients being treated with other antihypertensives)

Controlled hypotension in surgery, *by intravenous infusion*, max. 1.5 micrograms/kg/minute

Heart failure, *by intravenous infusion*, initially 10–15 micrograms/minute, increased every 5–10 minutes as necessary; usual range 10–200 micrograms/minute normally for max. 3 days

Sodium Nitroprusside (Non-proprietary) PoM
Intravenous solution, sodium nitroprusside 10 mg/mL. For dilution and use as an infusion, net price 5-mL vial = £6.64
Available from Faulding DBL

2.5.2

2.5.2 Centrally acting antihypertensive drugs

This group includes **methyldopa**, which has the advantage of being safe in asthmatics, in heart failure, and in pregnancy. Side-effects are minimised if the daily dose is kept below 1 g.

Clonidine has the disadvantage that sudden withdrawal may cause a hypertensive crisis. Reserpine and rauwolfia are no longer used in Britain.

Moxonidine, a centrally acting drug, has been introduced recently for mild to moderate essential hypertension. It may have a role when thiazides, beta-blockers, ACE inhibitors and calcium-channel blockers are not appropriate or have failed to control blood pressure.

CLONIDINE HYDROCHLORIDE

Indications: hypertension; migraine (section 4.7.4.2)

Cautions: must be withdrawn gradually to avoid hypertensive crisis; Raynaud's syndrome or other occlusive peripheral vascular disease; history of depression; avoid in porphyria (section 9.8.2); **interactions:** Appendix 1 (clonidine)

DRIVING. Drowsiness may affect performance of skilled tasks (e.g. driving); effects of alcohol may be enhanced

Side-effects: dry mouth, sedation, depression, fluid retention, bradycardia, Raynaud's phenomenon, headache, dizziness, euphoria, nocturnal unrest, rash, nausea, constipation, rarely impotence

Dose: *by mouth*, 50–100 micrograms 3 times daily, increased every second or third day; usual max. dose 1.2 mg daily

By slow intravenous injection, 150–300 micrograms; max. 750 micrograms in 24 hours

Catapres® (Boehringer Ingelheim) PoM
Tablets, both scored, clonidine hydrochloride 100 micrograms, net price 100-tab pack = £5.60; 300 micrograms, 100-tab pack = £13.04. Label: 3, 8
Injection, clonidine hydrochloride 150 micrograms/mL. Net price 1-mL amp = 29p
Dixarit® PoM (migraine), section 4.7.4.2

■ Modified release
Catapres® Perlongets (Boehringer Ingelheim) PoM
Capsules, m/r, red/yellow, clonidine hydrochloride 250 micrograms. Net price 56-cap pack = £11.11. Label: 3, 8, 25
Dose: usually 1 capsule in the evening; 2–3 capsules daily (1 morning and 1–2 evening) if necessary

denotes preparations that are considered to be less suitable for prescribing (see p. vi)

METHYLDOPA

Indications: hypertension; hypertensive crisis when immediate effect not necessary

Cautions: history of liver impairment (Appendix 2); renal impairment (Appendix 3); blood counts and liver-function tests advised; history of depression; positive direct Coombs' test in up to 20% of patients (may affect blood cross-matching); interference with laboratory tests; **interactions:** Appendix 1 (methyldopa)

DRIVING. Drowsiness may affect performance of skilled tasks (e.g. driving); effects of alcohol may be enhanced

ASTHMA. Presence of sulphites in ampoules may (especially in patients with asthma) lead to hypersensitivity (with bronchospasm and shock)

Contra-indications: depression, active liver disease, phaeochromocytoma; porphyria (section 9.8.2)

Side-effects: gastro-intestinal disturbances, dry mouth, stomatitis, sialadenitis; bradycardia, exacerbation of angina, postural hypotension, oedema; sedation, headache, dizziness, asthenia, myalgia, arthralgia, paraesthesia, nightmares, mild psychosis, depression, impaired mental acuity, parkinsonism, Bell's palsy; abnormal liver function tests, hepatitis, jaundice; pancreatitis; haemolytic anaemia; bone-marrow depression, leucopenia, thrombocytopenia, eosinophilia; hypersensitivity reactions including lupus erythematosus-like syndrome, drug fever, myocarditis, pericarditis; rashes (including toxic epidermal necrolysis); nasal congestion, failure of ejaculation, impotence, decreased libido, gynaecomastia, hyperprolactinaemia, amenorrhoea

Dose: *by mouth*, 250 mg 2–3 times daily, gradually increased at intervals of 2 or more days; max. dose 3 g daily; ELDERLY initially 125 mg twice daily, increased gradually; max. 2 g daily

By intravenous infusion, methyldopate hydrochloride 250–500 mg (in severe cases up to 1 g) every 6 hours if required

Methyldopa (Non-proprietary) PoM
Tablets, coated, methyldopa (anhydrous) 125 mg, net price 20 = 47p; 250 mg, 20 = 61p; 500 mg, 20 = £1.18. Label: 3, 8
Available from Cox, CP, Hillcross, Norton, Sovereign

Aldomet® (MSD) PoM
Tablets, all yellow, f/c, methyldopa (anhydrous) 125 mg, net price 20 = 34p; 250 mg, 20 = 63p; 500 mg, 20 = £1.27. Label: 3, 8
Injection, methyldopa hydrochloride 50 mg/mL. Net price 5-mL amp = £2.31

MOXONIDINE

Indications: mild to moderate essential hypertension

Cautions: renal impairment (see Appendix 3); avoid abrupt withdrawal (if concomitant treatment with beta-blocker has to be stopped, discontinue beta-blocker first, then moxonidine after few days); **interactions:** see Appendix 1 (moxonidine)

Contra-indications: history of angioedema; conduction disorders (sick sinus syndrome, sinoatrial block, second- or third-degree AV block); bradycardia; life-threatening arrhythmia; severe heart failure; severe coronary artery disease, unstable angina; severe liver disease or severe renal impairment; also on theoretical grounds: Raynaud's syndrome, intermittent claudication, epilepsy, depression, Parkinson's disease, glaucoma; pregnancy and breast-feeding

Side-effects: dry mouth; headache, fatigue, dizziness, nausea, sleep disturbance (rarely sedation), asthenia, vasodilatation; rarely skin reactions

Dose: 200 micrograms once daily in the morning, increased if necessary after 3 weeks to 400 micrograms daily in 1–2 divided doses; max. 600 micrograms daily in 2 divided doses (max. single dose 400 micrograms)

Physiotens® (Solvay) ▼ PoM
Tablets, f/c, moxonidine 200 micrograms (pink), net price 28-tab pack = £10.45; 400 micrograms (red), 28-tab pack = £14.26. Label: 3

2.5.3   Adrenergic neurone blocking drugs

Adrenergic neurone blocking drugs prevent the release of noradrenaline (norepinephrine) from postganglionic adrenergic neurones. Guanethidine also depletes the nerve endings of noradrenaline. These drugs do not control supine blood pressure and may cause postural hypotension. For this reason they have largely fallen from use, but may be necessary with other therapy in resistant hypertension.

GUANETHIDINE MONOSULPHATE

Indications: hypertensive crisis (but see section 2.5)

Cautions: postural hypotension may cause falls in elderly; coronary or cerebral arteriosclerosis, asthma, history of peptic ulceration; pregnancy; **interactions:** Appendix 1 (adrenergic neurone blockers)

Contra-indications: phaeochromocytoma, renal impairment (Appendix 3), heart failure

Side-effects: postural hypotension, failure of ejaculation, fluid retention, nasal congestion, headache, diarrhoea, drowsiness

Dose: *by intramuscular injection*, 10–20 mg, repeated after 3 hours if required

Ismelin® (Alliance) PoM
Injection, guanethidine monosulphate 10 mg/mL. Net price 1-mL amp = £1.56

DEBRISOQUINE

Indications: hypertension

Cautions; Contra-indications; Side-effects: see under Guanethidine Monosulphate (except diarrhoea)

Dose: 10 mg 1–2 times daily, increased by 10 mg every 3 days; usual range 20–60 mg daily (120 mg or higher in severe hypertension)

Debrisoquine (Cambridge) PoM
Tablets, scored, debrisoquine (as sulphate) 10 mg, net price 100-tab pack = £18.55

> ◣ denotes preparations that are considered to be less suitable for prescribing (see p. vi)

2.5.4 Alpha-adrenoceptor blocking drugs

Prazosin has post-synaptic alpha-blocking and vasodilator properties and rarely causes tachycardia. It may, however, cause a rapid reduction in blood pressure after the first dose and should be introduced with caution. **Doxazosin, indoramin,** and **terazosin** have properties similar to those of prazosin.

Alpha-blockers may be used with other antihypertensive drugs in the treatment of hypertension.

PROSTATIC HYPERPLASIA. Alfuzosin, doxazosin, indoramin, prazosin, tamsulosin and terazosin are indicated for benign prostatic hyperplasia (section 7.4.1).

DOXAZOSIN

Indications: hypertension; benign prostatic hyperplasia (section 7.4.1)

Cautions: care with initial dose (postural hypotension); hepatic impairment (Appendix 2); pregnancy and breast-feeding (Appendixes 4 and 5); **interactions:** Appendix 1 (alpha-blockers)

Side-effects: postural hypotension; dizziness, vertigo, headache, fatigue, asthenia, oedema, somnolence, nausea, rhinitis; less frequently abdominal discomfort, diarrhoea, vomiting, agitation, tremor, rash, pruritus; rarely blurred vision, epistaxis, haematuria, thrombocytopenia, purpura, leucopenia, hepatitis, jaundice, cholestasis, and urinary incontinence; isolated cases of priapism and impotence reported

Dose: hypertension, 1 mg daily, increased after 1–2 weeks to 2 mg once daily, and thereafter to 4 mg once daily, if necessary; max. 16 mg daily

Cardura® (Invicta) [PoM]
Tablets, doxazosin (as mesilate) 1 mg, net price 28-tab pack = £10.56; 2 mg, 28-tab pack = £14.08; 4 mg, 28-tab pack = £17.60

INDORAMIN

Indications: hypertension; benign prostatic hyperplasia (section 7.4.1)

Cautions: avoid alcohol (enhances rate and extent of absorption); control incipient heart failure with diuretics and digoxin; hepatic or renal impairment; elderly patients; Parkinson's disease; epilepsy (convulsions in *animal* studies); history of depression; **interactions:** Appendix 1 (alpha-blockers)

DRIVING. Drowsiness may affect performance of skilled tasks (e.g. driving); effects of alcohol may be enhanced

Contra-indications: established heart failure; patients receiving MAOIs

Side-effects: sedation; also dizziness, depression, failure of ejaculation, dry mouth, nasal congestion, extrapyramidal effects, weight gain

Dose: hypertension, initially 25 mg twice daily, increased by 25–50 mg daily at intervals of 2 weeks; max. daily dose 200 mg in 2–3 divided doses

Baratol® (Monmouth) [PoM]
Tablets, both f/c, indoramin (as hydrochloride) 25 mg (blue), net price 84-tab pack = £9.00; 50 mg (green, scored), 84-tab pack = £17.00. Label: 2

■ Prostatic hyperplasia
Doralese® [PoM] see section 7.4.1

PRAZOSIN

Indications: see under Dose

Cautions: first dose may cause collapse due to hypotension (therefore should be taken on retiring to bed); elderly; renal impairment (Appendix 3); pregnancy and breast-feeding; **interactions:** Appendix 1 (alpha-blockers)

Contra-indications: not recommended for congestive heart failure due to mechanical obstruction (e.g. aortic stenosis)

Side-effects: postural hypotension, drowsiness, weakness, dizziness, headache, lack of energy, nausea, palpitations; urinary frequency, incontinence and priapism reported

Dose: hypertension, 500 micrograms 2–3 times daily, the initial dose on retiring to bed at night (to avoid collapse, see Cautions); increased to 1 mg 2–3 times daily after 3–7 days; further increased if necessary to max. 20 mg daily

Congestive heart failure (but see section 2.5.5), 500 micrograms 2–4 times daily (initial dose at bedtime, see above), increasing to 4 mg daily in divided doses; maintenance 4–20 mg daily (but rarely used)

Raynaud's syndrome (but efficacy not established, see section 2.6.4.1), initially 500 micrograms twice daily (initial dose at bedtime, see above); maintenance 1–2 mg twice daily

Benign prostatic hyperplasia, section 7.4.1

Prazosin (Non-proprietary) [PoM]
Tablets, prazosin (as hydrochloride) 500 micrograms, net price 100-tab pack = £4.05; 1 mg, 100-tab pack = £5.06; 2 mg, 100-tab pack = £6.86; 5 mg, 100-tab pack = £14.85. Label: 3, counselling, see dose above
Available from APS, Ashbourne (*Alphavase®*), Cox, Hillcross, Norton

Hypovase® (Invicta) [PoM]
Tablets, prazosin (as hydrochloride) 500 micrograms, net price 56-tab pack = £2.09; 1 mg (orange, scored), 56-tab pack = £2.69; 2 mg (scored), 56-tab pack = £3.66; starter pack of 8 × 500-microgram tabs with 32 × 1-mg tabs = £2.52. Label: 3, counselling, see dose above

TERAZOSIN

Indications: mild to moderate hypertension; benign prostatic hyperplasia (section 7.4.1)

Cautions: first dose may cause collapse due to hypotension (within 30–90 minutes, therefore should be taken on retiring to bed) (may also occur with rapid dose increase); **interactions:** Appendix 1 (alpha-blockers)

Side-effects: dizziness, lack of energy, peripheral oedema; urinary frequency and priapism reported

Dose: hypertension, 1 mg at bedtime (compliance with bedtime dose important, see Cautions); dose doubled after 7 days if necessary; usual maintenance dose 2–10 mg once daily; more than 20 mg daily rarely improves efficacy

Hytrin® (Abbott) PoM
Tablets, terazosin (as hydrochloride) 2 mg (yellow), net price 28-tab pack = £8.07; 5 mg (tan), 28-tab pack = £13.07; 10 mg (blue), 28-tab pack = £26.59: starter pack of 7 × 1-mg tabs with 21 × 2-mg tabs = £13.00. Label: 3, counselling, see dose above

Phaeochromocytoma

Phenoxybenzamine is a powerful alpha-blocker with many side-effects. It is used with a beta-blocker in the short-term management of severe hypertensive episodes associated with phaeochromocytoma.
Phentolamine is a short-acting alpha-blocker used rarely as a suppression test for phaeochromocytoma.

PHENOXYBENZAMINE HYDROCHLORIDE

Indications: hypertensive episodes in phaeochromocytoma
Cautions: elderly; congestive heart failure; severe heart disease (see also Contra-indications); cerebrovascular disease (avoid if history of cerebrovascular accident); renal impairment; carcinogenic in *animals*; pregnancy; avoid in porphyria (section 9.8.2); avoid infusion in hypovolaemia; avoid extravasation (irritant to tissues)
Contra-indications: history of cerebrovascular accident; during recovery period after myocardial infarction (usually 3–4 weeks)
Side-effects: postural hypotension with dizziness and marked compensatory tachycardia, lassitude, nasal congestion, miosis, inhibition of ejaculation; rarely gastro-intestinal disturbances; decreased sweating and dry mouth after intravenous infusion; idiosyncratic profound hypotension within few minutes of starting infusion
Dose: see under preparations

Phenoxybenzamine (Goldshield) PoM
Injection concentrate, phenoxybenzamine hydrochloride 50 mg/mL. To be diluted before use. Net price 3 × 2-mL amp = £43.88 (hosp. only)
Dose: by intravenous infusion (preferably through large vein), adjunct in severe shock (but rarely used) and phaeochromocytoma, 1 mg/kg daily in 200 mL physiological saline over at least 2 hours; do not repeat within 24 hours (intensive care facilities needed)
CAUTION. Owing to risk of contact sensitisation doctors, nurses, and other health workers should avoid contamination of hands

Dibenyline® (Goldshield) PoM
Capsules, red/white, phenoxybenzamine hydrochloride 10 mg. Net price 30-cap pack = £10.84
Dose, phaeochromocytoma, 10 mg daily, increased by 10 mg daily; usual dose 1–2 mg/kg daily in 2 divided doses

PHENTOLAMINE MESILATE

Indications: hypertensive episodes due to phaeochromocytoma e.g. during surgery; diagnosis of phaeochromocytoma
Cautions: monitor blood pressure (avoid in hypotension), heart rate; renal impairment; gastritis, peptic ulcer; elderly; **interactions:** Appendix 1 (alpha-blockers)
ASTHMA. Presence of sulphites in ampoules may (especially in patients with asthma) lead to hypersensitivity (with bronchospasm and shock)

Contra-indications: hypotension; history of myocardial infarction; coronary insufficiency, angina, or other evidence of coronary artery disease
Side-effects: postural hypotension, tachycardia, dizziness; nausea and vomiting, diarrhoea, nasal congestion; also acute or prolonged hypotension, angina, chest pain, arrhythmias
Dose: hypertensive episodes, *by intravenous injection*, 2–5 mg repeated if necessary
Diagnosis of phaeochromocytoma, consult product literature

Rogitine® (Alliance) PoM
Injection, phentolamine mesilate 10 mg/mL. Net price 1-mL amp = £1.70

2.5.5 Drugs affecting the renin-angiotensin system

2.5.5.1   Angiotensin-converting enzyme inhibitors
2.5.5.2   Angiotensin-II receptor antagonists

Heart failure
The treatment of chronic heart failure aims to relieve symptoms, improve exercise tolerance, reduce the incidence of acute exacerbations and reduce mortality. An ACE inhibitor, given at an adequate dose, generally achieves these aims. Digoxin improves symptoms and exercise tolerance and reduces hospitalisation due to acute exacerbations but it does not reduce mortality. Diuretics are required to relieve symptoms in patients with fluid overload. The management of chronic systolic heart failure is covered below; optimal management of diastolic heart failure is less certain but digoxin should probably be avoided.

An ACE inhibitor (section 2.5.5.1) is generally advised for patients with asymptomatic left ventricular dysfunction or symptomatic heart failure.

Patients with fluid overload should also receive either a loop or a thiazide diuretic (with salt or fluid restriction where appropriate). A thiazide diuretic (section 2.2.1) may be of benefit in patients with mild heart failure and good renal function; thiazide diuretics are ineffective in patients with poor renal function (estimated creatinine clearance less than 30 mL/minute, see Appendix 3), and a loop diuretic (section 2.2.2) is preferred. If diuresis with a single diuretic is insufficient, a combination of a loop diuretic and a thiazide diuretic may be tried; addition of metolazone (section 2.2.1) may also be considered but the resulting diuresis may be profound and care is needed to avoid potentially dangerous electrolyte disturbances.

Digoxin (section 2.1) is given to patients with atrial fibrillation and also to those in sinus rhythm who remain symptomatic despite treatment with an ACE inhibitor and diuretic.

The aldosterone antagonist spironolactone (section 2.2.3) may be considered for patients with severe heart failure who are already receiving an ACE inhibitor and a diuretic and possibly digoxin; low doses of spironolactone (usually 25 mg daily) have been shown to reduce symptoms and mortality in these patients. Close monitoring of serum creatinine and potassium is necessary.

Patients who cannot tolerate ACE inhibitors or in whom they are contra-indicated may be given isosorbide dinitrate (section 2.6.1) with hydralazine (section 2.5.1), but this combination may be poorly tolerated. Angiotensin-II receptor antagonists (section 2.5.5.2), although not licensed for heart failure, may be useful alternatives for patients who, because of symptoms such as cough, cannot tolerate ACE inhibitors.

The beta-blocker carvedilol (section 2.4) is of value in selected patients with stable heart failure and left-ventricular systolic dysfunction; other beta-blockers such as bisoprolol and metoprolol [unlicensed indication] may also be beneficial. Treatment with a beta-blocker in heart failure should be initiated under specialist supervision.

2.5.5.1 Angiotensin-converting enzyme inhibitors

Angiotensin-converting enzyme inhibitors (ACE inhibitors) inhibit the conversion of angiotensin I to angiotensin II. They are effective and generally well tolerated.

HYPERTENSION. ACE inhibitors should be considered for hypertension when thiazides and beta-blockers are contra-indicated, not tolerated, or fail to control blood pressure; they are particularly indicated for hypertension in insulin-dependent diabetics with nephropathy (see also section 6.1.5). ACE inhibitors may cause very rapid falls of blood pressure in some patients particularly in those receiving diuretic therapy (see Cautions, below); the first dose should preferably be given at bedtime.

DIABETIC NEPHROPATHY. For comment on the role of ACE inhibitors in the management of diabetic nephropathy, see section 6.1.5.

HEART FAILURE. ACE inhibitors have a valuable role in all grades of heart failure, combined when appropriate with a diuretic and digoxin (section 2.5.5). Potassium supplements and potassium-sparing diuretics should be discontinued before introducing an ACE inhibitor because of the risk of hyperkalaemia. However, a low dose of spironolactone may be beneficial in severe heart failure (section 2.5.5) and can be used with an ACE inhibitor provided serum potassium is monitored carefully. Profound first-dose hypotension may occur when ACE inhibitors are introduced to patients with heart failure who are already taking a high dose of a loop diuretic (e.g. furosemide 80 mg daily or more). Temporary withdrawal of the loop diuretic reduces the risk, but may cause severe rebound pulmonary oedema. The ACE inhibitor should therefore be started at very low dosage (e.g. captopril 6.25 mg), with the patient recumbent and under close medical supervision, and with facilities to treat profound hypotension. In these circumstances and in other special risk groups (see below) the patient should be admitted to hospital for initiation.

MYOCARDIAL INFARCTION. ACE inhibitors are used in the immediate and long-term management of patients who have had a myocardial infarction, see section 2.10.1.

INITIATION IN HOSPITAL. ACE inhibitor therapy for heart failure should be initiated under close medical supervision (in hospital in severe heart failure). Initiation in hospital is also recommended for patients with mild to moderate heart failure:

- receiving multiple or high-dose diuretic therapy (e.g. more than 80 mg of furosemide daily or its equivalent);
- with hypovolaemia;
- with hyponatraemia (plasma-sodium concentration below 130 mmol/litre);
- with pre-existing hypotension (systolic blood pressure below 90 mmHg);
- with unstable heart failure;
- with renal impairment (plasma-creatinine concentration above 150 micromol/litre);
- receiving high-dose vasodilator therapy;
- aged 70 years or more.

RENAL EFFECTS. In patients with severe bilateral renal artery stenosis (or severe stenosis of the artery supplying a single functioning kidney), ACE inhibitors reduce or abolish glomerular filtration and are likely to cause severe and progressive renal failure. They are thus contra-indicated in patients known to have these forms of critical renovascular disease.

ACE inhibitor treatment is unlikely to have an adverse effect on overall renal function in patients with severe unilateral renal artery stenosis and a normal contralateral kidney, but glomerular filtration is likely to be reduced (or even abolished) in the affected kidney and the long-term consequences are unknown.

In general, ACE inhibitors are therefore best avoided in patients with known or suspected renovascular disease, unless the blood pressure cannot be controlled by other drugs. If they are used in these circumstances renal function needs to be monitored.

ACE inhibitors should also be used with particular caution in patients who may have undiagnosed and clinically silent renovascular disease. This includes patients with peripheral vascular disease or those with severe generalised atherosclerosis.

Renal function and electrolytes should be checked before starting ACE inhibitors and monitored during treatment (more frequently if features mentioned above present). Although ACE inhibitors now have a specialised role in some forms of renal disease they also occasionally cause impairment of renal function which may progress and become severe in other circumstances (at particular risk are the elderly).

Concomitant treatment with NSAIDs increases the risk of renal damage, and potassium-sparing diuretics (or potassium-containing salt substitutes) increase the risk of hyperkalaemia.

CAUTIONS. ACE inhibitors should be used with caution in patients receiving diuretics (**important:** see Concomitant diuretics, below); first doses may cause hypotension especially in patients taking diuretics, on a low-sodium diet, on dialysis, dehydrated or with heart failure (see above). They should also be used with caution in peripheral vascular disease or generalised atherosclerosis owing to risk of clinically silent renovascular disease (see also above). Renal function should be monitored before and during treatment, and the dose reduced in renal impairment (see also above and Appendix 3). The risk of agranulocytosis is possibly increased in collagen vascular disease (blood counts recommended). ACE inhibitors should be used with care (or avoided) in patients with a history of idiopathic or hereditary angioedema. Use ACE inhibitors with caution in breast-feeding (see Appendix 5). **Interactions:** Appendix 1 (ACE inhibitors)

ANAPHYLACTOID REACTIONS. To prevent anaphylactoid reactions, ACE inhibitors should be avoided during dialysis with high-flux polyacrylonitrile membranes and during low-density lipoprotein apheresis with dextran sulphate; they should also be withheld before desensitisation with wasp or bee venom

Concomitant diuretics. ACE inhibitors can cause very rapid falls of blood pressure in volume-depleted patients. Therefore, in these patients, any diuretic should be discontinued, or the dose reduced significantly, 2–3 days before initiation of an ACE inhibitor; however, in heart failure it may not be desirable to discontinue the diuretic (see notes above). If diuretic therapy cannot be stopped, medical supervision is recommended for at least 2 hours after administration of the first dose of the ACE inhibitor or until the blood pressure has stabilised.

CONTRA-INDICATIONS. ACE inhibitors are contra-indicated in patients with hypersensitivity to ACE inhibitors (including angioedema) and in known or suspected renovascular disease (see also above), aortic stenosis or outflow tract obstruction. ACE inhibitors should not be used in pregnancy (Appendix 4).

SIDE-EFFECTS. ACE inhibitors can cause profound hypotension (see Cautions) and renal impairment (see Renal effects above). They may also cause angioedema (onset may be delayed), rash (which may be associated with pruritus and urticaria), persistent dry cough, pancreatitis and upper respiratory-tract symptoms such as sinusitis, rhinitis and sore throat. Gastro-intestinal effects reported with ACE inhibitors include nausea, vomiting, dyspepsia, diarrhoea and constipation. Altered liver function tests, cholestatic jaundice and hepatitis have been reported. Blood dyscrasias including thrombocytopenia, leucopenia, neutropenia and haemolytic anaemia have also been reported. Other reported side-effects include headache, dizziness, fatigue, malaise, taste disturbance, paraesthesia, bronchospasm, fever, serositis, vasculitis, myalgia, arthralgia, positive antinuclear antibody, raised erythrocyte sedimentation rate, eosinophilia, leucocytosis and photosensitivity.

COMBINATION PRODUCTS. A number of products incorporating an ACE inhibitor with a thiazide diuretic are now available for the treatment of hypertension. Use of these combination products should be reserved for patients whose blood pressure has not responded to a thiazide diuretic or an ACE inhibitor alone.

Products combining an ACE inhibitor with a calcium-channel blocker are also available for the management of hypertension. Use of such a combination is rarely justified; the range of adverse effects may be increased considerably. A combination product should be considered only for those patients who have been stabilised on the individual components in the same proportions.

CAPTOPRIL

Indications: mild to moderate essential hypertension alone or with thiazide therapy and severe hypertension resistant to other treatment; congestive heart failure (adjunct—see section 2.5.5); following myocardial infarction, see dose; diabetic nephropathy (microalbuminuria greater than 30 mg/day) in insulin-dependent diabetes

Cautions: see notes above

Contra-indications: see notes above; porphyria (section 9.8.2)

Side-effects: see notes above; tachycardia, serum sickness, weight loss, stomatitis, maculopapular rash, photosensitivity, flushing and acidosis

Dose: hypertension, used alone, initially 12.5 mg twice daily; if used in addition to diuretic (see notes above), or in elderly, initially 6.25 mg twice daily (first dose at bedtime); usual maintenance dose 25 mg twice daily; max. 50 mg twice daily (rarely 3 times daily in severe hypertension)

Heart failure (adjunct), initially 6.25–12.5 mg under close medical supervision (see notes above); usual maintenance dose 25 mg 2–3 times daily; usual max. 150 mg daily

Prophylaxis after infarction in clinically stable patients with asymptomatic or symptomatic left ventricular dysfunction (radionuclide ventriculography or echocardiography undertaken before initiation), initially 6.25 mg, starting as early as 3 days after infarction, then increased over several weeks to 150 mg daily (if tolerated) in divided doses

Diabetic nephropathy, 75–100 mg daily in divided doses; if further blood pressure reduction required, other antihypertensives may be used in conjunction with captopril; in severe renal impairment, initially 12.5 mg twice daily (if concomitant diuretic therapy required, loop diuretic rather than thiazide should be chosen)

Captopril (Non-proprietary) ▣PoM▣
Tablets, captopril 12.5 mg, net price 56-tab pack = £7.08; 25 mg, 56-tab pack = £9.65; 50 mg, 56-tab pack = £12.35
Available from Berk (*Kaplon®*), Cox, CP, Galen, Generics, Genus, Goldshield (*Ecopace®*), Hillcross, Lagap, Norton (*Tensopril®*), Opus (*Hyteneze®*), Sovereign, Sterwin

Capoten® (Squibb) ▣PoM▣
Tablets, captopril 12.5 mg (scored), net price 56-tab pack = £10.56; 25 mg, 56-tab pack = £12.03, 84-tab pack = £18.05; 50 mg (scored), 56-tab pack = £20.50, 84-tab pack = £30.75 (also available as *Acepril®*)

■ With diuretic
Note. For mild to moderate hypertension in patients stabilised on the individual components in the same proportions

Co-zidocapt (Non-proprietary) ▣PoM▣
Tablets, co-zidocapt 12.5/25 (hydrochlorothiazide 12.5 mg, captopril 25 mg), net price 28-tab pack = £9.00
Available from Norton (*Capto-co®*)
Tablets, co-zidocapt 25/50 (hydrochlorothiazide 25 mg, captopril 50 mg), net price 28-tab pack = £11.31
Available from Cox, Norton (*Capto-co®*)

Capozide® (Squibb) PoM
LS tablets, scored, co-zidocapt 12.5/25 (hydrochlorothiazide 12.5 mg, captopril 25 mg). Net price 28-tab pack = £11.25
Tablets, scored, co-zidocapt 25/50 (hydrochlorothiazide 25 mg, captopril 50 mg). Net price 28-tab pack = £14.14 (also available as *Acezide®*)

CILAZAPRIL

Indications: essential and renovascular hypertension (but see notes above); congestive heart failure (adjunct—see section 2.5.5)
Cautions: see notes above
Contra-indications: see notes above; ascites
Side-effects: see notes above; dyspnoea and bronchitis
Dose: hypertension, initially 1–1.25 mg once daily (initial dose reduced in those receiving a diuretic, in the elderly, in renal impairment and in severe hepatic impairment—consult product literature); usual maintenance dose 2.5–5 mg once daily; max. 5 mg daily
Renovascular hypertension (see notes above), initially 250–500 micrograms once daily, then adjusted according to response
Heart failure (adjunct), initially 500 micrograms once daily under close medical supervision (see notes above), increased to 1 mg once daily; usual maintenance dose 1–2.5 mg daily; max. 5 mg daily

Vascace® (Roche) PoM
Tablets, f/c, cilazapril 500 micrograms (white), net price 28-tab pack = £3.92; 1 mg (yellow), 28-tab pack = £6.46; 2.5 mg (pink), 28-tab pack = £8.21; 5 mg (brown), 28-tab pack = £14.28

ENALAPRIL MALEATE

Indications: essential and renovascular hypertension (but see notes above); congestive heart failure (adjunct—see section 2.5.5); prevention of symptomatic heart failure and prevention of coronary ischaemic events in patients with left ventricular dysfunction
Cautions: see notes above
Contra-indications: see notes above; porphyria (section 9.8.2)
Side-effects: see notes above; also palpitations, arrhythmias, angina, chest pain, syncope, cerebrovascular accident, myocardial infarction; anorexia, ileus, stomatitis, hepatic failure; dermatological side-effects including erythema multiforme, Stevens-Johnson syndrome, toxic epidermal necrolysis, exfoliative dermatitis and pemphigus; confusion, depression, nervousness, asthenia, drowsiness, insomnia, blurred vision, tinnitus, sweating, flushing, impotence, alopecia, dyspnoea, asthma, pulmonary infiltrates and muscle cramps
Dose: hypertension, used alone, initially 5 mg once daily; if used in addition to diuretic (see notes above), in elderly patients, or in renal impairment, initially 2.5 mg daily; usual maintenance dose 10–20 mg once daily; in severe hypertension may be increased to max. 40 mg once daily
Heart failure (adjunct), asymptomatic left ventricular dysfunction, initially 2.5 mg daily under close medical supervision (see notes above); usual maintenance dose 20 mg daily in 1–2 divided doses

Enalapril Maleate (Non-proprietary) PoM
Tablets, enalapril maleate 2.5 mg, net price 28-tab pack = £5.35; 5 mg, 28-tab pack = £7.51; 10 mg, 28-tab pack = £10.53; 20 mg, 28-tab pack = £12.51
Available from Dexcel, Dominion (*Ednyt®*), Norton

Innovace® (MSD) PoM
Tablets, enalapril maleate 2.5 mg, net price 28-tab pack = £5.35; 5 mg (scored), 28-tab pack = £7.51; 10 mg (red), 28-tab pack = £10.53; 20 mg (peach), 28-tab pack = £12.51

■ With diuretic
Note. For mild to moderate hypertension in patients stabilised on the individual components in the same proportions
Innozide® (MSD) PoM
Tablets, yellow, scored, enalapril maleate 20 mg, hydrochlorothiazide 12.5 mg. Net price 28-tab pack = £13.90

FOSINOPRIL

Indications: hypertension; congestive heart failure (adjunct—see section 2.5.5)
Cautions: see notes above
Contra-indications: see notes above
Side-effects: see notes above; chest pain and musculoskeletal pain
Dose: hypertension, initially 10 mg daily, increased if necessary after 4 weeks; usual dose range 10–40 mg (doses over 40 mg not shown to increase efficacy); if used in addition to diuretic see notes above
Heart failure (adjunct), initially 10 mg daily under close medical supervision (see notes above); if initial dose well tolerated, may be increased to up to 40 mg once daily

Staril® (Squibb) PoM
Tablets, fosinopril sodium 10 mg, net price 28-tab pack = £12.04; 20 mg, 28-tab pack = £13.00

IMIDAPRIL HYDROCHLORIDE

Indications: essential hypertension
Cautions: see notes above
Contra-indications: see notes above
Side-effects: see notes above; dry mouth, glossitis, abdominal pain, ileus; bronchitis, dyspnoea; sleep disturbances, depression, confusion, blurred vision, tinnitus, impotence
Dose: initially 5 mg daily before food; if used in addition to diuretic (see notes above), in elderly, in patients with heart failure, angina or cerebrovascular disease, or in renal or hepatic impairment, initially 2.5 mg daily; if necessary increase dose at intervals of at least 3 weeks; usual maintenance dose 10 mg once daily; max. 20 mg daily (elderly, 10 mg daily)

Tanatril® (Trinity) ▼ PoM
Tablets, scored, imidapril hydrochloride 5 mg, net price 28-tab pack = £5.65; 10 mg, 28-tab pack = £6.39

LISINOPRIL

Indications: essential and renovascular hypertension (but see notes above); congestive heart failure (adjunct—see section 2.5.5); following myocardial infarction in haemodynamically stable patients; diabetic nephropathy in normotensive insulin-dependent and hypertensive non-insulin dependent diabetes mellitus

Cautions: see notes above

Contra-indications: see notes above

Side-effects: see notes above; tachycardia, cerebrovascular accident, myocardial infarction; dry mouth, confusion, mood changes, asthenia, sweating, impotence and alopecia

Dose: hypertension, initially 2.5 mg daily; usual maintenance dose 10–20 mg daily; max. 40 mg daily; if used in addition to diuretic see notes above

Heart failure (adjunct), initially 2.5 mg daily under close medical supervision (see notes above); usual maintenance dose 5–20 mg daily

Prophylaxis after myocardial infarction, systolic blood pressure over 120 mmHg, 5 mg within 24 hours, followed by further 5 mg 24 hours later, then 10 mg after a further 24 hours, and continuing with 10 mg once daily for 6 weeks (or continued if heart failure); systolic blood pressure 100–120 mmHg, initially 2.5 mg, increasing to maintenance dose of 5 mg once daily

Note. Should not be started after myocardial infarction if systolic blood pressure less than 100 mmHg; temporarily reduce maintenance dose to 5 mg and if necessary 2.5 mg daily if systolic blood pressure 100 mmHg or less during treatment; withdraw if prolonged hypotension occurs (systolic blood pressure less than 90 mmHg for more than 1 hour)

Diabetic nephropathy, initially 2.5 mg daily adjusted to achieve a sitting diastolic blood pressure below 75 mmHg in normotensive insulin-dependent diabetes and below 90 mmHg in hypertensive non-insulin dependent diabetes; usual dose range 10–20 mg daily

Carace® (Du Pont) PoM

Tablets, lisinopril 2.5 mg (blue), net price 28-tab pack = £7.30; 5 mg (scored), 28-tab pack = £9.15; 10 mg (yellow), 28-tab pack = £11.30; 20 mg (orange, scored), 28-tab pack = £12.78

Zestril® (Zeneca) PoM

Tablets, lisinopril (as dihydrate) 2.5 mg, net price 28-tab pack = £6.26; 5 mg (pink, scored), 28-tab pack = £7.86; 10 mg (pink), 28-tab pack = £9.70; 20 mg (red), 28-tab pack = £10.97

■ With diuretic

Note. For mild to moderate hypertension in patients stabilised on the individual components in the same proportions

Carace Plus® (Du Pont) PoM

Carace 10 Plus tablets, blue, lisinopril 10 mg, hydrochlorothiazide 12.5 mg. Net price 28-tab pack = £11.30

Carace 20 Plus tablets, yellow, scored, lisinopril 20 mg, hydrochlorothiazide 12.5 mg. Net price 28-tab pack = £12.78

Zestoretic® (Zeneca) PoM

Zestoretic 10 tablets, peach, lisinopril (as dihydrate) 10 mg, hydrochlorothiazide 12.5 mg. Net price 28-tab pack = £11.83

Zestoretic 20 tablets, lisinopril (as dihydrate) 20 mg, hydrochlorothiazide 12.5 mg. Net price 28-tab pack = £13.38

MOEXIPRIL HYDROCHLORIDE

Indications: essential hypertension

Cautions: see notes above

Contra-indications: see notes above

Side-effects: see notes above; arrhythmias, angina, chest pain, syncope, cerebrovascular accident, myocardial infarction; appetite and weight changes; dry mouth, photosensitivity, flushing, nervousness, mood changes, anxiety, drowsiness, sleep disturbance, tinnitus, influenza-like syndrome, sweating and dyspnoea

Dose: used alone, initially 7.5 mg once daily; if used in addition to diuretic (see notes above), with nifedipine, in elderly, in renal or hepatic impairment, initially 3.75 mg once daily; usual range 15–30 mg once daily; doses above 30 mg daily not shown to increase efficacy

Perdix® (Schwarz) PoM

Tablets, f/c, both pink, scored, moexipril hydrochloride 7.5 mg, net price 28-tab pack = £8.12; 15 mg, 28-tab pack = £9.36

PERINDOPRIL

Indications: essential and renovascular hypertension (but see notes above); congestive heart failure (adjunct—see section 2.5.5)

Cautions: see notes above

Contra-indications: see notes above

Side-effects: see notes above; asthenia, flushing, mood and sleep disturbances

Dose: hypertension, initially 2 mg daily (before food); usual maintenance dose 4 mg once daily; max. 8 mg daily; if used in addition to diuretic see notes above

Heart failure (adjunct), initial dose 2 mg in the morning under close medical supervision (see notes above); usual maintenance 4 mg once daily (before food)

Coversyl® (Servier) PoM

Tablets, perindopril erbumine (= tert-butylamine) 2 mg, net price 30-tab pack = £8.83; 4 mg (scored), 30-tab pack = £13.04

QUINAPRIL

Indications: essential hypertension; congestive heart failure (adjunct—see section 2.5.5)

Cautions: see notes above

Contra-indications: see notes above

Side-effects: see notes above; asthenia, chest pain, oedema, flatulence, nervousness, depression, insomnia, blurred vision, impotence, back pain and myalgia

Dose: hypertension, initially 10 mg once daily; with a diuretic, in elderly, or in renal impairment initially 2.5 mg daily; usual maintenance dose 20–40 mg daily in single or 2 divided doses; up to 80 mg daily has been given

Heart failure (adjunct), initial dose 2.5 mg under close medical supervision (see notes above); usual maintenance 10–20 mg daily in single or 2 divided doses; up to 40 mg daily has been given

Accupro® (Parke-Davis) PoM

Tablets, all brown, f/c, quinapril 5 mg, net price 28-tab pack = £7.17; 10 mg, 28-tab pack = £7.17; 20 mg, 28-tab pack = £8.99; 40 mg, 28-tab pack = £9.75

■ **With diuretic**

Note. For hypertension in patients stabilised on the individual components in the same proportions

Accuretic® (Parke-Davis) PoM

Tablets, pink, f/c, scored, quinapril 10 mg, hydrochlorothiazide 12.5 mg. Net price 28-tab pack = £9.79

RAMIPRIL

Indications: mild to moderate hypertension; congestive heart failure (adjunct—see section 2.5.5); following myocardial infarction in patients with clinical evidence of heart failure

Cautions: see notes above

Contra-indications: see notes above

Side-effects: see notes above; arrhythmias, angina, chest pain, syncope, cerebrovascular accident, myocardial infarction, loss of appetite, stomatitis, dry mouth, skin reactions including erythema multiforme and pemphigoid exanthema; precipitation or exacerbation of Raynaud's syndrome; conjunctivitis, onycholysis, confusion, nervousness, depression, anxiety, impotence, decreased libido, alopecia, bronchitis and muscle cramps

Dose: hypertension, initially 1.25 mg daily, increased at intervals of 1–2 weeks; usual range 2.5–5 mg once daily; max. 10 mg daily; if used in addition to diuretic see notes above
Heart failure (adjunct), initially 1.25 mg once daily under close medical supervision (see notes above), increased if necessary at intervals of 1–2 weeks; max. 10 mg daily (daily doses of 2.5 mg or more may be taken in 1–2 divided doses)
Prophylaxis after myocardial infarction (started in hospital 3 to 10 days after infarction), initially 2.5 mg twice daily, increased after 2 days to 5 mg twice daily; maintenance 2.5–5 mg twice daily

Note. If initial 2.5-mg dose not tolerated, give 1.25 mg twice daily for 2 days before increasing to 2.5 mg twice daily, then 5 mg twice daily; withdraw if 2.5 mg twice daily not tolerated

Tritace® (Hoechst Marion Roussel) PoM

Capsules, ramipril 1.25 mg (yellow/white), net price 28-cap pack = £5.30; 2.5 mg (orange/white), 28-cap pack = £7.51; 5 mg (red/white), 28-cap pack = £9.55; 10 mg (blue/white), 28-cap pack = £13.00

■ **With calcium-channel blocker**

Note. For hypertension in patients stabilised on the individual components in the same proportions, but combination with calcium-channel blocker not first-line treatment. For cautions, contra-indications and side-effects of felodipine, see section 2.6.2

Triapin® (Hoechst Marion Roussel) ▼ PoM ◤

Triapin® tablets, f/c, brown, ramipril 5 mg, felodipine 5 mg (m/r), net price 28-tab pack = £24.46. Label: 25

Triapin mite® tablets, f/c, orange, ramipril 2.5 mg, felodipine 2.5 mg (m/r), net price 28-tab pack = £19.37. Label: 25

TRANDOLAPRIL

Indications: mild to moderate hypertension; following myocardial infarction in patients with left ventricular dysfunction

Cautions: see notes above

Contra-indications: see notes above

Side-effects: see notes above; tachycardia, arrhythmias, angina, transient ischaemic attacks, cerebral haemorrhage, myocardial infarction; ileus, dry mouth; skin reactions including Stevens-Johnson syndrome, toxic epidermal necrolysis, psoriasis-like efflorescence; asthenia, alopecia, dyspnoea and bronchitis

Dose: hypertension, initially 500 micrograms once daily, increased at intervals of 2–4 weeks; usual range 1–2 mg once daily; max. 4 mg daily; if used in addition to diuretic see notes above
Prophylaxis after myocardial infarction (starting as early as 3 days after infarction), initially 500 micrograms daily, gradually increased to max. 4 mg once daily

Note. If symptomatic hypotension develops during titration, do not increase dose further; if possible, reduce dose of any adjunctive treatment and if this is not effective or feasible, reduce dose of trandolapril

Gopten® (Knoll) PoM

Capsules, trandolapril 500 micrograms (red/yellow), net price 14-cap pack = £4.09; 1 mg (red/orange), 28-cap pack = £10.33; 2 mg (red/red), 28-cap pack = £12.28

Odrik® (Hoechst Marion Roussel) PoM

Capsules, trandolapril 500 micrograms (red/yellow), net price 28-cap pack = £8.19; 1 mg (red/orange), 28-cap pack = £10.34; 2 mg (red/red), 28-cap pack = £12.29

■ **With calcium-channel blocker**

Note. For hypertension in patients stabilised on the individual components in the same proportions, but combination with calcium-channel blocker not first-line treatment. For cautions, contra-indications and side-effects of verapamil, see section 2.6.2

Tarka® (Knoll) ▼ PoM ◤

Capsules, pink, trandolapril 2 mg, verapamil hydrochloride 180 mg (m/r). Net price 28 cap-pack = £16.23. Label: 25

> ◤ denotes preparations that are considered to be less suitable for prescribing (see p. vi)

2.5.5.2   Angiotensin-II receptor antagonists

Losartan and **valsartan** are specific angiotensin-II receptor antagonists with many properties similar to those of the ACE inhibitors; **candesartan**, **irbesartan** and **telmisartan** have been introduced recently. However, unlike ACE inhibitors, they do not inhibit the breakdown of bradykinin and other kinins, and thus do not appear to cause the persistent dry cough which commonly complicates ACE inhibitor therapy. They are therefore a useful alternative for patients who have to discontinue an ACE inhibitor because of persistent cough. Beyond this their role in the management of hypertension remains to be established.

CAUTIONS. Angiotensin-II receptor antagonists should be used with caution in renal artery stenosis (see also Renal Effects, p. 89). Monitoring of plasma-potassium concentration is advised, particularly in the elderly and in patients with renal impairment; lower initial doses may be appropriate in these patients. **Interactions:** Appendix 1 (as for ACE inhibitors).

CONTRA-INDICATIONS. Angiotensin-II receptor antagonists, like the ACE inhibitors, should be avoided in pregnancy (see also Appendix 4).

SIDE-EFFECTS. Side-effects are usually mild. Symptomatic hypotension may occur, particularly in patients with intravascular volume depletion (e.g. those taking high-dose diuretics). Hyperkalaemia occurs occasionally; angioedema has also been reported with some angiotensin-II receptor antagonists.

CANDESARTAN CILEXETIL

Indications: hypertension (see also notes above)
Cautions: see notes above; hepatic and renal impairment (Appendixes 2 and 3), aortic and mitral valve stenosis
Contra-indications: see notes above; breast-feeding (Appendix 5), severe hepatic impairment and cholestasis
Side-effects: see notes above; also upper respiratory tract and influenza-like symptoms including rhinitis and pharyngitis; altered liver function tests, back pain, arthralgia, myalgia, nausea, headache, dizziness, rash also reported
Dose: initially 4 mg (2 mg in hepatic and renal impairment) once daily adjusted according to response; usual maintenance dose 8 mg once daily; max. 16 mg once daily

Amias® (Astra, Takeda) ▼ PoM
Tablets, candesartan cilexetil 2 mg, net price 7-tab pack = £2.99; 4 mg (scored), 7-tab pack = £3.24, 28-tab pack = £12.95; 8 mg (pink, scored), 28-tab pack = £14.95; 16 mg (pink, scored), 28-tab pack = £17.75

IRBESARTAN

Indications: hypertension (see also notes above)
Cautions: see notes above; also aortic and mitral valve stenosis
Contra-indications: see notes above; breast-feeding (Appendix 5)
Side-effects: see notes above; flushing, increase in plasma concentration of creatine kinase reported
Dose: 150 mg once daily, increased if necessary to 300 mg once daily (in haemodialysis or in elderly over 75 years, initial dose of 75 mg once daily may be used)

Aprovel® (Bristol-Myers, Sanofi-Synthelabo) ▼ PoM
Tablets, irbesartan 75 mg, net price 28-tab pack = £15.50; 150 mg, 28-tab pack = £17.22; 300 mg, 28-tab pack = £23.26

LOSARTAN POTASSIUM

Indications: hypertension (see also notes above)
Cautions: see notes above; hepatic and renal impairment (Appendixes 2 and 3)
Contra-indications: see notes above; breast-feeding (Appendix 5)

Side-effects: see notes above; diarrhoea, dizziness, taste disturbance, myalgia, migraine, urticaria, pruritus, rash, altered liver function tests; rarely hepatitis, anaemia (in severe renal disease or following renal transplant)
Dose: usually 50 mg once daily (elderly over 75 years, moderate to severe renal impairment, intravascular volume depletion, initially 25 mg once daily); if necessary increased after several weeks to 100 mg once daily

Cozaar® (MSD) PoM
Tablets, both f/c, losartan potassium 25 mg (Half Strength), net price 7-tab pack = £4.31; 50 mg (scored), 28-tab pack = £17.23

■ With diuretic
Note. For hypertension in patients stabilised on the individual components in the same proportions
Cozaar-Comp® (MSD) ▼ PoM
Tablets, f/c, yellow, losartan potassium 50 mg, hydrochlorothiazide 12.5 mg. Net price 28-tab pack = £17.23

TELMISARTAN

Indications: hypertension (see also notes above)
Cautions: see notes above; hepatic impairment (Appendix 2); aortic and mitral valve stenosis, obstructive hypertrophic cardiomyopathy; active gastric or duodenal ulceration or other gastro-intestinal disease (increased risk of gastro-intestinal bleeding)
Contra-indications: severe renal impairment; biliary obstruction; breast-feeding
Side-effects: see notes above; gastro-intestinal disturbances (rarely gastro-intestinal bleeding), pharyngitis, back pain; rarely anaemia, hyperuricaemia
Dose: 40 mg once daily, increased if necessary to 80 mg once daily

Micardis® (Boehringer Ingelheim) ▼ PoM
Tablets, telmisartan 40 mg, net price 28-tab pack = £12.60; 80 mg, 28-tab pack = £15.75

VALSARTAN

Indications: hypertension (see also notes above)
Cautions: see notes above; mild to moderate hepatic impairment (Appendix 2) and renal impairment (Appendix 3)
Contra-indications: see notes above; severe hepatic impairment (Appendix 2), cirrhosis, biliary obstruction, breast-feeding (Appendix 5)
Side-effects: see notes above; fatigue, rarely epistaxis; neutropenia reported
Dose: usually 80 mg once daily (elderly over 75 years, mild to moderate hepatic impairment, moderate to severe renal impairment, intravascular volume depletion, initially 40 mg once daily); if necessary increased after at least 4 weeks to 160 mg daily (80 mg daily in hepatic impairment)

Diovan® (Novartis) ▼ PoM
Capsules, valsartan 40 mg (grey), net price 7-cap pack = £3.35; 80 mg (grey/pink), 7-cap pack = £3.94 (hosp. only), 28-cap pack = £15.75; 160 mg (dark grey/pink), 7-cap pack = £4.92 (hosp. only), 28-cap pack = £19.69

2.5.6 Ganglion-blocking drugs

TRIMETAPHAN CAMSILATE

Indications: controlled hypotension in surgery

Cautions: hepatic or renal impairment, diabetes mellitus, elderly, cerebral or coronary vascular disease, adrenal insufficiency, Addison's disease, CNS degenerative disease

Contra-indications: severe arteriosclerosis, severe cardiac disease, pyloric stenosis, pregnancy

Side-effects: tachycardia and respiratory depression (particularly with muscle relaxants); constipation, increased intra-ocular pressure, pupillary dilatation

Dose: *by intravenous infusion*, 3–4 mg/minute initially, then adjusted according to response

Trimetaphan Camsilate (Cambridge) PoM
Injection, trimetaphan camsilate 50 mg/mL. Net price 5-mL amp = £17.42. For dilution and use as an infusion

2.5.7 Tyrosine hydroxylase inhibitors

Metirosine inhibits the enzyme tyrosine hydroxylase, and hence the synthesis of catecholamines. It is used in the pre-operative management of phaeochromocytoma, and long term in patients unsuitable for surgery; an alpha-adrenoceptor blocking drug (e.g. phenoxybenzamine, section 2.5.4) may also be required. Metirosine should **not** be used to treat essential hypertension.

METIROSINE

Indications: see notes above

Cautions: maintain high fluid intake and adequate blood volume; may impair ability to drive or operate machinery; **interactions:** Appendix 1 (metirosine)

Side-effects: sedation; extrapyramidal symptoms; diarrhoea (may be severe); hypersensitivity reactions

Dose: initially 250 mg 4 times daily, increased to max. of 4 g daily in divided doses; doses of 2–3 g daily should be given for 5–7 days before surgery

Demser® (MSD) PoM
Capsules, blue, metirosine 250 mg (hosp. only). Label: 2

2.6 Nitrates, calcium-channel blockers, and potassium-channel activators

2.6.1	Nitrates
2.6.2	Calcium-channel blockers
2.6.3	Potassium-channel activators
2.6.4	Peripheral and cerebral vasodilators

Nitrates, calcium-channel blockers and potassium-channel activators have a vasodilating effect. Vasodilators are known to act in heart failure either by arteriolar dilatation which reduces both peripheral vascular resistance and left ventricular pressure at systole and results in improved cardiac output, *or* venous dilatation which results in dilatation of capacitance vessels, increase of venous pooling, and diminution of venous return to the heart (decreasing left ventricular end-diastolic pressure).

Angina

Stable angina usually results from atherosclerotic plaques in the coronary arteries, whereas *unstable angina* is usually due to plaque rupture and may occur either in patients with a history of stable angina or in those with previously silent coronary artery disease. It is important to distinguish unstable from stable angina; unstable angina is usually characterised by new onset severe angina or sudden worsening of previously stable angina.

STABLE ANGINA. Acute attacks of stable angina should be managed with sublingual glyceryl trinitrate. If attacks occur more than twice a week, regular drug therapy is required and should be introduced in a stepwise manner according to response. Aspirin should be given to patients with angina; a dose of 75–150 mg daily is suitable. Revascularisation procedures may also be appropriate.

Patients with mild or moderate stable angina who do not have left ventricular dysfunction, may be managed effectively with sublingual glyceryl trinitrate and regular administration of a beta-blocker (section 2.4). If necessary a long-acting dihydropyridine calcium-channel blocker (section 2.6.2) and then a long-acting nitrate (section 2.6.1) may be added. For those without left ventricular dysfunction and in whom beta-blockers are inappropriate, diltiazem or verapamil may be given (section 2.6.2) and a long-acting nitrate (section 2.6.1) may be added if symptom control is not adequate. For those intolerant of standard treatment, or where standard treatment has failed, nicorandil may be tried.

For patients with left ventricular dysfunction a long-acting nitrate (section 2.6.1) should be used and a long-acting dihydropyridine calcium-channel blocker (section 2.6.2) may be added if necessary.

A statin (section 2.12) should be considered for those with an elevated plasma-cholesterol concentration.

UNSTABLE ANGINA. Patients with unstable angina should be admitted to hospital. The aims of management of unstable angina are to provide supportive care and pain relief during the acute attack and to prevent myocardial infarction and death.

Initial management. **Aspirin** (chewed or dispersed in water) is given for its antiplatelet effect at a dose of 300 mg (section 2.9). If aspirin is given before arrival at hospital, a note saying that it has been given should be sent with the patient.

Heparin (section 2.8.1) or the low molecular weight heparins **dalteparin** or **enoxaparin** (section 2.8.1) should also be given.

Nitrates (section 2.6.1) are used to relieve ischaemic pain. If sublingual glyceryl trinitrate is not effective, intravenous or buccal glyceryl trinitrate or intravenous isosorbide dinitrate is given.

Patients without contra-indications should receive intravenous or oral **beta-blockers** (section 2.4). In patients without left ventricular dysfunction and in whom beta-blockers are inappropriate, **diltiazem** or **verapamil** may be given (section 2.6.2).

Eptifibatide and **tirofiban** (section 2.9) have recently been introduced for the prevention of myocardial infarction in patients with unstable angina; they should be used under specialist supervision.

Revascularisation procedures are often appropriate for patients with unstable angina.

Long-term management. The importance of lifestyle changes, especially stopping smoking, should be emphasised. Patients should receive low-dose **aspirin** indefinitely—a dose of 75–150 mg daily is suitable. Use of a **statin** (section 2.12) should also be considered. The need for long-term angina treatment or for coronary angiography should be assessed. If there is continuing ischaemia, standard angina treatment should be continued; if not, antianginal treatment may be withdrawn cautiously at least 2 months after the acute attack.

2.6.1   Nitrates

Nitrates have a useful role in *angina* (for details on the management of stable angina, see section 2.6). Although they are potent coronary vasodilators, their principal benefit follows from a reduction in venous return which reduces left ventricular work. Unwanted effects such as flushing, headache, and postural hypotension may limit therapy, especially when angina is severe or when patients are unusually sensitive to the effects of nitrates.

Sublingual **glyceryl trinitrate** is one of the most effective drugs for providing rapid symptomatic relief of angina, but its effect lasts only for 20 to 30 minutes; the 300-microgram tablet is often appropriate when glyceryl trinitrate is first used. The *aerosol spray* provides an alternative method of rapid relief of symptoms for those who find difficulty in dissolving sublingual preparations. Duration of action may be prolonged by *modified-release* and *transdermal* preparations (but tolerance may develop, see below).

Isosorbide dinitrate is active *sublingually* and is a more stable preparation for those who only require nitrates infrequently. It is also effective by mouth for prophylaxis; although the effect is slower in onset, it may persist for several hours. Duration of action of up to 12 hours is claimed for *modified-release* preparations. The activity of isosorbide dinitrate may depend on the production of active metabolites, the most important of which is isosorbide mononitrate. **Isosorbide mononitrate** itself is also licensed for angina prophylaxis; modified-release formulations (for once daily administration) are available.

Glyceryl trinitrate or isosorbide dinitrate may be tried by *intravenous injection* when the sublingual form is ineffective in patients with chest pain due to myocardial infarction or severe ischaemia. Intravenous injections are also useful in the treatment of acute left ventricular failure.

TOLERANCE. Many patients on long-acting or transdermal nitrates rapidly develop tolerance (with reduced therapeutic effects). Reduction of blood-nitrate concentrations to low levels for 4 to 8 hours each day usually maintains effectiveness in such patients. If tolerance is suspected during the use of transdermal patches they should be left off for several consecutive hours in each 24 hours; in the case of modified-release tablets of isosorbide dinitrate (and conventional formulations of isosorbide mononitrate), the second of the two daily doses can be given after about 8 hours rather than after 12 hours. Conventional formulations of isosorbide mononitrate should not usually be given more than twice daily unless small doses are used; modified-release formulations of isosorbide mononitrate should only be given once daily, and used in this way do not produce tolerance.

GLYCERYL TRINITRATE

Indications: prophylaxis and treatment of angina; left ventricular failure

Cautions: severe hepatic or renal impairment; hypothyroidism, malnutrition, or hypothermia; recent history of myocardial infarction; metal-containing transdermal systems should be removed before cardioversion or diathermy; tolerance (see notes above); **interactions:** Appendix 1 (glyceryl trinitrate)

Contra-indications: hypersensitivity to nitrates; hypotensive conditions and hypovolaemia; hypertrophic obstructive cardiomyopathy, aortic stenosis, cardiac tamponade, constrictive pericarditis, mitral stenosis; marked anaemia, head trauma, cerebral haemorrhage, closed-angle glaucoma

Side-effects: throbbing headache, flushing, dizziness, postural hypotension, tachycardia (but paradoxical bradycardia has occurred)

INJECTION. Specific side-effects following injection (particularly if given too rapidly) include severe hypotension, nausea and retching, diaphoresis, apprehension, restlessness, muscle twitching, retrosternal discomfort, palpitations, abdominal pain, syncope; prolonged administration has been associated with methaemoglobinaemia

Dose: *sublingually,* 0.3–1 mg, repeated as required

By mouth, see under Preparations

By intravenous infusion, 10–200 micrograms/minute

■ Short-acting tablets and sprays

Glyceryl Trinitrate (Non-proprietary)

Sublingual tablets, glyceryl trinitrate 300 micrograms, net price 100 = £3.05; 500 micrograms, 100 = £1.30; 600 micrograms, 100 = £2.45. Label: 16

Note. Glyceryl trinitrate tablets should be supplied in glass containers of not more than 100 tablets, closed with a foil-lined cap, and containing no cotton wool wadding; they should be discarded after 8 weeks in use

Aerosol spray, glyceryl trinitrate 400 micrograms/metered dose. Net price 200-dose unit = £3.28

Dose: treatment or prophylaxis of angina, spray 1–2 doses under tongue and then close mouth

Available from Cox

Coro-Nitro Pump Spray® (Roche)

Aerosol spray, glyceryl trinitrate 400 micrograms/metered dose. Net price 200-dose unit = £3.13

Dose: treatment or prophylaxis of angina, spray 1–2 doses under tongue and then close mouth

Glytrin Spray® (Sterwin)

Aerosol spray, glyceryl trinitrate 400 micrograms/metered dose. Net price 200-dose unit = £3.65

Dose: treatment or prophylaxis of angina, spray 1–2 doses under tongue and then close mouth

Caution: flammable

GTN 300 mcg (Martindale)

Sublingual tablets, glyceryl trinitrate 300 micrograms. Net price 100 = £2.91. Label: 16

Nitrolingual Pumpspray® (Lipha)
Aerosol spray, glyceryl trinitrate 400 micrograms/
metered dose. Net price 200-dose unit = £3.65;
Duo Pack (250-dose unit and 75-dose unit) =
£6.22
Dose: treatment or prophylaxis of angina, spray 1–2
doses under tongue and then close mouth

Nitromin® (Servier)
Aerosol spray, glyceryl trinitrate 400 micrograms/
metered dose. Net price 180-dose unit = £2.92
Dose: treatment or prophylaxis of angina, spray 1–2
doses under tongue and then close mouth

■ Longer-acting tablets

Suscard® (Pharmax)
Buccal tablets, m/r, glyceryl trinitrate 1 mg, net
price 100-tab pack = £9.38; 2 mg, 100-tab pack =
£13.55; 3 mg, 100-tab pack = £19.56; 5 mg, 100-
tab pack = £26.63. Counselling, see administration below
Dose: treatment of angina, 2 mg as required (1 mg in
sensitive patients), increased to 3 mg if necessary;
prophylaxis 1–3 mg 3 times daily; 5 mg in severe angina
Unstable angina (adjunct), up to 5 mg with ECG monitoring
Congestive heart failure, 5 mg 3 times daily, increased to
10 mg 3 times daily in severe cases
Acute heart failure, 5 mg repeated until symptoms abate
ADMINISTRATION. Tablets have rapid onset of effect;
they are placed between upper lip and gum, and left to
dissolve; vary site to reduce risk of dental caries

Sustac® (Pharmax)
Tablets, m/r, all pink, glyceryl trinitrate 2.6 mg, net
price 90-tab pack = £5.12; 6.4 mg, 90-tab pack =
£7.38; 10 mg, 90-tab pack = £6.85. Label: 25
Dose: prophylaxis of angina, 2.6–12.8 mg 3 times daily
or 10 mg 2–3 times daily

■ Parenteral preparations

Note. Glass or polyethylene apparatus is preferable; loss of
potency will occur if PVC is used

Glyceryl Trinitrate (Non-proprietary) PoM
Injection, glyceryl trinitrate 5 mg/mL. To be
diluted before use. Net price 5-mL amp = £6.49;
10-mL amp = £12.98
Available from Faulding DBL

Nitrocine® (Schwarz) PoM
Injection, glyceryl trinitrate 1 mg/mL. To be
diluted before use or given undiluted with syringe
pump. Net price 10-mL amp = £7.90; 50-mL bottle = £18.51

Nitronal® (Lipha) PoM
Injection, glyceryl trinitrate 1 mg/mL. To be
diluted before use or given undiluted with syringe
pump. Net price 5-mL vial = £2.06; 50-mL vial =
£16.85

■ Transdermal preparations

Deponit® (Schwarz)
Patches, self-adhesive, transparent, glyceryl trinitrate, '5' patch (releasing approx. 5 mg/24
hours when in contact with skin), net price 28 =
£17.16; '10' patch (releasing approx. 10 mg/24
hours), 28 = £18.89
ADMINISTRATION: prophylaxis of angina, apply one '5'
or one '10' patch to lateral chest wall, upper arm, or
shoulder; replace every 24 hours, siting replacement
patch on different area; see also notes above

Minitran® (3M)
Patches, self-adhesive, transparent, glyceryl trinitrate, '5' patch (releasing approx. 5 mg/24
hours when in contact with skin), net price 30 =
£12.49; '10' patch (releasing approx. 10 mg/24
hours), 30 = £13.84; '15' patch (releasing approx.
15 mg/24 hours), 30 = £15.26
ADMINISTRATION: prophylaxis of angina, apply one '5'
patch to chest or upper arm; replace every 24 hours, siting replacement patch on different area; adjust dose
according to response; see also notes above
Maintenance of venous patency ('5' patch only), see literature

Nitro-Dur® (Schering-Plough)
Patches, self-adhesive, buff, glyceryl trinitrate,
'0.2 mg/h' patch (releasing approx. 5 mg/24 hours
when in contact with skin), net price 28 = £11.84;
'0.4 mg/h' patch (releasing approx. 10 mg/24
hours), 28 = £13.10; '0.6 mg/h' patch (releasing
approx. 15 mg/24 hours), 28 = £14.42
ADMINISTRATION: prophylaxis of angina, apply one
'0.2 mg/h' patch to chest or outer upper arm; replace
every 24 hours, siting replacement patch on different
area: adjust dose according to response; see also notes
above

Percutol® (Dominion)
Ointment, glyceryl trinitrate 2%. Net price 60 g =
£10.98. Counselling, see administration below
Excipients: include wool fat
ADMINISTRATION: prophylaxis of angina, usual dose 1–
2 inches of ointment measured on to *Applirule®*, and
applied (usually to chest, arm, or thigh) without rubbing
in and secured with surgical tape, every 3–4 hours as
required; to determine dose, ½ inch on first day then
increased by ½ inch/day until headache occurs, then
reduced by ½ inch
Note. Approx. 800 micrograms/hour absorbed from 1
inch of ointment

Transiderm-Nitro® (Novartis)
Patches, self-adhesive, pink, glyceryl trinitrate, '5'
patch (releasing approx. 5 mg/24 hours when in
contact with skin), net price 28 = £17.71; '10'
patch (releasing approx. 10 mg/24 hours), 28 =
£19.47
ADMINISTRATION: prophylaxis of angina, apply one '5'
or one '10' patch to lateral chest wall; replace every 24
hours, siting replacement patch on different area; max.
two '10' patches daily; see also notes above
Prophylaxis of phlebitis and extravasation ('5' patch
only), consult product literature

ISOSORBIDE DINITRATE

Indications: prophylaxis and treatment of angina;
left ventricular failure
Cautions; Contra-indications; Side-effects:
see under Glyceryl Trinitrate
Dose: *sublingually,* 5–10 mg
By mouth, daily in divided doses, angina 30–
120 mg, left ventricular failure 40–160 mg, up to
240 mg if required
By intravenous infusion, 2–10 mg/hour; higher
doses up to 20 mg/hour may be required

■ Short-acting tablets and sprays

Isosorbide Dinitrate (Non-proprietary)
Tablets, isosorbide dinitrate 10 mg, net price 20 =
22p; 20 mg, 20 = 42p
Available from Cox, Hillcross, Norton

Angitak® (Eastern)

Aerosol spray, isosorbide dinitrate 1.25 mg/
metered dose, net price 200-dose unit = £3.95

Dose: treatment or prophylaxis of angina, spray 1–3
doses under tongue whilst holding breath; allow 30 second interval between each dose

Isordil® (Monmouth)

Tablets (sublingual), pink, isosorbide dinitrate
5 mg. Net price 100-tab pack = £1.43. Label: 26

Tablets, both scored, isosorbide dinitrate 10 mg,
net price 112-tab pack = 75p; 30 mg, 112-tab pack
= £3.86

Sorbichew® (Stuart)

Tablets (chewable), green, scored, isosorbide
dinitrate 5 mg. Net price 100-tab pack = £1.51.
Label: 24

Sorbitrate® (Stuart)

Tablets, both scored, isosorbide dinitrate 10 mg
(yellow), net price 100-tab pack = £1.51; 20 mg
(blue), 100-tab pack = £2.10

■ Modified-release preparations

Cedocard Retard® (Pharmacia & Upjohn)

Retard-20 tablets, m/r, yellow, scored, isosorbide
dinitrate 20 mg. Net price 60-tab pack = £5.45.
Label: 25

Dose: prophylaxis of angina, 1 tablet every 12 hours

Retard-40 tablets, m/r, orange-red, scored, isosorbide dinitrate 40 mg. Net price 60-tab pack =
£10.59. Label: 25

Dose: prophylaxis of angina, 1–2 tablets every 12 hours

Isoket Retard® (Schwarz)

Retard-20 tablets, m/r, yellow, scored, isosorbide
dinitrate 20 mg. Net price 56-tab pack = £3.47.
Label: 25

Retard-40 tablets, m/r, orange, scored, isosorbide
dinitrate 40 mg. Net price 56-tab pack = £8.55.
Label: 25

Dose: prophylaxis of angina, 20–40 mg every 12 hours

Isordil Tembids® (Monmouth)

Capsules, m/r, blue/clear, isosorbide dinitrate
40 mg. Net price 56-cap pack = £8.70. Label: 25

Dose: prophylaxis of angina, 1 capsule 2–3 times daily

Sorbid SA® (Stuart)

Sorbid-20 SA capsules, m/r, red/yellow, isosorbide
dinitrate 20 mg. Net price 56-cap pack = £3.50.
Label: 25

Dose: prophylaxis of angina, 1–2 capsules twice daily

Sorbid-40 SA capsules, m/r, red/clear, isosorbide
dinitrate 40 mg. Net price 56-cap pack = £5.00.
Label: 25

Dose: prophylaxis of angina, 1–2 capsules twice daily

■ Parenteral preparations

Isoket® (Schwarz) [PoM]

Injection 0.05%, isosorbide dinitrate
500 micrograms/mL. To be diluted before use or
given undiluted with syringe pump. Net price 50-
mL bottle = £10.06

Injection 0.1%, isosorbide dinitrate 1 mg/mL. To
be diluted before use. Net price 10-mL amp =
£3.62; 50-mL bottle = £17.96; 100-mL bottle =
£25.98

Note. Glass or polyethylene infusion apparatus is preferable; loss of potency if PVC used

■ Transdermal preparations

Isocard® (Eastern)

Transdermal spray, isosorbide dinitrate, 30 mg/
metered dose. Net price 65-dose unit = £17.50.
Label: 10 patient information leaflet, counselling,
administration

Dose: prophylaxis of angina, initially (in those not
previously receiving nitrates) 1 spray daily for 3
days, increased if necessary to 2 sprays daily for 3
days and then to 2 sprays twice daily; usual dose,
1–2 sprays in the morning and at night if necessary
COUNSELLING. Apply to clean dry skin on the chest wall
holding can vertically. Spray each dose onto the chest
from a distance of about 20 cm and then rub in gently;
avoid contact with eyes; do not inhale

Caution: flammable

ISOSORBIDE MONONITRATE

Indications: prophylaxis of angina; adjunct in congestive heart failure

Cautions; Contra-indications; Side-effects:
see under Glyceryl Trinitrate

Dose: initially 20 mg 2–3 times daily *or* 40 mg
twice daily (10 mg twice daily in those who have
not previously received nitrates); up to 120 mg
daily in divided doses if required

Isosorbide Mononitrate (Non-proprietary)

Tablets, isosorbide mononitrate 10 mg, net price 56
= £2.08; 20 mg, 56 = £3.18; 40 mg, 56 = £6.38.
Label: 25

Various strengths available from APS, Ashbourne (*Isib®*),
Berk (*Dynamin®*), Cox, Dominion, Hillcross, Norton,
Opus (*Angeze®*)

Elantan® (Schwarz)

Elantan 10 tablets, scored, isosorbide mononitrate
10 mg. Net price 56 = £3.56; 84 = £5.34. Label: 25

[PoM] *Elantan 20 tablets*, scored, isosorbide
mononitrate 20 mg. Net price 56 = £4.64; 84 =
£6.59. Label: 25

[PoM] *Elantan 40 tablets*, scored, isosorbide
mononitrate 40 mg. Net price 56 = £7.56; 84 =
£11.35. Label: 25

Ismo® (Roche)

Ismo 10 tablets, isosorbide mononitrate 10 mg. Net
price 60-tab pack = £3.24. Label: 25

Ismo 20 tablets, isosorbide mononitrate 20 mg. Net
price 60-tab pack = £4.75. Label: 25

Ismo 40 tablets, isosorbide mononitrate 40 mg. Net
price 60-tab pack = £7.80. Label: 25

Isotrate® (Bioglan)

Tablets, isosorbide mononitrate 20 mg. Net price
60-tab pack = £7.09. Label: 25

Monit® (Sanofi-Synthelabo)

LS Tablets, isosorbide mononitrate 10 mg. Net
price 56-tab pack = £3.37. Label: 25

Tablets, scored, isosorbide mononitrate 20 mg. Net
price 56-tab pack = £4.30. Label: 25

Mono-Cedocard® (Pharmacia & Upjohn)

Mono-Cedocard 10 tablets, orange, scored, isosorbide mononitrate 10 mg. Net price 60-tab pack
= £3.51. Label: 25

Mono-Cedocard 20 tablets, scored, isosorbide
mononitrate 20 mg. Net price 60-tab pack =
£3.92. Label: 25

Mono-Cedocard 40 tablets, scored, isosorbide
mononitrate 40 mg. Net price 60-tab pack =
£8.71. Label: 25

■ Modified release

Chemydur® 60XL (Sovereign) [PoM]

Tablets, m/r, scored, ivory, isosorbide mononitrate 60 mg, net price 28-tab pack = £15.97. Label: 25

Dose: prophylaxis of angina, 1 tablet in the morning (half a tablet for 2–4 days to minimise possibility of headache), increased if necessary to 2 tablets

Elantan LA® (Schwarz)

Elantan LA 25 capsules, m/r, brown/white, enclosing white micropellets, isosorbide mononitrate 25 mg. Net price 28-cap pack = £6.69. Label: 25

Dose: prophylaxis of angina, 1 capsule in the morning, increased if necessary to 2 capsules

Elantan LA 50 capsules, m/r, brown/pink, enclosing white micropellets, isosorbide mononitrate 50 mg. Net price 28-cap pack = £10.79. Label: 25

Dose: prophylaxis of angina, 1 capsule daily in the morning, increased if necessary to 2 capsules

Imdur® (Astra)

Durules® (= tablets m/r), yellow, f/c, scored, isosorbide mononitrate 60 mg. Net price 28-tab pack = £11.14. Label: 25

Dose: prophylaxis of angina, 1 tablet in the morning (half a tablet if headache occurs), increased to 2 tablets if required

Isib 60XL® (Ashbourne)

Tablets, m/r, scored, ivory, isosorbide mononitrate 60 mg. Net price 28-tab pack = £9.47. Label: 25

Dose: prophylaxis of angina, 1 tablet in the morning (half a tablet for 2–4 days if headache occurs), increased if necessary to 2 tablets

Ismo Retard® (Roche)

Tablets, m/r, s/c, isosorbide mononitrate 40 mg. Net price 28-tab pack = £9.78. Label: 25

Dose: prophylaxis of angina, 1 tablet daily in morning

Isotard® (Galen)

Isotard 25XL capsules, m/r, brown/white, isosorbide mononitrate 25 mg, net price 28-cap pack = £6.05. Label: 25

Isotard 50XL capsules, m/r, brown/pink, isosorbide mononitrate 50 mg, net price 28-cap pack = £9.75. Label: 25

Isotard 25XL tablets, m/r, ivory, isosorbide mononitrate 25 mg, net price 28-tab pack = £10.99. Label: 25

Isotard 40XL tablets, m/r, ivory, isosorbide mononitrate 40 mg, net price 28-tab pack = £15.36. Label: 25

Isotard 50XL tablets, m/r, ivory, isosorbide mononitrate 50 mg, net price 28-tab pack = £16.49. Label: 25

Isotard 60XL tablets, m/r, ivory, isosorbide mononitrate 60 mg, net price 28-tab pack = £15.96. Label: 25

Dose: prophylaxis of angina, 25–60 mg daily in the morning (if headache occurs with 60-mg tablet, half a 60-mg tablet may be given for 2–4 days), increased if necessary to 50–120 mg daily

Note. Capsules also available as *Isodur XL®* (Galen)

¹MCR-50® (Pharmacia & Upjohn)

Capsules, m/r, containing white micropellets, isosorbide mononitrate 50 mg. Net price 28-cap pack = £10.52. Label: 25

Dose: prophylaxis of angina, 1 capsule in morning, increased to 2 capsules if required

1. Full product name Mono Cedocard Retard-50®

Modisal XL® (Lagap)

Tablets, m/r, ivory, isosorbide mononitrate 60 mg. Net price 28-tab pack = £15.97. Label: 25

Dose: prophylaxis of angina, 1 tablet daily in the morning (half a tablet for first 2–4 days to minimise possibility of headache), increased if necessary to 2 tablets once daily

Monit SR® (Sanofi-Synthelabo)

Tablets, m/r, s/c, isosorbide mononitrate 40 mg. Net price 28-tab pack = £10.24. Label: 25

Dose: prophylaxis of angina, 1 tablet daily in morning

Monomax SR® (Trinity) [PoM]

Capsules, m/r, isosorbide mononitrate 40 mg, net price 28-cap pack = £8.31; 60 mg, 28-cap pack = £9.03. Label: 25

Dose: prophylaxis of angina, 40 mg once daily, increased if necessary to 60 mg daily

Note. Also available as *Angeze SR®* (Opus)

Monosorb XL 60® (Dexcel) [PoM]

Tablets, m/r, f/c, isosorbide mononitrate 60 mg. Net price 28-tab pack = £16.70. Label: 25

Dose: prophylaxis of angina, 1 tablet daily in the morning (half a tablet for first 2–4 days to minimise possibility of headache), increased if necessary to 2 tablets

Note. Also available from Cox

■ With aspirin

Note. For prophylaxis of angina and secondary prevention of myocardial infarction; for cautions, contra-indications and side-effects of aspirin see section 2.9

Imazin® XL (Napp)

Tablets, aspirin 75 mg, isosorbide mononitrate 60 mg (m/r), net price 28-tab pack = £10.10. Label: 25, 32

Dose: 1 tablet in the morning, increased to 2 tablets if required

Forte tablets, aspirin 150 mg, isosorbide mononitrate 60 mg (m/r), net price 28-tab pack = £10.10. Label: 25, 32

Dose: 1 tablet in the morning

2.6.2 Calcium-channel blockers

Calcium-channel blockers (less correctly called 'calcium-antagonists') interfere with the inward displacement of calcium ions through the slow channels of active cell membranes. They influence the myocardial cells, the cells within the specialised conducting system of the heart, and the cells of vascular smooth muscle. Thus, myocardial contractility may be reduced, the formation and propagation of electrical impulses within the heart may be depressed, and coronary or systemic vascular tone may be diminished.

Calcium-channel blockers differ in their predilection for the various possible sites of action and, therefore, their therapeutic effects are disparate, with much greater variation than those of beta-blockers. There are important differences between verapamil, diltiazem, and the dihydropyridine calcium-channel blockers (amlodipine, felodipine, isradipine, lacidipine, lercanidipine, nicardipine, nifedipine, nimodipine, and nisoldipine). Verapamil and diltiazem should usually be **avoided** in *heart failure* because they may further depress cardiac function and cause clinically significant deterioration.

Verapamil is used for the treatment of *angina* (section 2.6), *hypertension*, and *arrhythmias* (section 2.3.2). It is a highly negatively inotropic calcium channel-blocker and it reduces cardiac output, slows the heart rate, and may impair atrioventricular conduction. It may precipitate heart failure, exacerbate conduction disorders, and cause hypotension at high doses and should **not** be used with beta-blockers (see p. 105). Constipation is the most common side-effect.

Nifedipine relaxes vascular smooth muscle and dilates coronary and peripheral arteries. It has more influence on vessels and less on the myocardium than does verapamil, and unlike verapamil has no anti-arrhythmic activity. It rarely precipitates heart failure because any negative inotropic effect is off-set by a reduction in left ventricular work. Short-acting formulations of nifedipine are not recommended for angina or long-term management of hypertension; their use may be associated with large variations in blood pressure and reflex tachycardia. **Nicardipine** has similar effects to those of nifedipine and may produce less reduction of myocardial contractility. **Amlodipine** and **felodipine** also resemble nifedipine and nicardipine in their effects and do not reduce myocardial contractility and they do not produce clinical deterioration in heart failure. They have a longer duration of action and can be given once daily. Nifedipine, nicardipine, amlodipine, and felodipine are used for the treatment of angina (section 2.6) or hypertension. All are valuable in forms of *angina associated with coronary vasospasm*. Side-effects associated with vasodilatation such as flushing and headache (which become less obtrusive after a few days), and ankle swelling (which may respond only partially to diuretics) are common.

Isradipine, **lacidipine**, **lercanidipine** and **nisoldipine** have similar effects to those of nifedipine and nicardipine; isradipine, lacidipine, and lercanidipine are only indicated for *hypertension* whereas nisoldipine is indicated for angina and hypertension.

Nimodipine is related to nifedipine but the smooth muscle relaxant effect preferentially acts on cerebral arteries. Its use is confined to prevention of *vascular spasm following subarachnoid haemorrhage*.

Diltiazem is effective in most forms of *angina* (section 2.6); the longer-acting formulation is also used for *hypertension*. It may be used in patients for whom beta-blockers are contra-indicated or ineffective. It has a less negative inotropic effect than verapamil and significant myocardial depression occurs rarely. Nevertheless because of the risk of bradycardia it should be used with caution in association with beta-blockers.

UNSTABLE ANGINA. Calcium-channel blockers do not reduce the risk of myocardial infarction in unstable angina. The use of diltiazem or verapamil should be reserved for patients resistant to treatment with beta-blockers.

WITHDRAWAL. There is some evidence that sudden withdrawal of calcium-channel blockers may be associated with an exacerbation of angina.

AMLODIPINE BESILATE

Indications: hypertension, prophylaxis of angina

Cautions: hepatic impairment; **interactions:** Appendix 1 (calcium-channel blockers)

Contra-indications: cardiogenic shock, unstable angina, significant aortic stenosis; pregnancy and breast-feeding

Side-effects: headache, oedema, fatigue, nausea, flushing, dizziness, gum hyperplasia, rashes (including rarely pruritus and very rarely erythema multiforme); rarely gastro-intestinal disturbances, palpitations, dyspnoea, drowsiness, mood changes, muscle cramps, myalgia, arthralgia, asthenia, impotence, urinary frequency, visual disturbances; also reported altered liver function tests, jaundice, gynaecomastia

Dose: hypertension or angina, initially 5 mg once daily; max. 10 mg once daily

Istin® (Pfizer) ▣PoM▣

Tablets, amlodipine (as besilate) 5 mg. Net price 28-tab pack = £11.85; 10 mg, 28-tab pack = £17.70

DILTIAZEM HYDROCHLORIDE

Indications: prophylaxis and treatment of angina; hypertension

Cautions: reduce dose in hepatic and renal impairment; heart failure or significantly impaired left ventricular function, bradycardia (avoid if severe), first degree AV block, or prolonged PR interval; **interactions:** Appendix 1 (calcium-channel blockers)

Contra-indications: severe bradycardia, left ventricular failure, second- or third-degree AV block (unless pacemaker fitted), sick sinus syndrome; pregnancy and breast-feeding (see Appendixes 4 and 5)

Side-effects: bradycardia, sino-atrial block, AV block, palpitations, dizziness, hypotension, malaise, asthenia, headache, hot flushes, gastro-intestinal disturbances, oedema (notably of ankles); rarely rashes (including erythema multiforme and exfoliative dermatitis), photosensitivity; altered liver function tests; hepatitis, gynaecomastia, gum hyperplasia, extrapyramidal symptoms, depression reported

Dose: angina, 60 mg 3 times daily (elderly initially twice daily); increased if necessary to 360 mg daily

Longer-acting formulations, see under preparations below

■ Standard formulations

Note. These formulations are licensed as generics and there is no requirement for brand name dispensing. Although their means of formulation has called for the strict designation 'modified-release' their duration of action corresponds to that of tablets requiring administration 3 times daily

Diltiazem (Non-proprietary) ▣PoM▣

Tablets, m/r (but see note above), diltiazem hydrochloride 60 mg. Net price 100 = £7.50. Label: 25
Available from Ashbourne (*Angiozem®*), Cox, Hillcross, Norton, Opus (*Optil®*)

Tildiem® (Sanofi-Synthelabo) ▣PoM▣

Tablets, m/r (but see note above), off-white, diltiazem hydrochloride 60 mg. Net price 90-tab pack = £10.35. Label: 25

■ **Longer-acting formulations**

Note. Different versions of modified-release preparations may not have the same clinical effect. To avoid confusion between these different formulations of diltiazem, prescribers should specify the brand to be dispensed

Adizem-SR® (Napp) PoM

Capsules, m/r, diltiazem hydrochloride 90 mg (white), net price 56-cap pack = £10.56; 120 mg (brown/white), 56-cap pack = £11.74; 180 mg (brown/white), 56-cap pack = £17.60. Label: 25

Tablets, m/r, f/c, scored, diltiazem hydrochloride 120 mg. Net price 56-tab pack = £17.32. Label: 25

Dose: mild to moderate hypertension, usually 120 mg twice daily (dose form not appropriate for initial dose titration)

Angina, initially 90 mg twice daily (elderly, dose form not appropriate for initial dose titration); increased to 180 mg twice daily if required

Adizem-XL® (Napp) PoM

Capsules, m/r, diltiazem hydrochloride 120 mg (pink/blue), net price 28-cap pack = £10.24; 180 mg (dark pink/blue), 28-cap pack = £11.61; 240 mg (red/blue), 28-cap pack = £12.90; 300 mg (maroon/blue), 28-cap pack = £10.24. Label: 25

Dose: angina and mild to moderate hypertension, initially 240 mg once daily, increased if necessary to 300 mg once daily; in elderly and in hepatic or renal impairment, initially 120 mg daily

Angitil SR® (Trinity) PoM

Capsules, m/r, diltiazem hydrochloride 90 mg (white), net price 56-cap pack = £8.45; 120 mg (brown), 56-cap pack = £9.39; 180 mg (brown), 56-cap pack = £14.08. Label: 25

Dose: angina and mild to moderate hypertension, initially 90 mg twice daily; increased if necessary to 120 mg or 180 mg twice daily

Note. Also available as *Optil® SR* (Opus)

Angitil XL® (Trinity) PoM

Capsules, m/r, diltiazem hydrochloride 240 mg (white), net price 28-cap pack = £10.15; 300 mg (yellow), 28-cap pack = £9.22. Label: 25

Dose: angina and mild to moderate hypertension, initially 240 mg once daily (elderly and in hepatic and renal impairment, dose form not appropriate for initial dose titration); increased if necessary to 300 mg once daily

Note. Also available as *Optil® XL* (Opus)

Calcicard CR® (Norton) PoM

Tablets, m/r, both f/c, diltiazem hydrochloride 90 mg, net price 56-tab pack = £11.06; 120 mg, 56-tab pack = £12.29. Label: 25

Dose: mild to moderate hypertension, initially 90 mg or 120 mg twice daily; up to 360 mg daily may be required; ELDERLY and in hepatic and renal impairment, initially 120 mg once daily; up to 240 mg daily may be required

Angina, initially 90 mg or 120 mg twice daily; up to 480 mg daily in divided doses may be required; ELDERLY and in hepatic and renal impairment, dose form not appropriate for initial dose titration; up to 240 mg daily may be required

Note. Also available as *Angiozem CR®* (Ashbourne)

Dilcardia SR® (Generics) PoM

Capsules, m/r, diltiazem hydrochloride 60 mg (pink/white), net price 100-cap pack = £14.82; 90 mg (pink/yellow), 56-cap pack = £11.06; 120 mg (pink/orange), 56-cap pack = £12.29. Label: 25

Dose: angina and mild to moderate hypertension, initially 90 mg twice daily; increased if necessary to 180 mg twice daily; ELDERLY and in hepatic or renal impairment, initially 60 mg twice daily, max. 90 mg twice daily

Dilzem SR® (Elan) PoM

Capsules, m/r, all beige, diltiazem hydrochloride 60 mg, net price 56-cap pack = £8.32; 90 mg, 56-cap pack = £11.23; 120 mg, 56-cap pack = £12.47. Label: 25

Dose: angina and mild to moderate hypertension, initially 90 mg twice daily (elderly 60 mg twice daily); up to 180 mg twice daily may be required

Dilzem XL® (Elan) PoM

Capsules, m/r, diltiazem hydrochloride 120 mg, net price 28-cap pack = £8.32; 180 mg, 28-cap pack = £11.40; 240 mg, 28-cap pack = £11.70. Label: 25

Dose: angina and mild to moderate hypertension, initially 180 mg once daily (elderly and in hepatic and renal impairment, 120 mg once daily); if necessary may be increased to 360 mg once daily

Slozem® (Lipha) PoM

Capsules, m/r, diltiazem hydrochloride 120 mg (pink/clear), net price 28-cap pack = £7.00; 180 mg (pink/clear), 28-cap pack = £7.80; 240 mg (red/clear), 28-cap pack = £8.20. Label: 25

Dose: angina and mild to moderate hypertension, initially 240 mg once daily (elderly and in hepatic and renal impairment, 120 mg once daily); if necessary may be increased to 360 mg once daily

Tildiem LA® (Sanofi-Synthelabo) PoM

Capsules, m/r, diltiazem hydrochloride 200 mg (pink/grey, containing white pellets), net price 28-cap pack = £11.61; 300 mg (white/yellow, containing white pellets), 28-cap pack = £12.80. Label: 25

Dose: angina and mild to moderate hypertension, initially 200 mg once daily before or with food, increased if necessary to 300–400 mg daily, max. 500 mg daily; ELDERLY and in hepatic or renal impairment, initially 200 mg daily, increased if necessary to 300 mg daily

Tildiem Retard® (Sanofi-Synthelabo) PoM

Tablets, m/r, diltiazem hydrochloride 90 mg, net price 56-tab pack = £11.06; 120 mg, 56-tab pack = £12.29. Label: 25

COUNSELLING. Tablet membrane may pass through gastro-intestinal tract unchanged, but being porous has no effect on efficacy

Dose: mild to moderate hypertension, initially 90 mg or 120 mg twice daily; increased if necessary to 360 mg daily in divided doses; ELDERLY and in hepatic or renal impairment, initially 120 mg once daily; increased if necessary to 120 mg twice daily

Angina, initially 90 mg or 120 mg twice daily; increased if necessary to 480 mg daily in divided doses; ELDERLY and in hepatic or renal impairment, dose form not appropriate for initial titration; up to 120 mg twice daily may be required

Viazem XL® (Du Pont) PoM

Capsules, m/r, diltiazem hydrochloride 120 mg (lavender), net price 28-cap pack = £8.82; 180 mg (white/blue-green), 28-cap pack = £8.82; 240 mg (blue-green/lavender), 28-cap pack = £9.22; 300 mg (white/lavender), 28-cap pack = £9.22; 360 mg (blue-green), 28-cap pack = £17.65. Label: 25

Dose: mild to moderate hypertension, titrate to usual maintenance dose of 300 mg once daily, adjusted according to response

ELDERLY and in hepatic or renal impairment, initially 120 mg once daily, adjusted according to response

Zemtard® (Galen) [PoM]

Zemtard 120XL capsules, m/r, brown/orange, diltiazem hydrochloride 120 mg, net price 28-cap pack = £7.65. Label: 25

Zemtard 180XL capsules, m/r, grey/pink, diltiazem hydrochloride 180 mg, net price 28-cap pack = £7.80. Label: 25

Zemtard 240XL capsules, m/r, blue, diltiazem hydrochloride 240 mg, net price 28-cap pack = £8.20. Label: 25

Zemtard 300XL capsules, m/r, white/blue, diltiazem hydrochloride 300 mg, net price 28-cap pack = £8.50. Label: 25

Dose: angina and mild to moderate hypertension, 180–300 mg once daily, increased if necessary to 360 mg once daily in hypertension and to 480 mg once daily in angina; ELDERLY and in hepatic or renal impairment, initially 120 mg once daily

FELODIPINE

Indications: hypertension, prophylaxis of angina

Cautions: withdraw if ischaemic pain occurs or existing pain worsens shortly after initiating treatment or if cardiogenic shock develops; severe left ventricular dysfunction; hepatic impairment; breast-feeding; avoid grapefruit juice (may affect metabolism); **interactions:** Appendix 1 (calcium-channel blockers)

Contra-indications: pregnancy; unstable angina; significant aortic stenosis; within 1 month of myocardial infarction

Side-effects: flushing, headache, palpitations, dizziness, fatigue, gravitational oedema, rash and pruritus, gum hyperplasia

Dose: hypertension, initially 5 mg (elderly 2.5 mg) daily in the morning; usual maintenance 5–10 mg once daily; doses above 20 mg daily rarely needed

Angina, initially 5 mg daily in the morning, increased if necessary to 10 mg once daily

Plendil® (Astra) [PoM]

Tablets, m/r, f/c, felodipine 2.5 mg, net price 28-tab pack = £6.09; 5 mg, 28-tab pack = £8.12; 10 mg, 28-tab pack = £10.92. Label: 25

ISRADIPINE

Indications: hypertension

Cautions: tight aortic stenosis; sick sinus syndrome (if pacemaker not fitted); reduce dose in hepatic or renal impairment; pregnancy (may prolong labour); avoid grapefruit juice (may affect metabolism); **interactions:** Appendix 1 (calcium-channel blockers)

Side-effects: headache, flushing, dizziness, tachycardia and palpitations, localised peripheral oedema; hypotension uncommon; rarely weight gain, fatigue, abdominal discomfort, rashes

Dose: 2.5 mg twice daily (1.25 mg twice daily in elderly, hepatic or renal impairment); increased if necessary after 3–4 weeks to 5 mg twice daily (exceptionally up to 10 mg twice daily); maintenance 2.5 or 5 mg once daily may be sufficient

Prescal® (Novartis) [PoM]

Tablets, yellow, scored, isradipine 2.5 mg. Net price 56-tab pack = £12.53

LACIDIPINE

Indications: hypertension

Cautions: cardiac conduction abnormalities; poor cardiac reserve; hepatic impairment; withdraw if ischaemic pain occurs shortly after initiating treatment or if cardiogenic shock develops; avoid grapefruit juice (may affect metabolism); **interactions:** Appendix 1 (calcium-channel blockers)

Contra-indications: aortic stenosis; pregnancy and breast-feeding; avoid within 1 month of myocardial infarction

Side-effects: headache, flushing, oedema, dizziness, palpitations; also asthenia, rash (including pruritus and erythema), gastro-intestinal disturbances, gum hyperplasia, muscle cramps, polyuria, chest pain (see Cautions); mood disturbances

Dose: initially 2 mg as a single daily dose, preferably in the morning; increased after 3–4 weeks to 4 mg daily, then if necessary to 6 mg daily

Motens® (Boehringer Ingelheim) [PoM]

Tablets, both f/c, lacidipine 2 mg, net price 28-tab pack = £10.23; 4 mg (scored), 28-tab pack = £15.30

LERCANIDIPINE HYDROCHLORIDE

Indications: mild to moderate hypertension

Cautions: hepatic and renal impairment (Appendixes 2 and 3); left ventricular dysfunction; sick sinus syndrome (if pacemaker not fitted); avoid grapefruit juice (may affect metabolism); **interactions:** Appendix 1 (calcium-channel blockers)

Contra-indications: aortic stenosis; unstable angina, uncontrolled heart failure; within 1 month of myocardial infarction; pregnancy and breast-feeding

Side-effects: flushing, peripheral oedema, palpitations, tachycardia, headache, dizziness, asthenia; also gastro-intestinal disturbances, hypotension, drowsiness, myalgia, polyuria, rash

Dose: initially 10 mg once daily; increased, if necessary, after at least 2 weeks to 20 mg daily

Zanidip® (Napp) ▼ [PoM]

Tablets, yellow, f/c, lercanidipine hydrochloride 10 mg, net price 28-tab pack = £9.74. Label: 22

NICARDIPINE HYDROCHLORIDE

Indications: prophylaxis of angina; mild to moderate hypertension

Cautions: withdraw if ischaemic pain occurs or existing pain worsens within 30 minutes of initiating treatment or increasing dose; congestive heart failure or significantly impaired left ventricular function; elderly; hepatic or renal impairment; avoid grapefruit juice (may affect metabolism); **interactions:** Appendix 1 (calcium-channel blockers)

Contra-indications: cardiogenic shock; advanced aortic stenosis; unstable or acute attacks of angina; pregnancy and breast-feeding; avoid within 1 month of myocardial infarction

Side-effects: dizziness, headache, peripheral oedema, flushing, palpitations, nausea; also gastro-intestinal disturbances, drowsiness, insomnia, tinnitus, hypotension, rashes, dyspnoea, paraesthesia, frequency of micturition; thrombocytopenia, depression and impotence reported

Dose: initially 20 mg 3 times daily, increased, after at least three days, to 30 mg 3 times daily (usual range 60–120 mg daily)

Cardene® (Yamanouchi) PoM

Capsules, nicardipine hydrochloride 20 mg (blue/white), net price 56-cap pack = £8.38; 30 mg (blue/pale blue), 56-cap pack = £9.73

■ Modified release

Cardene SR® (Yamanouchi) PoM

Capsules, m/r, nicardipine hydrochloride 30 mg, net price 56-cap pack = £9.68; 45 mg (blue), 56-cap pack = £13.44. Label: 25

Dose: mild to moderate hypertension, initially 30 mg twice daily; usual effective dose 45 mg twice daily (range 30–60 mg twice daily)

NIFEDIPINE

Indications: prophylaxis of angina; hypertension; Raynaud's phenomenon

Cautions: withdraw if ischaemic pain occurs or existing pain worsens shortly after initiating treatment; poor cardiac reserve; heart failure or significantly impaired left ventricular function (heart failure deterioration observed); severe hypotension; reduce dose in hepatic impairment; diabetes mellitus; may inhibit labour; pregnancy (Appendix 4); breast-feeding (Appendix 5); avoid grapefruit juice (may affect metabolism); **interactions:** Appendix 1 (calcium-channel blockers)

Contra-indications: cardiogenic shock; advanced aortic stenosis; within 1 month of myocardial infarction; unstable or acute attacks of angina; porphyria (section 9.8.2)

Side-effects: headache, flushing, dizziness, lethargy; tachycardia, palpitations; short-acting preparations may induce an exaggerated fall in blood pressure and reflex tachycardia which may lead to myocardial or cerebrovascular ischaemia; gravitational oedema, rash (erythema multiforme reported), pruritus, urticaria, nausea, constipation or diarrhoea, increased frequency of micturition, eye pain, visual disturbances, gum hyperplasia, paraesthesia, myalgia, tremor, impotence, gynaecomastia; depression, telangiectasia, cholestasis, jaundice reported

Dose: see preparations below

Adalat® (Bayer) PoM

Capsules, both orange, nifedipine 5 mg, net price 90-cap pack = £6.08; 10 mg, 90-cap pack = £7.74

Dose: angina prophylaxis (but not recommended, see notes above) and Raynaud's phenomenon, initially 5 mg 3 times daily, adjusted according to response to 20 mg 3 times daily

Hypertension, not recommended therefore no dose stated

Note. Nifedipine capsules also available from APS, Ashbourne (*Angiopine®*), Berk (*Calanif®*), Cox, CP, Hillcross, Norton

■ Modified release

Note. Different versions of modified-release preparations may not have the same clinical effect. To avoid confusion between these different formulations of nifedipine, prescribers should specify the brand to be dispensed. Modified-release formulations may not be suitable for dose titration in hepatic disease

Adalat® LA (Bayer) PoM

LA 20 tablets, m/r, pink, nifedipine 20 mg, net price 28-tab pack = £8.15. Label: 25

LA 30 tablets, m/r, pink, nifedipine 30 mg,net price 28-tab pack = £9.89. Label: 25

LA 60 tablets, m/r, pink, nifedipine 60 mg, net price 28-tab pack = £15.40. Label: 25

COUNSELLING. Tablet membrane may pass through gastro-intestinal tract unchanged, but being porous has no effect on efficacy

Dose: mild to moderate hypertension, 20 mg once daily, increased if necessary

Angina prophylaxis, 30 mg once daily, increased if necessary; max. 90 mg once daily

Caution: dose form not appropriate for use in hepatic impairment or where there is a history of oesophageal or gastro-intestinal obstruction, decreased lumen diameter of the gastro-intestinal tract, or inflammatory bowel disease (including Crohn's disease)

Adalat® Retard (Bayer) PoM

Retard 10 tablets, m/r, pink, nifedipine 10 mg. Net price 56-tab pack = £8.50. Label: 25

Retard 20 tablets, m/r, pink, nifedipine 20 mg. Net price 56-tab pack = £10.20. Label: 25

Dose: hypertension and angina prophylaxis, 10 mg twice daily, adjusted according to response to 40 mg twice daily

Adipine® MR (Trinity) PoM

Tablets, m/r, nifedipine 10 mg (apricot), net price 56-tab pack = £6.62; 20 mg (pink), 56-tab pack = £8.26. Label: 21, 25

Dose: hypertension and angina prophylaxis, 20 mg twice daily after food (initial titration 10 mg twice daily); max. 40 mg twice daily

Note. Also available as *Nimodrel MR®* (Opus)

Angiopine 40 LA® (Ashbourne) PoM

Tablets, m/r, brown, nifedipine 40 mg, net price 28-tab pack = £8.65. Label: 21, 25

Dose: hypertension, 40 mg once daily, increased if necessary to 80 mg once daily

Cardilate MR® (Norton) PoM

Tablets, m/r, nifedipine 10 mg (pink), net price 56-tab pack = £6.93; 20 mg (brown), net price 100-tab pack = £18.35. Label: 25

Dose: hypertension and angina prophylaxis, 20 mg twice daily (initial titration 10 mg twice daily); max. 80 mg daily

Note. Also available as *Angiopine MR®* (Ashbourne)

Coracten SR® (Medeva) PoM

Capsules, m/r, nifedipine 10 mg (grey/pink, enclosing yellow pellets), net price 60-cap pack = £7.15; 20 mg (pink/brown, enclosing yellow pellets), 60-cap pack = £9.97. Label: 25

Dose: hypertension and angina prophylaxis, one 20-mg capsule every 12 hours, adjusted within range 10–40 mg every 12 hours

Coracten XL® (Medeva) PoM

Capsules, m/r, nifedipine 30 mg (brown), net price 28-cap pack = £6.73; 60 mg (orange), 28-cap pack = £10.01. Label: 25

Dose: hypertension and angina prophylaxis, 30 mg once daily, increased if necessary; max. 90 mg once daily

Coroday MR® (Generics) PoM

Tablets, m/r, red, nifedipine 20 mg, net price 56-tab pack = £10.81. Label: 25

Dose: hypertension and angina prophylaxis, 20 mg every 12 hours, increased if necessary to 40 mg every 12 hours

Fortipine LA 40® (Goldshield) [PoM]
Tablets, m/r, red, nifedipine 40 mg, net price 30-tab pack = £8.00. Label: 21, 25
Dose: hypertension and angina prophylaxis, 40 mg once daily, increased if necessary to 80 mg daily in 1–2 divided doses

Hypolar® Retard 20 (Lagap) [PoM]
Tablets, m/r, red, f/c, nifedipine 20 mg. Net price 56-tab pack = £10.12. Label: 25
Dose: hypertension and angina prophylaxis, 20 mg twice daily, increased if necessary to 40 mg twice daily

Nifedipress® MR (Dexcel) [PoM]
Tablets, m/r, pink, nifedipine 10 mg, net price 56-tab pack = £9.93. Label: 25
Dose: hypertension and angina prophylaxis, initially 10 mg twice daily adjusted according to response to 40 mg twice daily

Nifedotard 20 MR® (Bartholomew Rhodes) [PoM]
Tablets, m/r, red, nifedipine 20 mg. Net price 56-tab pack = £10.62. Label: 25
Dose: hypertension and angina prophylaxis, 20 mg twice daily, increased if necessary to 40 mg twice daily

Nifopress® Retard (Goldshield) [PoM]
Tablets, m/r, pink, nifedipine 20 mg, net price 112-tab pack = £9.00. Label: 21, 25
Dose: mild to moderate hypertension, angina prophylaxis and Raynaud's phenomenon, usually 20 mg twice daily, adjusted according to response to 40 mg twice daily

Slofedipine® (Sterwin) [PoM]
Tablets, m/r, pink, nifedipine 20 mg, net price 56-tab pack = £10.32. Label: 25
Dose: hypertension and angina prophylaxis, initially 20 mg twice daily adjusted according to response to 40 mg twice daily

Slofedipine XL® (Sterwin) [PoM]
Tablets, m/r, brown, nifedipine 30 mg, net price 28-tab pack = £9.89; 60 mg, 28-tab pack = £14.71. Label: 25
Dose: hypertension and angina prophylaxis, 30 mg once daily, increased if necessary to 90 mg once daily
Caution: dose form not appropriate for use in hepatic impairment or where there is a history of oesophageal or gastro-intestinal obstruction, decreased lumen diameter of the gastro-intestinal tract, or inflammatory bowel disease (including Crohn's disease)

Tensipine MR® (Genus) [PoM]
Tablets, m/r, both pink, nifedipine 10 mg, net price 56-tab pack = £7.62; 20 mg, 56-tab pack = £9.51. Label: 21, 25
Dose: hypertension and angina prophylaxis, initially 10 mg twice daily adjusted according to response to 40 mg twice daily

Unipine XL® (Genus) [PoM]
Tablets, m/r, red, f/c, nifedipine 30 mg. Net price 28-tab pack = £9.51. Label: 22, 25
Dose: mild to moderate hypertension, 30 mg once daily, preferably in the morning, increased if necessary to 60 mg once daily

■ With atenolol
Section 2.4

NIMODIPINE

Indications: prevention and treatment of ischaemic neurological deficits following subarachnoid haemorrhage
Cautions: cerebral oedema or severely raised intracranial pressure; avoid concomitant administration of nimodipine tablets and infusion, other calcium-channel blockers, or beta-blockers; impaired renal function or nephrotoxic drugs; pregnancy; avoid grapefruit juice (may affect metabolism); **interactions:** Appendix 1 (calcium-channel blockers)

Side-effects: hypotension, variation in heart-rate, flushing, headache, gastro-intestinal disorders, nausea, and feeling of warmth; thrombocytopenia and ileus reported; transient increase in liver enzymes after intravenous administration

Dose: prevention, *by mouth*, 60 mg every 4 hours (total daily dose 360 mg), starting within 4 days of subarachnoid haemorrhage and continued for 21 days
Treatment, *by intravenous infusion* via central catheter, 1 mg/hour initially, increased after 2 hours to 2 mg/hour, providing no severe decrease in blood pressure; patients with unstable blood pressure or weighing less than 70 kg, 500 micrograms/hour initially or less if necessary; treatment should start as soon as possible and should continue for at least 5 days (max. 14 days); in the event of surgical intervention during treatment continue for at least 5 days after

Nimotop® (Bayer) [PoM]
Tablets, yellow, f/c, nimodipine 30 mg. Net price 100-tab pack = £38.85
Intravenous infusion, nimodipine 200 micrograms/mL; also contains ethanol 20% and macrogol '400' 17%. Net price 50-mL vial (with polyethylene infusion catheter) = £13.24
Note. Polyethylene or polypropylene apparatus should be used; PVC should be avoided

NISOLDIPINE

Indications: prophylaxis of angina, mild to moderate hypertension
Cautions: elderly; hypotension; avoid grapefruit juice (may affect metabolism); **interactions:** Appendix 1 (calcium-channel blockers)
Contra-indications: cardiogenic shock, aortic stenosis, unstable or acute attacks of angina; within 1 week of myocardial infarction; hepatic impairment (dose form not appropriate); pregnancy and breast-feeding
Side-effects: gravitational oedema, headache, flushing, tachycardia, palpitations; dizziness, asthenia, gastro-intestinal disturbances (including nausea, constipation); less frequently paraesthesia, myalgia, tremor, hypotension, weakness, dyspnoea, allergic skin reactions, increased frequency of micturition, liver enzyme disturbances; rarely exacerbation of angina, visual disturbances, gynaecomastia, gum hyperplasia
Dose: initially 10 mg daily, preferably before breakfast; if necessary increase at intervals of at least 1 week (usual maintenance in angina 20–40 mg once daily); max. 40 mg daily

Syscor MR® (Pharmax) [PoM]
Tablets, m/r, all f/c, yellow, nisoldipine 10 mg, net price 28-tab pack = £9.36; 20 mg, 28-tab pack = £13.10; 30 mg, 28-tab pack = £16.85. Label: 22, 25

VERAPAMIL HYDROCHLORIDE

Indications: see under Dose and preparations

Cautions: first-degree AV block; acute phase of myocardial infarction (avoid if bradycardia, hypotension, left ventricular failure); patients taking beta-blockers (**important:** see below); reduce dose in hepatic impairment; children, specialist advice only (section 2.3.2); pregnancy and breast-feeding; avoid grapefruit juice (may affect metabolism); **interactions:** Appendix 1 (calcium-channel blockers)

VERAPAMIL AND BETA-BLOCKERS. **Verapamil** injection should not be given to patients recently treated with beta-blockers because of the risk of hypotension and asystole. The suggestion that when verapamil injection has been given first, an interval of 30 minutes before giving a beta-blocker is sufficient has not been confirmed.

It may also be hazardous to give verapamil and a beta-blocker together by mouth (should only be contemplated if myocardial function well preserved).

Contra-indications: hypotension, bradycardia, second- and third-degree AV block, sick sinus syndrome, cardiogenic shock, sino-atrial block; history of heart failure or significantly impaired left ventricular function, even if controlled by therapy; atrial flutter or fibrillation complicating Wolff-Parkinson-White syndrome; porphyria (section 9.8.2)

Side-effects: constipation; less commonly nausea, vomiting, flushing, headache, dizziness, fatigue, ankle oedema; rarely reversible impairment of liver function, allergic reactions (erythema, pruritus, urticaria, angioedema, Stevens-Johnson syndrome); myalgia, arthralgia, paraesthesia, erythromelalgia; increased prolactin concentration; rarely gynaecomastia and gingival hyperplasia after long-term treatment; after intravenous administration or high doses, hypotension, heart failure, bradycardia, heart block, and asystole

Dose: *by mouth*, supraventricular arrhythmias (but see also Contra-indications), 40–120 mg 3 times daily
Angina, 80–120 mg 3 times daily
Hypertension, 240–480 mg daily in 2–3 divided doses

By slow intravenous injection over 2 minutes (3 minutes in elderly), 5–10 mg (preferably with ECG monitoring); in paroxysmal tachyarrhythmias a further 5 mg after 5–10 minutes if required

Verapamil (Non-proprietary) PoM
Tablets, coated, verapamil hydrochloride 40 mg, net price 20 = 33p; 80 mg, 20 = 58p; 120 mg, 20 = £1.12; 160 mg, 20 = £1.25
Various strengths available from APS, Berk (*Berkatens*®), Cox, Hillcross, Norton
Oral solution, sugar-free, verapamil hydrochloride 40 mg/5 mL available from Rosemont (special order)

Cordilox® (Baker Norton) PoM
Tablets, all yellow, f/c, verapamil hydrochloride 40 mg, net price 100-tab pack = £4.57; 80 mg, 100-tab pack = £9.15; 120 mg, 100-tab pack = £13.70; 160 mg, 56-tab pack = £12.77
Injection, verapamil hydrochloride 2.5 mg/mL, net price 2-mL amp = £1.11

Securon® (Knoll) PoM
Tablets, f/c, verapamil hydrochloride 40 mg, net price 100 = £4.57; 80 mg (scored), 100 = £9.14; 120 mg (scored), 60-tab pack = £7.67
Injection, verapamil hydrochloride 2.5 mg/mL. Net price 2-mL amp = £1.08

■ Modified release

Half Securon SR® (Knoll) PoM
Tablets, m/r, f/c, verapamil hydrochloride 120 mg. Net price 28-tab pack = £6.82. Label: 25
Dose: see *Securon SR*®

Securon SR® (Knoll) PoM
Tablets, m/r, pale green, f/c, scored, verapamil hydrochloride 240 mg. Net price 28-tab pack = £10.64. Label: 25
Dose: hypertension, 240 mg daily (new patients initially 120 mg), increased if necessary to max. 480 mg daily (doses above 240 mg daily as 2 divided doses)
Angina, 240 mg twice daily (may sometimes be reduced to once daily)
Prophylaxis after myocardial infarction where beta-blockers not appropriate (started at least 1 week after infarction), 360 mg daily in divided doses, given as 240 mg in the morning and 120 mg in the evening *or* 120 mg 3 times daily

Univer® (Elan) PoM
Capsules, m/r, verapamil hydrochloride 120 mg (yellow/dark blue), net price 28-cap pack = £7.51; 180 mg (yellow), 56-cap pack = £18.15; 240 mg (yellow/dark blue), 28-cap pack = £12.24. Label: 25
Dose: hypertension, 240 mg daily, max. 480 mg daily (new patients, initial dose 120 mg); angina, 360 mg daily, max. 480 mg daily

Verapress MR® (Dexcel) PoM
Tablets, m/r, pale green, f/c, verapamil hydrochloride 240 mg. Net price 28-tab pack = £10.64. Label: 25
Dose: hypertension, 1 tablet daily, increased to twice daily if necessary; angina, 1 tablet twice daily (may sometimes be reduced to once daily)
Note. Also available as *Cordilox*® *MR* (Norton), *Ethimil*® *MR* (Genus)

Vertab® SR 240 (Trinity) PoM
Tablets, m/r, pale green, f/c, scored, verapamil hydrochloride 240 mg, net price 28-tab pack = £8.63. Label: 25
Dose: mild to moderate hypertension, 240 mg daily, increased to twice daily if necessary; angina, 240 mg twice daily (may sometimes be reduced to once daily)

2.6.3 Potassium-channel activators

Nicorandil, a potassium-channel activator with a nitrate component, has both arterial and venous vasodilating properties and is indicated for the prevention and long-term treatment of angina. Nicorandil has similar efficacy to other antianginal drugs in controlling symptoms but there is little evidence about its efficacy in combination with other antianginal drugs.

NICORANDIL

Indications: prophylaxis and treatment of angina
Cautions: hypovolaemia; low systolic blood pressure; acute pulmonary oedema; acute myocardial infarction with acute left ventricular failure and

low filling pressures; pregnancy and breast-feeding; **interactions:** Appendix 1 (nicorandil)
DRIVING. Patients should be warned not to drive or operate machinery until it is established that their performance is unimpaired
Contra-indications: cardiogenic shock; left ventricular failure with low filling pressures; hypotension
Side-effects: headache (especially on initiation, usually transitory); cutaneous vasodilatation with flushing; nausea, vomiting, dizziness, weakness also reported; rarely oral ulceration and myalgia; at high dosage, reduction in blood pressure and/or increase in heart rate
Dose: initially 10 mg twice daily (if susceptible to headache 5 mg twice daily); usual dose 10–20 mg twice daily; up to 30 mg twice daily may be used

Ikorel® (Rhône-Poulenc Rorer) ▼ PoM
Tablets, both scored, nicorandil 10 mg, net price 60-tab pack = £8.65; 20 mg, 60-tab pack = £16.44

2.6.4   Peripheral and cerebral vasodilators

2.6.4.1	Peripheral vasodilators and related drugs
2.6.4.2	Cerebral vasodilators

2.6.4.1   Peripheral vasodilators and related drugs

Most serious peripheral vascular disorders, such as *intermittent claudication*, are due to occlusion of vessels, either by spasm or sclerotic plaques. Lifestyle changes including smoking cessation and exercise training are the most important measures in the conservative management of intermittent claudication. Low-dose aspirin (75–300 mg daily) should be given as long-term prophylaxis against cardiovascular events. **Naftidrofuryl** 200 mg 3 times daily may alleviate symptoms and improve pain-free walking distance in moderate disease, but it is not known whether naftidrofuryl has any effect on the outcome of the disease. Patients receiving naftidrofuryl should be assessed for improvement after 3–6 months. Inositol nicotinate, pentoxifylline (oxpentifylline) and cinnarizine are not established as being effective.

Management of *Raynaud's syndrome* includes avoidance of exposure to cold and stopping smoking. More severe symptoms may require vasodilator treatment, which is most often successful in primary Raynaud's syndrome. **Nifedipine** (section 2.6.2) is useful for reducing the frequency and severity of vasospastic attacks. Alternatively, **naftidrofuryl** may produce symptomatic improvement; **inositol nicotinate** (a nicotinic acid derivative) may also be considered. Cinnarizine, pentoxifylline (oxpentifylline), prazosin and moxisylyte (thymoxamine) are not established as being effective.

Vasodilator therapy is not established as being effective for *chilblains* (section 13.14).

▶ denotes preparations that are considered to be less suitable for prescribing (see p. vi)

CINNARIZINE ▭

Indications: peripheral vascular disease, Raynaud's syndrome
Cautions: see section 4.6
Contra-indications: see section 4.6
Side-effects: see section 4.6
Dose: initially, 75 mg 3 times daily; maintenance, 75 mg 2–3 times daily

Stugeron Forte® (Janssen-Cilag) ▭
Capsules, orange/ivory, cinnarizine 75 mg. Net price 100-cap pack = £5.50. Label: 2
Stugeron®: see section 4.6

MOXISYLYTE/THYMOXAMINE ▭

Indications: primary Raynaud's syndrome (short-term treatment); erectile dysfunction (section 7.4.5)
Cautions: diabetes mellitus
Contra-indications: active liver disease
Side-effects: nausea, diarrhoea, flushing, headache, dizziness; hepatic reactions including cholestatic jaundice and hepatitis reported to CSM
Dose: initially 40 mg 4 times daily, increased to 80 mg 4 times daily if poor initial response; discontinue after 2 weeks if no response

Opilon® (Hansam) PoM ▭
Tablets, yellow, f/c, moxisylyte 40 mg (as hydrochloride). Net price 112-tab pack = £79.98. Label: 21

NAFTIDROFURYL OXALATE

Indications: see under Dose
Side-effects: nausea, epigastric pain, rash, hepatitis, hepatic failure
Dose: peripheral vascular disease (see notes above), 100–200 mg 3 times daily; cerebral vascular disease, 100 mg 3 times daily

Naftidrofuryl (Non-proprietary) PoM
Capsules, naftidrofuryl oxalate 100 mg. Net price 84-cap pack = £8.12. Label: 25, 27
Available from Berk (*Stimlor®*), Cox
Praxilene® (Lipha) PoM
Capsules, pink, naftidrofuryl oxalate 100 mg. Net price 84-cap pack = £8.60. Label: 25, 27

NICOTINIC ACID DERIVATIVES ▭

Indications: peripheral vascular disease; hyperlipidaemia (section 2.12)
Side-effects: flushing, dizziness, nausea, vomiting, hypotension (more frequent with nicotinic acid than derivatives); occasional diabetogenic effect reported with nicotinic acid and nicotinyl alcohol; rarely associated with nodular changes to liver (monitor on prolonged high dosage)

Hexopal® (Sanofi-Synthelabo) ▭
Tablets, scored, inositol nicotinate 500 mg. Net price 20 = £4.07
Dose: 1 g 3 times daily, increased to 4 g daily if required
Tablets forte, scored, inositol nicotinate 750 mg. Net price 112-tab pack = £34.02
Dose: 1.5 g twice daily
Suspension, sugar-free, inositol nicotinate 1 g/5 mL. Net price 300 mL = £20.85
Dose: as for tablets (above)

PENTOXIFYLLINE/OXPENTIFYLLINE
▬◢

Indications: peripheral vascular disease
Cautions: hypotension, coronary artery disease; renal impairment, severe hepatic impairment; avoid in porphyria (section 9.8.2); **interactions:** Appendix 1 (pentoxifylline)
Contra-indications: cerebral haemorrhage, extensive retinal haemorrhage, acute myocardial infarction; pregnancy and breast-feeding
Side-effects: gastro-intestinal disturbances, dizziness, agitation, sleep disturbances, headache; rarely flushing, tachycardia, angina, hypotension, thrombocytopenia, intrahepatic cholestasis, hypersensitivity reactions including rash, pruritus and bronchospasm
Dose: 400 mg 2–3 times daily

Trental® (Borg) [PoM] ▬◢
Tablets, m/r, pink, s/c, pentoxifylline 400 mg. Net price 90-tab pack = £23.81. Label: 21, 25

Other preparations used in peripheral vascular disease

Rutosides (oxerutins, *Paroven®*) are not vasodilators and are not generally regarded as effective preparations as capillary sealants or for the treatment of cramps; side-effects include headache, flushing, rashes, mild gastro-intestinal disturbances.

Paroven® (Novartis Consumer Health) ▬◢
Capsules, yellow, oxerutins 250 mg. Net price 120-cap pack = £13.67
Dose: relief of symptoms of oedema associated with chronic venous insufficiency, 500 mg twice daily

2.6.4.2 Cerebral vasodilators

These drugs are claimed to improve mental function. Some improvements in performance of psychological tests have been reported but the drugs have not been shown clinically to be of much benefit in dementia.

CO-DERGOCRINE MESILATE ▬◢

A mixture in equal proportions of dihydroergocornine mesilate, dihydroergocristine mesilate, and (in the ratio 2 : 1) α- and β-dihydroergocryptine mesilates
Indications: adjunct in elderly patients with mild to moderate dementia
Cautions: severe bradycardia
Side-effects: gastro-intestinal disturbances, flushing, headache, rash, nasal congestion; dizziness and postural hypotension in hypertensive patients
Dose: 1.5 mg 3 times daily before meals *or* 4.5 mg once daily before a meal

Hydergine® (Novartis) [PoM] ▬◢
Tablets, co-dergocrine mesilate 1.5 mg (scored), net price 100-tab pack = £10.78; 4.5 mg, 28-tab pack = £10.78. Label: 22

▬◢ denotes preparations that are considered to be less suitable for prescribing (see p. vi)

2.7 Sympathomimetics

2.7.1	Inotropic sympathomimetics
2.7.2	Vasoconstrictor sympathomimetics
2.7.3	Cardiopulmonary resuscitation

The properties of sympathomimetics vary according to whether they act on alpha or on beta adrenergic receptors. Adrenaline (epinephrine) (section 2.7.3) acts on both alpha and beta receptors and increases both heart rate and contractility (beta$_1$ effects); it can cause peripheral vasodilation (a beta$_2$ effect) or vasoconstriction (an alpha effect).

2.7.1 Inotropic sympathomimetics

The cardiac stimulants **dobutamine** and **dopamine** act on beta$_1$ receptors in cardiac muscle, and increase contractility with little effect on rate. Dosage of dopamine is critical since although low doses induce vasodilatation and increase renal perfusion, higher doses (more than 5 micrograms per kg per minute) lead to vasoconstriction and may exacerbate heart failure.

Xamoterol also acts on beta$_1$ receptors but being a partial agonist it provokes only a modest stimulatory response at rest. **Important:** restricted to **mild heart failure only**, owing to deterioration in patients with moderate to severe heart failure, see p. 108.

Dopexamine acts on beta$_2$ receptors in cardiac muscle to produce its positive inotropic effect; and on peripheral dopamine receptors to increase renal perfusion; it is reported not to induce vasoconstriction.

Isoprenaline is less selective and increases both heart rate and contractility; it may prevent Stokes-Adams attacks, but insertion of a pacemaker is preferable. It is now only used as a short-term emergency treatment of heart block or severe bradycardia.

SHOCK. Shock is a medical emergency associated with a high mortality. The underlying causes of shock such as haemorrhage, sepsis or myocardial insufficiency should be corrected. The profound hypotension of shock must be treated promptly to prevent tissue hypoxia and organ failure. Volume replacement is essential to correct the hypovolaemia associated with haemorrhage and sepsis but may be detrimental in cardiogenic shock. Depending on haemodynamic status, cardiac output may be improved by the use of sympathomimetic inotropes such as adrenaline (epinephrine), dobutamine or dopamine (see notes above). In septic shock, when fluid replacement and inotropic support fail to maintain blood pressure, the vasoconstrictor noradrenaline (norepinephrine) (section 2.7.2) may be considered. In cardiogenic shock peripheral resistance is frequently high and to raise it further may worsen myocardial performance and exacerbate tissue ischaemia.

The use of sympathomimetic inotropes and vasoconstrictors should preferably be confined to the intensive care setting and undertaken with invasive haemodynamic monitoring.

For advice on the management of anaphylactic shock, see section 3.4.3.

DOBUTAMINE

Indications: inotropic support in infarction, cardiac surgery, cardiomyopathies, septic shock, and cardiogenic shock

Cautions: severe hypotension complicating cardiogenic shock; **interactions:** Appendix 1 (sympathomimetics)

Side-effects: tachycardia and marked increase in systolic blood pressure indicate overdosage

Dose: *by intravenous infusion*, 2.5–10 micrograms/kg/minute, adjusted according to response

Dobutrex® (Lilly) PoM
Strong sterile solution, dobutamine (as hydrochloride) 12.5 mg/mL. For dilution and use as an intravenous infusion. Net price 20-mL vial = £8.35
Note. Strong sterile solution containing dobutamine (as hydrochloride) 12.5 mg/mL also available in 20-mL amps from Phoenix

Posiject® (Boehringer Ingelheim) PoM
Strong sterile solution, dobutamine (as hydrochloride) 50 mg/mL. For dilution and use as an intravenous infusion. Net price 5-mL amp = £5.50

DOPAMINE HYDROCHLORIDE

Indications: cardiogenic shock in infarction or cardiac surgery

Cautions: correct hypovolaemia; low dose in shock due to acute myocardial infarction—see notes above; **interactions:** Appendix 1 (sympathomimetics)

Contra-indications: tachyarrhythmia, phaeochromocytoma

Side-effects: nausea and vomiting, peripheral vasoconstriction, hypotension, hypertension, tachycardia

Dose: *by intravenous infusion*, 2–5 micrograms/kg/minute initially (see notes above)

Dopamine (Non-proprietary) PoM
Sterile concentrate, dopamine hydrochloride 40 mg/mL, net price 5-mL amp = £3.00; 160 mg/mL, net price 5-mL amp = £14.75. For dilution and use as an intravenous infusion
Available from Antigen, Faulding DBL
Intravenous infusion, dopamine hydrochloride 1.6 mg/mL in glucose 5% intravenous infusion, net price 250-mL container (400 mg) = £11.69; 3.2 mg/mL, 250-mL container (800 mg) = £22.93 (both hosp. only)
Available from Abbott

Select-A-Jet® Dopamine (Medeva) PoM
Strong sterile solution, dopamine hydrochloride 40 mg/mL. Net price 5-mL vial = £4.14; 10-mL vial = £6.65; 20-mL vial = £11.86. For dilution and use as an intravenous infusion

---

DOPEXAMINE HYDROCHLORIDE

Indications: inotropic support and vasodilator in exacerbations of chronic heart failure and in heart failure associated with cardiac surgery

Cautions: myocardial infarction, recent angina, hypokalaemia, hyperglycaemia; correct hypovolaemia before starting, monitor blood pressure, pulse, plasma potassium, blood glucose; avoid abrupt withdrawal; **interactions:** Appendix 1 (sympathomimetics)

Contra-indications: left ventricular outlet obstruction such as hypertrophic cardiomyopathy or aortic stenosis; phaeochromocytoma, thrombocytopenia

Side-effects: tachycardia, other arrhythmias; also reported: nausea, vomiting, anginal pain, tremor, headache

Dose: *by intravenous infusion* into central or large peripheral vein, 500 nanograms/kg/minute, may be increased to 1 microgram/kg/minute and further increased up to 6 micrograms/kg/minute in increments of 0.5–1 microgram/kg/minute at intervals of not less than 15 minutes

Dopacard® (Elan) PoM
Strong sterile solution, dopexamine hydrochloride 10 mg/mL (1%). For dilution and use as an intravenous infusion. Net price 5-mL amp = £19.42
Note. Contact with metal in infusion apparatus should be minimised

---

ISOPRENALINE HYDROCHLORIDE

Indications: heart block, severe bradycardia

Cautions: ischaemic heart disease, diabetes mellitus, hyperthyroidism; **interactions:** Appendix 1 (sympathomimetics)

Side-effects: tachycardia, arrhythmias, hypotension, sweating, tremor, headache

Dose: *by intravenous infusion*, 0.5–10 micrograms/minute

Min-I-Jet® Isoprenaline (Medeva) PoM
Injection, isoprenaline hydrochloride 20 micrograms/mL. Net price 10-mL disposable syringe = £4.05

Saventrine IV® (Pharmax) PoM
Strong sterile solution, isoprenaline hydrochloride 1 mg/mL. For dilution and use as an intravenous infusion. Net price 2-mL amp = 42p

> ◢ denotes preparations that are considered to be less suitable for prescribing (see p. vi)

XAMOTEROL ◢

Indications: chronic mild heart failure (in patients not breathless at rest but limited by symptoms on exertion)

Cautions: withdraw if heart failure deteriorates; cardiac outflow obstruction, arrhythmias (maintain concurrent digoxin in atrial fibrillation), obstructive airways disease (withdraw if worsening, and reverse bronchospasm with inhaled bronchodilator such as salbutamol), reduce dose in renal impairment; pregnancy (toxicity in *animal* studies); **interactions:** Appendix 1 (xamoterol)

Contra-indications: moderate to severe heart failure; breast-feeding
HEART FAILURE. Xamoterol is contra-indicated in those:
- who are short of breath or fatigued at rest or limited on minimal exercise;
- with resting tachycardia (>90 beats per minute) or hypotension (systolic blood pressure <100 mmHg);
- with peripheral oedema, raised jugular venous pressure, enlarged liver, or third heart sound;
- with (or with history of) acute pulmonary oedema;
- who require treatment with furosemide in dose in excess of 40 mg daily (or equivalent);
- who require ACE inhibitor treatment

Side-effects: gastro-intestinal disturbances, headache, dizziness, bronchospasm, hypotension; also reported, chest pain, palpitations, muscle cramp, rashes

Dose: 200 mg daily for 1 week, then 200 mg twice daily

IMPORTANT. Treatment should be started in hospital after full assessment of severity of heart failure by exercise test

Corwin® (Stuart) PoM ◢
Tablets, yellow, f/c, xamoterol (as fumarate) 200 mg. Net price 56-tab pack = £25.94

◢ denotes preparations that are considered to be less suitable for prescribing (see p. vi)

2.7.2 Vasoconstrictor sympathomimetics

Vasoconstrictor sympathomimetics raise blood pressure transiently by acting on alpha-adrenergic receptors to constrict peripheral vessels. They are sometimes used as an emergency method of elevating blood pressure where other measures have failed (see also notes above).

The danger of vasoconstrictors is that although they raise blood pressure they do so at the expense of perfusion of vital organs such as the kidney.

Spinal and epidural anaesthesia may result in sympathetic block with resultant hypotension. Management may include intravenous fluids (which are usually given prophylactically), oxygen, elevation of the legs, and injection of a pressor drug such as ephedrine or methoxamine. As well as constricting peripheral vessels **ephedrine** also accelerates the heart rate (by acting on beta receptors). Use is made of this dual action of ephedrine to manage associated bradycardia (although intravenous injection of atropine sulphate 400 to 600 micrograms may also be required if bradycardia persists). When the hypotension occurs in association with tachycardia the pure alpha-adrenergic stimulant action of **methoxamine** is more appropriate.

EPHEDRINE HYDROCHLORIDE

Indications: see under Dose

Cautions: hyperthyroidism, diabetes mellitus, ischaemic heart disease, hypertension, angle-closure glaucoma, elderly, pregnancy (Appendix 4); may cause acute urine retention in prostatic hypertrophy; **interactions:** Appendix 1 (sympathomimetics)

Contra-indications: breast-feeding (Appendix 5)

Side-effects: nausea, vomiting, anorexia; tachycardia (sometimes bradycardia), arrhythmias, anginal pain, vasoconstriction with hypertension, vasodilation with hypotension, dizziness and flushing; dyspnoea; headache, anxiety, restlessness, confusion, psychoses, insomnia, tremor; difficulty in micturition, urine retention; sweating, hypersalivation; changes in blood-glucose concentration

Dose: reversal of hypotension from spinal or epidural anaesthesia, *by slow intravenous injection* of a solution containing ephedrine hydrochloride 3 mg/mL, 3–6 mg (max. 9 mg) repeated every 3–4 minutes to max. 30 mg

Ephedrine Hydrochloride (Non-proprietary) PoM
Injection, ephedrine hydrochloride 3 mg/mL, net price 10-mL amp = £2.70
Available from Aurum

METARAMINOL

Indications: acute hypotension (see notes above)

Cautions: see under Noradrenaline Acid Tartrate; longer duration of action than noradrenaline, see below

HYPERTENSIVE RESPONSE. Since metaraminol has a longer duration of action than noradrenaline (norepinephrine), an excessive vasopressor response may cause a prolonged rise in blood pressure

Contra-indications: see under Noradrenaline Acid Tartrate

Side-effects: see under Noradrenaline Acid Tartrate; tachycardia; fatal ventricular arrhythmia reported in Laennec's cirrhosis

Dose: *by intravenous infusion*, 15–100 mg in 500 mL, adjusted according to response

Aramine® (MSD) PoM
Injection, metaraminol 10 mg (as tartrate)/mL. Net price 1-mL amp = 57p

METHOXAMINE HYDROCHLORIDE

Indications: acute hypotension (see notes above)

Cautions: see under Noradrenaline Acid Tartrate; longer duration of action than noradrenaline, see below

HYPERTENSIVE RESPONSE. Since methoxamine has a longer duration of action than noradrenaline (norepinephrine), an excessive vasopressor response may cause a prolonged rise in blood pressure

Contra-indications: see under Noradrenaline Acid Tartrate

Side-effects: see under Noradrenaline Acid Tartrate

Dose: *by intramuscular injection*, 5–20 mg
By slow intravenous injection, 5–10 mg (rate 1 mg/ minute)

Vasoxine® (GlaxoWellcome) PoM
Injection, methoxamine hydrochloride 20 mg/mL. Net price 1-mL amp = 50p

NORADRENALINE ACID TARTRATE/ NOREPINEPHRINE BITARTRATE

Indications: see under preparations

Cautions: coronary, mesenteric, or peripheral vascular thrombosis; following myocardial infarction, Prinzmetal's variant angina, thyroid disease, diabetes mellitus; hypoxia or hypercapnia; appropriate blood volume replacement required; elderly; extravasation at injection site may cause necrosis; **interactions:** Appendix 1 (sympathomimetics)

Contra-indications: hypertension (monitor blood pressure and rate of flow frequently), pregnancy

Side-effects: hypertension, headache, bradycardia, arrhythmias, peripheral ischaemia

Dose: see under preparations

ADULT ADVANCED LIFE SUPPORT

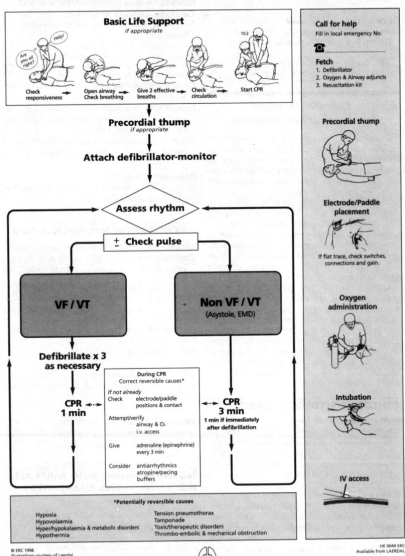

Basic Life Support
if appropriate

Check responsiveness → Open airway Check breathing → Give 2 effective breaths → Check circulation → Start CPR

Precordial thump
if appropriate

Attach defibrillator-monitor

Assess rhythm

± Check pulse

VF / VT

Non VF / VT
(Asystole, EMD)

Defibrillate x 3
as necessary

During CPR
Correct reversible causes*

If not already
Check   electrode/paddle positions & contact

Attempt/verify   airway & O₂
i.v. access

Give   adrenaline (epinephrine) every 3 min

Consider   antiarrhythmics
atropine/pacing
buffers

CPR
1 min

CPR
3 min
1 min if immediately after defibrillation

Potentially reversible causes

Hypoxia
Hypovolaemia
Hyper/hypokalaemia & metabolic disorders
Hypothermia

Tension pneumothorax
Tamponade
Toxic/therapeutic disorders
Thrombo-embolic & mechanical obstruction

Call for help
Fill in local emergency No.

Fetch
1. Defibrillator
2. Oxygen & Airway adjuncts
3. Resuscitation kit

Precordial thump

Electrode/Paddle placement

If flat trace, check switches, connections and gain.

Oxygen administration

Intubation

IV access

© ERC 1998
Illustrations courtesy of Laerdal

HE 0049 ERC
Available from LAERDAL

European Resuscitation Council

Levophed® (Abbott) PoM

Strong sterile solution, noradrenaline acid tartrate 2 mg/mL (equivalent to noradrenaline base 1 mg/mL). For dilution and use as an intravenous infusion. Net price 2-mL amp = £1.01; 4-mL amp = £1.50; 20-mL amp = £6.35

Dose: acute hypotension, *by intravenous infusion*, via central venous catheter, of a solution containing noradrenaline acid tartrate 80 micrograms/mL (equivalent to noradrenaline base 40 micrograms/mL) at an initial rate of 0.16–0.33 mL/minute, adjusted according to response

Levophed Special® (Abbott) PoM

Injection, noradrenaline acid tartrate 200 micrograms/mL (equivalent to noradrenaline base 100 micrograms/mL). Net price 2-mL amp = 98p

Dose: cardiac arrest, *by rapid intravenous or intracardiac injection*, 0.5 to 0.75 mL of a solution containing noradrenaline acid tartrate 200 micrograms/mL (equivalent to noradrenaline base 100 micrograms/mL)

PHENYLEPHRINE HYDROCHLORIDE

Indications: acute hypotension (see notes above)

Cautions: see under Noradrenaline Acid Tartrate; longer duration of action than noradrenaline, see below; severe coronary disease

HYPERTENSIVE RESPONSE. Since phenylephrine has a longer duration of action than noradrenaline (norepinephrine), an excessive vasopressor response may cause a prolonged rise in blood pressure

Contra-indications: see under Noradrenaline Acid Tartrate; severe hyperthyroidism

Side-effects: see under Noradrenaline Acid Tartrate; tachycardia or reflex bradycardia

Dose: *by subcutaneous or intramuscular injection*, 2–5 mg, followed if necessary by further doses of 1–10 mg

By slow intravenous injection of a 1 mg/mL solution, 100–500 micrograms repeated as necessary after at least 15 minutes

By intravenous infusion, initial rate up to 180 micrograms/minute reduced to 30–60 micrograms/minute according to response

Phenylephrine (Sovereign) PoM

Injection, phenylephrine hydrochloride 10 mg/mL (1%). Net price 1-mL amp = £5.00

2.7.3 Cardiopulmonary resuscitation

In *cardiac arrest* **adrenaline (epinephrine)** 1 in 10 000 (1 mg per 10 mL) is recommended in a dose of 10 mL by intravenous injection through a central line if one is in place but otherwise through a peripheral vein then flushed with 20 mL sodium chloride 0.9% injection (to expedite entry into the circulation). The procedure for cardiopulmonary resuscitation is given in the algorithm (see facing page) which reflects the recommendations of the European Resuscitation Council and the Resuscitation Council (UK). Other drugs used in cardiopulmonary resuscitation include **atropine** (section 15.1.3) and **calcium** (section 9.5.1.1).

For *acute anaphylaxis* see section 3.4.3.

ADRENALINE/EPINEPHRINE

Indications; Dose: see notes above

Cautions: ischaemic heart disease, diabetes mellitus, hyperthyroidism, hypertension; **interactions:** Appendix 1 (sympathomimetics)

Side-effects: anxiety, tremor, tachycardia, headache, cold extremities; in overdosage arrhythmias, cerebral haemorrhage, pulmonary oedema

Adrenaline/Epinephrine 1 in 10 000, Dilute (Non-proprietary) PoM

Injection, adrenaline (as acid tartrate) 100 micrograms/mL. 10-mL amp.

Available from Martindale (special order); also from Aurum (1-mL and 10-mL prefilled syringe), Medeva (*Min-I-Jet® Adrenaline* 3- and 10-mL disposable syringes)

2.8 Anticoagulants and protamine

2.8.1	Parenteral anticoagulants
2.8.2	Oral anticoagulants
2.8.3	Protamine sulphate

The main use of anticoagulants is to prevent thrombus formation or extension of an existing thrombus in the slower-moving venous side of the circulation, where the thrombus consists of a fibrin web enmeshed with platelets and red cells. They are therefore widely used in the prevention and treatment of *deep-vein thrombosis in the legs*.

Anticoagulants are of less use in preventing thrombus formation in arteries, for in faster-flowing vessels thrombi are composed mainly of platelets with little fibrin. They are used to prevent thrombi forming on *prosthetic heart valves*.

2.8.1 Parenteral anticoagulants

Heparin

Heparin initiates anticoagulation rapidly but has a short duration of action. It is now often referred to as being **standard** or **unfractionated heparin** to distinguish it from the **low molecular weight heparins** (see p. 113), which have a longer duration of action.

TREATMENT. For the initial treatment of *deep-vein thrombosis and pulmonary embolism* heparin is given as an *intravenous loading dose,* followed by *continuous intravenous infusion* (using an infusion pump) or by *intermittent subcutaneous injection*; the use of *intermittent intravenous injection* is no longer recommended. An oral anticoagulant (usually warfarin, section 2.8.2) is started at the same time as the heparin (which needs to be continued for at least 3 days, until the oral anticoagulant has taken effect). Laboratory monitoring is essential—preferably on a daily basis, determination of the activated partial thromboplastin time (APTT) being the most widely used technique. Heparin is also used in regimens for the management of *myocardial infarction* (see also section 2.10.1), the management of *unstable angina* (section 2.6), and the management of *acute peripheral arterial occlusion.*

PROPHYLAXIS. In patients undergoing *general surgery*, low-dose heparin by subcutaneous injection is widely advocated to *prevent postoperative deep-vein thrombosis and pulmonary embolism* in 'high risk' patients (i.e. those with obesity, malignant disease, history of deep-vein thrombosis or pulmonary embolism, patients over 40 years, or those with an established thrombophilic disorder or who are undergoing large or complicated surgical procedures); laboratory monitoring is not required with this *standard prophylactic regimen*.

To combat the increased risk in *major orthopaedic surgery* an *adjusted dose regimen* may be used (with monitoring) or *low molecular weight heparin* (see p. 113) may be selected.

EXTRACORPOREAL CIRCUITS. Heparin is also used in the maintenance of extracorporeal circuits in *cardiopulmonary bypass* and *haemodialysis*.

HAEMORRHAGE. If haemorrhage occurs it is usually sufficient to withdraw heparin, but if rapid reversal of the effects of heparin is required, protamine sulphate (section 2.8.3) is a specific antidote (but only partially reverses the effects of low molecular weight heparins).

HEPARIN

Indications: see under Dose

Cautions: hepatic and renal impairment (Appendix 2 and Appendix 3); pregnancy; hypersensitivity to low molecular weight heparins; spinal or epidural anaesthesia (risk of spinal haematoma); **interactions:** Appendix 1 (heparin)

THROMBOCYTOPENIA. Clinically important thrombocytopenia is immune-mediated, and does not usually develop until after 6 to 10 days; it may be complicated by thrombosis. Platelet counts are recommended for patients receiving heparin (including low molecular weight heparins) for longer than 5 days (heparin should be stopped immediately in those who develop thrombocytopenia). Patients requiring continued anticoagulation should preferably be given lepirudin or a heparinoid such as danaparoid

HYPERKALAEMIA. Inhibition of aldosterone secretion by heparin (including low molecular weight heparins) may result in hyperkalaemia; patients with diabetes mellitus, chronic renal failure, acidosis, raised plasma potassium or those taking potassium-sparing drugs seem to be more susceptible. The risk appears to increase with duration of therapy and the CSM has recommended that plasma potassium should be measured in patients at risk before starting heparin and monitored regularly thereafter, particularly if heparin is to be continued for more than 7 days

Contra-indications: haemophilia and other haemorrhagic disorders, thrombocytopenia, peptic ulcer, recent cerebral haemorrhage, severe hypertension, severe liver disease (including oesophageal varices), after major trauma or recent surgery (especially to eye or nervous system), hypersensitivity to heparin

Side-effects: haemorrhage (see notes above), skin necrosis, thrombocytopenia (see Cautions), hyperkalaemia (see Cautions), hypersensitivity reactions (including urticaria, angioedema, and anaphylaxis); osteoporosis after prolonged use (and rarely alopecia)

Dose: Treatment of deep-vein thrombosis and pulmonary embolism, *by intravenous injection*, loading dose of 5000 units (10 000 units in severe pulmonary embolism) followed by continuous *infusion* of 1000–2000 units/hour *or by subcutaneous injection* of 15 000 units every 12 hours (laboratory monitoring essential—preferably on a daily basis, and dose adjusted accordingly)

SMALL ADULT OR CHILD, lower loading dose *then*, 15–25 units/kg/hour *by intravenous infusion, or* 250 units/kg every 12 hours by *subcutaneous injection*

Unstable angina, acute peripheral arterial occlusion, as intravenous regimen for deep-vein thrombosis and pulmonary embolism, above

Prophylaxis in orthopaedic surgery, see notes above

Prophylaxis in general surgery (see notes above), *by subcutaneous injection*, 5000 units 2 hours before surgery, then every 8–12 hours for 7 days or until patient is ambulant (monitoring not needed); during pregnancy (with monitoring), 5000–10 000 units every 12 hours (**important:** not intended to cover prevention of prosthetic heart valve thrombosis in pregnancy which calls for separate specialist management)

MYOCARDIAL INFARCTION. For the prevention of *coronary re-occlusion after thrombolysis* heparin is used in a variety of regimens according to locally agreed protocols

For the prevention of *mural thrombosis* heparin is considered effective when given by *subcutaneous injection* of 12 500 units every 12 hours for at least 10 days

Prevention of clotting in extracorporeal circuits, consult product literature

> *Note.* Doses above reflect the guidelines of the British Society for Haematology; for doses of the low molecular weight heparins, see p. 113

Heparin Injection PoM (heparin sodium)
1000 units/mL, net price 1-mL amp = 19p; 5-mL amp = 57p; 5-mL vial = 46p
5000 units/mL, net price 1-mL amp = 37p; 5-mL amp = 99p; 5-mL vial = 92p
25 000 units/mL, net price 1-mL amp = £1.02; 5-mL vial = £3.44

Calciparine® (Sanofi-Synthelabo) PoM
Injection (subcutaneous only), heparin calcium 25 000 units/mL. Net price 0.2-mL syringe = 68p; 0.5-mL syringe = £1.46; 0.8-mL syringe = £1.76

Minihep® (Leo) PoM
Injection (subcutaneous only), heparin sodium 25 000 units/mL. Net price 0.2-mL amp = 39p

Minihep Calcium® (Leo) PoM
Injection (subcutaneous only), heparin calcium 25 000 units/mL. Net price 0.2-mL amp = 44p

Monoparin® (CP) PoM
Injection, heparin sodium (mucous) 1000 units/mL, net price 1-mL amp = 18p; 5-mL amp = 54p; 10-mL amp = 72p; 20-mL = £1.38; 5000 units/mL, 1-mL amp = 36p; 5-mL amp = 95p; 25 000 units/mL, 0.2-mL amp = 44p, 1-mL amp = 97p

Monoparin Calcium® (CP) PoM
Injection, heparin calcium 25 000 units/mL. Net price 0.2-mL amp = 47p

Multiparin® (CP) PoM
Injection, heparin sodium (mucous) 1000 units/mL, net price 5-mL vial = 46p; 5000 units/mL, 5-mL vial = 92p; 25 000 units/mL, 5-mL vial = £3.44

Pump-Hep® (Leo) PoM
Injection, heparin sodium (mucous) 1000 units/
mL. Net price 5-mL amp = 37p; 10-mL amp =
61p; 20-mL amp = 91p

Unihep® (Leo) PoM
Injection, heparin sodium (mucous) 1000 units/
mL, net price 1-mL amp = 13p; 5000 units/mL, 1-
mL amp = 26p; 10 000 units/mL, 1-mL amp =
42p; 25 000 units/mL, 1-mL amp = 99p

Uniparin Calcium® (CP) PoM
Injection (subcutaneous only), heparin calcium
25 000 units/mL. Net price 0.5-mL syringe = £1.50

Uniparin Forte® (CP) PoM
Injection (subcutaneous only), heparin sodium
25 000 units/mL. Net price 0.4-mL syringe = £1.53

Low molecular weight heparins

There is evidence that the low molecular weight
heparins, **certoparin**, **dalteparin**, **enoxaparin**, and
tinzaparin, are as effective and as safe as unfractionated heparin in the prevention of venous
thrombo-embolism; in orthopaedic practice they are
probably more effective. They have a longer duration of action than unfractionated heparin; *once-
daily subcutaneous* dosage means that they are convenient to use. The standard prophylactic regimen
does not require monitoring.

Some low molecular weight heparins are also
used in the treatment of deep-vein thrombosis,
pulmonary embolism, unstable coronary artery disease (section 2.6) and for the prevention of clotting
in extracorporeal circuits.

HAEMORRHAGE. See under Heparin.

CERTOPARIN

Indications: see notes above and under prepara-
tions
Cautions: see under Heparin
Contra-indications: see under Heparin
Side-effects: see under Heparin
Dose: see under preparation below

Alphaparin® (Grifols) PoM
Injection, certoparin 3000 units/0.3-mL
syringe, net price 1 syringe = £2.87
Dose: prophylaxis of deep-vein thrombosis, *by subcutaneous injection*, 3000 units 1–2 hours before surgery,
then 3000 units every 24 hours for 7–10 days (or until
the patient is mobile)

DALTEPARIN SODIUM

Indications: see notes above and under prepara-
tions
Cautions: see under Heparin
Contra-indications: see under Heparin
Side-effects: see under Heparin
Dose: see under preparations below

Fragmin® (Pharmacia & Upjohn) PoM
Injection (single-dose syringe), dalteparin sodium
12 500 units/mL, net price 0.2-mL (2500-unit)
syringe = £1.86; 25 000 units/mL, 0.2-mL (5000-
unit) syringe = £2.82, 0.4-mL (10 000-unit)
syringe = £5.64, 0.5-mL (12 500-unit) syringe =
£7.05, 0.6-mL (15 000-unit) syringe = £8.46,
0.72-mL (18 000-unit) syringe = £10.16
Dose: prophylaxis of deep-vein thrombosis, *by subcutaneous injection*, moderate risk, 2500 units 1–2 hours

before surgery then 2500 units every 24 hours for 5–7
days or longer; high risk, 2500 units 1–2 hours before
surgery, then 2500 units 8–12 hours later (*or* 5000 units
on the evening before surgery, then 5000 units on the
following evening), then 5000 units every 24 hours for
5–7 days or longer (5 weeks in hip replacement)
Treatment of deep-vein thrombosis, *by subcutaneous
injection*, as a single daily dose, body-weight 46–56 kg,
10 000 units daily; body-weight 57–68 kg, 12 500 units
daily; body-weight 69–82 kg, 15 000 units daily; body-
weight 83 kg and over, 18 000 units daily, with oral anticoagulant treatment until prothrombin complex concentration in therapeutic range (usually for at least 5 days);
monitoring of anti-factor Xa not usually required; for
patients at increased risk of haemorrhage, see below
Injection (for subcutaneous or intravenous use),
dalteparin sodium 2500 units/mL, net price 4-mL
(10 000-unit) amp = £5.12; 10 000 units/mL, 1-
mL (10 000-unit) amp = £5.12; 25 000 units/mL,
4-mL (100 000-unit) vial = £48.66
Dose: treatment of deep-vein thrombosis, *by subcutaneous injection*, 200 units/kg (max. 18 000 units) as a single daily dose (*or* 100 units/kg twice daily if increased
risk of haemorrhage) with oral anticoagulant treatment
until prothrombin complex concentration in therapeutic
range (usually for at least 5 days)
Note. For monitoring, blood should be taken 3–4 hours
after a dose (recommended plasma concentration of
anti-Factor Xa 0.5–1 unit/mL); monitoring not required
for once-daily treatment regimen and not generally necessary for twice-daily regimen
Unstable coronary artery disease, *by subcutaneous injection*, 120 units/kg every 12 hours (max. 10 000 units
twice daily) for 5–8 days
Prevention of clotting in extracorporeal circuits, consult
product literature
Injection (graduated syringe), dalteparin sodium
10 000 units/mL, net price 1-mL (10 000-unit)
syringe = £5.91
Dose: unstable coronary artery disease, *by subcutaneous
injection*, 120 units/kg every 12 hours (max. 10 000 units
twice daily) for 5–8 days

ENOXAPARIN

Indications: see notes above and under preparations
Cautions: see under Heparin
Contra-indications: see under Heparin
Side-effects: see under Heparin
Dose: see under preparation below

Clexane® (Rhône-Poulenc Rorer) PoM
Injection, enoxaparin 100 mg/mL. Net price 0.2-
mL syringe (20 mg, 2000 units) = £3.39; 0.4-mL
syringe (40 mg, 4000 units) = £4.52; 0.6-mL
syringe (60 mg, 6000 units) = £5.11; 0.8-mL
syringe (80 mg, 8000 units) = £5.81; 1-mL
syringe (100 mg, 10 000 units) = £7.19
Dose: prophylaxis of deep-vein thrombosis, *by subcutaneous injection, moderate risk*, 20 mg (2000 units) approx. 2
hours before surgery then 20 mg (2000 units) every 24
hours for 7–10 days; *high risk*, 40 mg (4000 units) 12 hours
before surgery then 40 mg (4000 units) every 24 hours for
7–10 days
Treatment of deep-vein thrombosis (with or without pulmonary embolism), *by subcutaneous injection*, 1.5 mg/kg
(150 units/kg) every 24 hours, usually for at least 5 days
(and until adequate oral anticoagulation established)
Unstable angina and non-Q-wave myocardial infarction, *by
subcutaneous injection*, 1 mg/kg (100 units/kg) every 12
hours usually for 2–8 days (minimum 2 days)
Prevention of clotting in extracorporeal circuits, consult
product literature

TINZAPARIN SODIUM

Indications: see notes above and under preparations

Cautions: see under Heparin

Contra-indications: see under Heparin

Side-effects: see under Heparin

Dose: see under preparations below

Innohep® (Leo) [PoM]
Injection, tinzaparin sodium 10 000 units/mL, net price 3500-unit (0.35-mL) syringe, = £2.98, 4500-unit (0.45-mL) syringe = £3.83, 20 000-unit (2-mL) vial = £11.36
Dose: prophylaxis of deep-vein thrombosis, *by subcutaneous injection*, general surgery, 3500 units 2 hours before surgery, then 3500 units every 24 hours for 7–10 days; orthopaedic surgery (high risk), 50 units/kg 2 hours before surgery, then 50 units/kg every 24 hours for 7–10 days *or* 4500 units 12 hours before surgery, then 4500 units every 24 hours for 7–10 days
Prevention of clotting in extracorporeal circuits, consult product literature
▼*Injection*, tinzaparin sodium 20 000 units/mL, net price 0.5-mL (10 000-unit) syringe = £9.65, 0.7-mL (14 000-unit) syringe = £13.51, 0.9-mL (18 000-unit) syringe = £17.37, 2-mL (40 000-unit) vial = £36.77
Dose: treatment of deep-vein thrombosis and of pulmonary embolism, *by subcutaneous injection*, 175 units/kg once daily for at least 6 days (and until adequate oral anticoagulation established)
Note. This treatment regimen does not require anticoagulation monitoring
ASTHMA. Presence of sulphites in formulation may (especially in patients with asthma) lead to hypersensitivity (with bronchospasm and shock)
Injection, tinzaparin sodium 1000 units/mL, net price 5-mL amp = £4.20
Dose: for prevention of clotting in extracorporeal circuits, consult product literature

Heparinoids

Danaparoid is a heparinoid used for prophylaxis of deep-vein thrombosis in patients undergoing general or orthopaedic surgery. Providing there is no evidence of cross-reactivity, it also has a role in patients who develop thrombocytopenia in association with heparin.

DANAPAROID SODIUM

Indications: prophylaxis of deep-vein thrombosis in general and orthopaedic surgery; thromboembolic disease requiring parenteral anticoagulation in patients with (or with a history of) heparin-induced thrombocytopenia

Cautions: hepatic and renal impairment (avoid for prophylaxis if severe); pregnancy and breast-feeding
ASTHMA. Presence of sulphite in ampoules may (especially in patients with asthma) lead to hypersensitivity (with bronchospasm and shock)

Contra-indications: see under Heparin; cross-reactivity to heparin-induced thrombocytopenia

Side-effects: haemorrhage (see notes above); thrombocytopenia (may be cross-reactivity with heparin); hypersensitivity reactions (including rash); liver enzyme changes; osteoporosis with excessive dosage; bruising or pain at injection site

Dose: prophylaxis of deep vein thrombosis, *by subcutaneous injection*, 750 units twice daily for 7–10 days; initiate treatment before operation (with last pre-operative dose 1–4 hours before surgery)
Heparin-induced thrombocytopenia, *by intravenous injection*, 2500 units (1250 units if body-weight less than 55 kg, 3750 units if over 90 kg), followed by *intravenous infusion* of 400 units/hour for 2 hours, *then* 300 units/hour for 2 hours, *then* 200 units/hour for 5 days; monitor anti-Xa activity in renal impairment and in patients over 90 kg (consult product literature)

Orgaran® (Durbin) [PoM]
Injection, danaparoid sodium 1250 units/mL, net price 0.6-mL amp (750 units) = £17.00

Hirudins

Lepirudin, a recombinant hirudin, has recently been introduced for anticoagulation in patients with heparin-associated thrombocytopenia type II who require parenteral antithrombotic treatment. The dose of lepirudin is adjusted according to activated partial thromboplastin time (APTT).

Desirudin, another recombinant hirudin has recently been introduced for the prophylaxis of deep-vein thrombosis in patients undergoing hip and knee replacement surgery.

DESIRUDIN

Indications: prophylaxis of deep-vein thrombosis in hip and knee replacement surgery

Cautions: renal impairment (avoid if severe; Appendix 3); hepatic impairment (avoid if severe; Appendix 2); recent bleeding or risk of bleeding (including recent major surgery, biopsy or puncture of large vessels, history of haemorrhagic stroke, intracranial or intraocular bleeding, cerebral ischaemic attack, haemorrhagic diathesis, concomitant use of oral anticoagulants)—monitor activated partial thromboplastin time

Contra-indications: active bleeding, irreversible coagulation disorders, severe uncontrolled hypertension, bacterial endocarditis; pregnancy and breast-feeding

Side-effects: bleeding manifestations; hypersensitivity reactions (including rash and urticaria); injection site reactions; very rarely anti-hirudin antibodies detected on re-exposure

Dose: *by subcutaneous injection* (preferably abdominal), 15 mg 5–15 minutes before surgery (after induction of regional block anaesthesia), then 15 mg twice daily for 9–12 days or until patient is ambulant (max. 12 days)

Revasc (Rhône-Poulenc Rorer) ▼ [PoM]
Injection, powder for reconstitution, desirudin, net price 15-mg vial (with diluent) = £11.50.

LEPIRUDIN

Indications: thromboembolic disease requiring parenteral anticoagulation in patients with heparin-associated thrombocytopenia type II

Cautions: renal impairment (Appendix 3); hepatic impairment (Appendix 2); recent bleeding or risk of bleeding including recent puncture of large vessels, organ biopsy, recent major surgery, stroke, haemorrhagic diathesis, severe uncontrolled hypertension, bacterial endocarditis; determine activated partial thromboplastin time 4 hours after start of treatment (or after infusion rate altered) and at least once daily thereafter

Contra-indications: pregnancy and breast-feeding

Side-effects: bleeding manifestations; reduced haemoglobin concentration without obvious source of bleeding; fever, hypersensitivity reactions (including rash); injection site reactions

Dose: initially *by slow intravenous injection* (of 5 mg/mL solution), 400 micrograms/kg followed by *continuous intravenous infusion* of 150 micrograms/kg/hour (max. 16.5 mg/hour), adjusted according to activated partial thromboplastin time, for 2–10 days (longer if necessary)

Refludan® (Hoechst Marion Roussel) ▼ PoM
Injection, powder for reconstitution, lepirudin. Net price 50-mg vial = £52.30

Heparin flushes

For maintaining patency of peripheral venous catheters, sodium chloride injection 0.9% is as effective as heparin flushes.

Canusal® (CP) PoM
Solution, heparin sodium 100 units/mL. Net price 2-mL amp = 29p. To maintain patency of catheters, cannulas, etc., 200 units flushed through every 4 hours or as required. Not for therapeutic use

Hep-Flush® (Leo) PoM
Solution, heparin sodium 100 units/mL. Net price 2-mL amp = 24p. To maintain patency of catheters, cannulas, etc., 200 units flushed through every 4–8 hours. Not for therapeutic use

Heplok® (Leo) PoM
Solution, heparin sodium 10 units/mL. Net price 5-mL amp = 28p. To maintain patency of catheters, cannulas, etc., 10–50 units flushed through every 4 hours. Not for therapeutic use

Hepsal® (CP) PoM
Solution, heparin sodium 10 units/mL. Net price 5-mL amp = 25p (glass), 30p (polypropylene). To maintain patency of catheters, cannulas, etc., 50 units flushed through every 4 hours or as required. Not for therapeutic use

---

Epoprostenol

Epoprostenol (prostacyclin) can be given to inhibit platelet aggregation during renal dialysis either alone or with heparin. Since its half-life is only about 3 minutes it must be given by continuous intravenous infusion. It is a potent vasodilator and therefore its side-effects include flushing, headache, and hypotension.

EPOPROSTENOL

Indications: see notes above
Cautions: anticoagulant monitoring required when given with heparin
Side-effects: see notes above; also bradycardia, pallor, sweating with higher doses
Dose: see product literature

Flolan® (GlaxoWellcome) PoM
Infusion, powder for reconstitution, epoprostenol (as sodium salt). Net price 500-microgram vial (with diluent) = £99.19

2.8.2   Oral anticoagulants

Oral anticoagulants antagonise the effects of vitamin K, and take at least 48 to 72 hours for the anticoagulant effect to develop fully; if an immediate effect is required, heparin must be given concomitantly.

USES. The main indication for an oral anticoagulant is *deep-vein thrombosis*. Patients with *pulmonary embolism* should also be treated, as should those with *atrial fibrillation who are at risk of embolisation* (see also section 2.3.1), and those with *mechanical prosthetic heart valves* (to prevent emboli developing on the valves); an antiplatelet drug may also be useful in these patients.

Warfarin is the drug of choice; **acenocoumarol (nicoumalone)** and **phenindione** are seldom used.

Oral anticoagulants should not be used in cerebral thrombosis or peripheral arterial occlusion as first-line therapy; aspirin (section 2.9) is more appropriate for reduction of risk in transient ischaemic attacks.

DOSE. Whenever possible, the base-line prothrombin time should be determined but the initial dose should not be delayed whilst awaiting the result.

The usual adult induction dose of warfarin is 10 mg[1] daily for 2 days (higher doses no longer recommended). The subsequent maintenance dose depends upon the prothrombin time, reported as INR (international normalised ratio). The daily maintenance dose of warfarin is usually 3 to 9 mg (taken at the **same time** each day). The indications and target INRs[2] currently recommended by the British Society for Haematology[3] are:

- INR 2–2.5 for prophylaxis of deep-vein thrombosis including surgery on high-risk patients;
- INR 2.5 for treatment of deep-vein thrombosis and pulmonary embolism (or for recurrence in patients no longer receiving warfarin), atrial fibrillation, cardioversion, dilated cardiomyopathy, mural thrombus following myocardial infarction, and rheumatic mitral valve disease;
- INR 3.5 for recurrent deep-vein thrombosis and pulmonary embolism (in patients currently receiving warfarin) and mechanical prosthetic heart valves.

---

1. First dose less than 10 mg if base-line prothrombin time prolonged, if liver-function tests abnormal, or if patient in cardiac failure, on parenteral feeding, less than average body weight, elderly, or receiving other drugs known to potentiate oral anticoagulants.
2. An INR which is within 0.5 units of the target value is generally satisfactory; larger deviations require dosage adjustment. Target values (rather than ranges) are now recommended (except for prophylaxis of deep-vein thrombosis where a range is still recommended).
3. Guidelines on Oral Anticoagulation: third edition. *Br J Haematol* 1998; **101**: 374–87

MONITORING. It is essential that the INR be determined daily or on alternate days in early days of treatment, *then* at longer intervals (depending on response[4]) *then* up to every 12 weeks

HAEMORRHAGE. The main adverse effect of all oral anticoagulants is haemorrhage. Checking the INR and omitting doses when appropriate is essential; if the anticoagulant is stopped but not reversed, the INR should be measured 1–2 days later to ensure that it is falling. The following recommendations of the British Society for Haematology are based on the result of the INR and whether there is major or minor bleeding; the recommendations apply to patients taking warfarin:

- Major bleeding—stop warfarin; give phytomenadione (vitamin K$_1$) 5 mg by slow intravenous injection; give prothrombin complex concentrate (factors II, VII, IX and X) 50 units/kg *or* (if no concentrate available) fresh frozen plasma 15 mL/kg
- INR > 8.0, no bleeding or minor bleeding—stop warfarin, restart when INR < 5.0; if there are other risk factors for bleeding give phytomenadione (vitamin K$_1$) 0.5 mg by slow intravenous injection or 5 mg by mouth (for partial reversal of anticoagulation give smaller oral doses of phytomenadione e.g. 0.5–2.5 mg using the intravenous preparation orally); repeat dose of phytomenadione if INR still too high after 24 hours
- INR 6.0–8.0, no bleeding or minor bleeding—stop warfarin, restart when INR < 5.0
- INR < 6.0 but more than 0.5 units above target value—reduce dose or stop warfarin, restart when INR < 5.0
- Unexpected bleeding at therapeutic levels—always investigate possibility of underlying cause e.g. unsuspected renal or gastro-intestinal tract pathology

PREGNANCY. Oral anticoagulants are teratogenic and should not be given in the first trimester of pregnancy. Women at risk of pregnancy should be warned of this danger since stopping warfarin before the sixth week of gestation may largely avoid the risk of fetal abnormality. Oral anticoagulants cross the placenta with risk of placental or fetal haemorrhage, especially during the last few weeks of pregnancy and at delivery. Therefore, if at all possible, oral anticoagulants should be avoided in pregnancy, especially in the first and third trimesters. Difficult decisions may have to be made, particularly in women with prosthetic heart valves or with a history of recurrent venous thrombosis or pulmonary embolism.

TREATMENT BOOKLETS. Anticoagulant treatment booklets should be issued to patients, and are available for distribution to local healthcare professionals from Health Authorities and also from:

England:	Scotland:
The Stationery Office	The Stationery Office
Broadway	21, South Gyle Crescent
Chadderton	Edinburgh EH12 9EB
Oldham	
Lancs OL9 6QH	

Northern Ireland Office
Central Services Agency
27 Adelaide St
Belfast BT2 8FH

These booklets include advice for patients on anticoagulant treatment.

---

4. Change in patient's clinical condition, particularly associated with liver disease, intercurrent illness, or drug administration, necessitates more frequent testing. See also **interactions**, Appendix 1 (warfarin). Major changes in diet (especially involving salads and vegetables) and in alcohol consumption may also affect warfarin control.

WARFARIN SODIUM

Indications: prophylaxis of embolisation in rheumatic heart disease and atrial fibrillation; prophylaxis after insertion of prosthetic heart valve; prophylaxis and treatment of venous thrombosis and pulmonary embolism; transient ischaemic attacks

Cautions: hepatic or renal disease (Appendixes 2 and 3), recent surgery; breast-feeding (Appendix 5); **interactions:** Appendix 1 (warfarin)

Contra-indications: pregnancy (see notes above), peptic ulcer, severe hypertension, bacterial endocarditis

Side-effects: haemorrhage—see notes above for British Society for Haematology recommendations; other side-effects reported include hypersensitivity, rash, alopecia, diarrhoea, unexplained drop in haematocrit, 'purple toes', skin necrosis, jaundice, hepatic dysfunction; also nausea, vomiting, and pancreatitis

Dose: see notes above

Warfarin (Non-proprietary) ▣PoM▣
Tablets, warfarin sodium 0.5 mg (white), net price 28-tab pack = £1.00; 1 mg (brown), 20 = 88p; 3 mg (blue), 20 = £1.36; 5 mg (pink), 20 = £2.16.
Label: 10 anticoagulant card
Available from APS, Cox, Goldshield (*Marevan*®), Hillcross, Norton

ACENOCOUMAROL/NICOUMALONE

Indications: see under Warfarin Sodium
Cautions: see under Warfarin Sodium
Contra-indications: see under Warfarin Sodium
Side-effects: see under Warfarin Sodium
Dose: 8–12 mg on 1st day; 4–8 mg on 2nd day; maintenance dose usually 1–8 mg daily

Sinthrome® (Alliance) ▣PoM▣
Tablets, acenocoumarol 1 mg. Net price 20 = 95p.
Label: 10 anticoagulant card

PHENINDIONE

Indications: prophylaxis of embolisation in rheumatic heart disease and atrial fibrillation; prophylaxis after insertion of prosthetic heart valve; prophylaxis and treatment of venous thrombosis and pulmonary embolism

Cautions: see under Warfarin Sodium; **interactions:** Appendix 1 (phenindione)

Contra-indications: see under Warfarin Sodium; avoid breast-feeding

Side-effects: see under Warfarin Sodium; also hypersensitivity reactions including rashes, exfoliative dermatitis, exanthema, fever, leucopenia, agranulocytosis, eosinophilia, diarrhoea, renal and hepatic damage; urine coloured pink or orange

Dose: 200 mg on day 1; 100 mg on day 2; maintenance dose usually 50–150 mg daily

Dindevan® (Goldshield) ▣PoM▣
Tablets, phenindione 10 mg, net price 20 = 68p; 25 mg (green), 20 = 95p; 50 mg, 20 = £1.21.
Label: 10 anticoagulant card, 14 (urine pink or orange)

2.8.3   Protamine sulphate

Although protamine sulphate is used to counteract overdosage with heparin, if used in excess it has an anticoagulant effect.

PROTAMINE SULPHATE

(Protamine Sulfate)

Indications; Cautions: see above; also if increased risk of allergic reaction to protamine (includes previous treatment with protamine or protamine insulin, allergy to fish, men who are infertile or who have had a vasectomy)

Side-effects: nausea, vomiting, lassitude, flushing, hypotension, bradycardia, dyspnoea; hypersensitivity reactions (including angioedema, anaphylaxis) reported

Dose: *by intravenous injection* over approx. 10 minutes, 1 mg neutralises 80–100 units heparin when given within 15 minutes of heparin; if longer time, less protamine required as heparin rapidly excreted; max. 50 mg

Protamine Sulphate (Non-proprietary) PoM
Injection, protamine sulphate 10 mg/mL, net price 5-mL amp = 98p, 10-mL amp = £2.20
Available from Medeva, Sovereign

Prosulf® (CP) PoM
Injection, protamine sulphate 10 mg/mL. Net price 5-mL amp = 96p (glass), £1.20 (polypropylene)

2.9   Antiplatelet drugs

By decreasing platelet aggregation, these drugs may inhibit thrombus formation on the arterial side of the circulation, where thrombi are formed by platelet aggregation and anticoagulants have little effect.

Encouraging results have been obtained using **aspirin** 75–300 mg daily for the *secondary* prevention of thrombotic cerebrovascular or cardiovascular disease. Aspirin is used to reduce mortality after myocardial infarction (section 2.10.1). Low doses of aspirin (such as 75 or 100 mg daily) are also given following bypass surgery. For details on the use of aspirin in atrial fibrillation see section 2.3.1, for stable angina see section 2.6 and for intermittent claudication see section 2.6.4.1.

Clopidogrel and **ticlopidine** have recently been introduced for the prevention of ischaemic events in patients with a history of symptomatic ischaemic disease.

Dipyridamole is used by mouth as an adjunct to oral anticoagulation for prophylaxis of thromboembolism associated with prosthetic heart valves. Modified-release preparations are licensed for secondary prevention of ischaemic stroke and transient ischaemic attacks.

Abciximab is a monoclonal antibody which inhibits platelet aggregation and thrombus formation. It is indicated for use by specialist physicians as an adjunct to heparin and aspirin for the prevention of ischaemic complications in high-risk patients undergoing, or scheduled for, percutaneous transluminal coronary angioplasty. Abciximab should be used once only.

Eptifibatide and **tirofiban** have been introduced recently; they inhibit platelet aggregation by binding to platelet glycoprotein IIb/IIIa receptors. They are licensed for use with heparin and aspirin to prevent early myocardial infarction in patients with unstable angina or non-Q-wave myocardial infarction. They should be used by specialists.

For use of epoprostenol, see section 2.8.1.

ABCIXIMAB

Indications: prevention of ischaemic cardiac complications in patients undergoing percutaneous coronary intervention; short-term prevention (1 month) of myocardial infarction in patients with unstable angina not responding to conventional treatment and who are scheduled for percutaneous coronary intervention (use under specialist supervision)

Cautions: measure baseline prothrombin time, activated partial thromboplastin time, platelet count, haemoglobin and haematocrit; monitor haemoglobin and haematocrit 12 hours and 24 hours after start of treatment and platelet count 2–4 hours and 24 hours after start of treatment; concomitant use of drugs that increase risk of bleeding; discontinue if uncontrollable serious bleeding occurs or emergency cardiac surgery needed; consult product literature for details of procedures to minimise bleeding; pregnancy (Appendix 4)

Contra-indications: active internal bleeding, major surgery, intracranial or intraspinal surgery or trauma within last 2 months, stroke within last 2 years; intracranial neoplasm, arteriovenous malformation or aneurysm, severe hypertension, haemorrhagic diathesis, thrombocytopenia, vasculitis, hypertensive or diabetic retinopathy; severe hepatic or renal impairment (Appendixes 2 and 3); breast-feeding

Side-effects: bleeding manifestations; nausea, vomiting, hypotension, bradycardia, chest pain, back pain, headache, fever, puncture site pain, thrombocytopenia; rarely cardiac tamponade, adult respiratory distress, hypersensitivity reactions

Dose: ADULT initially *by intravenous injection* over 1 minute, 250 micrograms/kg, then *by intravenous infusion,* 125 nanograms/kg/minute (max. 10 micrograms/minute); for prevention of ischaemic complications start 10–60 minutes before percutaneous coronary intervention and continue infusion for 12 hours; for unstable angina start up to 24 hours before possible percutaneous coronary intervention and continue infusion for 12 hours after intervention

ReoPro® (Lilly) ▼ PoM
Injection, abciximab 2 mg/mL, net price 5-mL vial = £280.00

ASPIRIN (antiplatelet)

(Acetylsalicylic Acid)

Indications: prophylaxis of cerebrovascular disease or myocardial infarction (see section 2.10.1 and notes above)

Cautions: asthma; uncontrolled hypertension; pregnancy (but see Appendix 4); **interactions:** Appendix 1 (aspirin)

Contra-indications: children under 12 years and in breast-feeding (Reye's syndrome, section 4.7.1); active peptic ulceration; haemophilia and other bleeding disorders

Side-effects: bronchospasm; gastro-intestinal haemorrhage (occasionally major), also other haemorrhage (e.g. subconjunctival)

Dose: see notes above

¹**Aspirin** (Non-proprietary) PoM
Dispersible tablets, aspirin 75 mg, net price 20 = 10p; 300 mg, see section 4.7.1. Label: 13, 21, 32
Tablets, e/c, aspirin 75 mg, net price 56-tab pack = £3.13; 300 mg, see section 4.7.1. Label: 5, 25, 32
Available from Ashbourne (*PostMI 75EC*®), Galen, Lagap

Angettes 75® (Bristol-Myers)
Tablets, aspirin 75 mg. Net price 28-tab pack = 94p. Label: 32

Caprin® (Sinclair) PoM
Tablets, e/c, pink, aspirin 75 mg, net price 56-tab pack = £3.08; 300 mg, see section 4.7.1. Label: 5, 25, 32

Disprin CV® (R&C)
Tablets, both m/r, aspirin 100 mg, net price 28-tab pack = £1.68; 300 mg, 28-tab pack = £1.99. Label: 25, 32

Nu-Seals® **Aspirin** (Lilly) PoM
Tablets, e/c, aspirin 75 mg, net price 28-tab pack = £1.55, 56-tab pack = £3.09; 300 mg, see section 4.7.1. Label: 5, 25, 32
Note. Tablets may be chewed at diagnosis for rapid absorption

■ With isosorbide mononitrate
Section 2.6.1

CLOPIDOGREL

Indications: prevention of atherosclerotic events in patients with history of symptomatic atherosclerotic disease (ischaemic stroke, myocardial infarction or established peripheral arterial disease)

Cautions: avoid for first few days after myocardial infarction and for 7 days after ischaemic stroke; not recommended in unstable angina, coronary artery bypass grafting and percutaneous transluminal coronary angioplasty; patients at risk of increased bleeding from trauma, surgery or other pathological conditions; discontinue 7 days before elective surgery if antiplatelet effect not desirable; liver impairment (Appendix 2), renal impairment; pregnancy (Appendix 4); **interactions:** Appendix 1 (clopidogrel)

Contra-indications: active bleeding, breast-feeding

Side-effects: haemorrhage (including gastro-intestinal and intracranial); other side-effects reported include abdominal discomfort, nausea, vomiting, diarrhoea, constipation, gastric and duodenal ulceration; headache, dizziness, vertigo, paraesthesia; rash, pruritus; hepatic and biliary disorders, neutropenia, isolated report of aplastic anaemia

Dose: 75 mg once daily

Plavix® (Bristol-Myers, Sanofi-Synthelabo) ▼ PoM
Tablets, pink, f/c, clopidogrel (as hydrogen sulphate) 75 mg, net price 28-tab pack = £35.31

1. Aspirin tablets 75 mg may be sold to the public in packs of up to 100 tablets; for details relating to other strengths see section 4.7.1 and *Medicines, Ethics and Practice*, No. 23, London, Pharmaceutical Press, 2000 (and subsequent editions as available)

DIPYRIDAMOLE

Indications: see notes above and under preparations

Cautions: rapidly worsening angina, aortic stenosis, recent myocardial infarction, heart failure; may exacerbate migraine; hypotension; **interactions:** Appendix 1 (dipyridamole)

Side-effects: gastro-intestinal effects, dizziness, myalgia, throbbing headache, hypotension, hot flushes and tachycardia; rarely worsening symptoms of coronary heart disease, hypersensitivity reactions such as rash and urticaria, increased bleeding during or after surgery

Dose: *by mouth*, 300–600 mg daily in 3–4 divided doses before food
Modified-release preparations, see under preparation below
By intravenous injection, diagnostic only, consult product literature

Dipyridamole (Non-proprietary) PoM
Tablets, coated, dipyridamole 25 mg, net price 20 = 47p; 100 mg, 20 = £1.13; 84 = £4.73. Label: 22
Available from APS, Ashbourne (*Cerebrovase*®), Cox, Hillcross, Norton
Oral suspension, dipyridamole 50 mg/5 ml. Available from Rosemont (sugar-free, special order)

Persantin® (Boehringer Ingelheim) PoM
Tablets, both s/c, dipyridamole 25 mg (orange), net price 84-tab pack = £1.70; 100 mg, 84-tab pack = £4.73. Label: 22
Injection, dipyridamole 5 mg/mL. Net price 2-mL amp = 11p

■ Modified release

Persantin® **Retard** (Boehringer Ingelheim) PoM
Capsules, m/r, red/orange containing yellow pellets, dipyridamole 200 mg. Net price 60-cap pack = £9.75. Label: 21, 25
Dose: secondary prevention of ischaemic stroke and transient ischaemic attacks (used alone or with aspirin), adjunct to oral anticoagulation for prophylaxis of thromboembolism associated with prosthetic heart valves, 200 mg twice daily preferably with food
Note. Dispense in original container (pack contains a desiccant) and discard any capsules remaining 6 weeks after opening

■ With aspirin
For cautions, contra-indications and side-effects of aspirin, see under Aspirin, above

Asasantin® **Retard** (Boehringer Ingelheim) ▼ PoM
Capsules, red/yellow, aspirin 25 mg, dipyridamole 200 mg (m/r), net price 60-cap pack = £9.75. Label: 21, 25
Dose: secondary prevention of ischaemic stroke and transient ischaemic attacks, 1 capsule twice daily
Note: Dispense in original container (pack contains a desiccant) and discard any capsules remaining 6 weeks after opening

EPTIFIBATIDE

Indications: prevention of early myocardial infarction in patients with unstable angina or non-Q-wave myocardial infarction and with last episode of chest pain within 24 hours (use under specialist supervision)

Cautions: renal impairment (Appendix 3); risk of bleeding, concomitant drugs that increase risk of bleeding—discontinue immediately if uncontrolled serious bleeding; measure baseline prothrombin time, activated partial thromboplastin time, platelet count, haemoglobin, haematocrit and serum creatinine; monitor haemoglobin, haematocrit and platelets within 6 hours after start of treatment then at least once daily; discontinue if thrombolytic therapy, intra-aortic balloon pump or emergency cardiac surgery necessary; pregnancy (Appendix 4)

Contra-indications: abnormal bleeding within 30 days, major surgery or severe trauma within 6 weeks, stroke within last 30 days or any history of haemorrhagic stroke, intracranial disease (aneurysm, neoplasm or arteriovenous malformation), severe hypertension, haemorrhagic diathesis, increased prothrombin time or INR, thrombocytopenia, significant hepatic impairment; breast-feeding

Side-effects: bleeding manifestations

Dose: initially *by intravenous injection*, 180 micrograms/kg, then *by intravenous infusion* 2 micrograms/kg/minute for up to 72 hours (up to 96 hours if percutaneous coronary intervention during treatment)

Integrilin® (Schering-Plough) ▼ PoM
Injection, eptifibatide 2 mg/mL, net price 10-mL (20-mg) vial = £16.80
Infusion, eptifibatide 750 micrograms/mL, net price 100-mL (75-mg) vial = £52.80

TICLOPIDINE HYDROCHLORIDE

Indications: prophylaxis of major ischaemic events in patients with a history of ischaemic stroke, reversible ischaemic neurological deficit or transient ischaemic attack, and in patients with intermittent claudication (initiate in hospital)

Cautions: hepatic impairment (Appendix 2); renal impairment (Appendix 3); monitor full blood count before treatment and every 2 weeks for first 3 months (and within 2 weeks of discontinuation if before 3 months)—discontinue if neutropenia or thrombocytopenia develop; discontinue at least 10 days before elective surgery; pregnancy (Appendix 4) and breast-feeding (Appendix 5); **interactions:** Appendix 1 (ticlopidine)
BLOOD DISORDERS AND JAUNDICE. Patients and their carers should be told how to recognise signs of blood disorders or jaundice and advised to seek immediate medical attention if symptoms such as fever, sore throat, mouth ulcers, purpura, bruising or bleeding develop

Contra-indications: haemorrhagic diathesis; recent bleeding or risk of bleeding including acute haemorrhagic stroke and active gastroduodenal ulcer; history of leucopenia, thrombocytopenia or agranulocytosis

Side-effects: bleeding manifestations; blood disorders including neutropenia, agranulocytosis, rarely bone marrow aplasia, pancytopenia, thrombotic thrombocytopenic purpura and isolated cases of thrombocytopenia; nausea, diarrhoea (discontinue if severe and persistent); elevated liver enzymes, rarely hepatitis, cholestatic jaundice; increased serum cholesterol and triglyceride concentrations; hypersensitivity reactions including angioedema, vasculitis, lupus syndrome and nephropathy; rashes, pruritus

Dose: 250 mg twice daily

Ticlid (Sanofi-Synthelabo) ▼ PoM
Tablets, f/c, ticlopidine hydrochloride 250 mg, net price 60-tab pack = £100.00. Label: 21

TIROFIBAN

Indications: prevention of early myocardial infarction in patients with unstable angina or non-Q-wave myocardial infarction and with last episode of chest pain within 12 hours (use under specialist supervision)

Cautions: renal impairment (Appendix 3); hepatic impairment (avoid if severe; Appendix 2); major surgery or severe trauma within 3 months (avoid if within 6 weeks); traumatic or protracted cardiopulmonary resuscitation, organ biopsy or lithotripsy within last 2 weeks; risk of bleeding including active peptic ulcer within 3 months; acute pericarditis, aortic dissection, haemorrhagic retinopathy, vasculitis, haematuria, faecal occult blood; severe heart failure, cardiogenic shock, anaemia; puncture of non-compressible vessel within 24 hours; concomitant drugs that increase risk of bleeding (including within 48 hours after thrombolytic); monitor platelet count, haemoglobin and haematocrit before treatment, 2–6 hours after start of treatment and then at least once daily; discontinue if thrombolytic therapy, intra-aortic balloon pump or emergency cardiac surgery necessary; discontinue immediately if serious bleeding uncontrolled by pressure occurs; pregnancy (Appendix 4)

Contra-indications: abnormal bleeding within 30 days, stroke within 30 days or any history of haemorrhagic stroke, intracranial disease (aneurysm, neoplasm or arteriovenous malformation), severe hypertension, haemorrhagic diathesis, increased prothrombin time or INR, thrombocytopenia; breast-feeding

Side-effects: bleeding manifestations; reversible thrombocytopenia

Dose: *by intravenous infusion*, initially 400 nanograms/kg/minute for 30 minutes, then 100 nanograms/kg/minute for at least 48 hours (continue during and for 12–24 hours after percutaneous coronary intervention); max. duration of treatment 108 hours

Aggrastat® (MSD) ▼ PoM
Concentrate for intravenous infusion, tirofiban (as hydrochloride) 250 micrograms/mL. For dilution before use, net price 50-mL (12.5-mg) vial = £151.06

2.10   Myocardial infarction and fibrinolysis

2.10.1   Management of myocardial infarction
2.10.2   Fibrinolytic drugs

2.10.1   Management of myocardial infarction

Local guidelines for the management of myocardial infarction should be followed where they exist

These notes give an overview of the initial and long-term management of myocardial infarction. The aims of management are to provide supportive care and pain relief, to promote revascularisation and to reduce mortality. Oxygen, diamorphine and nitrates provide initial support and pain relief; thrombolytics and aspirin promote revascularisation; long-term use of aspirin, beta-blockers, ACE inhibitors and statins help to reduce mortality further.

INITIAL MANAGEMENT. **Oxygen** (section 3.6) should be administered unless the patient has severe chronic obstructive airways disease.

The pain (and anxiety) of myocardial infarction is managed with slow intravenous injection of **diamorphine** (section 4.7.2); an antiemetic such as metoclopramide (or, if left ventricular function is not compromised, cyclizine) by intravenous injection should also be given (section 4.6).

Aspirin (chewed or dispersed in water) is given for its antiplatelet effect (section 2.9); a dose of 150–300 mg is suitable. If aspirin is given prior to arrival at hospital, a note saying that it has been given should be sent with the patient.

Thrombolytic drugs (alteplase, anistreplase, reteplase or streptokinase, section 2.10.2) are given to patients without contra-indications who present within 12 hours of a myocardial infarction; use after 12 hours requires specialist advice. **Streptokinase** remains the drug of choice although antibodies appear after 4 days and streptokinase or anistreplase should not therefore be used again after this time.

Nitrates (section 2.6.1) are used to relieve ischaemic pain. If sublingual glyceryl trinitrate is not effective, intravenous glyceryl trinitrate or isosorbide dinitrate is given.

Early intravenous administration of some **beta-blockers** (section 2.4) has been shown to be of benefit and patients without contra-indications should receive **atenolol** by intravenous injection at a dose of 5 mg over 5 minutes, and the dose repeated once after 10–15 minutes; **metoprolol** by intravenous injection is an alternative.

ACE inhibitors (section 2.5.5.1) are also of benefit to patients who have no contra-indications; in normotensive patients treatment with an ACE inhibitor can be started within 24 hours of the myocardial infarction and continued for at least 5–6 weeks (see below for long-term treatment).

LONG-TERM MANAGEMENT. **Aspirin** (section 2.9) should be given to all patients, unless contraindicated, at a dose of 75–150 mg daily.

Beta-blockers (section 2.4) should be given to all patients in whom they are not contra-indicated and continued for at least 2–3 years. Acebutolol, metoprolol, propranolol and timolol are suitable.

Although other calcium-channel blockers (section 2.6.2) have no place in routine management, **verapamil** may be useful in patients in whom beta-blockers are inappropriate.

ACE inhibitors (section 2.5.5.1) are recommended for any patient with evidence of left ventricular dysfunction.

Nitrates (section 2.6.1) are used for patients with angina.

Statins are beneficial in preventing recurrent coronary events, particularly for patients at high risk because of other factors (section 2.12).

2.10.2   Fibrinolytic drugs

Fibrinolytic drugs act as thrombolytics by activating plasminogen to form plasmin, which degrades fibrin and so breaks up thrombi.

Streptokinase is used in the treatment of *life-threatening venous thrombosis*, and in *pulmonary embolism*, but treatment must be started promptly.

The value of thrombolytic drugs for the treatment of *myocardial infarction* has been established (section 2.10.1). **Streptokinase, alteplase,** and **anistreplase** have all been shown to reduce mortality; **reteplase** has been licensed recently for acute myocardial infarction. Thrombolytic drugs are indicated for any patient with acute myocardial infarction for whom the benefit is believed to outweigh the risk of treatment. Trials have shown that the benefit is greatest in those with ECG changes that include ST segment elevation especially in those with anterior infarction. Patients should not be excluded on account of age alone because mortality in this group is high and the percentage reduction in mortality is the same as in younger patients.

CAUTIONS. Risk of bleeding including that from venepuncture or invasive procedures, any external chest compression, pregnancy (see Appendix 4), abdominal aneurysm or conditions in which thrombolysis might give rise to embolic complications such as enlarged left atrium with atrial fibrillation (risk of dissolution of clot and subsequent embolisation), diabetic retinopathy (very small risk of retinal bleeding), recent or concurrent anticoagulant therapy.

CONTRA-INDICATIONS. Recent haemorrhage, trauma, or surgery (including dental extraction), coagulation defects, bleeding diatheses, aortic dissection, coma, history of cerebrovascular disease especially recent events or with any residual disability, recent symptoms of possible peptic ulceration, heavy vaginal bleeding, severe hypertension, active pulmonary disease with cavitation, acute pancreatitis, severe liver disease, oesophageal varices; also in the case of streptokinase or anistreplase, previous allergic reactions to either drug.

Prolonged persistence of antibodies to streptokinase and anistreplase may reduce the effectiveness of subsequent treatment, therefore neither drug should be used again beyond 4 days of first administration.

SIDE-EFFECTS. Side-effects of thrombolytics are mainly nausea and vomiting and bleeding. When thrombolytics are used in myocardial infarction, reperfusion arrhythmias may occur. Hypotension may also occur and can usually be controlled by elevating the patient's legs, or by reducing the rate of infusion or stopping it temporarily. Back pain has been reported. Bleeding is usually limited to the site of injection, but intracerebral haemorrhage or bleeding from other sites may occur. Serious bleeding calls for discontinuation of the thrombolytic and may require administration of coagulation factors and antifibrinolytic drugs (aprotinin or tranexamic acid). Streptokinase and anistreplase may cause allergic reactions (including rash, flushing and uveitis) and anaphylaxis has been reported (for details of management see Allergic Emergencies, section 3.4.3). Guillain-Barré syndrome has been reported rarely after streptokinase treatment.

ALTEPLASE

(rt-PA, tissue-type plasminogen activator)

Indications: acute myocardial infarction (see notes above); pulmonary embolism

Cautions: see notes above

Contra-indications: see notes above

Side-effects: see notes above

Dose:

Myocardial infarction, accelerated regimen (initiated within 6 hours), 15 mg by *intravenous injection*, followed by *intravenous infusion* of 50 mg over 30 minutes, then 35 mg over 60 minutes (total dose 100 mg over 90 minutes); lower doses in patients less than 65 kg

Myocardial infarction, initiated within 6–12 hours, 10 mg by *intravenous injection*, followed by *intravenous infusion* of 50 mg over 60 minutes, then 4 *infusions* each of 10 mg over 30 minutes (total dose 100 mg over 3 hours; max. 1.5 mg/kg in patients less than 65 kg)

Pulmonary embolism, 10 mg by *intravenous injection* over 1–2 minutes followed by *intravenous infusion* of 90 mg over 2 hours; max. 1.5 mg/kg in patients less than 65 kg

Actilyse® (Boehringer Ingelheim) [PoM]

Injection, powder for reconstitution, alteplase 10 mg (5.8 million units)/vial, net price per vial (with diluent) = £150.00; 20 mg (11.6 million units)/vial (with diluent and transfer device) = £200.00; 50 mg (29 million units)/vial (with diluent, transfer device, and infusion bag) = £375.00

ANISTREPLASE

(APSAC)

Indications: acute myocardial infarction (see notes above)

Cautions: see notes above

Contra-indications: see notes above

Side-effects: see notes above

Dose: *by intravenous injection*, 30 units over 4–5 minutes; treatment should be initiated as soon as possible and preferably within 6 hours

Eminase® (Monmouth) [PoM]

Injection, powder for reconstitution, anistreplase. Net price 30-unit vial = £495.00 (also available in injection pack with 5-mL amp water for injections and disposable syringe and needle)

RETEPLASE

Indications: acute myocardial infarction (see notes above)

Cautions: see notes above

Contra-indications: see notes above

Side-effects: see notes above

Dose: *by intravenous injection,* 10 units over not more than 2 minutes, followed after 30 minutes by a further 10 units

Rapilysin® (Roche) ▼ [PoM]

Injection, powder for reconstitution, reteplase 10 units (1.16 g)/vial, net price pack of 2 vials (with 2 prefilled syringes of diluent and transfer device) = £716.25

STREPTOKINASE

Indications: deep-vein thrombosis, pulmonary embolism, acute arterial thromboembolism, central retinal venous or arterial thrombosis, thrombosed arteriovenous shunts; acute myocardial infarction (section 2.10.1); topical use, see section 13.11.7

Cautions: see notes above

Contra-indications: see notes above

Side-effects: see notes above

Dose: *by intravenous infusion*, 250 000 units over 30 minutes, then 100 000 units every hour for up to 12–72 hours according to condition with monitoring of clotting parameters (consult product literature)

Myocardial infarction, 1 500 000 units over 60 minutes

Thrombosed arteriovenous shunts and intracoronary use in myocardial infarction, consult product literature

Streptokinase (Non-proprietary) [PoM]

Injection, powder for reconstitution, streptokinase, net price 100 000-unit vial = £10.00; 250 000-unit vial = £15.00; 750 000-unit vial = £40.00; 1.5 million-unit vial = £85.00

Available from Braun

Kabikinase® (Pharmacia & Upjohn) [PoM]

Injection, powder for reconstitution, streptokinase, net price 250 000-unit vial = £14.33; 750 000-unit vial = £38.20; 1.5 million-unit vial = £81.18

Streptase® (Hoechst Marion Roussel) [PoM]

Injection, powder for reconstitution, streptokinase, net price 250 000-unit vial = £17.11; 750 000-unit vial = £44.86; 1.5 million-unit vial = £89.72 (hosp. only)

2.11 Antifibrinolytic drugs and haemostatics

Fibrin dissolution can be impaired by the administration of **tranexamic acid**, which inhibits fibrinolysis. It may be useful to prevent bleeding (e.g. in prostatectomy and dental extraction in haemophilia) and can be particularly useful in menorrhagia. Tranexamic acid may also be used in hereditary angioedema, epistaxis and in thrombolytic overdose.

Desmopressin (see section 6.5.2) is used in the management of mild to moderate haemophilia.

Aprotinin is a proteolytic enzyme inhibitor acting on plasmin and kallidinogenase (kallikrein). It is indicated for patients at high risk of major blood loss during and after open heart surgery with extracorporeal circulation and for patients in whom optimal blood conservation during open heart surgery is an absolute priority; it is also indicated for the treatment of life-threatening haemorrhage due to hyperplasminaemia (occasionally observed during the mobilisation and dissection of malignant tumours, in acute promyelocytic leukaemia, and following thrombolytic therapy).

Etamsylate (ethamsylate) reduces capillary bleeding in the presence of a normal number of platelets. It does not act by fibrin stabilisation, but probably by correcting abnormal platelet adhesion.

APROTININ

Indications: see notes above

Side-effects: occasionally hypersensitivity reactions and localised thrombophlebitis

Dose: *by slow intravenous injection or infusion* Open heart surgery, loading dose, 2 000 000 units (200 mL) after induction of anaesthesia and before sternotomy—initial 50 000 units (5 mL) *by slow intravenous injection* over several minutes (to detect allergy), remainder *by intravenous infusion* over 20 minutes; maintenance dose, *by intravenous infusion* 500 000 units (50 mL) every hour until end of operation (or early postoperative period in septic endocarditis); pump prime, 2 000 000 units (200 mL) in priming volume of extracorporeal circuit; in septic endocarditis 3 000 000 units (300 mL) added to pump prime

Hyperplasminaemia, *by slow intravenous injection or by infusion* initially, 500 000 units (50 mL) to 1 000 000 units (100 mL) at max. rate 10 mL/min; followed if necessary by 200 000 units (20 mL) every hour until bleeding stops

Trasylol® (Bayer) PoM

Injection, aprotinin 10 000 kallikrein inactivator units/mL. Net price 50-mL vial = £20.53

Note. Aprotinin injection containing 10 000 kallikrein inactivator units/mL also available from Paines & Byrne

ETAMSYLATE

(Ethamsylate)

Indications: see under preparations

Contra-indications: porphyria (see section 9.8.2)

Side-effects: nausea, headache, rashes

Dose: see below

Dicynene® (Delandale) PoM

Tablets, scored, etamsylate 500 mg, net price 100-tab pack = £22.13

Dose: short-term treatment of blood loss in menorrhagia, 500 mg 4 times daily during menstruation

Injection, etamsylate 125 mg/mL. Net price 2-mL amp = 82p

Dose: prophylaxis and treatment of periventricular haemorrhage in low birth-weight infants, by intramuscular or intravenous injection, 12.5 mg/kg every 6 hours

IMPORTANT. The ampoules currently available contain a total of 250 mg in 2 mL volume therefore **small fraction only** required for neonatal use

TRANEXAMIC ACID

Indications: see notes above

Cautions: renal impairment (Appendix 3); massive haematuria (avoid if risk of ureteric obstruction); pregnancy (Appendix 4); regular eye examinations and liver function tests in long-term treatment of hereditary angioedema

Note. Requirement for regular eye examinations during long-term treatment is based on unsatisfactory evidence

Contra-indications: thromboembolic disease

Side-effects: nausea, vomiting, diarrhoea (reduce dose); disturbances in colour vision (discontinue) and thromboembolic events reported rarely; giddiness on rapid intravenous injection

Dose: *by mouth*, local fibrinolysis, 15–25 mg/kg 2–3 times daily

Menorrhagia (initiated when heavy bleeding has started), 1–1.5 g 3–4 times daily for 3–4 days

Hereditary angioedema, 1–1.5 g 2–3 times daily

By slow intravenous injection, local fibrinolysis, 0.5–1 g 3 times daily

Cyklokapron® (Pharmacia & Upjohn) PoM

Tablets, f/c, scored, tranexamic acid 500 mg. Net price 60-tab pack = £14.30

Syrup, sugar-free, tranexamic acid 500 mg/5 mL. Net price 300 mL = £14.90

Injection, tranexamic acid 100 mg/mL. Net price 5-mL amp = £1.29

Blood products

FACTOR VIIa (RECOMBINANT)

Recombinant factor VIIa is used in patients with inhibitors to factors VIII and IX

Available from Novo Nordisk (*NovoSeven®* ▼)

FACTOR VIII FRACTION, DRIED

(Human Antihaemophilic Fraction, Dried)

Dried factor VIII fraction is prepared from human plasma by a suitable fractionation technique

Indications: control of haemorrhage in haemophilia A

Cautions: intravascular haemolysis after large or frequently repeated doses in patients with blood groups A, B, or AB—less likely with high potency concentrates

Side-effects: allergic reactions including chills, fever; hyperfibrinogenaemia occurred after massive doses with earlier products but less likely since fibrinogen content has now been substantially reduced

Available from BPL (*Replenate®*, *8Y®*), Centeon (*Monoclate-P®*), Grifols (*Alphanate®*), SNBTS (*Liberate®*, High Potency Factor VIII Concentrate)

Note. Preparation of recombinant human antihaemophilic factor VIII (octocog alfa) available from Bayer (*Kogenate®*), Hyland Immuno (*Recombinate®*), Wyeth (*ReFacto®* ▼)

FACTOR VIII INHIBITOR BYPASSING FRACTION

Preparations with factor VIII inhibitor bypassing activity are prepared from human plasma

Human Factor VIII Inhibitor Bypassing Fraction (*FEIBA*, Hyland Immuno) is used in patients with factor VIII inhibitors

Note. A porcine preparation of antihaemophilic factor for patients with inhibitors to human factor VIII is available from Speywood (*Hyate C®*)

FACTOR IX FRACTION, DRIED

Dried factor IX fraction is prepared from human plasma by a suitable fractionation technique; it may also contain clotting factors II, VII, and X.

Indications: congenital factor IX deficiency (haemophilia B)

Cautions: risk of thrombosis—principally with former low purity products

Contra-indications: disseminated intravascular coagulation

Side-effects: allergic reactions, including chills, fever

Available from BPL (Dried Factor IX Fraction, Heat-Treated; *Replenine®-VF*), Centeon (*Mononine®*), Grifols (*AlphaNine®*), SNBTS (Human Factor IX Concentrate, Heat Treated; *HT Defix®*)

Note. Preparation of recombinant coagulation factor IX (nonocog alfa) available from Hyland Immuno (*Bene-FIX®* ▼)

FRESH FROZEN PLASMA

Fresh frozen plasma is prepared from the supernatant liquid obtained by centrifugation of one donation of whole blood

Indications: to replace coagulation factors or other plasma proteins where their concentration or functional activity is critically reduced, e.g. to reverse warfarin effect

Cautions: avoid in circulatory overload; need for compatibility

Side-effects: allergic reactions including chills, fever, bronchospasm; adult respiratory distress syndrome

Available from Regional Blood Transfusion Services and BPL

Note. A preparation of solvent/detergent treated human plasma (frozen) is available from Octapharma (*Octaplas®* ▼)

2.12   Lipid-regulating drugs

Lowering the concentration of low density lipoprotein (LDL) cholesterol and raising high density lipoprotein (HDL) cholesterol reduces the progression of coronary atherosclerosis and may even induce regression.

There is evidence that lowering LDL-cholesterol by 25 to 35% is effective in both the primary and secondary prevention of clinical manifestations of coronary heart disease. Therefore, treatment with a lipid-regulating drug should be considered in patients with coronary heart disease and it should also be considered in those at high risk of developing it because of multiple risk factors (including smoking, hypertension, diabetes mellitus, and a family history of premature coronary heart disease). Treatment with statins (see Statins, below) has been shown to reduce myocardial infarction, coronary deaths and overall mortality and they are the drugs of choice in patients with a high risk of coronary heart disease. Any drug therapy must be combined with strict adherence to diet, maintenance of near-ideal body weight and, if appropriate, reduction of blood pressure and cessation of smoking.

A number of conditions, some familial, are characterised by very high plasma concentrations of cholesterol, or triglycerides, or both. Statins are drugs of first choice for treating hypercholesterolaemia, fibrates for treating hypertriglyceridaemia, and statins or fibrates can be used, either alone or together, to treat mixed hyperlipidaemia.

Severe hyperlipidaemia often requires a combination of lipid-regulating drugs such as an anion-exchange resin with a fibrate, a statin, or nicotinic acid; such treatment should generally be under specialist supervision. Combinations of a statin with nicotinic acid or a fibrate carry an increased risk of side-effects (including rhabdomyolysis) and should be used with caution.

> **Muscle effects.** The CSM has advised that rhabdomyolysis associated with lipid-regulating drugs such as the fibrates and statins appears to be rare (approx. 1 case in every 100 000 treatment years) but may be increased in those with renal impairment and possibly in those with hypothyroidism. Concomitant treatment with ciclosporin (cyclosporin) may increase plasma-statin concentration and the risk of muscle toxicity; concomitant treatment with a fibrate and a statin may also be associated with an increased risk of serious muscle toxicity.

Anion-exchange resins

Colestyramine (cholestyramine) and **colestipol** are anion-exchange resins used in the management of hypercholesterolaemia. They act by binding bile acids, preventing their reabsorption; this promotes hepatic conversion of cholesterol into bile acids; the resultant increased LDL-receptor activity of liver cells increases the breakdown of LDL-cholesterol. Thus both compounds effectively reduce LDL-cholesterol but can aggravate hypertriglyceridaemia.

CAUTIONS. Anion-exchange resins interfere with the absorption of fat-soluble vitamins; supplements of vitamins A, D and K may be required when treatment is prolonged. **Interactions:** Appendix 1 (colestyramine and colestipol).

SIDE-EFFECTS. As colestyramine and colestipol are not absorbed, gastro-intestinal side-effects predominate. Constipation is common, but diarrhoea has occurred, as have nausea, vomiting, and gastro-intestinal discomfort. An increased bleeding tendency has been reported due to hypoprothrombinaemia associated with vitamin K deficiency.

COUNSELLING. Other drugs should be taken at least 1 hour before or 4–6 hours after colestyramine or colestipol to reduce possible interference with absorption.

COLESTYRAMINE

(Cholestyramine)

Indications: hyperlipidaemias, particularly type IIa, in patients who have not responded adequately to diet and other appropriate measures; primary prevention of coronary heart disease in men aged 35–59 years with primary hypercholesterolaemia who have not responded to diet and other appropriate measures; pruritus associated with partial biliary obstruction and primary biliary cirrhosis; diarrhoeal disorders (section 1.5)

Cautions: see notes above; pregnancy and breast-feeding

Contra-indications: complete biliary obstruction (not likely to be effective)

Side-effects: see notes above; hyperchloraemic acidosis reported on prolonged use

Dose: lipid reduction (after initial introduction over 3–4 weeks) 12–24 g daily in water (or other suitable liquid) in single or up to 4 divided doses; up to 36 g daily if necessary

Pruritus, 4–8 g daily in water (or other suitable liquid)

Diarrhoeal disorders, see section 1.5

CHILD 6–12 years, see product literature

Colestyramine (Non-proprietary) [PoM]
Powder, colestyramine (anhydrous) 4 g/sachet, net price 180-sachet pack = £63.18. Label: 13, counselling, avoid other drugs at same time (see notes above)
Excipients: include aspartame (section 9.4.1)
Available from Dominion, Genus

Questran® (Bristol-Myers) [PoM]
Powder, orange, colestyramine (anhydrous) 4 g/sachet. Net price 60-sachet pack = £21.06. Label: 13, counselling, avoid other drugs at same time (see notes above)

Questran Light® (Bristol-Myers) [PoM]
Powder, orange, colestyramine (anhydrous) 4 g/sachet, net price 60-sachet pack = £22.11. Label: 13, counselling, avoid other drugs at same time (see notes above)
Excipients: include aspartame (section 9.4.1)

COLESTIPOL HYDROCHLORIDE

Indications: hyperlipidaemias, particularly type IIa, in patients who have not responded adequately to diet and other appropriate measures
Cautions: see notes above; pregnancy
Side-effects: see notes above
Dose: 5 g 1–2 times daily in liquid increased if necessary at intervals of 1–2 months to max. of 30 g daily (in single or 2 divided doses)

Colestid® (Pharmacia & Upjohn) [PoM]
Granules, yellow, colestipol hydrochloride 5 g/sachet. Net price 30 sachets = £11.98. Label: 13, counselling, avoid other drugs at same time (see notes above)
Colestid Orange, granules, yellow/orange, colestipol hydrochloride 5 g/sachet, with aspartame. Net price 30 sachets = £11.98. Label: 13, counselling, avoid other drugs at same time (see notes above)

Fibrates

Clofibrate, **bezafibrate**, **ciprofibrate**, **fenofibrate**, and **gemfibrozil** can be regarded as broad-spectrum lipid-modulating agents in that although their main action is to decrease serum triglycerides they also tend to reduce LDL-cholesterol and to raise HDL-cholesterol.

All can cause a myositis-like syndrome (see also CSM advice above), especially in patients with impaired renal function. In addition, clofibrate predisposes to gallstones by increasing biliary cholesterol excretion; it is therefore only indicated in patients who have had a cholecystectomy.

BEZAFIBRATE

Indications: hyperlipidaemias of types IIa, IIb, III, IV and V in patients who have not responded adequately to diet and other appropriate measures
Cautions: renal impairment (Appendix 3—see also under Myotoxicity below); **interactions:** Appendix 1 (fibrates)
MYOTOXICITY. Special care needed in patients with renal disease, as progressive increases in serum creatinine concentration or failure to follow dosage guidelines may result in myotoxicity (rhabdomyolysis); discontinue if myotoxicity suspected or creatine kinase concentration increases significantly

Contra-indications: severe hepatic impairment, hypoalbuminaemia, primary biliary cirrhosis, gall bladder disease, nephrotic syndrome, pregnancy and breast-feeding
Side-effects: gastro-intestinal (e.g. nausea, anorexia, gastric pain), pruritus, urticaria, impotence; also headache, dizziness, vertigo, fatigue, hair loss; myotoxicity (with myasthenia or myalgia)—special risk in renal impairment (see Cautions); also reported, anaemia, leucopenia, thrombocytopenia
Dose: see preparations below

Bezalip® (Roche) [PoM]
Tablets, f/c, bezafibrate 200 mg. Net price 100-tab pack = £9.84. Label: 21
Dose: 200 mg 3 times daily with or after food

Bezalip-Mono® (Roche) [PoM]
Tablets, m/r, f/c, bezafibrate 400 mg. Net price 28-tab pack = £8.12. Label: 21, 25
Dose: 1 tablet daily after food (dose form not appropriate in renal impairment)

CIPROFIBRATE

Indications: hyperlipidaemias of types IIa, IIb, III, and IV in patients who have not responded adequately to diet
Cautions; Contra-indications; Side-effects: see under Bezafibrate
Dose: 100 mg daily

Modalim® (Sanofi-Synthelabo) [PoM]
Tablets, scored, ciprofibrate 100 mg. Net price 28-tab pack = £13.38

CLOFIBRATE

Indications: hyperlipidaemias of types IIb, III, IV and V in patients who have not responded adequately to diet and other appropriate measures (but see also notes above)
Cautions; Contra-indications: see under Bezafibrate and notes above
Side-effects: see under Bezafibrate; also cholesterol cholelithiasis
Dose: over 65 kg, 2 g daily (50–65 kg, 1.5 g daily) in 2 or 3 divided doses

Atromid-S® (Zeneca) [PoM]
Capsules—discontinued

FENOFIBRATE

Indications: hyperlipidaemias of types IIa, IIb, III, IV, and V in patients who have not responded adequately to diet and other appropriate measures
Cautions: see under Bezafibrate; renal impairment (Appendix 3); liver function tests recommended every 3 months for first year
Contra-indications: severe renal or hepatic impairment, existing gall bladder disease; pregnancy and breast-feeding
Side-effects: see under Bezafibrate; also reported rash, photosensitivity, raised serum transaminases, hepatitis
Dose: see preparations below

Lipantil® (Fournier) PoM

Lipantil® Micro 67 capsules, yellow, fenofibrate (micronised) 67 mg, net price 90-cap pack = £23.30. Label: 21

Dose: initially 3 capsules daily in divided doses; usual range 2–4 capsules daily; CHILD 1 capsule/20 kg daily

Lipantil® Micro 200 capsules, orange, fenofibrate (micronised) 200 mg, net price 28-cap pack = £21.75. Label: 21

Dose: initially 1 capsule daily (dose form not appropriate for children or in renal impairment)

Lipantil® Micro 267 capsules, orange/cream, fenofibrate (micronised) 267 mg, net price 28-cap pack = £21.75. Label: 21

Dose: severe hyperlipidaemia, 1 capsule daily (dose form not appropriate for children or in renal impairment)

Note. For an equivalent therapeutic effect, 100 mg previously available non-micronised fenofibrate ≡ 67 mg micronised fenofibrate

GEMFIBROZIL

Indications: hyperlipidaemias of types IIa, IIb, III, IV and V in patients who have not responded adequately to diet and other appropriate measures; primary prevention of coronary heart disease in men aged 40–55 years with hyperlipidaemias that have not responded to diet and other appropriate measures

Cautions: lipid profile, blood counts, and liver-function tests before initiating long-term treatment; renal impairment; **interactions:** Appendix 1 (fibrates)

Contra-indications: alcoholism, hepatic impairment, gallstones; pregnancy and breast-feeding

Side-effects: gastro-intestinal disturbances; also rash, dermatitis, pruritus, urticaria, impotence, headache, dizziness, blurred vision, cholestatic jaundice, angioedema, laryngeal oedema, atrial fibrillation, pancreatitis, myasthenia, myopathy, rhabdomyolysis, painful extremities, myalgia accompanied by increases in creatine kinase

Dose: 1.2 g daily, usually in 2 divided doses; range 0.9–1.5 g daily

Gemfibrozil (Non-proprietary) PoM

Capsules, gemfibrozil 300 mg, net price 112-cap pack = £23.56

Available from Berk (*Emfib®*)

Tablets, gemfibrozil 600 mg, net price 30-tab pack = £15.91

Available from Norton

Lopid® (Parke-Davis) PoM

'300' capsules, white/maroon, gemfibrozil 300 mg. Net price 112-cap pack = £29.64

'600' tablets, f/c, gemfibrozil 600 mg. Net price 56-tab pack = £29.64

Ispaghula

Ispaghula husk, a form of soluble fibre, can be used as an adjunct to a lipid-lowering diet in patients with mild to moderate hypercholesterolaemia. It probably acts by reducing reabsorption of bile acids; plasma triglycerides remain unchanged.

ISPAGHULA

Indications: primary hypercholesterolaemia in patients with cholesterol concentration of 6.5–7.8 mmol/litre who have not responded adequately to dietary control; constipation, see section 1.6.1

Cautions: maintain adequate fluid intake; diabetes mellitus

Contra-indications: intestinal obstruction, faecal impaction, colonic atony

Side-effects: flatulence, abdominal bloating, particularly on starting treatment (if necessary, reduce dosage to once daily for few days); gastrointestinal obstruction or impaction

Dose: see under preparation below

Fybozest Orange® (R&C)

Granules, effervescent, sugar-free, ispaghula husk. Net price 265-g tub (with measure) = £6.43. Label: 13, counselling, see below

Note. Contains aspartame 50 mg/3.5-g dose (section 9.4.1) also, sodium 0.4 mmol/3.5-g dose and potassium 0.7 mmol/3.5-g dose

Dose: 3.5 g (1 measure) in at least 150 mL water twice daily; for earlier onset of cholesterol reduction (under medical supervision only), initially 5.25 g (1½ measures) twice daily for 2–3 months

COUNSELLING. Preparations that swell in contact with liquid should always be carefully swallowed with water and should not be taken immediately before going to bed

Statins

The statins (**atorvastatin, cerivastatin, fluvastatin, pravastatin** and **simvastatin**) competitively inhibit 3-hydroxy-3-methylglutaryl coenzyme A (HMG CoA) reductase, an enzyme involved in cholesterol synthesis, especially in the liver. They are more effective than anion-exchange resins in lowering LDL-cholesterol but less effective than the fibrates in reducing triglycerides and raising HDL-cholesterol.

Statins produce important reductions in coronary events, in all cardiovascular events, and in total mortality in patients aged up to 75 years with coronary heart disease (history of angina or acute myocardial infarction) and with a total serum-cholesterol concentration of 5 mmol/litre or greater. Statins should also be considered for patients who have had coronary artery bypass surgery or angioplasty, or who have other clinically overt atherosclerotic disease such as cerebrovascular disease (non-haemorrhagic stroke or transient ischaemic attacks) or peripheral vascular disease because these patients are at risk of major coronary events. Statins also reduce the incidence of non-haemorrhagic stroke when used for secondary prevention in coronary heart disease.

Statins have a role in primary prevention of coronary events in patients at increased risk. Risk of coronary events is not accurately predicted from cholesterol concentrations alone and methods that take into account factors such as smoking, hypertension and diabetes mellitus should be used to estimate risk. A statin should be considered for patients with a total serum-cholesterol concentration of 5 mmol/litre or greater and a coronary heart disease risk[1] of 30% or greater over 10 years, for primary prevention following a trial of lifestyle measures and other appropriate interventions.

The Joint British recommendations on prevention of coronary heart disease in clinical practice (British Cardiac Society, British Hyperlipidaemia Association, British Hypertension Society. *Heart* 1998; **80**(suppl 2): S1–29) recommend a target total serum-cholesterol concentration less than 5 mmol/litre (LDL cholesterol less than 3 mmol/litre) in both primary and secondary prevention of coronary heart disease[2]. Dietary and lifestyle measures to reduce coronary risk should also be instigated, along with treatment of hypertension (section 2.5) and use of aspirin where appropriate (section 2.9).

CAUTIONS. Statins should be used with caution in those with a history of liver disease or with a high alcohol intake (use should be avoided in active liver disease). Liver-function tests should be carried out before and within 1–3 months of starting treatment and thereafter at intervals of 6 months for 1 year, unless indicated sooner by symptoms or signs suggestive of hepatotoxicity. Treatment should be discontinued if serum transaminase concentration rises to, and persists at, 3 times the upper limit of the reference range. Patients should be advised to report unexplained muscle pain (see Muscle Effects below). **Interactions:** Appendix 1 (statins).

CONTRA-INDICATIONS. Statins are contra-indicated in those with active liver disease and in pregnancy (adequate contraception should be ensured during treatment and for 1 month afterwards) and breast-feeding (see Appendixes 4 and 5).

SIDE-EFFECTS. Reversible myositis is a rare but significant side-effect of the statins (see also Muscle Effects, p. 123 and below). The statins also cause headache, altered liver-function tests (rarely hepatitis) and gastro-intestinal effects including abdominal pain, flatulence, diarrhoea, nausea and vomiting.

MUSCLE EFFECTS. Myalgia, myositis and myopathy have been reported with the statins; if the creatine kinase concentration is markedly elevated (> 10 times upper limit of normal), and myopathy is suspected or diagnosed, treatment should be discontinued. There is an increased incidence of myopathy if the statins are given with a fibrate, with lipid-lowering doses of nicotinic acid, or with immunosuppressants such as ciclosporin (cyclosporin); close monitoring of liver function and, if symptomatic, of creatine kinase is required in patients receiving these drugs. Rhabdomyolysis with acute renal impairment secondary to myoglobinuria has also been reported.

COUNSELLING. Advise patient to report promptly unexplained muscle pain, tenderness, weakness.

1. Coronary heart disease risk may be determined using the Joint British Societies' 'Cardiac Risk Assessor' computer program or chart (British Cardiac Society, British Hyperlipidaemia Association, British Hypertension Society. *Heart* 1998; **80**(suppl 2): S1–29)

2. The Standing Medical Advisory Committee has recommended that the dose of statin should be adjusted to achieve a 20–25% reduction in total serum-cholesterol concentration in those at high risk (e.g. previous myocardial infarction) whose total cholesterol is less than 6.3 mmol/litre before treatment

ATORVASTATIN

Indications: primary hypercholesterolaemia, heterozygous familial hypercholesterolaemia, homozygous familial hypercholesterolaemia or combined (mixed) hyperlipidaemia in patients who have not responded adequately to diet and other appropriate measures

Cautions: see notes above

Contra-indications: see notes above

Side-effects: see notes above; also insomnia, angioedema, anorexia, asthenia, paraesthesia, peripheral neuropathy, alopecia, pruritus, rash, impotence, chest pain, hypoglycaemia and hyperglycaemia reported; hypersensitivity reactions (including anaphylaxis) and thrombocytopenia reported rarely

Dose: primary hypercholesterolaemia and combined hyperlipidaemia, usually 10 mg once daily Familial hypercholesterolaemia, initially 10 mg daily, increased at intervals of 4 weeks to 40 mg once daily; if necessary, further increased to max. 80 mg once daily (or combined with anion-exchange resin in heterozygous familial hypercholesterolaemia)

Lipitor® (Parke-Davis) ▼ PoM
Tablets, all f/c, atorvastatin (as calcium trihydrate) 10 mg, net price 28-tab pack = £18.88; 20 mg, 28-tab pack = £30.60; 40 mg 28-tab pack = £47.04. Counselling, muscle effects, see notes above

CERIVASTATIN SODIUM

Indications: primary hypercholesterolaemia (types IIa and IIb) in patients who have not responded adequately to dietary control

Cautions: see notes above; renal impairment

Contra-indications: see notes above

Side-effects: see notes above; also insomnia, arthralgia, asthenia, paraesthesia, vertigo, rash, eye disorders; hypersensitivity reactions reported rarely

Dose: initially 100 micrograms once daily in the evening, increased by increments of 100 micrograms at intervals of not less than 4 weeks to max. 300 micrograms once daily (200 micrograms daily in moderate to severe renal impairment)

Lipobay® (Bayer) ▼ PoM
Tablets, all f/c, cerivastatin sodium 100 micrograms (yellow), net price 28-tab pack = £12.95; 200 micrograms (light yellow-brown), net price 28-tab pack = £17.35; 300 micrograms (yellow-brown), net price 28-tab pack = £18.20. Counselling, muscle effects, see notes above

FLUVASTATIN

Indications: primary hypercholesterolaemia (hyperlipidaemia type IIa) in patients with total cholesterol concentration of 6.5 mmol/litre or greater who have not responded adequately to dietary control; adjunct to diet in retarding progression of coronary atherosclerosis in primary hypercholesterolaemia and concomitant coronary heart disease

Cautions: see notes above

Contra-indications: see notes above; also severe renal impairment

Side-effects: see notes above; also insomnia

Dose: initially 20–40 mg daily in the evening; usual range 20–40 mg daily in the evening, adjusted at intervals of 4 weeks; up to 40 mg twice daily may be required

Lescol® (Novartis) PoM

Capsules, fluvastatin (as sodium salt) 20 mg (brown/yellow), net price 28-cap pack = £12.72; 40 mg (brown/orange), 28-cap pack = £12.72, 56-cap pack = £25.44. Counselling, muscle effects, see notes above

PRAVASTATIN SODIUM

Indications: primary hypercholesterolaemia in patients who have not responded adequately to dietary control; adjunct to diet to slow progression of coronary atherosclerosis and reduce incidence of cardiac events in patients with hypercholesterolaemia and atherosclerotic coronary artery disease; adjunct to diet in hypercholesterolaemia without clinically evident coronary heart disease; prevention of stroke, recurrent coronary events (including myocardial infarction), or need for revascularisation procedure in patients with previous myocardial infarction or unstable angina and total serum cholesterol concentration greater than 4.8 mmol/litre (or LDL-cholesterol greater than 3.2 mmol/litre) (see also notes above)

Cautions: see notes above

Contra-indications: see notes above

Side-effects: see notes above; also rash, chest pain, fatigue

Dose: usual range 10–40 mg once daily at night, adjusted at intervals of not less than 4 weeks

Lipostat® (Squibb) PoM

Tablets, all yellow, pravastatin sodium 10 mg, net price 28-tab pack = £16.18; 20 mg, 28-tab pack = £29.69; 40 mg, 28-tab pack = £29.69. Counselling, muscle effects, see notes above

SIMVASTATIN

Indications: primary hypercholesterolaemia, heterozygous familial hypercholesterolaemia or combined (mixed) hyperlipidaemia in patients who have not responded adequately to diet and other appropriate measures; prevention of coronary events, need for revascularisation procedures, and to slow progression of coronary atherosclerosis in patients with coronary heart disease and total cholesterol concentration of 5.5 mmol/litre or greater (see also notes above)

Cautions: see notes above; severe renal impairment (Appendix 3)

Contra-indications: see notes above; also porphyria (see section 9.8.2)

Side-effects: see notes above; also rash, alopecia, anaemia, dizziness, paraesthesia, peripheral neuropathy, hepatitis, jaundice, pancreatitis; hypersensitivity syndrome (including angioedema) reported rarely

Dose: hyperlipidaemia, 10 mg daily at night, adjusted at intervals of not less than 4 weeks; usual range 10–40 mg once daily at night

Coronary heart disease, initially 20 mg once daily at night

Note. Max. 10 mg daily with concomitant ciclosporin, fibrate or lipid-lowering dose of nicotinic acid

Zocor® (MSD) PoM

Tablets, all f/c, simvastatin 10 mg (peach), net price 28-tab pack = £18.03; 20 mg (tan), 28-tab pack = £29.69; 40 mg (red), 28-tab pack = £29.69. Counselling, muscle effects, see notes above

Nicotinic acid group

The value of **nicotinic acid** is limited by its side-effects, especially vasodilatation. In doses of 1.5 to 3 g daily it lowers both cholesterol and triglyceride concentrations by inhibiting synthesis; it also increases HDL-cholesterol. **Acipimox** seems to have fewer side-effects but may be less effective in its lipid-modulating capabilities.

ACIPIMOX

Indications: hyperlipidaemias of types IIa, IIb, and IV in patients who have not responded adequately to diet and other appropriate measures

Cautions: renal impairment (Appendix 3)

Contra-indications: peptic ulcer; pregnancy and breast-feeding

Side-effects: vasodilatation, flushing, itching, rashes, urticaria, erythema; heartburn, epigastric pain, nausea, diarrhoea, headache, malaise, dry eyes; rarely angioedema, bronchospasm, anaphylaxis

Dose: usually 500–750 mg daily in divided doses

Olbetam® (Pharmacia & Upjohn) PoM

Capsules, brown/pink, acipimox 250 mg. Net price 90-cap pack = £36.87. Label: 21

NICOTINIC ACID

Indications: see notes above

Cautions: diabetes mellitus, gout, liver disease, peptic ulcer; **interactions:** Appendix 1 (nicotinic acid)

Contra-indications: pregnancy, breast-feeding

Side-effects: flushing, dizziness, headache, palpitations, pruritus (prostaglandin-mediated symptoms can be reduced by low initial doses taken with meals, or by taking aspirin 75 mg 30 minutes before the dose); nausea, vomiting; rarely impaired liver function and rashes

Dose: initially 100–200 mg 3 times daily (see above), gradually increased over 2–4 weeks to 1–2 g 3 times daily

[1]**Nicotinic Acid Tablets,** PoM nicotinic acid 50 mg, net price 100 = £8.48. Label: 21

1. May be sold to the public unless max. daily dose exceeds 600 mg or if intended for treatment of hyperlipidaemia

Fish oils

A fish-oil preparation (*Maxepa*®), rich in omega-3 marine triglycerides, is useful in the treatment of severe hypertriglyceridaemia; however, it can sometimes aggravate hypercholesterolaemia.

OMEGA-3 MARINE TRIGLYCERIDES

Indications: reduction of plasma triglycerides in patients with severe hypertriglyceridaemia judged to be at special risk of ischaemic heart disease or pancreatitis, in conjunction with dietary and other methods (see notes above)

Side-effects: occasional nausea and belching

Dose: see under preparations below

Maxepa® (Seven Seas)

Capsules, 1 g (approx. 1.1 mL) concentrated fish oils containing, as percentage of total fatty acid composition, eicosapentaenoic acid 18%, docosa-hexaenoic acid 12%. Vitamin A content less than 100 units/g, vitamin D content less than 10 units/g. Net price 200-cap pack = £27.28. Label: 21
Dose: 5 capsules twice daily with food

Liquid, golden-coloured, concentrated fish oils containing, as percentage of total fatty acid composition, eicosapentaenoic acid 18% w/w, docosa-hexaenoic acid 12% w/w. Vitamin A content less than 100 units/g, vitamin D content less than 10 units/g. Net price 150 mL = £20.46. Label: 21
Dose: 5 mL twice daily with food

2.13   Local sclerosants

Ethanolamine oleate and sodium tetradecyl sulphate are used in sclerotherapy of varicose veins, and phenol is used in haemorrhoids (section 1.7.3).

ETHANOLAMINE OLEATE

(Monoethanolamine Oleate)

Indications: sclerotherapy of varicose veins

Cautions: extravasation may cause necrosis of tissues

Contra-indications: inability to walk, acute phlebitis, oral contraceptive use, obese legs

Side-effects: allergic reactions (including anaphylaxis)

Ethanolamine Oleate Injection, PoM ethanolamine oleate 5%. Net price 5-mL amp = £1.97
Available from Medeva
Dose: by slow injection into empty isolated segment of vein, 2–5 mL divided between 3–4 sites; repeated at weekly intervals

SODIUM TETRADECYL SULPHATE

Indications: sclerotherapy of varicose veins

Cautions; Contra-indications; Side-effects: see under Ethanolamine Oleate

Fibro-Vein® (STD Pharmaceutical) PoM
Injection, sodium tetradecyl sulphate 0.2%, net price 5-mL amp = £2.20; 0.5%, 2-mL amp =

£1.35; 1%, 2-mL amp = £1.46; 3%, 2-mL amp = £1.64, 5-mL vial = £3.15
Dose: by slow injection into empty isolated segment of vein, 0.1–1 mL according to site and condition being treated (consult product literature)

3: Respiratory system

3.1 Bronchodilators

Asthma

For tables outlining the management of chronic asthma and acute severe asthma see p. 130 and p. 131.

Chronic obstructive pulmonary disease

Chronic obstructive pulmonary disease (chronic bronchitis and emphysema) may be helped by an inhaled short-acting **beta$_2$-adrenoceptor stimulant** (section 3.1.1.1) used as required *or* when the airways obstruction is more severe, by a regular inhaled **antimuscarinic bronchodilator** (section 3.1.2) *or* both if necessary. Although many patients are treated with an inhaled corticosteroid its role in chronic obstructive pulmonary disease is not clear at present. A limited trial of high-dose inhaled corticosteroid *or* an oral corticosteroid is recommended for patients with moderate airflow obstruction to determine the extent of the airway reversibility and to ensure that asthma has not been overlooked.

For the management of infections in bronchitis see Table 1, section 5.1.

3.1.1 Adrenoceptor stimulants
(Sympathomimetics)

3.1.1.1 Selective beta$_2$-adrenoceptor
stimulants
3.1.1.2 Other adrenoceptor stimulants

The selective beta$_2$-adrenoceptor stimulants (selective beta$_2$-stimulants, selective beta$_2$-agonists) (section 3.1.1.1) such as salbutamol or terbutaline (preferably given by aerosol inhalation) are the safest and most effective beta-stimulants for asthma. They are recommended over the less selective beta-adrenoceptor stimulants such as orciprenaline (section 3.1.1.2), which should be avoided whenever possible.

Adrenaline (epinephrine) (which has both alpha- and beta-adrenoceptor stimulant properties) is used in the emergency management of allergic and anaphylactic reactions (section 3.4.3).

Start at **step most appropriate** to initial severity; **'rescue' course** of prednisolone at **any time** or **any step**

Chronic asthma: adults and schoolchildren

Step 1: occasional relief bronchodilators

Inhaled short-acting beta$_2$ stimulant as required (up to once daily)

Note. Move to step 2 if needed more than once daily (or night-time symptoms); check compliance, inhaler technique

Step 2: regular inhaled preventer therapy

Inhaled short-acting beta$_2$ stimulant as required
> *plus*
Either regular standard-dose[1] inhaled corticosteroid
Or regular cromoglicate or nedocromil (but change to inhaled corticosteroid if control not achieved)

Note. Higher dose of inhaled corticosteroid may be required to gain initial control; some individuals benefit from doubling for short period to cover an exacerbation

Step 3: high-dose inhaled corticosteroids or standard-dose inhaled corticosteroids + long-acting inhaled beta$_2$ stimulant

Inhaled short-acting beta$_2$ stimulant as required
> *plus*
Either regular high-dose[2] inhaled corticosteroid
Or regular standard-dose[1] inhaled corticosteroid *plus* regular inhaled long-acting beta$_2$ stimulant (salmeterol 50 micrograms twice daily *or* in those over 18 years, formoterol 12 micrograms twice daily)

Note. In few who have problems with high-dose inhaled corticosteroid use standard-dose inhaled corticosteroid with *either* inhaled long-acting beta$_2$ stimulant option *or* regular modified-release oral theophylline *or try* regular cromoglicate or nedocromil

Step 4: high-dose inhaled corticosteroids + regular bronchodilators

Inhaled short-acting beta$_2$ stimulant as required
> with
Regular high-dose[2] inhaled corticosteroid
>> *plus sequential therapeutic trial of one or more of*
>> Inhaled long-acting beta$_2$ stimulant
>> Modified-release oral theophylline
>> Inhaled ipratropium or, in adults, oxitropium
>> Modified-release oral beta$_2$ stimulant
>> High-dose inhaled bronchodilators
>> Cromoglicate or nedocromil

Step 5: regular corticosteroid tablets

Inhaled short-acting beta$_2$ stimulant as required
> with
Regular high-dose[2] inhaled corticosteroid *and* one or more long-acting bronchodilators (see step 4)
> *plus*
Regular prednisolone tablets (as single daily dose)

Note. In addition to regular prednisolone, continue high-dose inhaled corticosteroid (in exceptional cases may exceed licensed doses); these patients should normally be referred to an asthma clinic

Stepping down

Review treatment every 3–6 months; if control achieved stepwise reduction may be possible; if treatment started recently at step 4 or 5 (or contained corticosteroid tablets) reduction may take place after short interval; in other patients a 1–3 month or longer period of stability needed before slow stepwise reduction is undertaken

---

1. Standard-dose inhaled corticosteroids are beclometasone dipropionate or budesonide 100–400 micrograms twice daily *or* fluticasone propionate 50–200 micrograms twice daily
2. High-dose inhaled corticosteroids are beclometasone dipropionate or budesonide 0.8–2 mg daily (in divided doses) *or* fluticasone propionate 0.4–1 mg daily (in divided doses); use a large-volume spacer

Chronic asthma: children under 5 years

Step 1: occasional relief bronchodilators

Short-acting beta$_2$ stimulant as required (not more than once daily)

Note. Whenever possible inhaled (less effective and more side-effects when given by mouth); check compliance, technique and that inhaler device is appropriate

Step 2: regular inhaled preventer therapy

Inhaled short-acting beta$_2$ stimulant as required
> *plus*
Either regular inhaled cromoglicate (powder or metered-dose inhaler via large-volume spacer)
Or regular inhaled corticosteroid in standard paediatric dose[3]
>> *Consider for stabilisation*
>> 5-day course of soluble prednisolone tablets[5] *or* temporary doubling of dose of inhaled corticosteroid

Note. Try cromoglicate for 4–6 weeks. For inhaled corticosteroids assess effect on symptoms after 1 month and adjust doses; if control not adequate consider doubling dose of inhaled corticosteroid for 1 month (alternatively give 5-day course of soluble prednisolone tablets or consider introducing other treatments before increasing dose of inhaled corticosteroid for long periods)

Step 3: increased-dose inhaled corticosteroids

Inhaled short-acting beta$_2$ stimulant as required
> *plus*
Regular inhaled corticosteroid in high paediatric dose[4]
>> *Consider*
>> Short course of soluble prednisolone tablets[5]
>> Regular inhaled long-acting beta$_2$ stimulant *or* regular modified-release oral theophylline

Note. Long-acting beta$_2$ stimulant should probably be reserved for supplementing treatment in child already receiving cromoglicate or a corticosteroid; modified-release oral theophylline may be helpful (particularly for nocturnal symptoms), but has appreciable side-effects in up to one-third of children (plasma- or salivary-concentration monitoring recommended)

Step 4: high-dose inhaled corticosteroid + regular bronchodilators

Inhaled short-acting beta$_2$ stimulant as required
> with
Regular inhaled corticosteroid in high dose (beclometasone dipropionate or budesonide up to 2 mg daily *via* large-volume spacer)
>> *Consider* (as in step 3)
>> Short course of soluble prednisolone[5]
>> Regular inhaled long-acting beta$_2$ stimulant
>> Regular modified-release oral theophylline
>> *Also* nebulised beta$_2$ stimulant

Stepping down

Regularly review need for treatment

---

3. Standard paediatric dose of inhaled corticosteroid is beclometasone dipropionate or budesonide up to 400 micrograms daily (in divided doses) *or* fluticasone propionate up to 200 micrograms daily (in divided doses); initial dose according to age, weight and severity of asthma; use a large-volume spacer
4. High paediatric dose of inhaled corticosteroid is beclometasone dipropionate or budesonide up to 800 micrograms daily (in divided doses) *or* fluticasone propionate up to 500 micrograms daily (in divided doses); use a large-volume spacer
5. Doses of prednisolone tablets are child under 1 year 1–2 mg/kg daily, 1–5 years 20 mg daily; rescue courses usually for 1–3 days

Based on tables in: British Thoracic Society and others. The British Guidelines on Asthma Management. *Thorax* 1997; **52** (suppl): S1–S21. Reproduced with permission of BMJ Specialist Journals

MANAGEMENT OF ACUTE SEVERE ASTHMA IN GENERAL PRACTICE

Uncontrolled asthma in adults

— Speech normal
— Pulse <110 beats/minute
— Respiration <25 breaths/minute
— Peak flow >50% of predicted or best

Treat at home but response to treatment **must** be assessed before doctor leaves

Treatment:
Nebulised salbutamol 5 mg or nebulised terbutaline 10 mg
Monitor response 15–30 minutes after nebulisation
If peak flow 50–75% of predicted or best give:
   Oral prednisolone 30–60 mg
   and step up usual treatment
Alternatively if peak flow >75% of predicted or best:
   Step up usual treatment

Follow up
Monitor symptoms and peak flow
Set up self management plan
Review in surgery within 48 hours
Modify treatment at review according to guidelines for chronic asthma (see opposite page)

Important: regard each emergency consultation as being for **acute severe asthma** until shown otherwise.

Important: failure to respond adequately **at any time** requires immediate referral to hospital.

Acute severe asthma in adults

— Cannot complete sentences
— Pulse ≥110 beats/minute
— Respiration ≥25 breaths/minute
— Peak flow ≤50% of predicted or best

Seriously consider hospital admission if more than one of above features present

Treatment:
Oxygen 40–60% if available
Nebulised salbutamol 5 mg or nebulised terbutaline 10 mg
Oral prednisolone 30–60 mg or i/v hydrocortisone 200 mg
Monitor response 15–30 minutes after nebulisation
If any signs of acute asthma persist:
   Arrange hospital admission
   While awaiting ambulance repeat nebulised beta₂ stimulant and give with nebulised ipratropium 500 micrograms or give subcutaneous terbutaline (or salbutamol)
   or give slow intravenous aminophylline 250 mg (**important:** not if taking an oral theophylline)
Alternatively if symptoms have improved, respiration and pulse settling, and peak flow >50% of predicted or best:
   Step up usual treatment and continue prednisolone

Follow up
Monitor symptoms and peak flow
Set up self management plan
Review in surgery within 24 hours
Modify treatment at review (see opposite page)

Life-threatening asthma in adults

— Silent chest
— Cyanosis
— Bradycardia or exhaustion
— Peak flow <33% of predicted or best
Arrange IMMEDIATE hospital admission

Treatment:
Oral prednisolone 30–60 mg or i/v hydrocortisone 200 mg (immediately)
Oxygen-driven nebuliser in ambulance
Nebulised beta₂ stimulant with nebulised ipratropium or subcutaneous terbutaline (or salbutamol)
or slow intravenous aminophylline 250 mg (**important:** not if taking an oral theophylline)
STAY WITH PATIENT UNTIL AMBULANCE ARRIVES

1. If no nebuliser available give 2 puffs of beta₂ stimulant using large-volume spacer and repeat 10–20 times

Important patients with severe or life-threatening attacks may not be distressed and may not have all these abnormalities; the presence of any should alert doctor.

Important: do not give bolus aminophylline to patient already taking an oral theophylline.

Acute episodes or exacerbations of asthma in young children in primary care

Mild/moderate episode in young children
— short-acting beta₂ stimulant via large-volume dose inhaler via large-volume spacer (and face mask in very young), up to 10 puffs (1 puff every 15–30 seconds); alternatively give by nebuliser every 3–4 hours
— if favourable response (respiratory rate reduced, reduced use of accessory muscles, improved 'behaviour' pattern), repeat inhaled beta₂ stimulant every 3–4 hours; consider doubling dose of inhaled corticosteroids

— if beta₂ stimulant still required every 3–4 hours after 12 hours, start short course of oral prednisolone for 1–3 days (under 1 year 1–2 mg/kg daily; 1–5 years 20 mg daily)

If unresponsive or relapse within 3–4 hours:
— immediately refer to hospital
— increase frequency of beta₂ stimulant (give as frequently as needed)
— start oral prednisolone
— give high-flow oxygen via face mask

Signs of acute asthma in children

Acute severe asthma:
— too breathless to talk
— too breathless to feed
— respiration >50 breaths/minute (≥40/minute in children over 5 years)
— pulse >140 beats/minute (≥120 beats/minute in children over 5 years)
— in younger children, use of accessory muscles of breathing
— in older children, peak flow ≤50% of predicted or best

Life-threatening features:
— cyanosis, silent chest, or poor respiratory effort
— fatigue or exhaustion
— agitation or reduced level of consciousness
— in older children, peak flow <33% of predicted or best

3.1.1.1   Selective beta$_2$-adrenoceptor stimulants

Most mild to moderate symptoms of asthma respond rapidly to aerosol administration of a selective short-acting beta$_2$-adrenoceptor stimulant such as salbutamol or terbutaline. If beta$_2$-adrenoceptor stimulant inhalation is needed more than once daily prophylactic treatment should be considered, using a stepped approach as outlined on p. 130. However in more severe exacerbations a short course of an oral corticosteroid may be necessary to bring the asthma under control (section 3.2). Treatment of patients with acute severe asthma or airways obstruction (see also below) is safer in hospital where oxygen and resuscitation facilities are immediately available (see also Acute Severe Asthma table, p. 131).

There are some differences among the various selective beta$_2$-adrenoceptor stimulant drugs. **Salbutamol** and **terbutaline** are available in the widest range of formulations. **Fenoterol** may be less beta$_2$-selective than salbutamol.

Salmeterol and **formoterol** (**eformoterol**) are longer-acting beta$_2$-adrenoceptor stimulants which are administered by inhalation on a twice-daily basis. They are not indicated for the relief of an acute attack. Salmeterol or formoterol should be added to existing corticosteroid therapy and **not** replace it. Salmeterol and formoterol can be useful in nocturnal asthma.

REGULAR TREATMENT. Short-acting beta$_2$-adrenoceptor stimulants should not be prescribed on a regular basis in patients with mild or moderate asthma since several studies show that regular treatment provides no clinical benefit (compared with placebo). In contrast, the longer acting beta$_2$-adrenoceptor stimulants, salmeterol and formoterol when taken regularly have shown clear benefit compared to placebo and to regular treatment with short-acting beta$_2$-adrenoceptor stimulants.

INHALATION. Administration by inhalation delivers the drug directly to the bronchi and is therefore effective in smaller doses; inhalation is preferred to administration by tablets or oral liquid because it provides relief more rapidly and causes fewer side-effects (such as tremor and nervous tension).

Pressurised (aerosol) inhalation (using a metered dose inhaler) is an effective and convenient method of administration for mild to moderate airways obstruction. The duration of action of an aerosol inhalation depends on the drug that it contains and the dose administered. With recommended doses salbutamol, terbutaline and fenoterol will usually last for 3 to 5 hours, and salmeterol and formoterol for around 12 hours.

CFC-FREE INHALERS. Chlorofluorocarbon (CFC) propellants in pressurised aerosol inhalers are being replaced by hydrofluoroalkane (HFA) propellants. Patients receiving CFC-free inhalers should be reassured about the efficacy of the new inhalers and counselled that the aerosol may feel and taste different; any difficulty with the new inhaler should be discussed with the doctor or pharmacist.

CSM advice. The CSM has requested doctors to report any adverse reaction to the new HFA-containing inhalers and to include the brand name of the inhaler on the yellow card.

Patients should be given careful instruction on the use of their pressurised (aerosol) inhalers and it is important to check that they continue to use them correctly because inadequate technique may be mistaken for drug failure. It should be emphasised that they must inhale slowly and hold their breath for 10 seconds after inhalation.

Most patients can be successfully taught to use pressurised (aerosol) inhalers but some patients, particularly the elderly, the arthritic, and small children experience difficulty using them; some patients are unable to synchronise their breathing with the administration of aerosol. For such patients *breath-actuated aerosol inhalers* and *spacing devices* (section 3.1.5) are available. Alternatively *dry powder inhalers*, activated by the patient's inspiration, are of value; some occasionally cause coughing. Patients who are changed from an aerosol inhaler to a dry powder inhaler may notice a lack of sensation in the mouth and throat previously associated with each actuation.

The **dose** in terms of the number of inhalations at one time, the frequency, and the maximum number of inhalations allowed in 24 hours should be **stated explicitly** to the patient. High doses of beta$_2$-stimulants can be dangerous in some patients. Excessive use is usually an indication of **inadequately treated** asthma and should be treated with preventative medication such as an inhaled corticosteroid. Patients should be advised to seek medical advice when they fail to obtain their usual degree of symptomatic relief because this usually indicates a worsening of the asthma and may require alternative medication (see Chronic Asthma table, p. 130).

Respirator (or *nebuliser*) *solutions* of salbutamol and terbutaline are used for the treatment of acute asthma both in hospital and in general practice. They are administered over a period of 5–10 minutes from a nebuliser, usually driven by oxygen in hospital. An electric compressor is most suitable for domiciliary use but these are costly and not currently prescribable under the NHS. Patients with a severe attack of asthma should have oxygen if possible during nebulisation since beta$_2$-adrenoceptor stimulants can cause an increase in arterial hypoxaemia. For patients with chronic bronchitis and hypercapnia, however, oxygen can be dangerous, and the nebuliser should be driven by air. The dose prescribed by nebuliser is substantially higher than that prescribed by metered dose inhaler. Patients should therefore be warned that it is dangerous to exceed the stated dose and that if they fail to respond to the usual dose of their respirator solution they should seek medical advice. See also guidelines in section 3.1.5.

ORAL. *Oral preparations* are available for patients who cannot manage the inhaled route. They are sometimes used for children, although the inhaled route is better and most children can use one or other of the inhalation devices. Oral preparations have a slower onset but a slightly more prolonged action than the aerosol inhalers. The longer-acting preparations may be of value in nocturnal asthma as an alternative to modified-release theophylline preparations (section 3.1.3).

PARENTERAL. *Intravenous* and occasionally *subcutaneous* injections of salbutamol and terbutaline are given for severe bronchospasm. Although some patients with chronic asthma are treated with a beta$_2$-adrenoceptor stimulant by subcutaneous injection on a regular basis, the evidence of benefit is uncertain and it may be difficult to withdraw such treatment once started; patients supplied with either adrenaline (epinephrine) injection or a selective beta$_2$-adrenoceptor stimulant injection for severe attacks should be advised to attend hospital immediately after using the injection for further assessment.

CHILDREN. Selective beta$_2$-adrenoceptor stimulants are useful even in children under the age of 18 months. They are most effective by the *inhaled route*, but an inhalation device may be needed (with the technique carefully checked). They may also be administered as tablets or oral liquids although administration by inhalation is preferred. In severe attacks *nebulisation* using a selective beta$_2$-adrenoceptor stimulant or ipratropium is advisable (see also Asthma tables, pp. 130–1).

PREGNANCY AND BREAST-FEEDING. It is particularly important that asthma should be well controlled during pregnancy; where this is achieved asthma has no important effects on pregnancy, labour, or the fetus.

Inhalation has particular advantages as a means of drug administration during pregnancy because the therapeutic action can be achieved without the need for plasma drug concentrations liable to have a pharmacological effect on the fetus.

Severe exacerbations of asthma can have an adverse effect on pregnancy and should be treated promptly with conventional therapy, including oral or parenteral administration of corticosteroids and nebulisation of a selective beta$_2$-adrenoceptor stimulant; prednisolone is the preferred corticosteroid for oral administration since very little of the drug reaches the fetus.

Although theophylline has been given without adverse effects during pregnancy or breast-feeding there have been occasional reports of toxicity in the fetus and neonate.

Acute severe asthma

Severe asthma can be fatal and **must** be treated promptly and energetically. It is characterised by persistent dyspnoea poorly relieved by bronchodilators, exhaustion, a high pulse rate (usually over 110/minute), and a very low peak expiratory flow. As asthma becomes more severe, wheezing may be absent. Such patients should be given oxygen (if available) and a large dose of a **corticosteroid** (section 6.3.2)—for adults, prednisolone 30–60 mg by mouth *or* hydrocortisone 200 mg (preferably as sodium succinate) intravenously; for children, prednisolone 1–2 mg/kg (1–4 years max. 20 mg, 5–15 years max. 40 mg) by mouth *or* hydrocortisone 100 mg (preferably as sodium succinate) intravenously; if the patient experiences vomiting, the parenteral route may be preferred for the first dose. Patients should also be given **salbutamol** or **terbutaline** by nebuliser with oxygen if available. For a table outlining the management of acute severe asthma, see p. 131.

If there is little response the following additional treatment should be considered: **ipratropium** by nebuliser (section 3.1.2), **aminophylline** by slow intravenous injection if the patient has not already been receiving theophylline (section 3.1.3), or administer the beta$_2$-selective adrenoceptor stimulant by the intravenous route.

Further treatment of these patients is safer in hospital where resuscitation facilities are immediately available. Treatment should **never** be delayed for investigations, patients should **never** be sedated, and the possibility of a pneumothorax should also be considered.

If the patient deteriorates despite appropriate pharmacological treatment, intermittent positive pressure ventilation may be needed temporarily.

SALBUTAMOL

Indications: asthma and other conditions associated with reversible airways obstruction; premature labour (section 7.1.3)

Cautions: hyperthyroidism, myocardial insufficiency, arrhythmias, susceptibility to QT-interval prolongation, hypertension, pregnancy and breast-feeding (but appropriate to use, see notes above); diabetes—especially intravenous administration to diabetics (monitor blood glucose; ketoacidosis reported); see also notes above; **interactions:** Appendix 1 (sympathomimetics, beta$_2$)

HYPOKALAEMIA. The CSM has advised that potentially serious hypokalaemia may result from beta$_2$-adrenoceptor stimulant therapy. Particular caution is required in severe asthma, because this effect may be potentiated by concomitant treatment with theophylline and its derivatives, corticosteroids, and diuretics, and by hypoxia. Plasma-potassium concentration should therefore be monitored in severe asthma

Side-effects: fine tremor (usually hands), nervous tension, headache, peripheral vasodilatation, arrhythmias, palpitations, tachycardia (seldom troublesome when given by aerosol inhalation); sleep and behavioural disturbances in children; rarely muscle cramps; hypokalaemia after high doses (for **CSM** advice see under Cautions); hypersensitivity reactions including paradoxical bronchospasm, urticaria, and angioedema reported; slight pain on intramuscular injection

Dose: *by mouth*, 4 mg (elderly and sensitive patients initially 2 mg) 3–4 times daily; max. single dose 8 mg (but unlikely to provide much extra benefit or to be tolerated); CHILD under 2 years 100 micrograms/kg 4 times daily [unlicensed]; 2–6 years 1–2 mg 3–4 times daily, 6–12 years 2 mg

By subcutaneous or intramuscular injection, 500 micrograms, repeated every 4 hours if necessary

By slow intravenous injection, 250 micrograms, repeated if necessary

By intravenous infusion, initially 5 micrograms/minute, adjusted according to response and heart-rate usually in range 3–20 micrograms/minute, or more if necessary; CHILD 1 month–12 years 0.1–1 microgram/kg/minute [unlicensed]

By aerosol inhalation, 100–200 micrograms (1–2 puffs); for persistent symptoms up to 3–4 times daily (but see also Chronic Asthma table); CHILD 100 micrograms (1 puff), increased to 200 micrograms (2 puffs) if necessary; for persistent symptoms up to 3–4 times daily

Prophylaxis in exercise-induced bronchospasm, 200 micrograms (2 puffs); CHILD 100 micrograms (1 puff)

By inhalation of powder (*Ventolin Rotacaps®, Ventodisks®*; for *Ventolin Accuhaler®* and *Asmasal®* dose see under preparation), 200–400 micrograms; for persistent symptoms up to 3–4 times daily (but see also Chronic Asthma table); CHILD 200 micrograms

Prophylaxis in exercise-induced bronchospasm (*powder*), 400 micrograms; CHILD 200 micrograms
Note. Bioavailability appears to be lower, so recommended doses for dry powder inhalers are twice those in a metered inhaler

By inhalation of nebulised solution, chronic bronchospasm unresponsive to conventional therapy and severe acute asthma, ADULT and CHILD over 18 months 2.5 mg, repeated up to 4 times daily; may be increased to 5 mg if necessary, but medical assessment should be considered since alternative therapy may be indicated; CHILD under 18 months, clinical efficacy uncertain (transient hypoxaemia may occur—consider supplemental oxygen)

■ Oral

Salbutamol (Non-proprietary) PoM
Tablets, salbutamol (as sulphate) 2 mg, net price 20 = 16p; 4 mg, 20 = 29p
Available from APS, Berk (Asmaven®), Cox, Hillcross, Norton
Oral solution, salbutamol (as sulphate) 2 mg/5 mL. Net price 150 mL = 72p

Ventmax® SR (Trinity) PoM
Capsules, m/r, salbutamol (as sulphate) 4 mg (green/grey), net price 56-cap pack = £8.97; 8 mg (white), 56-cap pack = £10.76. Label: 25
Dose: 8 mg twice daily; CHILD 3–12 years 4 mg twice daily

Ventolin® (A&H) PoM
Syrup, sugar-free, salbutamol (as sulphate) 2 mg/5 mL. Net price 150 mL = 71p

Volmax® (DF) PoM
Tablets, m/r, salbutamol (as sulphate) 4 mg, net price 56-tab pack = £10.55; 8 mg, 56-tab pack = £12.66. Label: 25
Dose: 8 mg twice daily; CHILD 3–12 years 4 mg twice daily

■ Parenteral

Salbutamol (Non-proprietary) PoM
Injection, salbutamol (as sulphate)
100 micrograms/mL, net price 50-mL vial = £5.25
Available from Aurum

Ventolin® (A&H) PoM
Injection, salbutamol (as sulphate) 50 micrograms/mL, net price 5-mL amp = 57p; 500 micrograms/mL, 1-mL amp = 43p
Solution for intravenous infusion, salbutamol (as sulphate) 1 mg/mL. Dilute before use. Net price 5-mL amp = £3.08

■ Inhalation

COUNSELLING. Advise patients not to exceed prescribed dose and to follow manufacturer's directions; if a previously effective dose of inhaled salbutamol fails to provide at least 3 hours relief, a doctor's advice should be obtained as soon as possible.
Patients receiving CFC-free inhalers should be reassured about their efficacy and counselled that aerosol may feel and taste different

Salbutamol (Non-proprietary) PoM
Aerosol inhalation, salbutamol 100 micrograms/metered inhalation, net price 200-dose unit =

£1.96. Counselling, dose
Available from APS, Ashbourne (*Maxivent®*), Berk (*Asmaven®*), Cox, Hillcross, Norton
Note. Vortex-based aerosol inhalers releasing salbutamol 100 micrograms/metered inhalation also available from Medeva (*Asmasal Spacehaler®*)
Excipients: include CFC propellants
Nebuliser solution, salbutamol (as sulphate) 1 mg/mL, net price 20 × 2.5 mL (2.5 mg) = £5.64; 2 mg/mL, 20 × 2.5 mL (5 mg) = £11.50. May be diluted with sterile sodium chloride 0.9%
Available from Ashbourne (*Maxivent Steripoules®*), Baker Norton (*Salamol Steri-Neb®*), Galen, Generics

Aerolin® Autohaler (3M) PoM
Aerosol inhalation, salbutamol (as sulphate) 100 micrograms/metered inhalation. Net price 200-dose breath-actuated unit = £10.04. Counselling, dose
Excipients: include CFC propellants

Airomir® (3M) PoM
Aerosol inhalation, salbutamol (as sulphate) 100 micrograms/metered inhalation, net price 200-dose unit = £1.97. Counselling, dose, change to CFC-free inhaler
Excipients: include HFA-134a (a non-CFC propellant), alcohol
Also available as *Salbulin®* (3M)
Note. Can be supplied against a generic prescription but if 'CFC-free' not specified will be reimbursed at price for CFC-containing inhaler
Autohaler (breath-actuated aerosol inhalation), salbutamol (as sulphate) 100 micrograms/metered inhalation, net price 200-dose unit = £6.02. Counselling, dose, change to CFC-free inhaler
Excipients: include HFA-134a (a non-CFC propellant), alcohol

Asmasal Clickhaler® (Medeva) PoM
Dry powder for inhalation, salbutamol (as sulphate) 95 micrograms/metered inhalation, net price 200-dose unit = £6.32. Counselling, dose
Dose: acute bronchospasm 1–2 puffs
Persistent symptoms, 2 puffs 3–4 times daily
Prophylaxis in exercise-induced bronchospasm, 2 puffs

Ventodisks® (A&H) PoM
Dry powder for inhalation, disks containing 8 blisters of salbutamol (as sulphate) 200 micrograms/blister, net price 14 disks with *Diskhaler®* device = £6.40; 5-disk refill = £2.53 (hosp. only), 14-disk refill = £5.89; 400 micrograms/blister, 14 disks with *Diskhaler®* device = £10.82; 5-disk refill = £3.87 (hosp. only), 14-disk refill = £10.30. Counselling, dose

Ventolin® (A&H) PoM
Accuhaler® (dry powder for inhalation), disk containing 60 blisters of salbutamol (as sulphate) 200 micrograms/blister with *Accuhaler®* device, net price = £5.00. Counselling, dose
Dose: by inhalation of powder, 200 micrograms; for persistant symptoms up to 4 times daily (but see also Chronic Asthma table); CHILD 200 micrograms
Prophylaxis in allergen- or exercise-induced bronchospasm, 200 micrograms
Easi-Breathe® aerosol inhalation, salbutamol 100 micrograms/metered inhalation, net price 200-dose breath-actuated unit = £6.30. Counselling, dose
Excipients: include CFC propellants
Evohaler® ▼ *aerosol inhalation*, salbutamol (as sulphate) 100 micrograms/metered inhalation, net price 200-dose unit = £2.30. Counselling, dose, change to CFC-free inhaler
Excipients: include HFA-134a (a non-CFC propellant)
Note. Can be supplied against a generic prescription but if CFC-free not specified will be reimbursed at price for CFC-containing inhaler

Nebules® (for use with nebuliser), salbutamol (as sulphate) 1 mg/mL, net price 20×2.5 mL (2.5 mg) = £3.38; 2 mg/mL, 20×2.5 mL (5 mg) = £6.90. May be diluted with sterile sodium chloride 0.9% if administration time in excess of 10 minutes is required

Respirator solution (for use with a nebuliser or ventilator), salbutamol (as sulphate) 5 mg/mL. Net price 20 mL = £2.44 (hosp. only). May be diluted with sterile sodium chloride 0.9%

Rotacaps® (dry powder for inhalation; for use with *Ventolin Rotahaler®*), salbutamol (as sulphate), 200 micrograms (light-blue/clear), net price 112-cap pack = £5.33; 400 micrograms (dark-blue/clear), 112-cap pack = £9.01. Counselling, dose

■ Compound preparations

For some **compound preparations** containing salbutamol, see section 3.1.4

■ Inhaler devices
Section 3.1.5

Chronic Asthma table, see p. 130
Acute Severe Asthma table, see p. 131

TERBUTALINE SULPHATE

Indications: see under Salbutamol; premature labour (section 7.1.3)

Cautions: see under Salbutamol

Side-effects: see under Salbutamol

Dose: *by mouth,* initially 2.5 mg 3 times daily for 1–2 weeks, then up to 5 mg 3 times daily
CHILD 75 micrograms/kg 3 times daily; 7–15 years 2.5 mg 2–3 times daily

By subcutaneous, intramuscular, or slow intravenous injection, 250–500 micrograms up to 4 times daily; CHILD 2–15 years 10 micrograms/kg to a max. of 300 micrograms

By continuous intravenous infusion as a solution containing 3–5 micrograms/mL, 1.5–5 micrograms/minute for 8–10 hours; reduce dose for children

By aerosol inhalation, adults and children 250–500 micrograms (1–2 puffs); for persistent symptoms up to 3–4 times daily (but see also Chronic Asthma table)

By inhalation of powder (*Turbohaler®*), 500 micrograms (1 inhalation); for persistent symptoms up to 4 times daily (but see also Chronic Asthma table)

By inhalation of nebulised solution, 5–10 mg 2–4 times daily; additional doses may be necessary in severe acute asthma; CHILD, up to 3 years 2 mg, 3–6 years 3 mg; 6–8 years 4 mg, over 8 years 5 mg, 2–4 times daily

■ Oral and parenteral

Bricanyl® (Astra) PoM
Tablets, scored, terbutaline sulphate 5 mg. Net price 20 = 74p
Syrup, sugar-free, terbutaline sulphate 1.5 mg/5 mL. Net price 300 mL = £2.36
Injection, terbutaline sulphate 500 micrograms/mL. Net price 1-mL amp = 27p; 5-mL amp = £1.27

Bricanyl SA® (Astra) PoM
Tablets, m/r, terbutaline sulphate 7.5 mg. Net price 20 = £1.55. Label: 25
Dose: 7.5 mg twice daily

Monovent® (Lagap) PoM
Syrup, sugar-free, terbutaline sulphate 1.5 mg/5 mL. Net price 300 mL = £2.15

■ Inhalation
COUNSELLING. Advise patients not to exceed prescribed dose and to follow manufacturer's directions; if a previously effective dose of inhaled terbutaline fails to provide at least 3 hours relief, a doctor's advice should be obtained as soon as possible

Terbutaline Sulphate (Non-proprietary) PoM
Nebuliser solution, terbutaline sulphate 2.5 mg/mL, net price 20 × 2 mL (5 mg) = £5.49. May be diluted with sterile sodium chloride 0.9%
Available from Galen

Bricanyl® (Astra) PoM
Aerosol inhalation, terbutaline sulphate 250 micrograms/metered inhalation. Net price 400-dose unit = £5.31; 400-dose unit with *Spacer* device (collapsible extended mouthpiece) = £7.21. Counselling, dose
Excipients: include CFC propellants
Turbohaler® (= dry powder inhaler), terbutaline sulphate 500 micrograms/inhalation. Net price 100-dose unit = £7.96. Counselling, dose
Respules® (= single-dose units for nebulisation), terbutaline sulphate 2.5 mg/mL. Net price 20 × 2-mL units (5-mg) = £3.67
Respirator solution (for use with a nebuliser or ventilator), terbutaline sulphate 10 mg/mL. Net price 20 mL = £2.64. Before use dilute with sterile sodium chloride 0.9%

■ Inhaler devices
Section 3.1.5

BAMBUTEROL HYDROCHLORIDE

Note. Bambuterol is a pro-drug of terbutaline

Indications: asthma and other conditions associated with reversible airways obstruction

Cautions: see under Salbutamol; renal impairment (Appendix 3); avoid in cirrhosis, severe hepatic impairment; manufacturer advises avoid in pregnancy

Side-effects: see under Salbutamol

Dose: 20 mg once daily at bedtime if patient has previously tolerated beta₂-adrenoceptor stimulants; other patients, initially 10 mg once daily at bedtime, increased if necessary after 1–2 weeks to 20 mg once daily; CHILD not recommended

Bambec® (Astra) PoM
Tablets, both scored, bambuterol hydrochloride 10 mg, net price 28-tab pack = £10.95; 20 mg, 28-tab pack = £13.14

FENOTEROL HYDROBROMIDE

Indications: reversible airways obstruction

Cautions: see under Salbutamol

Side-effects: see under Salbutamol

Dose: *by aerosol inhalation,* 100–200 micrograms (1–2 puffs *Berotec® '100'*) 1–3 times daily, and see also *Berotec® '200'* below (but see also Chronic Asthma table); CHILD 6–12 years 100 micrograms (1 puff *Berotec® '100'*) 1–3 times daily
Persistent bronchospasm not adequately controlled by *Berotec® '100'*, *by aerosol inhalation,* 400 micrograms (2 puffs *Berotec® '200'*) 1–3 times daily; not more than 400 micrograms (2 puffs *Berotec® '200'*) every 6 hours; max. 1.6 mg daily (**important:** see also Chronic Asthma table); CHILD under 16 years, not recommended
COUNSELLING. Advise patients not to exceed prescribed dose and to follow manufacturer's directions; if a previously effective dose of inhaled fenoterol fails to provide at least 3 hours relief, a doctor's advice should be obtained as soon as possible

Berotec® (Boehringer Ingelheim) [PoM]

'100' aerosol inhalation, fenoterol hydrobromide 100 micrograms/metered inhalation. Net price 200-dose unit = £2.36. Counselling, dose
Excipients: include CFC propellants

'200' aerosol inhalation, fenoterol hydrobromide 200 micrograms/metered inhalation. Net price 200-dose unit = £2.78. Counselling, dose
Excipients: include CFC propellants

Note. Only for persistent bronchospasm inadequately controlled by *Berotec® '100'*

■ Compound preparations

For some **compound preparations** containing fenoterol, see section 3.1.4

FORMOTEROL FUMARATE/ EFORMOTEROL FUMARATE

Indications: reversible airways obstruction (including nocturnal asthma and prevention of exercise-induced bronchospasm) in patients requiring long-term regular bronchodilator therapy, who should normally also be receiving regular and adequate doses of inhaled anti-inflammatory drugs (e.g. corticosteroids and/or sodium cromoglicate) or oral corticosteroids; see also Chronic Asthma table, p. 130

Note. Formoterol is not for immediate relief of acute attacks and existing corticosteroid therapy should not be reduced or withdrawn

Cautions: see under Salbutamol and notes above; severe liver cirrhosis; pregnancy (Appendix 4 and notes above); avoid in breast-feeding

Side-effects: see under Salbutamol; oropharyngeal and conjunctival irritation, eyelid oedema, taste disturbances, rash, insomnia, nausea and pruritus also reported; **important:** potential for paradoxical bronchospasm (calling for discontinuation and alternative therapy)

Dose: see under preparations below

COUNSELLING. Advise patients that formoterol should **not** be used for relief of acute attacks, not to exceed prescribed dose, and to follow manufacturer's directions; if a previously effective dose of inhaled formoterol fails to provide adequate relief, a doctor's advice should be obtained as soon as possible

Foradil® (Novartis) ▼ [PoM]

Dry powder for inhalation, formoterol fumarate 12 micrograms/capsule, net price 56-dose unit (with inhaler device) = £24.00, 14-dose unit (with inhaler device) = £6.00 (hosp. only). Counselling, dose

Dose: by inhalation of powder, 12 micrograms twice daily, increased to 24 micrograms twice daily in more severe airways obstruction; CHILD under 18 years not recommended

Oxis® (Astra) ▼ [PoM]

Turbohaler® (= dry powder inhaler), formoterol fumarate 6 micrograms/inhalation, net price 56-dose unit = £24.80; 12 micrograms/inhalation, 60-dose unit = £24.80. Counselling, dose

Dose: by inhalation of powder, 6–12 micrograms once or twice daily, increased to 24 micrograms twice daily in more severe airways obstruction; CHILD under 12 years not recommended

REPROTEROL HYDROCHLORIDE

Indications: reversible airways obstruction
Cautions: see under Salbutamol
Side-effects: see under Salbutamol
Dose: *by aerosol inhalation*, 0.5–1 mg (1–2 puffs); persistent symptoms, up to 3 times daily (but see also Chronic Asthma table); CHILD 6–12 years 500 micrograms (1 puff)

COUNSELLING. Advise patients not to exceed prescribed dose and to follow manufacturer's directions; if a previously effective dose of inhaled reproterol fails to provide at least 3 hours relief, a doctor's advice should be obtained as soon as possible

Bronchodil® (ASTA Medica) [PoM]

Aerosol inhalation, reproterol hydrochloride 500 micrograms/metered inhalation. Net price 400-dose unit = £7.01. Counselling, dose
Excipients: include CFC propellants

SALMETEROL

Indications: reversible airways obstruction (including nocturnal asthma and prevention of exercise-induced bronchospasm) in patients requiring long-term regular bronchodilator therapy, who should normally also be receiving regular and adequate doses of inhaled anti-inflammatory drugs (e.g. corticosteroids and/or, in children, sodium cromoglicate) or oral corticosteroids; see also Chronic Asthma table, p. 130

Note. CSM has emphasised that salmeterol is not for immediate relief of acute attacks and that existing corticosteroid therapy should not be reduced or withdrawn

Cautions: see under Salbutamol and notes above
Side-effects: see under Salbutamol; significant incidence of paradoxical bronchospasm—may be clinically important in severe or deteriorating asthma

Dose: *by inhalation*, 50 micrograms (2 puffs or 1 blister) twice daily; up to 100 micrograms (4 puffs or 2 blisters) twice daily in more severe airways obstruction; CHILD under 4 years not recommended, over 4 years, 50 micrograms (2 puffs or 1 blister) twice daily

COUNSELLING. Advise patients that salmeterol should **not** be used for relief of acute attacks, not to exceed prescribed dose, and to follow manufacturer's directions; if a previously effective dose of inhaled salmeterol fails to provide adequate relief, a doctor's advice should be obtained as soon as possible

Serevent® (A&H) [PoM]

Accuhaler® (dry powder for inhalation), disk containing 60 blisters of salmeterol (as xinafoate (= hydroxynaphthoate)) 50 micrograms/blister with *Accuhaler®* device, net price = £28.60. Counselling, dose

Aerosol inhalation, salmeterol (as xinafoate (= hydroxynaphthoate)) 25 micrograms/metered inhalation, net price 60-dose unit = £14.30 (hosp. only), 120-dose unit = £28.60. Counselling, dose
Excipients: include CFC propellants

Diskhaler® (dry powder for inhalation), disks containing 4 blisters of salmeterol (as xinafoate (= hydroxynaphthoate)) 50 micrograms/blister, net price 14 disks with *Diskhaler®* device = £29.97, 5-disk refill = £9.99 (hosp. only), 14-disk refill = £29.40. Counselling, dose

TULOBUTEROL HYDROCHLORIDE

Indications: reversible airways obstruction

Cautions: see under Salbutamol; mild renal impairment (avoid if severe); pregnancy

Contra-indications: moderate to severe renal impairment; acute liver failure, chronic liver disease

Side-effects: see under Salbutamol

Dose: 2 mg twice daily; increased if necessary to 2 mg 3 times daily; CHILD 6–10 years 0.5–1 mg twice daily; over 10 years, 1–2 mg twice daily

Respacal® (UCB Pharma) PoM

Tablets, f/c, scored, tulobuterol hydrochloride 2 mg. Net price 60-tab pack = £12.54

Syrup, sugar-free, tulobuterol hydrochloride 1 mg/ 5 mL. Net price 150 mL = £4.48

3.1.1.2 Other adrenoceptor stimulants

Ephedrine and the partially selective orciprenaline are less suitable and less safe for use as bronchodilators than the selective beta$_2$-adrenoceptor stimulants, because they are more likely to cause arrhythmias and other side-effects. They should be avoided whenever possible.

Adrenaline (epinephrine) injection (1 in 1000) is used in the emergency treatment of acute allergic and anaphylactic reactions (section 3.4.3).

EPHEDRINE HYDROCHLORIDE ▃

Indications: reversible airways obstruction, but see notes above

Cautions: hyperthyroidism, diabetes mellitus, ischaemic heart disease, hypertension, renal impairment, elderly; prostatic hypertrophy (risk of acute retention); interaction with MAOIs a disadvantage; **interactions:** Appendix 1 (sympathomimetics)

Side-effects: tachycardia, anxiety, restlessness, insomnia common; also tremor, arrhythmias, dry mouth, cold extremities

Dose: 15–60 mg 3 times daily; CHILD up to 1 year 7.5 mg 3 times daily, 1–5 years 15 mg 3 times daily, 6–12 years 30 mg 3 times daily

[1] **Ephedrine Hydrochloride** (Non-proprietary) PoM ▃

Tablets, ephedrine hydrochloride 15 mg, net price 28 = £1.63; 30 mg, 28 = £1.69

Elixir, ephedrine hydrochloride 15 mg/5 mL in a suitable flavoured vehicle, containing alcohol 12%. Net price 100 mL = 85p

1. For exemptions see *Medicines, Ethics and Practice*, No. 23, London, Pharmaceutical Press, 2000 (and subsequent editions as available)

For a list of **cough and decongestant preparations on sale to the public**, including those containing ephedrine, see section 3.9.2

▃ denotes preparations that are considered to be less suitable for prescribing (see p. vi)

ORCIPRENALINE SULPHATE ▃

Indications: reversible airways obstruction, but see notes above

Cautions: see under Salbutamol (section 3.1.1.1) and notes above; **interactions:** Appendix 1 (sympathomimetics)

Side-effects: see under Salbutamol (section 3.1.1.1) and notes above

Dose: *by mouth*, 20 mg 4 times daily; CHILD up to 1 year 5–10 mg 3 times daily, 1–3 years 5–10 mg 4 times daily, 3–12 years 40–60 mg daily in divided doses

By aerosol inhalation, 0.75–1.5 mg (1–2 puffs) repeated if necessary after not less than 30 minutes to max. 9 mg (12 puffs) daily; CHILD up to 6 years 750 micrograms (1 puff) up to 4 times daily, 6–12 years 0.75–1.5 mg (1–2 puffs) up to 4 times daily

COUNSELLING. Advise patients not to exceed prescribed dose and to follow manufacturer's directions; if a previously effective dose of inhaled orciprenaline fails to provide at least 3 hours relief, a doctor's advice should be obtained as soon as possible

Alupent® (Boehringer Ingelheim) PoM ▃

Tablets, scored, orciprenaline sulphate 20 mg. Net price 100-tab pack = £3.80

Syrup, sugar-free, orciprenaline sulphate 10 mg/ 5 mL. Net price 300 mL = £2.26

Aerosol inhalation, orciprenaline sulphate 750 micrograms/metered inhalation. Net price 300-dose vial with mouthpiece = £2.90; refill vial = £2.66. Counselling, dose

Excipients: include CFC propellants

3.1.2 Antimuscarinic bronchodilators

Ipratropium or **oxitropium** may be used by inhalation in the management of chronic asthma in patients who already require high-dose inhaled corticosteroids (see Chronic Asthma table, p. 130). Ipratropium by nebulisation may be added to other standard treatment in life-threatening asthma or where acute asthma fails to improve with standard therapy (see Acute Severe Asthma table, p. 131).

Antimuscarinic bronchodilators are regarded as being more effective in relieving bronchoconstriction associated with chronic obstructive pulmonary disease than in relieving asthma. The aerosol inhalation of ipratropium has a maximum effect 30–60 minutes after use; its duration of action is 3 to 6 hours and bronchodilation can usually be maintained with treatment 3 times a day. **Oxitropium** has a similar action to that of ipratropium.

IPRATROPIUM BROMIDE

Indications: reversible airways obstruction, particularly in chronic bronchitis

Cautions: glaucoma (standard doses unlikely to be harmful but see below); prostatic hypertrophy; pregnancy

GLAUCOMA. *Acute angle-closure glaucoma* has been reported in patients given nebulised ipratropium, particularly when used in association with nebulised salbutamol (and possibly other beta$_2$-adrenoceptor stimulants). Special caution is needed to protect patient's eyes from nebulised drug

Side-effects: dry mouth occasionally reported; rarely urinary retention, constipation

Dose: *by aerosol inhalation*, 20–40 micrograms, in early treatment up to 80 micrograms at a time, 3–4 times daily; CHILD up to 6 years 20 micrograms 3 times daily, 6–12 years 20–40 micrograms 3 times daily

By inhalation of powder, 40 micrograms 3–4 times daily (may be doubled in less responsive patients); CHILD under 12 years, not recommended

By inhalation of nebulised solution, 100–500 micrograms up to 4 times daily; CHILD 1 month–3 years 62.5–250 micrograms up to 3 times daily [unlicensed]; 3–14 years 100–500 micrograms up to 3 times daily. Dilution of solution is adjusted according to equipment and length of administration. Because paradoxical bronchospasm has occurred, *first dose* should be inhaled under medical supervision

COUNSELLING. Advise patient not to exceed prescribed dose and to follow manufacturer's directions

Ipratropium Bromide (Non-proprietary) PoM
Nebuliser solution, ipratropium bromide 250 micrograms/mL, net price 20 × 1-mL (250-microgram) unit-dose vials = £6.23, 60 × 1-mL = £18.52; 20 × 2-mL (500-microgram) = £7.30, 60 × 2-mL = £21.69. If dilution is necessary use only sterile sodium chloride 0.9%
Available from Galen, Generics

Atrovent® (Boehringer Ingelheim) PoM
Aerocaps® (dry powder for inhalation; for use with *Atrovent Aerohaler®*), green, ipratropium bromide 40 micrograms, net price pack of 100 caps with *Aerohaler®* = £14.53; 100 caps = £10.53. Counselling, dose
Aerosol inhalation, ipratropium bromide 20 micrograms/metered inhalation, net price 200-dose unit = £4.21. Counselling, dose
Excipients: include CFC propellants
Autohaler® (= breath-actuated aerosol inhalation), ipratropium bromide 20 micrograms/metered inhalation, net price 200-dose unit = £9.39. Counselling, dose
Excipients: include CFC propellants
Forte aerosol inhalation, ipratropium bromide 40 micrograms/metered inhalation, net price 200-dose unit = £6.22. Counselling, dose
Excipients: include CFC propellants
Nebuliser solution, isotonic, ipratropium bromide 250 micrograms/mL, net price 20 × 1-mL unit-dose vials = £6.82; 20 × 2-mL vials = £8.00. If dilution is necessary use only sterile sodium chloride 0.9%
Note. One Atrovent Aerocap® is equivalent to 2 puffs of Atrovent® metered aerosol inhalation *or* 1 puff of *Atrovent Forte®* metered aerosol inhalation

Ipratropium Steri-Neb® (Baker Norton) PoM
Nebuliser solution, isotonic, ipratropium bromide 250 micrograms/mL, net price 20 × 1-mL (250-microgram) unit-dose vials = £5.53; 20 × 2-mL (500-microgram) = £6.48. If dilution is necessary use only sterile sodium chloride 0.9%

Respontin® (A&H) PoM
Nebuliser solution, isotonic, ipratropium bromide 250 micrograms/mL, net price 20 × 1-mL (250-microgram) unit-dose vials = £5.44; 20 × 2-mL (500-microgram) = £6.40. If dilution is necessary use only sterile sodium chloride 0.9%
For some **compound preparations** containing ipratropium, see section 3.1.4

OXITROPIUM BROMIDE

Indications: reversible airways obstruction, particularly in chronic bronchitis
Cautions: see under Ipratropium Bromide
Side-effects: see under Ipratropium Bromide; rarely blurring of vision
Dose: *by aerosol inhalation*, 200 micrograms (2 puffs) 2–3 times daily; CHILD not recommended
COUNSELLING. Advise patient not to exceed prescribed dose and to follow manufacturer's directions

Oxivent® (Boehringer Ingelheim) PoM
Aerosol inhalation, oxitropium bromide 100 micrograms/metered inhalation. Net price 200-dose unit = £6.69. Counselling, dose
Excipients: include CFC propellants
Autohaler® (= breath-actuated aerosol inhalation), oxitropium bromide 100 micrograms/metered inhalation. Net price 200-dose unit = £15.72. Counselling, dose
Excipients: include CFC propellants

3.1.3   Theophylline

Theophylline is a bronchodilator used for reversible airways obstruction. It may have an additive effect when used in conjunction with small doses of beta$_2$-adrenoceptor stimulants; the combination may increase the risk of side-effects, including hypokalaemia (for CSM advice see p. 133).

Theophylline is metabolised in the liver; there is considerable variation in its half-life particularly in smokers, in patients with hepatic impairment or heart failure, or if certain drugs are taken concurrently. The half-life is *increased* in heart failure, cirrhosis, viral infections, in the elderly, and by drugs such as cimetidine, ciprofloxacin, erythromycin, fluvoxamine, and oral contraceptives. The half-life is *decreased* in smokers and in chronic alcoholism, and by drugs such as phenytoin, carbamazepine, rifampicin, and barbiturates. For other interactions of theophylline see Appendix 1.

These differences in half-life are important because theophylline has a narrow margin between the therapeutic and toxic dose. In most subjects a plasma-theophylline concentration of between 10–20 mg/litre is usually required for satisfactory bronchodilation although a plasma-theophylline concentration of 10 mg/litre (or less) may be effective. Adverse effects can occur within the range 10–20 mg/litre and both the frequency and severity increase at concentrations above 20 mg/litre.

Theophylline modified-release preparations are usually able to produce adequate plasma concentrations for up to 12 hours. When given as a single dose at night they have a useful role in controlling nocturnal asthma and early morning wheezing. The use of *rapid-release* oral theophylline preparations has declined because of the high incidence of side-effects associated with rapid absorption.

Theophylline is given by injection as **aminophylline**, a mixture of theophylline with ethylenediamine, which is 20 times more soluble than theophylline alone. Aminophylline must be given by **very slow** intravenous injection (over at least 20 minutes); it is too irritant for intramuscular use.

Intravenous aminophylline has a role in the treatment of severe attacks of asthma that do not respond rapidly to a nebulised beta$_2$-adrenoceptor stimulant (see also Acute Severe Asthma table,

p. 131). Measurement of plasma theophylline concentrations may be helpful, and is **essential** if aminophylline is to be given to patients who have been taking oral theophylline preparations, as serious side-effects such as convulsions and arrhythmias can occasionally occur before the appearance of other symptoms of toxicity.

Aminophylline injection was formerly also used in the treatment of left ventricular failure but has been superseded for this purpose by diuretics (section 2.2.1 and section 2.2.2) and the opioid analgesics (section 4.7.2). However, it may have a role in patients with heart failure who are also suffering from asthma and bronchitis, where opioids are contra-indicated, though care is needed in those with increased myocardial excitability.

THEOPHYLLINE

Indications: reversible airways obstruction, acute severe asthma; for guidelines see also Asthma tables (pp.130–1)

Cautions: cardiac disease, hypertension, hyperthyroidism, peptic ulcer, hepatic impairment (reduce dose), epilepsy, pregnancy and breast-feeding, elderly, fever; **CSM** advice on hypokalaemia risk, p. 133; avoid in porphyria (section 9.8.2); **interactions:** Appendix 1 (theophylline) and notes above

Side-effects: tachycardia, palpitations, nausea, gastro-intestinal disturbances, headache, insomnia, arrhythmias, and convulsions especially if given rapidly by intravenous injection; **overdosage:** see Emergency Treatment of Poisoning, p. 25

Dose: see below

Note. Plasma theophylline concentration for optimum response 10–20 mg/litre (55–110 micromol/litre); narrow margin between therapeutic and toxic dose, see also notes above

Nuelin® (3M)

Tablets, scored, theophylline 125 mg. Net price 90-tab pack = £3.29. Label: 21
Dose: 125 mg 3–4 times daily after food, increased to 250 mg if required; CHILD 7–12 years 62.5–125 mg 3–4 times daily
Liquid, brown, theophylline hydrate (as sodium glycinate) 60 mg/5 mL. Net price 300 mL = £2.93. Label: 21
Dose: 120–240 mg 3–4 times daily after food; CHILD 2–6 years 60–90 mg, 7–12 years 90–120 mg, 3–4 times daily

■ Modified release
Note. The Council of the Royal Pharmaceutical Society of Great Britain advises pharmacists that if a general practitioner prescribes a modified-release, oral theophylline preparation without specifying a brand name, the pharmacist should contact the prescriber and agree the brand to be dispensed. Additionally, it is essential that a patient discharged from hospital should be maintained on the brand on which that patient was stabilised as an in-patient.

Lasma® (Pharmax)

Tablets, m/r, scored, theophylline 300 mg. Net price 60-tab pack = £5.41. Label: 25
Dose: 300 mg every 12 hours (increased after 1 week to 450 mg every 12 hours in patients over 70 kg); adjust dose by 150-mg increments as required
Total daily dose may be given as single dose at night when nocturnal symptoms predominate (daytime symptoms then controlled with inhaled bronchodilators)

Nuelin SA® (3M)

SA tablets, m/r, theophylline 175 mg. Net price 60-tab pack = £3.43. Label: 25
Dose: 175–350 mg every 12 hours; CHILD over 6 years 175 mg every 12 hours
SA 250 tablets, m/r, scored, theophylline 250 mg. Net price 60-tab pack = £4.80. Label: 25
Dose: 250–500 mg every 12 hours; CHILD over 6 years 125–250 mg every 12 hours

Slo-Phyllin® (Lipha)

Capsules, all m/r, theophylline 60 mg (white/clear, enclosing white pellets), net price 56-cap pack = £1.83; 125 mg (brown/clear, enclosing white pellets), 56-cap pack = £2.31; 250 mg (blue/clear, enclosing white pellets), 56-cap pack = £2.88. Label: 25 *or* counselling, see below
Dose: 250–500 mg every 12 hours; CHILD, every 12 hours, 2–6 years 60–120 mg, 7–12 years 125–250 mg
COUNSELLING. Swallow whole with fluid *or* swallow enclosed granules with soft food (e.g. yoghurt)

Theo-Dur® (Astra)

Tablets, m/r, both scored, theophylline 200 mg, net price 20 = £1.21; 300 mg, 20 = £1.75. Label: 25
Dose: 300 mg every 12 hours, adjust dose by 100–150-mg steps as required; CHILD up to 35 kg 100 mg, over 35 kg 200 mg, every 12 hours
For nocturnal asthma, total daily requirement may be given as single evening dose

Uniphyllin Continus® (Napp)

Tablets, m/r, all scored, theophylline 200 mg, net price 56-tab pack = £3.87; 300 mg, 56-tab pack = £5.89; 400 mg, 56-tab pack = £6.99. Label: 25
Dose: 200 mg every 12 hours increased after 1 week to 300 mg every 12 hours; over 70 kg 200–300 mg every 12 hours increased after 1 week to 400 mg every 12 hours
May be appropriate to give larger evening or morning dose to achieve optimum therapeutic effect when symptoms most severe; in patients whose night- or daytime symptoms persist despite other therapy, who are not currently receiving theophylline, total daily requirement may be added as single evening or morning dose
CHILD over 7 years, 9 mg/kg twice daily; some children with chronic asthma may require 10–16 mg/kg every 12 hours

For a list of **cough and decongestant preparations on sale to the public,** including those containing theophylline, see section 3.9.2

AMINOPHYLLINE

Note. Aminophylline is a stable mixture or combination of theophylline and ethylenediamine; the ethylenediamine confers greater solubility in water

Indications: reversible airways obstruction, acute severe asthma

Cautions: see under Theophylline

Side-effects: see under Theophylline; also allergy to ethylenediamine can cause urticaria, erythema, and exfoliative dermatitis

Dose: see under preparations, below

Note. Plasma theophylline concentration for optimum response 10–20 mg/litre (55–110 micromol/litre); narrow margin between therapeutic and toxic dose, see also notes above

Aminophylline (Non-proprietary)

Tablets, aminophylline 100 mg, net price 20 = 71p. Label: 21

Dose: by mouth, 100–300 mg, 3–4 times daily, after food

Injection, aminophylline 25 mg/mL, net price 10-mL amp = 65p PoM

Available from Antigen, Medeva (*Min-I-Jet®*), Phoenix

Dose: deteriorating acute severe asthma **not** previously treated with theophylline, *by slow intravenous injection* over at least 20 minutes, 250–500 mg (5 mg/kg), then as for acute severe asthma; CHILD 5 mg/kg, then as for acute severe asthma

Acute severe asthma, *by intravenous infusion*, 500 micrograms/kg/hour, adjusted according to plasma-theophylline concentration; CHILD 6 months–9 years 1 mg/kg/hour, 10–16 years 800 micrograms/kg/hour, adjusted according to plasma-theophylline concentration

Note. Patients taking oral theophylline or aminophylline should not normally receive intravenous aminophylline unless plasma-theophylline concentration is available to guide dosage

■ Modified release

Note. Advice about modified-release theophylline preparations on p. 139 also applies to modified-release aminophylline preparations

Phyllocontin Continus® (Napp)

Tablets, m/r, yellow, f/c, aminophylline hydrate 225 mg. Net price 56-tab pack = £3.14. Label: 25

Dose: 1 tablet twice daily initially, increased after 1 week to 2 tablets twice daily

Forte tablets, m/r, yellow, f/c, aminophylline hydrate 350 mg. Net price 56-tab pack = £5.21. Label: 25

Note. Forte tablets are for smokers and other patients with decreased theophylline half-life (see notes above)

Paediatric tablets, m/r, peach, aminophylline hydrate 100 mg. Net price 56-tab pack = £2.02. Label: 25

Dose: CHILD over 3 years, 6 mg/kg twice daily initially, increased after 1 week to 12 mg/kg twice daily; some children with chronic asthma may require 13–20 mg/kg every 12 hours

Note. Modified-release tablets containing aminophylline 225 mg also available from Ashbourne (*Amnivent® 225 SR*), Norton (*Norphyllin® SR*)

3.1.4   Compound bronchodilator preparations

In general, patients are best treated with single-ingredient preparations, such as a selective beta₂-adrenoceptor stimulant (section 3.1.1.1) or ipratropium bromide (section 3.1.2), so that the dose of each drug can be adjusted. This flexibility is lost with combinations, although those in which both components are effective may have a role when compliance is a problem.

For **cautions, contra-indications** and **side-effects** see under individual drugs.

> ◢ denotes preparations that are considered to be less suitable for prescribing (see p. vi)

Combivent® (Boehringer Ingelheim) PoM ◢

Aerosol inhalation, ipratropium bromide 20 micrograms, salbutamol (as sulphate) 100 micrograms/metered inhalation. Net price 200-dose unit = £6.45. Counselling, dose

Excipients: include CFC propellants

Dose: bronchospasm associated with chronic obstructive pulmonary disease, 2 puffs 4 times daily; CHILD under 12 years not recommended

Nebuliser solution, isotonic, ipratropium bromide 500 micrograms, salbutamol (as sulphate) 2.5 mg/2.5-mL vial, net price 60 unit-dose vials = £33.00

Dose: bronchospasm in chronic obstructive pulmonary disease, *by inhalation of nebulised solution*, 1 vial 3–4 times daily; CHILD under 12 years not recommended

GLAUCOMA. In addition to other potential side-effects acute angle-closure glaucoma has been reported with nebulised ipratropium—for details, see p. 137

Duovent® (Boehringer Ingelheim) PoM ◢

Aerosol inhalation, fenoterol hydrobromide 100 micrograms, ipratropium bromide 40 micrograms/metered inhalation. Net price 200-dose unit with mouthpiece = £5.18 (extension tube also available). Counselling, dose

Excipients: include CFC propellants

Dose: reversible airways obstruction in asthma, bronchitis and emphysema, 1–2 puffs 3–4 times daily; CHILD over 6 years 1 puff 3 times daily

Autohaler® (= breath-actuated aerosol inhalation), fenoterol hydrobromide 100 micrograms, ipratropium bromide 40 micrograms/metered inhalation. Net price 200-dose unit = £10.18. Counselling, dose

Excipients: include CFC propellants

Dose: reversible airways obstruction in asthma, bronchitis and emphysema, 1–2 puffs 3–4 times daily; CHILD over 6 years 1 puff 3 times daily

Nebuliser solution, isotonic, fenoterol hydrobromide 1.25 mg, ipratropium bromide 500 micrograms/4-mL vial, net price 20 unit-dose vials = £11.00

Dose: acute severe asthma or acute exacerbation of chronic asthma, *by inhalation of nebulised solution*, 1 vial (4 mL); may be repeated up to max. 4 vials in 24 hours; CHILD under 14 years, not recommended

GLAUCOMA. In addition to other potential side-effects acute angle-closure glaucoma has been reported with nebulised ipratropium—for details, see p. 137

■ Preparations on sale to the public

For **compound bronchodilator preparations** on sale to the public, see p. 161

3.1.5   Peak flow meters, inhaler devices and nebulisers

Peak flow meters

Measurement of peak flow is particularly helpful for patients who are 'poor perceivers' and hence slow to detect deterioration in their asthma, and for those with moderate or severe asthma. Patients must be given clear guidelines as to the action they should take if their peak flow falls below a certain level. Patients can be encouraged to adjust some of their own treatment (within specified limits) according to changes in peak flow rate.

Ferraris Pocketpeak® (Ferraris)
Peak flow meter, standard (90–710 litres/minute), net price = £6.53, low range (40–370 litres/minute) = £6.53, replacement mouthpiece = 38p (for adult or child)

Mini-Wright® (Clement Clarke)
Peak flow meter, standard (60 to 800 litres/minute), net price = £6.86, low range (30 to 400 litres/minute) = £6.90, replacement mouthpiece = 38p (for adult or child)

Vitalograph® (Vitalograph)
Peak flow meter, standard (50 to 750 litres/minute), now called *Asmaplan®*, net price = £6.65, low range (25 to 280 litres/minute) = £6.65, replacement mouthpiece = 40p (for adult or child)

Rotahaler® (A&H)
Breath-actuated device for use with *Rotacaps®*. Available as *Becotide Rotahaler®*, *Ventolin Rotahaler®*, and *Ventide Rotahaler®*. Net price = 78p

Spinhaler® (Rhône-Poulenc Rorer)
Breath-actuated device for use with *Intal Spincaps®*. Net price = £1.92

Volumatic® (A&H)
Spacer inhaler, large-volume device. For use with *Becloforte®*, *Becotide®*, *Flixotide®*, *Serevent®*, *Ventide®*, and *Ventolin®* inhalers, net price = £2.75; with paediatric mask = £2.75

Inhaler devices

A variety of *spacing devices* is now available for use with *pressurised (aerosol) inhalers* (metered dose inhalers). By providing a space between inhaler and mouth, they reduce the velocity of the aerosol and subsequent impaction on the oropharynx; in addition they allow more time for evaporation of the propellant so that a larger proportion of the particles can be inhaled and deposited in the lungs; also co-ordination of inspiration with actuation of the aerosol is less important. The size of the spacer is important and the larger spacing devices with a one-way valve (*Nebuhaler®*, *Volumatic®*) are the most effective. Spacing devices are particularly useful for patients with poor inhalation technique, for children, for patients requiring higher doses, for nocturnal asthma, and for patients prone to develop candidiasis with inhaled corticosteroids.

Alternatively *dry powder inhalers*, activated by the patient's inspiration, are of value; some occasionally cause coughing.

USE AND CARE OF SPACER DEVICES. Patients should inhale from the spacer devices as soon as possible after actuation since the drug aerosol is very short-lived; single-dose actuation is recommended. The device is cleansed once a week by washing, rinsing and then allowing to dry in air (wiping should be avoided since any electrostatic charge may affect drug delivery). Spacer devices should be replaced every 6–12 months.

Able Spacer® (Clement Clarke)
Spacer device, small-volume device. For use with pressurised (aerosol) inhalers, net price = £4.20; mask (small, medium, or large) NHS = £4.75

AeroChamber® (3M)
Spacer device, medium-volume device. For use with *Airomir®*, *Salbulin®*, and *Qvar®* inhalers, net price standard device (blue) = £4.28, with mask (blue) = £7.14; child device (yellow) with mask = £7.14; infant device (orange) with mask = £7.14

Babyhaler® (A&H) NHS
Spacer device for paediatric use with *Becotide®-50* and *Ventolin®* inhalers. Net price = £11.34

E-Z Spacer® (Vitalograph) NHS
Spacer device, large-volume, collapsible device. For use with pressurised (aerosol) inhalers, price (direct from manufacturer) = £22.50

Haleraid® (GlaxoWellcome) NHS
Device to place over standard inhalers as aid to operation by patients with impaired strength in hands (e.g. with arthritis). Available as *Haleraid®-120* for 120-dose inhalers and *Haleraid®-200* for 200-dose inhalers. Net price = 80p

Nebuhaler® (Astra)
Spacer inhaler, large-volume device. For use with *Bricanyl®* and *Pulmicort®* refill canisters, net price = £4.28; with paediatric mask = £4.28

Nebulisers

In England and Wales nebulisers and compressors are not available on the NHS (but they are free of VAT); some nebulisers (but not compressors) are available on form GP10A in Scotland (for details consult Scottish Drug Tariff).

Nebulisers convert a solution of a drug into an aerosol for inhalation. They are used to deliver higher doses of drug to the airways than is usual with standard inhalers. The main indications for use of a nebuliser are:

- To deliver a beta-adrenoceptor stimulant or ipratropium to a patient with an *acute exacerbation* of asthma or of airway obstruction

- To deliver a beta-adrenoceptor stimulant or ipratropium on a *regular basis* to a patient with severe asthma or reversible airways obstruction who has been shown to benefit from regular treatment with higher doses

- To deliver *prophylactic medication* such as cromoglicate or a corticosteroid to a patient unable to use other inhalational devices (particularly a young child)

- To deliver an antibiotic (such as colistin) to a patient with chronic purulent infection (as in cystic fibrosis or bronchiectasis)

- To deliver pentamidine for the prophylaxis and treatment of pneumocystis pneumonia to a patient with AIDS.

The proportion of a nebuliser solution that reaches the lungs depends on the type of nebuliser and although it can be as high as 30% it is more frequently close to 10% and sometimes below 10%. The remaining solution is left in the nebuliser as residual volume or it is deposited in the mouthpiece and tubing. The extent to which the nebulised solution is deposited in the airways or alveoli depends on particle size. Particles with a mass median diameter of 1–5 microns are deposited in the airways and are therefore appropriate for asthma whereas a particle size of 1–2 microns is needed for alveolar deposition of pentamidine to combat pneumocystis infection. The type of nebuliser is therefore chosen according to the deposition required and according to the viscosity of the solution (antibiotic solutions usually being more viscous).

Some jet nebulisers are able to increase drug output during inspiration and hence increase efficiency.

The patient should be aware that the dose of a bronchodilator given by nebulisation is usually **much higher** than that from an aerosol inhaler; see below for British Thoracic Society guidelines.

The British Thoracic Society has advised that nebulised bronchodilators may be given to patients with chronic persistent asthma or those with sudden catastrophic severe asthma (brittle asthma). In chronic asthma, nebulised bronchodilators should only be used to relieve persistent daily wheeze (see Chronic Asthma table p. 130). The British Thoracic Society has further recommended that the use of nebulisers in chronic persistent asthma should only be considered:

- After a review of the diagnosis
- If the airflow obstruction is significantly reversible by bronchodilators without unacceptable side-effects
- After the patient has been using the usual hand-held inhaler correctly
- After a larger dose of bronchodilator from a hand-held inhaler (with a spacer if necessary) has been tried for at least 2 weeks
- If the patient is complying with the prescribed dose and frequency of anti-inflammatory treatment including regular use of high-dose inhaled corticosteroid

Before prescribing, a home trial should preferably be undertaken to monitor peak flow for up to 2 weeks on standard treatment and up to 2 weeks on nebulised treatment. If prescribed patients must:

- Have clear instructions from doctor, specialist nurse or pharmacist on the use of the nebuliser and on peak-flow monitoring
- Be instructed not to treat acute attacks at home without also seeking help
- Receive an education program
- Have regular follow up including peak-flow monitoring and be seen by doctor, specialist nurse or physiotherapist

■ Jet nebulisers

Jet nebulisers utilise the Venturi principle for nebulisation; they are more widely used than ultrasonic nebulisers. Most jet nebulisers require an optimum gas flow rate of 6–8 litres/minute and in hospital can be driven by piped air or oxygen. Domiciliary oxygen cylinders do not provide an adequate flow rate therefore for domiciliary use an electrical compressor is used.

For patients with *chronic bronchitis and hypercapnia*, oxygen can be dangerous and the nebuliser should be driven by air (see also p. 132).

> **Important:** the Department of Health has reminded users of the need to use the correct grade of tubing when connecting a nebuliser to a medical gas supply or compressor.

Medix All Nebuliser® (Medix) DHS

Jet nebuliser, disposable; for use with bronchodilators, antimuscarinics, corticosteroids, and antibiotics, replacement recommended every 2–3 months if used 4 times a day. Compatible with **AC 2000 Hi Flo**® DHS, **World Traveller Hi Flo**® DHS, and **Econoneb**® DHS. Net price 5 = £7.50

Medix Antibiotic Circuit® (Medix) DHS

Jet nebuliser, closed-system; for use with antibiotics and other respiratory drugs. Compatible with **AC 2000 Hi Flo**® DHS, **Econoneb**® DHS, and **Turboneb**® DHS. Net price 1 = £7.30

Medix System® (Medix) DHS

Jet nebuliser, consisting of mouthpiece, tubing, and nebuliser chamber. Net price 1 = £2.80; mask kits with tubing and nebuliser chamber also available, net price 1 (adult) = £2.90; 1 (child) = £2.90

Pari LC Plus Filter® (Pari) DHS

Jet nebuliser, closed system, non-disposable, for hospital or home use with low flow compressors; supplied with filter/valve set. Compatible with **Pari TurboBoy**® DHS and **Pari JuniorBoy**® DHS compressors. Net price 1 = £19.90, replacement filters 100 = £33.30

Pari LC Plus® (Pari) DHS

Jet nebuliser, non-disposable, for hospital or home use with low flow compressors; for use with bronchodilators, antibiotics, and corticosteroids, replacement recommended yearly if used 4 times a day. Compatible with **Pari TurboBoy**® DHS, **Pari JuniorBoy**® DHS and **Pari WalkBoy**® DHS compressors. Net price 1 = £13.90

Pari Baby® (Pari) DHS

Jet nebuliser, non-disposable, for hospital or home use with low flow compressors; for use with bronchodilators, antibiotics and corticosteroids; replacement recommended yearly if used 4 times a day. Compatible with **Pari TurboBoy**® DHS, **Pari JuniorBoy**® DHS, **Pari WalkBoy**® DHS compressors. Available separately for children aged less than 1 year, 1–4 years or 4–7 years. Net price 1 (with connection hose) = £25.00

Sidestream Durable® (Medic-Aid) DHS

Jet nebuliser, non-disposable, for home use; for use with bronchodilators; yearly replacement recommended if 4 six-minute treatments used per day. Compatible with **CR50**® DHS, **Freeway Lite**® DHS and **Porta-Neb 50**® DHS (depending on nebulising solution). Net price 10 pack = £94.50; patient pack with **CR50**® DHS compressor = £98.50. **Disposable Sidestream**® DHS nebuliser also available

Note. This has been developed to replace the **System 22 Acorn**® DHS

Ventstream® (Medic-Aid) DHS

Jet nebuliser, closed-system, for use with low flow compressors, compatible with **CR50**® DHS, **Porta-Neb 50**® DHS, and **Freeway Lite**® DHS compressors; for use with antibiotics, bronchodilators, and corticosteroids, replacement recommended yearly if used 3 times a day. Net price 1 with filter = £27.00; 10-pack with filter = £250.00; 1 without filter = £23.00; 10-pack without filter = £215.00; patient pack with **CR 50**® DHS compressor = £119.95

■ Home compressors with nebulisers

AC 2000 HI FLO® (Medix) DHS

Portable, home use, containing 1 **Jet Nebuliser**® DHS set with mouthpiece, 1 adult or 1 child mask, 1 spare inlet filter, filter spanner. Mains operated. Nebulises bronchodilators and antibiotics. Net price 1 = £105.00; carrying case available

Aquilon® (Henleys) DHS

Portable, home use, with 1 adult or 1 child mask and tubing. Mains operated; for use with bronchodilators, corticosteroids and antibiotics. Net price = £81.00

Econoneb® (Medix) DHS

Home, clinic and hospital use, used with 1 **Jet Nebuliser**® DHS set with mouthpiece, 1 adult or 1 child mask, 1 spare inlet filter, filter spanner. Compatible with all types of jet nebuliser sets and also the **Micro Cirrus**® DHS nebuliser (recommended for alveolar deposition). Nebulises bronchodilators, corticosteroids, and antibiotics. Mains operated. Net price 1 = £99.00

Freeway Lite® (Medic-Aid) DHS

Portable, containing 1 **Sidestream Durable**® DHS reusable nebuliser, 1 adult or 1 child mask, 1 mouthpiece, 1 Coiled Duratube®, 2 filters. Net price 1 = £149.00 with carrying case. **Freeway Lite Luxury**® DHS contains additional battery. Net price 1 = £198.00

Also compatible with **Ventstream**® DHS closed system nebuliser

M-Flo® (Medix) DHS

Portable, home use, containing 1 **Jet Nebuliser**® DHS set with mouthpiece, spare inlet filter, filter spanner. Mains operated. Nebulises bronchodilators and corticosteroids. Net price 1 = £95.00

Medi-Neb® (Timesco) DHS

Range of compressors all supplied with adult and child mask, vapourising chamber, and PVC tubing, including: **Medi-Neb Elite**® DHS, *home use*. Mains operated. Net price 1 = £84.96. **Medi-Neb Companion**® DHS, *portable*. Mains/car battery operated. Net price 1 = £104.95 (includes car battery adaptor and carrying case). **Medi-**

Neb Companion Plus® [NHS], *portable*. Mains/battery operated. Net price 1 = £144.96 (includes rechargeable battery, car battery adaptor, and carrying case). **Medi-Neb Tempest®** [NHS], *home/hospital use*. Mains operated. Net price 1 = £94.96

All used for nebulising antibiotics and bronchodilators

Pari TurboBoy® (Pari) [NHS]

Portable, for hospital or home use, containing **Pari LC Plus** [NHS] with connection tube and mains cable. Filter replacement recommended every 12 months or 550 hours of use. Compatible with **Pari LC Plus®** [NHS], **Pari LC Plus Filter®** [NHS], and **Pari Baby®** [NHS] nebulisers. Net price = £109.00

Pari JuniorBoy® (Pari) [NHS]

Portable, for hospital or home use, containing **Pari LC Plus** [NHS] with connection tube and mains cable. Filter replacement recommended every 12 months or 550 hours of use. Compatible with **Pari LC Plus®** [NHS], **Pari LC Plus Filter®** [NHS], and **Pari Baby®** [NHS] nebulisers. Net price = £119.00

Pari WalkBoy® (Pari) [NHS]

Portable, containing 1 **Pari LC Plus®** [NHS] nebuliser with connection tube, mains cable, rechargeable battery and carrying bag. Compatible with **Pari LC Plus®** [NHS] and **Pari Baby®** [NHS] nebulisers. Net price 1 = £219.00; car cigarette lighter adapter = £63.00

Porta-Neb® (Medic-Aid) [NHS]

Portable, containing 1 **Sidestream Durable®** [NHS] reusable nebuliser, 1 adult or 1 child mask, 1 Duratube® supply tubing, 4 spare filters. Mains operated; for use with bronchodilators. Net price 1 = £109.50; carrying case available
Also compatible with **Ventstream®** [NHS] closed-system nebuliser; for use with antibiotics, bronchodilators, and corticosteroids

Pulmo-Aide® (De Vilbiss) [NHS]

Home, clinic use, containing disposable nebuliser set, mouthpiece, mask, mains lead, tubing, thumb-valve. For use with bronchodilators. Net price 1 = £99.50. **Pulmo-Aide Escort®** [NHS], *portable*, containing disposable nebuliser set, transformer, rechargeable battery, AC to DC adapter charger, DC lead with car adapter, and carrying case. For use with bronchodilators. Net price 1 = £198.50. **Pulmo-Aide AP50®** [NHS], *home, clinic, hospital use*. Net price 1 = £180.00, 1 with anti-pollution kit = £188.50. **Pulmo-Aide Sunmist®** [NHS], *home use*, containing nebuliser set, mouthpiece, face mask, mains lead. Net price 1 = £84.25

SunMist® (De Vilbiss) [NHS]

Home, clinic and hospital use, with mouthpiece. Mains operated. Net price = £89.50. **SunMist Plus®** [NHS], *home, clinic and hospital use*, with mouthpiece, higher flow rate. Mains operated. Net price = £107.50

Tourer® (Henleys) [NHS]

Portable, home use. Mains/car battery operated; for use with bronchodilators, corticosteroids and antibiotics. Net price = £118.50, rechargeable battery pack = £54.00

Ultima® (Henleys) [NHS]

Portable, home use. Rechargable or mains/car battery operated. Nebulises bronchodilators and corticosteroids. Net price = £184.00 (includes case)

World Traveller HI FLO® (Medix) [NHS]

Portable, containing 1 **Jet Nebuliser®** [NHS] set with mouthpiece, 1 adult or 1 child mask, 1 spare inlet filter, filter spanner. Battery/mains operated; rechargeable battery pack available. Nebulises bronchodilators, corticosteroids, and antibiotics. Net price 1 excluding battery = £145.00; 1 with battery = £199.00; carrying case available

■ Compressors

System 22 CR50® (Medic-Aid) [NHS]

Home, clinic and hospital use. Mains operated. Net price 1 = £89.50. Also compatible with **Ventstream®** [NHS], and **Sidestream Durable®** [NHS]

System 22 CR60® (Medic-Aid) [NHS]

Hospital use, high flow compressor. Mains operated. Net price = £199.90. Also compatible with **System 22 Antibiotic Tee®** [NHS] for nebulisation of high viscosity drugs such as antibiotics

Turboneb® (Medix) [NHS]

Hospital use, high flow compressor. Mains operated. Net price 1 = £125.00. Also compatible with **Medix Antibiotic Circuit®** [NHS] for nebulisation of respiratory drugs in particular viscous antibiotics

■ Ultrasonic nebulisers

Ultrasonic nebulisers produce an aerosol by ultrasonic vibration of the drug solution and therefore do not require a gas flow

AeroSonic® (De Vilbiss) [NHS]

Portable, containing 1 controlling unit, chamber assembly, carrying case, AC to DC adapter/charger, DC lead, 1 mouthpiece with check valve and adapter. Net price 1 = £250.00

F16 Wave® (Parkside) [NHS]

Portable, delivery rate adjustable to suit user. Mains/car battery operated or rechargeable battery pack (supplied). Net price = £125.00

Omron U1 MicroAir® (Hutchings) [NHS]

Portable. Battery operated/mains adaptor. Net price = £325.00

Omron NE U07® (Hutchings) [NHS]

Portable. Mains operated or rechargeable battery pack. Net price = £166.00 (mains version), £253.00 (rechargeable version)

Sonix 2000® (Medix) [NHS]

Portable, delivery rate adjustable to suit user. Supplied with carrying case and DC lead. Mains/car battery operated; rechargeable battery pack available. Net price 1 excluding battery = £150.00, 1 with battery = £215.00

Ultra Neb 2000® (De Vilbiss) [NHS]

Hospital, clinic and home use, delivery rate adjustable. Supplied with stand. Net price = £1125.50

Nebuliser diluent

Nebulisation may be carried out using an undiluted nebuliser solution or it may require dilution beforehand. The usual diluent is sterile sodium chloride 0.9% (physiological saline).

Sodium Chloride (Non-proprietary) [PoM]

Nebuliser solution, sodium chloride 0.9%, net price 20×2.5 mL = £3.66
Available from Baker Norton (*Saline Steri-Neb®*), Galen (*Saline Steripoule®*)

3.2   Corticosteroids

Corticosteroids are effective in *asthma*; they reduce airway inflammation (and hence reduce oedema and secretion of mucus into the airway).

Patients with *chronic obstructive pulmonary disease* usually show little or no response to corticosteroids. Whether inhaled corticosteroids reduce the decline in lung function in chronic obstructive pulmonary disease has not yet been established. Some patients with asthma, however, may be clinically indistinguishable from those with chronic obstructive pulmonary disease except that they will respond to a trial course of corticosteroids.

INHALATION. Inhaled corticosteroids are recommended for prophylactic treatment of asthma when patients are using a beta$_2$-stimulant more than once daily (see Chronic Asthma table). They have many fewer side-effects than those associated with systemic administration (section 6.3.2), but nevertheless these need to be borne in mind, including the potential of higher inhaled doses to induce adrenal suppression and to have effects on bone metabolism (for further details see below); the lowest effective dose should be used. The growth retardation in children associated with oral corticosteroid therapy does not appear to be a significant problem with recommended doses of inhaled therapy; however, the CSM recommends that the height of children receiving prolonged treatment is monitored. If growth is slowed, referral to a paediatrician should be considered.

Corticosteroid *aerosol inhalations* must be used regularly to obtain maximum benefit; alleviation of symptoms usually occurs 3 to 7 days after initiation. **Beclometasone** (beclomethasone) **dipropionate, budesonide** and **fluticasone propionate** appear to be equally effective; fluticasone achieves the same effect as the other two with half the dose (when given by an equivalent delivery system). Doses for CFC-free corticosteroid inhalers may be different from those that contain CFCs.

If a beta$_2$-adrenoceptor stimulant is to be used at the same time as an inhaled corticosteroid it should be used first to help increase the penetration of the inhaled corticosteroid.

Patients who have been taking long-term oral corticosteroids can often be transferred to an inhaled corticosteroid but the transfer must be done slowly, with gradual reduction in dose of oral corticosteroid, and at a time when the asthma is well controlled.

High-dose aerosol inhalations are available for patients who only have a partial response to standard inhalers. The maximum doses for high-dose corticosteroid inhalations are associated with some adrenal suppression (section 6.3.2), therefore patients on high doses should be given a 'steroid card' and may need corticosteroid cover during an episode of stress (e.g. an operation). Systemic therapy may also be necessary during episodes of infection or increased bronchoconstriction where higher doses are needed and access of inhaled drug to small airways may be reduced; patients may need a reserve supply of tablets.

Inhaled corticosteroids have considerably fewer systemic effects than oral corticosteroids, but adverse effects have been reported including a small increased risk of glaucoma with prolonged high doses of inhaled corticosteroids; cataracts have also been reported with inhaled corticosteroids. Effects on bone metabolism can be detected following inhalation of higher doses of beclometasone, budesonide and fluticasone. Although there is no firm evidence that this may lead to increased osteoporosis in the future, it is sensible to ensure that the dose of inhaled corticosteroid is no higher than necessary to keep a patient's asthma under good control. The dose may therefore be reduced cautiously when the asthma has been well controlled for a few weeks as long as the patient knows that it is necessary to reinstate it should the asthma deteriorate or the peak flow rate fall.

Corticosteroids are preferably inhaled from aerosol inhalers using large-volume 'spacer devices' (section 3.1.5) particularly if high doses are required. Spacer devices increase airway deposition and reduce oropharyngeal deposition, resulting in a marked reduction in the incidence of candidiasis. *Dry powder inhalers* are actuated by the patient's inhalation and are particularly useful for patients who are unable to use the aerosol inhalers. Patients who are changed from an aerosol inhaler to a dry

powder inhaler may notice a lack of sensation in the mouth and throat previously associated with each actuation.

Budesonide and fluticasone propionate are both available as suspension for nebulisation.

ORAL. *Acute attacks* of asthma should be treated with short courses of oral corticosteroids starting with a high dose, e.g. prednisolone 30 to 60 mg (30 to 40 mg usually adequate) daily for a few days, gradually reducing once the attack has been controlled. Patients whose asthma has deteriorated rapidly usually respond quickly to corticosteroids, which can then be tailed down over a few days; more gradual reduction is necessary in those whose asthma has deteriorated gradually. For use of corticosteroids in the emergency treatment of *acute severe asthma* see table on p. 131.

In *chronic continuing asthma*, when the response to other anti-asthma drugs has been relatively small, continued administration of oral corticosteroids may be necessary; in such cases high doses of inhaled corticosteroids should be continued so that oral requirements are reduced to a minimum. Oral corticosteroids should normally be taken as a single dose in the morning to reduce the disturbance to circadian cortisol secretion. Dosage should always be titrated to the lowest dose which controls symptoms. Regular peak flow measurements often help both patient and doctor to adjust the dose optimally. Prednisolone is available as tablets of 1 mg as well as 5 mg, and the smaller tablets may conveniently be used to adjust the maintenance dosage to the minimum necessary.

Alternate-day administration has not been very successful in the management of asthma in adults as they tend to deteriorate during the second 24 hours. If an attempt is made to introduce this, pulmonary function should be monitored carefully over the 48 hours.

PARENTERAL. For the use of hydrocortisone injection in the emergency treatment of acute severe asthma, see Acute Severe Asthma table, p. 131.

BECLOMETASONE DIPROPIONATE
(Beclomethasone Dipropionate)

Indications: chronic asthma not controlled by short-acting beta$_2$ stimulants (see also Chronic Asthma table p. 130)

Cautions: see notes above; also active or quiescent tuberculosis; may need to reinstate systemic therapy during periods of stress or when airways obstruction or mucus prevent drug access to smaller airways

PARADOXICAL BRONCHOSPASM. The potential for paradoxical bronchospasm (calling for discontinuation and alternative therapy) should be borne in mind—if mild it may be prevented by inhalation of a beta$_2$-adrenoceptor stimulant (or by transfer from an aerosol inhalation to a dry powder inhalation)

Side-effects: see notes above; also hoarseness and candidiasis of mouth or throat (usually only with large doses); rarely hypersensitivity reactions including rash and angioedema

CANDIDIASIS. Candidiasis can be reduced by using spacer, see notes above, and responds to antifungal lozenges (section 12.3.2) without discontinuation of therapy—rinsing the mouth with water (or cleaning child's teeth) after inhalation of a dose may also be helpful

Dose: Standard dose inhalers

By aerosol inhalation, 200 micrograms twice daily *or* 100 micrograms 3–4 times daily (in more severe cases initially 600–800 micrograms daily); CHILD 50–100 micrograms 2–4 times daily

By inhalation of powder, 200 micrograms 3–4 times daily *or* 400 micrograms twice daily; CHILD 100 micrograms 2–4 times daily *or* 200 micrograms twice daily

High dose inhalers

By aerosol inhalation, 500 micrograms twice daily *or* 250 micrograms 4 times daily; if necessary may be increased to 500 micrograms 4 times daily; CHILD not recommended

By inhalation of powder, 400 micrograms twice daily; if necessary may be increased to 800 micrograms twice daily; CHILD not recommended

■ Standard-dose inhalers

Beclometasone (Non-proprietary) PoM

Aerosol inhalation, beclometasone dipropionate 50 micrograms/metered inhalation, net price 200-dose unit = £4.72; 100 micrograms/metered inhalation, 200-dose unit = £8.57; 200 micrograms/metered inhalation, 200-dose unit = £19.61. Label: 8, counselling, dose

Available from Baker Norton (*Beclazone®*), Generics and 3M (*Filair®*); vortex-based aerosol inhalers releasing beclometasone dipropionate 50 micrograms/metered inhalation and 100 micrograms/metered inhalation available from Medeva (*Asmabec Spacehaler®*)

Excipients: include CFC propellants

AeroBec® (3M) PoM

AeroBec 50 Autohaler® (breath-actuated aerosol inhalation), beclometasone dipropionate 50 micrograms/metered inhalation, net price 200-dose unit = £10.51. Label: 8, counselling, dose

Excipients: include CFC propellants

AeroBec 100 Autohaler® (breath-actuated aerosol inhalation), beclometasone dipropionate 100 micrograms/metered inhalation, net price 200-dose unit = £12.89. Label: 8, counselling, dose

Excipients: include CFC propellants

Asmabec Clickhaler® (Medeva) PoM

Dry powder for inhalation, beclometasone dipropionate 50 micrograms/metered inhalation, net price 200-dose unit = £7.18; 100 micrograms/metered inhalation, 200-dose unit = £10.55. Label: 8, counselling, dose

Dose: by inhalation of powder, 400 micrograms daily, in 2–4 divided doses (in more severe cases initially 600–800 micrograms daily, in 2–4 divided doses); CHILD 50–100 micrograms 2–4 times daily

Becodisks® (A&H) PoM

Dry powder for inhalation, disks containing 8 blisters of beclometasone dipropionate 100 micrograms/blister, net price 14 disks with *Diskhaler®* device = £10.99, 5-disk refill = £3.93 (hosp. only), 14-disk refill = £10.42; 200 micrograms/blister, 14 disks with *Diskhaler®* device = £20.90, 5-disk refill = £7.46 (hosp. only), 14-disk refill = £20.33; 400 micrograms/blister, 7 disks with *Diskhaler®* device = £20.90, 7-disk refill = £20.33. Label: 8, counselling, dose

Becotide® (A&H) PoM

Becotide®-50 aerosol inhalation, beclometasone dipropionate 50 micrograms/metered inhalation.

Net price 80-dose unit = £1.91 (hosp. only), 200-dose unit = £5.43. Label: 8, counselling, dose

Becotide®-100 aerosol inhalation, beclometasone dipropionate 100 micrograms/metered inhalation. Net price 80-dose unit = £3.82 (hosp. only), 200-dose unit = £10.32. Label: 8, counselling, dose

Becotide®-200 aerosol inhalation, beclometasone dipropionate 200 micrograms/metered inhalation. Net price 200-dose unit = £19.61. Label: 8, counselling, dose, 10 steroid card

Note. Becotide®-200 not indicated for children

Excipients: all include CFC propellants

Easi-Breathe® aerosol inhalation, beclometasone dipropionate 50 micrograms/metered inhalation, net price 200-dose breath-actuated unit = £4.34; 100 micrograms/metered inhalation, 200-dose breath-actuated unit = £8.24. Label: 8, counselling, dose

Excipients: include CFC propellants

Rotacaps® (dry powder for inhalation; for use with *Becotide Rotahaler®*), beclometasone dipropionate 100 micrograms (buff/clear), net price 112-cap pack = £8.47; 200 micrograms (brown/clear), 112-cap pack = £16.07; 400 micrograms (dark brown/clear), 112-cap pack = £30.54. Label: 8, counselling, dose

Qvar® (3M) ▼ PoM

Qvar® 50 aerosol inhalation, beclometasone dipropionate 50 micrograms/metered inhalation, net price 200-dose unit = £7.87. Label: 8, counselling, dose

Qvar® 100 aerosol inhalation, beclometasone dipropionate 100 micrograms/metered inhalation, net price 200-dose unit = £17.21. Label: 8, counselling, dose, 10 steroid card

Qvar 50 Autohaler® (breath-actuated aerosol inhalation), beclometasone dipropionate 50 micrograms/metered inhalation, net price 200-dose unit = £7.87. Label: 8, counselling, dose

Qvar 100 Autohaler® (breath-actuated aerosol inhalation), beclometasone dipropionate 100 micrograms/metered inhalation, net price 200-dose unit = £17.21. Label: 8, counselling, dose, 10 steroid card

Excipients: include HFA-134a (a non-CFC propellant), ethanol

Dose: by aerosol inhalation, 50–200 micrograms twice daily, if necessary may be increased to max. 400 micrograms twice daily; CHILD not recommended

Note. When transferring a patient from a CFC-containing inhaler (asthma well-controlled), initially a 100-microgram metered dose of *Qvar®* should be substituted for:
• 200–250 micrograms of beclometasone dipropionate or budesonide
• 100 micrograms of fluticasone

When transferring a patient from a CFC-containing inhaler (asthma poorly-controlled), initially a 100-microgram metered dose of *Qvar®* should be substituted for 100 micrograms of beclometasone dipropionate, budesonide or fluticasone

---

CFC-FREE INHALERS. Chlorofluorocarbon (CFC) propellants in pressurised aerosol inhalers are being replaced by hydrofluoroalkane (HFA) propellants. Patients receiving CFC-free inhalers should be reassured about the efficacy of the new inhalers and counselled that the aerosol may feel and taste different; any difficulty with the new inhaler should be discussed with the doctor or pharmacist.

CSM advice. The CSM has requested doctors to report any adverse reaction to the new HFA-containing inhalers and to include the brand name of the inhaler on the yellow card.

■ High-dose inhalers

Note. High-dose inhalers not indicated for children

Beclometasone (Non-proprietary) PoM

Aerosol inhalation, beclometasone dipropionate 250 micrograms/metered inhalation, net price 200-dose unit = £18.57. Label: 8, counselling, dose, 10 steroid dose

Available from Baker Norton (*Beclazone*®), Generics and 3M (*Filair Forte*®); vortex-based aerosol inhalers releasing beclometasone dipropionate 250 micrograms/metered inhalation available from Medeva (*Asmabec Spacehaler*®)

Excipients: include CFC propellants

AeroBec Forte® (3M) PoM

Aerosol inhalation, beclometasone dipropionate 250 micrograms/metered inhalation, net price 200-inhalation breath-actuated unit (*Autohaler*®) = £23.97. Label: 8, counselling, dose, 10 steroid card

Excipients: include CFC propellants

Asmabec Clickhaler® (Medeva) PoM

Dry powder for inhalation, beclometasone dipropionate 250 micrograms/metered inhalation, net price 100-dose unit = £13.24. Label: 8, counselling, dose, 10 steroid card

Dose: by inhalation of powder, 500 micrograms twice daily *or* 250 micrograms 4 times daily; if necessary may be increased to 500 micrograms 4 times daily; CHILD not recommended

Becloforte® (A&H) PoM

Aerosol inhalation, beclometasone dipropionate 250 micrograms/metered inhalation. Net price 80-dose unit = £8.82 (hosp. only), 200-dose unit = £23.10; 200-puff unit with spacer device (*Becloforte Integra*®) = £23.10; 200-dose refill for use with *Becloforte Integra*® = £18.02. Label: 8, counselling, dose, 10 steroid card

Excipients: include CFC propellants

Easi-Breathe® aerosol inhalation, beclometasone dipropionate 250 micrograms/metered inhalation, net price 200-dose breath-actuated unit = £18.02. Label: 8, counselling, dose, 10 steroid card

Excipients: include CFC propellants

Dry powder for inhalation, disks containing 8 blisters of beclometasone dipropionate 400 micrograms/blister, net price 14 disks with *Diskhaler*® device = £39.70; 14-disk refill = £39.13. Label: 8, counselling, dose, 10 steroid card

Qvar® (3M) PoM

See under standard-dose inhalers

> ◢ denotes preparations that are considered to be less suitable for prescribing (see p. vi)

■ Compound preparations

(Not recommended)

Ventide® (A&H) PoM ◢

Aerosol inhalation, beclometasone dipropionate 50 micrograms, salbutamol 100 micrograms/metered inhalation. Net price 200-dose unit = £5.42. Label: 8, counselling, dose

Excipients: include CFC propellants

Dose: maintenance, 2 puffs 3–4 times daily; CHILD 1–2 puffs 3–4 times daily

Paediatric Rotacaps® (dry powder for inhalation; for use with *Ventide Rotahaler*®), light grey/clear, beclometasone dipropionate 100 micrograms, salbutamol (as sulphate) 200 micrograms. Net price 112-cap pack = £12.68. Label: 8, counselling, dose

Dose: by inhalation of powder, 1 *Paediatric Rotacap*® 2–4 times daily

Rotacaps® (dry powder for inhalation; for use with *Ventide Rotahaler*®), dark grey/clear, beclometasone dipropionate 200 micrograms, salbutamol (as sulphate) 400 micrograms. Net price 112-cap pack = £23.01. Label: 8, counselling, dose

Dose: by inhalation of powder, 1 *Rotacap*® 3–4 times daily

■ Inhaler devices

See section 3.1.5

BUDESONIDE

Indications: see under Beclometasone Dipropionate
Cautions: see under Beclometasone Dipropionate
Side-effects: see under Beclometasone Dipropionate
Dose: see preparations below

Pulmicort® (Astra) PoM

LS aerosol inhalation, budesonide 50 micrograms/metered inhalation. Net price 200-dose unit with standard or *Spacer* inhaler = £6.66. Label: 8, counselling, dose

Excipients: include CFC propellants

Aerosol inhalation, budesonide 200 micrograms/metered inhalation. Net price 200-dose unit with standard or *Spacer* inhaler = £19.00; 100-dose unit with standard inhaler = £7.60 (hosp. only). Label: 8, counselling, dose, 10 steroid card

Excipients: include CFC propellants

Dose: by aerosol inhalation, 200 micrograms twice daily; may be reduced in well-controlled asthma to not less than 200 micrograms daily; in severe asthma dose may be increased to 1.6 mg daily; CHILD 50–400 micrograms twice daily; in severe asthma may be increased to 800 micrograms daily

Turbohaler® (= dry powder inhaler), budesonide 100 micrograms/inhalation, net price 200-dose unit = £18.50; 200 micrograms/inhalation, 100-dose unit = £18.50; 400 micrograms/inhalation, 50-dose unit = £18.50. Label: 8, counselling, dose, 10 steroid card

Dose: by inhalation of powder, when starting treatment, during periods of severe asthma, and while reducing or discontinuing oral corticosteroid, 0.2–1.6 mg daily in 2 divided doses; in less severe cases 200–400 micrograms once daily (each evening); patients already controlled on inhaled beclometasone dipropionate or budesonide administered twice daily may be transferred to once-daily dosing (each evening) at the same equivalent total daily dose (up to 800 micrograms once daily); CHILD under 12 years 200–800 micrograms daily in 2 divided doses (800 micrograms daily in severe asthma) *or* 200–400 micrograms once daily (each evening)

Respules® (= single-dose units for nebulisation), budesonide 250 micrograms/mL, net price 20 × 2-mL (500-microgram) unit = £32.00; 500 micrograms/mL, 20 × 2-mL (1-mg) unit = £44.64. May be diluted with sterile sodium chloride 0.9%. Label: 8, counselling, dose, 10 steroid card

Dose: by inhalation of nebulised suspension, when starting treatment, during periods of severe asthma, and while reducing or discontinuing oral corticosteroids, 1–2 mg twice daily (may be increased further in very severe asthma); CHILD 3 months–12 years, 0.5–1 mg twice daily

Maintenance, usually half above doses

Croup, 2 mg as a single dose (*or* as two 1-mg doses separated by 30 minutes)

■ Inhaler devices

Section 3.1.5

FLUTICASONE PROPIONATE

Indications: see under Beclometasone Dipropionate
Cautions: see under Beclometasone Dipropionate
Side-effects: see under Beclometasone Dipropionate
Dose: see preparations below

Flixotide® (A&H) [PoM]

Accuhaler® (dry powder for inhalation), disk containing 60 blisters of fluticasone propionate 50 micrograms/blister with *Accuhaler®* device, net price = £6.86; 100 micrograms/blister with *Accuhaler®* device = £9.60; 250 micrograms/blister with *Accuhaler®* device = £22.86; 500 micrograms/blister with *Accuhaler®* device = £38.86. Label: 8, counselling, dose; 250- and 500-microgram strengths also label 10 steroid card

Note. Flixotide Accuhaler® 250 micrograms and 500 micrograms are not indicated for children

Dose: by inhalation of powder, ADULT and CHILD over 16 years, 100–250 micrograms twice daily, increased according to severity of asthma to 1 mg twice daily; CHILD 4–16 years, 50–100 micrograms twice daily adjusted as necessary

Aerosol inhalation, fluticasone propionate 25 micrograms/metered inhalation, net price 120-dose unit = £6.86; 50 micrograms/metered inhalation, 120-dose unit = £11.43; 125 micrograms/metered inhalation, 60-dose unit = £11.43 (hosp. only), 120-dose unit = £22.86; 250 micrograms/metered inhalation, 60-dose unit = £19.43 (hosp. only), 120-dose unit = £38.86. Label: 8, counselling, dose; 250-microgram strength also label 10 steroid card

Excipients: include CFC propellants

Note. Flixotide® 125 micrograms and 250 micrograms inhalers not indicated for children

Dose: by aerosol inhalation, ADULT and CHILD over 16 years, 100–250 micrograms twice daily, increased according to severity of asthma to 1 mg twice daily; CHILD 4–16 years, 50–100 micrograms twice daily adjusted as necessary

Diskhaler® (dry powder for inhalation), fluticasone propionate 50 micrograms/blister, net price 14 disks of 4 blisters with *Diskhaler®* device = £8.23, 14-disk refill = £7.66; 100 micrograms/blister, 14 disks of 4 blisters with *Diskhaler®* device = £12.80, 14-disk refill = £12.23; 250 micrograms/blister, 14 disks of 4 blisters with *Diskhaler®* device = £24.23, 5-disk refill = £8.65 (hosp. only), 14-disk refill = £23.66; 500 micrograms/blister, 14 disks of 4 blisters with *Diskhaler®* device = £40.23, 5-disk refill = £14.37 (hosp. only), 14-disk refill = £39.66. Label: 8, counselling, dose; 250- and 500-microgram strengths also label 10 steroid card

Note. Flixotide Diskhaler® 250 micrograms and 500 micrograms are not indicated for children

Dose: by inhalation of powder, ADULT and CHILD over 16 years, 100–250 micrograms twice daily, increased according to severity of asthma to 1 mg twice daily; CHILD 4–16 years, 50–100 micrograms twice daily adjusted as necessary

Nebules® (= single-dose units for nebulisation) fluticasone propionate 250 micrograms/mL, net price 10 × 2-mL (500-microgram) unit = £10.04; 1 mg/mL, 10 × 2-mL (2-mg) unit = £40.16. May be diluted with sterile sodium chloride 0.9%. Label: 8, counselling, dose, 10 steroid card

Dose: by inhalation of nebulised suspension, ADULT and CHILD over 16 years, 0.5–2 mg twice daily

■ Compound preparations

Seretide® (A&H) ▼ [PoM]

Seretide 100 Accuhaler® (dry powder for inhalation), disk containing 60 blisters of fluticasone propionate 100 micrograms, salmeterol (as xinafoate) 50 micrograms/blister with *Accuhaler®* device, net price = £33.54. Label: 8, counselling, dose

Dose: by inhalation of powder, ADULT and CHILD over 4 years, 1 blister twice daily

Seretide 250 Accuhaler® (dry powder for inhalation), disk containing 60 blisters of fluticasone propionate 250 micrograms, salmeterol (as xinafoate) 50 micrograms/blister with *Accuhaler®* device, net price = £39.41. Label: 8, counselling, dose, 10 steroid card

Dose: by inhalation of powder, ADULT and CHILD over 12 years, 1 blister twice daily

Seretide 500 Accuhaler® (dry powder for inhalation), disk containing 60 blisters of fluticasone propionate 500 micrograms, salmeterol (as xinafoate) 50 micrograms/blister with *Accuhaler®* device, net price = £66.98. Label: 8, counselling, dose, 10 steroid card

Dose: by inhalation of powder, ADULT and CHILD over 12 years, 1 blister twice daily

3.3   Cromoglicate, related therapy and leukotriene receptor antagonists

3.3.1   Cromoglicate and related therapy

Regular inhalation of **sodium cromoglicate** (sodium cromoglycate) can reduce the incidence of asthma attacks and allow dosage reduction of bronchodilators and oral corticosteroids. In general, prophylaxis with sodium cromoglicate is less effective in adults than prophylaxis with corticosteroid inhalations (see Chronic Asthma table, p. 130) but in the long term corticosteroid inhalations may be associated with more side-effects. Children may respond better than adults although there is less evidence of efficacy in those under the age of 4 years. Sodium cromoglicate is of no value in the treatment of acute attacks of asthma.

Sodium cromoglicate is of value in the prevention of exercise-induced asthma, a single dose being inhaled half-an-hour beforehand.

The mode of action of sodium cromoglicate is not completely understood. It may be of value in asthma with an allergic basis but, in practice, it is difficult to predict who will benefit, therefore it is reasonable to try it for a period of 4 to 6 weeks. Dose frequency is adjusted according to response but is usually 3 to 4 times a day initially; this may subsequently be reduced.

If inhalation of the dry powder form of sodium cromoglicate causes bronchospasm a selective beta$_2$-adrenoceptor stimulant such as salbutamol or terbutaline should be inhaled a few minutes beforehand. The nebuliser solution is an alternative means of delivery for children who cannot manage the dry powder inhaler or the aerosol.

Nedocromil has a pharmacological action similar to that of sodium cromoglicate.

SODIUM CROMOGLICATE
(Sodium Cromoglycate)

Indications: prophylaxis of asthma; food allergy (section 1.5); allergic conjunctivitis (section 11.4.2); allergic rhinitis (section 12.2.1)

Side-effects: coughing, transient bronchospasm, and throat irritation due to inhalation of powder (see also notes above)

Dose: *by aerosol inhalation*, ADULT and CHILD, 10 mg (2 puffs) 4 times daily, increased in severe cases or during periods of risk to 6–8 times daily; additional doses may also be taken before exercise; maintenance 5 mg (1 puff) 4 times daily

By inhalation of powder (Spincaps®), ADULT and CHILD, 20 mg 4 times daily, increased in severe cases to 8 times daily; additional doses may also be taken before exercise

By inhalation of nebulised solution, ADULT and CHILD, 20 mg 4 times daily, increased in severe cases to 6 times daily

COUNSELLING. Regular use is necessary

Sodium Cromoglicate (Non-proprietary) PoM
Aerosol inhalation, sodium cromoglicate 5 mg/metered inhalation. Net price 112-dose unit = £15.30. Label: 8
Available from Baker Norton (*Cromogen®*)
Excipients: include CFC propellants
Nebuliser solution, sodium cromoglicate 10 mg/mL. Net price 60 × 2-mL unit-dose vials = £11.58
Available from Baker Norton (*Cromogen Steri-Neb®*)

Cromogen Easi-Breathe® (Baker Norton) PoM
Aerosol inhalation, sodium cromoglicate 5 mg/metered inhalation. Net price 112-dose breath-actuated unit = £13.91. Label: 8
Excipients: include CFC propellants

Intal® (Rhône-Poulenc Rorer) PoM
Aerosol inhalation, sodium cromoglicate 5 mg/metered inhalation. Net price 112-puff unit = £19.09; 2 × 112-puff unit with spacer device (*Syncroner®*) = £37.98; also available with large volume spacer inhaler (*Fisonair®*), complete unit = £22.06. Label: 8
Excipients: include CFC propellants
Spincaps®, yellow/clear, sodium cromoglicate 20 mg. Net price 112-cap pack = £16.60. Label: 8
Spinhaler insufflator® (for use with Intal Spincaps). Net price = £1.92
Nebuliser solution, sodium cromoglicate 10 mg/mL. Net price 2-mL amp = 34p. For use with power-operated nebuliser

■ Compound preparations
Note. The compound inhalation of sodium cromoglicate with a beta-adrenoceptor stimulant is not recommended as the inhalation is liable to be used inappropriately for relief of bronchospasm rather than for its prophylactic effect

Aerocrom® (Castlemead) PoM ◾◼
Aerosol inhalation, sodium cromoglicate 1 mg, salbutamol (as sulphate) 100 micrograms/metered inhalation, net price 200-puff unit = £34.42; 200-puff unit with spacer device (*Syncroner®*) = £34.42. Label: 8
Excipients: include CFC propellants
Dose: by aerosol inhalation, 2 inhalations 4 times daily; CHILD, not recommended

---

◾◼ denotes preparations that are considered to be less suitable for prescribing (see p. vi)

NEDOCROMIL SODIUM

Indications: prophylaxis of asthma

Side-effects: see under Sodium Cromoglicate; also headache, nausea, vomiting, dyspepsia, abdominal pain (mild and transient); bitter taste (masked by mint flavour)

Dose: *by aerosol inhalation*, ADULT and CHILD over 6 years 4 mg (2 puffs) 4 times daily, when control achieved may be possible to reduce to twice daily

COUNSELLING. Regular use is necessary

Tilade® (Pantheon) PoM
Aerosol inhalation, nedocromil sodium 2 mg/metered inhalation. Net price 2 × 56-puff mint-flavoured units = £42.98; 2 × 112-puff unit with spacer device (*Syncroner®*) = £85.96. Label: 8
Excipients: include CFC propellants

Related therapy

Antihistamines are of no value in the treatment of bronchial asthma. **Ketotifen** is an antihistamine with an action said to resemble that of sodium cromoglicate, but it has proved disappointing.

KETOTIFEN

Indications: see notes above

Cautions: previous anti-asthmatic treatment should be continued for a minimum of 2 weeks after initiation of ketotifen treatment; pregnancy and breast-feeding (see Appendixes 4 and 5); **interactions:** Appendix 1 (antihistamines)—also, manufacturer advises avoid with oral antidiabetics (fall in thrombocyte count reported)

DRIVING. Drowsiness may affect performance of skilled tasks (e.g. driving); effects of alcohol enhanced

Side-effects: drowsiness, dry mouth, slight dizziness; CNS stimulation, weight gain also reported

Dose: 1 mg twice daily with food increased if necessary to 2 mg twice daily; initial treatment in readily sedated patients 0.5–1 mg at night; CHILD over 2 years 1 mg twice daily

Zaditen® (Novartis) PoM
Capsules, ketotifen (as hydrogen fumarate) 1 mg. Net price 56-cap pack = £7.60. Label: 2, 8, 21
Tablets, scored, ketotifen (as hydrogen fumarate) 1 mg. Net price 60-tab pack = £8.14. Label: 2, 8, 21
Elixir, ketotifen (as hydrogen fumarate) 1 mg/5 mL. Net price 300 mL = £9.64. Label: 2, 8, 21

3.3.2   Leukotriene receptor antagonists

The leukotriene receptor antagonists, montelukast and zafirlukast, block the effects of cysteinyl leukotrienes in the airways.

Montelukast is indicated for add-on therapy in mild to moderate asthma which is not adequately controlled with an inhaled corticosteroid and a short-acting beta$_2$-stimulant used as required. It may also be used to prevent exercise-induced bronchospasm.

Zafirlukast has been introduced recently and is indicated for the prophylaxis of asthma.

The **CSM** has advised that leukotriene receptor antagonists should not be used to relieve an attack of acute severe asthma and that their use does not necessarily allow a reduction in existing corticosteroid treatment.

CHURG-STRAUSS SYNDROME. Churg-Strauss syndrome (characterised by a history of asthma, and often rhinitis and sinusitis, with systemic vasculitis and eosinophilia) has been reported in association with the use of leukotriene receptor antagonists; in many cases the reaction followed the reduction or withdrawal of oral corticosteroid therapy. The CSM has advised that in patients prescribed leukotriene receptor antagonists prescribers should be alert to the development of eosinophilia, vasculitic rash, worsening pulmonary symptoms, cardiac complications or peripheral neuropathy.

MONTELUKAST

Indications: adjunctive therapy in prophylaxis of mild to moderate and exercise-induced asthma inadequately controlled by inhaled corticosteroid and short-acting beta$_2$-stimulant as needed

Cautions: pregnancy (Appendix 4) and breast-feeding (Appendix 5); Churg-Strauss syndrome, see notes above; **interactions:** Appendix 1 (leukotriene antagonists)

Side-effects: gastro-intestinal disturbances; dry mouth; hypersensitivity reactions including anaphylaxis, angioedema and skin reactions; asthenia, dizziness, headache, insomnia; upper respiratory-tract infection, fever; arthralgia, myalgia

Dose: 10 mg daily at bedtime; CHILD 6–14 years 5 mg daily at bedtime

Singulair® (MSD) ▼ PoM
Chewable tablets, pink, montelukast (as sodium salt) 5 mg, net price 28-tab pack = £25.69. Label: 23, 24
Excipients: contains aspartame equivalent to phenylalanine 842 micrograms per tablet (section 9.4.1)
Tablets, beige, f/c, montelukast (as sodium salt) 10 mg, net price 28-tab pack = £25.69

ZAFIRLUKAST

Indications: prophylaxis of asthma

Cautions: elderly, pregnancy (Appendix 4), renal impairment (Appendix 3); Churg-Strauss syndrome, see notes above; **interactions:** Appendix 1 (leukotriene antagonists)

Contra-indications: hepatic impairment (Appendix 2); breast-feeding (Appendix 5)

Side-effects: gastro-intestinal disturbances; headache; bleeding disorders; hypersensitivity reactions including angioedema and skin reactions; rarely raised liver enzymes and very rarely agranulocytosis; also respiratory-tract infection in the elderly

Dose: 20 mg twice daily; CHILD under 12 years, not recommended

Accolate® (Zeneca) ▼ PoM
Tablets, f/c, zafirlukast 20 mg, net price 56-tab pack = £25.69. Label: 23

3.4 Antihistamines, hyposensitisation, and allergic emergencies

3.4.1   Antihistamines
3.4.2   Hyposensitisation
3.4.3   Allergic emergencies

3.4.1   Antihistamines

All antihistamines are of potential value in the treatment of nasal allergies, particularly seasonal allergic rhinitis (hay fever), and may be of some value in vasomotor rhinitis. They reduce rhinorrhoea and sneezing but are usually less effective for nasal congestion.

Oral antihistamines are also of some value in preventing urticaria and are used to treat urticarial rashes, pruritus, and insect bites and stings; they are also used in drug allergies. Injections of chlorphenamine (chlorpheniramine) or promethazine are used as an adjunct to adrenaline (epinephrine) in the emergency treatment of anaphylaxis and angioedema (section 3.4.3). For the use of antihistamines (including cinnarizine, cyclizine, dimenhydrinate, and promethazine teoclate) in nausea and vomiting, see section 4.6. Buclizine is included as an antiemetic in a preparation for migraine (section 4.7.4.1). For reference to the use of antihistamines for occasional insomnia, see section 4.1.1.

Antihistamines differ in their duration of action and incidence of drowsiness and antimuscarinic effects. Many older antihistamines are relatively short acting but some (e.g. promethazine) act for up to 12 hours, while most of the newer non-sedating antihistamines are long acting.

All older antihistamines cause sedation but **alimemazine (trimeprazine)**, **dimenhydrinate** and **promethazine** (section 4.6) may be more sedating whereas **chlorphenamine (chlorpheniramine)**, **cyclizine** (section 4.6), and **mequitazine** may be less so. This sedating activity is sometimes used to alleviate the pruritus associated with some allergies. There is little evidence that any one of the older, 'sedating' antihistamines is superior to another and patients vary widely in their responses.

Non-sedating antihistamines such as **acrivastine**, **cetirizine**, **fexofenadine**, **loratadine**, **mizolastine**, and **terfenadine** cause less sedation and psychomotor impairment than the older antihistamines because they penetrate the blood brain barrier only to a slight extent. **Fexofenadine**, an active metabolite of terfenadine, has been introduced recently.

CAUTIONS AND CONTRA-INDICATIONS. Antihistamines should be used with caution in prostatic hypertrophy, urinary retention, glaucoma, and hepatic disease (mizolastine and terfenadine in particular should be **avoided** in significant hepatic impairment); caution may also be required in epilepsy. Children and the elderly are more susceptible to side-effects. See Appendix 4 and Appendix 5 for information on antihistamines in pregnancy and breast-feeding. Many antihistamines should be avoided in porphyria although some (e.g. chlorphenamine (chlorpheniramine) and cetirizine) are thought to be safe (section 9.8.2). **Interactions:** Appendix 1 (antihistamines); **important:** see also under Terfenadine.

SIDE-EFFECTS. Drowsiness is a significant side-effect with most of the older antihistamines (although paradoxical stimulation may occur rarely, especially in high dosage or in children and the elderly) but this side-effect may diminish after a few days of continued treatment; drowsiness is considerably less of a problem with the newer antihistamines (see also notes above). Side-effects that are more common with the older antihistamines include headache, psychomotor impairment, and antimuscarinic effects such as urinary retention, dry mouth, blurred vision, and gastro-intestinal disturbances.

Other side-effects of antihistamines reported include palpitations and arrhythmias (**important:** see especially risks associated with *terfenadine*, see below), hypotension, hypersensitivity reactions (including bronchospasm, angioedema, and anaphylaxis), rashes and photosensitivity reactions, extrapyramidal effects, confusion, depression, sleep disturbances, tremor, convulsions, sweating, myalgia, paraesthesia, blood disorders, liver dysfunction, and hair loss.

Non-sedating antihistamines

DRIVING. Although drowsiness is rare, nevertheless patients should be advised that it can occur and may affect performance of skilled tasks (e.g. driving); excess alcohol should be avoided.

ACRIVASTINE

Indications: symptomatic relief of allergy such as hay fever, urticaria
Cautions: see notes above
Contra-indications: see notes above; avoid in renal impairment
Side-effects: see notes above; incidence of sedation and antimuscarinic effects low
Dose: 8 mg 3 times daily; CHILD under 12 years, not recommended; ELDERLY not recommended

[1]**Semprex®** (GlaxoWellcome) [PoM]
Capsules, arrivastine 8 mg. Net price 84-cap pack = £4.81. Counselling, driving
1. Capsules can be sold to the public for the treatment of hayfever and allergic skin conditions in adults and children over 12 years provided packs do not contain over 10 days' supply (*Benadryl® Allergy Relief*)

CETIRIZINE HYDROCHLORIDE

Indications: symptomatic relief of allergy such as hay fever, urticaria
Cautions: see notes above; halve dose in renal impairment
Contra-indications: pregnancy and breast-feeding
Side-effects: see notes above; incidence of sedation and antimuscarinic effects low
Dose: ADULT and CHILD over 6 years, 10 mg daily *or* 5 mg twice daily; CHILD 2–6 years, hayfever, 5 mg daily *or* 2.5 mg twice daily

[1]**Zirtek®** (UCB Pharma) [PoM]
Tablets, f/c, scored, cetirizine hydrochloride 10 mg. Net price 30-tab pack = £8.73. Counselling, driving
Oral solution, sugar-free, cetirizine hydrochloride 5 mg/5 mL. Net price 200 mL = £6.10. Counselling, driving
1. Tablets can be sold to the public for adults and children over 12 years provided packs do not contain more than 10 days' supply (*Zirtek 7® [NHS]*)

FEXOFENADINE HYDROCHLORIDE

Indications: see under preparations below
Cautions: see notes above; pregnancy
Contra-indications: breast-feeding
Side-effects: see notes above; dizziness
Dose: see under preparations below

Telfast® 120 (Hoechst Marion Roussel) ▼ [PoM]
Tablets, f/c, peach, fexofenadine hydrochloride 120 mg. Net price 30-tab pack = £7.40. Counselling, driving
Dose: symptomatic relief of seasonal allergic rhinitis, 120 mg once daily; CHILD under 12 years, not recommended

Telfast® 180 (Hoechst Marion Roussel) ▼ [PoM]
Tablets, f/c, peach, fexofenadine hydrochloride 180 mg. Net price 30-tab pack = £9.63. Counselling, driving
Dose: symptomatic relief of chronic idiopathic urticaria, 180 mg once daily; CHILD under 12 years, not recommended

LORATADINE

Indications: symptomatic relief of allergy such as hay fever, urticaria
Cautions: see notes above
Contra-indications: see notes above; pregnancy (Appendix 4) and breast-feeding (Appendix 5)
Side-effects: see notes above; incidence of sedation and antimuscarinic effects low
Dose: ADULT and CHILD over 6 years 10 mg daily; CHILD 2–5 years 5 mg daily

[1]**Clarityn®** (Schering-Plough) [PoM]
Tablets, scored, loratadine 10 mg. Net price 30-tab pack = £7.57. Counselling, driving
Syrup, yellow, loratadine 5 mg/5 mL. Net price 100 mL = £7.57. Counselling, driving
1. Tablets and syrup can be sold to the public provided packs do not contain more than 10 days' supply (*Clarityn Allergy® [NHS]*); another brand on sale to the public is *Boots Hayfever Relief All Day®*

MIZOLASTINE

Indications: symptomatic relief of allergy such as hayfever, urticaria
Cautions: see notes above
Contra-indications: see notes above; cardiac disease, hypokalaemia, pregnancy and breast-feeding
Side-effects: see notes above; may cause weight gain
Dose: 10 mg daily; CHILD under 12 years, not recommended

Mistamine® (Galderma) ▼ [PoM]
Tablets, m/r, mizolastine 10 mg, net price 30-tab pack = £8.55. Label: 25. Counselling, driving
Mizollen® (Sanofi-Synthelabo) ▼ [PoM]
Tablets, m/r, scored, mizolastine 10 mg, net price 30-tab pack = £8.55. Label: 25. Counselling, driving

TERFENADINE

Indications: symptomatic relief of allergy such as allergic rhinitis, urticaria
Cautions: see notes above; pregnancy and breast-feeding

Contra-indications: see notes above; avoid grapefruit juice (may inhibit metabolism of terfenadine); **important:** see also Arrhythmias, below ARRHYTHMIAS. Rare hazardous arrhythmias are associated with terfenadine particularly in association with increased terfenadine blood concentration. Recommendations include:

- not to exceed recommended dose
- avoid in significant hepatic impairment
- avoid in hypokalaemia (or other electrolyte imbalance)
- avoid in known or suspected prolonged QT interval
- avoid concomitant administration of drugs that prolong the QT interval or inhibit the metabolism of terfenadine, or those liable to produce electrolyte imbalance or are potentially arrhythmogenic; for details, see **interactions**: Appendix 1 (antihistamines)
- discontinue if syncope occurs and evaluate for potential arrhythmias

Side-effects: see notes above; incidence of sedation and antimuscarinic effects low; erythema multiforme and galactorrhoea reported; **important:** ventricular arrhythmias (including torsades de pointes) have followed excessive dosage, see also Arrhythmias above

Dose: allergic rhinitis and conjunctivitis, ADULT and CHILD over 50 kg, 60 mg daily increased if necessary to 120 mg daily in single or 2 divided doses; CHILD 3–12 years and under 50 kg (suspension only) 1 mg/kg daily increased if necessary to 1 mg/kg twice daily

Allergic skin disorders, ADULT and CHILD over 50 kg, 120 mg daily in single or 2 divided doses; CHILD 3–12 years and under 50 kg (suspension only) 1 mg/kg twice daily

Terfenadine (Non-proprietary) PoM
Tablets, terfenadine 60 mg, net price 60-tab pack = £4.02. Counselling, driving
Note. May be difficult to obtain

Sedating antihistamines

DRIVING. Drowsiness may affect performance of skilled tasks (e.g. driving); sedating effects enhanced by alcohol.

ALIMEMAZINE TARTRATE/
TRIMEPRAZINE TARTRATE

Indications: urticaria and pruritus, premedication
Cautions: see notes above; see also under Chlorpromazine Hydrochloride, section 4.2.1
Contra-indications: see notes above; pregnancy and breast-feeding; see also under Chlorpromazine Hydrochloride, section 4.2.1
Side-effects: see notes above; see also under Chlorpromazine Hydrochloride, section 4.2.1
Dose: 10 mg 2–3 times daily, in severe cases up to max. 100 mg daily has been used; ELDERLY 10 mg 1–2 times daily; CHILD under 2 years not recommended, over 2 years 2.5–5 mg 3–4 times daily
Premedication, CHILD 2–7 years up to 2 mg/kg 1–2 hours before operation

Vallergan® (Castlemead) PoM
Tablets, blue, f/c, alimemazine tartrate 10 mg. Net price 28-tab pack = £3.24. Label: 2
Syrup, straw-coloured, alimemazine tartrate 7.5 mg /5 mL. Net price 100 mL = £3.70. Label: 2
Syrup forte, alimemazine tartrate 30 mg/5 mL. Net price 100 mL = £5.72. Label: 2

AZATADINE MALEATE

Indications: symptomatic relief of allergy such as hay fever, urticaria
Cautions: see notes above
Contra-indications: see notes above; pregnancy and breast-feeding
Side-effects: see notes above
Dose: 1 mg, increased if necessary to 2 mg, twice daily; CHILD under 1 year not recommended, 1–6 years 250 micrograms twice daily, 6–12 years 0.5–1 mg twice daily

Optimine® (Schering-Plough)
Syrup, azatadine maleate 500 micrograms/5 mL. Net price 120 mL = £1.39. Label: 2

BROMPHENIRAMINE MALEATE

Indications: symptomatic relief of allergy such as hay fever, urticaria
Cautions: see notes above
Contra-indications: see notes above
Side-effects: see notes above
Dose: 4–8 mg 3–4 times daily; CHILD up to 3 years 0.4–1 mg/kg daily in 4 divided doses, 3–6 years 2 mg 3–4 times daily, 6–12 years 2–4 mg 3–4 times daily

Dimotane® (Wyeth)
Tablets, peach, scored, brompheniramine maleate 4 mg. Net price 28-tab pack = 83p. Label: 2
Elixir, yellow-green, brompheniramine maleate 2 mg/5 mL. Net price 200 mL = £1.42. Label: 2
Dimotane LA® (Wyeth)
Tablets, m/r, peach, s/c, brompheniramine maleate 12 mg. Net price 28-tab pack = £1.25. Label: 2, 25
Dose: 12–24 mg twice daily; CHILD 6–12 years 12 mg at bedtime, increased if necessary to 12 mg twice daily
For a list of **cough and decongestant preparations on sale to the public,** including those containing brompheniramine, see section 3.9.2.

CHLORPHENAMINE MALEATE/
CHLORPHENIRAMINE MALEATE

Indications: symptomatic relief of allergy such as hay fever, urticaria; emergency treatment of anaphylactic reactions (section 3.4.3)
Cautions: see notes above; injections may be irritant
Contra-indications: see notes above
Side-effects: see notes above; exfoliative dermatitis and tinnitus reported; injections may cause transient hypotension or CNS stimulation
Dose: *by mouth,* 4 mg every 4–6 hours, max. 24 mg daily; CHILD under 1 year not recommended, 1–2 years 1 mg twice daily; 2–5 years 1 mg every 4–6 hours, max. 6 mg daily; 6–12 years 2 mg every 4–6 hours, max. 12 mg daily

By subcutaneous or intramuscular injection, 10–20 mg, repeated if required; max. 40 mg in 24 hours

By slow intravenous injection over 1 minute, 10–20 mg

Chlorphenamine/Chlorpheniramine (Non-proprietary)

Tablets, chlorphenamine maleate 4 mg, net price 20 = 8p. Label: 2

Available from APS, Cox, Hillcross

Injection [PoM], chlorphenamine maleate 10 mg/mL, net price 1-mL amp = 50p

Available from Link (*Piriton®*)

Piriton® (Stafford-Miller)

Tablets, ivory, chlorphenamine maleate 4 mg. Net price 20 = 19p. Label: 2

Syrup, chlorphenamine maleate 2 mg/5 mL. Net price 150 mL = £2.16. Label: 2

Note. In addition to *Piriton Allergy®* [NHS], proprietary brands of chlorphenamine maleate tablets on sale to the public include *Boots Allergy Relief®*, *Calimal®*

For a list of **cough and decongestant preparations on sale to the public**, including those containing chlorphenamine, see section 3.9.2

CLEMASTINE

Indications: symptomatic relief of allergy such as hay fever, urticaria

Cautions: see notes above; pregnancy and breast-feeding

Contra-indications: see notes above

Side-effects: see notes above

Dose: 1 mg twice daily, increased up to 6 mg daily if required; CHILD under 1 year not recommended, 1–3 years 250–500 micrograms twice daily; 3–6 years 500 micrograms twice daily; 6–12 years 0.5–1 mg twice daily

Tavegil® (Novartis)

Tablets, scored, clemastine (as hydrogen fumarate) 1 mg. Net price 60-tab pack = £2.46. Label: 2

Elixir, sugar-free, clemastine (as hydrogen fumarate) 500 micrograms/5 mL. Net price 150 mL = 96p. Label: 2

Note. In addition to *Tavegil®*, proprietary brands of clemastine hydrogen fumarate on sale to the public include *Aller-eze®* [NHS]; it is also on sale to the public combined with phenylpropanolamine (*Aller-eze Plus®* [NHS])

CYPROHEPTADINE HYDROCHLORIDE

Indications: symptomatic relief of allergy such as hay fever, urticaria; migraine

Cautions: see notes above; pregnancy

Contra-indications: see notes above; breast-feeding

Side-effects: see notes above; may cause weight gain

Dose: allergy, usual dose 4 mg 3–4 times daily; usual range 4–20 mg daily, max. 32 mg daily; CHILD under 2 years not recommended, 2–6 years 2 mg 2–3 times daily, max. 12 mg daily; 7–14 years 4 mg 2–3 times daily, max. 16 mg daily

Migraine, 4 mg with a further 4 mg after 30 minutes if necessary; maintenance, 4 mg every 4–6 hours

Periactin® (MSD)

Tablets, scored, cyproheptadine hydrochloride 4 mg. Net price 30 = 86p. Label: 2

DIPHENHYDRAMINE HYDROCHLORIDE

Indications: see under Preparations

Cautions: see notes above

Contra-indications: see notes above

Side-effects: see notes above

Preparations

Proprietary brands of diphenhydramine hydrochloride on sale to the public to aid relief of temporary sleep disturbance in adults include *Medinex®* (diphenhydramine hydrochloride 10 mg/5 mL), *Nytol®* [NHS] (diphenhydramine hydrochloride tablets 25 mg and 50 mg), and *Panadol Night®* (diphenhydramine hydrochloride 25 mg and paracetamol 500 mg, for relief of temporary sleeplessness and night-time pain)

For a list of **cough and decongestant preparations on sale to the public**, including those containing diphenhydramine, see section 3.9.2

DIPHENYLPYRALINE HYDROCHLORIDE

Cautions: see notes above

Contra-indications: see notes above

Side-effects: see notes above

Preparations

For a list of **cough and decongestant preparations on sale to the public**, including those containing diphenylpyraline, see section 3.9.2

DOXYLAMINE

Cautions: see notes above

Contra-indications: see notes above

Side-effects: see notes above

Preparations

Ingredient of **cough and decongestant preparations** (section 3.9.2.) and of **compound analgesics** (section 4.7.1.) on sale to the public

---

HYDROXYZINE HYDROCHLORIDE

Indications: pruritus, anxiety (short-term)

Cautions: see notes above; renal impairment (Appendix 3)

Contra-indications: see notes above; pregnancy and breast-feeding

Side-effects: see notes above

Dose: pruritus, initially 25 mg at night increased if necessary to 25 mg 3–4 times daily; CHILD 6 months–6 years initially 5–15 mg daily increased if necessary to 50 mg daily in divided doses; over 6 years initially 15–25 mg daily increased if necessary to 50–100 mg daily in divided doses

Anxiety (adults only), 50–100 mg 4 times daily

Atarax® (Pfizer) [PoM]

Tablets, both s/c, hydroxyzine hydrochloride 10 mg (orange), net price 84-tab pack = £1.52; 25 mg (green), 28-tab pack = £1.02. Label: 2

Ucerax® (UCB Pharma) [PoM]

Tablets [NHS], f/c, scored, hydroxyzine hydrochloride 25 mg, net price 25-tab pack = 91p. Label: 2

Syrup, hydroxyzine hydrochloride 10 mg/5 mL. Net price 200-mL pack = £1.91. Label: 2

MEQUITAZINE

Indications: symptomatic relief of allergy such as hay fever, urticaria

Cautions: see notes above

Contra-indications: see notes above; pregnancy

Side-effects: see notes above

Dose: 5 mg twice daily; CHILD under 12 years, not recommended

Primalan® (Rhône-Poulenc Rorer) PoM
Tablets, mequitazine 5 mg. Net price 56-tab pack = £2.80. Label: 2

PHENIRAMINE MALEATE

Cautions: see notes above

Contra-indications: see notes above

Side-effects: see notes above

Preparations
For a list of **cough and decongestant preparations on sale to the public**, including those containing pheniramine, see section 3.9.2

PROMETHAZINE HYDROCHLORIDE

Indications: symptomatic relief of allergy such as hay fever, urticaria, premedication; emergency treatment of anaphylactic reactions (section 3.4.3); sedation (section 4.1.1); motion sickness (section 4.6)

Cautions: see notes above; intramuscular injection may be painful

Contra-indications: see notes above

Side-effects: see notes above

Dose: *by mouth*, 25 mg at night increased to 25 mg twice daily if necessary *or* 10–20 mg 2–3 times daily; CHILD under 2 years not recommended, 2–5 years 5–15 mg daily in 1–2 divided doses, 5–10 years 10–25 mg daily in 1–2 divided doses
Premedication, CHILD under 2 years not recommended, 2–5 years 15–20 mg, 5–10 years 20–25 mg
By deep intramuscular injection, 25–50 mg; max. 100 mg; CHILD 5–10 years 6.25–12.5 mg
Premedication, 25–50 mg 1 hour before operation; CHILD 5–10 years, 6.25–12.5 mg
By slow intravenous injection in emergencies, 25–50 mg as a solution containing 2.5 mg/mL in water for injections; max. 100 mg

Phenergan® (Rhône-Poulenc Rorer)
Tablets, both blue, f/c, promethazine hydrochloride 10 mg, net price 56-tab pack = £1.43; 25 mg, 56-tab pack = £2.13. Label: 2
Elixir, sugar-free, golden, promethazine hydrochloride 5 mg/5 mL. Net price 100 mL = £1.35. Label: 2
Injection PoM, promethazine hydrochloride 25 mg/mL. Net price 1-mL amp = 49p
Promethazine hydrochloride injection 25 mg/mL (1-mL and 2-mL ampoules) also available from Antigen
Note. Proprietary brands of promethazine hydrochloride on sale to the public include *Phenergan Nightime®* (promethazine hydrochloride tablets 25 mg, for occasional insomnia in adults), *Sominex®* NHS (promethazine hydrochloride tablets 20 mg, for occasional insomnia in adults) and *Q-Mazine®* (promethazine hydrochloride 5 mg/5 mL for urticaria and other skin conditions in children)
For a list of **cough and decongestant preparations on sale to the public**, including those containing promethazine, see section 3.9.2

TRIPROLIDINE HYDROCHLORIDE

Cautions: see notes above

Contra-indications: see notes above

Side-effects: see notes above

Preparations
For a list of **cough and decongestant preparations on sale to the public**, including those containing triprolidine, see section 3.9.2

3.4.2   Hyposensitisation

Except for wasp and bee sting allergy, specific hyposensitisation with allergen extract vaccines has usually shown little benefit in asthma. Hyposensitisation may be effective in allergic rhinitis if sensitisation to a particular allergen can be proven. However, the benefit of hyposensitisation needs to be balanced against the significant risk of anaphylaxis, particularly in patients with asthma (see CSM advice below).

Diagnostic skin tests are unreliable and can only be used in conjunction with a detailed history of allergen exposure.

CSM advice. After re-examination of the efficacy and safety of desensitising vaccines, the CSM has concluded that they should only be used for the following indications:

- Seasonal allergic hay fever (which has not responded to anti-allergy drugs) caused by pollens, using licensed products only—patients with *asthma* should not be treated with desensitising vaccines as they are more likely to develop severe adverse reactions.
- Hypersensitivity to wasp and bee venoms—since reactions can be life-threatening, *asthma* is not an absolute contra-indication. There is inadequate evidence of benefit from desensitisation to other allergens such as house dust, house dust mite, animal danders and foods and desensitisation is **not** recommended. Desensitising vaccines should be avoided in pregnant women, in children under five years old, and in those taking beta-blockers.

Bronchospasm usually develops within 1 hour and anaphylaxis within 30 minutes of injection. Therefore patients need to be monitored for 1 hour after injection. If symptoms or signs of hypersensitivity develop (e.g. rash, urticaria, bronchospasm, faintness), **even when mild**, the patient should be observed until these have **resolved completely**.

For details of the management of anaphylactic shock, see section 3.4.3.

BEE AND WASP ALLERGEN EXTRACTS

Each set usually contains vials for the administration of graded amounts to patients undergoing hyposensitisation. Maintenance sets containing vials at the highest strength are also available. Product literature must be consulted for details of allergens, vial strengths, and administration

Indications: hypersensitivity to wasp or bee venom (see notes above)

Cautions: see notes above including CSM advice; manufacturers recommend that patients should be warned not to eat a heavy meal before the injection

CSM advice. The CSM has advised that facilities for cardiopulmonary resuscitation must be immediately available and patients monitored closely for one hour after each injection, for full details see above.

Contra-indications: pregnancy, febrile conditions, inadequately controlled asthma
Side-effects: allergic reactions, especially in small children
Dose: *by subcutaneous injection*, see product literature

Pharmalgen® (ALK) [PoM]
Bee venom extract (*Apis mellifera*) or wasp venom extract (*Vespula* spp.). Net price initial treatment set = £62.59 (bee), £76.73 (wasp); maintenance treatment set = £72.82 (bee), £93.67 (wasp)

3.4.3   Allergic emergencies

Adrenaline (epinephrine) provides physiological reversal of the immediate symptoms (such as laryngeal oedema, bronchospasm, and hypotension) associated with hypersensitivity reactions such as *anaphylaxis* and *angioedema*. See below for full details of adrenaline administration and for adjunctive treatment.

Anaphylaxis

Anaphylactic shock requires prompt energetic treatment of *laryngeal oedema, bronchospasm,* and *hypotension*. Atopic individuals are particularly susceptible. Insect bites are a recognised risk (in particular wasp and bee stings). Certain foods, including eggs, fish, cow's milk protein, peanuts, and nuts may also precipitate anaphylaxis. Medicinal products particularly associated with anaphylaxis include blood products, vaccines, hyposensitising (allergen) preparations, antibiotics, aspirin and other NSAIDs, iron injections, heparin, and neuromuscular blocking drugs. In the case of drugs, anaphylaxis is more likely after parenteral administration; resuscitation facilities must always be available for injections associated with special risk. Anaphylactic reactions may also be associated with *additives and excipients* in foods and medicines; some oils, such as arachis (peanut) oil, may be contaminated with allergenic proteins from their original source—it is wise to check the full formula of preparations which may contain allergenic fats or oils (including those for topical application, particularly if they are intended for use in the mouth or for application to the nasal mucosa).

First-line treatment includes securing the airway, restoration of blood pressure (laying the patient flat, raising the feet), and administration of **adrenaline (epinephrine)** injection. This is given **intramuscularly** in a dose of 0.5–1 mg (0.5–1 mL adrenaline injection 1 in 1000); a dose of 300 micrograms (0.3 mL adrenaline injection 1 in 1000) may be appropriate for *immediate self-administration*. The dose is repeated every 10 minutes, according to blood pressure and pulse, until improvement occurs [important: possible need for *intravenous route* using *dilute solution*, see below]. **Oxygen** administration is also of primary importance. An antihistamine (e.g. **chlorphenamine (chlorpheniramine)**, given by slow intravenous injection in a dose of 10–20 mg, see p. 151) is a useful adjunctive treatment,

given after adrenaline injection and continued for 24 to 48 hours to prevent relapse. In patients on non-cardioselective beta-blockers severe anaphylaxis may not respond to adrenaline injection, calling for addition of **salbutamol** by intravenous injection.

Continuing deterioration requires further treatment including intravenous fluids (section 9.2.2), intravenous aminophylline (see p. 140) or a nebulised beta$_2$-adrenoceptor stimulant (such as salbutamol or terbutaline, see p.133 and p. 135); in addition to oxygen, assisted respiration and possibly emergency tracheotomy may be necessary.

An intravenous corticosteroid e.g. **hydrocortisone** (as sodium succinate) in a dose of 100–300 mg (section 6.3.2) is of secondary value in the initial management of anaphylactic shock because the onset of action is delayed for several hours, but should be given to prevent further deterioration in severely affected patients.

When a patient is so ill that there is doubt as to the adequacy of the circulation, the initial injection of adrenaline may need to be given as a *dilute solution by the intravenous route*, for details of cautions, dose and strength, see under Intravenous Adrenaline (Epinephrine), below.

Some patients with severe allergy to insect stings or foods are encouraged to carry pre-filled adrenaline syringes (e.g. *EpiPen®*) for *self-administration* during periods of risk.

Angioedema

Angioedema is dangerous if *laryngeal oedema* is present. In this circumstance adrenaline (epinephrine) injection and oxygen should be given as described under Anaphylaxis (see above); antihistamines and corticosteroids should also be given (see again above). Tracheal intubation and other measures may be necessary.

The administration of C$_1$ esterase inhibitor (in fresh frozen plasma or in partially purified form) may terminate acute attacks of *hereditary angioedema*, but is not practical for long-term prophylaxis.

Intramuscular adrenaline (epinephrine)

The *intramuscular route* is the *first choice route* for the administration of adrenaline (epinephrine) in the management of anaphylactic shock. Adrenaline has a rapid onset of action after intramuscular administration and in the shocked patient its absorption from the intramuscular site is faster and more reliable than from the subcutaneous site (the intravenous route should be reserved for extreme emergency when there is doubt as to the adequacy of the circulation, for details of cautions, dose and strength see under Intravenous Adrenaline (Epinephrine), below).

Patients with severe allergy should ideally be instructed in the self-administration of adrenaline by intramuscular injection (for details see under

Self-administration of Adrenaline (Epinephrine), below).

Prompt injection of adrenaline is of paramount importance and the recommendations in the following table avoid the need for dosage calculations in children.

Volume of adrenaline (epinephrine) injection 1 in 1000 (1 mg/mL) for **intramuscular** injection (or subcutaneous injection but not generally recommended) in anaphylactic shock

Age	Volume of adrenaline 1 in 1000
Under 1 year	0.05 mL
1 year	0.1 mL
2 years	0.2 mL[1]
3–4 years	0.3 mL[1]
5 years	0.4 mL[1]
6–12 years	0.5 mL[1]
Adult	0.5–1 mL

These doses may be repeated every 10 minutes, according to blood pressure and pulse, until improvement occurs (may be repeated several times).

1. Suitable for robust children in these age groups; for underweight children use half these doses.

Intravenous adrenaline (epinephrine)

Where the patient is severely ill and there is real doubt about adequacy of the circulation and absorption from the intramuscular injection site, adrenaline (epinephrine) may be given by **slow intravenous injection** in a dose of 500 micrograms (5 mL of the dilute 1 in 10 000 adrenaline injection) given at a rate of 100 micrograms (1 mL of the dilute 1 in 10 000 adrenaline injection) per minute, *stopping when a response has been obtained*; children can be given a dose of 10 micrograms/kg (0.1 mL/kg of the dilute 1 in 10 000 adrenaline injection) by **slow** *intravenous injection* over several minutes. Great vigilance is needed to ensure that the *correct strength* is used; anaphylactic shock kits need to make a *very clear distinction* between the 1 in 10 000 strength and the 1 in 1000 strength. It is also important that, where intramuscular injection might still succeed, time should not be wasted seeking intravenous access.

For reference to the use of the intravenous route for *cardiac resuscitation*, see section 2.7.3.

Self-administration of adrenaline (epinephrine)

Individuals who are at considerable risk of anaphylaxis need to carry adrenaline (epinephrine) with them at all times and need to be *instructed in advance* how to inject it. In addition, the packs need to be labelled so that in the case of rapid collapse someone else is able to administer the adrenaline. It is important to ensure that an adequate supply is provided to treat symptoms until medical assistance is available.

Some patients may best be able to cope with a pre-assembled syringe fitted with a needle suitable for very rapid administration (if necessary by a bystander). *EpiPen®* consists of a fully assembled syringe and needle delivering a dose of 300 micrograms of adrenaline by *intramuscular injection*; a 150-microgram version (*EpiPen® Jr*) is also available for use in children. Other products for the immediate treatment of anaphylaxis are available but are not licensed for use in the UK. *Anapen® Adult* is a fully assembled device that delivers 300 micrograms of adrenaline *by intramuscular injection*; a 150-microgram version (*Anapen® Junior*) is also available. *Anapen®* is available on a named-patient basis from Allerayde. *Ana-Guard®* is a pre-filled syringe that delivers two 300-microgram doses of adrenaline *by subcutaneous or intramuscular injection*; it can be adjusted to administer smaller doses for children. *Ana-Kit®* includes a similar pre-filled adrenaline syringe, chewable tablets of chlorphenamine maleate (chlorpheniramine maleate) 2 mg, 2 sterile pads impregnated with 70% isopropyl alcohol, and a tourniquet. *Ana-Guard®* and *Ana-Kit®* are available on a named-patient basis from IDIS.

ADRENALINE/EPINEPHRINE

Indications: emergency treatment of acute anaphylaxis; angioedema; cardiopulmonary resuscitation (section 2.7.3)

Cautions: hyperthyroidism, diabetes mellitus, ischaemic heart disease, hypertension, elderly patients

INTERACTIONS. Severe anaphylaxis in patients on non-cardioselective beta-blockers may not respond to adrenaline injection calling for intravenous injection of salbutamol (see p. 133). Patients on tricyclic antidepressants are considerably more susceptible to arrhythmias calling for a much reduced dose of adrenaline. Other **interactions**, see Appendix 1 (sympathomimetics).

Side-effects: anxiety, tremor, tachycardia, arrhythmias, cold extremities; also hypertension (risk of cerebral haemorrhage) and pulmonary oedema (on excessive dosage or extreme sensitivity); nausea, vomiting, sweating, weakness, and dizziness also reported

Dose: acute anaphylaxis, *by intramuscular (or subcutaneous) injection* of 1 in 1000 (1 mg/mL) solution, see notes and table above

Acute anaphylaxis when there is doubt as to the adequacy of the circulation, *by slow intravenous injection* of 1 in 10 000 (100 micrograms/mL) solution (extreme caution), see notes above

IMPORTANT. Intravenous route should be used with **extreme care**, see notes above

■ Intramuscular or subcutaneous

Adrenaline/Epinephrine 1 in 1000 (Non-proprietary) PoM

Injection, adrenaline (as acid tartrate) 1 mg/mL, net price 0.5-mL amp = 43p; 1-mL amp = 36p

Available from Antigen, BCM Specials, Hillcross, Martindale, Medeva, Phoenix; also available from Aurum (1-mL prefilled syringe)

Min-I-Jet® Adrenaline (Medeva) PoM

Injection, adrenaline (as hydrochloride) 1 in 1000 (1 mg/mL). Net price 1 mL (with 25 gauge × 0.25 inch needle for subcutaneous injection) = £7.37, 1 mL (with 21 gauge × 1.5 inch needle for intramuscular injection) = £3.91 (both disposable syringes)

■ Intravenous

Extreme caution, see notes above

Adrenaline/Epinephrine 1 in 10 000, Dilute
(Non-proprietary) PoM

Injection, adrenaline (as acid tartrate)
100 micrograms/mL. 10-mL amp.
Available from Martindale (special order); also from
Aurum (1-mL and 10-mL prefilled syringe) and Medeva
(*Min-I-Jet® Adrenaline* 3- and 10-mL disposable
syringes)

■ Intramuscular injection for self-administration

EpiPen® (ALK) PoM

EpiPen® Auto-injector 0.3 mg (delivering a single
dose of adrenaline 300 micrograms), adrenaline
1 mg/mL (1 in 1000), net price 2-mL *Auto-injector* = £23.50
Note. 1.7 mL of the solution remains in the *Auto-injector*
after use
Dose: by intramuscular injection, ADULT and CHILD
over 30 kg, 300 micrograms repeated after 15 minutes as
necessary
Epipen® Jr Auto-injector 0.15 mg (delivering a single dose of adrenaline 150 micrograms), adrenaline 500 micrograms/mL (1 in 2000), net price 2-
mL *Auto-injector* = £23.50
Note. 1.7 mL of the solution remains in the *Auto-injector*
after use
Dose: by intramuscular injection, CHILD 15–30 kg,
10 micrograms/kg repeated after 10 minutes as necessary

3.5   Respiratory stimulants and pulmonary surfactants

3.5.1   Respiratory stimulants
3.5.2   Pulmonary surfactants

3.5.1   Respiratory stimulants

Respiratory stimulants (analeptic drugs) have a limited place in the treatment of ventilatory failure in
patients with chronic obstructive pulmonary disease. They are effective only when given by intravenous injection or infusion and have a short
duration of action. Their use has largely been
replaced by ventilatory support including nasal
intermittent positive pressure ventilation. However,
occasionally when ventilatory support is contra-
indicated and in patients with hypercapnic respiratory failure who are becoming drowsy or comatose, respiratory stimulants in the short term may
arouse patients sufficiently to co-operate and clear
their secretions.

Respiratory stimulants can also be harmful in
respiratory failure since they stimulate non-respiratory as well as respiratory muscles. They should
only be given under **expert supervision** in hospital
and must be combined with active physiotherapy.
There is at present no oral respiratory stimulant
available for long-term use in chronic respiratory
failure.

Doxapram (section 15.1.7) is given by continuous intravenous infusion. Frequent arterial blood

gas studies and pH measurements are necessary
during treatment to ensure the correct dosage (for
full details see section 15.1.7).

Nikethamide (now discontinued by most suppliers) is not recommended because the effective
doses are close to those causing toxic effects, especially convulsions.

3.5.2   Pulmonary surfactants

Pulmonary surfactants are used in the management
of respiratory distress syndrome (hyaline membrane disease) in preterm infants.

BERACTANT

Indications: treatment of respiratory distress
syndrome in preterm infants who are intubated
and receiving mechanical ventilation, whose heart
rate and arterial oxygenation are continuously
monitored

Cautions: continuous monitoring required to
avoid hyperoxaemia (due to rapid improvement
in arterial oxygen concentration)

Side-effects: pulmonary haemorrhage reported

Dose: *by endotracheal tube*, phospholipid 100 mg/
kg equivalent to a volume of 4 mL/kg, preferably
within 8 hours of birth; may be repeated within 48
hours at intervals of at least 6 hours for up to 4
doses

Survanta® (Abbott) PoM
Suspension, beractant (bovine lung extract) providing phospholipid 25 mg/mL, with lipids and
proteins, Net price 8-mL vial = £306.43

COLFOSCERIL PALMITATE

Indications: see under Beractant (also prophylaxis
of respiratory distress syndrome)

Cautions: see under Beractant

Side-effects: may increase incidence of pulmonary haemorrhage; obstruction of endotracheal
tube by mucous secretions

Dose: *by endotracheal tube*, treatment, 67.5 mg/
kg; if still intubated, may be repeated after 12
hours; prophylaxis, first dose soon after birth, if
still intubated may be repeated 12 and 24 hours
later

Exosurf Neonatal® (GlaxoWellcome) PoM
Suspension, colfosceril palmitate 108 mg for
reconstitution with 8 mL water for injections
(when reconstituted, contains 67.5 mg/5 mL). Net
price per vial (with endotracheal tube connectors)
= £306.43

PORACTANT ALFA

Indications: treatment of respiratory distress
syndrome or hyaline membrane disease in
neonates over 700 g (also prophylaxis of respiratory distress syndrome)

Cautions: see under Beractant

Side-effects: transient depression of cerebro-elec-
trical activity

Dose: *by endotracheal tube*, treatment, 100–200 mg/kg; further doses of 100 mg/kg may be repeated at 12-hour intervals if still intubated; prophylaxis, 100–200 mg/kg soon after birth (preferably within 15 minutes); further doses of 100 mg/kg may be repeated 6–12 hours after the first dose and again 12 hours later if still intubated; max. total dose 300–400 mg/kg

Curosurf® (Serono) PoM
Suspension, poractant alfa (porcine lung phospholipid fraction) 80 mg/mL. Net price 1.5-mL vial = £400.00; 3-mL vial = £800.00

PUMACTANT

Indications: see under Beractant (also prophylaxis of respiratory distress syndrome)
Cautions: see under Beractant
Side-effects: obstruction of endotracheal tube
Dose: *by endotracheal tube*, 100 mg as soon as possible after intubation; may be repeated after 1 hour and again at 24 hours if still intubated

Alec® (Britannia) PoM
Suspension, pumactant 100 mg (synthetic lung phospholipids) for reconstitution with 1.2 mL cold sterile sodium chloride 0.9%. Net price per vial (with syringe and catheter) = £150.00

3.6 Oxygen

Oxygen should be regarded as a drug. It is prescribed for hypoxaemic patients to increase alveolar oxygen tension and decrease the work of breathing necessary to maintain a given arterial oxygen tension. The concentration depends on the condition being treated; an inappropriate concentration may have serious or even lethal effects.

High concentration oxygen therapy, with concentrations of up to 60% for short periods, is safe in conditions such as pneumonia, pulmonary thromboembolism, and fibrosing alveolitis. In such conditions low arterial oxygen (P_aO_2) is usually associated with low or normal arterial carbon dioxide (P_aCO_2), therefore there is little risk of hypoventilation and carbon dioxide retention.

In acute severe asthma, the arterial carbon dioxide (P_aCO_2) is usually subnormal but as asthma deteriorates it may rise steeply (particularly in children). These patients usually require high concentrations of oxygen and if the arterial carbon dioxide (P_aCO_2) remains high despite other treatment intermittent positive pressure ventilation needs to be considered urgently. Where facilities for blood gas measurements are not immediately available, for example while transferring the patient to hospital, 35% to 50% oxygen delivered through a conventional mask is recommended. Exceptionally, asthma is diagnosed in patients with a long history of chronic bronchitis and probable respiratory failure; in these patients a lower concentration (24% to 28%) may be needed to limit oxygen-induced reduction of respiratory drive.

Low concentration oxygen therapy (controlled oxygen therapy) is reserved for patients with ventilatory failure due to chronic obstructive pulmonary disease or other causes. The concentration should not exceed 28% and in some patients a concentration above 24% may be excessive. The aim is to provide the patient with just enough oxygen to improve hypoxaemia without worsening pre-existing carbon dioxide retention and respiratory acidosis. Treatment should be initiated in hospital as repeated blood gas measurements are required to estimate the correct concentration.

DOMICILIARY OXYGEN. Oxygen should only be prescribed for patients in the home after careful evaluation in hospital by respiratory experts; it should never be prescribed on a placebo basis.

Patients should be **advised of the fire risks** when receiving oxygen therapy.

Intermittent oxygen therapy

Oxygen is occasionally prescribed for intermittent use for episodes of hypoxaemia of short duration, for example asthma. It is important, however, that the patient does not rely on oxygen instead of obtaining medical help or taking more specific treatment.

Alternatively, intermittent oxygen may be prescribed for patients with advanced irreversible respiratory disorders to increase mobility and capacity for exercise and to ease discomfort, for example in chronic obstructive pulmonary disease. Appropriate patients may be prescribed portable equipment through the hospital service, refillable from cylinders in the home.

Under the NHS oxygen may be supplied by pharmacy contractors as **oxygen cylinders**. Oxygen flow can be adjusted as the cylinders are equipped with an oxygen flow meter with 'medium' (2 litres/minute) and 'high' (4 litres/minute) settings. The Health Authorities have lists of pharmacy contractors who provide domiciliary oxygen services.

Patients are supplied with either constant or variable performance masks. The *Intersurgical 010 28%* or *Ventimask Mk IV 28%* are constant performance masks and provide a nearly constant supply of oxygen (28%) over a wide range irrespective of the patient's breathing pattern. The variable performance masks include the *Intersurgical 005 Mask* and the *Venticaire Mask*; the concentration of oxygen supplied to the patient varies with the rate of flow of oxygen and with the patient's breathing pattern.

PORTABLE OXYGEN CYLINDERS. Portable oxygen sets are not prescribable on the NHS since the fitting is not compatible with the Drug Tariff oxygen equipment. However, Medigas and BOC supply a portable oxygen cylinder called a 'PD oxygen cylinder', which has the same bull-nose fitting as the normal domiciliary headsets (prescriptions must therefore specify 'PD oxygen cylinder'). The PD oxygen cylinder holds about 300 litres of oxygen which will last approximately 2 hours at a standard flow rate of 2 litres/minute.

Long-term oxygen therapy

Long-term administration of oxygen (at least 15 hours daily) prolongs survival in patients with chronic obstructive pulmonary disease.

The Royal College of Physicians have produced guidelines for oxygen therapy (*Domiciliary oxygen therapy services: Clinical guidelines and advice for prescribers*; June 1999). Assessment for long-term oxygen therapy requires measurement of arterial blood gas tensions. Measurements should be taken on 2 occasions at least 3 weeks apart to demonstrate clinical stability, and not sooner than 4 weeks after an acute exacerbation of the disease. The guidelines recommend that long-term oxygen therapy should be considered for patients with:

- chronic obstructive pulmonary disease with P_aO_2 < 7.3 kPa when breathing air during a period of clinical stability;
- chronic obstructive pulmonary disease with P_aO_2 7.3–8 kPa in the presence of secondary polycythaemia, nocturnal hypoxaemia, peripheral oedema or evidence of pulmonary hypertension;
- interstitial lung disease with P_aO_2 < 8 kPa and in patients with P_aO_2 > 8 kPa with disabling dyspnoea;
- cystic fibrosis when P_aO_2 < 7.3 kPa *or* if P_aO_2 7.3–8 kPa in the presence of secondary polycythaemia, nocturnal hypoxaemia, pulmonary hypertension or peripheral oedema;
- pulmonary hypertension, without parenchymal lung involvement when P_aO_2 < 8 kPa;
- neuromuscular or skeletal disorders, after specialist assessment;
- obstructive sleep apnoea despite continuous positive airways pressure therapy, after specialist assessment;
- pulmonary malignancy or other terminal disease with disabling dyspnoea;
- heart failure with daytime P_aO_2 < 7.3 kPa (on air) or with nocturnal hypoxaemia;
- paediatric respiratory disease, after specialist assessment.

Increased respiratory depression is seldom a problem in patients with stable respiratory failure treated with low concentrations of oxygen although it may occur during exacerbations; patients and relatives should be warned to call for medical help if drowsiness or confusion occur.

Oxygen concentrators are more economical for patients requiring oxygen for long periods, and in England and Wales are now prescribable on the NHS on a regional tendering basis (see below). A concentrator was formerly only provided for a patient who required oxygen for 15 hours a day but it has been found to be cost-effective to provide one for a patient requiring it for 8 hours a day (or 21 cylinders per month).

Prescribing arrangements for oxygen concentrators

Prescribe concentrator and accessories (face mask, nasal cannula, and humidifier) on form FP10. Specify amount of oxygen required (hours per day) and flow rate. If required, prescribe back-up oxygen set and cylinder at same time. Inform patient that the supplier will be in contact to make arrangements and that the prescription form is to be given to the person who installs the concentrator.

Inform supplier by telephone (see table below) that a concentrator has been prescribed. The sup-

plier will send written confirmation of the order to the prescriber, the patient, and the Health Authority.

Follow the same procedure if a back-up oxygen set and cylinder are required later.

Health Authority regional group	Supplier
South Western London South (includes Kent, Surrey, and Sussex)	BOC gases *to order:* Dial 0800 136603
Eastern London North North Western and North Wales West Midlands	De Vilbiss Medequip Ltd *to order:* Dial 0800 020202
Central and South Wales Northern Yorkshire (South and West) and Humberside	Oxygen Therapy Co Ltd *to order:* Dial 0800 373580

In **Scotland** refer the patient for assessment by a respiratory consultant. If the need for a concentrator is confirmed the consultant will arrange for the provision of a concentrator through the Common Services Agency.

3.7   Mucolytics

Mucolytics are sometimes prescribed to facilitate expectoration by reducing sputum viscosity in chronic asthma and bronchitis. Few patients, however, have been shown to derive much benefit from them although they do render sputum less viscid. Steam inhalation with postural drainage, is good expectorant therapy in bronchiectasis and some chronic bronchitics.

For reference to the newly introduced dornase alfa, see below.

CARBOCISTEINE

Indications: reduction of sputum viscosity

Contra-indications: active peptic ulceration

Side-effects: occasional gastro-intestinal irritation, rashes

Dose: 750 mg 3 times daily initially, then 1.5 g daily in divided doses; CHILD 2–5 years 62.5–125 mg 4 times daily, 6–12 years 250 mg 3 times daily

* **Carbocisteine Capsules** (Non-proprietary) NHS PoM

Capsules, carbocisteine 375 mg. Net price 30-cap pack = £4.48

* **Carbocisteine Syrup** (Non-proprietary) NHS PoM

Oral liquid, carbocisteine 125 mg/5 mL, net price 300 mL = £4.91; 250 mg/5 mL, 300 mL = £6.28

* NHS except, for patients under the age of 18 years and in whom any condition which, through damage or disease, affects the airways and has required a tracheostomy and endorsed 'SLS'

Note. The brand name *Mucodyne®* NHS (Rhône-Poulenc Rorer) is used for carbocisteine preparations; capsules and 250 mg/5 mL strength of syrup contain tartrazine

MECYSTEINE HYDROCHLORIDE

(Methyl Cysteine Hydrochloride)

Indications: reduction of sputum viscosity

Dose: 100–200 mg 3–4 times daily before meals reduced to 200 mg twice daily after 6 weeks; CHILD over 5 years 100 mg 3 times daily

Prophylaxis, 100–200 mg 2–3 times every other day during winter months

Visclair® (Sinclair) NHS

Tablets, yellow, s/c, e/c, mecysteine hydrochloride 100 mg. Net price 20 = £3.66. Label: 5, 22, 25

Dornase alfa

Dornase alfa is a genetically engineered version of a naturally occurring human enzyme which cleaves extracellular deoxyribonucleic acid (DNA); it is used in cystic fibrosis. It is administered by inhalation using a jet nebuliser (section 3.1.5).

DORNASE ALFA

Phosphorylated glycosylated recombinant human deoxyribonuclease 1 (rhDNase)

Indications: management of cystic fibrosis patients with a forced vital capacity (FVC) of greater than 40% of predicted to improve pulmonary function

Cautions: pregnancy (Appendix 4)

Side-effects: pharyngitis, voice changes, chest pain; occasionally laryngitis, rashes, urticaria, conjunctivitis

Dose: *by inhalation of nebulised solution* (by jet nebuliser), 2500 units (2.5 mg) once daily (patients over 21 years may benefit from twice daily dosage); CHILD under 5 years not recommended

Pulmozyme® (Roche) PoM

Nebuliser solution, dornase alfa 1000 units (1 mg)/mL. Net price 2.5-mL (2500 units) vial = £19.47

Note. For use undiluted with jet nebulisers only; ultrasonic nebulisers are unsuitable

---

3.8   Aromatic inhalations

Inhalations containing volatile substances such as eucalyptus oil are traditionally used and although the vapour may contain little of the additive it encourages deliberate inspiration of warm moist air which is often comforting in bronchitis; boiling water should not be used owing to the risk of scalding. Inhalations are also used for the relief of nasal obstruction in acute rhinitis or sinusitis.

CHILDREN. The use of strong aromatic decongestants (applied as rubs or to pillows) is not advised for infants under the age of 3 months. Mothers with young infants in whom nasal obstruction with mucus is a problem can readily be taught appropriate techniques of suction aspiration.

Benzoin Tincture, Compound, BP

(Friars' Balsam)

Tincture, balsamic acids approx. 4.5%. Label: 15

Directions for use: add one teaspoonful to a pint of hot, **not** boiling, water and inhale the vapour

Menthol and Eucalyptus Inhalation, BP 1980

Inhalation, racementhol or levomenthol 2 g, eucalyptus oil 10 mL, light magnesium carbonate 7 g, water to 100 mL

Directions for use: add one teaspoonful to a pint of hot, **not** boiling, water and inhale the vapour

Karvol® (Crookes) NHS

Inhalation capsules, levomenthol 35.55 mg, with chlorobutanol, pine oils, terpineol, and thymol. Net price 10-cap pack = £1.27; 20-cap pack = £2.27

Inhalation solution, levomenthol 7.92 mg, with chlorobutanol, pine oils, terpineol, and thymol. Net price 12-mL dropper bottle = £1.63

Administration: express into handkerchief or add to a pint of hot, **not** boiling, water the contents of 1 capsule or 6 drops of solution; avoid in infants under 3 months

---

3.9   Cough preparations

3.9.1   Cough suppressants

3.9.2   Expectorant and demulcent cough preparations

3.9.1   Cough suppressants

Cough is usually a symptom of an underlying disorder e.g. asthma (section 3.1.1), gastro-oesophageal reflux disease (section 1.1.3), and 'post-nasal drip'; where there is no identifiable cause, cough suppressants may be useful, for example if sleep is disturbed. They may cause sputum retention and this may be harmful in patients with chronic bronchitis and bronchiectasis.

Codeine may be effective but it is constipating and can cause dependence; **dextromethorphan** and **pholcodine** have fewer side-effects.

Sedating antihistamines, such as diphenhydramine, are used as the cough suppressant component of many compound cough preparations on sale to the public; all tend to cause drowsiness which may reflect their main mode of action.

CHILDREN. The use of cough suppressants containing codeine or similar opioid analgesics is not generally recommended in children and should be avoided altogether in those under 1 year of age.

CODEINE PHOSPHATE

Indications: dry or painful cough; diarrhoea (section 1.4.2); pain (section 4.7.2)

Cautions: asthma; hepatic and renal impairment; history of drug abuse; see also notes above and section 4.7.2; **interactions:** Appendix 1 (opioid analgesics)

Contra-indications: liver disease, ventilatory failure

Side-effects: constipation, respiratory depression in sensitive patients or if given large doses

¹ **Codeine Linctus, BP** PoM

Linctus (= oral solution), codeine phosphate 15 mg/
5 mL. Net price 100 mL = 41p (diabetic, 75p)

Dose: 5–10 mL 3–4 times daily; CHILD (but not generally recommended) 5–12 years, 2.5–5 mL

Available from APS, Cox, Galen (*Galcodine®*, sugar-
free), Norton

Note. BP directs that when Diabetic Codeine Linctus is
prescribed, Codeine Linctus formulated with a vehicle
appropriate for administration to diabetics, whether or
not labelled 'Diabetic Codeine Linctus', shall be dispensed or supplied

1. Can be sold to the public provided the maximum single
dose does not exceed 5 mL

Codeine Linctus, Paediatric, BP

Linctus (= oral solution), codeine phosphate 3 mg/
5 mL. Net price 100 mL = 21p

Dose: CHILD (but not generally recommended) 1–5
years 5 mL 3–4 times daily

Available from Galen (*Galcodine® Paediatric*, sugar-
free), Medeva

Note. BP directs that Paediatric Codeine Linctus may be
prepared extemporaneously by diluting Codeine Linctus
with a suitable vehicle in accordance with the manufacturer's instructions

For a list of **cough and decongestant preparations on
sale to the public**, including those containing codeine, see
section 3.9.2

PHOLCODINE

Indications: dry or painful cough

Cautions: see under Codeine Phosphate

Contra-indications: see under Codeine Phosphate

Side-effects: see under Codeine Phosphate

Pholcodine Linctus, BP

Linctus (= oral solution), pholcodine 5 mg/5 mL in
a suitable flavoured vehicle, containing citric acid
monohydrate 1%. Net price 100 mL = 24p

Dose: 5–10 mL 3–4 times daily; CHILD (but not generally recommended) 5–12 years 2.5–5 mL

Available from APS, Boehringer Ingelheim (*Pavacol-D®*,
sugar-free), Galen (*Galenphol®*, sugar-free), Norton

Pholcodine Linctus, Strong, BP

Linctus (= oral solution), pholcodine 10 mg/5 mL
in a suitable flavoured vehicle, containing citric
acid monohydrate 2%. Net price 100 mL = 33p

Dose: 5 mL 3–4 times daily

Available from APS (sugar-free), Norton

Galenphol® (Galen)

Paediatric linctus (= oral solution), orange, sugar-
free, pholcodine 2 mg/5 mL. Net price 90-mL
pack = £1.11

Dose: CHILD (but not generally recommended) 1–5
years 5 mL 3 times daily; 6–12 years 5–10 mL

For a list of **cough and decongestant preparations on
sale to the public**, including those containing pholcodine,
see section 3.9.2

Palliative care

Diamorphine and methadone have been used to
control distressing cough in terminal lung cancer
although morphine is now preferred (see Prescribing in Palliative Care, p. 13). In other circumstances they are contra-indicated because they
induce sputum retention and ventilatory failure as
well as causing opioid dependence. Methadone
linctus should be avoided because it has a long
duration of action and tends to accumulate.

METHADONE HYDROCHLORIDE

Indications: cough in terminal disease

Cautions: see notes in section 4.7.2

Contra-indications: see notes in section 4.7.2

Side-effects: see notes in section 4.7.2; longer-acting than morphine therefore effects may be cumulative

Dose: see below

Methadone Linctus CD ▰

Linctus (= oral solution), methadone hydrochloride
2 mg/5 mL in a suitable vehicle with a tolu flavour. Label: 2

Dose: 2.5–5 mL every 4–6 hours, reduced to twice daily
on prolonged use

▰ denotes preparations that are considered to
be less suitable for prescribing (see p. vi)

MORPHINE HYDROCHLORIDE

Indications: cough in terminal disease (see also
Prescribing in Palliative Care p. 12)

Cautions: see notes in section 4.7.2

Contra-indications: see notes in section 4.7.2

Side-effects: see notes in section 4.7.2

Dose: initially 5 mg every 4 hours

Preparations

Section 4.7.2

3.9.2   Expectorant and demulcent cough preparations

Expectorants are claimed to promote expulsion of
bronchial secretions but there is no evidence that
any drug can specifically facilitate expectoration.
The assumption that sub-emetic doses of expectorants, such as ammonium chloride, ipecacuanha,
and squill promote expectoration is a myth. However, a simple expectorant mixture may serve a useful placebo function and has the advantage of being
inexpensive.

Demulcent cough preparations contain soothing
substances such as syrup or glycerol and certainly
some patients believe that such preparations relieve
a dry irritating cough. Preparations such as **simple
linctus** have the advantage of being harmless and
inexpensive; **paediatric simple linctus** is particularly useful in children and sugar-free versions are
available.

Compound cough preparations are on sale to
the public; the rationale for some is dubious.

Ammonia and Ipecacuanha Mixture, BP

Mixture, ammonium bicarbonate 200 mg, liquorice
liquid extract 0.5 mL, ipecacuanha tincture
0.3 mL, concentrated camphor water 0.1 mL, concentrated anise water 0.05 mL, double-strength
chloroform water 5 mL, water to 10 mL. It should
be recently prepared

Dose: 10–20 mL 3–4 times daily

Simple Linctus, BP

Linctus (= oral solution), citric acid monohydrate 2.5% in a suitable vehicle with an anise flavour.
Net price 100 mL = 18p
Dose: 5 mL 3–4 times daily
A sugar-free version is available from Pinewood and various wholesalers.

Simple Linctus, Paediatric, BP

Linctus (= oral solution), citric acid monohydrate 0.625% in a suitable vehicle with an anise flavour. Net price 100 mL = 16p
Dose: CHILD 5–10 mL 3–4 times daily
A sugar-free version is available from Pinewood and various wholesalers.

Systemic cough and decongestant preparations on sale to the public, together with their significant ingredients.

Important: in overdose contact **Poisons Information Services** (p. 19) for full details of the ingredients.

Actifed® (pseudoephedrine, triprolidine), **Actifed Compound Linctus**® (dextromethorphan, pseudoephedrine, triprolidine), **Actifed Expectorant**® (guaifenesin, pseudoephedrine, triprolidine), **Adult Meltus**® **Expectorant with Decongestant** (guaifenesin, pseudoephedrine, menthol), **Advil Cold and Sinus**® (ibuprofen, pseudoephedrine), **Baby Meltus**® (dilute acetic acid), **Beechams All-In-One**® (guaifenesin, paracetamol, phenylephrine), **Beechams Flu-Plus Caplets**® (paracetamol, phenylephrine), **Beechams Hot Lemon**®, **Hot Lemon and Honey**®, **Hot Blackcurrant**®, **Beechams Powders Capsules**® **with Decongestant** (paracetamol, phenylephrine), **Benylin Chesty Cough**® (ammonium chloride, diphenhydramine, menthol), **Benylin Children's Chesty Coughs**® (guaifenesin), **Benylin Children's Night Coughs**® (diphenhydramine, menthol), **Benylin Children's Dry Coughs**® (pholcodine), **Benylin Children's Coughs and Colds**® (dextromethorphan, triprolidine), **Benylin with Codeine**® (codeine, diphenhydramine, menthol), **Benylin Cough and Congestion**® (dextromethorphan, diphenhydramine, menthol, pseudoephedrine), **Benylin Dry Cough**® (dextromethorphan, diphenhydramine, menthol), **Benylin Four Flu**® (diphenhydramine, paracetamol, pseudoephedrine), **Benylin Non-drowsy for Chesty Coughs**® (guaifenesin, menthol), **Benylin Non-drowsy for Dry Coughs**® (dextromethorphan), **Benylin Sugar-free for Children**® (diphenhydramine, menthol), **Benylin Day and Night Cold and Flu Relief**® (*day tablets,* paracetamol, phenylpropanolamine, *night tablets,* paracetamol, diphenhydramine), **Boots Bronchial Cough Mixture**® (ammonium carbonate, ammonium chloride, guaifenesin), **Boots Catarrh Cough Syrup**® (codeine, creosote), **Boots Children's 1 Year Plus Chesty Cough Syrup**® (guaifenesin), **Boots Children's 1 Year Plus Decongestant Syrup**® (pseudoephedrine), **Boots Children's 1 Year Plus Night Time Cough Syrup**® (diphenhydramine, pholcodine), **Boots Children's 2 Years Plus Cough and Cold Syrup with Decongestant**® (guaifenesin, pseudoephedrine), **Boots Children's 3 Months Plus Simple Cough Linctus**® (glycerol), **Boots Children's 6 Months Plus Cough and Congestion Syrup**® (ephedrine, ipecacuanha), **Boots Cold Relief Tablets**® (paracetamol, phenylephrine), **Boots Decongestant Tablets**® (pseudoephedrine), **Bronalin Decongestant Elixir**® (pseudoephedrine), **Bronalin Dry Cough**® (dextromethorphan, pseudoephedrine), **Bronalin Expectorant**® (ammonium chloride, guaifenesin), **Bronalin Junior Linctus**® (diphenhydramine), **Buttercup Syrup Traditional**® (squill), **Buttercup Honey and Lemon**® **and Blackcurrant**® (ipecacuanha, menthol)

Cabdrivers® (dextromethorphan, menthol), **CAM**® (ephedrine), **Catarrh-Ex**® (paracetamol, pseudoephedrine), **Coldrex Hot Lemon Powders**® **and Tab-**

lets® (paracetamol, phenylephrine), **Contac 400**® (phenylpropanolamine, chlorphenamine (chlorpheniramine)), **Contac CoughCaps**® (dextromethorphan), **Covonia Bronchial Balsam**® (dextromethorphan, menthol), **Covonia for Children**® (dextromethorphan, menthol), **Covonia Mentholated Cough Mixture**® (liquorice, menthol, squill), **Covonia Night Time Formula**® (dextromethorphan, diphenhydramine)

Day Nurse®, **Day Nurse Hot**® (dextromethorphan, paracetamol, phenylpropanolamine), **Dimotane Elixir**®, **Tablets**® **and Dimotane LA**® (brompheniramine), **Dimotane Expectorant**® (brompheniramine, guaifenesin, pseudoephedrine), **Dimotane Co**® **and Dimotane Co Paediatric**® (brompheniramine, codeine, pseudoephedrine), **Dimotane Plus**® **and Dimotane Plus Paediatric**® (brompheniramine, pseudoephedrine), **Dimotapp**®, **Dimotapp Paediatric**®, **and Dimotapp LA**® (brompheniramine, phenylephrine, phenylpropanolamine), **Do-Do Expectorant**® (guaifenesin), **Do-Do Chesteze**® (ephedrine, theophylline), **Dristan Tablets**® (aspirin, chlorphenamine, phenylephrine)

ES Bronchial® (ammonium bicarbonate, ipecacuanha, senna, squill), **Eskornade**® (diphenylpyraline, phenylpropanolamine), **Expulin**® (chlorphenamine (chlorpheniramine), menthol, pholcodine, pseudoephedrine), **Expulin Chesty Cough**® (guaifenesin, menthol), **Expulin Decongestant for Babies and Children**® (chlorphenamine (chlorpheniramine), ephedrine, menthol), **Expulin Dry**® (menthol, pholcodine), **Expulin Paediatric**® (chlorphenamine (chlorpheniramine), menthol, pholcodine)

Famel Expectorant® (guaifenesin), **Famel Original**® (codeine, creosote), **Fennings Little Healers**® (ipecacuanha), **Franol**® **and Franol Plus**® (both ephedrine, theophylline)

Galcodine® (codeine), **Galcodine Paediatric**® (codeine), **Galenphol**® (pholcodine), **Galenphol Paediatric**® (pholcodine), **Galenphol Strong**® (pholcodine), **Galloway's**® (ipecacuanha, squill), **Galpseud**® (pseudoephedrine), **Galpseud Plus**® (chlorphenamine (chlorpheniramine), pseudoephedrine), **Gee's Linctus**® (opium, squill, tolu), **Guanor Expectorant**® (ammonium chloride, diphenhydramine, menthol)

Haymine® (chlorphenamine (chlorpheniramine), ephedrine), **Hill's Balsam Adult Expectorant**® (ipecacuanha, pholcodine), **Hill's Balsam Cough Suppressant**® (pholcodine), **Histalix**® (ammonium chloride, diphenhydramine, menthol)

Jackson's All Fours® (guaifenesin), **Junior Meltus Dry Cough**® (dextromethorphan, pseudoephedrine), **Junior Meltus Expectorant**® (guaifenesin)

Lemsip Lemcaps®, **Lemsip Flu Strength**®, **Lemsip Lemon**® **or Blackcurrant**®, **Lemsip Menthol Extra**® (all paracetamol, phenylephrine), **Lemsip Chesty Cough**® (guaifenesin), **Lemsip Power +**® (ibuprofen, pseudoephedrine), **Liqufruta Garlic**® (guaifenesin)

Medised® (paracetamol, promethazine), **Melo**® (ipecacuanha), **Meltus Baby**® (dilute acetic acid), **Meltus Dry Cough**® (dextromethorphan, pseudoephedrine), **Meltus Expectorant**®, **Meltus Honey and Lemon**® (guaifenesin), **Mu-Cron Tablets**® (paracetamol, phenylpropanolamine)

Night Nurse® (dextromethorphan, paracetamol, promethazine), **Nirolex for Chesty Coughs with Decongestant**® (guaifenesin, pseudoephedrine), **Nirolex Chesty Cough Linctus**® (guaifenesin), **Nirolex Day Cold Comfort**® (paracetamol, pholcodine, pseudoephedrine), **Nirolex Dry Cough Linctus**® (glycerol), **Nirolex for Dry Coughs with Decongestant**® (dextromethorphan, pseudoephedrine), **Nirolex for Night Time Coughs**® (diphenhydramine, pholcodine), **Numark Cold Relief Powders**® (paracetamol), **Nurofen Cold and Flu**® (ibuprofen, pseudoephedrine), **Nurse Sykes Balsam**® (guaifenesin)

Pavacol D® (pholcodine), **Pulmo Bailly**® (codeine, guaiacol)

Robitussin Chesty Cough® (guaifenesin), **Robitussin Chesty Cough with Congestion**® (guaifenesin, pseudoephedrine), **Robitussin Dry Cough**® (dextromethorphan), **Robitussin Junior Persistant Cough**® (dextromethorphan), **Robitussin Night-Time**® (brompheniramine, codeine, pseudoephedrine)

Sinutab® (paracetamol, phenylpropanolamine), **SP Cold Relief Capsules**® (paracetamol, phenylephrine), **Strepsils Cough Lozenges**® (dextromethorphan), **Sudafed**® (pseudoephedrine), **Sudafed Co**® (paracetamol, pseudoephedrine), **Sudafed Expectorant**® (guaifenesin, pseudoephedrine), **Sudafed Linctus**® (dextromethorphan, pseudoephedrine), **Sudafed Plus**® (pseudoephedrine, triprolidine)

Throaties Family Cough Linctus® (ipecacuanha), **Tixylix Catarrh**® (diphenhydramine, menthol), **Tixylix Chesty Cough**® (guaifenesin), **Tixylix Cough and Cold**® (chlorphenamine (chlorpheniramine), pholcodine, pseudoephedrine), **Tixylix Daytime**® (pholcodine), **Tixylix Night-time**® (pholcodine, promethazine), **Tixymol**® (paracetamol), Triogesic® (paracetamol, phenylpropanolamine), **Triominic**® (pheniramine, phenylpropanolamine)

Uniflu with Gregovite C® (codeine, diphenhydramine, paracetamol, phenylephrine)

Venos for Dry Coughs®, **Venos Expectorant**® (guaifenesin), **Venos Honey and Lemon**®, **Vicks Medinite**® (dextromethorphan, doxylamine, ephedrine, paracetamol), **Vicks Vaposyrup for Tickly Coughs**® (honey, menthol), **Vicks Vaposyrup Chesty Cough**® (guaifenesin), **Vicks Vaposyrup Dry Cough**® (dextromethorphan)

3.10   Systemic nasal decongestants

Nasal decongestants for administration by mouth may not be as effective as preparations for local application (section 12.2.2) but they do not give rise to rebound nasal congestion on withdrawal. Some systemic nasal decongestants can have unwanted sympathomimetic effects. **Pseudoephedrine** is available over-the-counter; it has few sympathomimetic effects.

Systemic decongestants should be used with caution in diabetes, hypertension, hyperthyroidism, and ischaemic heart disease and **avoided** in patients taking monoamine oxidase inhibitors; **interactions:** Appendix 1 (sympathomimetics).

The main ingredients in systemic nasal decongestant preparations are shown in the list of cough and decongestant preparations on sale to the public (section 3.9.2). Many preparations also contain antihistamines which may cause drowsiness and affect the ability to drive or operate machinery.

PSEUDOEPHEDRINE HYDROCHLORIDE

Indications: see notes above

Cautions: see under Ephedrine Hydrochloride (section 3.1.1.2)

Side-effects: see under Ephedrine Hydrochloride (section 3.1.1.2)

Dose: see preparations below

Galpseud® (Galen) ▬
Tablets, pseudoephedrine hydrochloride 60 mg. Net price 20 = 87p
Dose: 1 tablet 4 times daily

Linctus, orange, sugar-free, pseudoephedrine hydrochloride 30 mg/5 mL. Net price 140 mL = £1.70
Dose: 10 mL 3 times daily; CHILD 2–6 years 2.5 mL, 6–12 years 5 mL

Sudafed® (Warner Lambert) ▬
Tablets, red, f/c, pseudoephedrine hydrochloride 60 mg. Net price 20 = 96p
Dose: 1 tablet every 4–6 hours (up to 4 times daily)
Elixir, red, pseudoephedrine hydrochloride 30 mg/5 mL. Net price 100 mL = £1.40
Dose: 10 mL every 4–6 hours (up to 4 times daily); CHILD 2–5 years 2.5 mL, 6–12 years 5 mL

> ▬ denotes preparations that are considered to be less suitable for prescribing (see p. vi)

■ Preparations on sale to the public
For a list of **cough and decongestant preparations on sale to the public**, including those containing pseudoephedrine, see p. 161

4: Central nervous system

4.1   Hypnotics and anxiolytics

4.1.1   Hypnotics
4.1.2   Anxiolytics
4.1.3   Barbiturates

Most anxiolytics ('sedatives') will induce sleep when given at night and most hypnotics will sedate when given during the day. Prescribing of these drugs is widespread but dependence (both physical and psychological) and tolerance occurs. This may lead to difficulty in withdrawing the drug after the patient has been taking it regularly for more than a few weeks (see Dependence and Withdrawal, below). Hypnotics and anxiolytics should therefore, be reserved for short courses to alleviate acute conditions after causal factors have been established.

Benzodiazepines are the most commonly used anxiolytics and hypnotics; they act at benzodiazepine receptors which are associated with gamma-aminobutyric acid (GABA) receptors. Older drugs such as meprobamate and barbiturates (section 4.1.3) are **not** recommended—they have more side-effects and interactions than benzodiazepines and are much more dangerous in overdosage.

PARADOXICAL EFFECTS. A paradoxical increase in hostility and aggression may be reported by patients taking benzodiazepines. The effects range from talkativeness and excitement, to aggressive and antisocial acts. Adjustment of the dose (up or down) usually attenuates the impulses. Increased anxiety and perceptual disorders are other paradoxical effects. Increased hostility and aggression after barbiturates and alcohol usually indicates intoxication.

DRIVING. Hypnotics and anxiolytics may impair judgement and increase reaction time, and so affect ability to drive or operate machinery; they increase the effects of alcohol. Moreover the hangover effects of a night dose may impair driving on the following day.

DEPENDENCE AND WITHDRAWAL. Withdrawal of a benzodiazepine should be gradual because abrupt withdrawal may produce confusion, toxic psychosis, convulsions, or a condition resembling delirium tremens. Abrupt withdrawal of an older drug, such as a barbiturate (section 4.1.3), may be even more likely to have serious effects.

The benzodiazepine withdrawal syndrome may not develop until up to 3 weeks after stopping a long-acting benzodiazepine, but may occur within a few hours in the case of a short-acting one. It is characterised by insomnia, anxiety, loss of appetite and of body-weight, tremor, perspiration, tinnitus, and perceptual disturbances. These symptoms may be similar to the original complaint and encourage further prescribing; some symptoms may continue for weeks or months after stopping benzodiazepines entirely.

A benzodiazepine can be withdrawn in steps of about one-eighth (range one-tenth to one-quarter) of the daily dose every fortnight. A suggested withdrawal protocol for patients who have difficulty is as follows:

1. Transfer patient to equivalent daily dose of diazepam[1] preferably taken at night
2. Reduce diazepam dose in fortnightly steps of 2 or 2.5 mg; if withdrawal symptoms occur, maintain this dose until symptoms improve
3. Reduce dose further, if necessary in smaller fortnightly steps[2]; it is better to reduce too slowly rather than too quickly
4. Stop completely; time needed for withdrawal can vary from about 4 weeks to a year or more

Counselling may help; beta-blockers should **only** be tried if other measures fail; antidepressants should **only** be used if clinical depression present; **avoid** antipsychotics (which may aggravate withdrawal symptoms)

CSM advice

1. Benzodiazepines are indicated for the short-term relief (two to four weeks only) of anxiety that is severe, disabling or subjecting the individual to unacceptable distress, occurring alone or in association with insomnia or short-term psychosomatic, organic or psychotic illness.

2. The use of benzodiazepines to treat short-term 'mild' anxiety is inappropriate and unsuitable.

3. Benzodiazepines should be used to treat insomnia only when it is severe, disabling, or subjecting the individual to extreme distress.

4.1.1   Hypnotics

Before a hypnotic is prescribed the cause of the insomnia should be established and, where possible, underlying factors should be treated. However, it should be noted that some patients have unrealistic sleep expectations, and others understate their alcohol consumption which is often the cause of the insomnia.

Transient insomnia may occur in those who normally sleep well and may be due to extraneous factors such as noise, shift work, and jet lag. If a hypnotic is indicated one that is rapidly eliminated should be chosen, and only one or two doses should be given.

Short-term insomnia is usually related to an emotional problem or serious medical illness. It may last for a few weeks and may recur; a hypnotic can be useful but should not be given for more than three weeks (preferably only one week). Intermittent use is desirable with omission of some doses. A rapidly eliminated drug is generally appropriate.

1. Approximate equivalent doses, diazepam 5 mg
   ≡ chlordiazepoxide 15 mg
   ≡ loprazolam 0.5–1 mg
   ≡ lorazepam 500 micrograms
   ≡ lormetazepam 0.5–1 mg
   ≡ nitrazepam 5 mg
   ≡ oxazepam 15 mg
   ≡ temazepam 10 mg
2. Steps may be adjusted according to initial dose and duration of treatment and can range from diazepam 500 micrograms (one-quarter of a 2-mg tablet) to 2.5 mg

Chronic insomnia is rarely benefited by hypnotics and is more often due to mild dependence caused by injudicious prescribing. Psychiatric disorders such as anxiety, depression, and abuse of drugs and alcohol are common causes. Sleep disturbance is very common in depressive illness and early wakening is often a useful pointer. The underlying psychiatric complaint should be treated, adapting the drug regimen to alleviate insomnia. For example, amitriptyline, prescribed for depression, will also help to promote sleep if it is taken at night. Other causes of insomnia include daytime cat-napping and physical causes such as pain, pruritus, and dyspnoea.

Hypnotics should **not** be prescribed indiscriminately and routine prescribing is undesirable. They should be reserved for short courses in the acutely distressed. Tolerance to their effects develops within 3 to 14 days of continuous use and long-term efficacy cannot be assured. A major drawback of long-term use is that withdrawal causes rebound insomnia and precipitates a withdrawal syndrome (section 4.1).

Where prolonged administration is unavoidable hypnotics should be discontinued as soon as feasible and the patient warned that sleep may be disturbed for a few days before normal rhythm is re-established; broken sleep with vivid dreams and increased REM (rapid eye movement) may persist for several weeks.

CHILDREN. The prescribing of hypnotics to children, except for occasional use such as for night terrors and somnambulism (sleep-walking), is not justified.

ELDERLY. Hypnotics should be avoided in the elderly, who are at risk of becoming ataxic and confused and so liable to fall and injure themselves.

Benzodiazepines

Benzodiazepines used as hypnotics include **nitrazepam**, **flunitrazepam**, and **flurazepam** which have a prolonged action and may give rise to residual effects on the following day; repeated doses tend to be cumulative.

Loprazolam, **lormetazepam**, and **temazepam** act for a shorter time and they have little or no hangover effect. Withdrawal phenomena however are more common with the short-acting benzodiazepines.

Benzodiazepine anxiolytics such as **diazepam** given as a single dose at night may also be used as hypnotics.

For general guidelines on benzodiazepine prescribing see section 4.1.2 and for benzodiazepine withdrawal see section 4.1.

NITRAZEPAM

Indications: insomnia (short-term use)

Cautions: respiratory disease, muscle weakness, history of drug or alcohol abuse, marked personality disorder, pregnancy and breast-feeding (Appendixes 4 and 5); reduce dose in elderly and debilitated, and in hepatic (avoid if severe) and renal impairment (Appendixes 2 and 3); avoid prolonged use (and abrupt withdrawal thereafter); porphyria (section 9.8.2); **interactions:** Appendix 1 (anxiolytics and hypnotics)

DRIVING. Drowsiness may persist the next day and affect performance of skilled tasks (e.g. driving); effects of alcohol enhanced

Contra-indications: respiratory depression; acute pulmonary insufficiency; severe hepatic impairment, myasthenia gravis, sleep apnoea syndrome; not for phobic or obsessional states and not for use alone to treat depression (or anxiety associated with depression) or chronic psychosis

Side-effects: drowsiness and lightheadedness the next day; confusion and ataxia (especially in the elderly); amnesia may occur; dependence; see also under Diazepam (section 4.1.2); **overdosage:** see Emergency Treatment of Poisoning, p. 24

Dose: 5–10 mg at bedtime; ELDERLY (or debilitated) 2.5–5 mg; CHILD not recommended

Nitrazepam (Non-proprietary) PoM
Tablets, nitrazepam 5 mg, net price 20 = 88p. Label: 19
Available from APS, Cox, CP, DDSA (*Remnos®* NHS), ICN (*Mogadon®* NHS), Norton
Oral suspension, nitrazepam 2.5 mg/5 mL. Net price 150 mL = £5.30. Label: 19
Available from Norgine (*Somnite®* NHS)

FLUNITRAZEPAM
Indications: insomnia (short-term use)
Cautions: see under Nitrazepam
Contra-indications: see under Nitrazepam
Side-effects: see under Nitrazepam
Dose: 0.5–1 mg at bedtime; max. 2 mg; ELDERLY (or debilitated) 500 micrograms (max. 1 mg); CHILD not recommended

Rohypnol® (Roche) NHS CD
Tablets, grey-green, f/c, scored, flunitrazepam 1 mg. Net price 30-tab pack = £4.41. Label: 19
WARNING. Flunitrazepam tablets may be particularly subject to abuse

FLURAZEPAM
Indications: insomnia (short-term use)
Cautions: see under Nitrazepam
Contra-indications: see under Nitrazepam
Side-effects: see under Nitrazepam
Dose: 15–30 mg at bedtime; ELDERLY (or debilitated) 15 mg; CHILD not recommended

Dalmane® (ICN) NHS PoM
Capsules, flurazepam (as hydrochloride), 15 mg (grey/yellow), net price 30-cap pack = £2.92; 30 mg (black/grey), 30-cap pack = £3.75. Label: 19

LOPRAZOLAM
Indications: insomnia (short-term use)
Cautions: see under Nitrazepam
Contra-indications: see under Nitrazepam
Side-effects: see under Nitrazepam
Dose: 1 mg at bedtime, increased to 1.5 or 2 mg if required; ELDERLY (or debilitated) 0.5–1 mg; CHILD not recommended

Loprazolam (Non-proprietary) PoM
Tablets, loprazolam 1 mg (as mesilate). Net price 28-tab pack = £4.46. Label: 19
Available from Hoechst Marion Roussel (previously *Dormonoct®* NHS)

LORMETAZEPAM
Indications: insomnia (short-term use)
Cautions: see under Nitrazepam
Contra-indications: see under Nitrazepam
Side-effects: see under Nitrazepam; shorter acting
Dose: 0.5–1.5 mg at bedtime; ELDERLY (or debilitated) 500 micrograms; CHILD not recommended

Lormetazepam (Non-proprietary) PoM
Tablets, lormetazepam 500 micrograms, net price 20 = 53p; 1 mg, 20 = 99p. Label: 19
Available from APS, Cox, Genus, Norton, Wyeth

TEMAZEPAM
Indications: insomnia (short-term use); see also section 15.1.4.1 for peri-operative use
Cautions: see under Nitrazepam
Contra-indications: see under Nitrazepam
Side-effects: see under Nitrazepam; shorter acting
Dose: 10–20 mg at bedtime, exceptional circumstances 30–40 mg; ELDERLY (or debilitated) 10 mg at bedtime, exceptional circumstances 20 mg; CHILD not recommended

[1] **Temazepam** (Non-proprietary) CD
Gel-filled capsules NHS (soft gelatin), temazepam 10 mg, net price 20 = 37p; 15 mg, 20 = 62p; 20 mg, 20 = 60p; 30 mg, 20 = £1.24. Label: 19
WARNING. Gel-filled capsules may be particularly subject to abuse; gangrene has followed abuse by injection
Tablets, temazepam 10 mg, net price 20 = 68p; 20 mg, 20 = £1.20. Label: 19
Available from APS, Cox, Generics, Hillcross, Lagap, Norton
Oral solution, temazepam 10 mg/5 mL, net price 300 mL = £9.95. Label: 19
Available from Generics (sugar-free), Hillcross (sugar-free), Lagap, Pharmacia & Upjohn (sugar-free), Rosemont (sugar-free)
1. See p. 7 for prescribing requirements for temazepam

Zolpidem and zopiclone

Zopiclone is a cyclopyrrolone and **zolpidem** is an imidazopyridine. Although neither are benzodiazepines both act on the same receptors (or receptor sub-types) as benzodiazepines. Both have a short duration of action with little or no hangover effect. As with other hypnotics they should not be used for long-term treatment.

ZOLPIDEM TARTRATE
Indications: insomnia (short-term use)
Cautions: depression, history of drug or alcohol abuse, hepatic impairment (reduce dose, avoid if severe); renal impairment; elderly; avoid prolonged use (and abrupt withdrawal thereafter); **interactions:** Appendix 1 (anxiolytics and hypnotics)
DRIVING. Drowsiness may persist the next day and affect performance of skilled tasks (e.g. driving); effects of alcohol enhanced
Contra-indications: obstructive sleep apnoea, acute pulmonary insufficiency, respiratory depression, myasthenia gravis, severe hepatic impairment, psychotic illness, pregnancy and breast-feeding
Side-effects: diarrhoea, nausea, vomiting, vertigo, dizziness, headache, drowsiness, asthenia; dependence, memory disturbances, nightmares, nocturnal restlessness, depression, confusion, perceptual disturbances or diplopia, tremor, ataxia, falls reported
Dose: 10 mg at bedtime; ELDERLY (or debilitated) 5 mg; CHILD not recommended

Stilnoct® (Sanofi-Synthelabo) PoM
Tablets, both f/c, zolpidem tartrate 5 mg, net price
28-tab pack = £3.08; 10 mg, 28-tab pack = £4.48.
Label: 19

ZOPICLONE

Indications: insomnia (short-term use)
Cautions: hepatic (avoid if severe) and renal
impairment (Appendixes 2 and 3); elderly; history of drug abuse, psychiatric illness; avoid prolonged use (and abrupt withdrawal thereafter);
interactions: Appendix 1 (anxiolytics and hypnotics)
DRIVING. Drowsiness may persist the next day and affect
performance of skilled tasks (e.g. driving); effects of
alcohol enhanced
Contra-indications: myasthenia gravis, respiratory failure, severe sleep apnoea syndrome,
severe hepatic impairment; pregnancy and breast-
feeding
Side-effects: bitter or metallic taste; gastro-intestinal disturbances including nausea and vomiting,
dry mouth; irritability, confusion, depressed
mood; drowsiness, dizziness, lightheadedness,
and incoordination, headache; dependence;
hypersensitivity reactions reported (including
urticaria and rashes); hallucinations, nightmares,
amnesia, and behavioural disturbances (including
aggression) reported
Dose: 7.5 mg at bedtime; ELDERLY initially 3.75 mg
at bedtime increased if necessary; CHILD not recommended

Zopiclone (Non-proprietary) PoM
Tablets, zopiclone 3.75 mg, net price 28-tab pack =
£3.08; 7.5 mg, 28-tab pack = £4.59. Label: 19
Available from Cox, Generics, Norton, Opus (*Zileze®*)
Zimovane® (Rhône-Poulenc Rorer) PoM
Tablets, f/c, zopiclone 3.75 mg (*Zimovane® LS*,
blue), net price 28-tab pack = £3.08; 7.5 mg, 28-
tab pack = £4.48. Label: 19

Chloral and derivatives

Chloral hydrate and derivatives were formerly
popular hypnotics for children (but the use of hypnotics in children is not usually justified). There is
no convincing evidence that they are particularly
useful in the elderly and their role as hypnotics is
now very limited. **Triclofos** causes fewer gastro-
intestinal disturbances than chloral hydrate.

CHLORAL HYDRATE

Indications: insomnia (short-term use)
Cautions: respiratory disease, history of drug or
alcohol abuse, marked personality disorder;
reduce dose in elderly and debilitated; avoid prolonged use (and abrupt withdrawal thereafter);
avoid contact with skin and mucous membranes;
interactions: Appendix 1 (anxiolytics and hypnotics)
DRIVING. Drowsiness may persist the next day and affect
performance of skilled tasks (e.g. driving); effects of
alcohol enhanced
Contra-indications: cardiac disease, gastritis,
hepatic or renal impairment; pregnancy and
breast-feeding; not recommended in porphyria

Side-effects: gastric irritation (nausea and vomiting reported), abdominal distention and flatulence; also vertigo, ataxia, staggering gait, rashes,
headache, light headedness, malaise, ketonuria,
excitement, nightmares, delirium (especially in
the elderly), eosinophilia, reduction in white cell
count; dependence (may be associated with gastritis and renal damage) on prolonged use
Dose: insomnia, 0.5–1 g (max. 2 g) with plenty of
water at bedtime; CHILD 30–50 mg/kg up to a
max. single dose of 1 g

Chloral Mixture, BP PoM
(Chloral Oral Solution)
Mixture, chloral hydrate 500 mg/5 mL in a suitable
vehicle. Extemporaneous preparations should be
recently prepared according to the following formula: chloral hydrate 1 g, syrup 2 mL, water to
10 mL. Net price 100 mL = 43p. Label: 19, 27
Dose: 5–20 mL; CHILD 1–5 years 2.5–5 mL, 6–12 years
5–10 mL, taken well diluted with water at bedtime

Chloral Elixir, Paediatric, BP PoM
(Chloral Oral Solution, Paediatric)
Elixir, chloral hydrate 4% in a suitable vehicle
with a blackcurrant flavour. Extemporaneous
preparations should be recently prepared according to the following formula: chloral hydrate
200 mg, water 0.1 mL, blackcurrant syrup 1 mL,
syrup to 5 mL. Net price 100 mL = 95p. Label: 1,
27
Dose: up to 1 year 5 mL, taken well diluted with water at
bedtime

Welldorm® (S&N Hlth.) PoM
Tablets, blue-purple, f/c, cloral betaine 707 mg
(≡ chloral hydrate 414 mg). Net price 30-tab pack
= £2.43. Label: 19, 27
Dose: 1–2 tablets with water or milk at bedtime, max. 5
tablets (2 g chloral hydrate) daily
Elixir, red, chloral hydrate 143 mg/5 mL. Net price
150-mL pack = £2.05. Label: 19, 27
Dose: 15–45 mL (0.4–1.3 g chloral hydrate) with water
or milk, at bedtime, max. 70 mL (2 g chloral hydrate)
daily; CHILD 1–1.75 mL/kg (30–50 mg/kg chloral
hydrate), max. 35 mL (1 g chloral hydrate) daily

TRICLOFOS SODIUM

Indications: insomnia (short-term use)
Cautions: see Chloral Hydrate
Contra-indications: see Chloral Hydrate
Side-effects: see Chloral Hydrate, less gastric irri-
tation
Dose: see under preparation below

Triclofos Oral Solution, BP PoM
(Triclofos Elixir)
Oral solution, triclofos sodium 500 mg/5 mL. Net
price 100 mL = £11.54. Label: 19
Available from Norton
Dose: 10–20 mL (1–2 g triclofos sodium) at bedtime;
CHILD up to 1 year 25–30 mg/kg, 1–5 years 2.5–5 mL
(250–500 mg triclofos sodium), 6–12 years 5–10 mL
(0.5–1 g triclofos sodium)

> denotes preparations that are considered to
> be less suitable for prescribing (see p. vi)

Clomethiazole

Clomethiazole (chlormethiazole) may be a useful hypnotic for elderly patients because of its freedom from hangover but, as with all hypnotics, routine administration is undesirable and dependence occurs. It is indicated for use as a hypnotic only in the elderly (and for *very short-term use* in younger adults to attenuate alcohol withdrawal symptoms, see section 4.10).

Clomethiazole is licensed for use as an intravenous infusion to maintain sleep during surgery carried out under regional anaesthesia, but is no longer used for this purpose.

CLOMETHIAZOLE
(Chlormethiazole)

Indications: see under Dose; status epilepticus (section 4.8.2); alcohol withdrawal (also section 4.10); sedation during regional anaesthesia; eclampsia, see product literature

Cautions: cardiac and respiratory disease (confusional state may indicate hypoxia); history of drug abuse; marked personality disorder; elderly; excessive sedation may occur (particularly with higher doses); hepatic impairment (especially if severe since sedation can mask hepatic coma); renal impairment; avoid prolonged use (and abrupt withdrawal thereafter); **interactions:** Appendix 1 (anxiolytics and hypnotics).

SPECIAL CAUTIONS FOR INTRAVENOUS INFUSION. Resuscitation facilities must be available; maintain clear airway (risk of mechanical obstruction in deep sedation); *rapid infusion* to be given only under direct medical supervision (risk of apnoea and hypotension—special care in those susceptible to cerebral or cardiac complications, e.g. elderly); during *continuous infusion* sleep induced may lapse into deep unconsciousness and patient must be kept under close and constant observation; if patient becomes unconscious, stop infusion, secure airway, assist respiration by giving oxygen, using artificial ventilation if necessary—on recovery of consciousness, restart infusion at a slower rate; *prolonged infusion* may lead to accumulation and delay recovery, may also cause electrolyte imbalance (infusion contains Na⁺ 32 mmol/litre and no other electrolytes)

DRIVING. Drowsiness may persist the next day and affect performance of skilled tasks (e.g. driving); effects of alcohol enhanced

Contra-indications: acute pulmonary insufficiency; alcohol-dependent patients who continue to drink

Side-effects: nasal congestion and irritation (increased nasopharyngeal and bronchial secretions), conjunctival irritation, headache; rarely, paradoxical excitement, confusion, dependence, gastro-intestinal disturbances, rash, urticaria, bullous eruption, anaphylaxis, alterations in liver enzymes; on *intravenous infusion*, localised thrombophlebitis, tachycardia and transient fall in blood pressure (apnoea and hypotension on rapid infusion, see Cautions)

Dose: *by mouth*, severe insomnia in the elderly (short-term use), 1–2 capsules (*or* 5–10 mL syrup) at bedtime; CHILD not recommended

Restlessness and agitation in the elderly, 1 capsule (*or* 5 mL syrup) 3 times daily

Alcohol withdrawal, initially 2–4 capsules, if necessary repeated after some hours;

day 1 (first 24 hours), 9–12 capsules in 3–4 divided doses;

day 2, 6–8 capsules in 3–4 divided doses;

day 3, 4–6 capsules in 3–4 divided doses; then gradually reduced over days 4–6; total treatment for not more than 9 days

Note. For an equivalent therapeutic effect 1 capsule ≡ 5 mL syrup

By intravenous infusion, acute alcohol withdrawal, when oral administration not practicable, as a 0.8% solution of clomethiazole edisilate, initially 3–7.5 mL (24–60 mg)/minute until shallow sleep induced (from which patient can be easily awakened) then reduced to 0.5–1 mL (4–8 mg)/minute to achieve lowest possible rate to maintain shallow sleep and adequate spontaneous respiration; urgent deep sedation (direct medical supervision only) 40–100 mL (320–800 mg) over 3–5 minutes then reduced to maintenance as indicated above

IMPORTANT. See special cautions for intravenous infusion under Cautions (above)

Heminevrin® (Astra) [PoM]

Capsules, grey-brown, clomethiazole base 192 mg in an oily basis. Net price 60-cap pack = £4.34. Label: 19

Syrup, sugar-free, clomethiazole edisilate 250 mg/5 mL. Net price 300-mL pack = £3.63. Label: 19

Intravenous infusion 0.8%, clomethiazole edisilate 8 mg/mL. Net price 500-mL bottle = £5.12

Antihistamines

Some **antihistamines** such as diphenhydramine (section 3.4.1) and promethazine are on sale to the public for occasional insomnia; their prolonged duration of action may often lead to drowsiness the following day. The sedative effect of antihistamines may diminish after a few days of continued treatment; antihistamines are associated with headache, psychomotor impairment and antimuscarinic effects.

Promethazine is also popular for use in children, but the use of hypnotics in children is not usually justified.

PROMETHAZINE HYDROCHLORIDE

Indications: night sedation and insomnia (short-term use); other indications (section 3.4.1, section 4.6)

Cautions: section 3.4.1

Contra-indications: section 3.4.1

Side-effects: section 3.4.1

Dose: *by mouth,* 25 mg at bedtime increased to 50 mg if necessary; CHILD under 2 years not recommended, 2–5 years 15–20 mg, 5–10 years 20–25 mg, at bedtime

Preparations
Section 3.4.1

◢ denotes preparations that are considered to be less suitable for prescribing (see p. vi)

Alcohol

Alcohol is a poor hypnotic because its diuretic action interferes with sleep during the latter part of the night. With chronic use, alcohol disturbs sleep patterns and causes insomnia; **interactions:** Appendix 1 (alcohol).

4.1.2   Anxiolytics

Benzodiazepine anxiolytics can be effective in alleviating definite anxiety states and they are widely prescribed. Although there has been a tendency to prescribe these drugs to almost anyone with stress-related symptoms, unhappiness, or minor physical disease, their use in many situations is unjustified. In particular, they are not appropriate for treating depression, phobic or obsessional states, or chronic psychosis. In bereavement, psychological adjustment may be inhibited by benzodiazepines. In children anxiolytic treatment should be used only to relieve acute anxiety (and related insomnia) caused by fear (e.g. before surgery).

Anxiolytic treatment should be limited to the lowest possible dose for the shortest possible time (see CSM advice, section 4.1). Dependence is particularly likely in patients with a history of alcohol or drug abuse and in patients with marked personality disorders.

Anxiolytics, particularly the benzodiazepines, have been termed 'minor tranquillisers'. This term is misleading because not only do they differ markedly from the antipsychotic drugs ('major tranquillisers') but their use is by no means minor. Antipsychotics, in low doses, are also sometimes used in severe anxiety for their sedative action but long-term use should be avoided in view of a possible risk of tardive dyskinesia (section 4.2.1). The use of antihistamines (e.g. hydroxyzine, section 3.4.1) for their sedative effect in anxiety is not considered to be appropriate.

Benzodiazepines

Benzodiazepines are indicated for the *short-term relief of severe anxiety* but long-term use should be avoided (see p. 163). Diazepam, alprazolam, bromazepam, chlordiazepoxide, clobazam, and clorazepate have a sustained action. Shorter-acting compounds such as **lorazepam** and **oxazepam** may be preferred in patients with hepatic impairment but they carry a greater risk of withdrawal symptoms.

Diazepam or lorazepam are very occasionally administered intravenously for the *control of panic attacks*. This route is the most rapid but the procedure is not without risk (section 4.8.2) and should be used only when alternative measures have failed. The intramuscular route has no advantage over the oral route.

For guidelines on benzodiazepine withdrawal, see p. 163.

DIAZEPAM

Indications: short-term use in anxiety or insomnia, adjunct in acute alcohol withdrawal; status epilepticus (section 4.8.2); febrile convulsions (section 4.8.3); muscle spasm (section 10.2.2); perioperative use (section 15.1.4.1)

Cautions: respiratory disease, muscle weakness (special care in myasthenia gravis), history of drug or alcohol abuse, marked personality disorder, pregnancy and breast-feeding (Appendixes 4 and 5); reduce dose in elderly and debilitated, and in hepatic impairment (avoid if severe, Appendix 2), renal impairment (Appendix 3); avoid prolonged use (and abrupt withdrawal thereafter); special precautions for intravenous injection (section 4.8.2); porphyria (section 9.8.2); **interactions:** Appendix 1 (anxiolytics and hypnotics)

DRIVING. Drowsiness may affect performance of skilled tasks (e.g. driving); effects of alcohol enhanced

Contra-indications: respiratory depression; acute pulmonary insufficiency; sleep apnoea syndrome; severe hepatic impairment; not for phobic or obsessional states, not for chronic psychosis; should not be used alone in depression or in anxiety with depression; myasthenia gravis

Side-effects: drowsiness and lightheadedness the next day; confusion and ataxia (especially in the elderly); amnesia may occur; dependence; paradoxical increase in aggression (see also section 4.1); muscle weakness; *occasionally:* headache, vertigo, hypotension, salivation changes, gastrointestinal disturbances, rashes, visual disturbances, dysarthria, tremor, changes in libido, incontinence, urinary retention; blood disorders and jaundice reported; skin reactions; on intravenous injection, pain, thrombophlebitis, and rarely apnoea; raised liver enzymes; **overdosage:** see Emergency Treatment of Poisoning, p. 24

Dose: *by mouth,* anxiety, 2 mg 3 times daily increased if necessary to 15–30 mg daily in divided doses; ELDERLY (or debilitated) half adult dose

Insomnia associated with anxiety, 5–15 mg at bedtime

CHILD night terrors and somnambulism, 1–5 mg at bedtime

By intramuscular injection or slow intravenous injection (into a large vein, at a rate of not more than 5 mg/minute), for severe acute anxiety, control of acute panic attacks, and acute alcohol withdrawal, 10 mg, repeated if necessary after not less than 4 hours

Note. Only use intramuscular route when oral and intravenous routes not possible; special precautions for intravenous injection see section 4.8.2

By intravenous infusion—section 4.8.2

By rectum as rectal solution, acute anxiety and agitation, 500 micrograms/kg repeated after 12 hours as required; ELDERLY 250 micrograms/kg; CHILD not recommended

CHILD febrile convulsions, see p. 234

By rectum as suppositories, anxiety when oral route not appropriate, 10–30 mg (higher dose divided); dose form not appropriate for less than 10 mg

Diazepam (Non-proprietary) PoM
Tablets, diazepam 2 mg, net price 20 =14p; 5 mg, 20 = 23p; 10 mg, 20 =35p. Label: 2 *or* 19
Available from APS, Cox, DDSA (*Tensium* NHS), Norton, Ranbaxy (*Rimapam* NHS), Roche (*Valium* NHS)
Oral solution, diazepam 2 mg/5 mL, net price 100 mL = £2.28. Label: 2 *or* 19
Available from Cox, Lagap (*Dialar* NHS)
Strong oral solution, diazepam 5 mg/5 mL, net price 100-mL pack = £3.07. Label: 2 *or* 19 NHS
Available from Lagap (*Dialar* NHS)
Injection (solution), diazepam 5 mg/mL. Do not dilute (except for intravenous infusion). Net price 2-mL amp = 25p
Available from CP, Roche (*Valium*), Phoenix
Injection (emulsion), diazepam 5 mg/mL. For intravenous injection or infusion. Net price 2-mL amp = 76p
Available from Dumex (*Diazemuls*)

Rectal tubes (= rectal solution), diazepam 2 mg/mL, net price 1.25-mL (2.5-mg) tube = 90p, 2.5-mL (5-mg) tube = £1.27; 4 mg/mL, 2.5-mL (10-mg) tube = £1.62, 5-mL (20-mg) tube = £2.92
Available from CP (*Diazepam Rectubes®* 2.5 mg, 5 mg, 10 mg, 20 mg), Dumex (*Stesolid®* 5 mg, 10 mg), Lagap
Suppositories, diazepam 10 mg, net price 6 = £6.51. Label: 2 *or* 19
Available from Sinclair (*Valclair®*)

ALPRAZOLAM

Indications: anxiety (short-term use)
Cautions: see under Diazepam
Contra-indications: see under Diazepam
Side-effects: see under Diazepam
Dose: 250–500 micrograms 3 times daily (elderly or debilitated 250 micrograms 2–3 times daily), increased if necessary to a total of 3 mg daily; CHILD not recommended

Xanax® (Pharmacia & Upjohn) NHS PoM
Tablets, both scored, alprazolam 250 micrograms, net price 60-tab pack = £2.75; 500 micrograms (pink), 60-tab pack = £5.27. Label: 2

BROMAZEPAM

Indications: anxiety (short-term use)
Cautions: see under Diazepam
Contra-indications: see under Diazepam
Side-effects: see under Diazepam
Dose: 3–18 mg daily in divided doses; ELDERLY (or debilitated) half adult dose; max. (in exceptional circumstances in hospitalised patients) 60 mg daily in divided doses; CHILD not recommended

Lexotan® (Roche) NHS PoM
Tablets, both scored, bromazepam 1.5 mg (lilac), net price 60-tab pack = £5.47; 3 mg (pink), 60-tab pack = £6.93. Label: 2

CHLORDIAZEPOXIDE

Indications: anxiety (short-term use); adjunct in acute alcohol withdrawal (section 4.10)
Cautions: see under Diazepam
Contra-indications: see under Diazepam
Side-effects: see under Diazepam
Dose: anxiety, 10 mg 3 times daily increased if necessary to 60–100 mg daily in divided doses; ELDERLY (or debilitated) half adult dose; CHILD not recommended
Note. The doses stated above refer equally to chlordiazepoxide and to its hydrochloride

Chlordiazepoxide (Non-proprietary) PoM
Capsules, chlordiazepoxide hydrochloride 5 mg, net price 20 = 81p; 10 mg, 20 = £1.17. Label: 2
Various strengths available from APS, Cox, DDSA (*Tropium®* NHS), Hillcross, ICN (*Librium®* NHS), Lagap
Chlordiazepoxide Hydrochloride (Non-proprietary) PoM
Tablets, chlordiazepoxide hydrochloride 5 mg, net price 20 = 79p; 10 mg, 20 = £1.09; 25 mg, 20 = 70p. Label: 2

CLORAZEPATE DIPOTASSIUM

Indications: anxiety (short-term use)
Cautions: see under Diazepam
Contra-indications: see under Diazepam
Side-effects: see under Diazepam
Dose: 7.5–22.5 mg daily in 2–3 divided doses *or* a single dose of 15 mg at bedtime; ELDERLY (or debilitated) half adult dose; CHILD not recommended

Tranxene® (Boehringer Ingelheim) NHS PoM
Capsules, clorazepate dipotassium 7.5 mg (maroon/grey), net price 20-cap pack = £2.66; 15 mg (pink/grey), 20-cap pack = £2.78. Label: 2 *or* 19

LORAZEPAM

Indications: short-term use in anxiety or insomnia; status epilepticus (section 4.8.2); peri-operative (section 15.1.4.1)
Cautions: see under Diazepam; short acting
Contra-indications: see under Diazepam
Side-effects: see under Diazepam
Dose: *by mouth*, anxiety, 1–4 mg daily in divided doses; ELDERLY (or debilitated) half adult dose
Insomnia associated with anxiety, 1–2 mg at bedtime; CHILD not recommended
By intramuscular or slow intravenous injection (into a large vein), acute panic attacks, 25–30 micrograms/kg, repeated every 6 hours if necessary; CHILD not recommended
Note. Only use intramuscular route when oral and intravenous routes not possible

Lorazepam (Non-proprietary) PoM
Tablets, lorazepam 1 mg, net price 20 = 27p; 2.5 mg, 20 = 39p. Label: 2 *or* 19
Available from APS, CP, Genus, Norton, Wyeth (*Ativan®* NHS)
Injection, lorazepam 4 mg/mL. Net price 1-mL amp = 40p
For intramuscular injection it should be diluted with an equal volume of water for injections or physiological saline (but only use when oral and intravenous routes not possible)
Available from Wyeth (*Ativan®*)

OXAZEPAM

Indications: anxiety (short-term use)
Cautions: see under Diazepam; short acting
Contra-indications: see under Diazepam
Side-effects: see under Diazepam
Dose: anxiety, 15–30 mg (elderly or debilitated 10–20 mg) 3–4 times daily; CHILD not recommended
Insomnia associated with anxiety, 15–25 mg (max. 50 mg) at bedtime; CHILD not recommended

Oxazepam (Non-proprietary) PoM
Tablets, oxazepam 10 mg, net price 20 = 25p; 15 mg, 20 = 24p; 30 mg, 20 = 42p. Label: 2
Available from most generic manufacturers

Buspirone

Buspirone is thought to act at specific serotonin ($5HT_{1A}$) receptors. Response to treatment may take up to 2 weeks. It does not alleviate the symptoms of benzodiazepine withdrawal. Therefore a patient taking a benzodiazepine still needs to have the benzodiazepine withdrawn gradually; it is advisable to do this before starting buspirone. The dependence and abuse liability of buspirone has not yet been established.

BUSPIRONE HYDROCHLORIDE

Indications: anxiety (short-term use)
Cautions: does not alleviate benzodiazepine withdrawal (see notes above); history of hepatic or renal impairment; **interactions:** Appendix 1 (anxiolytics and hypnotics)
DRIVING. May affect performance of skilled tasks (e.g. driving); effects of alcohol may be enhanced
Contra-indications: epilepsy, severe hepatic or renal impairment, pregnancy and breast-feeding

Side-effects: nausea, dizziness, headache, nervousness, lightheadedness, excitement; rarely tachycardia, palpitations, chest pain, drowsiness, confusion, dry mouth, fatigue, and sweating

Dose: initially 5 mg 2–3 times daily, increased as necessary every 2–3 days; usual range 15–30 mg daily in divided doses; max. 45 mg daily; CHILD not recommended

Buspirone Hydrochloride (Non-proprietary) PoM
Tablets, buspirone hydrochloride 5 mg, net price 100-tab pack = £31.20; 10 mg, 100-tab pack = £46.80. Counselling, driving
Available from Bartholomew Rhodes

Buspar® (Bristol-Myers) PoM
Tablets, buspirone hydrochloride 5 mg, net price 126-tab pack = £39.31; 10 mg, 100-tab pack = £46.80. Counselling, driving

---

Beta-blockers

Beta-blockers (e.g. propranolol, oxprenolol) (section 2.4) do not affect psychological symptoms, such as worry, tension, and fear, but they do reduce autonomic symptoms, such as palpitations and tremor; they do not reduce non-autonomic symptoms, such as muscle tension. Beta-blockers are therefore indicated for patients with predominantly somatic symptoms; this, in turn, may prevent the onset of worry and fear. Patients with predominantly psychological symptoms may obtain no benefit.

Meprobamate

Meprobamate is **less effective** than the benzodiazepines, more hazardous in overdosage, and can also induce dependence. It is **not** recommended.

MEPROBAMATE ◪

Indications: short-term use in anxiety, but see notes above

Cautions: respiratory disease, muscle weakness, epilepsy (may induce seizures), history of drug or alcohol abuse, marked personality disorder, pregnancy; elderly and debilitated; hepatic and renal impairment; avoid prolonged use, abrupt withdrawal may precipitate convulsions; **interactions:** Appendix 1 (anxiolytics and hypnotics)
DRIVING. Drowsiness may affect performance of skilled tasks (e.g. driving); effects of alcohol enhanced

Contra-indications: acute pulmonary insufficiency; respiratory depression; porphyria (section 9.8.2); breast-feeding

Side-effects: see under Diazepam, but incidence greater and drowsiness most common side-effect; also gastro-intestinal disturbances, hypotension, paraesthesia, weakness, CNS effects including headache, paradoxical excitement, disturbances of vision; rarely agranulocytosis and rashes

Dose: 400 mg 3–4 times daily; elderly patients half adult dose or less; CHILD not recommended

Meprobamate (Non-proprietary) CD ◪
Tablets, scored, meprobamate 400 mg. Net price 84-tab pack = £5.62. Label: 2
Available from Genus

Equagesic® CD ◪
Section 4.7.1

4.1.3   Barbiturates

The intermediate-acting **barbiturates** have a place only in the treatment of severe intractable insomnia in patients **already taking** barbiturates; they should be **avoided** in the elderly. The long-acting barbiturates, phenobarbital and methylphenobarbital, are still sometimes of value in epilepsy (section 4.8.1) but their use as sedatives is unjustified. The very short-acting barbiturate thiopental is used in anaesthesia (section 15.1.1).

BARBITURATES

Indications: severe intractable insomnia **only** in patients already taking barbiturates; see also notes above

Cautions: avoid use where possible; dependence and tolerance readily occur; abrupt withdrawal may precipitate serious withdrawal syndrome (rebound insomnia, anxiety, tremor, dizziness, nausea, convulsions, delirium, and death); repeated doses are cumulative and may lead to excessive sedation; respiratory disease, renal disease, hepatic impairment; **interactions:** Appendix 1 (barbiturates and primidone)
DRIVING. Drowsiness may persist the next day and affect performance of skilled tasks (e.g. driving); effects of alcohol enhanced

Contra-indications: insomnia caused by pain; porphyria (section 9.8.2), pregnancy, breast-feeding; children, young adults, elderly and debilitated patients, also patients with history of drug or alcohol abuse

Side-effects: include hangover with drowsiness, dizziness, ataxia, respiratory depression, hypersensitivity reactions, headache, particularly in elderly; paradoxical excitement and confusion occasionally precede sleep; **overdosage:** see Emergency Treatment of Poisoning, p. 24

Dose: see under preparations below

Amytal® (Flynn) CD ◪
Tablets, amobarbital (amylobarbitone) 50 mg, net price 20 = £1.84. Label: 19
Dose: 100–200 mg at bedtime (**important:** but see also contra-indications)

Sodium Amytal® (Flynn) CD
Capsules ◪, both blue, amobarbital (amylobarbitone) sodium 60 mg, net price 20 = £3.43; 200 mg, 20 = £6.75. Label: 19
Dose: 60–200 mg at bedtime (**important:** but see also contra-indications)

Injection, powder for reconstitution, amobarbital (amylobarbitone) sodium. Net price 500-mg vial = £28.83. For specialised use in procedures in **expert epilepsy centres only**
Dose: by deep intramuscular injection into large muscle, preferably gluteal, (max. 5 mL at any one site) or by slow intravenous injection (max. 50 mg/minute), 0.25–1 g; max. single dose, intramuscular 500 mg, intravenous 1 g

Soneryl® (Concord) CD ◪
Tablets, pink, scored, butobarbital (butobarbitone) 100 mg. Net price 56-tab pack = £10.65. Label: 19
Dose: 100–200 mg at bedtime (**important:** but see also contra-indications)

◪ denotes preparations that are considered to be less suitable for prescribing (see p. vi)

■ Preparations containing secobarbital (quinal-barbitone)

Note. Secobarbital (quinalbarbitone) is in schedule 2 of the Misuse of Drugs Regulations 1985; receipt and supply must therefore be recorded in the CD register.

Seconal Sodium® (Flynn) CD ▭

Capsules, both orange, secobarbital (quinalbarbitone) sodium 50 mg, net price 20 = £5.30; 100 mg, 20 = £6.96. Label: 19

Dose: 100 mg at bedtime (**important:** but see also contra-indications)

Tuinal® (Flynn) CD ▭

Capsules, orange/blue, a mixture of amobarbital (amylobarbitone) sodium 50 mg, secobarbital (quinalbarbitone) sodium 50 mg. Net price 20 = £3.88. Label: 19

Dose: 1–2 capsules at bedtime (**important:** but see also contra-indications)

Note. Prescriptions need only specify 'Tuinal capsules'

4.2 Drugs used in psychoses and related disorders

4.2.1 Antipsychotic drugs
4.2.2 Antipsychotic depot injections
4.2.3 Antimanic drugs

Advice of Royal College of Psychiatrists on doses above BNF upper limit

Unless otherwise stated, doses in the BNF are licensed doses—any higher dose is therefore **unlicensed** (for an explanation of the significance of this, see p. 1).

1. Consider alternative approaches including adjuvant therapy and newer or atypical neuroleptics such as clozapine.
2. Bear in mind risk factors, including obesity—particular caution is indicated in older patients especially those over 70.
3. Consider potential for drug interactions—see **interactions:** Appendix 1 (antipsychotics).
4. Carry out ECG to exclude untoward abnormalities such as prolonged QT interval; repeat ECG periodically and reduce dose if prolonged QT interval or other adverse abnormality develops.
5. Increase dose slowly and not more often than once weekly.
6. Carry out regular pulse, blood pressure, and temperature checks; ensure that patient maintains adequate fluid intake.
7. Consider high-dose therapy to be for limited period and review regularly; abandon if no improvement after 3 months (return to standard dosage).

Important: When prescribing an antipsychotic for administration on an emergency basis, the intramuscular dose should be **lower** than the corresponding oral dose (owing to absence of first-pass effect), particularly if the patient is very active (increased blood flow to muscle considerably increases the rate of absorption). The prescription should specify the dose for **each route** and should **not** imply that the same dose can be given by mouth or by intramuscular injection. The dose of antipsychotic for emergency use should be reviewed at least **daily.**

4.2.1 Antipsychotic drugs

Antipsychotic drugs are also known as 'neuroleptics' and (misleadingly) as 'major tranquillisers'. Antipsychotic drugs generally tranquillise without impairing consciousness and without causing paradoxical excitement but they should not be regarded merely as tranquillisers. For conditions such as schizophrenia the tranquillising effect is of secondary importance.

In the short term they are used to quieten disturbed patients whatever the underlying psychopathology, which may be schizophrenia, brain damage, mania, toxic delirium, or agitated depression. Antipsychotic drugs are used to alleviate severe anxiety but this too should be a short-term measure. Some antipsychotic drugs (e.g. chlorpromazine, thioridazine, flupentixol) also have some antidepressant effect.

SCHIZOPHRENIA. Antipsychotic drugs relieve florid psychotic symptoms such as thought disorder, hallucinations, and delusions, and prevent relapse. Although they are usually less effective in apathetic withdrawn patients, they sometimes appear to have an activating influence. For example, haloperidol may restore an acutely ill schizophrenic, who was previously withdrawn or even mute and akinetic, to normal activity and social behaviour. Patients with acute schizophrenia generally respond better than those with chronic symptoms.

Long-term treatment of a patient with a definite diagnosis of schizophrenia may be necessary even after the first episode of illness in order to prevent the manifest illness from becoming chronic. Withdrawal of drug treatment requires careful surveillance because the patient who appears well on medication may suffer a disastrous relapse if treatment is withdrawn inappropriately. In addition the need for continuation of treatment may not become immediately evident because relapse is often delayed for several weeks after cessation of treatment.

Antipsychotic drugs are considered to act by interfering with dopaminergic transmission in the brain by blocking dopamine receptors, which may give rise to the extrapyramidal effects described below, and also to hyperprolactinaemia. Antipsychotic drugs may also affect cholinergic, alpha-adrenergic, histaminergic, and serotonergic receptors.

SIDE-EFFECTS. Extrapyramidal symptoms are the most troublesome. They are caused most frequently by the piperazine phenothiazines (fluphenazine, perphenazine, prochlorperazine, and trifluoperazine), the butyrophenones (benperidol, droperidol and haloperidol), and the depot preparations. They are easy to recognise but cannot be accurately predicted because they depend partly on the dose and partly on the type of drug, and on patient susceptibility. They consist of *parkinsonian symptoms* (including tremor) which may occur gradually, *dystonia* (abnormal face and body movements) which may appear after only a few doses, *akathisia* (restlessness) which may resemble an exacerbation of the condition being treated, and *tardive dyskinesia* (which usually takes longer to develop).

Parkinsonian symptoms remit if the drug is withdrawn and may be suppressed by the administration of **antimuscarinic** drugs (section 4.9.2). Routine administration of such drugs is **not** justified as not all patients are affected and because tardive dyskinesia may be unmasked or worsened by them. Furthermore, these drugs are sometimes abused for their mood-altering effects. Tardive dyskinesia is of particular concern because it may be irreversible on withdrawing therapy and treatment is usually ineffective. It occurs fairly frequently in patients (especially the elderly) on long-term therapy and with high dosage, and the treatment of such patients must be carefully and regularly reviewed. Tardive dyskinesia may also occur occasionally after short-term treatment with low dosage.

Hypotension and *interference with temperature regulation* are dose-related side-effects and are liable to cause dangerous falls and hypothermia in the elderly; very serious consideration should be given before prescribing these drugs for patients over 70 years of age.

Neuroleptic malignant syndrome (hyperthermia, fluctuating level of consciousness, muscular rigidity and autonomic dysfunction with pallor, tachycardia, labile blood pressure, sweating, and urinary incontinence) is a rare but potentially fatal side-effect of some drugs. Drugs for which it has been reported in the UK include haloperidol, chlorpromazine, and flupentixol decanoate. Discontinuation of drug therapy is essential as there is no proven effective treatment but bromocriptine and dantrolene have been used. The syndrome, which usually lasts for 5–10 days after drug discontinuation, may be unduly prolonged if depot preparations have been used.

Overdosage: see Emergency Treatment of Poisoning, p. 24.

CLASSIFICATION OF ANTIPSYCHOTICS. The **phenothiazine** derivatives can be divided into 3 main groups.

Group 1: chlorpromazine, levomepromazine (methotrimeprazine), and promazine, generally characterised by pronounced sedative effects and moderate antimuscarinic and extrapyramidal side-effects.

Group 2: pericyazine, pipotiazine, and thioridazine, generally characterised by moderate sedative effects, marked antimuscarinic effects, but fewer extrapyramidal side-effects than groups 1 or 3.

Group 3: fluphenazine, perphenazine, prochlorperazine, and trifluoperazine, generally characterised by fewer sedative effects, fewer antimuscarinic effects, but more pronounced extrapyramidal side-effects than groups 1 and 2.

Drugs of other chemical groups tend to resemble the phenothiazines of *group 3*. They include the **butyrophenones** (benperidol, droperidol, and haloperidol); **diphenylbutylpiperidines** (pimozide); **thioxanthenes** (flupentixol and zuclopenthixol); **substituted benzamides** (sulpiride); **oxypertine**; and **loxapine**.

For details of the newer antipsychotic drugs amisulpride, clozapine, olanzapine, quetiapine, risperidone, sertindole, and zotepine, see under Atypical antipsychotics below.

CHOICE. As indicated above, the various drugs differ somewhat in predominant actions and side-effects. Selection is influenced by the degree of sedation required and the patient's susceptibility to extrapyramidal side-effects. However, the differences between antipsychotic drugs are less important than the great variability in patient response; moreover, tolerance to these secondary effects usually develops. The atypical antipsychotics are better tolerated and may be appropriate if extrapyramidal side-effects are a particular concern (see under Atypical antipsychotics, below). Clozapine is used

for schizophrenia when other antipsychotics are ineffective or not tolerated.

Prescribing of more than one antipsychotic at the same time is **not** recommended; it may constitute a hazard and there is no significant evidence that side-effects are minimised.

Chlorpromazine is still widely used despite the wide range of adverse effects associated with it. It has a marked sedating effect and is useful for treating violent patients without causing stupor. Agitated states in the elderly can be controlled without confusion, a dose of 10 to 25 mg once or twice daily usually being adequate.

Flupentixol (flupenthixol) and **pimozide** (see CSM advice p. 176) are less sedating than chlorpromazine.

Sulpiride in high doses controls florid positive symptoms, but in lower doses it has an alerting effect on apathetic withdrawn schizophrenics.

Fluphenazine, haloperidol, and **trifluoperazine** are also of value but their use is limited by the high incidence of extrapyramidal symptoms. Haloperidol may be preferred for the rapid control of hyperactive psychotic states. It is less hypotensive than chlorpromazine and is therefore also popular for agitation in the elderly, despite the high incidence of extrapyramidal side-effects.

Thioridazine was formerly popular for treating the elderly as there is a reduced incidence of extrapyramidal symptoms. However, there is a high incidence of antimuscarinic effects and possibly an increased risk of cardiotoxicity.

Promazine is not sufficiently active by mouth to be used as an antipsychotic drug.

Loxapine causes relatively little sedation; in overdosage it has a high potential for serious neurological and cardiac toxicity.

OTHER USES. Nausea and vomiting (section 4.6), choreas, motor tics (section 4.9.3), and intractable hiccup (see under Chlorpromazine Hydrochloride and under Haloperidol). **Benperidol** is used in deviant antisocial sexual behaviour but its value is not established.

Equivalent doses of oral antipsychotics
These equivalences are intended **only** as an approximate guide; individual dosage instructions should **also** be checked; patients should be carefully monitored after **any** change in medication

Antipsychotic	Daily dose
Chlorpromazine	100 mg
Clozapine	50 mg[1]
Haloperidol	2–3 mg[2]
Loxapine	10–20 mg
Pimozide	2 mg[3]
Risperidone	0.5–1 mg
Sulpiride	200 mg
Thioridazine	100 mg
Trifluoperazine	5 mg

1. The prescribing of clozapine needs to comply with the Clozaril Patient Monitoring Service, see p. 179
2. In specialist psychiatric units where very high doses are required the equivalent dose of haloperidol might be up to 10 mg
3. See also the CSM warning concerning pimozide dose, p. 176

IMPORTANT. These equivalences must **not** be extrapolated beyond the max. dose for the drug.

WITHDRAWAL. Withdrawal of antipsychotic drugs after long-term therapy should always be gradual and closely monitored to avoid the risk of acute withdrawal syndromes or rapid relapse.

DOSAGE. After an initial period of stabilisation, in most patients, the long half-life of antipsychotic drugs allows the total daily oral dose to be given as a single dose. For the advice of The Royal College of Psychiatrists on doses above the BNF upper limit, see p. 171.

CHLORPROMAZINE HYDROCHLORIDE

WARNING. Owing to the risk of contact sensitisation, pharmacists, nurses, and other health workers should avoid direct contact with chlorpromazine; tablets should not be crushed and solutions should be handled with care

Indications: see under Dose; antiemetic in palliative care (section 4.6)

Cautions: cardiovascular and cerebrovascular disease, respiratory disease, parkinsonism, epilepsy (possibly avoid), acute infections, pregnancy, breast-feeding, renal and hepatic impairment (avoid if severe), history of jaundice, leucopenia (blood counts if unexplained infection or fever); hypothyroidism, myasthenia gravis, prostatic hypertrophy, angle-closure glaucoma; caution in elderly particularly in very hot or very cold weather; avoid abrupt withdrawal; patients should remain supine and the blood pressure monitored for 30 minutes after intramuscular injection; **interactions:** Appendix 1 (antipsychotics)

DRIVING. Drowsiness may affect performance of skilled tasks (e.g. driving); effects of alcohol enhanced

Contra-indications: coma caused by CNS depressants; bone-marrow depression; avoid in phaeochromocytoma

Side-effects: extrapyramidal symptoms (reversed by dose reduction or antimuscarinic drugs) and, on prolonged administration, occasionally tardive dyskinesia; hypothermia (occasionally pyrexia), drowsiness, apathy, pallor, nightmares, insomnia, depression, and, more rarely, agitation, EEG changes, convulsions; nasal congestion; antimuscarinic symptoms such as dry mouth, constipation, difficulty with micturition, and blurred vision; cardiovascular symptoms such as hypotension, tachycardia, and arrhythmias; ECG changes; respiratory depression; endocrine effects such as menstrual disturbances, galactorrhoea, gynaecomastia, impotence, and weight gain; sensitivity reactions such as agranulocytosis, leucopenia, leucocytosis, and haemolytic anaemia, photosensitisation (more common with chlorpromazine than with other antipsychotics), contact sensitisation and rashes, jaundice (including cholestatic) and alterations in liver function; neuroleptic malignant syndrome; lupus erythematosus-like syndrome reported; with prolonged high dosage, corneal and lens opacities and purplish pigmentation of the skin, cornea, conjunctiva, and retina; intramuscular injection may be painful, cause hypotension and tachycardia (see Cautions), and give rise to nodule formation; **overdosage:** see Emergency Treatment of Poisoning, p. 24

Dose: *by mouth*,
  Schizophrenia and other psychoses, mania, short-term adjunctive management of severe anxiety, psychomotor agitation, excitement, and violent or dangerously impulsive behaviour initially 25 mg 3 times daily (*or* 75 mg at night), adjusted according to response, to usual maintenance dose of 75–300 mg daily (but up to 1 g daily may be required in psychoses); ELDERLY (or debilitated) third to half adult dose; CHILD (childhood schizophrenia and autism) 1–5 years 500 micrograms/kg every 4–6 hours (max. 40 mg daily); 6–12 years third to half adult dose (max. 75 mg daily)

  Intractable hiccup, 25–50 mg 3–4 times daily

By deep intramuscular injection, (for relief of acute symptoms but see also Cautions and Side-effects), 25–50 mg every 6–8 hours; CHILD, 1–5 years 500 micrograms/kg every 6–8 hours (max. 40 mg daily); 6–12 years 500 micrograms/kg every 6–8 hours (max. 75 mg daily)

  Induction of hypothermia (to prevent shivering), *by deep intramuscular injection*, 25–50 mg every 6–8 hours; CHILD 1–12 years, initially 0.5–1 mg/kg, followed by maintenance 500 micrograms/kg every 4–6 hours

By rectum in suppositories as chlorpromazine base 100 mg every 6–8 hours [unlicensed]

  Note. For equivalent therapeutic effect 100 mg chlorpromazine base given *rectally* as a suppository ≡ 20–25 mg chlorpromazine hydrochloride *by intramuscular injection* ≡ 40–50 mg of chlorpromazine base or hydrochloride *by mouth*

Chlorpromazine (Non-proprietary) ▣PoM▣
Tablets, coated, chlorpromazine hydrochloride 10 mg, net price 20 = 26p; 25 mg, 20 = 31p; 50 mg, 20 = 62p; 100 mg, 20 = £1.03. Label: 2, 11
Available from Antigen, APS, DDSA (*Chloractil®*), Hillcross, Norton
Oral solution, chlorpromazine hydrochloride 25 mg/5 mL, net price 150 mL = £1.34, 100 mg/5 mL, 150 mL = £3.00. Label: 2, 11
Available from Hillcross, Rosemont
Injection, chlorpromazine hydrochloride 25 mg/mL, net price 1-mL amp = 32p; 2-mL amp = 30p
Available from Antigen
Suppositories, chlorpromazine 100 mg. Label: 2, 11
'Special order' [unlicensed] product; contact Martindale or regional hospital manufacturing unit

Largactil® (Hawgreen) ▣PoM▣
Tablets, all off-white, f/c, chlorpromazine hydrochloride 10 mg. Net price 56-tab pack = 71p; 25 mg, 56-tab pack = 98p; 50 mg, 56-tab pack = £2.05; 100 mg, 56-tab pack = £3.81. Label: 2, 11
Syrup, brown, chlorpromazine hydrochloride 25 mg/5 mL. Net price 100-mL pack = £1.11. Label: 2, 11
Suspension forte, orange, sugar-free, chlorpromazine hydrochloride 100 mg (as embonate)/5 mL. Net price 100-mL pack = £2.56. Label: 2, 11
Injection, chlorpromazine hydrochloride 25 mg/mL. Net price 2-mL amp = 67p

---

BENPERIDOL

Indications: control of deviant antisocial sexual behaviour (but see notes above)
Cautions: see under Haloperidol
Contra-indications: see under Haloperidol
Side-effects: see under Haloperidol
Dose: 0.25–1.5 mg daily in divided doses, adjusted according to the response; ELDERLY (or debilitated) initially half adult dose; CHILD not recommended

Anquil® (Janssen-Cilag) PoM
Tablets, benperidol 250 micrograms. Net price
100-tab pack = £26.13. Label: 2

DROPERIDOL

Indications: see under Dose
Cautions: see under Haloperidol
Contra-indications: see under Haloperidol
Side-effects: see under Haloperidol
Dose: *by mouth*, tranquillisation and emergency
control in mania, 5–20 mg repeated every 4–8
hours if necessary (elderly, initially half adult
dose); CHILD, 0.5–1 mg daily
By intramuscular injection, up to 10 mg repeated
every 4–6 hours if necessary (elderly, initially
half adult dose); CHILD, 0.5–1 mg daily
By intravenous injection, 5–15 mg repeated every
4–6 hours if necessary (elderly, initially half adult
dose)
Cancer chemotherapy-induced nausea and vomiting, *by intramuscular or intravenous injection*,
1–10 mg 30 minutes before starting therapy, followed by *continuous intravenous infusion* of 1–
3 mg/hour *or* 1–5 mg *by intramuscular or intravenous injection* every 1–6 hours as necessary;
CHILD *by intramuscular or intravenous injection*,
20–75 micrograms/kg
Premedication, *by intramuscular injection*, up to
10 mg 60 minutes before operation; CHILD 200–
500 micrograms/kg

Droleptan® (Janssen-Cilag) PoM
Tablets, yellow, scored, droperidol 10 mg. Net
price 50-tab pack = £12.30. Label: 2
Oral liquid, sugar-free, droperidol 1 mg/mL. Net
price 100-mL pack (with graduated cap) = £4.47;
500-mL pack = £21.25. Label: 2
Injection, droperidol 5 mg/mL. Net price 2-mL
amp = 90p

FLUPENTIXOL

(Flupenthixol)
Indications: schizophrenia and other psychoses,
particularly with apathy and withdrawal but not
mania or psychomotor hyperactivity; depression,
section 4.3.4
Cautions: see under Chlorpromazine Hydrochloride; avoid in porphyria (section 9.8.2)
Contra-indications: see under Chlorpromazine
Hydrochloride; senile confusional states, excitable and overactive patients
Side-effects: see under Chlorpromazine Hydrochloride but less sedating; extrapyramidal symptoms more frequent (25% of patients)
Dose: psychosis, initially 3–9 mg twice daily
adjusted according to the response; max. 18 mg
daily; ELDERLY (or debilitated) initially quarter to
half adult dose; CHILD not recommended
Depression, see section 4.3.4

Depixol® (Lundbeck) PoM
Tablets, yellow, s/c, flupentixol 3 mg (as dihydrochloride). Net price 20 = £2.99. Label: 2
Depot injection (flupentixol decanoate): section
4.2.2

FLUPHENAZINE HYDROCHLORIDE

Indications: see under Dose
Cautions: see under Chlorpromazine Hydrochloride
Contra-indications: see under Chlorpromazine
Hydrochloride; depression
Side-effects: see under Chlorpromazine Hydrochloride, but less sedating and fewer antimuscarinic or hypotensive symptoms; extrapyramidal
symptoms, particularly dystonic reactions and
akathisia, more frequent
Dose: schizophrenia and other psychoses, mania,
initially 2.5–10 mg daily in 2–3 divided doses,
adjusted according to response to 20 mg daily;
doses above 20 mg daily (10 mg in elderly) only
with special caution; CHILD not recommended
Short-term adjunctive management of severe
anxiety, psychomotor agitation, excitement, and
violent or dangerously impulsive behaviour, initially 1 mg twice daily, increased as necessary to
2 mg twice daily; CHILD not recommended

Moditen® (Sanofi-Synthelabo) PoM
Tablets, all s/c, fluphenazine hydrochloride 1 mg
(pink), net price 20 = £1.06; 2.5 mg (yellow), 20 =
£1.33; 5 mg, 20 = £1.77. Label: 2

Modecate® PoM
Section 4.2.2

HALOPERIDOL

Indications: see under Dose; motor tics, section
4.9.3
Cautions: see under Chlorpromazine Hydrochloride
Contra-indications: see under Chlorpromazine
Hydrochloride; basal ganglia disease
Side-effects: see under Chlorpromazine Hydrochloride but less sedating and fewer antimuscarinic or hypotensive symptoms; pigmentation
and photosensitivity reactions rare; extrapyramidal symptoms, particularly dystonic reactions
and akathisia more frequent especially in thyrotoxic patients; rarely weight loss
Dose: *by mouth*,
Schizophrenia and other psychoses, mania, short-
term adjunctive management of psychomotor agitation, excitement, and violent or dangerously
impulsive behaviour, initially 1.5–3 mg 2–3 times
daily *or* 3–5 mg 2–3 times daily in severely
affected or resistant patients; in resistant schizophrenia up to 100 mg (rarely 120 mg) daily may
be needed; adjusted according to response to lowest effective maintenance dose (as low as 5–
10 mg daily); ELDERLY (or debilitated) initially
half adult dose; CHILD initially 25–
50 micrograms/kg daily (in 2 divided doses) to a
max. of 10 mg; adolescents up to 30 mg daily
(exceptionally 60 mg)
Short-term adjunctive management of severe
anxiety, adults 500 micrograms twice daily;
CHILD not recommended
Intractable hiccup, 1.5 mg 3 times daily adjusted
according to response; CHILD not recommended
By intramuscular injection, 2–10 mg, subsequent
doses being given every 4–8 hours according to
response (up to every hour if necessary) to total
max. 60 mg; severely disturbed patients may
require initial dose of up to 30 mg; CHILD not recommended
Nausea and vomiting, 0.5–2 mg

Haloperidol (Non-proprietary) PoM
Tablets, haloperidol 1.5 mg, net price 20 = 90p; 5 mg, 20 = £2.50; 10 mg, 20 = £4.66; 20 mg, 20 = £8.51. Label: 2

Dozic® (Rosemont) PoM
Oral liquid, sugar-free, haloperidol 1 mg/mL. Net price 100-mL pack = £7.30. Label: 2

Haldol® (Janssen-Cilag) PoM
Tablets, both scored, haloperidol 5 mg (blue), net price 20 = £1.65; 10 mg (yellow), 20 = £3.21. Label: 2
Oral liquid, sugar-free, haloperidol 2 mg/mL. Net price 100-mL pack (with pipette) = £5.08. Label: 2
Injection, haloperidol 5 mg/mL. Net price 1-mL amp = 33p
Depot injection (haloperidol decanoate): section 4.2.2

Serenace® (Baker Norton) PoM
Capsules, green, haloperidol 500 micrograms. Net price 20 = 65p. Label: 2
Tablets, haloperidol 1.5 mg, net price 20 = £1.16; 5 mg (pink), 20 = £3.27; 10 mg (pale pink), 20 = £5.87; 20 mg (dark pink), 20 = £10.58. Label: 2
Oral liquid, sugar-free, haloperidol 2 mg/mL. Net price 100-mL pack = £8.77. Label: 2
Injection, haloperidol 5 mg/mL, net price 1-mL amp = 59p; 10 mg/mL, 2-mL amp = £2.03

LEVOMEPROMAZINE/ METHOTRIMEPRAZINE

Indications: see under Dose
Cautions: see under Chlorpromazine Hydrochloride
Contra-indications: see under Chlorpromazine Hydrochloride
Side-effects: see under Chlorpromazine Hydrochloride but more sedating
ELDERLY. Risk of postural hypotension particularly in patients over 50 years—not recommended for ambulant patients over 50 years unless risk of hypotensive reaction has been assessed
Dose: *by mouth*, schizophrenia, initially 25–50 mg daily in divided doses increased as necessary; bedpatients initially 100–200 mg daily usually in 3 divided doses, increased if necessary to 1 g daily; ELDERLY, see Cautions
Adjunctive treatment in palliative care (including management of pain and associated restlessness, distress, or vomiting), 12.5–50 mg every 4–8 hours
By intramuscular injection or by intravenous injection (by intravenous injection after dilution with an equal volume of sodium chloride 0.9% injection), adjunct in palliative care, 12.5–25 mg (severe agitation up to 50 mg) every 6–8 hours if necessary
By continuous subcutaneous infusion, adjunct in palliative care (via syringe driver), diluted in a suitable volume of sodium chloride 0.9% injection, see Prescribing in Palliative Care, p. 14; CHILD (experience limited), 0.35–3 mg/kg daily

Nozinan® (Link) PoM
Tablets, scored, levomepromazine maleate 25 mg. Net price 20 = £3.41. Label: 2
Injection, levomepromazine hydrochloride 25 mg/mL. Net price 1-mL amp = £1.85

LOXAPINE

Indications: acute and chronic psychoses
Cautions: see under Chlorpromazine Hydrochloride; avoid in porphyria (section 9.8.2)
Contra-indications: see under Chlorpromazine Hydrochloride
Side-effects: see under Chlorpromazine Hydrochloride; nausea and vomiting, weight gain or loss, dyspnoea, ptosis, hyperpyrexia, flushing and headache, paraesthesia, and polydipsia also reported
Dose: initially 20–50 mg daily in 2 divided doses, increased as necessary over 7–10 days to 60–100 mg daily (max. 250 mg) in 2–4 divided doses, then adjusted to usual maintenance dose of 20–100 mg daily; CHILD not recommended

Loxapac® (Lederle) PoM
Capsules, loxapine (as succinate) 10 mg (yellow/green), net price 56-cap pack = £5.33; 25 mg (light green/dark green), 56-cap pack = £10.67; 50 mg (blue/dark green), 28-cap pack = £9.60. Label: 2

OXYPERTINE

Indications: see under Dose
Cautions: see under Chlorpromazine Hydrochloride
Contra-indications: see under Chlorpromazine Hydrochloride
Side-effects: see under Chlorpromazine Hydrochloride, but extrapyramidal symptoms less frequent; agitation and hyperactivity with low doses and sedation with high doses; occasionally photophobia
Dose: schizophrenia and other psychoses, mania, short-term adjunctive management of psychomotor agitation, excitement, and violent or dangerously impulsive behaviour, initially 80–120 mg daily in divided doses adjusted according to the response; max. 300 mg daily; CHILD not recommended
Short-term adjunctive management of severe anxiety, initially 10 mg 3–4 times daily preferably after food; max. 60 mg daily; CHILD not recommended

Oxypertine (Sanofi-Synthelabo) PoM
Capsules, oxypertine 10 mg. Net price 20 = £2.12. Label: 2
Tablets, scored, oxypertine 40 mg. Net price 20 = £6.64. Label: 2

PERICYAZINE
(Periciazine)

Indications: see under Dose
Cautions: see under Chlorpromazine Hydrochloride
Contra-indications: see under Chlorpromazine Hydrochloride
Side-effects: see under Chlorpromazine Hydrochloride, but more sedating; hypotension commonly occurs when treatment initiated

Dose: schizophrenia and other psychoses, initially 75 mg daily in divided doses increased at weekly intervals by steps of 25 mg according to response; usual max. 300 mg daily (elderly initially 15–30 mg daily)

Short-term adjunctive management of severe anxiety, psychomotor agitation, and violent or dangerously impulsive behaviour, initially 15–30 mg (elderly 5–10 mg) daily divided into 2 doses, taking the larger dose at bedtime, adjusted according to response

CHILD (severe mental or behavioural disorders only), initially, 500 micrograms daily for 10-kg child, increased by 1 mg for each additional 5 kg to max. total daily dose of 10 mg; dose may be gradually increased according to response but maintenance should not exceed twice initial dose INFANT under 1 year not recommended

Neulactil® (JHC) PoM

Tablets, all yellow, scored, pericyazine 2.5 mg, net price 84-tab pack = £7.69; 10 mg, 84-tab pack = £20.79. Label: 2

Syrup forte, brown, pericyazine 10 mg/5 mL. Net price 100-mL pack = £10.07. Label: 2

PERPHENAZINE

Indications: see Dose; anti-emetic, section 4.6

Cautions: see under Chlorpromazine Hydrochloride; not indicated for agitation and restlessness in the elderly

Contra-indications: see under Chlorpromazine Hydrochloride

Side-effects: see under Chlorpromazine Hydrochloride, but less sedating; extrapyramidal symptoms, especially dystonia, more frequent, particularly at high dosage

Dose: schizophrenia and other psychoses, mania, short-term adjunctive management of anxiety, severe psychomotor agitation, excitement, and violent or dangerously impulsive behaviour, initially 4 mg 3 times daily adjusted according to the response; max. 24 mg daily; ELDERLY quarter to half adult dose (but see Cautions); CHILD under 14 years not recommended

Fentazin® (Goldshield) PoM

Tablets, both s/c, perphenazine 2 mg, net price 20 = £3.73; 4 mg, 20 = £4.39. Label: 2

PIMOZIDE

Indications: see under Dose

Cautions: see under Chlorpromazine Hydrochloride; following reports of sudden unexplained death, the CSM recommends ECG before treatment in all patients, periodic ECGs at doses over 16 mg daily and review of need for pimozide if repolarisation changes develop (close supervision and preferably dose reduction advised)—for additional CSM warnings see also below

ADDITIONAL CSM WARNING. In addition to the advice above, the CSM also recommends that patients on pimozide should have an annual ECG (if the QT interval is prolonged treatment should be reviewed and either withdrawn or dose reduced under close supervision) and that pimozide should **not** be given with other antipsychotic drugs (including depot preparations), tricyclic antidepressants or other drugs which prolong the QT interval, such as certain antimalarials, anti-arrhythmic drugs and certain antihistamines (terfenadine) and should **not** be given with drugs which cause electrolyte disturbances (especially diuretics)

Contra-indications: see under Chlorpromazine Hydrochloride; history of arrhythmias or congenital QT prolongation; breast-feeding

Side-effects: see under Chlorpromazine Hydrochloride, but less sedating; serious arrhythmias reported

Dose: schizophrenia, initially 2 mg daily, increased according to response in steps of 2–4 mg at intervals of not less than 1 week; usual dose range 2–20 mg daily; ELDERLY half usual starting dose; CHILD not recommended

Monosymptomatic hypochondriacal psychosis, paranoid psychosis, initially 4 mg daily, increased according to response in steps of 2–4 mg at intervals of not less than 1 week; max. 16 mg daily; ELDERLY half usual starting dose; CHILD not recommended

Orap® (Janssen-Cilag) PoM

Tablets, all scored, pimozide 2 mg, net price 20 = £3.17; 4 mg (green), 20 = £6.13; 10 mg, 20 = £11.76. Label: 2

PROCHLORPERAZINE

Indications: see under Dose; anti-emetic (section 4.6)

Cautions: see under Chlorpromazine Hydrochloride

Contra-indications: see under Chlorpromazine Hydrochloride; children (but see section 4.6 for use as anti-emetic)

Side-effects: see under Chlorpromazine Hydrochloride, but less sedating; extrapyramidal symptoms, particularly dystonic reactions, more frequent

Dose: *by mouth*, schizophrenia and other psychoses, mania, prochlorperazine maleate or mesilate, 12.5 mg twice daily for 7 days adjusted at intervals of 4–7 days to usual dose of 75–100 mg daily according to response; CHILD not recommended

Short-term adjunctive management of severe anxiety, 15–20 mg daily in divided doses; max. 40 mg daily; CHILD not recommended

By deep intramuscular injection, psychoses, mania, prochlorperazine mesilate 12.5–25 mg 2–3 times daily; CHILD not recommended

By rectum in suppositories, psychoses, mania, the equivalent of prochlorperazine maleate 25 mg 2–3 times daily; CHILD not recommended

Preparations
Section 4.6

PROMAZINE HYDROCHLORIDE

Indications: see under Dose

Cautions: see under Chlorpromazine Hydrochloride

Contra-indications: see under Chlorpromazine Hydrochloride

Side-effects: see under Chlorpromazine Hydrochloride

Dose: *by mouth*, short-term adjunctive management of psychomotor agitation, 100–200 mg 4 times daily; CHILD not recommended

Agitation and restlessness in elderly, 25–50 mg 4 times daily

By intramuscular injection, short-term adjunctive management of psychomotor agitation, 50 mg (25 mg in elderly or debilitated), repeated if necessary after 6–8 hours; CHILD not recommended

Promazine (Non-proprietary) PoM
Tablets ⬛, coated, promazine hydrochloride 25 mg, net price 20 = 44p; 50 mg, 20 = 80p. Label: 2
Available from Biorex
Oral solution ⬛, promazine hydrochloride 25 mg/5 mL, net price 150 mL = £1.60; 50 mg/5 mL, 150 mL = £1.60. Label: 2
Available from Rosemont
Suspension ⬛, yellow, promazine hydrochloride (as embonate) 50 mg/5 mL. Net price 150 mL = £1.68. Label: 2
Available from Genus
Injection, promazine hydrochloride 50 mg/mL. Net price 1-mL amp = 30p

---

⬛ denotes preparations that are considered to be less suitable for prescribing (see p. vi)

SULPIRIDE

Indications: schizophrenia
Cautions: see under Chlorpromazine Hydrochloride; reduce dose (preferably avoid) in renal impairment
Contra-indications: see under Chlorpromazine Hydrochloride; breast-feeding; porphyria (section 9.8.2)
Side-effects: see under Chlorpromazine Hydrochloride, but less sedating; structurally distinct from chlorpromazine hence not associated with jaundice or skin reactions
Dose: 200–400 mg twice daily; max. 800 mg daily in predominantly negative symptoms, and 2.4 g daily in mainly positive symptoms; ELDERLY, lower initial dose, increased gradually according to response; CHILD under 14 years not recommended

Sulpiride (Non-proprietary) PoM
Tablets, sulpiride 200 mg, net price 100-tab pack = £18.23; 400 mg, 100-tab pack = £38.00. Label: 2
Available from Cox, CP, Norton
Dolmatil® (Sanofi-Synthelabo) PoM
Tablets, both scored, sulpiride 200 mg, net price 100-tab pack = £14.50; 400 mg (f/c), 100-tab pack = £38.00. Label: 2
Sulparex® (Bristol-Myers) PoM
Tablets, scored, sulpiride 200 mg. Net price 100-tab pack = £20.03. Label: 2
Sulpitil® (Pharmacia & Upjohn) PoM
Tablets, scored, sulpiride 200 mg. Net price 28-tab pack = £5.36; 112-tab pack = £21.42. Label: 2

THIORIDAZINE

Indications: see under Dose
Cautions: see under Chlorpromazine Hydrochloride; monitor for visual defects on prolonged use; avoid in porphyria (section 9.8.2)
Contra-indications: see under Chlorpromazine Hydrochloride
Side-effects: see under Chlorpromazine Hydrochloride, but less sedating and extrapyramidal symptoms and hypothermia rarely occur; more likely to induce hypotension and possibly increased risk of cardiotoxicity and prolongation of QT interval; pigmentary retinopathy (with reduced visual acuity, brownish colouring of vision, and impaired night vision) occurs rarely with high doses; sexual dysfunction, particularly retrograde ejaculation, may occur

Dose: schizophrenia and other psychoses, mania, 150–600 mg daily (initially in divided doses); max. 800 mg daily (hospital patients only) for up to 4 weeks
Short-term adjunctive management of psychomotor agitation, excitement, violent or dangerously impulsive behaviour, 75–200 mg daily
Short-term adjunctive management of severe anxiety, and agitation and restlessness in the elderly, 30–100 mg daily
CHILD (severe mental or behavioural problems only) 1–5 years 1 mg/kg daily, 5–12 years 75–150 mg daily (in severe cases, up to 300 mg daily)

Thioridazine (Non-proprietary) PoM
Tablets, coated, thioridazine hydrochloride 25 mg, net price 20 = 43p; 50 mg, 20 = 85p; 100 mg, 20 = £1.67. Label: 2
Available from Cox, DDSA (*Rideril®*), Hillcross, Norton
Oral solution, thioridazine (as hydrochloride) 25 mg/5 mL. Net price 500-mL = £3.06. Label: 2
Available from Hillcross, Rosemont
Melleril® (Novartis) PoM
Tablets, all f/c, thioridazine hydrochloride 10 mg, net price 84-tab pack = 92p; 25 mg, 84-tab pack = £1.52; 50 mg, 84-tab pack = £2.95; 100 mg, 84-tab pack = £5.70. Label: 2
Suspension 25 mg/5 mL, thioridazine 25 mg/5 mL, net price 300 mL = £1.79. Label: 2
Suspension 100 mg/5 mL, thioridazine 100 mg/5 mL, net price 300 mL = £6.53. Label: 2
Note. These suspensions should not be diluted but the two preparations may be mixed with each other to provide intermediate strengths
Syrup, orange, thioridazine (as hydrochloride) 25 mg/5 mL, net price 300 mL = £1.81. Label: 2

TRIFLUOPERAZINE

Indications: see under Dose; anti-emetic (section 4.6)
Cautions: see under Chlorpromazine Hydrochloride; children
Contra-indications: see under Chlorpromazine Hydrochloride
Side-effects: see under Chlorpromazine Hydrochloride but less sedating, and hypotension, hypothermia, and antimuscarinic side-effects occur less frequently; extrapyramidal symptoms, particularly dystonic reactions and akathisia, are more frequent (particularly when the daily dose exceeds 6 mg)
Dose: *by mouth* (reduce initial doses in elderly by at least half)
Schizophrenia and other psychoses, short-term adjunctive management of psychomotor agitation, excitement, and violent or dangerously impulsive behaviour, initially 5 mg twice daily, *or* 10 mg daily in modified-release form, increased by 5 mg after 1 week, then at intervals of 3 days, according to the response; CHILD up to 12 years, initially up to 5 mg daily in divided doses, adjusted according to response, age, and body-weight
Short-term adjunctive management of severe anxiety, 2–4 mg daily in divided doses *or* 2–4 mg daily in modified-release form, increased if necessary to 6 mg daily; CHILD 3–5 years up to 1 mg daily, 6–12 years up to 4 mg daily

Trifluoperazine (Non-proprietary) [PoM]

Tablets, coated, trifluoperazine (as hydrochloride) 1 mg, net price 20 = 59p; 5 mg, 20 = 75p. Label: 2
Available from most generic manufacturers

Oral solution, trifluoperazine (as hydrochloride) 5 mg/5 mL. Net price 200-mL = £11.50. Label: 2
Available from Rosemont (sugar-free)

Stelazine® (Goldshield) [PoM]

Tablets, both blue, f/c, trifluoperazine (as hydrochloride) 1 mg, net price 20 = 61p; 5 mg, 20 = 87p. Label: 2

Spansules® (= capsules m/r), all clear/yellow, enclosing dark blue, light blue, and white pellets, trifluoperazine (as hydrochloride) 2 mg, net price 60-cap pack = £4.36; 10 mg, 30-cap pack = £2.83; 15 mg, 30-cap pack = £4.27. Label: 2, 25

Syrup, yellow, sugar-free, trifluoperazine (as hydrochloride) 1 mg/5 mL. Net price 200-mL pack = £2.95. Label: 2

ZUCLOPENTHIXOL ACETATE

Indications: short-term management of acute psychosis, mania, or exacerbations of chronic psychosis

Cautions: see under Chlorpromazine Hydrochloride; avoid in porphyria (section 9.8.2)

Contra-indications: see under Chlorpromazine Hydrochloride

Side-effects: see under Chlorpromazine Hydrochloride

Dose: *by deep intramuscular injection* into the gluteal muscle or lateral thigh, 50–150 mg (elderly 50–100 mg), if necessary repeated after 2–3 days (1 additional dose may be needed 1–2 days after the first injection); max. cumulative dose 400 mg per course and max. 4 injections; max. duration of treatment 2 weeks—if maintenance treatment necessary change to an oral antipsychotic 2–3 days after last injection, *or* to a longer acting antipsychotic depot injection given concomitantly with last injection of zuclopenthixol acetate; CHILD not recommended

Clopixol Acuphase® (Lundbeck) [PoM]

Injection (oily), zuclopenthixol acetate 50 mg/mL. Net price 1-mL amp = £5.20; 2-mL amp = £10.03

ZUCLOPENTHIXOL DIHYDROCHLORIDE

Indications: schizophrenia and other psychoses, particularly when associated with agitated, aggressive, or hostile behaviour

Cautions: see under Chlorpromazine Hydrochloride; should not be used in apathetic or withdrawn states; avoid in porphyria (section 9.8.2)

Contra-indications: see under Chlorpromazine Hydrochloride

Side-effects: see under Chlorpromazine Hydrochloride

Dose: initially 20–30 mg daily in divided doses, increasing to a max. of 150 mg daily if necessary; usual maintenance dose 20–50 mg daily; ELDERLY (or debilitated) initially quarter to half adult dose; CHILD not recommended

Clopixol® (Lundbeck) [PoM]

Tablets, all f/c, zuclopenthixol (as dihydrochloride) 2 mg (pink), net price 20 = 64p; 10 mg (light brown), 20 = £1.73; 25 mg (brown), 20 = £3.47. Label: 2

Depot injection (zuclopenthixol decanoate): section 4.2.2

Atypical antipsychotics

The 'atypical antipsychotics' **amisulpride**, **clozapine**, **olanzapine**, **quetiapine**, **risperidone**, and **zotepine** may be better tolerated than other antipsychotics; extrapyramidal symptoms and prolactin elevation may be less frequent than with older antipsychotics.

Clozapine is indicated for the treatment of schizophrenia only in patients unresponsive to, or intolerant of, conventional antipsychotic drugs. It can cause agranulocytosis and its use is restricted to patients registered with the Clozaril Patient Monitoring Service (see under Clozapine, below).

Risperidone is indicated for psychoses in which both positive and negative symptoms are prominent.

Olanzapine is effective in maintaining clinical improvement in patients who have responded to initial treatment.

Quetiapine is indicated for the treatment of both positive and negative symptoms. It should be used with caution in cardiovascular disease because it may prolong the QT interval; it is occasionally associated with neutropenia.

Amisulpride is indicated for both positive and negative symptoms of schizophrenia.

Sertindole has been suspended following reports of arrhythmias and sudden cardiac death. It remains available on a named-patient basis for patients already stabilised on the drug in whom other antipsychotics are inappropriate.

CAUTIONS. Atypical antipsychotics should be used with caution in patients with cardiovascular disease, history of epilepsy, and Parkinson's disease; **interactions:** Appendix 1 (antipsychotics)
DRIVING. Atypical antipsychotics may affect performance of skilled tasks (e.g. driving); effects of alcohol enhanced

SIDE-EFFECTS. Side-effects of the atypical antipsychotics include weight gain, dizziness, postural hypotension (especially during initial dose titration) which may be associated with syncope or reflex tachycardia in some patients, extrapyramidal symptoms (which are usually mild and transient and respond to dose reduction or to antimuscarinic drugs), occasionally tardive dyskinesia on long-term administration; neuroleptic malignant syndrome has been reported rarely.

AMISULPRIDE

Indications: schizophrenia; see also notes above

Cautions: see notes above; renal impairment (Appendix 3), elderly (risk of hypotension or sedation); **interactions:** Appendix 1 (antipsychotics)

Contra-indications: pregnancy and breast-feeding, phaeochromocytoma, prolactin-dependent tumours

Side-effects: see notes above; insomnia, anxiety, agitation, drowsiness, gastro-intestinal disorders such as constipation, nausea, vomiting, and dry mouth, hyperprolactinaemia (with galactorrhoea, amenorrhoea, gynaecomastia, breast pain, sexual dysfunction), occasionally bradycardia, seizures; QT interval prolongation reported

Dose: acute psychotic episode, 400–800 mg daily in divided doses, adjusted according to response; max. 1.2 g daily

Predominently negative symptoms, 50–300 mg daily; CHILD under 15 years, not recommended

Note. Doses up to 300 mg may be administered once daily

Solian® (Sanofi-Synthelabo) ▼ PoM
Tablets, scored, amisulpride 50 mg, net price 60-tab pack = £16.45, 90-tab pack = £24.69; 200 mg, net price 60-tab pack = £60.00, 90-tab pack = £90.00. Label: 2

CLOZAPINE

Indications: schizophrenia in patients unresponsive to, or intolerant of, conventional antipsychotic drugs

Cautions: see notes above; initiation must be in hospital in-patients; leucocyte and differential blood counts must be normal before starting treatment and must be monitored weekly for first 18 weeks then at least fortnightly—patients who have received clozapine for 1 year or more and have stable blood counts may have their blood monitoring reduced to every 4 weeks (continue monitoring for 4 weeks after discontinuation); avoid drugs which depress leucopoiesis (Appendix 1) and taper off conventional neuroleptic before starting; withdraw treatment permanently if leucocyte count falls below 3000/mm³ or absolute neutrophil count falls below 1500/mm³; patients should report any symptoms of infection immediately; mild to moderate renal impairment (Appendix 3); prostatic hypertrophy, angle-closure glaucoma; **interactions:** Appendix 1 (antipsychotics)

WITHDRAWAL. On planned withdrawal reduce dose gradually over 1–2 weeks to avoid risk of rebound psychosis. If abrupt withdrawal necessary observe patient carefully

GASTRO-INTESTINAL OBSTRUCTION. Following reports of adverse reactions resembling gastro-intestinal obstruction, it is recommended that clozapine should be used with caution in patients receiving concomitant treatment with drugs known to cause constipation (e.g. drugs with antimuscarinic effects) or in patients with a history of colonic disease or previous bowel surgery. Patients receiving clozapine should be monitored for constipation and laxatives prescribed as required.

Contra-indications: severe cardiac failure; hepatic impairment (Appendix 2), severe renal impairment (Appendix 3); history of drug-induced neutropenia or agranulocytosis; bone marrow disorders; alcoholic and toxic psychoses; history of circulatory collapse or paralytic ileus; drug intoxication; coma or severe CNS depression; uncontrolled epilepsy; pregnancy and breast-feeding

Side-effects: see notes above; neutropenia and potentially fatal agranulocytosis (**important:** see Cautions), fever (rule out underlying infection or agranulocytosis), drowsiness, anxiety, agitation, confusion, fatigue, blurred vision, dry mouth, constipation, paralytic ileus (see Gastro-intestinal obstruction, above), nausea and vomiting, dysphagia, headache, dizziness, hypersalivation, urinary incontinence and retention, priapism, impaired temperature regulation, liver enzyme abnormalities (asymptomatic elevation common during early stages of treatment), hepatitis, jaundice (discontinue immediately), rarely fulminant hepatic necrosis; arrhythmias, pericarditis, myocarditis, cardiomyopathy, delirium; tachycardia, rarely circulatory collapse with cardiac and respiratory arrest (but hypertension also reported), acute pancreatitis; thromboembolism, hyperglycaemia, rash, elevated plasma-creatine kinase concentration, interstitial nephritis, parotid gland enlargement also reported

Dose: (close medical supervision on initiation—risk of collapse due to hypotension) 12.5 mg once or twice on first day then 25–50 mg on second day then increased gradually (if well tolerated) in steps of 25–50 mg over 14–21 days to 300 mg daily in divided doses (larger dose at night, up to 200 mg daily may be taken as a single dose at bedtime); if necessary may be further increased in steps of 50–100 mg once (preferably) or twice weekly; usual antipsychotic dose 200–450 mg daily (max. 900 mg daily); subsequent adjustment to usual maintenance of 150–300 mg; CHILD not recommended

Note. Restarting after *interval of more than 2 days*, 12.5 mg once or twice on first day (but may be feasible to increase more quickly than on initiation)—unless previous respiratory or cardiac arrest with initial dosing in which case extreme caution

ELDERLY AND SPECIAL RISK GROUPS. In *elderly*, 12.5 mg once on first day—subsequent adjustments restricted to 25 mg daily; in *cardiovascular disease, hepatic* or *renal impairment* or if history of *epilepsy*, 12.5 mg on first day—subsequent adjustments slowly and in small steps (if epileptic seizures (see also Cautions), suspend for 24 hours and resume at lower dose)

Clozaril® (Novartis) PoM
Tablets, both yellow, clozapine 25 mg (scored), net price 28-tab pack = £12.52, 84-tab pack (hosp. only) = £37.54; 100 mg, 28-tab pack = £50.05, 84-tab pack (hosp. only) = £150.15. Label: 2, 10
patient information leaflet
Note. Patient, prescriber, and supplying pharmacist must be registered with the Clozaril Patient Monitoring Service—takes several days to do this

OLANZAPINE

Indications: schizophrenia

Cautions: see notes above; pregnancy, prostatic hypertrophy, paralytic ileus, hepatic impairment (Appendix 2), renal impairment (Appendix 3), diabetes mellitus, low leucocyte or neutrophil count, bone marrow depression, hypereosinophilic disorders, myeloproliferative disease; concomitant administration of drugs that prolong QT interval (especially in elderly); **interactions:** Appendix 1 (antipsychotics)

Contra-indications: angle-closure glaucoma; breast-feeding

Side-effects: see notes above; mild, transient antimuscarinic effects; drowsiness, increased appetite, peripheral oedema, hyperprolactinaemia (but clinical manifestations rare), occasionally blood dyscrasias, transient asymptomatic elevation of liver enzymes, rarely photosensitivity and elevated creatine kinase concentration

Dose: 10 mg daily adjusted to usual range of 5–20 mg daily; doses of 15 mg daily or greater only after reassessment; CHILD and ADOLESCENT under 18 years not recommended

Note. When one or more factors present that might result in slower metabolism (e.g. female gender, elderly, non-smoker) consider lower initial dose and more gradual dose increase

Zyprexa® (Lilly) ▼ [PoM]

Tablets, f/c, olanzapine 2.5 mg, net price 28-tab pack = £31.70; 5 mg, 28-tab pack = £48.78; 7.5 mg, 56-tab pack = £146.34; 10 mg, 28-tab pack = £97.56, 56-tab pack = £195.11. Label: 2

QUETIAPINE

Indications: schizophrenia, see also notes above

Cautions: see notes above; pregnancy, hepatic impairment (Appendix 2), renal impairment (Appendix 3), elderly, concomitant administration of drugs that prolong QT interval (especially in elderly), cerebrovascular disease; **interactions:** Appendix 1 (antipsychotics)

Contra-indications: breast-feeding

Side-effects: see notes above; drowsiness, dyspepsia, constipation, dry mouth, asymptomatic liver enzyme abnormalities, mild asthenia, rhinitis, tachycardia; anxiety, fever, myalgia, rash; leucopenia, neutropenia and occasionally, eosinophilia reported; elevated plasma-triglyceride and cholesterol concentrations, reduced plasma-thyroid hormone concentrations; possible QT interval prolongation

Dose: 25 mg twice daily on day 1, 50 mg twice daily on day 2, 100 mg twice daily on day 3, 150 mg twice daily on day 4, then adjusted according to response, usual range 300–450 mg daily in 2 divided doses; max. 750 mg daily; ELDERLY initially 25 mg daily, increased in steps of 25–50 mg daily

Seroquel® (Zeneca) ▼ [PoM]

Tablets, f/c, quetiapine (as fumarate) 25 mg (peach), net price 60-tab pack = £28.20; 100 mg (yellow), 60-tab pack = £113.10; 150 mg (yellow), 60-tab pack = £113.10; 200 mg (white), 60-tab pack = £113.10; starter pack of 6 × 25-mg tabs, 2 × 100-mg tabs, and 2 × 150-mg tabs = £10.36. Label: 2

RISPERIDONE

Indications: acute and chronic psychoses, see also notes above

Cautions: see notes above; pregnancy, breast-feeding (Appendix 5); hepatic impairment (Appendix 2), renal impairment (Appendix 3), concomitant administration of drugs that prolong QT interval; **interactions:** Appendix 1 (antipsychotics)

Side-effects: see notes above; insomnia, agitation, anxiety, headache, drowsiness, impaired concentration, fatigue, blurred vision, constipation, nausea and vomiting, dyspepsia, abdominal pain, hyperprolactinaemia (with galactorrhoea, menstrual disturbances, amenorrhoea, gynaecomastia), sexual dysfunction, priapism, urinary

incontinence, liver enzyme abnormalities, tachycardia, hypertension, skin rash, rhinitis; neutropenia and thrombocytopenia have been reported; rarely, water intoxication with hyponatraemia, abnormal temperature regulation, seizures

Dose: 2 mg in 1–2 divided doses on first day *then* 4 mg in 1–2 divided doses on second day (slower titration appropriate in some patients); usual dose range 4–6 mg daily; doses above 10 mg daily only if benefit considered to outweigh risk (max. 16 mg daily); ELDERLY (or in hepatic or renal impairment) initially 500 micrograms twice daily increased in steps of 500 micrograms twice daily to 1–2 mg twice daily; CHILD under 15 years not recommended

Risperdal® (Janssen-Cilag, Organon) [PoM]

Tablets, f/c, scored, risperidone 1 mg (white), net price 20-tab pack = £13.45, 60-tab pack = £40.35; 2 mg (orange), 60-tab pack = £79.56; 3 mg (yellow), 60-tab pack = £117.00; 4 mg (green), 60-tab pack = £154.44; 6 mg (yellow), 28-tab pack = £109.20. Label: 2

Liquid, risperidone 1 mg/mL, net price 100 mL = £65.00. Label: 2

Note. Liquid may be diluted with mineral water, orange juice or black coffee (should be taken immediately)

SERTINDOLE

Indications: schizophrenia, see also notes above

Cautions: see notes above; mild or moderate hepatic impairment (Appendix 2); diabetes; correct hypokalaemia or hypomagnesaemia before treatment; monitor ECG during treatment; monitor blood pressure during dose titration and early maintenance therapy (risk of postural hypotension); **interactions:** Appendix 1 (antipsychotics)

Contra-indications: see notes above; pregnancy and breast-feeding, severe hepatic impairment, QT interval prolongation (ECG required before treatment); concomitant administration of drugs which prolong QT interval or cause hypokalaemia (see interactions)

Side-effects: see notes above; prolonged QT interval, peripheral oedema, dry mouth, rhinitis, nasal congestion, dyspnoea, paraesthesia, abnormal ejaculation (decreased volume); rarely seizures, hyperglycaemia

Dose: initially 4 mg daily increased in steps of 4 mg at intervals of 4–5 days to usual maintenance of 12–20 mg as a single daily dose; max. 24 mg daily; ELDERLY and in hepatic impairment consider slower dose titration and lower maintenance dose

Serdolect® (Lundbeck) ▼ [PoM]

Tablets—Product suspended (see notes above); available only on a named-patient basis for patients stabilised on sertindole in whom other antipsychotics have previously failed

ZOTEPINE

Indications: schizophrenia

Cautions: see notes above; personal or close family history of epilepsy; withdrawal of concomitantly prescribed CNS depressants; QT interval prolongation (ECG required before treatment), concomitant administration of drugs which prolong QT interval or cause hypokalaemia; hepatic impairment (Appendix 2); renal impairment (Appendix 3); prostatic hypertrophy, urinary retention, angle-closure glaucoma, paralytic ileus, pregnancy; **interactions:** Appendix 1 (antipsychotics)

Contra-indications: acute intoxication with CNS depressants; high doses of concomitantly prescribed antipsychotics; acute gout (avoid for 3 weeks after resolution of episode), history of nephrolithiasis; breast-feeding

Side-effects: see notes above; constipation, dyspepsia, dry mouth, liver enzyme abnormalities, tachycardia, QT interval prolongation, rhinitis, agitation, anxiety, depression, asthenia, headache, EEG abnormalities, insomnia, drowsiness, hyperthermia or hypothermia, increased salivation, blood dyscrasias (including leucocytosis, leucopenia), raised erythrocyte sedimentation rate, blurred vision, sweating; less frequently anorexia, diarrhoea, nausea and vomiting, abdominal pain, hypertension, influenza-like syndrome, cough, dyspnoea, confusion, convulsions, decreased libido, speech disorder, vertigo, hyperprolactinaemia, anaemia, thrombocythaemia, increased serum-creatinine, hypoglycaemia and hyperglycaemia, hyperlipidaemia, hypouricaemia, oedema, thirst, impotence, urinary incontinence, arthralgia, myalgia, conjunctivitis, acne, dry skin, rash; rarely bradycardia, epistaxis, abdominal enlargement, amnesia, ataxia, coma, delirium, hypaesthesia, myoclonus, thrombocytopenia, abnormal ejaculation, urinary retention, menstrual irregularities, myasthenia, alopecia, photosensitivity

Dose: initially 25 mg 3 times daily increased according to response at intervals of 4 days to max. 100 mg 3 times daily; ELDERLY initially 25 mg twice daily increased according to response to max. 75 mg twice daily; CHILD and ADOLESCENT under 18 years not recommended

Zoleptil® (Orion) ▼ PoM

Tablets, s/c, zotepine 25 mg, net price 30-tab pack = £14.33, 90-tab pack = £42.98; 50 mg (yellow), 30-tab pack = £19.10, 90-tab pack = £57.30; 100 mg (pink), 30-tab pack = £31.52, 90-tab pack = £99.00. Label: 2

4.2.2 Antipsychotic depot injections

Long-acting depot injections are used for maintenance therapy especially when compliance with oral treatment is unreliable. However, they may give rise to a higher incidence of extrapyramidal reactions than oral preparations.

ADMINISTRATION. Depot antipsychotics are administered by deep intramuscular injection at intervals of 1 to 4 weeks. Patients should first be given a small test-dose as undesirable side-effects are prolonged. In general not more than 2–3 mL of oily injection should be administered at any one site; correct injection technique (including the use

of z-track technique) and rotation of injection sites are essential. If the dose needs to be reduced to alleviate side-effects, it is important to recognise that the plasma-drug concentration may not fall for some time after reducing the dose, therefore it may be a month or longer before side-effects subside.

> DOSAGE. Individual responses to neuroleptic drugs are very variable and to achieve optimum effect, dosage and dosage interval must be titrated according to the patient's response. For the advice of The Royal College of Psychiatrists on doses above the BNF upper limit, see p. 171

Equivalent doses of depot antipsychotics
These equivalences are intended **only** as an approximate guide; individual dosage instructions should **also** be checked; patients should be carefully monitored after **any** change in medication

Antipsychotic	Dose (mg)	Interval
Flupentixol decanoate	40	2 weeks
Fluphenazine decanoate	25	2 weeks
Haloperidol (as decanoate)	100	4 weeks
Pipotiazine palmitate	50	4 weeks
Zuclopenthixol decanoate	200	2 weeks

IMPORTANT. These equivalences must **not** be extrapolated beyond the max. dose for the drug

CHOICE. There is no clear-cut division in the use of these drugs, but **zuclopenthixol** may be suitable for the treatment of agitated or aggressive patients whereas **flupentixol** can cause over-excitement in such patients. The incidence of extrapyramidal reactions is similar for all these drugs.

CAUTIONS. Treatment requires careful monitoring for optimum effect; extrapyramidal symptoms occur frequently. When transferring from oral to depot therapy, dosage by mouth should be gradually phased out.

CONTRA-INDICATIONS. Do not use in children, confusional states, coma caused by CNS depressants, parkinsonism, intolerance to antipsychotics.

SIDE-EFFECTS. Pain may occur at injection site and occasionally erythema, swelling, and nodules. For side-effects of specific antipsychotics see under the relevant monograph.

FLUPENTIXOL DECANOATE
(Flupenthixol Decanoate)

Indications: maintenance in schizophrenia and other psychoses

Cautions: see under Chlorpromazine Hydrochloride (section 4.2.1) and notes above; an alternative antipsychotic may be necessary if symptoms such as aggression or agitation appear; avoid in porphyria (section 9.8.2)

Contra-indications: see under Chlorpromazine Hydrochloride (section 4.2.1) and notes above

Side-effects: see under Chlorpromazine Hydrochloride (section 4.2.1) and notes above, but may have a mood elevating effect; extrapyramidal symptoms usually appear 1–3 days after administration and continue for about 5 days but may be delayed

Dose: *by deep intramuscular injection* into the gluteal muscle, test dose 20 mg, then after at least 7 days 20–40 mg repeated at intervals of 2–4 weeks, adjusted according to response; max. 400 mg weekly; usual maintenance dose 50 mg every 4 weeks to 300 mg every 2 weeks; ELDERLY initially quarter to half adult dose; CHILD not recommended

Depixol® (Lundbeck) PoM
Injection (oily), flupentixol decanoate 20 mg/mL. Net price 1-mL amp = £1.63; 2-mL amp = £2.73

Depixol Conc.® (Lundbeck) PoM
Injection (oily), flupentixol decanoate 100 mg/mL. Net price 0.5-mL amp = £3.67; 1-mL amp = £6.72

Depixol Low Volume® (Lundbeck) PoM
Injection (oily), flupentixol decanoate 200 mg/mL. Net price 1-mL amp = £20.99

FLUPHENAZINE DECANOATE

Indications: maintenance in schizophrenia and other psychoses

Cautions: see under Chlorpromazine Hydrochloride (section 4.2.1) and notes above

Contra-indications: see under Chlorpromazine Hydrochloride (section 4.2.1) and notes above; severely depressed states

Side-effects: see under Chlorpromazine Hydrochloride (section 4.2.1) and notes above; extrapyramidal symptoms usually appear a few hours after the dose has been administered and continue for about 2 days but may be delayed

Dose: *by deep intramuscular injection* into the gluteal muscle, test dose 12.5 mg (6.25 mg in elderly), then after 4–7 days 12.5–100 mg repeated at intervals of 14–35 days, adjusted according to response; CHILD not recommended

Modecate® (Sanofi-Synthelabo) PoM
Injection (oily), fluphenazine decanoate 25 mg/mL. Net price 0.5-mL amp = £1.35; 1-mL amp = £2.35; 1-mL syringe = £2.72; 2-mL amp = £4.62; 2-mL syringe = £4.93; 10-mL vial = £23.45
Excipients: include sesame oil
Note. Fluphenazine decanoate injection also available from Antigen, Berk, Faulding DBL, Hillcross—at least some versions contain sesame oil

Modecate Concentrate® (Sanofi-Synthelabo) PoM
Injection (oily), fluphenazine decanoate 100 mg/mL. Net price 0.5-mL amp = £4.66; 1-mL amp = £9.10
Excipients: include sesame oil
Note. Fluphenazine decanoate injection also available from Antigen, Berk, Faulding DBL, Hillcross—at least some versions contain sesame oil

HALOPERIDOL DECANOATE

Indications: maintenance in schizophrenia and other psychoses

Cautions: see under Haloperidol (section 4.2.1) and notes above

Contra-indications: see under Haloperidol (section 4.2.1) and notes above

Side-effects: see under Haloperidol (section 4.2.1) and notes above

Dose: *by deep intramuscular injection* into the gluteal muscle, haloperidol (as decanoate), initially 50 mg every 4 weeks, if necessary increasing after 2 weeks by 50-mg increments to 300 mg every 4 weeks; higher doses may be needed in some patients; ELDERLY, initially 12.5–25 mg every 4 weeks; CHILD not recommended

Haldol Decanoate® (Janssen-Cilag) PoM
Injection (oily), haloperidol (as decanoate) 50 mg/mL, net price 1-mL amp = £4.35; 100 mg/mL, 1-mL amp = £5.77
Excipients: include sesame oil

PIPOTIAZINE PALMITATE

(Pipothiazine Palmitate)

Indications: maintenance in schizophrenia and other psychoses

Cautions: see under Chlorpromazine Hydrochloride (section 4.2.1) and notes above

Contra-indications: see under Chlorpromazine Hydrochloride (section 4.2.1) and notes above

Side-effects: see under Chlorpromazine Hydrochloride (section 4.2.1) and notes above

Dose: *by deep intramuscular injection* into the gluteal muscle, test dose 25 mg, then a further 25–50 mg after 4–7 days, then adjusted according to response at intervals of 4 weeks; usual maintenance range 50–100 mg (max. 200 mg) every 4 weeks; ELDERLY initially 5–10 mg; CHILD not recommended

Piportil Depot® (JHC) PoM
Injection (oily), pipotiazine palmitate 50 mg/mL. Net price 1-mL amp = £11.31; 2-mL amp = £18.51

ZUCLOPENTHIXOL DECANOATE

Indications: maintenance in schizophrenia and other psychoses, particularly with aggression and agitation

Cautions: see under Chlorpromazine Hydrochloride (section 4.2.1) and notes above; avoid in porphyria (section 9.8.2)

Contra-indications: see under Chlorpromazine Hydrochloride (section 4.2.1) and notes above

Side-effects: see under Chlorpromazine Hydrochloride (section 4.2.1) and notes above but less sedating

Dose: *by deep intramuscular injection* into the gluteal muscle, test dose 100 mg, followed after 7–28 days by 100–200 mg or more, followed by 200–400 mg at intervals of 2–4 weeks, adjusted according to response; max. 600 mg weekly; CHILD not recommended

Clopixol® (Lundbeck) PoM
Injection (oily), zuclopenthixol decanoate 200 mg/mL. Net price 1-mL amp = £3.39

Clopixol Conc.® (Lundbeck) PoM
Injection (oily), zuclopenthixol decanoate 500 mg/mL. Net price 1-mL amp = £8.00

4.2.3   Antimanic drugs

Drugs are used in mania both to control acute attacks and also to prevent their recurrence.

Benzodiazepines

Use of benzodiazepines (section 4.1) may be helpful in the initial stages of treatment until lithium achieves its full effect; they should not be used for long periods because of the risk of dependence.

Antipsychotic drugs

In an acute attack of mania, treatment with an antipsychotic drug (section 4.2.1) is usually required because it may take a few days for lithium to exert its antimanic effect. Lithium may be given concurrently with the antipsychotic drug, and treatment with the antipsychotic gradually tailed off as lithium becomes effective. Alternatively, lithium therapy may be commenced once the patient's mood has been stabilised with the antipsychotic. However, high doses of haloperidol, fluphenazine, or flupentixol may be hazardous when used with lithium; irreversible toxic encephalopathy has been reported.

Carbamazepine

Carbamazepine (section 4.8.1) may be used for the prophylaxis of manic-depressive illness in patients unresponsive to lithium; it seems to be particularly effective in patients with rapid cycling manic-depressive illness (4 or more affective episodes per year).

Lithium

Lithium salts are used in the prophylaxis and treatment of mania, in the prophylaxis of bipolar disorder (manic-depressive disorder) and in the prophylaxis of recurrent depression (unipolar illness or unipolar depression). Lithium is unsuitable for children.

The decision to give prophylactic lithium usually requires *specialist advice*, and must be based on careful consideration of the likelihood of recurrence in the individual patient, and the benefit weighed against the risks. In long-term use lithium has been associated with thyroid disorders and mild cognitive and memory impairment. Long-term treatment should therefore be undertaken only with careful assessment of risk and benefit, and with regular monitoring of thyroid function. The need for continued therapy should be assessed regularly and patients should be maintained on lithium after 3–5 years only if benefit persists.

SERUM CONCENTRATIONS. Lithium salts have a narrow therapeutic/toxic ratio and should therefore not be prescribed unless facilities for monitoring serum-lithium concentrations are available. There seem few if any reasons for preferring one or other of the salts of lithium available. Doses are adjusted to achieve serum-lithium concentration of 0.4–1 mmol/litre (lower end of the range for maintenance therapy and elderly patients) on samples taken 12 hours after the preceding dose. It is important to determine the optimum range for each individual patient.

Overdosage, usually with serum-lithium concentration of over 1.5 mmol/litre, may be fatal and toxic effects include tremor, ataxia, dysarthria, nystagmus, renal impairment, and convulsions. If these potentially hazardous signs occur, treatment should be stopped, serum-lithium concentrations redetermined, and steps taken to reverse lithium toxicity. In mild cases withdrawal of lithium and administration of generous amounts of sodium and fluid will reverse the toxicity. Serum-lithium concentration in excess of 2 mmol/litre require urgent treatment as indicated under Emergency Treatment of Poisoning, p. 24. When toxic concentrations are reached there may be a delay of 1 or 2 days before maximum toxicity occurs.

INTERACTIONS. Lithium toxicity is made worse by sodium depletion, therefore concurrent use of diuretics (particularly thiazides) is hazardous and should be avoided. For other **interactions** with lithium, see Appendix 1 (lithium).

WITHDRAWAL. While there is no clear evidence of withdrawal or rebound psychosis, abrupt discontinuation of lithium increases the risk of relapse. If lithium is to be discontinued, the dose should be reduced gradually over a period of a few weeks and patients should be warned of possible relapse if discontinued abruptly.

> LITHIUM CARDS. A lithium treatment card available from pharmacies tells patients how to take lithium preparations, what to do if a dose is missed, and what side-effects to expect. It also explains why regular blood tests are important and warns that some medicines and illnesses can change serum-lithium concentration
>
> Cards may be obtained from NPA Services, 38–42 St. Peter's St, St. Albans, Herts AL1 3NP.

LITHIUM CARBONATE

Indications: treatment and prophylaxis of mania, bipolar disorder, and recurrent depression (see also notes above); aggressive or self-mutilating behaviour

Cautions: measure serum-lithium concentration regularly (every 3 months on stabilised regimens), monitor thyroid function; maintain adequate sodium and fluid intake; avoid in renal impairment, cardiac disease, and conditions with sodium imbalance such as Addison's disease; reduction in dose or discontinuation may be necessary in diarrhoea, vomiting and intercurrent infection (especially when associated with profuse sweating); caution in pregnancy (Appendix 4), breast-feeding, elderly (reduce dose), diuretic treatment, myasthenia gravis; surgery (section 15.1); if possible avoid abrupt withdrawal (see notes above); **interactions:** Appendix 1 (lithium)

COUNSELLING. Patients should maintain an adequate fluid intake and should avoid dietary changes which might reduce or increase sodium intake; lithium treatment cards are available from pharmacies (see above)

Note. **Different preparations vary widely in bioavailability**; a change in the preparation used requires the same precautions as initiation of treatment

Side-effects: gastro-intestinal disturbances, fine tremor, polyuria and polydipsia; also weight gain and oedema (may respond to dose reduction); signs of intoxication are blurred vision, increasing gastro-intestinal disturbances (anorexia, vomiting, diarrhoea), muscle weakness, increased CNS disturbances (mild drowsiness and sluggishness increasing to giddiness with ataxia, coarse tremor, lack of co-ordination, dysarthria), and require withdrawal of treatment; with severe **overdosage** (serum-lithium concentration above 2 mmol/litre) hyperreflexia and hyperextension of limbs, convulsions, toxic psychoses, syncope, oliguria, circulatory failure, coma, and occasionally, death; goitre, raised antidiuretic hormone concentration, hypothyroidism, hypokalaemia, ECG changes, exacerbation of psoriasis, and kidney changes may also occur; see also Emergency Treatment of Poisoning, p. 24

Dose: see under preparations below, adjusted to achieve a serum-lithium concentration of 0.4–1 mmol/litre 12 hours after a dose on the fourth to seventh day of treatment, then every week until dosage has remained constant for 4 weeks and every 3 months thereafter; doses are initially divided throughout the day, but once daily administration is preferred when serum-lithium concentration stabilised

Note. Lithium carbonate 200 mg ≡ lithium citrate 509 mg

Camcolit® (Norgine) [PoM]
Camcolit 250® tablets, f/c, scored, lithium carbonate 250 mg (Li+ 6.8 mmol), net price 20 = 58p. Label: 10 lithium card, counselling, see above

Camcolit 400® tablets, m/r, f/c, scored, lithium carbonate 400 mg (Li+ 10.8 mmol), net price 20 = 77p. Label: 10 lithium card, 25, counselling, see above

Dose (serum monitoring, see above):
Treatment, initially 1–1.5 g daily; prophylaxis, initially 300–400 mg daily; CHILD not recommended

Note. Camcolit 400® also available as *Lithonate®* (Berk)

Liskonum® (SmithKline Beecham) [PoM]
Tablets, m/r, f/c, scored, lithium carbonate 450 mg (Li+ 12.2 mmol), net price 60-tab pack = £2.82. Label: 10 lithium card, 25, counselling, see above

Dose (serum monitoring, see above):
Treatment, initially 450–675 mg twice daily (elderly initially 225 mg twice daily); prophylaxis, initially 450 mg twice daily (elderly 225 mg twice daily); CHILD not recommended

Priadel® (Sanofi-Synthelabo) [PoM]
Tablets, both m/r, scored, lithium carbonate 200 mg (Li+ 5.4 mmol), net price 20 = 50p; 400 mg (Li+ 10.8 mmol), 20 = 82p. Label: 10 lithium card, 25, counselling, see above

Dose (serum monitoring, see above):
Treatment and prophylaxis, initially 0.4–1.2 g daily as a single dose or in 2 divided doses (elderly or patients less than 50 kg, 400 mg daily); CHILD not recommended

Liquid, see under Lithium Citrate, below

LITHIUM CITRATE

Indications: see under Lithium Carbonate and notes above

Cautions: see under Lithium Carbonate and notes above

COUNSELLING. Patients should maintain an adequate fluid intake and should avoid dietary changes which might reduce or increase sodium intake; lithium treatment cards are available from pharmacies (see above)

Side-effects: see under Lithium Carbonate and notes above

Dose: see under preparations below, adjusted to achieve serum-lithium concentration of 0.4–1 mmol/litre as described under Lithium Carbonate

Note. **Different preparations vary widely in bioavailability**; a change in the preparation used requires the same precautions as initiation of treatment

Note. Lithium carbonate 200 mg ≡ lithium citrate 509 mg

Li-Liquid® (Rosemont) [PoM]
Oral solution, sugar-free, lithium citrate 509 mg/5 mL (Li+ 5.4 mmol/5 mL), yellow, net price 150-mL pack = £6.16; 1.018 g/5 mL (Li+ 10.8 mmol/5 mL), orange, 150-mL pack = £12.32. Label: 10 lithium card, counselling, see above

Dose (plasma monitoring, see above):
Treatment and prophylaxis, initially 1.018–3.054 g daily in 2 divided doses (elderly or patients less than 50 kg, initially 509 mg twice daily); CHILD not recommended

Litarex® (Dumex) [PoM]
Tablets, m/r, lithium citrate 564 mg (Li+ 6 mmol). Net price 20 = 69p. Label: 10 lithium card, 25, counselling, see above

Dose (plasma monitoring, see above):
Treatment and prophylaxis, initially 564 mg twice daily; CHILD not recommended

Priadel® (Delandale) [PoM]
Tablets, see under Lithium Carbonate, above

Liquid, sugar-free, lithium citrate 520 mg/5 mL (approx. Li+ 5.4 mmol/5 mL), net price 150-mL pack = £6.58. Label: 10 lithium card, counselling, see above

Dose (plasma monitoring, see above):
Treatment and prophylaxis, initially 1.04–3.12 g daily in 2 divided doses (elderly or patients less than 50 kg, 520 mg twice daily); CHILD not recommended

4.3   Antidepressant drugs

4.3.1	Tricyclic and related antidepressant drugs
4.3.2	Monoamine-oxidase inhibitors (MAOIs)
4.3.3	Selective serotonin re-uptake inhibitors
4.3.4	Other antidepressant drugs

Tricyclic and related antidepressants and the selective serotonin re-uptake inhibitors (SSRIs) and related antidepressants are preferred to the traditional MAOIs because they are more effective and do not show the dangerous interactions with some *foods* and have fewer of the dangerous interactions with *drugs* that are characteristic of the traditional MAOIs.

The choice between **older tricyclics** (e.g. amitriptyline) and **related drugs** (e.g. maprotiline) depends mainly on the lower incidence of antimuscarinic side-effects associated with the related ones, such as less dry mouth and constipation; the related ones may also be associated with a lower risk of cardiotoxicity in overdosage; however, some have additional side-effects (for further details see section 4.3.1).

The **SSRIs** also have fewer antimuscarinic side-effects than the **older tricyclics** and they also seem to be less cardiotoxic in overdosage. Therefore, although not more effective, they may be preferred where there is a major risk of overdosage. The SSRIs do, however, have characteristic side-effects of their own. Hence, drowsiness, dry mouth and cardiotoxicity may be less of a problem, but gastro-intestinal side-effects such as nausea and vomiting may be more common.

A number of antidepressants cannot be accommodated easily into the existing classification; these are included in section 4.3.4.

See section 4.2.3 for references to the role of **lithium** and **carbamazepine** in depression or in bipolar disorder.

Where the depression is very severe **electroconvulsive therapy** may be indicated.

Prescribing more than one antidepressant at the same time is **not** recommended. It may constitute a hazard and there is no evidence that side-effects are minimised.

Compound preparations of an antidepressant and an anxiolytic are **not** recommended because the dosage of the individual components should be adjusted separately. Whereas antidepressants are given continuously over several months, anxiolytics are prescribed on a **short-term** basis.

It should be noted that although anxiety is often present in depressive illness and may be the presenting symptom, the use of antipsychotics or anxiolytics may mask the true diagnosis. They should therefore be used with caution (but are useful adjuncts in agitated depression).

> **CSM advice (hyponatraemia)**. Hyponatraemia (usually in the elderly and possibly due to inappropriate secretion of antidiuretic hormone) has been associated with all types of antidepressants and should be considered in all patients who develop drowsiness, confusion or convulsions while taking an antidepressant.

MANAGEMENT. The patient must be assessed frequently, especially in the early weeks of treatment, to detect any suicidal tendencies. Limited quantities of antidepressant drugs should be prescribed at any one time since antidepressant drugs and in particular tricyclic antidepressants are dangerous in overdosage. Some of the newer drugs seem less dangerous in overdose than the older tricyclics.

Treatment should be continued for 2 weeks before suppression of symptoms can be expected and thereafter should be maintained at the optimum level for at least 4–6 months after the depression has resolved. Treatment should not be withdrawn prematurely, otherwise symptoms are likely to recur. The natural history of depressive illness suggests that remission usually occurs after 3 months to a year or more. In recurrent depression, prophylactic maintenance therapy with an effective dose may need to be continued for several years.

In patients who do not respond to antidepressants, the diagnosis, dosage, compliance, and possible continuation of psychosocial or physical aggravating causes should all be carefully reviewed; other drug treatment may be successful.

WITHDRAWAL. Gastro-intestinal symptoms of nausea, vomiting, and anorexia, accompanied by headache, giddiness, 'chills', and insomnia, and sometimes by hypomania, panic-anxiety, and extreme motor restlessness may occur if an antidepressant (particularly an MAOI) is stopped suddenly after regular administration for 8 weeks or more. Reduction in dosage should preferably be carried out gradually over a period of about 4 weeks. SSRIs and in particular paroxetine have been associated with a specific withdrawal syndrome (section 4.3.3).

4.3.1 Tricyclic and related antidepressant drugs

This section covers tricyclic antidepressants and also 1-, 2-, and 4-ring structured drugs with broadly similar properties.

These drugs are most effective for treating moderate to severe *endogenous depression* associated with psychomotor and physiological changes such as loss of appetite and sleep disturbances; improvement in sleep is usually the first benefit of therapy. Since there may be an interval of 2 weeks before the antidepressant action takes place electroconvulsive treatment may be required in severe depression when delay is hazardous or intolerable.

Some tricyclic antidepressants are also effective in the management of *panic disorder*.

For reference to the role of some tricyclic antidepressants in some forms of *neuralgia*, see section 4.7.3, and in *nocturnal enuresis* in children, see section 7.4.2.

DOSAGE. About 10 to 20% of patients fail to respond to tricyclic and related antidepressant drugs and inadequate dosage may account for some of these failures. It is important to use doses that are sufficiently high for effective treatment but not so high as to cause toxic effects. Low doses should be used for initial treatment in the **elderly** (see under Side-effects, below).

In most patients the long half-life of tricyclic antidepressant drugs allows **once-daily** administration, usually at night; the use of modified-release preparations is therefore unnecessary.

CHOICE. Tricyclic and related antidepressant drugs can be roughly divided into those with additional sedative properties and those which are less so. Agitated and anxious patients tend to respond best to the sedative compounds whereas withdrawn and apathetic patients will often obtain most benefit from the less sedating ones. Those with **sedative** properties include amitriptyline, clomipramine, dosulepin (dothiepin), doxepin, maprotiline, mianserin, trazodone, and trimipramine. Those with **less sedative** properties include amoxapine, imipramine, lofepramine, nortriptyline, and viloxazine. Protriptyline has a **stimulant** action.

Imipramine and **amitriptyline** are well established and relatively safe and effective, but nevertheless have more marked antimuscarinic or cardiac side-effects than compounds such as **doxepin, mianserin, trazodone,** and **viloxazine**; this may be important in individual patients. **Lofepramine** also has a lower incidence of antimuscarinic and sedative side-effects and may be less dangerous in overdosage; it is, however, associated with hepatic toxicity. **Amoxapine** is related to the antipsychotic loxapine and its side-effects include tardive dyskinesia.

For a comparison of tricyclic and related antidepressants with SSRIs and related antidepressants and MAOIs, see section 4.3.

SIDE-EFFECTS. *Arrhythmias* and *heart block* occasionally follow the use of tricyclic antidepressants, particularly amitriptyline, and may be a factor in the sudden death of patients with cardiac disease. They are also sometimes associated with *convulsions* (and should be prescribed with special caution in epilepsy as they lower the convulsive threshold); maprotiline has particularly been associated with convulsions. *Hepatic* and *haematological* reactions may occur and have been particularly associated with mianserin.

Other side-effects of tricyclic and related antidepressants include *drowsiness, dry mouth, blurred vision, constipation,* and *urinary retention* (all attributed to antimuscarinic activity), and sweating. The patient should be encouraged to persist with treatment as some tolerance to these side-effects seems to develop. They are reduced if low doses are given initially and then gradually increased, but this must be balanced against the need to obtain a full therapeutic effect as soon as possible. Gradual introduction of treatment is particularly important in the elderly, who, because of the hypotensive effects of these drugs, are prone to attacks of *dizziness* or even *syncope*. Another side-effect to which the elderly are particularly susceptible is *hyponatraemia* (see CSM advice on p. 185).

Neuroleptic malignant syndrome (section 4.2.1) may, very rarely, arise in the course of antidepressant treatment.

Limited quantities of tricyclic antidepressants should be prescribed at any one time because they are dangerous in overdosage. For advice on **overdosage** see Emergency Treatment of Poisoning, p. 23.

WITHDRAWAL. If possible tricyclic and related antidepressants should be withdrawn slowly (see also section 4.3).

INTERACTIONS. A tricyclic or related antidepressant (or an SSRI or related antidepressant) should not be started until 2 weeks after stopping an MAOI (3 weeks if starting clomipramine or imipramine). Conversely, an MAOI should not be started until at least 7–14 days after a tricyclic or related antidepressant (3 weeks in the case of clomipramine or imipramine) has been stopped. For guidance relating to the reversible monoamine oxidase inhibitor, moclobemide, see p. 191. For other tricyclic antidepressant **interactions**, see Appendix 1 (antidepressants, tricyclic).

Tricyclic antidepressants

AMITRIPTYLINE HYDROCHLORIDE

Indications: depressive illness, particularly where sedation is required; nocturnal enuresis in children (section 7.4.2)

Cautions: cardiac disease (particularly with arrhythmias, see Contra-indications below), history of epilepsy, pregnancy and breast-feeding (Appendixes 4 and 5), elderly, hepatic impairment (avoid if severe), thyroid disease, phaeochromocytoma, history of mania, psychoses (may aggravate psychotic symptoms), angle-closure glaucoma, history of urinary retention, concurrent electroconvulsive therapy; if possible avoid abrupt withdrawal; anaesthesia (increased risk of arrhythmias and hypotension, see surgery section 15.1); porphyria (section 9.8.2); see section 7.4.2 for additional nocturnal enuresis warnings; **interactions:** Appendix 1 (antidepressants, tricyclic) DRIVING. Drowsiness may affect performance of skilled tasks (e.g. driving); effects of alcohol enhanced

Contra-indications: recent myocardial infarction, arrhythmias (particularly heart block), not indicated in manic phase, severe liver disease

Side-effects: dry mouth, sedation, blurred vision (disturbance of accommodation, increased intraocular pressure), constipation, nausea, difficulty with micturition; cardiovascular side-effects (such as ECG changes, arrhythmias, postural hypotension, tachycardia, syncope, particularly with high doses); sweating, tremor, rashes and hypersensitivity reactions (including urticaria, photosensitivity), behavioural disturbances (particularly children), hypomania or mania, confusion (particularly elderly), interference with sexual function, blood sugar changes; increased appetite and weight gain (occasionally weight loss); endocrine side-effects such as testicular enlargement, gynaecomastia, galactorrhoea; also convulsions (see also Cautions), movement disorders and dyskinesias, fever, agranulocytosis, leucopenia, eosinophilia, purpura, thrombocytopenia, hyponatraemia (may be due to inappropriate antidiuretic hormone secretion) see CSM advice, p. 185, abnormal liver function tests (jaundice); for a general outline of side-effects see also notes above; **overdosage:** see Emergency Treatment of Poisoning, p. 23

Dose: depression, initially 75 mg (elderly and adolescents 30–75 mg) daily in divided doses *or* as a single dose at bedtime increased gradually as necessary to max. 150 mg; CHILD under 16 years not recommended for depression
Nocturnal enuresis, CHILD 7–10 years 10–20 mg, 11–16 years 25–50 mg at night; max. period of treatment (including gradual withdrawal) 3 months—full physical examination before further course

Amitriptyline (Non-proprietary) PoM
Tablets, coated, amitriptyline hydrochloride 10 mg, net price 20 = 17p; 25 mg, 20 = 17p; 50 mg, 20 =70p. Label: 2
Available from Antigen, APS, Cox, DDSA (*Elavil®*)
Oral solution, amitriptyline (as hydrochloride) 25 mg/5 mL, net price 200 mL = £13.00; 50 mg/5 mL, 200 mL = £18.00. Label: 2
Available from Rosemont (sugar-free)

Lentizol® (Parke-Davis) PoM ▱

Capsules, m/r, both enclosing white pellets, amitriptyline hydrochloride 25 mg (pink), net price 56-cap pack = £2.58; 50 mg (pink/red), 56-cap pack = £4.79. Label: 2, 25

■ Compound preparations

Triptafen® (Goldshield) PoM ▱

Tablets, pink, s/c, amitriptyline hydrochloride 25 mg, perphenazine 2 mg. Net price 20 = £4.25. Label: 2

Triptafen-M® (Goldshield) PoM ▱

Tablets, pink, s/c, amitriptyline hydrochloride 10 mg, perphenazine 2 mg. Net price 20 = £3.80. Label: 2

AMOXAPINE

Indications: depressive illness

Cautions: see under Amitriptyline Hydrochloride

Contra-indications: see under Amitriptyline Hydrochloride

Side-effects: see under Amitriptyline Hydrochloride; tardive dyskinesia reported; menstrual irregularities, breast enlargement, and galactorrhoea reported in women

Dose: initially 100–150 mg daily in divided doses *or* as a single dose at bedtime increased as necessary to max. 300 mg daily; ELDERLY initially 25 mg twice daily increased as necessary after 5–7 days to max. 50 mg 3 times daily; CHILD under 16 years not recommended

Asendis® (Lederle) PoM

Tablets, amoxapine 50 mg (orange, scored), net price 84-tab pack = £15.25; 100 mg (blue, scored), 56-tab pack = £16.95. Label: 2

CLOMIPRAMINE HYDROCHLORIDE

Indications: depressive illness, phobic and obsessional states; adjunctive treatment of cataplexy associated with narcolepsy

Cautions: see under Amitriptyline Hydrochloride

Contra-indications: see under Amitriptyline Hydrochloride

Side-effects: see under Amitriptyline Hydrochloride

Dose: *by mouth*, initially 10 mg daily, increased gradually as necessary to 30–150 mg daily in divided doses *or* as a single dose at bedtime; max. 250 mg daily; ELDERLY initially 10 mg daily increased to 30–50 mg daily; CHILD not recommended

Phobic and obsessional states, initially 25 mg daily (elderly 10 mg daily) increased over 2 weeks to 100–150 mg daily; CHILD not recommended

Adjunctive treatment of cataplexy associated with narcolepsy, initially 10 mg daily gradually increased until satisfactory response (range 10–75 mg daily)

By intramuscular injection, initially 25–50 mg daily, increased by 25 mg daily to 100–150 mg daily; CHILD not recommended

By intravenous infusion (careful monitoring) initially to assess tolerance, 25–50 mg, then increase by 25 mg daily to usual dose of 100 mg daily for 7–10 days—see product literature for details; CHILD not recommended

Clomipramine (Non-proprietary) PoM

Capsules, clomipramine hydrochloride 10 mg, net price 20 = 52p; 25 mg, 20 = £1.52; 50 mg, 20 = £2.81. Label: 2

Available from APS, Berk (*Tranquax®*), Cox, Generics, Hillcross, Norton

Anafranil® (Novartis) PoM

Capsules, clomipramine hydrochloride 10 mg (yellow/caramel), net price 84-cap pack = £2.75; 25 mg (orange/caramel), 84-cap pack = £5.40; 50 mg (grey/caramel), 56-cap pack = £6.85. Label: 2

Syrup, clomipramine hydrochloride 25 mg/5 mL. Net price 150-mL pack = £7.23. Label: 2

Injection, clomipramine hydrochloride 12.5 mg/mL. Net price 2-mL amp = 47p

Anafranil SR® (Novartis) PoM ▱

Tablets, m/r, grey-red, f/c, clomipramine hydrochloride 75 mg. Net price 28-tab pack = £7.51. Label: 2, 25

> ▰ denotes preparations that are considered to be less suitable for prescribing (see p. vi)

DOSULEPIN HYDROCHLORIDE/ DOTHIEPIN HYDROCHLORIDE

Indications: depressive illness, particularly where sedation is required

Cautions: see under Amitriptyline Hydrochloride

Contra-indications: see under Amitriptyline Hydrochloride

Side-effects: see under Amitriptyline Hydrochloride

Dose: initially 75 mg (elderly 50–75 mg) daily in divided doses *or* as a single dose at bedtime, increased gradually as necessary to 150 mg daily (elderly 75 mg may be sufficient); up to 225 mg daily in some circumstances (e.g. hospital use); CHILD not recommended

Dosulepin/Dothiepin (Non-proprietary) PoM

Capsules, dosulepin hydrochloride 25 mg, net price 20 = 74p. Label: 2

Available from APS, Ashbourne (*Dothapax®*), Berk (*Prepadine®*), Cox, Generics, Hillcross, Kent, Lagap, Norton, Sanofi-Synthelabo, Sovereign

Tablets, dosulepin hydrochloride 75 mg, net price 28-tab pack = £3.34. Label: 2

Available from APS, Ashbourne (*Dothapax®*), Berk (*Prepadine®*), Cox, Generics, Hillcross, Kent, Lagap, Norton, Sanofi-Synthelabo, Sovereign

Prothiaden® (Knoll) PoM

Capsules, red/red-brown, dosulepin hydrochloride 25 mg. Net price 20 = £1.05. Label: 2

Tablets, red, s/c, dosulepin hydrochloride 75 mg. Net price 28-tab pack = £4.20. Label: 2

DOXEPIN

Indications: depressive illness, particularly where sedation is required; skin (section 13.3)

Cautions: see under Amitriptyline Hydrochloride

Contra-indications: see under Amitriptyline Hydrochloride; breast-feeding (see Appendix 5)

Side-effects: see under Amitriptyline Hydrochloride

Dose: initially 75 mg daily in divided doses *or* as a single dose at bedtime, increased as necessary to max. 300 mg daily in 3 divided doses (up to 100 mg may be given as a single dose); ELDERLY initially 10–50 mg daily, range of 30–50 mg daily may be adequate; CHILD not recommended

Sinequan® (Pfizer) [PoM]
Capsules, doxepin (as hydrochloride) 10 mg
(orange), net price 56-cap pack = £1.21; 25 mg
(orange/blue), 28-cap pack = 87p; 50 mg (blue),
28-cap pack = £1.43; 75 mg (yellow/blue), 28-cap
pack = £2.26. Label: 2

IMIPRAMINE HYDROCHLORIDE

Indications: depressive illness; nocturnal enuresis
in children (see section 7.4.2)
Cautions: see under Amitriptyline Hydrochloride
Contra-indications: see under Amitriptyline
Hydrochloride
Side-effects: see under Amitriptyline Hydrochloride, but less sedating
Dose: depression, initially up to 75 mg daily in
divided doses increased gradually to 150–200 mg
(up to 300 mg in hospital patients); up to 150 mg
may be given as a single dose at bedtime; ELD-
ERLY initially 10 mg daily, increased gradually to
30–50 mg daily; CHILD not recommended for
depression
Nocturnal enuresis, CHILD 7 years 25 mg, 8–11
years 25–50 mg, over 11 years 50–75 mg at bedtime; max. period of treatment (including gradual
withdrawal) 3 months—full physical examination
before further course

Imipramine (Non-proprietary) [PoM]
Tablets, coated, imipramine hydrochloride 10 mg,
net price 20 = 31p; 25 mg, 20 = 31p. Label: 2
Tofranil® (Novartis) [PoM]
Tablets, red-brown, s/c, imipramine hydrochloride
25 mg, net price 84-tab pack = £3.05. Label: 2
Syrup, imipramine hydrochloride 25 mg/5 mL. Net
price 150-mL pack = £3.11. Label: 2

LOFEPRAMINE

Indications: depressive illness
Cautions: see under Amitriptyline Hydrochloride
Contra-indications: see under Amitriptyline
Hydrochloride; hepatic and severe renal impairment
Side-effects: see under Amitriptyline Hydrochloride, but less sedating; hepatic disorders
reported
Dose: 140–210 mg daily in divided doses; ELDERLY
may respond to lower doses; CHILD not recommended

Lofepramine (Non-proprietary) [PoM]
Tablets, lofepramine 70 mg (as hydrochloride). Net
price 56-tab pack = £10.61. Label: 2
Available from Cox, Hillcross, Lagap
Oral suspension, lofepramine 70 mg/5 mL (as
hydrochloride). Net price 200 mL = £27.10.
Label: 2
Available from Rosemont (*Lomont®*, sugar-free)
Gamanil® (Merck) [PoM]
Tablets, f/c, brown-violet, lofepramine 70 mg (as
hydrochloride). Net price 56-tab pack = £9.40.
Label: 2

NORTRIPTYLINE

Indications: depressive illness; nocturnal enuresis
in children (section 7.4.2)
Cautions: see under Amitriptyline Hydrochloride;
manufacturer advises plasma-nortriptyline con-

centration monitoring if dose above 100 mg daily,
but evidence of practical value uncertain
Contra-indications: see under Amitriptyline
Hydrochloride
Side-effects: see under Amitriptyline Hydrochloride, but less sedating
Dose: depression, low dose initially increased as
necessary to 75–100 mg daily in divided doses *or*
as a single dose (max. 150 mg daily); ADOLES-
CENT and ELDERLY 30–50 mg daily in divided
doses; CHILD not recommended for depression
Nocturnal enuresis, CHILD 7 years 10 mg, 8–11
years 10–20 mg, over 11 years 25–35 mg, at
night; max period of treatment (including gradual
withdrawal) 3 months—full physical examination
and ECG before further course

Allegron® (Dista) [PoM]
Tablets, nortriptyline (as hydrochloride) 10 mg, net
price 20 = £2.28; 25 mg (orange, scored), 20 =
£4.63. Label: 2

■ Compound preparations
Motipress® (Sanofi-Synthelabo) [PoM] ◤
Tablets, yellow, s/c, fluphenazine hydrochloride
1.5 mg, nortriptyline 30 mg (as hydrochloride).
Net price 28-tab pack = £2.83. Label: 2
Motival® (Sanofi-Synthelabo) [PoM] ◤
Tablets, pink, s/c, fluphenazine hydrochloride
500 micrograms, nortriptyline 10 mg (as hydro-
chloride). Net price 20 = 70p. Label: 2

◤ denotes preparations that are considered to
be less suitable for prescribing (see p. vi)

PROTRIPTYLINE HYDROCHLORIDE

Indications: depressive illness, particularly with
apathy and withdrawal
Cautions: see under Amitriptyline Hydrochloride
Contra-indications: see under Amitriptyline
Hydrochloride
Side-effects: see under Amitriptyline Hydrochloride but less sedating; anxiety, agitation,
tachycardia, and hypotension more common;
rashes associated with photosensitisation (avoid
direct sunlight); daily dose above 20 mg in elderly
(increased risk of cardiovascular side-effects)
Dose: initially 10 mg 3–4 times daily (elderly 5 mg
3 times daily initially), increased gradually up to
60 mg daily in divided doses according to
response; if insomnia, last dose not after 4 p.m.;
CHILD under 16 years not recommended

Concordin® (MSD) [PoM]
Tablets, both f/c, protriptyline hydrochloride 5 mg
(pink), net price 30-tab pack = 66p. Label: 2, 11

TRIMIPRAMINE

Indications: depressive illness, particularly where
sedation is required
Cautions: see under Amitriptyline Hydrochloride
Contra-indications: see under Amitriptyline
Hydrochloride
Side-effects: see under Amitriptyline Hydrochloride
Dose: initially 50–75 mg daily, increased as necessary to 150–300 mg daily; ELDERLY initially 10–
25 mg 3 times daily, maintenance half adult dose
may be sufficient; CHILD not recommended

Surmontil® (Futuna) [PoM]
Capsules, green/white, trimipramine 50 mg (as maleate). Net price 28-cap pack = £8.51. Label: 2
Tablets, trimipramine (as maleate) 10 mg, net price 28-tab pack = £3.84, 84-tab pack = £11.49; 25 mg, 28-tab pack = £5.06, 84-tab pack = £15.16. Label: 2

Related antidepressants

MAPROTILINE HYDROCHLORIDE

Indications: depressive illness, particularly where sedation is required
Cautions: see under Amitriptyline Hydrochloride
Contra-indications: see under Amitriptyline Hydrochloride; history of epilepsy
Side-effects: see under Amitriptyline Hydrochloride, antimuscarinic effects may occur less frequently but rashes common and increased risk of convulsions at higher dosage
Dose: initially 25–75 mg (elderly 30 mg) daily in 3 divided doses *or* as a single dose at bedtime, increased gradually as necessary to max. 150 mg daily; CHILD not recommended

Ludiomil® (Novartis) [PoM]
Tablets, all f/c, maprotiline hydrochloride 10 mg (pale yellow), net price 28-tab pack = 98p; 25 mg (greyish-red), 28-tab pack = £2.11; 50 mg (light orange), 28-tab pack = £4.18; 75 mg (brownish-orange), 28-tab pack = £6.21. Label: 2
Excipients: include gluten

MIANSERIN HYDROCHLORIDE

Indications: depressive illness, particularly where sedation is required
Cautions: see under Amitriptyline Hydrochloride; **interactions:** Appendix 1 (mianserin)
BLOOD COUNTS. A full **blood count** is recommended every 4 weeks during the first 3 months of treatment; subsequent clinical monitoring should continue and treatment should be stopped and a full blood count obtained if *fever, sore throat, stomatitis,* or other signs of infection develop.
Contra-indications: see under Amitriptyline Hydrochloride
Side-effects: see under Amitriptyline Hydrochloride; leucopenia, agranulocytosis and aplastic anaemia (particularly in the elderly); jaundice; arthritis, arthralgia; fewer and milder antimuscarinic and cardiovascular effects
Dose: initially 30–40 mg (elderly 30 mg) daily in divided doses *or* as a single dose at bedtime, increased gradually as necessary; usual dose range 30–90 mg; CHILD not recommended

Mianserin (Non-proprietary) [PoM]
Tablets, mianserin hydrochloride 10 mg, net price 20 = £2.47; 20 mg, 20 = £5.06; 30 mg, 20 = £7.35. Label: 2, 25
Available from Cox, Norton

TRAZODONE HYDROCHLORIDE

Indications: depressive illness, particularly where sedation is required
Cautions: see under Amitriptyline Hydrochloride; **interactions:** Appendix 1 (trazodone)
Contra-indications: see under Amitriptyline Hydrochloride

Side-effects: see under Amitriptyline Hydrochloride but fewer antimuscarinic and cardiovascular effects; rarely priapism (discontinue immediately)
Dose: initially 150 mg (elderly 100 mg) daily in divided doses after food *or* as a single dose at bedtime; may be increased to 300 mg daily; hospital patients up to max. 600 mg daily in divided doses; CHILD not recommended

Molipaxin® (Hoechst Marion Roussel) [PoM]
Capsules, trazodone hydrochloride 50 mg (violet/green), net price 84-cap pack = £17.31; 100 mg (violet/fawn), 56-cap pack = £20.38. Label: 2, 21
Tablets, pink, f/c, trazodone hydrochloride 150 mg. Net price 28-tab pack = £11.62. Label: 2, 21
Liquid, sugar-free, trazodone hydrochloride 50 mg/5 mL. Net price 150 mL = £7.74. Label: 2, 21
CR tablets ▬, m/r, blue, f/c, trazodone hydrochloride 150 mg. Net price 28-tab pack = £11.62. Label: 2, 21, 25
Dose: initially 1 tablet daily (elderly, dose form not appropriate for initial dose titration), increased if necessary to 2 tablets daily (up to 4 tablets daily in hospital patients); CHILD not recommended

VILOXAZINE HYDROCHLORIDE

Indications: depressive illness
Cautions: see under Amitriptyline Hydrochloride; **interactions:** Appendix 1 (viloxazine)
Contra-indications: see under Amitriptyline Hydrochloride
Side-effects: see under Amitriptyline Hydrochloride, but less sedating and antimuscarinic and cardiovascular side-effects are fewer and milder; nausea and headache may occur
Dose: 300 mg daily (preferably as 200 mg in the morning and 100 mg at midday), increased gradually as necessary; max. 400 mg daily; last dose not later than 6 p.m.; ELDERLY 100 mg daily initially, half adult maintenance dose may be sufficient; CHILD under 14 years not recommended

Vivalan® (Zeneca) [PoM]
Tablets, f/c, viloxazine 50 mg (as hydrochloride). Net price 20 = £1.23. Label: 2

4.3.2 Monoamine-oxidase inhibitors
(MAOIs)

Monoamine-oxidase inhibitors are used much less frequently than tricyclic and related antidepressants, or SSRIs and related antidepressants because of the dangers of dietary and drug interactions and the fact that it is easier to prescribe MAOIs when tricyclic antidepressants have been unsuccessful than vice versa. **Tranylcypromine** is the most **hazardous** of the MAOIs because of its stimulant action. The drugs of choice are **phenelzine** or **isocarboxazid** which are less stimulant and therefore safer.

Phobic patients and depressed patients with atypical, hypochondriacal, or hysterical features are said to respond best to MAOIs. However, MAOIs should be tried in any patients who are refractory to treatment with other antidepressants as there is occasionally a dramatic response. Response to treatment may be delayed for 3 weeks or more and may take an additional 1 or 2 weeks to become maximal.

WITHDRAWAL. If possible MAOIs should be withdrawn slowly (see also section 4.3).

INTERACTIONS. MAOIs inhibit monoamine oxidase, thereby causing an accumulation of amine neurotransmitters. The metabolism of some amine drugs such as *indirect-acting sympathomimetics* (present in many cough and decongestant preparations, see section 3.10) is also inhibited and their pressor action may be potentiated; the pressor effect of tyramine (in some foods, such as cheese, pickled herring, broad bean pods, and *Bovril®*, *Oxo®*, *Marmite®* or any similar meat or yeast extract or fermented soya bean extract) may also be dangerously potentiated. These interactions may cause a dangerous rise in blood pressure. An early warning symptom may be a throbbing headache. Patients should be advised to eat only fresh foods and avoid food that is suspected of being stale or 'going off'. This is especially important with meat, fish, poultry or offal; game should be avoided. The danger of interaction persists for up to 2 weeks after treatment with MAOIs is discontinued. Patients should also avoid alcoholic drinks or de-alcoholised (low alcohol) drinks.

Other antidepressants should **not** be started for 2 weeks after treatment with MAOIs has been stopped (3 weeks if starting clomipramine or imipramine). Some psychiatrists use selected tricyclics in conjunction with MAOIs but this is hazardous, indeed potentially lethal, except in experienced hands and there is no evidence that the combination is more effective than when either constituent is used alone. The combination of tranylcypromine with clomipramine is particularly **dangerous**.

Conversely, an MAOI should not be started until 2 weeks (tranylcypramine manufacturer specifies at least 1 week) after a *tricyclic or related antidepressant* has been stopped.

In addition, an MAOI should not be started for at least 2 weeks after a previous MAOI has been stopped (then started at a reduced dose).

For other interactions with MAOIs including those with opioid analgesics (notably pethidine), see Appendix 1 (MAOIs). For guidance on interactions relating to the reversible monoamine oxidase inhibitor, moclobemide, see p. 191; for guidance on interactions relating to SSRIs, see p. 191.

PHENELZINE

Indications: depressive illness

Cautions: diabetes mellitus, cardiovascular disease, epilepsy, blood disorders, concurrent electroconvulsive therapy; elderly (great caution); monitor blood pressure to detect hypotensive responses (postural hypotension) and hypertensive responses (discontinue if palpitations or frequent headaches); if possible avoid abrupt withdrawal; severe hypertensive reactions to certain drugs and foods; avoid in agitated patients; porphyria (see section 9.8.2); pregnancy and breast-feeding; surgery (see section 15.1); **interactions:** Appendix 1 (MAOIs)

DRIVING. Drowsiness may affect performance of skilled tasks (e.g. driving)

Contra-indications: hepatic impairment or abnormal liver function tests (see Appendix 2), cerebrovascular disease, phaeochromocytoma; not indicated in manic phase

Side-effects: adverse effects commonly associated with phenelzine and other MAOIs include postural hypotension (especially in elderly) and dizziness; other side-effects include drowsiness, insomnia, headache, weakness and fatigue, dryness of mouth, constipation and other gastrointestinal disturbances, oedema, myoclonic movement, hyperreflexia, elevated liver enzymes; agitation and tremors, nervousness, euphoria, arrhythmias, blurred vision, nystagmus, difficulty in micturition, sweating, convulsions, rashes, purpura, leucopenia, sexual disturbances, and weight gain with inappropriate appetite may also occur; psychotic episodes with hypomanic behaviour, confusion, and hallucinations, may be induced in susceptible persons; jaundice has been reported and, on rare occasions, fatal progressive hepatocellular necrosis; paraesthesia, peripheral neuritis, peripheral neuropathy may be due to pyridoxine deficiency; for CSM advice on possible hyponatraemia, see p. 185 (hypernatraemia also reported)

Dose: 15 mg 3 times daily, increased if necessary to 4 times daily after 2 weeks (hospital patients, max. 30 mg 3 times daily), then reduced gradually to lowest possible maintenance dose (15 mg on alternate days may be adequate); CHILD not recommended

Nardil® (Hansam) [PoM]
Tablets, orange, f/c, phenelzine 15 mg (as sulphate). Net price 20 = £3.99. Label: 3, 10 patient information leaflet

---

ISOCARBOXAZID

Indications: depressive illness

Cautions: see under Phenelzine

Contra-indications: see under Phenelzine

Side-effects: see under Phenelzine

Dose: initially 30 mg daily in single or divided doses until improvement occurs (increased after 4 weeks if necessary to max. 60 mg daily for 4–6 weeks under close supervision), then reduced to usual maintenance dose 10–20 mg daily (but up to 40 mg daily may be required); ELDERLY 5–10 mg daily; CHILD not recommended

Isocarboxazid (Cambridge) [PoM]
Tablets, pink, scored, isocarboxazid 10 mg. Net price 50 = £24.29. Label: 3, 10 patient information leaflet

 denotes preparations that are considered to be less suitable for prescribing (see p. vi)

TRANYLCYPROMINE

Indications: depressive illness

Cautions: see under Phenelzine

Contra-indications: see under Phenelzine; hyperthyroidism

Side-effects: see under Phenelzine; insomnia if given in evening; hypertensive crises with throbbing headache requiring discontinuation of treatment more frequent than with other MAOIs; liver damage less frequent than with phenelzine

Dose: initially 10 mg twice daily not later than 3 p.m., increasing the second daily dose to 20 mg after 1 week if necessary; doses above 30 mg daily under close supervision only; usual maintenance dose 10 mg daily; CHILD not recommended

Parnate® (SK&F) [PoM] [▭]

Tablets, red, s/c, tranylcypromine 10 mg (as sulphate). Net price 28-tab pack = £1.27. Label: 3, 10 patient information leaflet

Note. The future availability of *Parnate®* is uncertain; prescribers should seek alternative treatment

Reversible MAOIs

Moclobemide is indicated for major depression only; it is reported to act by reversible inhibition of monoamine oxidase type A (it is therefore termed a RIMA). It should be reserved as a second-line treatment.

INTERACTIONS. Moclobemide is claimed to cause less potentiation of the pressor effect of tyramine than the traditional (irreversible) MAOIs, but patients should avoid consuming large amounts of tyramine-rich food (such as mature cheese, yeast extracts and fermented soya bean products).

The risk of drug interactions is also claimed to be less but patients still need to avoid sympathomimetics such as ephedrine, pseudoephedrine, and phenylpropanolamine. In addition, moclobemide should not be given with another antidepressant. Owing to its short duration of action no treatment-free period is required after it has been stopped but it should not be started until at least a week after a tricyclic or related antidepressant or an SSRI has been stopped (2 weeks in the case of paroxetine and sertraline, and at least 5 weeks in the case of fluoxetine), or for at least a week after an MAOI has been stopped. For other interactions, see Appendix 1 (moclobemide).

MOCLOBEMIDE

Indications: depressive illness; social phobia

Cautions: avoid in agitated or excited patients (or give with sedative for up to 2–3 weeks), thyrotoxicosis, hepatic impairment (Appendix 2), may provoke manic episodes in bipolar disorders, pregnancy and breast-feeding (patient information leaflet advises avoid); **interactions:** see notes above and Appendix 1 (moclobemide)

Contra-indications: acute confusional states, phaeochromocytoma

Side-effects: sleep disturbances, dizziness, gastrointestinal disorders, headache, restlessness, agitation; paraesthesia, dry mouth, visual disturbances, oedema, skin reactions, confusional states reported; rarely raised liver enzymes, galactorrhoea; for CSM advice on possible hyponatraemia, see p. 185

Dose: depression, initially 300 mg daily usually in divided doses after food, adjusted according to response; usual range 150–600 mg daily; CHILD not recommended

Social phobia, initially 300 mg daily increased on fourth day to 600 mg daily in 2 divided doses, continued for 8–12 weeks to assess efficacy; CHILD not recommended

Manerix® (Roche) [PoM]

Tablets, yellow, f/c, scored, moclobemide 150 mg, net price 30-tab pack = £10.03; 300 mg, 30-tab pack = £15.04. Label: 10 patient information leaflet, 21

4.3.3 Selective serotonin re-uptake inhibitors

Citalopram, fluoxetine, fluvoxamine, paroxetine, and **sertraline** selectively inhibit the re-uptake of serotonin (5-hydroxytryptamine, 5-HT); they are termed selective serotonin re-uptake inhibitors (SSRIs) and appear to be effective antidepressants. For a general comment on the management of depression and on the comparison between *tricyclic and related antidepressants* and the *SSRIs and related antidepressants*, see section 4.3.

CAUTIONS. SSRIs should be used with caution in patients with epilepsy (avoid if poorly controlled, discontinue if convulsions develop), concurrent electroconvulsive therapy (prolonged seizures reported with fluoxetine), history of mania, cardiac disease, history of bleeding disorders, hepatic and renal impairment (Appendixes 2 and 3), pregnancy and breast-feeding (Appendixes 4 and 5). SSRIs may also impair performance of skilled tasks (e.g. driving). Abrupt withdrawal of SSRIs should be avoided (associated with headache, nausea, paraesthesia, dizziness and anxiety); **interactions:** see below and Appendix 1 (antidepressants, SSRI).

INTERACTIONS. An SSRI or related antidepressant should not be started until 2 weeks after stopping an MAOI. Conversely, an MAOI should not be started until at least a week after an SSRI or related antidepressant has been stopped (2 weeks in the case of paroxetine and sertraline, at least 5 weeks in the case of fluoxetine). For guidance relating to the reversible monoamine oxidase inhibitor, moclobemide, see above. For other SSRI antidepressant interactions, see Appendix 1 (antidepressants, SSRI).

CONTRA-INDICATIONS. SSRIs should not be used if the patient enters a manic phase.

SIDE-EFFECTS. SSRIs are considered to be less sedating and have fewer antimuscarinic and cardiotoxic effects than tricyclic antidepressants (section 4.3). Side-effects of the SSRIs include gastro-intestinal effects (dose related; fairly common—include nausea, vomiting, dyspepsia, abdominal pain, diarrhoea, constipation), anorexia with weight loss (increased appetite and weight gain also reported with citalopram) and hypersensitivity reactions; other side-effects include dry mouth, nervousness, anxiety, headache, insomnia, tremor, dizziness, asthenia, drowsiness, convulsions (see Cautions above), sexual dysfunction, sweating, purpura, hypomania or mania (see Cautions above), movement disorders and dyskinesias, hyponatraemia (may be due to inappropriate antidiuretic hormone secretion—see CSM warning, section 4.3). Suicidal ideation has been linked with some SSRIs particularly fluoxetine but causality has not been established.

CITALOPRAM

Indications: depressive illness, panic disorder
Cautions: see notes above
Contra-indications: see notes above
Side-effects: see notes above; palpitations, tachycardia, postural hypotension, coughing, yawning, confusion, impaired concentration, amnesia, migraine, hypersensitivity reactions (including rash, pruritus, myalgia), paraesthesia, visual disturbances, taste disturbance, increased salivation, rhinitis, tinnitus, micturition disorders also reported
Dose: depressive illness, 20 mg daily as a single dose in the morning or evening increased if necessary to max. 60 mg daily (ELDERLY max. 40 mg daily); CHILD not recommended
Panic disorder, initially 10 mg daily increased to 20 mg after 7 days, usual dose 20–30 mg daily; max. 60 mg daily (ELDERLY max. 40 mg daily); CHILD not recommended

Cipramil® (Lundbeck) PoM
Tablets, f/c, citalopram (as hydrobromide) 10 mg, net price 28-tab pack = £9.73; 20 mg (scored), 28-tab pack = £16.19; 40 mg, 28-tab pack = £27.37. Counselling, driving
Oral drops, sugar-free, citalopram (as hydrochloride) 40 mg/mL, net price 15 mL = £21.68. Counselling, driving, administration
Excipients: include alcohol
Note. Mix with water, orange juice, or apple juice before taking

FLUOXETINE

Indications: see under Dose
Cautions: see notes above
DRIVING. May impair performance of skilled tasks (e.g. driving)
Contra-indications: see notes above
Side-effects: see notes above; possible changes in blood sugar, hypersensitivity reactions (**important:** see also below), fever, neuroleptic malignant syndrome-like event; abnormal liver function tests reported; also reported (no causal relationship established): abnormal bleeding, aplastic anaemia, cerebrovascular accident, ecchymoses, eosinophilic pneumonia, gastrointestinal haemorrhage, hyperprolactinaemia, haemolytic anaemia, pancreatitis, pancytopenia, thrombocytopenia, thrombocytopenic purpura, vaginal bleeding on withdrawal, violent behaviour; hair loss also reported
HYPERSENSITIVITY. Angioedema, urticaria, and other allergic reactions including anaphylaxis have been reported (discontinue if rash occurs, may be warning of impending serious systemic reaction, possibly associated with vasculitis); pharyngitis and rarely pulmonary inflammation or fibrosis (with dyspnoea only warning sign) also reported; other possible hypersensitivity signs include arthralgia, myalgia, serum sickness
Dose: depressive illness, 20 mg daily; CHILD not recommended
Bulimia nervosa, 60 mg daily; CHILD not recommended
Obsessive-compulsive disorder, initially 20 mg daily, dose increase may be considered if no response after several weeks, but may be increased potential for side-effects; max. 60 mg daily; CHILD not recommended
Premenstrual dysphoric disorder, 20 mg daily for 6 months then reassess for benefit before continuing
LONG DURATION OF ACTION. Consider the long half-life of fluoxetine when adjusting dosage (or in overdosage)

Fluoxetine (Non-proprietary) PoM
Capsules, fluoxetine (as hydrochloride) 20 mg, net price 30-cap pack = £19.84. Counselling, driving
Available from CP, Lagap, Norton, Sovereign
Prozac® (Dista) PoM
Capsules, fluoxetine (as hydrochloride) 20 mg (green/yellow), net price 30-cap pack = £19.84, 98-cap pack = £64.80; 60 mg (yellow), 30-cap pack = £59.51. Counselling, driving
Liquid, fluoxetine (as hydrochloride) 20 mg/5 mL. Net price 70-mL pack = £18.52. Counselling, driving

FLUVOXAMINE MALEATE

Indications: depressive illness, obsessive-compulsive disorder
Cautions: see notes above
CSM ADVICE. The CSM has advised that concomitant use of fluvoxamine and theophylline or aminophylline should usually be avoided; see also **interactions:** Appendix 1 (antidepressants, SSRIs)
Contra-indications: see notes above
Side-effects: see notes above; palpitations, tachycardia (may also cause bradycardia), rarely postural hypotension, confusion, hallucinations, ataxia, rarely abnormal liver function tests, usually symptomatic (discontinue treatment), hypersensitivity reactions (including rash, pruritus, arthralgia, myalgia, photosensitivity, anaphylactoid reactions), galactorrhoea
Dose: initially 100 mg daily increased if necessary to max. 300 mg daily (over 100 mg in divided doses); CHILD not recommended
Note. If no improvement in obsessive-compulsive disorder within 10 weeks, treatment should be reconsidered

Fluvoxamine Maleate (Non-proprietary) PoM
Tablets, fluvoxamine maleate 50 mg, net price 60-tab pack = £19.00; 100 mg, 30-tab pack = £19.00. Counselling, driving
Available from Norton
Faverin® (Solvay) PoM
Tablets, f/c, scored, fluvoxamine maleate 50 mg, net price 60-tab pack = £19.00; 100 mg, 30-tab pack = £19.00. Counselling, driving

PAROXETINE

Indications: depressive illness, obsessive-compulsive disorder, panic disorder; social phobia
Cautions: see notes above
IMPORTANT. During initial treatment of panic disorder, there is potential for worsening of panic symptoms
CSM ADVICE. Extrapyramidal reactions (including orofacial dystonias) and withdrawal syndrome are reported to the CSM more commonly with paroxetine than with other SSRIs
Contra-indications: see notes above
Side-effects: see notes above; postural hypotension reported, hypersensitivity reactions

(including rash, urticaria, pruritus, angioedema), abnormal liver function tests

Dose: depressive illness, usually 20 mg each morning, if necessary increased gradually in increments of 10 mg to max. 50 mg daily (elderly, 40 mg daily); CHILD not recommended

Obsessive-compulsive disorder, initially 20 mg each morning, if necessary increased gradually in weekly increments of 10 mg to usual dose 40 mg daily (max. 60 mg daily, max. in elderly 40 mg daily); CHILD not recommended

Panic disorder, initially 10 mg each morning, if necessary increased gradually in weekly increments of 10 mg to usual dose of 40 mg daily (max. 50 mg daily, max. in elderly 40 mg daily); CHILD not recommended

Social phobia, initially 20 mg in the morning; if no improvement after at least 2 weeks, increase in steps of 10 mg at intervals of at least 1 week (max. 50 mg daily, max. in elderly 40 mg daily); CHILD not recommended

Seroxat® (SmithKline Beecham) PoM
Tablets, both f/c, scored, paroxetine (as hydrochloride) 20 mg, net price 30-tab pack = £17.76; 30 mg (blue), 30-tab pack = £31.16. Label: 21, counselling, driving
Liquid, orange, sugar-free, paroxetine (as hydrochloride) 10 mg/5 mL. Net price 150-mL pack = £20.77. Label: 21, counselling, driving

SERTRALINE

Indications: depressive illness, obsessive compulsive disorder

Cautions: see notes above

Contra-indications: see notes above

Side-effects: see notes above; tachycardia, confusion, amnesia, hallucinations, aggressive behaviour, psychosis, hypersensitivity reactions (including rash, erythema multiforme, photosensitivity, angioedema, arthralgia, myalgia), abnormal liver function tests, pancreatitis, hepatitis, jaundice, liver failure, galactorrhoea, menstrual irregularities, paraesthesia; also reported (no causal relationship established) thrombocytopenia, cutaneous bleeding abnormalities including ecchymoses and purpura

Dose: depressive illness, initially 50 mg daily, increased if necessary by increments of 50 mg over several weeks to max. 200 mg daily, then reduced to usual maintenance of 50 mg daily; CHILD not recommended
Obsessive-compulsive disorder, initially 50 mg daily, increased if necessary by increments of 50 mg over several weeks; usual dose range 50–200 mg daily; CHILD not recommended

Lustral® (Pfizer) PoM
Tablets, sertraline (as hydrochloride) 50 mg, net price 28-tab pack = £16.20; 100 mg, 28-tab pack = £26.51. Counselling, driving

4.3.4 Other antidepressant drugs

The thioxanthene **flupentixol** (*Fluanxol®*) has antidepressant properties, and low doses (1 to 3 mg daily) are given by mouth for this purpose. Flupen-

tixol is also used for the treatment of psychoses (section 4.2.1 and section 4.2.2)

Mirtazapine, a presynaptic α_2-antagonist, increases central noradrenergic and serotonergic neurotransmission. It has few antimuscarinic effects, but causes sedation during initial treatment.

Nefazodone inhibits re-uptake of serotonin and also selectively blocks serotonin receptors.

Reboxetine, a selective inhibitor of noradrenaline re-uptake, has been introduced for the treatment of depressive illness.

Tryptophan appears to benefit some patients with resistant depression when given as adjunctive therapy but tryptophan products have been associated with the eosinophilia-myalgia syndrome; *Optimax®* (Merck) is available for patients for whom no alternative treatment is suitable.

Venlafaxine is a serotonin and noradrenaline re-uptake inhibitor (SNRI); it lacks the sedative and antimuscarinic effects of the tricyclic antidepressants.

FLUPENTIXOL

(Flupenthixol)

Indications: depressive illness (short-term use); psychoses (section 4.2.1)

Cautions: cardiovascular disease (including cardiac disorders and cerebral arteriosclerosis), senile confusional states, parkinsonism, renal and hepatic disease; avoid in excitable and overactive patients; porphyria (section 9.8.2); **interactions:** Appendix 1 (antipsychotics)
DRIVING. Drowsiness may affect performance of skilled tasks (e.g. driving); effects of alcohol enhanced

Side-effects: restlessness, insomnia; hypomania reported; rarely dizziness, tremor, visual disturbances, headache, hyperprolactinaemia, extrapyramidal symptoms

Dose: initially 1 mg (elderly 500 micrograms) in the morning, increased after 1 week to 2 mg (elderly 1 mg) if necessary. Max. 3 mg (elderly 2 mg) daily, doses above 2 mg (elderly 1 mg) being divided in 2 portions, second dose not after 4 p.m. Discontinue if no response after 1 week at max. dosage; CHILD not recommended
COUNSELLING. Although drowsiness may occur, can also have an alerting effect so should not be taken in the evening

Fluanxol® (Lundbeck) PoM
Tablets, both red, s/c, flupentixol (as dihydrochloride) 500 micrograms, net price 60-tab pack = £3.10; 1 mg, 60-tab pack = £5.23. Label: 2, counselling, administration

MIRTAZAPINE

Indications: depressive illness

Cautions: epilepsy, hepatic or renal impairment, cardiac disorders, hypotension, history of urinary retention, angle-closure glaucoma, diabetes mellitus, psychoses (may aggravate psychotic symptoms), history of bipolar depression, avoid abrupt withdrawal; manufacturer advises avoid in pregnancy and in breast-feeding; **interactions:** Appendix 1 (mirtazapine)
BLOOD DISORDERS. Patients should be advised to report any fever, sore throat, stomatitis or other signs of infection during treatment. Blood count should be performed and the drug stopped immediately if blood dyscrasia suspected

Side-effects: increased appetite and weight gain, sedation, less commonly elevated liver enzymes, jaundice (discontinue treatment); rarely oedema, postural hypotension, exanthema, tremor, myoclonus; reversible agranulocytosis (see Cautions above), leucopenia, granulocytosis

Dose: initially 15 mg daily at bedtime increased according to response up to 45 mg daily as a single dose at bedtime or in 2 divided doses; CHILD not recommended

Zispin® (Organon) ▼ PoM

Tablets, scored, red/brown, mirtazapine 30 mg. Net price 28-tab pack = £22.92. Label: 2, 25

NEFAZODONE HYDROCHLORIDE

Indications: depressive illness

Cautions: epilepsy, concurrent electroconvulsive therapy (no studies), history of mania or hypomania, elderly (especially female), hepatic and renal impairment (lower end of dose range), pregnancy; **interactions:** Appendix 1 (nefazodone)

DRIVING. May impair performance of skilled tasks (e.g. driving)

Contra-indications: breast-feeding

Side-effects: asthenia, dry mouth, nausea, somnolence, dizziness; less frequently, chills, fever, postural hypotension, constipation, lightheadedness, paraesthesia, confusion, ataxia, amblyopia and other minor visual disturbances; rarely syncope

Dose: initially 50–100 mg twice daily increased after 5–7 days to 200 mg twice daily, may be gradually increased if necessary to max. 300 mg twice daily (ELDERLY usual max. 100–200 mg twice daily); ADOLESCENT and CHILD under 18 years not recommended

Dutonin® (Bristol-Myers) ▼ PoM

Tablets, both scored, nefazodone hydrochloride 100 mg (white), net price 56-tab pack = £16.80; 200 mg (yellow), 56-tab pack = £16.80; treatment initiation pack consisting of 14 × 50 mg (pink) tablets, 14 × 100 mg tablets and 28 × 200 mg tablets = £16.80. Label: 3

REBOXETINE

Indications: depressive illness

Cautions: severe renal impairment (Appendix 3), hepatic impairment (Appendix 2), history of cardiovascular disease and epilepsy, bipolar disorders, urinary retention, prostatic hypertrophy, glaucoma; **interactions:** Appendix 1 (reboxetine)

Contra-indications: pregnancy (Appendix 4) and breast-feeding (Appendix 5)

Side-effects: insomnia, sweating, dizziness, postural hypotension, vertigo, paraesthesia, impotence, dysuria, urinary retention (mainly in men), dry mouth, constipation, tachycardia; lowering of plasma-potassium concentration on prolonged administration in the elderly

Dose: 4 mg twice daily increased if necessary after 3–4 weeks to 10 mg daily in divided doses, max. 12 mg daily; CHILD and ELDERLY not recommended

Edronax® (Pharmacia & Upjohn) ▼ PoM

Tablets, scored, reboxetine (as mesilate) 4 mg. Net price 60-tab pack = £18.91. Counselling, driving

TRYPTOPHAN

(L-Tryptophan)

Indications: restricted to use by hospital specialists *only* for patients with severe and disabling depressive illness of more than 2 years continuous duration, *only* after an adequate trial of standard antidepressant drug treatment, and *only* as an adjunct to other antidepressant medication

Cautions: eosinophilia-myalgia syndrome has been reported with tryptophan-containing products therefore close and regular surveillance required; monitor eosinophil count, haematological changes and muscle symptomatology; pregnancy and breast-feeding; **interactions:** Appendix 1 (tryptophan)

Contra-indications: history of eosinophilia-myalgia syndrome following use of tryptophan

Side-effects: drowsiness, nausea, headache, lightheadedness; eosinophilia-myalgia syndrome, see Cautions

Dose: 1 g 3 times daily; max. 6 g daily; ELDERLY lower dose may be appropriate especially where renal or hepatic impairment; CHILD not recommended

Optimax® (Merck) ▼ PoM

Tablets, scored, tryptophan 500 mg. Net price 84-tab pack = £16.30. Label: 3

Important. Patient and prescriber must be registered with the *Optimax®* Information and Clinical Support (OPTICS) Unit. A **safety questionnaire** is sent to the prescriber after **3** and **6 months** of treatment and **every 6 months** thereafter. The information is reviewed by the CSM—it is **important** that the questionnaires should be completed

VENLAFAXINE

Indications: depressive illness

Cautions: history of myocardial infarction or unstable heart disease, blood pressure monitoring advisable with doses of more than 200 mg daily, history of epilepsy, hepatic or renal impairment (Appendixes 2 and 3), history of drug abuse, avoid abrupt withdrawal (if taken for more than 1 week withdraw over at least 1 week); **interactions:** Appendix 1 (venlafaxine)

DRIVING. May affect performance of skilled tasks (e.g. driving)

SKIN REACTIONS. Patients should be advised to contact doctor if rash, urticaria or related allergic reaction develops

Contra-indications: severe hepatic or renal impairment; pregnancy and breast-feeding

Side-effects: nausea, headache, insomnia, somnolence, dry mouth, dizziness (and occasionally hypotension), constipation, asthenia, sweating, nervousness, convulsions (discontinue); other side-effects reported include anorexia, dyspepsia, abdominal pain, anxiety, sexual dysfunction, visual disturbances, vasodilatation, vomiting, tremor, abnormal dreams, paraesthesia, chills, hypertension (see Cautions, above), palpitations, weight changes, agitation, hypertonia, rash (see Skin reactions, above); hyponatraemia, reversible increase in liver enzymes, and alterations in serum cholesterol also reported

Dose: initially 75 mg daily in 2 divided doses increased if necessary after several weeks to 150 mg daily in 2 divided doses

Severely depressed or hospitalised patients, initially 150 mg daily in 2 divided doses increased if necessary in steps of up to 75 mg every 2–3 days to max. 375 mg daily then gradually reduced; ADOLESCENT and CHILD under 18 years not recommended

Efexor® (Wyeth) PoM

Tablets, both peach, venlafaxine (as hydrochloride) 37.5 mg, net price 56-tab pack = £23.97; 50 mg, 42-tab pack = £23.97; 75 mg, 56-tab pack = £39.97. Label: 21, counselling, driving, skin reactions

Efexor® XL (Wyeth) PoM

Capsules, m/r, venlafaxine (as hydrochloride) 75 mg (peach), net price 28-cap pack = £23.97, 150 mg (orange), 28-cap pack = £39.97. Label: 21, 25, counselling, driving, skin reactions

Dose: 75 mg daily as a single dose, increased if necessary after at least 2 weeks to 150 mg once daily; max. 225 mg once daily; ADOLESCENT and CHILD under 18 years not recommended

4.4   Central nervous system stimulants

Central nervous system stimulants include the **amphetamines** (notably dexamfetamine) **and related drugs** (e.g. methylphenidate). They have very few indications and in particular, should **not** be used to treat depression, obesity, senility, debility, or for relief of fatigue.

Caffeine is a weak stimulant present in tea and coffee. It is included in many analgesic preparations (section 4.7.1) but does not contribute to their analgesic or anti-inflammatory effect. Over-indulgence may lead to a state of anxiety.

The **amphetamines** have a limited field of usefulness and their use should be **discouraged** as they may cause dependence and psychotic states. They have **no place** in the management of **depression** or **obesity**.

Patients with *narcolepsy* may derive benefit from treatment with dexamfetamine.

Dexamfetamine (dexamphetamine) and **methylphenidate** have been advocated (under specialist supervision) for the management of *hyperactive children*; beneficial effects have been described. However, they must be used very selectively since they retard growth and the effect of long-term therapy has not been evaluated.

Modafinil is used for the treatment of narcolepsy; dependence with long-term use cannot be excluded and it should therefore be used with caution

DEXAMFETAMINE SULPHATE

(Dexamphetamine Sulphate)

Indications: narcolepsy, adjunct in the management of refractory hyperkinetic states in children (under specialist supervision)

Cautions: mild hypertension (contra-indicated if moderate or severe)—monitor blood pressure; history of epilepsy (discontinue if convulsions occur); monitor growth in children (see also below); avoid abrupt withdrawal; data on safety and efficacy of long-term use not complete; porphyria (see section 9.8.2); **interactions:** Appendix 1 (sympathomimetics)

SPECIAL CAUTIONS IN CHILDREN. Monitor height and weight as growth retardation may occur during prolonged therapy (drug free periods may allow catch-up in growth but withdraw slowly to avoid inducing depression or renewed hyperactivity). In psychotic children may exacerbate behavioural disturbances and thought disorder

Contra-indications: cardiovascular disease including moderate to severe hypertension (caution if mild), hyperexcitability or agitated states, hyperthyroidism, history of drug or alcohol abuse, glaucoma, predisposition to tics or Tourette syndrome (discontinue if tics occur), pregnancy and breast-feeding

DRIVING. May affect performance of skilled tasks (e.g. driving); effects of alcohol unpredictable

Side-effects: insomnia, restlessness, irritability and excitabilitiy, nervousness, night terrors, euphoria, tremor, dizziness, headache; convulsions (see also Cautions); dependence and tolerance, sometimes psychosis; anorexia, gastrointestinal symptoms, growth retardation in children (see also under Cautions); dry mouth, sweating, tachycardia (and anginal pain), palpitations, increased blood pressure; visual disturbances; cardiomyopathy reported with chronic use; central stimulants have provoked choreoathetoid movements, tics and Tourette syndrome in predisposed individuals (see also Contra-indications above); **overdosage:** see Emergency Treatment of Poisoning, p. 24

Dose: narcolepsy, 10 mg (elderly, 5 mg) daily in divided doses increased by 10 mg (elderly, 5 mg) daily at intervals of 1 week to a max. of 60 mg daily

Hyperkinesia, CHILD under 6 years not recommended, over 6 years 5–10 mg daily, increased if necessary by 5 mg at intervals of 1 week to usual max. 20 mg daily (older children have received max. 40 mg daily)

Dexedrine® (Medeva) CD

Tablets, scored, dexamfetamine sulphate 5 mg. Net price 28-tab pack = 96p. Counselling, driving

METHYLPHENIDATE HYDROCHLORIDE

Indications: part of a comprehensive treatment programme for attention-deficit hyperactivity disorder when remedial measures alone prove insufficient (under specialist supervision)

Cautions: see under Dexamfetamine Sulphate; manufacturer recommends periodic complete and differential blood and platelet counts; **interactions:** Appendix 1 (sympathomimetics)

Contra-indications: see under Dexamfetamine Sulphate

Side-effects: see under Dexamfetamine Sulphate; rash, urticaria, fever, arthralgia, alopecia, exfoliative dermatitis, erythema multiforme, thrombo-

cytopenic   purpura,   thrombocytopenia,
leucopenia

Dose: CHILD under 6 years not recommended, over
6 years, initially 5 mg 1–2 times daily, increased
if necessary at weekly intervals by 5–10 mg daily
to max. 60 mg daily in divided doses; discontinue
if no response after 1 month, also discontinue
periodically to assess child's condition (usually
finally discontinued during or after puberty)

EVENING DOSE. If effect wears off in evening (with
rebound hyperactivity) a dose at bedtime may be appropriate (establish need with trial bedtime dose)

Ritalin® (Novartis) CD
Tablets, scored, methylphenidate hydrochloride
10 mg, net price 30-tab pack = £5.57

MODAFINIL

Indications: narcolepsy

Cautions: hepatic impairment (Appendix 2); renal
impairment (Appendix 3); monitor blood pressure
and heart rate in hypertensive patients (but see
below); possibility of dependence; **interactions:**
Appendix 1 (modafinil)

Contra-indications: pregnancy and breast-feeding; moderate to severe hypertension; history of
left ventricular hypertrophy or ischaemic ECG
changes, chest pain, arrhythmia, mitral valve prolapse associated with CNS stimulant use

Side-effects: anorexia, abdominal pain, headache,
personality disorder, CNS stimulation including
insomnia, excitation, euphoria, nervousness, dry
mouth, palpitation, tachycardia, hypertension,
tremor; gastro-intestinal disturbances (including
nausea, gastric discomfort); rashes, pruritus,
rarely buccofacial dyskinesia, dose-related
increase in alkaline phosphatase

Dose: 200–400 mg daily, *either* in 2 divided doses
morning and at noon *or* as a single dose in the
morning; ELDERLY initiate at 100 mg daily; CHILD
not recommended

Provigil® (Cephalon) ▼ PoM
Tablets, modafinil 100 mg. Net price 30-tab pack =
£60.00

Cocaine

Cocaine is a drug of addiction which causes central
nervous stimulation. Its clinical use is mainly as a
topical local anaesthetic (section 15.2). It has been
included in analgesic elixirs for the relief of pain in
palliative care but this use is obsolete. For management of cocaine poisoning, see p. 24.

4.5   Drugs used in the treatment of obesity

4.5.1   Anti-obesity drugs acting on the gastro-
intestinal tract

4.5.2   Centrally acting appetite suppressants

Obesity is associated with many health problems
including cardiovascular disease, diabetes mellitus,
gallstones and osteoarthritis. Factors that aggravate

obesity may include depression, other psychosocial
problems, and drug treatment.

The main treatment of the obese patient is a suitable diet, carefully explained to the patient, with
appropriate support and encouragement; the patient
should also be advised to increase physical activity.
Smoking cessation (while maintaining body
weight) may be worthwhile before attempting
supervised weight loss since cigarette smoking may
be more harmful than obesity. Attendance at groups
(e.g. 'weight-watchers') helps some individuals.

An anti-obesity drug should be considered only
for those with a body mass index (BMI, individual's
body-weight divided by the square of the individual's height) of 30 kg/m² or greater in whom at least
3 months of managed care involving supervised
diet, exercise and behaviour modification fails to
achieve a realistic reduction in weight. If risk factors are present (such as established diabetes mellitus, coronary heart disease, hypertension, and
obstructive sleep apnoea) then it may be appropriate to prescribe a drug to individuals with a BMI of
28 kg/m² or greater (if permitted by the marketing
authorisation). Drugs should **never** be used as the
sole element of treatment. The individual should be
monitored on a regular basis; drug treatment should
be discontinued if weight loss is less than 5% after
the first 12 weeks or if the individual regains weight
at any time whilst receiving drug treatment.

Severe obesity should be managed in an appropriate setting by staff who have been trained in the
management of obesity; the patient should receive
advice on diet and lifestyle modification and be
monitored for changes in weight as well as in blood
pressure, blood lipids and other associated conditions.

Combination therapy involving more than one
anti-obesity drug is **contra-indicated** until further
information about efficacy and long-term safety is
available.

Thyroid hormones have **no** place in the treatment
of obesity except in biochemically proven hypothyroid patients. The use of diuretics, chorionic
gonadotrophin, or amphetamines is **not** appropriate
for weight reduction.

4.5.1   Anti-obesity drugs acting on the gastro-intestinal tract

Orlistat, a pancreatic lipase inhibitor, reduces the
absorption of dietary fat. It is licensed for use in
conjunction with a mildly hypocaloric diet in those
with a body mass index (BMI) of 30 kg/m² or
greater; it may also be considered in those with a
BMI of 28 kg/m² or greater and associated risk factors. Treatment with orlistat should be started only
if diet alone has previously produced a weight loss
of 2.5 kg over a period of 4 consecutive weeks.
Some of the weight loss in patients taking orlistat
probably results from subjects reducing their fat
intake to avoid severe gastro-intestinal effects
including steatorrhoea.

The most commonly used bulk-forming drug is
methylcellulose. It is claimed to reduce intake by
producing a feeling of satiety but there is little evidence to support this claim.

METHYLCELLULOSE

Indications: adjunct in obesity (but see notes above); other indications (section 1.6.1)

Cautions: maintain adequate fluid intake

Contra-indications: gastro-intestinal obstruction

Side-effects: flatulence, abdominal distension, intestinal obstruction

Dose: see under preparations below

COUNSELLING. Preparations that swell in contact with liquid should always be carefully swallowed with water and should not be taken immediately before going to bed

Celevac® (Monmouth)

Tablets, pink, methylcellulose '450' 500 mg. Net price 112-tab pack = £2.69. Counselling, see above and dose

Dose: adjunct in obesity (but see notes above), 3 tablets, chewed or crushed, with a tumblerful of liquid half an hour before food or when hungry

ORLISTAT

Indications: adjunct in obesity (see notes above)

Cautions: diabetes mellitus; may impair absorption of fat-soluble vitamins; **interactions:** Appendix 1 (orlistat)

MULTIVITAMINS. If a multivitamin supplement is required, it should be taken at least 2 hours after orlistat dose or at bedtime

Contra-indications: chronic malabsorption syndrome; cholestasis; pregnancy and breast-feeding

Side-effects: liquid oily stools, faecal urgency, flatulence, less frequently abdominal and rectal pain (gastro-intestinal effects minimised by reduced fat diet); headache; menstrual irregularities; anxiety, fatigue

Dose: 120 mg taken immediately before, during, or up to 1 hour after each main meal (up to max. 360 mg daily); max. period of treatment 2 years; CHILD not recommended

Note. If a meal is missed or contains no fat, the dose of orlistat should be omitted

Xenical® (Roche) ▼ PoM

Capsules, turquoise, orlistat 120 mg, net price 84-cap pack = £41.16

4.5.2 Centrally acting appetite suppressants

Appetite suppressants are used as adjuncts to other methods in an appropriate setting (section 4.5). Patients prescribed these drugs should be reviewed at least at monthly intervals and a careful record kept of all treatment with appetite suppressant drugs. The patient's general practitioner should be kept informed of details of treatment and progress, if the prescription is initiated by another physician.

Dexfenfluramine and fenfluramine have been withdrawn following reports of valvular heart disease associated with their use.

Phentermine is a catecholaminergic drug with minor sympathomimetic and stimulant effects; it is licensed for use as an adjunct to the treatment of selected patients with moderate to severe obesity. Rapid weight relapse frequently occurs after short-term use of an appetite suppressant and since the use of phentermine is restricted to 12 weeks or less,

this drug is not recommended for the routine management of severe obesity.

As with dexfenfluramine and fenfluramine, phentermine is associated with the rare but serious risk of pulmonary hypertension which may be insidious. Patients should be advised to report any dyspnoea or deterioration in exercise tolerance when the drug should be discontinued immediately.

CHILDREN. Centrally acting appetite suppressants should be avoided in children because of the possibility of growth suppression.

PHENTERMINE ◿

Indications: not recommended, see notes above

Cautions: mild hypertension (avoid if moderate to severe), diabetes mellitus, history of anxiety or depression; **interactions:** Appendix 1 (sympathomimetics)

DRIVING. May impair performance of skilled tasks (e.g. driving); effects of alcohol unpredictable

Contra-indications: cardiovascular disease (including moderate to severe hypertension), glaucoma, hyperthyroidism, epilepsy, unstable personality, history of psychiatric illness; history of drug or alcohol abuse; pregnancy (congenital malformations reported with related drugs) and breast-feeding

Side-effects: see notes above; dry mouth, headache, rashes, euphoria and dependence; also insomnia, restlessness, nervousness, agitation, nausea, vomiting, dizziness, depression, psychosis, hallucinations, palpitations and tachycardia, hypertension, constipation, urinary frequency, facial oedema

Dose: 15–30 mg at breakfast time for 4–6 weeks; max. period of treatment should not exceed 3 months; ELDERLY and CHILD not recommended

Duromine® (3M) CD ◿

Capsules, both m/r, phentermine (as resin complex) 15 mg (green/grey), net price 30-cap pack = £1.09; 30 mg (maroon/grey), 30-cap pack = £1.43. Label: 25, counselling, driving

Ionamin® (CHS) CD ◿

Capsules, both m/r, phentermine (as resin complex) 15 mg (grey/yellow), net price 20 = £1.11; 30 mg (yellow), 20 = £1.38. Label: 25, counselling, driving

◿ denotes preparations that are considered to be less suitable for prescribing (see p. vi)

4.6 Drugs used in nausea and vertigo

Anti-emetics should be prescribed only when the cause of vomiting is known, particularly in children, otherwise the symptomatic relief that they produce may delay diagnosis. Anti-emetics are unnecessary and sometimes harmful when the cause can be treated, e.g. as in diabetic ketoacidosis, or in excessive digoxin or antiepileptic dosage.

If antinauseant drug treatment is indicated the choice of drug depends on the aetiology of vomiting.

Vestibular disorders

The most effective drug for the prevention of *motion sickness* is **hyoscine**. Adverse effects (drowsiness, blurred vision, dry mouth, urinary retention) are more frequent than with the antihistamines but are not generally prominent at the doses employed. **Antihistamines** are slightly less effective, but are generally better tolerated. There is no evidence that any one antihistamine is superior to another but their duration of action and incidence of adverse effects (drowsiness and antimuscarinic effects) differ. If a sedative effect is desired **promethazine** and **dimenhydrinate** are useful, but generally a slightly less sedating antihistamine such as **cyclizine** or **cinnarizine** is preferred. **Metoclopramide** and the **phenothiazines** (except the antihistamine phenothiazine promethazine), which act selectively on the chemoreceptor trigger zone, are ineffective in motion sickness.

Vertigo and nausea associated with *Ménière's disease* and *middle-ear surgery* may be difficult to treat. **Hyoscine, antihistamines,** and **phenothiazines** (such as prochlorperazine) are effective in the prophylaxis and treatment of such conditions. **Cinnarizine** and **betahistine** have been promoted as specific treatments for Ménière's disease. In the acute attack **cyclizine** or **prochlorperazine** may be given rectally or by intramuscular injection.

Treatment of vertigo in its chronic forms is seldom fully effective but antihistamines (such as dimenhydrinate) or phenothiazines (such as prochlorperazine) may help.

For advice to avoid the inappropriate prescribing of drugs (notably phenothiazines) for dizziness in the elderly, see Prescribing for the Elderly, p. 16.

Vomiting of pregnancy

Nausea in the first trimester of pregnancy does **not** require drug therapy. On rare occasions if vomiting is severe, an antihistamine or a phenothiazine (e.g. promethazine) may be required. If symptoms have not settled in 24 to 48 hours then a specialist opinion should be sought.

Symptomatic relief of nausea from underlying disease

The **phenothiazines** are dopamine antagonists and act centrally by blocking the chemoreceptor trigger zone. They are of considerable value for the prophylaxis and treatment of nausea and vomiting associated with diffuse neoplastic disease, radiation sickness, and the emesis caused by drugs such as opioid analgesics, general anaesthetics, and cytotoxic drugs. **Prochlorperazine, perphenazine,** and **trifluoperazine** are less sedating than **chlorpromazine** but severe dystonic reactions sometimes occur, especially in children. Other antipsychotic drugs including droperidol, haloperidol, and levomepromazine (methotrimeprazine) (see section 4.2.1) are also used for the relief of nausea.

Metoclopramide is an effective anti-emetic with a spectrum of activity closely resembling that of the phenothiazines but it has a peripheral action on the gut in addition to its central effect and therefore may be superior to the phenothiazines in the emesis associated with gastroduodenal, hepatic, and biliary disease. As with the phenothiazines, metoclopramide may induce acute dystonic reactions with facial and skeletal muscle spasms and oculogyric crises. These are more common in the young (especially girls and young women) and the very old, usually occur shortly after starting treatment, and subside within 24 hours of stopping the drug. Injection of an antiparkinsonian drug such as procyclidine (section 4.9.2) will abort attacks. The high-dose preparation of metoclopramide has been used for the prevention of nausea and vomiting associated with cytotoxic drug therapy.

Domperidone is used for the relief of nausea and vomiting, especially when associated with cytotoxic drug therapy. It has the advantage over metoclopramide and the phenothiazines of being less likely to cause central effects such as sedation and dystonic reactions because it does not readily cross the blood-brain barrier. It may be given for the treatment of levodopa- and bromocriptine-induced vomiting in parkinsonism (section 4.9.1). Domperidone acts at the chemoreceptor trigger zone and so is unlikely to be effective in motion sickness and other vestibular disorders.

Antihistamines are active in most of these conditions, but are not usually drugs of choice.

Nabilone is a synthetic cannabinoid with antiemetic properties, reported to be superior to prochlorperazine. Side-effects occur frequently with standard doses.

Granisetron, ondansetron and **tropisetron** are specific (5HT$_3$) serotonin antagonists. They have a valuable role in the management of nausea and vomiting in patients receiving cytotoxics (section 8.1).

CYTOTOXIC CHEMOTHERAPY. For *anti-emetic regimens* used in the management of nausea and vomiting induced by cytotoxic chemotherapy, see section 8.1.

Antihistamines

CINNARIZINE

Indications: vestibular disorders, such as vertigo, tinnitus, nausea, and vomiting in Ménière's disease; motion sickness; vascular disease (section 2.6.4)

Cautions: see under Cyclizine; high doses in hypotension; avoid in porphyria (section 9.8.2)

Contra-indications: see under Cyclizine

Side-effects: see under Cyclizine; allergic skin reactions, fatigue; rarely, extrapyramidal symptoms in elderly on prolonged therapy

Dose: vestibular disorders, 30 mg 3 times daily; CHILD 5–12 years half adult dose

Motion sickness, 30 mg 2 hours before travel then 15 mg every 8 hours during journey if necessary; CHILD 5–12 years half adult dose

Cinnarizine (Non-proprietary)
Tablets, cinnarizine 15 mg. Net price 20 = £1.18.
Label: 2
Available from APS, Ashbourne (*Cinazière®*), Cox, Hillcross, Norton

Stugeron® (Janssen-Cilag)
Tablets, scored, cinnarizine 15 mg. Net price 20 = 75p. Label: 2
Stugeron Forte®: see section 2.6.4

CYCLIZINE

Indications: nausea, vomiting, vertigo, motion sickness, labyrinthine disorders
Cautions: see section 3.4.1; severe heart failure; may counteract haemodynamic benefits of opioids; **interactions:** Appendix 1 (antihistamines)
DRIVING. Drowsiness may affect performance of skilled tasks (e.g. driving); effects of alcohol enhanced
Contra-indications: see section 3.4.1
Side-effects: see section 3.4.1; drowsiness, occasional dry mouth and blurred vision
Dose: *by mouth*, cyclizine hydrochloride 50 mg up to 3 times daily; CHILD 6–12 years 25 mg
By intramuscular or intravenous injection, cyclizine lactate 50 mg 3 times daily

Valoid® (GlaxoWellcome)
Tablets, scored, cyclizine hydrochloride 50 mg. Net price 20 = 95p. Label: 2
Injection [PoM], cyclizine lactate 50 mg/mL. Net price 1-mL amp = 54p

DIMENHYDRINATE

Indications: nausea, vomiting, vertigo, motion sickness, labyrinthine disorders
Cautions: see under Cyclizine; avoid in porphyria (section 9.8.2)
Contra-indications: see under Cyclizine
Side-effects: see under Cyclizine
Dose: 50–100 mg 2–3 times daily; CHILD 1–6 years 12.5–25 mg, 7–12 years 25–50 mg
Motion sickness, first dose 30 minutes before journey

Dramamine® (Pharmacia & Upjohn)
Tablets, scored, dimenhydrinate 50 mg, net price 100-tab pack = £5.13. Label: 2

MECLOZINE HYDROCHLORIDE

Indications: see under preparations
Cautions: see under Cyclizine
Contra-indications: see under Cyclizine
Side-effects: see under Cyclizine

Preparations
A proprietary brand of meclozine hydrochloride tablets 12.5 mg (*Sea-legs®*) is on sale to the public for motion sickness

PROMETHAZINE HYDROCHLORIDE

Indications: nausea, vomiting, vertigo, labyrinthine disorders, motion sickness; other indications (section 3.4.1, section 4.1.1, section 15.1.4.1)
Cautions: see under Cyclizine; avoid in porphyria (section 9.8.2)
Contra-indications: see under Cyclizine
Side-effects: see under Cyclizine but more sedating; intramuscular injection may be painful

Dose: motion sickness prevention, 20–25 mg at bedtime on night before travelling, repeat following morning if necessary; CHILD under 2 years not recommended, 2–5 years, 5 mg at night and following morning if necessary; 5–10 years, 10 mg at night and following morning if necessary

Preparations
Section 3.4.1

PROMETHAZINE TEOCLATE

Indications: nausea, vertigo, labyrinthine disorders, motion sickness (acts longer than the hydrochloride)
Cautions: see under Promethazine Hydrochloride
Contra-indications: see under Promethazine Hydrochloride
Side-effects: see under Promethazine Hydrochloride
Dose: 25–75 mg, max. 100 mg, daily; CHILD 5–10 years, 12.5–37.5 mg daily
Motion sickness prevention, 25 mg at bedtime on night before travelling *or* 25 mg 1–2 hours before travelling; CHILD 5–10 years, half adult dose
For severe vomiting in pregnancy, 25 mg at bedtime, increased if necessary to a max. of 100 mg daily (but see also Vomiting of Pregnancy in notes above)

Avomine® (Manx)
Tablets, scored, promethazine teoclate 25 mg. Net price 10-tab pack = £1.06; 28-tab pack = £3.05. Label: 2

Phenothiazines and related drugs

CHLORPROMAZINE HYDROCHLORIDE

Indications: nausea and vomiting of terminal illness (where other drugs have failed or are not available); other indications (section 4.2.1 and section 15.1.4.1)
Cautions: see section 4.2.1
Contra-indications: see section 4.2.1
Side-effects: see section 4.2.1
Dose: *by mouth*, 10–25 mg every 4–6 hours; CHILD 500 micrograms/kg every 4–6 hours (1–5 years max. 40 mg daily, 6–12 years max. 75 mg daily)
By deep intramuscular injection 25 mg initially then 25–50 mg every 3–4 hours until vomiting stops; CHILD 500 micrograms/kg every 6–8 hours (1–5 years max. 40 mg daily, 6–12 years max. 75 mg daily)
By rectum in suppositories, chlorpromazine 100 mg every 6–8 hours [unlicensed]

Preparations
Section 4.2.1

PERPHENAZINE

Indications: severe nausea, vomiting (see notes above); other indications (section 4.2.1)
Cautions: see Perphenazine (section 4.2.1)
Contra-indications: see Perphenazine (section 4.2.1)

Side-effects: see Perphenazine (section 4.2.1); extrapyramidal symptoms particularly in young adults, elderly, and debilitated

Dose: 4 mg 3 times daily, adjusted according to response; max. 24 mg daily (chemotherapy-induced); ELDERLY quarter to half adult dose; CHILD under 14 years not recommended

Preparations

Section 4.2.1

PROCHLORPERAZINE

Indications: severe nausea, vomiting, vertigo, labyrinthine disorders (see notes above); other indications, section 4.2.1

Cautions: see under Chlorpromazine Hydrochloride (section 4.2.1); oral route only for children (avoid if less than 10 kg); elderly (see notes above)

Contra-indications: see under Chlorpromazine Hydrochloride (section 4.2.1)

Side-effects: see under Chlorpromazine Hydrochloride (section 4.2.1); extrapyramidal symptoms, particularly in children, elderly, and debilitated

Dose: *by mouth*, nausea and vomiting, prochlorperazine maleate or mesilate, acute attack, 20 mg initially then 10 mg after 2 hours; prevention 5–10 mg 2–3 times daily; CHILD (over 10 kg only) 250 micrograms/kg 2–3 times daily
Labyrinthine disorders, 5 mg 3 times daily, gradually increased if necessary to 30 mg daily in divided doses, then reduced after several weeks to 5–10 mg daily; CHILD not recommended

By deep intramuscular injection, nausea and vomiting, 12.5 mg when required followed if necessary after 6 hours by an oral dose, as above; CHILD not recommended

By rectum in suppositories, nausea and vomiting, 25 mg followed if necessary after 6 hours by oral dose, as above; *or* due to migraine, 5 mg 3 times daily; CHILD not recommended

Prochlorperazine (Non-proprietary) PoM
Tablets, prochlorperazine maleate 5 mg, net price 20 = £1.29. Label: 2
Available from Ashbourne (Prozière®), Cox, Generics, Hillcross, Norton

Stemetil® (Castlemead) PoM
Tablets, prochlorperazine maleate 5 mg (off-white), net price 84-tab pack = £6.65; 25 mg (scored), 56-tab pack = £11.73. Label: 2
Syrup, straw-coloured, prochlorperazine mesilate 5 mg/5 mL. Net price 100-mL pack = £3.74. Label: 2
Eff sachets, granules, effervescent, sugar-free, prochlorperazine mesilate 5 mg/sachet. Net price 21-sachet pack = £6.95. Label: 2, 13
Injection, prochlorperazine mesilate 12.5 mg/mL. Net price 1-mL amp = 59p
Suppositories, prochlorperazine maleate (as prochlorperazine), 5 mg, net price 10 = £9.40; 25 mg, 10 = £12.32. Label: 2

■ Buccal preparation

Buccastem® (R&C) PoM
Tablets (buccal), pale yellow, prochlorperazine maleate 3 mg. Net price 5 × 10-tab pack = £5.75. Label: 2, counselling, administration, see under Dose below
Dose: 1–2 tablets twice daily; tablets are placed high between upper lip and gum and left to dissolve; CHILD not recommended

TRIFLUOPERAZINE

Indications: severe nausea and vomiting (see notes above); other indications (section 4.2.1)

Cautions: see under Trifluoperazine (section 4.2.1)

Contra-indications: see under Trifluoperazine (section 4.2.1)

Side-effects: see under Trifluoperazine (section 4.2.1); extrapyramidal symptoms, particularly in children, elderly, and debilitated

Dose: 2–4 mg daily in divided doses *or* as a single dose of a modified-release preparation; max. 6 mg daily; CHILD 3–5 years up to 1 mg daily, 6–12 years up to 4 mg daily

Preparations

Section 4.2.1

Domperidone and metoclopramide

DOMPERIDONE

Indications: see under Dose
CHILDREN. Use in children is restricted to nausea and vomiting following cytotoxics or radiotherapy

Cautions: pregnancy and breast-feeding; not recommended for routine prophylaxis of post-operative vomiting or for chronic administration; **interactions:** Appendix 1 (domperidone)

Side-effects: raised prolactin concentrations (possible galactorrhoea and gynaecomastia), reduced libido reported; rashes and other allergic reactions; acute dystonic reactions reported

Dose: *by mouth*, acute nausea and vomiting, (including nausea and vomiting induced by levodopa and bromocriptine), 10–20 mg every 4–8 hours; max. period of treatment 12 weeks; CHILD, nausea and vomiting following cytotoxic therapy or radiotherapy only, 200–400 micrograms/kg every 4–8 hours
Functional dyspepsia, 10–20 mg 3 times daily before food and 10–20 mg at night; max. period of treatment 12 weeks; CHILD not recommended

By rectum in suppositories, nausea and vomiting, 30–60 mg every 4–8 hours; CHILD over 2 years (following cytotoxic therapy or radiotherapy only), body-weight 10–15 kg max. 15 mg twice daily, body-weight 15.5–25 kg max. 30 mg twice daily, body-weight 25.5–35 kg max. 30 mg 3 times daily, body-weight 35.5–45 kg max. 30 mg 4 times daily; since dose needs to be divided throughout day, suppositories may be cut in half for younger children

¹ **Domperidone** (Non-proprietary) PoM

Tablets, 10 mg (as maleate), net price 30-tab pack = £2.59; 100-tab pack = £8.55

Available from CP, Generics, Hillcross, Sterwin

1. Domperidone can be sold to the public (provided packs do not contain more than 100 mg) for the relief of post-prandial symptoms of excessive fullness, nausea, epi-gastric bloating and belching occasionally accompanied by epigastric discomfort and heartburn (max. single dose 10 mg, max. daily dose 40 mg); a proprietary brand (*Motilium® 10*) is on sale to the public

Motilium® (Sanofi-Synthelabo) PoM

Tablets, f/c, domperidone 10 mg (as maleate). Net price 30-tab pack = £2.46; 100-tab pack = £8.21

Suspension, sugar-free, domperidone 5 mg/5 mL. Net price 200-mL pack = £1.80

Suppositories, domperidone 30 mg. Net price 10 = £2.65

■ Compound preparations (for migraine), section 4.7.4.1

METOCLOPRAMIDE HYDROCHLORIDE

Indications: adults, nausea and vomiting, particularly in gastro-intestinal disorders (section 1.2) and treatment with cytotoxics or radiotherapy; migraine (section 4.7.4.1)

PATIENTS UNDER 20 YEARS. Use restricted to severe intractable vomiting of known cause, vomiting of radiotherapy and cytotoxics, aid to gastro-intestinal intubation, pre-medication

Cautions: hepatic and renal impairment; elderly, young adults, and children (measure dose accurately, preferably with a pipette); may mask underlying disorders such as cerebral irritation; avoid for 3–4 days following gastro-intestinal surgery, may cause acute hypertensive response in phaeochromocytoma; pregnancy and breast-feeding; porphyria (see section 9.8.2); **interactions:** Appendix 1 (metoclopramide)

Side-effects: extrapyramidal effects (especially in children/young adults), hyperprolactinaemia, occasionally tardive dyskinesia on prolonged administration; also reported, drowsiness, restlessness, diarrhoea, depression, neuroleptic malignant syndrome; cardiac conduction abnormalities reported following intravenous administration

Dose: *by mouth, or by intramuscular injection or by intravenous injection* over 1–2 minutes, 10 mg (5 mg in young adults 15–19 years under 60 kg) 3 times daily; CHILD up to 1 year (up to 10 kg) 1 mg twice daily, 1–3 years (10–14 kg) 1 mg 2–3 times daily, 3–5 years (15–19 kg) 2 mg 2–3 times daily, 5–9 years (20–29 kg) 2.5 mg 3 times daily, 9–14 years (30 kg and over) 5 mg 3 times daily

Note. Daily dose of metoclopramide should not normally exceed 500 micrograms/kg, particularly for children and young adults (restricted use, see above)

For diagnostic procedures, as a single dose 5–10 minutes before examination, 10–20 mg (10 mg in young adults 15–19 years); CHILD under 3 years 1 mg, 3–5 years 2 mg, 5–9 years 2.5 mg, 9–14 years 5 mg

Metoclopramide (Non-proprietary) PoM

Tablets, metoclopramide hydrochloride 10 mg, net price 28-tab pack = £2.60

Available from Antigen, APS, Ashbourne (*Gastroflux®*), Berk (*Primperan®*), Cox, CP, Norton

Oral solution, metoclopramide hydrochloride 5 mg/5 mL, net price 100-mL pack = £1.10

Available from Berk (*Primperan®*, sugar-free), Lagap, Rosemont (sugar-free)

Injection, metoclopramide hydrochloride 5 mg/ mL, net price 2-mL amp = 20p

Available from Antigen, Phoenix

Maxolon® (Monmouth) PoM

Tablets, scored, metoclopramide hydrochloride 5 mg, net price 84-tab pack = £4.69; 10 mg, 84-tab pack = £9.38, 100-tab pack = £11.17

Syrup, sugar-free, metoclopramide hydrochloride 5 mg/5 mL. Net price 200-mL pack = £3.83

Paediatric liquid, sugar-free, metoclopramide hydrochloride 1 mg/mL. Net price 15-mL pack with pipette = £1.51. Counselling, use of pipette

Injection, metoclopramide hydrochloride 5 mg/ mL. Net price 2-mL amp = 27p

■ High-dose (with cytotoxic chemotherapy only)

Maxolon High Dose® (Monmouth) PoM

Injection, metoclopramide hydrochloride 5 mg/ mL. Net price 20-mL amp = £2.67.

For dilution and use as an intravenous infusion in nausea and vomiting associated with cytotoxic chemotherapy only

Dose: by continuous intravenous infusion (preferred method), initially (before starting chemotherapy), 2–4 mg/kg over 15–20 minutes, then 3–5 mg/kg over 8–12 hours; max. in 24 hours, 10 mg/kg

By intermittent intravenous infusion, initially (before starting chemotherapy), up to 2 mg/kg over at least 15 minutes then up to 2 mg/kg over at least 15 minutes every 2 hours; max. in 24 hours, 10 mg/kg

Note. Injection of metoclopramide hydrochloride 5 mg/ mL also available in 20-mL ampoules from Phoenix

■ Modified-release preparations

Note. All unsuitable for patients under 20 years

Gastrobid Continus® (Napp) PoM ▱

Tablets, m/r, metoclopramide hydrochloride 15 mg. Net price 56-tab pack = £9.70. Label: 25

Dose: patients over 20 years, 1 tablet twice daily

Gastromax® (Pfizer) PoM ▱

Capsules, m/r, orange/yellow, enclosing white to light beige pellets, metoclopramide hydrochloride 30 mg. Net price 28-cap pack = £11.55. Label: 22, 25

Dose: patients over 20 years, 1 capsule daily

Maxolon SR® (Monmouth) PoM ▱

Capsules, m/r, clear, enclosing white granules, metoclopramide hydrochloride 15 mg. Net price 56-cap pack = £7.01. Label: 25

Dose: patients over 20 years, 1 capsule twice daily

■ Compound preparations (for migraine), section 4.7.4.1

5HT₃ antagonists

GRANISETRON

Indications: see under Dose
Cautions: pregnancy and breast-feeding

Side-effects: constipation, headache, rash; transient increases in liver enzymes; hypersensitivity reactions reported

Dose: nausea and vomiting induced by cytotoxic chemotherapy or radiotherapy, *by mouth*, 1–2 mg within 1 hour before start of treatment, then 2 mg daily in 1–2 divided doses during treatment; when intravenous infusion also used, max. combined total 9 mg in 24 hours; CHILD 20 micrograms/kg (max. 1 mg) within 1 hour before start of treatment, then 20 micrograms/kg (max. 1 mg) twice daily for up to 5 days during treatment

By intravenous injection (diluted in 15 mL sodium chloride 0.9% and given over not less than 30 seconds) *or by intravenous infusion* (over 5 minutes, see Appendix 6), prevention, 3 mg before start of cytotoxic therapy (up to 2 additional 3-mg doses may be given within 24 hours); treatment, as for prevention (the two additional doses must not be given less than 10 minutes apart); max. 9 mg in 24 hours; CHILD, *by intravenous infusion*, (over 5 minutes), prevention, 40 micrograms/kg (max. 3 mg) before start of cytotoxic therapy; treatment, as for prevention—one additional dose of 40 micrograms/kg (max. 3 mg) may be given within 24 hours (not less than 10 minutes after initial dose)

Postoperative nausea and vomiting, *by intravenous injection* (diluted to 5 mL and given over 30 seconds), prevention, 1 mg before induction of anaesthesia; treatment, 1 mg, given as for prevention; max. 2 mg in one day; CHILD not recommended

Kytril® (SmithKline Beecham) PoM

Tablets, f/c, granisetron (as hydrochloride) 1 mg, net price 10-tab pack = £91.43; 2 mg, 5-tab pack = £91.43

Paediatric liquid, sugar-free, granisetron (as hydrochloride) 1 mg/5 mL, net price 30 mL = £54.86

Sterile solution, granisetron (as hydrochloride) 1 mg/mL, for dilution and use as injection or infusion, net price 1-mL vial = £12.00, 3-mL amp = £36.00

ONDANSETRON

Indications: see under Dose

Cautions: pregnancy and breast-feeding; moderate or severe hepatic impairment (max. 8 mg daily)

Side-effects: constipation; headache, sensation of warmth or flushing, hiccups; occasional alterations in liver enzymes; hypersensitivity reactions reported; occasional transient visual disturbances and dizziness following intravenous administration; involuntary movements, seizures, chest pain, arrhythmias, hypotension and bradycardia also reported; suppositories may cause rectal irritation

Dose: moderately emetogenic chemotherapy or radiotherapy, *by mouth*, 8 mg 1–2 hours before treatment *or by rectum*, 16 mg 1–2 hours before treatment *or by intramuscular injection or slow intravenous injection*, 8 mg immediately before treatment

then by mouth, 8 mg every 12 hours for up to 5 days *or by rectum*, 16 mg daily for up to 5 days

Severely emetogenic chemotherapy, *by intramuscular injection or slow intravenous injection*, 8 mg immediately before treatment, where necessary followed by 8 mg at intervals of 2–4 hours for 2 further doses (*or* followed by 1 mg/hour *by con-*

tinuous intravenous infusion for up to 24 hours) *then by mouth*, 8 mg every 12 hours for up to 5 days *or by rectum*, 16 mg daily for up to 5 days

alternatively, by intravenous infusion over at least 15 minutes, 32 mg immediately before treatment *or by rectum*, 16 mg 1–2 hours before treatment *then by mouth*, 8 mg every 12 hours for up to 5 days *or by rectum*, 16 mg daily for up to 5 days

Note. Efficacy may be enhanced by addition of a single dose of dexamethasone sodium phosphate 20 mg by intravenous injection

CHILD, *by slow intravenous injection or by intravenous infusion* over 15 minutes, 5 mg/m^2 immediately before chemotherapy then, 4 mg *by mouth* every 12 hours for up to 5 days

Prevention of postoperative nausea and vomiting, *by mouth*, 16 mg 1 hour before anaesthesia *or* 8 mg 1 hour before anaesthesia followed by 8 mg at intervals of 8 hours for 2 further doses

alternatively, by intramuscular or slow intravenous injection, 4 mg at induction of anaesthesia; CHILD over 2 years, *by slow intravenous injection*, 100 micrograms/kg (max. 4 mg) before, during, or after induction of anaesthesia

Treatment of postoperative nausea and vomiting, *by intramuscular or slow intravenous injection*, 4 mg; CHILD over 2 years, *by slow intravenous injection*, 100 micrograms/kg (max. 4 mg)

Zofran® (GlaxoWellcome) PoM

Tablets, both yellow, f/c, ondansetron (as hydrochloride) 4 mg, net price 30-tab pack = £116.03; 8 mg, 10-tab pack = £77.36

Oral lyophilisates (Zofran Melt®), ondansetron 4 mg, net price 10-tab pack = £38.68; 8 mg, 10-tab pack = £77.36. Counselling, administration

COUNSELLING. Tablets should be placed on the tongue, allowed to disperse and swallowed

Excipients: include aspartame (section 9.4.1)

Syrup, sugar-free, ondansetron (as hydrochloride) 4 mg/5 mL. Net price 50-mL pack = £38.68

Injection, ondansetron (as hydrochloride) 2 mg/mL, net price 2-mL amp = £6.45; 4-mL amp = £12.89

Suppositories, ondansetron 16 mg. Net price 5 = £77.35

TROPISETRON

Indications: see under Dose

Cautions: uncontrolled hypertension (has been aggravated by doses higher than recommended); cardiac conduction disorders; arrhythmias, concomitant administration of drugs that prolong QT interval; pregnancy and breast-feeding; **interactions:** Appendix 1 (tropisetron)

DRIVING. Dizziness or drowsiness may affect performance of skilled tasks (e.g. driving)

Side-effects: constipation, diarrhoea, abdominal pain; headache, dizziness, fatigue; hypersensitivity reactions reported (including facial flushing, urticaria, chest tightness, dyspnoea, bronchospasm and hypotension); collapse, syncope, bradycardia, cardiovascular collapse also reported (causal relationship not established)

Dose: prevention of nausea and vomiting induced by cytotoxic chemotherapy, *by slow intravenous injection or by intravenous infusion*, 5 mg shortly before chemotherapy, then 5 mg *by mouth* every morning at least 1 hour before food for 5 days; CHILD over 2 years, *by intravenous injection* over at least 1 minute or *by intravenous infusion*, 200 micrograms/kg (max. 5 mg) shortly before chemotherapy, then 200 micrograms/kg daily for 4 days; CHILD 25 kg and over, *by intravenous injection* over at least 1 minute or *by intravenous infusion*, 5 mg shortly before chemotherapy, then *by mouth* (preferably) or *by intravenous injection* over at least 1 minute or *by intravenous infusion*, 5 mg daily for 5 days

Postoperative nausea and vomiting, *by slow intravenous injection* or *by intravenous infusion*, prevention, 2 mg shortly before induction of anaesthesia; treatment, 2 mg within 2 hours of the end of anaesthesia

Navoban® (Novartis) PoM

Capsules, white/yellow, tropisetron (as hydrochloride) 5 mg, net price 5-cap pack = £53.86; 50-cap pack = £538.60. Label: 23

Injection, tropisetron (as hydrochloride), 1 mg/mL, net price 2-mL amp = £4.86, 5-mL amp = £12.16

Cannabinoid

NABILONE

Indications: nausea and vomiting caused by cytotoxic chemotherapy, unresponsive to conventional anti-emetics (under close observation, preferably in in-patient setting)

Cautions: history of psychiatric disorder; elderly; hypertension; heart disease; adverse effects on mental state can persist for 48–72 hours after stopping; **interactions:** Appendix 1 (nabilone)

DRIVING. Drowsiness may affect performance of skilled tasks (e.g. driving); effects of alcohol enhanced

Contra-indications: severe hepatic impairment; pregnancy and breast-feeding

Side-effects: drowsiness, vertigo, euphoria, dry mouth, ataxia, visual disturbance, concentration difficulties, sleep disturbance, dysphoria, hypotension, headache and nausea; also confusion, disorientation, hallucinations, psychosis, depression, decreased coordination, tremors, tachycardia, decreased appetite, and abdominal pain

BEHAVIOURAL EFFECTS. Patients should be made aware of possible changes of mood and other adverse behavioural effects

Dose: patients over 18 years, initially 1 mg twice daily, increased if necessary to 2 mg twice daily, throughout each cycle of cytotoxic therapy and, if necessary, for 48 hours after the last dose of each cycle; max. 6 mg daily given in 3 divided doses. The first dose should be taken the night before initiation of cytotoxic treatment and the second dose 1–3 hours before the first dose of cytotoxic drug; ADOLESCENT and CHILD under 18 years not recommended

Nabilone (Cambridge) PoM

Capsules, blue/white, nabilone 1 mg. Net price 20-cap pack = £114.40 (hosp. only). Label: 2, counselling, behavioural effects

Hyoscine

HYOSCINE HYDROBROMIDE

(Scopolamine Hydrobromide)

Indications: motion sickness; premedication (section 15.1.3)

Cautions: elderly, urinary retention, cardiovascular disease, gastro-intestinal obstruction, hepatic or renal impairment; porphyria (see section 9.8.2); pregnancy and breast-feeding; **interactions:** Appendix 1 (antimuscarinics)

DRIVING. Drowsiness may affect performance of skilled tasks (e.g. driving) and may persist for up to 24 hours or longer after removal of patch: effects of alcohol enhanced

Contra-indications: closed-angle glaucoma

Side-effects: drowsiness, dry mouth, dizziness, blurred vision, difficulty with micturition

Dose: motion sickness, *by mouth*, 300 micrograms 30 minutes before start of journey followed by 300 micrograms every 6 hours if required; max. 3 doses in 24 hours; CHILD 4–10 years 75–150 micrograms, over 10 years 150–300 micrograms

Note. Proprietary brands of hyoscine hydrobromide tablets (*Joy-rides®, Kwells®*) are on sale to the public for motion sickness

Injection, see section 15.1.3

Scopoderm TTS® (Novartis) PoM

Patch, self-adhesive, pink, releasing hyoscine approx. 1 mg/72 hours when in contact with skin. Net price 2 = £4.50. Label: 19, counselling, see below

Administration: motion sickness prevention, apply 1 patch to hairless area of skin behind ear 5–6 hours before journey; replace if necessary after 72 hours, siting replacement patch behind other ear; CHILD under 10 years not recommended

COUNSELLING. Explain accompanying instructions to patient and in particular emphasise advice to wash hands after handling and to wash application site after removing, and to use one at a time

Other drugs for Ménière's disease

Betahistine has been promoted as a specific treatment for Ménière's disease.

BETAHISTINE DIHYDROCHLORIDE

Indications: vertigo, tinnitus and hearing loss associated with Ménière's disease

Cautions: asthma, history of peptic ulcer; pregnancy and breast-feeding; **interactions:** Appendix 1 (betahistine)

Contra-indications: phaeochromocytoma

Side-effects: gastro-intestinal disturbances; headache, rashes and pruritus reported

Dose: initially 16 mg 3 times daily, preferably with food; maintenance 24–48 mg daily; CHILD not recommended

Betahistine Dihydrochloride (Non-proprietary)
PoM

Tablets, betahistine dihydrochloride 8 mg, net price 120-tab pack = £9.00; 16 mg, 84-tab pack = £16.39. Label: 21
Available from Cox, Generics, Norton

Serc® (Solvay) PoM
Tablets, betahistine dihydrochloride 8 mg (*Serc®-8*), net price 120-tab pack = £10.04; 16 mg (*Serc®-16*), 84-tab pack = £14.06. Label: 21

4.7   Analgesics

4.7.1	Non-opioid analgesics
4.7.2	Opioid analgesics
4.7.3	Neuropathic pain
4.7.4	Antimigraine drugs

The non-opioid drugs (section 4.7.1), paracetamol and aspirin (and other NSAIDs), are particularly suitable for pain in musculoskeletal conditions, whereas the opioid analgesics (section 4.7.2) are more suitable for moderate to severe visceral pain.

PAIN IN PALLIATIVE CARE. For advice on pain relief in palliative care see Prescribing in Palliative Care, p. 12.

PAIN IN SICKLE-CELL DISEASE. The pain of mild sickle-cell crises is managed with paracetamol, an NSAID, codeine, or dihydrocodeine. Severe crises may require the use of morphine or diamorphine; concomitant use of an NSAID may potentiate analgesia and allow lower doses of the opioid to be used. Pethidine should be avoided if possible because accumulation of a neurotoxic metabolite can precipitate seizures; the relatively short half-life of pethidine necessitates frequent injections.

DYSMENORRHOEA. Use of an oral contraceptive prevents the pain of dysmenorrhoea which is generally associated with ovulatory cycles. If treatment is necessary paracetamol or an NSAID (section 10.1.1) will generally provide adequate relief of pain. The vomiting and severe pain associated with dysmenorrhoea in women with endometriosis may call for an antiemetic (in addition to an analgesic). Antispasmodics (such as alverine citrate, section 1.2) have been advocated for dysmenorrhoea but the antispasmodic action does not generally provide significant relief. Hyoscine butylbromide (section 1.2) has also been advocated for its antispasmodic action despite the fact that its absorption following oral administration is extremely poor.

4.7.1   **Non-opioid analgesics**

Aspirin is indicated for headache, transient musculoskeletal pain, dysmenorrhoea and pyrexia. In inflammatory conditions, most physicians prefer anti-inflammatory treatment with another NSAID which may be better tolerated and more convenient for the patient. Aspirin is used increasingly for its antiplatelet properties (section 2.9). Aspirin tablets or dispersible aspirin tablets are adequate for most purposes as they act rapidly.

Gastric irritation may be a problem; it is minimised by taking the dose after food. Enteric coated preparations are available, but have a slow onset of action and are therefore unsuitable for single-dose analgesic use (though their prolonged action may be useful for night pain).

Aspirin interacts significantly with a number of other drugs and its interaction with warfarin is a **special hazard**, see **interactions:** Appendix 1 (aspirin).

Paracetamol is similar in efficacy to aspirin, but has no demonstrable anti-inflammatory activity; it is less irritant to the stomach and for that reason is now generally preferred to aspirin, particularly in the elderly. **Overdosage** with paracetamol is particularly dangerous as it may cause hepatic damage which is sometimes not apparent for 4 to 6 days (see Emergency Treatment of Poisoning, p. 21). **Benorilate** (section 10.1.1) is an aspirin–paracetamol ester.

Nefopam may have a place in the relief of persistent pain unresponsive to other non-opioid analgesics. It causes little or no respiratory depression, but sympathomimetic and antimuscarinic side-effects may be troublesome.

Non-steroidal anti-inflammatory analgesics (NSAIDs, section 10.1.1) are particularly useful for the treatment of patients with chronic disease accompanied by pain and inflammation. Some of them are also used in the short-term treatment of mild to moderate pain including transient musculoskeletal pain but paracetamol is now often preferred, particularly in the elderly (see also p. 16). They are also suitable for the relief of pain in *dysmenorrhoea* and to treat pain caused by *secondary bone tumours*, many of which produce lysis of bone and release prostaglandins (see Prescribing in Palliative Care, p. 12). NSAIDs including ketorolac are also used for peri-operative analgesia (section 15.1.4.2).

Compound analgesic preparations

Compound analgesic preparations containing paracetamol or aspirin with a *low dose* of an opioid analgesic (e.g. 8 mg of codeine phosphate per compound tablet) are commonly used, but the advantages have not been substantiated. The low dose of the opioid may be enough to cause opioid side-effects (in particular, constipation) and can complicate the treatment of **overdosage** (see p. 23) yet may not provide significant additional relief of pain.

Compound analgesic preparations containing a *full dose* of the opioid component (e.g. 30 mg of codeine phosphate per compound tablet) carry the full range of opioid side-effects (including nausea, vomiting, severe constipation, drowsiness, respiratory depression, and risk of dependence on long-term administration). For details of the **side-effects, cautions** and **contra-indications** of opioid analgesics, see p. 210 (**important**: the elderly are particularly susceptible to opioid side-effects and should receive lower doses).

In general, when assessing pain, it is necessary to weigh up carefully whether there is a need for a non-opioid and an opioid analgesic to be taken simultaneously.

Caffeine is a weak stimulant that is often included, in small doses, in analgesic preparations. It is claimed that the addition of caffeine may enhance the analgesic effect, but the alerting effect, mild habit-forming effect and possible provocation of headache may not always be desirable. Moreover, in excessive dosage or on withdrawal caffeine may itself induce headache.

ASPIRIN

(Acetylsalicylic Acid)

Indications: mild to moderate pain, pyrexia; see also section 10.1.1; antiplatelet (section 2.9)

Cautions: asthma, allergic disease, impaired renal or hepatic function (avoid if severe), dehydration, pregnancy; elderly; G6PD-deficiency (section 9.1.5); **interactions:** Appendix 1 (aspirin)

Contra-indications: children under 12 years and in breast-feeding (Reye's syndrome, see below); gastro-intestinal ulceration, haemophilia; not for treatment of gout

HYPERSENSITIVITY. Aspirin and other NSAIDs are **contra-indicated** in patients with a history of hypersensitivity to aspirin or any other NSAID—*which includes those* in whom attacks of *asthma, angioedema, urticaria or rhinitis* have been precipitated by aspirin or any other NSAID

REYE'S SYNDROME. Owing to an association with Reye's syndrome the CSM has recommended that aspirin-containing preparations should no longer be given to children under the age of 12 years, unless specifically indicated, e.g. for juvenile arthritis (Still's disease). It is **important** to advise families that aspirin is not a suitable medicine for children with minor illness.

Side-effects: generally mild and infrequent but high incidence of gastro-intestinal irritation with slight asymptomatic blood loss, increased bleeding time, bronchospasm and skin reactions in hypersensitive patients. Prolonged administration, see section 10.1.1. **Overdosage:** see Emergency Treatment of Poisoning, p. 21

Dose: 300–900 mg every 4–6 hours when necessary; max. 4 g daily; CHILD not recommended (see notes above)

Aspirin (Non-proprietary)

Tablets PoM [1], aspirin 300 mg. Net price 20 =16p. Label: 21, 32

Available from most generic manufacturers

Tablets PoM [1], e/c, aspirin 300 mg, net price 100-tab pack = £3.53; 75 mg, see section 2.9. Label: 5, 25, 32

Available from Ashbourne, Galen

Dispersible tablets PoM [1], aspirin 300 mg, net price 20 = 9p; 75 mg, see section 2.9. Label: 13, 21, 32

Available from most generic manufacturers

Note. BP directs that when no strength is stated the 300-mg strength should be dispensed, and that when soluble aspirin tablets are prescribed, dispersible aspirin tablets shall be dispensed.

Suppositories, aspirin 300 mg, net price 10 = £9.13. Label: 32

Dose: 2–3 suppositories inserted every 4 hours when necessary (max. 12 suppositories in 24 hours); CHILD not recommended (see above)

Available from Aurum (who also supply a 150-mg strength)

Caprin® (Sinclair)

Tablets PoM [1], e/c, f/c, pink, aspirin 300 mg, net price 30-tab pack = £1.66, 100-tab pack = £4.89; 75 mg, see section 2.9. Label: 5, 25, 32

Nu-Seals® Aspirin (Lilly)

Tablets PoM [1], e/c, aspirin 300 mg, net price 100-tab pack = £5.80; 75 mg, see section 2.9. Label: 5, 25, 32

■ With codeine phosphate 8 mg

[1]Co-codaprin (Non-proprietary) PoM ▨

Tablets, co-codaprin 8/400 (codeine phosphate 8 mg, aspirin 400 mg). Net price 20 = 34p. Label: 21, 32

Dose: 1–2 tablets every 4–6 hours when necessary; max. 8 tablets daily

Dispersible tablets, co-codaprin 8/400 (codeine phosphate 8 mg, aspirin 400 mg). Net price 20 = 71p. Label: 13, 21, 32

Dose: 1–2 tablets in water every 4–6 hours; max. 8 tablets daily

Available from Cox

When co-codaprin tablets or dispersible tablets are prescribed and no strength is stated tablets, or dispersible tablets, respectively, containing codeine phosphate 8 mg and aspirin 400 mg should be dispensed

▨ denotes preparations that are considered to be less suitable for prescribing (see p. vi)

■ Other compound preparations

Aspav® (Cox) PoM ▨

Dispersible tablets, aspirin 500 mg, papaveretum 7.71 mg (providing the equivalent of 5 mg of anhydrous morphine). Net price 100-tab pack = £15.33. Label: 2, 13, 21, 32

Dose: 1–2 tablets in water every 4–6 hours if necessary; max. 8 tablets daily

Equagesic® (Wyeth) NHS CD ▨

Tablets, pink/white/yellow, ethoheptazine citrate 75 mg, meprobamate 150 mg, aspirin 250 mg. Net price 100-tab pack = £5.40. Label: 2, 21, 32

Dose: muscle pain, 1–2 tablets 3–4 times daily

■ Preparations on sale to the public

For a list of **preparations** containing aspirin and paracetamol **on sale to the public**, see p. 208.

PARACETAMOL

(Acetaminophen)

Indications: mild to moderate pain, pyrexia

Cautions: hepatic and renal impairment, alcohol dependence; **interactions:** Appendix 1 (paracetamol)

1. May be sold to the public provided packs contain no more than 32 capsules or tablets; pharmacists can sell multiple packs up to a total quantity of 100 capsules or tablets in justifiable circumstances; for details see *Medicines, Ethics and Practice*, No. 23, London, Pharmaceutical Press, 2000 (and subsequent editions as available)

Side-effects: side-effects rare, but rashes, blood disorders; acute pancreatitis reported after prolonged use; **important:** liver damage (and less frequently renal damage) following **overdosage**, see Emergency Treatment of Poisoning, p. 21

Dose: *by mouth*, 0.5–1 g every 4–6 hours to a max. of 4 g daily; CHILD 2 months 60 mg for post-immunisation pyrexia; otherwise under 3 months (on doctor's advice only), 10 mg/kg (5 mg/kg if jaundiced); 3 months–1 year 60–120 mg, 1–5 years 120–250 mg, 6–12 years 250–500 mg; these doses may be repeated every 4–6 hours when necessary (max. of 4 doses in 24 hours)

For full Joint Committee on Vaccination and Immunisation recommendation on post-immunisation pyrexia, see section 14.1

Rectal route, see below

Paracetamol (Non-proprietary)

Tablets PoM[1], paracetamol 500 mg. Net price 20 = 12p. Label: 29, 30

Available from APS, Cox, Norton, Sterling Health (*Panadol*® NHS)

Soluble Tablets (= Dispersible tablets) PoM[2], paracetamol 500 mg. Net price 60-tab pack = £2.75. Label: 13, 29, 30

Available from Sterling Health (*Panadol Soluble*® NHS)

Paediatric Soluble Tablets (=Paediatric dispersible tablets), paracetamol 120 mg. Net price 24-tab pack = 82p. Label: 13, 30

Available from R&C (*Disprol*® Soluble *Paracetamol* NHS)

Paediatric Oral Solution (= Paediatric Elixir), paracetamol 120 mg/5 mL. Net price 100 mL = 29p. Label: 30

Note. Sugar-free versions are available and can be ordered by specifying 'sugar-free' on the prescription.

Available from Berk, Norton, Rosemont (*Paldesic*® NHS), Wallace Mfg (*Salzone*® NHS)

Oral Suspension 120 mg/5 mL (= Paediatric Mixture), paracetamol 120 mg/5 mL. Net price 100 mL = 43p. Label: 30

Note. BP directs that when Paediatric Paracetamol Oral Suspension or Paediatric Paracetamol Mixture is prescribed Paracetamol Oral Suspension 120 mg/5 mL should be dispensed; sugar-free versions can be ordered by specifying 'sugar-free' on the prescription

Available from Cupal (*Medinol*® *Paediatric*, sugar-free), Norton, R&C (*Disprol*® *Paediatric*, sugar-free), Rosemont (*Paldesic*®), Sterling Health (*Panadol*®, sugar-free), Warner Lambert (*Calpol*® *Paediatric*, *Calpol*® *Paediatric* sugar-free)

Oral Suspension 250 mg/5 mL (= Mixture), paracetamol 250 mg/5 mL. Net price 100 mL = 75p. Label: 30

Available from Cupal (*Medinol*® *Over 6* NHS), Hillcross, Rosemont (*Paldesic*®), Warner Wellcome (*Calpol*® *6 Plus* NHS)

Suppositories, paracetamol 60 mg, net price 10 = £9.96; 125 mg, 10 = £11.50; 250 mg, 10 = £23.00; 500 mg, 10 = £10.25. Label: 30

Dose: by rectum, ADULT and CHILD over 12 years 0.5–1 g up to 4 times daily, CHILD 1–5 years 125–250 mg, 6–12 years 250–500 mg

Available from Astra (*Alvedon*®, 60 mg, 125 mg, 250 mg), Aurum (120 mg, 240 mg, 500 mg)

▨ denotes preparations that are considered to be less suitable for prescribing (see p. vi)

■ Co-codamol 8/500

When co-codamol tablets, dispersible (or effervescent) tablets, or capsules are prescribed and **no strength is stated** tablets, dispersible (or effervescent) tablets, or capsules, respectively, containing codeine phosphate **8 mg** and paracetamol **500 mg** should be dispensed.

Co-codamol 8/500 PoM[2] (Non-proprietary) ▨

Tablets, co-codamol 8/500 (codeine phosphate 8 mg, paracetamol 500 mg) Net price 20 = 35p. Label: 29, 30

Dose: 1–2 tablets every 4–6 hours; max. 8 tablets daily; CHILD 6–12 years ½–1 tablet

Available from APS, Cox, CP, Galen, (*Parake*® NHS), Generics, Norton, Sterling Health (*Panadeine*® NHS), Sterwin

Effervescent or *dispersible tablets*, co-codamol 8/500 (codeine phosphate 8 mg, paracetamol 500 mg). Net price 20 = 73p. Label: 13, 29, 30

Dose: 1–2 tablets in water every 4–6 hours, max. 8 tablets daily; CHILD 6–12 years ½–1 tablet, max 4 daily

Available from Lagap, Roche Consumer Health (*Paracodol*® NHS), Sterwin

Note. The Drug Tariff allows tablets of co-codamol labelled 'dispersible' to be dispensed against an order for 'effervescent' and *vice versa*

Capsules, co-codamol 8/500 (codeine phosphate 8 mg, paracetamol 500 mg). Net price 30 = £2.58. Label: 29, 30

Dose: 1–2 capsules every 4 hours; max. 8 capsules daily

Available from Roche Consumer Health (*Paracodol*® NHS)

■ Co-codamol 30/500

When co-codamol tablets, dispersible (or effervescent) tablets, or capsules are prescribed and **no strength is stated** tablets, dispersible (or effervescent) tablets, or capsules, respectively, containing codeine phosphate **8 mg** and paracetamol **500 mg** should be dispensed (see preparations above).

See warnings and notes on p. 204 (**important:** special care in elderly—reduce dose)

Co-codamol 30/500 (Non-proprietary) PoM ▨

Tablets, co-codamol 30/500 (codeine phosphate 30 mg, paracetamol 500 mg), net price 100-tab pack = £7.53. Label: 2, 29, 30

Dose: 1–2 tablets every 4 hours; max. 8 tablets daily; CHILD not recommended

Available from CP

Kapake® (Galen) PoM ▨

Tablets, scored, co-codamol 30/500 (codeine phosphate 30 mg, paracetamol 500 mg). Net price 30-tab pack = £2.26 (hosp. only), 100-tab pack = £7.53. Label: 2, 29, 30

Dose: 1–2 tablets every 4 hours; max. 8 tablets daily; CHILD not recommended

Capsules, co-codamol 30/500 (codeine phosphate 30 mg, paracetamol 500 mg), net price 100-cap pack = £7.53. Label: 2, 29, 30

Dose: 1–2 capsules every 4 hours; max. 8 capsules daily; CHILD not recommended

1. May be sold to the public provided packs contain no more than 32 capsules or tablets; pharmacists can sell multiple packs up to a total quantity of 100 capsules or tablets in justifiable circumstances; for details see *Medicines, Ethics and Practice*, No. 23, London, Pharmaceutical Press, 2000 (and subsequent editions as available)

2. May be sold to the public under certain circumstances; for exemptions see *Medicines, Ethics and Practice*, No. 23, London, Pharmaceutical Press, 2000 (and subsequent editions as available)

Sachets (Kapake Insts®), co-codamol 30/500 (codeine phosphate 30 mg, paracetamol 500 mg), net price 30-sachet pack (hosp. only) = £2.56, 100-sachet pack = £8.53. Label: 2, 13, 29, 30

Dose: 1–2 sachets every 4 hours; max. 8 sachets daily; CHILD not recommended

Solpadol® (Sanofi-Synthelabo) PoM ▄▄▄

Caplets (= tablets), co-codamol 30/500 (codeine phosphate 30 mg, paracetamol 500 mg). Net price 100-tab pack = £7.90. Label: 2, 29, 30

Dose: 2 tablets every 4 hours; max. 8 daily; CHILD not recommended

Capsules, grey/purple, co-codamol 30/500 (codeine phosphate 30 mg, paracetamol 500 mg). Net price 100-cap pack = £7.90. Label: 2, 29, 30

Dose: 1–2 capsules every 4 hours; max. 8 capsules daily; CHILD not recommended

Effervescent tablets, co-codamol 30/500 (codeine phosphate 30 mg, paracetamol 500 mg). Contains Na$^+$ 18.6 mmol/tablet; avoid in *renal impairment*. Net price 100-tab pack = £9.48. Label: 2, 13, 29, 30

Dose: 2 tablets in water every 4 hours; max. 8 daily; CHILD not recommended

Tylex® (Schwarz) PoM ▄▄▄

Capsules, co-codamol 30/500 (codeine phosphate 30 mg, paracetamol 500 mg). Net price 100-cap pack = £8.21. Label: 2, 29, 30

Dose: 1–2 capsules every 4 hours; max. 8 capsules daily; CHILD not recommended

Effervescent tablets, co-codamol 30/500 (codeine phosphate 30 mg, paracetamol 500 mg). Contains Na$^+$ 13.6 mmol/tablet; avoid in *renal impairment*. Net price 90-tab pack = £8.15. Label: 2, 13, 29, 30

Note. Contains aspartame 25 mg/tablet (see section 9.4.1)

Dose: 1–2 tablets in water every 4 hours; max. 8 tablets daily; CHILD not recommended

■ Co-codamol 60/1000

See warnings and notes on p. 204 (**important:** special care in elderly—reduce dose)

Kapake® (Galen) PoM ▄▄▄

Sachets (Kapake Insts®), co-codamol 60/1000 (codeine phosphate 60 mg, paracetamol 1 g), net price 50-sachet pack = £8.53. Label: 2, 13, 30

Dose: 1 sachet every 4 hours; max. 4 sachets daily; CHILD not recommended

■ With methionine (co-methiamol)

A mixture of methionine and paracetamol; methionine has no analgesic activity but may prevent paracetamol-induced liver toxicity if overdose taken

Paradote® (Penn)

Tablets, f/c, co-methiamol 100/500 (DL-methionine 100 mg, paracetamol 500 mg). Net price 24-tab pack = £1.05, 96-tab pack = £2.77. Label: 29, 30

Dose: 2 tablets every 4 hours; max. 8 tablets daily; CHILD 12 years and under, not recommended

▄▄▄ denotes preparations that are considered to be less suitable for prescribing (see p. vi)

■ With dihydrocodeine tartrate 10 mg

See notes on p. 204

Co-dydramol (Non-proprietary) PoM ▄▄▄

Tablets, scored, co-dydramol 10/500 (dihydrocodeine tartrate 10 mg, paracetamol 500 mg). Net price 20 = 51p. Label: 21, 29, 30

Dose: 1–2 tablets every 4–6 hours; max. 8 tablets daily; CHILD not recommended

Available from APS, Cox, CP, Galen (*Galake®* NHS), Generics, Norton, Sterwin

When co-dydramol tablets are prescribed and no strength is stated tablets containing dihydrocodeine tartrate 10 mg and paracetamol 500 mg should be dispensed.

Note. Tablets containing paracetamol 500 mg and dihydrocodeine 7.46 mg (*Paramol®* NHS) are on sale to the public. The name *Paramol®* was formerly applied to a brand of co-dydramol tablets

■ With dihydrocodeine tartrate 20 or 30 mg

See warnings and notes on p. 204 (**important:** special care in elderly—reduce dose)

Remedeine® (Napp) PoM ▄▄▄

Tablets, paracetamol 500 mg, dihydrocodeine tartrate 20 mg. Net price 112-tab pack = £11.66. Label: 2, 21, 29, 30

Dose: 1–2 tablets every 4–6 hours; max. 8 tablets daily; CHILD not recommended

Effervescent tablets, paracetamol 500 mg, dihydrocodeine tartrate 20 mg. Contains Na$^+$ 15.2 mmol/tablet; avoid in *renal impairment*. Net price 56-tab pack = £7.06. Label: 2, 13, 21, 29, 30

Dose: 1–2 tablets every 4–6 hours; max. 8 tablets daily; CHILD not recommended

Forte tablets, paracetamol 500 mg, dihydrocodeine tartrate 30 mg. Net price 56-tab pack = £7.20. Label: 2, 21, 29, 30

Dose: 1–2 tablets every 4–6 hours; max. 8 tablets daily; CHILD not recommended

Forte effervescent tablets, paracetamol 500 mg, dihydrocodeine tartrate 30 mg. Contains Na$^+$ 15.2 mmol/tablet; avoid in *renal impairment*. Net price 56-tab pack = £8.74. Label: 2, 13, 21, 29, 30

Dose: 1–2 tablets every 4–6 hours; max. 8 tablets daily; CHILD not recommended

■ Other compound preparations

See warnings and notes on p. 204 (**important:** special care in elderly—reduce dose)

Co-proxamol (Non-proprietary) PoM ▄▄▄

Tablets, co-proxamol 32.5/325 (dextropropoxyphene hydrochloride 32.5 mg, paracetamol 325 mg). Net price 20 = 30p. Label: 2, 10 patient information leaflet (if available), 29, 30

Dose: 2 tablets 3–4 times daily; max. 8 tablets daily; CHILD not recommended

Available from APS, Berk, Cox (*Cosalgesic®* NHS), Dista (*Distalgesic®* NHS), Norton, Sterwin

When co-proxamol tablets are prescribed and no strength is stated tablets containing dextropropoxyphene hydrochloride 32.5 mg and paracetamol 325 mg should be dispensed.

Fortagesic® (Sanofi-Synthelabo) NHS CD ▄▄▄

Tablets, pentazocine 15 mg (as hydrochloride), paracetamol 500 mg. Net price 100-tab pack = £7.00. Label: 2, 21, 29, 30

Dose: 2 tablets up to 4 times daily; CHILD 7–12 years 1 tablet every 4 hours, max. 4 tablets daily

■ Preparations on Sale to the Public

The following is a list of preparations on sale to the public that contain aspirin or **paracetamol, alone** or with **other ingredients**. Other significant ingredients (such as codeine and caffeine) are listed. For details of preparations containing ibuprofen on sale to the public, see section 10.1.1.

Important: in overdose contact **Poisons Information Services** (p. 19) for full details of the ingredients

Alka-Seltzer® (aspirin), **Alka-Seltzer**® XS (aspirin, caffeine, paracetamol), **Anadin**® (aspirin, caffeine), **Anadin Cold Control**® (paracetamol, caffeine, phenylephrine), **Anadin Cold Control Flu Strength**® (paracetamol, phenylephrine), **Anadin Extra**®, **Anadin Extra Soluble**® (both aspirin, caffeine, paracetamol), **Anadin Maximum Strength**® (aspirin, caffeine), **Anadin Paracetamol**® (paracetamol), **Andrews Answer**® (paracetamol, caffeine), **Angettes 75**® (aspirin), **Askit**® (aspirin, aloxiprin = polymeric product of aspirin, caffeine), **Aspro**® (aspirin), **Aspro Clear**® (aspirin)

Bayer Aspirin® (aspirin), **Beechams-All-In-One**®, (paracetamol, guaifenesin, phenylephrine), **Beechams Cold & Flu**® (paracetamol, phenylephrine), **Beechams Flu-Plus Powder**®, **Beechams Hot Lemon**®, **Hot Lemon and Honey**®, **Hot Blackcurrant**® (all paracetamol, phenylephrine), **Beechams Flu-Plus Caplets**® (paracetamol, caffeine, phenylephrine), **Beechams Powders**® (aspirin, caffeine), **Beechams Powders Capsules**® **With Decongestant** (paracetamol, caffeine, phenylephrine), **Beecham Aspirin**®, **Beechams Powders Tablets**® (both aspirin), **Benylin 4 Flu**® (paracetamol, diphenhydramine, pseudoephedrine), **Benylin Day and Night**® (day tablets, paracetamol, phenylpropanolamine, night tablets, paracetamol, diphenhydramine), **Boots Back Pain Relief**® (aspirin), **Boots Children's Cold Relief**®, **Boots Cold & Flu Relief Tablets**® (paracetamol, caffeine, phenylephrine), **Boots Children's Pain Relief Syrup**® (paracetamol), **Boots Cold Relief Hot Blackcurrant**®, **Hot Lemon**® (paracetamol), **Boots Dental Pain Relief**® (paracetamol, dihydrocodeine), **Boots Headache and Indigestion Relief**® (paracetamol, caffeine), **Boots Headache Relief**® (aspirin, paracetamol, caffeine), **Boots Migraine Relief**® (codeine, paracetamol), **Boots Night-Cold Comfort**® (diphenhydramine, paracetamol, pholcodine, pseudoephedrine), **Boots Pain Relief Tablets**® (paracetamol, caffeine), **Boots Sinus Pain Relief**® (paracetamol, caffeine, phenylephrine), **Boots Tension Headache Relief**® (paracetamol, caffeine, codeine, doxylamine)

Calpol Infant®, **Calpol 6 Plus**®, **Calpol Paediatric**® (all paracetamol), **Caprin**® (aspirin), **Catarrh-Ex**® (paracetamol, caffeine, phenylephrine), **Codis 500**® (aspirin, codeine), **Coldrex Blackcurrant Powders**®, **Hot Lemon Powders**® (both paracetamol, phenylephrine), **Coldrex Tablets**® (paracetamol, caffeine, phenylephrine), **Mrs. Cullen's**® (aspirin), **Cupanol Over 6**®, **Cupanol Under 6**® (both paracetamol)

Day Nurse® (paracetamol, dextromethorphan, phenylpropanolamine), **De Witt's Analgesic Pills**® (paracetamol, caffeine), **Disprin**®, **Disprin CV**®, **Disprin Direct**® (all aspirin), **Disprin Extra**® (aspirin, paracetamol), **Disprol**® (paracetamol), **Dristan Tablets**® (aspirin, caffeine, chlorphenamine, phenylephrine)

Fanalgic® (paracetamol), **Feminax**® (paracetamol, caffeine, codeine, hyoscine), **Fennings Children's Cooling Powders**® (paracetamol), **Flurex Bedtime**® (paracetamol, diphenhydramine, pseudoephedrine), **Fynnon**® **Calcium Aspirin** (aspirin)

Hedex® (paracetamol), **Hedex Extra**® (paracetamol, caffeine), **Hedex Headcold Caplets**® (paracetamol, caffeine, phenylephrine), **Hedex Headcold Powders**® (paracetamol, phenylephrine), **Hill's Balsam Flu Strength Hot Lemon Powders**® (paracetamol)

Infadrops® (paracetamol)

Lem-Plus Capsules® (paracetamol, caffeine, phenylephrine), **Lem-Plus Powders**® (paracetamol), **Lemsip Lemcaps**® (paracetamol, caffeine, phenylephrine), **Lemsip Cool Lemon**®, **Lemsip Flu Strength**®, **Lemsip Lemon**® or **Blackcurrant**®, **Lemsip Max Strength**®, **Lemsip Menthol**

Extra® (all paracetamol, phenylephrine), **Lemsip Flu Strength Nightime**® (paracetamol, chlorphenamine, dextromethorphan, phenylpropanolamine)

Maximum Strength Aspro Clear® (aspirin), **Medinol**® (paracetamol), **Medised**® (paracetamol, promethazine), **Midrid**® (paracetamol, isometheptene mucate), **Migraleve**® (pink tablets, paracetamol, codeine, buclizine, yellow tablets, paracetamol, codeine), **Miradol**® (paracetamol), **Mu-Cron Tablets**® (paracetamol, phenylpropanolamine)

Night Nurse® (paracetamol, dextromethorphan, promethazine), **Nirolex Day Cold Comfort**® (paracetamol, pholcodine, pseudoephedrine), **Nurse Sykes' Powders**® (aspirin, caffeine, paracetamol)

Paldesic® (paracetamol), **Panadeine**® (paracetamol, codeine), **Panadol**®, **Panadol Baby and Infant**® (both paracetamol), **Panadol Extra**® (paracetamol, caffeine), **Panadol Junior**® (paracetamol), **Panadol Night**® (paracetamol, diphenhydramine), **Panadol Ultra**® (paracetamol, codeine), **Panaleve Junior**®, **Panaleve 6+**® (both paracetamol), **Paracets**® (paracetamol), **Paraclear Extra Strength**® (paracetamol, caffeine), **Paraclear**® (paracetamol), **Paracodol**® (paracetamol, codeine), **Paramin**® (paracetamol), **Paramol**® (paracetamol, dihydrocodeine), **Phensic**® (aspirin, caffeine), **Placidex**® (paracetamol), **Powerin**® (aspirin, caffeine, paracetamol), **Propain**® (paracetamol, caffeine, codeine, diphenhydramine)

Resolve® (paracetamol)

Salzone® (paracetamol), **Sinutab**® (paracetamol, phenylpropanolamine), **Sinutab Nightime**® (paracetamol, phenylpropanolamine, phenyltoloxamine), **Solpadeine**® (paracetamol, caffeine, codeine), **Solpadeine Max**® (paracetamol, codeine), **SP Cold Relief Capsules**® (paracetamol, caffeine, phenylephrine), **Sudafed-Co**® (paracetamol, pseudoephedrine), **Syndol**® (paracetamol, caffeine, codeine, doxylamine)

Tixymol® (paracetamol), **Toptabs**® (aspirin, caffeine), **Tramil**® **500** (paracetamol), **Triogesic**® (paracetamol, phenylpropanolamine)

Uniflu with Gregovite C® (aspirin, caffeine, codeine, diphenhydramine, phenylephrine)

Veganin® (aspirin, paracetamol, codeine), **Vicks Medinite**® (paracetamol, dextromethorphan, doxylamine, ephedrine)

NEFOPAM HYDROCHLORIDE

Indications: moderate pain

Cautions: hepatic or renal disease, elderly, urinary retention; pregnancy and breast-feeding; **interactions:** Appendix 1 (nefopam)

Contra-indications: convulsive disorders; not indicated for myocardial infarction

Side-effects: nausea, nervousness, urinary retention, dry mouth, lightheadedness; less frequently vomiting, blurred vision, drowsiness, sweating, insomnia, tachycardia, headache; confusion and hallucinations also reported; may colour urine (pink)

Dose: by mouth, initially 60 mg (elderly, 30 mg) 3 times daily, adjusted according to response; usual range 30–90 mg 3 times daily; CHILD not recommended

By intramuscular injection, 20 mg every 6 hours; CHILD not recommended

Note. Nefopam hydrochloride 20 mg by injection ≡ 60 mg by mouth

Acupan® (3M) [PoM]
Tablets, f/c, nefopam hydrochloride 30 mg. Net price 90-tab pack = £10.93. Label: 2, 14
Injection, nefopam hydrochloride 20 mg/mL. Net price 1-mL amp = 69p

4.7.2   Opioid analgesics

Opioid analgesics are usually used to relieve moderate to severe pain particularly of visceral origin. Repeated administration may cause dependence and tolerance, but this is no deterrent in the control of pain in terminal illness, for guidelines see Prescribing in Palliative Care, p. 12.

SIDE-EFFECTS. Opioid analgesics share many side-effects though qualitative and quantitative differences exist. The most common include nausea, vomiting, constipation, and drowsiness. Larger doses produce respiratory depression and hypotension. **Overdosage**, see Emergency Treatment of Poisoning, p. 23.

INTERACTIONS. See Appendix 1 (opioid analgesics) (**important**: special hazard with *pethidine and possibly other opioids* and MAOIs).

DRIVING. Drowsiness may affect performance of skilled tasks (e.g. driving); effects of alcohol enhanced.

CHOICE. **Morphine** remains the most valuable opioid analgesic for severe pain although it frequently causes nausea and vomiting. It is the standard against which other opioid analgesics are compared. In addition to relief of pain, morphine also confers a state of euphoria and mental detachment.

Morphine is the opioid of choice for the oral treatment of *severe pain in palliative care*. It is given regularly every 4 hours (or every 12 or 24 hours as modified-release preparations). For guidelines on dosage adjustment in palliative care, see p. 12.

Buprenorphine has both opioid agonist and antagonist properties and may precipitate withdrawal symptoms, including pain, in patients dependent on other opioids. It has abuse potential and may itself cause dependence. It has a much longer duration of action than morphine and sublingually is an effective analgesic for 6 to 8 hours. Vomiting may be a problem. Unlike most opioid analgesics its effects are only partially reversed by naloxone.

Codeine is effective for the relief of mild to moderate pain but is too constipating for long-term use.

Dextromoramide is less sedating than morphine and has a short duration of action.

Diphenoxylate (in combination with atropine, as co-phenotrope) is used in acute diarrhoea (see section 1.4.2).

Dipipanone used alone is less sedating than morphine but the only preparation available contains an anti-emetic and is therefore not suitable for regular regimens in palliative care (see p. 14).

Dextropropoxyphene given alone is a very mild analgesic somewhat less potent than codeine. Combinations of dextropropoxyphene with paracetamol (co-proxamol) or aspirin have little more analgesic effect than paracetamol or aspirin alone. An important disadvantage of co-proxamol is that **overdosage** (which may be combined with alcohol) is complicated by respiratory depression and acute heart failure due to the dextropropoxyphene and by hepatotoxicity due to the paracetamol. Rapid treatment is essential (see Emergency Treatment of Poisoning, p. 23).

Diamorphine (heroin) is a powerful opioid analgesic. It may cause less nausea and hypotension than morphine. In *palliative care* the greater solubility of diamorphine allows effective doses to be injected in smaller volumes and this is important in the emaciated patient.

Dihydrocodeine has an analgesic efficacy similar to that of codeine. The dose of dihydrocodeine by mouth is usually 30 mg every 4 hours; doubling the dose to 60 mg may provide some additional pain relief but this may be at the cost of more nausea and vomiting. A 40-mg tablet is now also available.

Alfentanil, **fentanyl** and **remifentanil** are used by injection for intra-operative analgesia (section 15.1.4.3); fentanyl is available in a transdermal drug delivery system as a self-adhesive patch which is changed every 72 hours.

Meptazinol is claimed to have a low incidence of respiratory depression. It has a reported length of action of 2 to 7 hours with onset within 15 minutes.

Methadone is less sedating than morphine and acts for longer periods. In prolonged use, methadone should not be administered more often than twice daily to avoid the risk of accumulation and opioid overdosage. Methadone may be used instead of morphine in the occasional patient who experiences excitation (or exacerbation of pain) with morphine.

Nalbuphine has a similar efficacy to that of morphine for pain relief, but may have fewer side-effects and less abuse potential. Nausea and vomiting occur less than with other opioids but respiratory depression is similar to that with morphine.

Oxycodone is used as the pectinate in suppositories (special order from BCM Specials) for the control of *pain in palliative care*.

Pentazocine has both agonist and antagonist properties and precipitates withdrawal symptoms, including pain in patients dependent on other opioids. By injection it is more potent than dihydrocodeine or codeine, but hallucinations and thought disturbances may occur. It is not recommended and, in particular, should be avoided after myocardial infarction as it may increase pulmonary and aortic blood pressure as well as cardiac work.

Pethidine produces prompt but short-lasting analgesia; it is less constipating than morphine, but even in high doses is a less potent analgesic. It is not suitable for severe continuing pain. It is used for analgesia in labour; however, other opioids, such as morphine or diamorphine, are often preferred for obstetric pain.

Phenazocine is effective in severe pain and has less tendency to increase biliary pressure than other opioid analgesics. It can be administered sublingually if nausea and vomiting are a problem.

Tramadol is claimed to produce analgesia by two mechanisms: an opioid effect and an enhancement of serotoninergic and adrenergic pathways. It is reported to have fewer of the typical opioid side-effects (notably, less respiratory depression, less constipation and less addiction potential); psychiatric reactions have been reported.

POSTOPERATIVE ANALGESIA. The use of intra-operative opioids affects the prescribing of post-operative analgesics and in many cases delays the need for a postoperative analgesic. A postoperative opioid analgesic should be given with care since it may potentiate any residual respiratory depression (for the treatment of opioid-induced respiratory depression, see section 15.1.7). Non-opioid analgesics are also used for postoperative pain (section 15.1.4.2).

Morphine and **papaveretum** are used most widely. **Tramadol** is not as effective in severe pain as other opioid analgesics. **Buprenorphine** may antagonise the analgesic effect of previously administered opioids and is generally not recommended. **Pethidine** is metabolised to norpethidine which may accumulate, particularly in renal impairment; norpethidine stimulates the central nervous system and may cause convulsions. **Meptazinol** and **nalbuphine** are rarely used.

Opioids are also given epidurally [unlicensed route] in the postoperative period but are associated with side-effects such as pruritus, urinary retention, nausea and vomiting; respiratory depression can be delayed, particularly with morphine.

For details of patient-controlled analgesia (PCA) to relieve postoperative pain, consult hospital protocols. Formulations specifically designed for PCA are available (*Pharma-Ject® Morphine Sulphate*)

ADDICTS. Although caution is necessary addicts (and ex-addicts) may be treated with analgesics in the same way as other people when there is a real clinical need. Doctors are reminded that they do not require a special licence to prescribe opioid analgesics for addicts for relief of pain due to organic disease or injury.

MORPHINE SALTS

Indications: see notes above and under Dose; acute diarrhoea (section 1.4.2); cough in terminal care (section 3.9.1)

Cautions: hypotension, hypothyroidism, asthma (avoid during attack) and decreased respiratory reserve, prostatic hypertrophy; pregnancy and breast-feeding; may precipitate coma in hepatic impairment (reduce dose or avoid but many such patients tolerate morphine well); reduce dose or avoid in renal impairment (see also Appendix 3), elderly and debilitated (reduce dose); convulsive disorders, dependence (severe withdrawal symptoms if withdrawn abruptly); use of cough suppressants containing opioid analgesics not generally recommended in children and should be avoided altogether in those under at least 1 year; **interactions:** Appendix 1 (opioid analgesics)

PALLIATIVE CARE. In the control of pain in terminal illness these cautions should not necessarily be a deterrent to the use of opioid analgesics

Contra-indications: avoid in acute respiratory depression, acute alcoholism and where risk of paralytic ileus; not indicated for acute abdomen; also avoid in raised intracranial pressure or head injury (in addition to interfering with respiration, affect pupillary responses vital for neurological assessment); avoid injection in phaeochromocytoma (risk of pressor response to histamine release)

Side-effects: nausea and vomiting (particularly in initial stages), constipation, and drowsiness; larger doses produce respiratory depression and hypotension; other side-effects include difficulty with micturition, ureteric or biliary spasm, dry

mouth, sweating, headache, facial flushing, vertigo, bradycardia, tachycardia, palpitations, postural hypotension, hypothermia, hallucinations, dysphoria, mood changes, dependence, miosis, decreased libido or potency, rashes, urticaria and pruritus; **overdosage:** see Emergency Treatment of Poisoning, p. 23; for reversal of opioid-induced respiratory depression, see section 15.1.7.

Dose: acute pain, *by subcutaneous injection* (not suitable for oedematous patients) *or by intramuscular injection*, 10 mg every 4 hours if necessary (15 mg for heavier well-muscled patients); CHILD up to 1 month 150 micrograms/kg, 1–12 months 200 micrograms/kg, 1–5 years 2.5–5 mg, 6–12 years 5–10 mg

By slow intravenous injection, quarter to half corresponding intramuscular dose

Premedication, *by subcutaneous or intramuscular injection*, up to 10 mg 60–90 minutes before operation; CHILD, *by intramuscular injection*, 150 micrograms/kg

Postoperative pain, *by subcutaneous or intramuscular injection*, 10 mg every 2–4 hours if necessary (15 mg for heavier well-muscled patients); CHILD up to 1 month 150 micrograms/kg, 1–12 months 200 micrograms/kg, 1–5 years 2.5–5 mg, 6–12 years 5–10 mg

Note. In the postoperative period, the patient should be closely monitored for pain relief as well as for side-effects especially respiratory depression

Patient controlled analgesia (PCA), consult hospital protocols

Myocardial infarction, *by slow intravenous injection* (2 mg/minute), 10 mg followed by a further 5–10 mg if necessary; elderly or frail patients, reduce dose by half

Acute pulmonary oedema, *by slow intravenous injection* (2 mg/minute) 5–10 mg

Chronic pain, *by mouth or by subcutaneous injection* (not suitable for oedematous patients) *or by intramuscular injection*, 5–20 mg regularly every 4 hours; dose may be increased according to needs; oral dose should be approx. double corresponding intramuscular dose and approximately triple corresponding intramuscular *diamorphine* dose (see also Prescribing in Palliative Care, p. 12); *by rectum*, as suppositories, 15–30 mg regularly every 4 hours

Note. The doses stated above refer equally to morphine hydrochloride, sulphate, and tartrate; see below for doses of **modified-release** preparations.

■ Oral solutions

Note. For advice on transfer from oral solutions of morphine to modified-release preparations of morphine, see Prescribing in Palliative Care, p. 12

Morphine Oral Solutions PoM or CD

Oral solutions of morphine can be prescribed by writing the formula:

Morphine hydrochloride 5 mg
Chloroform water to 5 mL

Note. The proportion of morphine hydrochloride may be altered when specified by the prescriber; if above 13 mg per 5 mL the solution becomes **CD**. For sample prescription see Controlled Drugs and Drug Dependence, p. 7. It is usual to adjust the strength so that the dose volume is 5 or 10 mL.

Oramorph® (Boehringer Ingelheim)

Oramorph® oral solution PoM, morphine sulphate 10 mg/5 mL. Net price 100-mL pack = £2.08; 300-mL pack = £5.79; 500-mL pack = £8.73. Label: 2

Oramorph® Unit Dose Vials 10 mg PoM (oral vials), sugar-free, morphine sulphate 10 mg/5-mL vial, net price 25 vials = £3.31. Label: 2

Oramorph® Unit Dose Vials 30 mg CD (oral vials), sugar-free, morphine sulphate 30 mg/5-mL vial, net price 25 vials = £9.30. Label: 2

Oramorph® concentrated oral solution CD, sugar-free, morphine sulphate 100 mg/5 mL. Net price 30-mL pack = £5.82; 120-mL pack = £21.74 (both with calibrated dropper). Label: 2

Oramorph® Unit Dose Vials 100 mg CD (oral vials), sugar-free, morphine sulphate 100 mg/5-mL vial, net price 25 vials = £31.00. Label: 2

Sevredol® (Napp)

Oral solution PoM, morphine sulphate 10 mg/5 mL, net price 100 mL = £1.99, 300 mL = £5.53, 500 mL = £8.34. Label: 2

Concentrated oral solution CD, morphine sulphate 20 mg/mL, net price 30 mL = £5.56, 120 mL = £20.76 (both with dropper or oral syringe). Label: 2

■ Tablets

Sevredol® (Napp) CD

Tablets, f/c, scored, morphine sulphate 10 mg (blue), net price 56-tab pack = £6.03; 20 mg (pink), 56-tab pack = £12.05; 50 mg (pale green), 56-tab pack = £30.13. Label: 2

Dose: severe pain uncontrolled by weaker opioid, 10–50 mg every 4 hours (dose adjusted according to need and tolerance); CHILD 3–5 years, 5 mg; 6–12 years, 5–10 mg

■ Modified release

Morcap® SR (Sanofi-Synthelabo) CD

Capsules, m/r, clear enclosing ivory and brown pellets, morphine sulphate 20 mg, net price 30-cap pack = £5.71, 60-cap pack = £11.42; 50 mg, 30-cap pack = £13.84, 60-cap pack = £27.68; 100 mg, 30-cap pack = £27.68, 60-cap pack = £55.37. Label: 2, counselling, see below

Dose: adjusted according to daily morphine requirements, for further advice on determining dose, see Prescribing in Palliative Care, p. 12; dosage requirements may need to be reviewed if the brand is altered

COUNSELLING. Swallow whole or open capsule and sprinkle contents on soft food

Note. Prescription must also specify 'capsules' (i.e. 'Morcap SR capsules')

MST Continus® (Napp) CD

Tablets, m/r, f/c, morphine sulphate 5 mg (white), net price 60-tab pack = £4.30; 10 mg (brown), 60-tab pack = £7.17; 15 mg (green), 60-tab pack = £12.57; 30 mg (purple), 60-tab pack = £17.22; 60 mg (orange), 60-tab pack = £33.58; 100 mg (grey), 60-tab pack = £53.16; 200 mg (green), 60-tab pack = £106.34. Label: 2, 25

Suspension (= sachet of granules to mix with water), m/r, pink, morphine sulphate 20 mg/sachet, net price 30-sachet pack = £27.31; 30 mg/sachet, 30-sachet pack = £28.38; 60 mg/sachet, 30-sachet pack = £56.77; 100 mg/sachet, 30-

sachet pack = £94.61; 200 mg/sachet pack, 30-sachet pack = £189.22. Label: 2, 13

Dose: adjusted according to daily morphine requirements, for further advice on determining dose, see Prescribing in Palliative Care, p. 12; dosage requirements may need to be reviewed if the brand is altered

Note. Prescriptions must also specify 'tablets' or 'suspension' (i.e. 'MST Continus tablets' or 'MST Continus suspension').

MXL® (Napp) CD

Capsules, m/r, morphine sulphate 30 mg (light blue), net price 28-cap pack = £11.73; 60 mg (brown), 28-cap pack = £16.07; 90 mg (pink), 28-cap pack = £23.70; 120 mg (green), 28-cap pack = £31.34; 150 mg (blue), 28-cap pack = £39.17; 200 mg (red-brown), 28-cap pack = £49.62. Label: 2, counselling, see below

Dose: adjusted according to daily morphine requirements, for further advice on determining dose, see Prescribing in Palliative Care, p. 12; dosage requirements may need to be reviewed if the brand is altered

COUNSELLING. Swallow whole or open capsule and sprinkle contents on soft food

Note. Prescriptions must also specify 'capsules' (i.e. 'MXL capsules')

Oramorph® SR (Boehringer Ingelheim) CD

Tablets, m/r, f/c, morphine sulphate 10 mg (buff), net price 60-tab pack = £5.75; 30 mg (violet), 60-tab pack = £13.80; 60 mg (orange), 60-tab pack = £26.89; 100 mg (grey), 60-tab pack = £42.59. Label: 2, 25

Dose: adjusted according to daily morphine requirements, for further advice on determining dose, see Prescribing in Palliative Care, p. 12; dosage requirements may need to be reviewed if the brand is altered

Note. Prescriptions must also specify 'tablets' (i.e. 'Oramorph SR tablets')

Zomorph® (Link) CD

Capsules, m/r, morphine sulphate 10 mg (yellow/clear enclosing pale yellow pellets), net price 60-cap pack = £4.31; 30 mg (pink/clear enclosing pale yellow pellets), 60-cap pack = £10.33; 60 mg (orange/clear enclosing pale yellow pellets), 60-cap pack = £20.15; 100 mg (white/clear enclosing pale yellow pellets), 60-cap pack = £31.90; 200 mg (clear enclosing pale yellow pellets), 60-cap pack = £63.79. Label: 2, counselling, see below

Dose: adjusted according to daily morphine requirements, for further advice on determining doses, see Prescribing in Palliative Care, p. 12; dosage requirements may need to be reviewed if the brand is altered

COUNSELLING. Swallow whole or open capsule and sprinkle contents on soft food

Note. Prescriptions must also specify 'capsules' (i.e. 'Zomorph capsules')

■ Injections

Morphine Sulphate (Non-proprietary) CD

Injection, morphine sulphate 10, 15, 20, and 30 mg/mL, net price 1- and 2-mL amp (all) = 66–99p

Intravenous infusion, morphine sulphate 1 mg/mL, net price 50-mL vial = £4.75; 2 mg/mL, 50-mL vial = £4.85

Available from Aurum, Faulding DBL

Min-I-Jet® Morphine Sulphate (IMS) CD

Injection, morphine sulphate 10 mg/mL, net price 2-mL disposable syringe = £10.85

Morphine and Atropine Injection (Non-proprietary) CD
Injection, morphine sulphate 10 mg, atropine sulphate 600 micrograms/mL. Net price 1-mL amp = £4.65
Dose: premedication, by subcutaneous injection, 0.5–1 mL

■ Injection with anti-emetic
CAUTION. In myocardial infarction cyclizine may aggravate severe heart failure and counteract the haemodynamic benefits of opioids, see section 4.6. **Not recommended** in palliative care, see p. 14
Cyclimorph® (GlaxoWellcome) CD
Cyclimorph-10® Injection, morphine tartrate 10 mg, cyclizine tartrate 50 mg/mL. Net price 1-mL amp = £1.28
Dose: by subcutaneous, intramuscular, or intravenous injection, 1 mL, repeated not more often than every 4 hours, with not more than 3 doses in any 24-hour period
Cyclimorph-15® Injection, morphine tartrate 15 mg, cyclizine tartrate 50 mg/mL. Net price 1-mL amp = £1.33
Dose: by subcutaneous, intramuscular, or intravenous injection, 1 mL, repeated not more often than every 4 hours, with not more than 3 doses in any 24-hour period

■ Suppositories
Morphine (Non-proprietary) CD
Suppositories, morphine hydrochloride or sulphate 10 mg, net price 12 = £6.12; 15 mg, 12 = £5.38; 20 mg, 12 = £7.45; 30 mg, 12 = £8.34. Label: 2
Available from Aurum, Martindale, Medeva
Note. Both the strength of the suppositories and the morphine salt contained in them must be specified by the prescriber

BUPRENORPHINE

Indications: moderate to severe pain; peri-operative analgesia; opioid dependence (section 4.10)
Cautions: see under Morphine Salts and notes above; effects only partially reversed by naloxone; **interactions:** Appendix 1 (opioid analgesics)
Contra-indications: see under Morphine Salts and notes above
Side-effects: see under Morphine Salts and notes above; can give rise to mild withdrawal symptoms in patients dependent on opioids
Dose: moderate to severe pain, *by sublingual administration*, initially 200–400 micrograms every 8 hours, increasing if necessary to 200–400 micrograms every 6–8 hours; CHILD over 6 months, 16–25 kg, 100 micrograms; 25–37.5 kg, 100–200 micrograms; 37.5–50 kg, 200–300 micrograms
By intramuscular or slow intravenous injection, 300–600 micrograms every 6–8 hours; CHILD over 6 months 3–6 micrograms/kg every 6–8 hours (max. 9 micrograms/kg)
Premedication, *by sublingual administration*, 400 micrograms
By intramuscular injection, 300 micrograms
Intra-operative analgesia, *by slow intravenous injection*, 300–450 micrograms

Temgesic® (Schering-Plough) CD
Tablets (sublingual), buprenorphine (as hydrochloride), 200 micrograms, net price 50-tab pack = £5.73; 400 micrograms, 50-tab pack = £11.46. Label: 2, 26
Injection, buprenorphine (as hydrochloride) 300 micrograms/mL, net price 1-mL amp = 53p

CODEINE PHOSPHATE

Indications: mild to moderate pain; diarrhoea (section 1.4.2); cough suppression (section 3.9.1)
Cautions: see under Morphine Salts and notes above; use of cough suppressants containing codeine or similar opioid analgesics not generally recommended in children and should be avoided altogether in those under 1 year; **interactions:** Appendix 1 (opioid analgesics)
Contra-indications: see under Morphine Salts and notes above
Side-effects: see under Morphine Salts and notes above
Dose: *by mouth*, 30–60 mg every 4 hours when necessary, to a max. of 240 mg daily; CHILD 1–12 years, 3 mg/kg daily in divided doses
By intramuscular injection, 30–60 mg every 4 hours when necessary

Codeine Phosphate (Non-proprietary)
Tablets PoM, codeine phosphate 15 mg, net price 20 = 52p; 30 mg, 20 = £1.57; 60 mg, 20 = £1.35. Label: 2
Note. As for schedule 2 controlled drugs, travellers needing to take codeine phosphate preparations abroad may require a doctor's letter explaining why they are necessary
Syrup PoM, codeine phosphate 25 mg/5 mL. Net price 100 mL = 90p. Label: 2
Injection CD, codeine phosphate 60 mg/mL. Net price 1-mL amp = £1.85
Codeine Linctuses
Section 3.9.1

Note. Codeine is an ingredient of some compound analgesic preparations, section 4.7.1 and section 10.1.1 (*Codafen Continus®*)

DEXTROMORAMIDE

Indications: severe pain
Cautions: see under Morphine Salts and notes above; only short duration of action (2–3 hours); **interactions:** Appendix 1 (opioid analgesics)
Contra-indications: see under Morphine Salts and notes above; obstetric analgesia (increased risk of neonatal depression)
Side-effects: see under Morphine Salts and notes above
Dose: *by mouth*, 5 mg increasing to 20 mg, when required
By rectum in suppositories, 10 mg when required

Palfium® (Roche) CD
Tablets, both scored, dextromoramide (as tartrate) 5 mg, net price 60-tab pack = £4.45; 10 mg (peach), 60-tab pack = £8.80. Label: 2
Suppositories, dextromoramide 10 mg (as tartrate). Net price 10 = £2.19. Label: 2

DEXTROPROPOXYPHENE HYDROCHLORIDE

Indications: mild to moderate pain
Cautions: see under Morphine Salts and notes above; compound preparations special hazard in overdose, see notes above; **interactions:** Appendix 1 (opioid analgesics)

Contra-indications: see under Morphine Salts and notes above; those who are suicidal or addiction prone; porphyria (section 9.8.2)

Side-effects: see under Morphine Salts and notes above; occasional hepatotoxicity; convulsions reported in overdose

Dose: 65 mg every 6–8 hours when necessary; CHILD not recommended

Note. 65 mg dextropropoxyphene hydrochloride ≡ 100 mg dextropropoxyphene napsilate

Dextropropoxyphene (Non-proprietary) PoM
Capsules, the equivalent of dextropropoxyphene hydrochloride 65 mg (as napsilate). Net price 20 = £1.64. Label: 2

Available from Lilly (Doloxene® NHS)

Note. Dextropropoxyphene is an ingredient of some compound analgesic preparations, section 4.7.1

DIAMORPHINE HYDROCHLORIDE
(Heroin Hydrochloride)

Indications: see notes above; acute pulmonary oedema

Cautions: see under Morphine Salts and notes above; **interactions:** Appendix 1 (opioid analgesics)

Contra-indications: see under Morphine Salts and notes above

Side-effects: see under Morphine Salts and notes above

Dose: acute pain, *by subcutaneous or intramuscular injection*, 5 mg repeated every 4 hours if necessary (up to 10 mg for heavier well-muscled patients)
By slow intravenous injection, quarter to half corresponding intramuscular dose

Myocardial infarction, *by slow intravenous injection* (1 mg/minute), 5 mg followed by a further 2.5–5 mg if necessary; elderly or frail patients, reduce dose by half

Acute pulmonary oedema, *by slow intravenous injection* (1 mg/minute) 2.5–5 mg

Chronic pain, *by mouth or by subcutaneous or intramuscular injection*, 5–10 mg regularly every 4 hours; dose may be increased according to needs; intramuscular dose should be approx. half corresponding oral dose, and approx. one third corresponding oral *morphine* dose—see also Prescribing in Palliative Care, p. 12; *by subcutaneous infusion* (using syringe driver), see Prescribing in Palliative Care, p. 14

Diamorphine (Non-proprietary) CD
Tablets, diamorphine hydrochloride 10 mg. Net price 100-tab pack = £12.92. Label: 2
Available from Aurum

Injection, powder for reconstitution, diamorphine hydrochloride. Net price 5-mg amp = £1.38, 10-mg amp = £1.70, 30-mg amp = £1.82, 100-mg amp = £5.07, 500-mg amp = £22.91
Available from Berk (*Diagesil®*), CP, Hillcross, Medeva

Diamorphine Linctus CD
See section 3.9.1

DIHYDROCODEINE TARTRATE

Indications: moderate to severe pain

Cautions: see under Morphine Salts and notes above; **interactions:** Appendix 1 (opioid analgesics)

Contra-indications: see under Morphine Salts and notes above

Side-effects: see under Morphine Salts and notes above

Dose: *by mouth*, 30 mg every 4–6 hours when necessary (see also notes above); CHILD over 4 years 0.5–1 mg/kg every 4–6 hours
By deep subcutaneous or intramuscular injection, up to 50 mg repeated every 4–6 hours if necessary; CHILD over 4 years 0.5–1 mg/kg every 4–6 hours

Dihydrocodeine (Non-proprietary)
Tablets PoM, dihydrocodeine tartrate 30 mg. Net price 20 = £1.15. Label: 2, 21
Available from most generic manufacturers

Oral solution PoM, dihydrocodeine tartrate 10 mg/5 mL. Net price 150 mL = £2.80. Label: 2, 21
Available from Martindale

Injection CD, dihydrocodeine tartrate 50 mg/mL. Net price 1-mL amp = £1.94
Available from Aurum

DF 118 Forte® (Martindale) PoM
Tablets, dihydrocodeine tartrate 40 mg. Net price 100-tab pack = £11.51. Label: 2, 21
Dose: severe pain, 40–80 mg 3 times daily; max. 240 mg daily; CHILD not recommended

■ Modified release

DHC Continus® (Napp) PoM
Tablets, m/r, dihydrocodeine tartrate 60 mg, net price 56-tab pack = £6.28; 90 mg, 56-tab pack = £9.89; 120 mg, 56-tab pack = £13.21. Label: 2, 25
Dose: chronic severe pain, 60–120 mg every 12 hours; CHILD not recommended

Note. Dihydrocodeine is an ingredient of some compound analgesic preparations, see section 4.7.1

DIPIPANONE HYDROCHLORIDE

Indications: moderate to severe pain

Cautions: see under Morphine Salts and notes above; **interactions:** Appendix 1 (opioid analgesics)

Contra-indications: see under Morphine Salts and notes above

Side-effects: see under Morphine Salts and notes above

Dose: see preparation below

Diconal® (GlaxoWellcome) CD
Tablets, pink, scored, dipipanone hydrochloride 10 mg, cyclizine hydrochloride 30 mg. Net price 50-tab pack = £7.59. Label: 2
Dose: acute pain, 1 tablet gradually increased to 3 tablets every 6 hours; CHILD not recommended
CAUTION. **Not recommended** in palliative care, see p. 14

FENTANYL

Indications: chronic intractable pain due to cancer, see below; other indications (section 15.1.4.3)

Cautions: see under Morphine Salts and notes above; **interactions:** Appendix 1 (opioid analgesics)

FEVER OR EXTERNAL HEAT. Monitor patients for increased side-effects if fever present (increased absorption possible); avoid exposing application site to external heat (may also increase absorption)

Contra-indications: see under Morphine Salts and notes above

Side-effects: see under Morphine Salts and notes above; local reactions such as rash, erythema and itching reported

Administration: see under preparation, below

LONG DURATION OF ACTION. In view of the long duration of action, patients who have experienced severe side-effects should be monitored for up to 24 hours after patch removal

Durogesic® (Janssen-Cilag) CD

Patches, self-adhesive, transparent, fentanyl, '25' patch (releasing approx. 25 micrograms/hour for 72 hours), net price 5 = £28.97; '50' patch (releasing approx. 50 micrograms/hour for 72 hours), 5 = £54.11; '75' patch (releasing approx. 75 micrograms/hour for 72 hours), 5 = £75.43; '100' patch (releasing approx. 100 micrograms/hour for 72 hours), 5 = £92.97. Label: 2

ADMINISTRATION: apply to dry, non-irritated, non-irradiated, non-hairy skin on torso or upper arm, removing after 72 hours and siting replacement patch on a different area (avoid using the same area for several days). Patients who have not previously received a strong opioid analgesic, initial dose, one '25 micrograms/hour' patch replaced after 72 hours; patients who have received a strong opioid analgesic, initial dose based on previous 24-hour opioid requirement (oral morphine sulphate 90 mg over 24 hours ≈ one '25 micrograms/hour' patch, consult product literature for details); CHILD not recommended

Note. When starting, evaluation of the analgesic effect should **not** be made before the system has been worn for **24 hours** (to allow for the gradual increase in plasma-fentanyl concentration)—previous analgesic therapy should be phased out gradually from time of first patch application; dose adjustment should normally be carried out in 72-hour steps of '25 micrograms/hour'. More than one patch may be used at a time for doses greater than '100 micrograms/hour' (but applied at *same time* to avoid confusion)—consider additional or alternative analgesic therapy if dose required exceeds 300 micrograms/hour (**important:** it may take 17 hours or longer for the plasma-fentanyl concentration to decrease by 50%, therefore replacement opioid therapy should be initiated at a low dose, increasing gradually).

HYDROMORPHONE HYDROCHLORIDE

Indications: severe pain in cancer

Cautions: see Morphine Salts and notes above; **interactions:** Appendix 1 (opioid analgesics)

Contra-indications: see Morphine Salts and notes above

Side-effects: see under Morphine Salts and notes above

Dose: see under preparations below

Palladone® (Napp) CD

Capsules, hydromorphone hydrochloride 1.3 mg (orange/clear), net price 56-cap pack = £8.28; 2.6 mg (red/clear), 56-cap pack = £16.56. Label: 2, counselling, see below

Dose: 1.3 mg every 4 hours, increased if necessary according to severity of pain; CHILD under 12 years not recommended

COUNSELLING. Swallow whole or open capsule and sprinkle contents on soft food

Palladone® **SR** (Napp) CD

Capsules, m/r, hydromorphone hydrochloride 2 mg (yellow/clear), net price 56-cap pack = £17.59; 4 mg (pale blue/clear), 56-cap pack = £24.10; 8 mg (pink/clear), 56-cap pack = £47.01; 16 mg (brown/clear), 56-cap pack = £89.31; 24 mg (dark blue/clear), 56-cap pack = £133.99. Label: 2, counselling, see below

Dose: 4 mg every 12 hours, increased if necessary according to severity of pain; CHILD under 12 years not recommended

COUNSELLING. Swallow whole or open capsule and sprinkle contents on soft food

MEPTAZINOL

Indications: moderate to severe pain, including postoperative and obstetric pain and renal colic; peri-operative analgesia, see section 15.1.4.3

Cautions: see under Morphine Salts and notes above; effects only partially reversed by naloxone; **interactions:** Appendix 1 (opioid analgesics)

Contra-indications: see under Morphine Salts and notes above

Side-effects: see under Morphine Salts and notes above

Dose: *by mouth*, 200 mg every 3–6 hours as required; CHILD not recommended

By intramuscular injection, 75–100 mg every 2–4 hours if necessary; obstetric analgesia, 100–150 mg according to patient's weight (2 mg/kg); CHILD not recommended

By slow intravenous injection, 50–100 mg every 2–4 hours if necessary; CHILD not recommended

Meptid® (Monmouth) PoM

Tablets, orange, f/c, meptazinol 200 mg, net price 112-tab pack = £24.57. Label: 2

Injection, meptazinol 100 mg (as hydrochloride)/mL, net price 1-mL amp = £1.92

METHADONE HYDROCHLORIDE

Indications: severe pain, see notes above; cough in terminal disease (section 3.9.1); adjunct in treatment of opioid dependence (section 4.10)

Cautions: see under Morphine Salts and notes above; **interactions:** Appendix 1 (opioid analgesics)

Contra-indications: see under Morphine Salts and notes above

Side-effects: see under Morphine Salts and notes above

Dose: *by mouth or by subcutaneous or intramuscular injection*, 5–10 mg every 6–8 hours, adjusted according to response; CHILD not recommended

Methadone (Non-proprietary) CD
Tablets, scored, methadone hydrochloride 5 mg. Net price 50 = £3.11. Label: 2
Available from Martindale (*Physeptone®*)
Injection, methadone hydrochloride, 10 mg/mL, net price 1-mL amp = 86p, 2-mL amp = £1.55, 3.5-mL amp = £1.78, 5-mL amp = £1.92
Available from CP, Martindale (*Physeptone®*)

NALBUPHINE HYDROCHLORIDE

Indications: moderate to severe pain; premedication; peri-operative analgesia; myocardial infarction

Cautions: see under Morphine Salts and notes above; **interactions:** Appendix 1 (opioid analgesics)

Contra-indications: see under Morphine Salts and notes above

Side-effects: see under Morphine Salts and notes above

Dose: moderate to severe pain, *by subcutaneous, intramuscular, or intravenous injection*, 10–20 mg for 70 kg patient, adjusted as required; CHILD up to 300 micrograms/kg repeated once or twice as necessary

Premedication, *by subcutaneous, intramuscular, or intravenous injection*, 100–200 micrograms/kg

Induction, *by intravenous injection*, 0.3–1 mg/kg over 10–15 minutes

Intra-operative analgesia, *by intravenous injection*, 250–500 micrograms/kg at 30-minute intervals

Myocardial infarction, *by slow intravenous injection*, 10–20 mg repeated after 30 minutes if necessary

Nubain® (Du Pont) PoM
Injection, nalbuphine hydrochloride 10 mg/mL. Net price 1-mL amp = 69p, 2-mL amp = £1.08

PAPAVERETUM

IMPORTANT. Do **not** confuse with papaverine (section 7.4.5)

A mixture of 253 parts of morphine hydrochloride, 23 parts of papaverine hydrochloride and 20 parts of codeine hydrochloride

REFORMULATION. *BP* includes the following explanation concerning the reformulation of papaveretum: *papaveretum injection* contains the three alkaloids *morphine*, *papaverine* and *codeine*; in reformulating the injection to remove *noscapine*, the amounts of the other three alkaloids have been maintained; thus the total amount of material per mL has decreased. Before reformulation the *lower strength injection* (which provides *the equivalent of 5 mg of the major component, morphine*) contained 10 mg per mL of the four-component material; it now contains *7.7 mg of papaveretum per mL*. Likewise, before reformulation the *higher strength injection* (which provides *the equivalent of 10 mg of morphine*) contained 20 mg per mL of the four-component material; it now contains *15.4 mg of papaveretum per mL*.

The **CSM** has advised that to avoid confusion the figures of 7.7 mg/mL or 15.4 mg/mL should be used for prescribing purposes.

Indications: postoperative analgesia; premedication

Cautions: see Morphine Salts and notes above

Contra-indications: see Morphine Salts and notes above

Side-effects: see Morphine Salts and notes above

Dose: *by subcutaneous, intramuscular, or intravenous injection*, 7.7–15.4 mg repeated every 4 hours if necessary (ELDERLY initially 7.7 mg); CHILD up to 1 month 115.5 micrograms/kg, 1–12 months 115.5–154 micrograms/kg, 1–12 years 154–231 micrograms/kg

INTRAVENOUS DOSE. In general the intravenous dose should be 25–50% of the corresponding subcutaneous or intramuscular dose

Papaveretum (Non-proprietary) CD
Injection, papaveretum 7.7 mg/mL (providing the equivalent of 5 mg of anhydrous morphine/mL), net price 1-mL amp = 92p; 15.4 mg/mL (providing the equivalent of 10 mg of anhydrous morphine/mL), 1-mL amp = £1.00
Available from Martindale
Note. The name *Omnopon®* was formerly used for papaveretum preparations.

■ With hyoscine
Papaveretum and Hyoscine Injection CD
papaveretum 15.4 mg (providing the equivalent of 10 mg of anhydrous morphine), hyoscine hydrobromide 400 micrograms/mL. Net price 1-mL amp = £1.72
Dose: premedication, by subcutaneous or intramuscular injection, 0.5–1 mL
Available from Martindale

■ With aspirin
Section 4.7.1

▰ denotes preparations that are considered to be less suitable for prescribing (see p. vi)

PENTAZOCINE ▰

Indications: moderate to severe pain, but see notes above

Cautions: see under Morphine Salts and notes above; avoid in porphyria (section 9.8.2); **interactions:** Appendix 1 (opioid analgesics)

Contra-indications: see under Morphine Salts and notes above; patients dependent on opioids and in arterial or pulmonary hypertension and heart failure

Side-effects: see under Morphine Salts and notes above; occasional hallucinations

Dose: *by mouth*, pentazocine hydrochloride 50 mg every 3–4 hours preferably after food (range 25–100 mg); CHILD 6–12 years 25 mg

By subcutaneous, intramuscular, or intravenous injection, moderate pain, pentazocine 30 mg, severe pain 45–60 mg every 3–4 hours when necessary; CHILD over 1 year, *by subcutaneous or intramuscular injection*, up to 1 mg/kg, *by intravenous injection* up to 500 micrograms/kg

By rectum in suppositories, pentazocine 50 mg up to 4 times daily; CHILD not recommended

Pentazocine (Non-proprietary) CD ▰
Capsules, pentazocine hydrochloride 50 mg. Net price 20 = £3.93. Label: 2, 21
Tablets, pentazocine hydrochloride 25 mg. Net price 20 = £1.51. Label: 2, 21
Injection, pentazocine 30 mg (as lactate)/mL. Net price 1-mL amp = £1.67; 2-mL amp = £3.21
Suppositories, pentazocine 50 mg (as lactate). Net price 20 = £19.93. Label: 2
Note. The brand name *Fortral®* NHS (Sanofi-Synthelabo) is used for all the above preparations of pentazocine

PETHIDINE HYDROCHLORIDE

Indications: moderate to severe pain, obstetric analgesia; peri-operative analgesia

Cautions: see under Morphine Salts and notes above; not suitable for severe continuing pain; **interactions:** Appendix 1 (opioid analgesics)

Contra-indications: see under Morphine Salts and notes above; severe renal impairment

Side-effects: see under Morphine Salts and notes above; convulsions reported in **overdosage**

Dose: acute pain, *by mouth*, 50–150 mg every 4 hours; CHILD 0.5–2 mg/kg

By subcutaneous or intramuscular injection, 25–100 mg, repeated after 4 hours; CHILD, *by intramuscular injection*, 0.5–2 mg/kg

By slow intravenous injection, 25–50 mg, repeated after 4 hours

Obstetric analgesia, *by subcutaneous or intramuscular injection*, 50–100 mg, repeated 1–3 hours later if necessary; max. 400 mg in 24 hours

Premedication, *by intramuscular injection*, 25–100 mg 1 hour before operation; CHILD 0.5–2 mg/kg

Postoperative pain, *by subcutaneous or intramuscular injection*, 25–100 mg, every 2–3 hours if necessary; CHILD, *by intramuscular injection*, 0.5–2 mg/kg

Note. In the postoperative period, the patient should be closely monitored for pain relief as well as for side-effects especially respiratory depression

Pethidine (Non-proprietary) CD

Tablets, pethidine hydrochloride 50 mg, net price 20 = £1.97. Label: 2

Available from Martindale

Injection, pethidine hydrochloride 50 mg/mL, net price 1-mL amp = 53p, 2-mL amp = 47p; 10 mg/mL, 5-mL amp = £1.40, 10-mL amp = £1.47

Various strengths available from Martindale

Pamergan P100® (Martindale) CD [image]

Injection, pethidine hydrochloride 50 mg, promethazine hydrochloride 25 mg/mL. Net price 2-mL amp = 70p

Dose: by intramuscular injection, premedication, 2 mL 60–90 minutes before operation; CHILD 8–12 years 0.75 mL, 13–16 years 1 mL

Obstetric analgesia, 1–2 mL every 4 hours if necessary

Severe pain, 1–2 mL every 4–6 hours if necessary

Note. Although usually given intramuscularly, may be given intravenously after dilution to at least 10 mL with water for injections

PHENAZOCINE HYDROBROMIDE

Indications: severe pain

Cautions: see under Morphine Salts and notes above; **interactions:** Appendix 1 (opioid analgesics)

Contra-indications: see under Morphine Salts and notes above

Side-effects: see under Morphine Salts and notes above

Dose: *by mouth or sublingually*, 5 mg every 4–6 hours when necessary; single doses may be increased to 20 mg; CHILD not recommended

Narphen® (Napp) CD

Tablets, phenazocine hydrobromide 5 mg. Net price 100-tab pack = £27.23. Label: 2

TRAMADOL HYDROCHLORIDE

Indications: moderate to severe pain

Cautions: see under Morphine Salts and notes above; history of epilepsy (convulsions reported, usually after rapid intravenous injection); manufacturer advises avoid in pregnancy and breast-feeding; not suitable as substitute in opioid-dependent patients; **interactions:** Appendix 1 (opioid analgesics)

GENERAL ANAESTHESIA. Not recommended for analgesia during potentially very light planes of general anaesthesia (possibly increased operative recall reported)

Contra-indications: see under Morphine Salts and notes above

Side-effects: see under Morphine Salts and notes above; hypotension and occasionally hypertension; anaphylaxis, hallucinations, and confusion reported

Dose: *by mouth*, 50–100 mg not more often than every 4 hours; total of more than 400 mg daily by mouth not usually required; CHILD not recommended

By intramuscular injection or by intravenous injection (over 2–3 minutes) *or by intravenous infusion*, 50–100 mg every 4–6 hours

Postoperative pain, 100 mg initially then 50 mg every 10–20 minutes if necessary during first hour to total max. 250 mg (including initial dose) in first hour, *then* 50–100 mg every 4–6 hours; max. 600 mg daily; CHILD not recommended

Tramadol Hydrochloride (Non-proprietary) PoM

Capsules, tramadol hydrochloride 50 mg. Net price 100-cap pack = £15.59. Label: 2

Available from Cox, Galen (*Tramake®*), Generics, Genus, Norton, Sovereign, Tillomed

Tramake Insts® (Galen) PoM

Sachets, effervescent powder, sugar-free, lemon-flavoured, tramadol hydrochloride 50 mg (contains Na^+ 9.7 mmol/sachet), net price 60-sachet pack = £8.95; 100 mg (contains Na^+ 14.6 mmol/sachet), 60-sachet pack = £17.90. Label: 2, 13

Excipients: include aspartame (section 9.4.1)

Zamadol® (ASTA Medica) PoM

Capsules, tramadol hydrochloride 50 mg, net price 100-cap pack = £14.52. Label: 2

Injection, tramadol hydrochloride 50 mg/mL, net price 2-mL amp = £1.18

Zydol® (Searle) PoM

Capsules, green/yellow, tramadol hydrochloride 50 mg. Net price 100-cap pack = £16.91. Label: 2

Soluble tablets, tramadol hydrochloride 50 mg, net price 20-tab pack = £3.05, 100-tab pack = £15.23. Label: 2, 13

Injection, tramadol hydrochloride 50 mg/mL. Net price 2-mL amp = £1.24

■ Modified release

Zamadol® SR (ASTA Medica) PoM

Capsules, m/r, tramadol hydrochloride 50 mg (green), net price 60-cap pack = £8.21; 100 mg, net price 60-cap pack = £16.43; 150 mg (dark green), 60-cap pack = £24.64; 200 mg (yellow), 60-cap pack = £32.85. Label: 2

Dose: 50–100 mg twice daily increased if necessary to 150–200 mg twice daily; total of more than 400 mg daily not usually required; CHILD under 12 years not recommended

COUNSELLING. Swallow whole or open capsule and swallow contents immediately without chewing

Zydol SR® (Searle) [PoM]

Tablets, m/r, f/c, tramadol hydrochloride 100 mg, net price 60-tab pack = £18.26; 150 mg (beige), 60-tab pack = £27.39; 200 mg (orange), 60-tab pack = £36.52. Label: 2, 25

Dose: 100 mg twice daily increased if necessary to 150–200 mg twice daily; total of more than 400 mg daily not usually required; CHILD not recommended

Zydol XL® (Searle) [PoM]

Tablets, m/r, f/c, tramadol hydrochloride 150 mg, net price 30-tab pack = £15.22; 200 mg, 30-tab pack = £20.29; 300 mg, 30-tab pack = £30.44; 400 mg, 30-tab pack = £40.59. Label: 2, 25

Dose: 150 mg daily increased if necessary; more than 400 mg once daily not usually required; CHILD not recommended

4.7.3 Neuropathic pain

Neuropathic pain occurs as a result of damage to neural tissue.

Patients with neuropathic pain (including central pain, phantom limb pain, causalgia, and reflex sympathetic dystrophy) are generally managed with a tricyclic antidepressant; certain antiepileptic or anti-arrhythmic drugs are used as adjuncts to antidepressants. Neuropathic pain may respond only partially to opioid analgesics, which may be considered when other measures fail.

Corticosteroids may also be used for compression neuropathies.

Nerve blocks may be considered for control of localised pain. Transcutaneous electrical nerve stimulation (TENS) may also provide useful relief of localised pain; central electrical stimulation of the spinal cord may help in more widespread pain. Preliminary trials have shown **gabapentin** [unlicensed] to be of benefit in some forms of neuropathic pain.

Ketamine (section 15.1.1), a N-methyl-D-aspartic acid (NMDA) antagonist, may also be useful in some forms of neuropathic pain [unlicensed indication; specialist use only].

The management of trigeminal neuralgia, postherpetic neuralgia, atypical facial pain, and temporomandibular joint dysfunction are outlined below; for the management of neuropathic pain in **palliative care**, see p. 13; for the management of **diabetic neuropathy**, see section 6.1.5.

Trigeminal neuralgia

Carbamazepine (section 4.8.1), taken during the acute stages of trigeminal neuralgia, reduces the frequency and severity of attacks. It has no effect on other forms of headache. Plasma-carbamazepine concentration should be monitored when high doses are given. Occasionally extreme dizziness occurs; treatment should be started with a small dose and increased slowly.

Some cases of trigeminal neuralgia respond to **phenytoin** (section 4.8.1) given alone or with carbamazepine. A combination of phenytoin and carbamazepine is required only in refractory cases or in those unable to tolerate high doses of carbamazepine.

Postherpetic neuralgia

Postherpetic neuralgia may follow acute herpes zoster infection (shingles), particularly in the elderly. Attempts at preventing the development of postherpetic neuralgia have not been particularly effective. Treatment is therefore based on managing the neuralgia once it develops. **Amitriptyline** may be used early in the acute phase, initially at 10–25 mg daily at night and the dose increased gradually to about 75 mg daily [unlicensed indication]. Where amitriptyline fails to manage the pain adequately, the addition of the antiepileptics **sodium valproate** or **carbamazepine** may improve control [unlicensed indications].

A topical analgesic preparation containing capsaicin 0.075% (section 10.3.2) is licensed for use in postherpetic neuralgia. It produces an intense burning sensation during the initial treatment period.

Atypical facial pain

Chronic oral and facial pain (e.g. atypical facial pain or arthritic pain) may call for prolonged use of conventional analgesics or of other appropriate drugs. Tricyclic antidepressants may be useful for facial pain [unlicensed indication] particularly if associated with depression.

Temporomandibular joint dysfunction

Temporomandibular joint dysfunction can be related to anxiety in some patients who may clench or grind their teeth (bruxism) during the day or night; the patient should be referred to a dental surgeon. The muscle spasm (which may be the main source of pain) can be treated empirically with an overlay appliance which provides a free sliding occlusion and may also interfere with grinding. In addition, diazepam may be helpful but should be prescribed only on a short-term basis during the acute phase. Analgesics such as aspirin or ibuprofen may also be tried.

4.7.4 Antimigraine drugs

4.7.4.1	Treatment of the acute migraine attack
4.7.4.2	Prophylaxis of migraine

4.7.4.1 Treatment of the acute migraine attack

Acute attacks of migraine may be relieved by analgesics or a specific treatment such as the use of a $5HT_1$ agonist or ergotamine. An anti-emetic may also be given if nausea and vomiting are features.

Analgesics

Most migraine headaches respond to analgesics such as **aspirin** or **paracetamol** (section 4.7.1) but since peristalsis is often reduced during migraine attacks the medication may not be sufficiently well absorbed to be effective; dispersible or effervescent preparations should therefore preferably be used.

The NSAID **tolfenamic acid** is licensed specifically for the treatment of acute attack of migraine; **diclofenac potassium**, **flurbiprofen**, **ibuprofen**, and **naproxen sodium** (section 10.1.1) are also licensed for use in migraine.

5HT₁ agonists

Sumatriptan is a 5HT₁ agonist; it is of considerable value in the treatment of an acute attack. It may be used during the established headache phase of an attack and should be regarded as preferred treatment in those who fail to respond to conventional analgesics. Sumatriptan is also of value in cluster headache.

Naratriptan, rizatriptan and **zolmitriptan** have been introduced recently; they are claimed to have better absorption than sumatriptan.

CAUTIONS. 5HT₁ agonists should be used with caution in conditions which predispose to coronary artery disease (pre-existing cardiac disease, see Contra-indications below); hepatic impairment (see Appendix 2); pregnancy and breast-feeding. 5HT₁ agonists are recommended as monotherapy and should not be taken concurrently with other acute migraine therapies.

CONTRA-INDICATIONS. 5HT₁ agonists should not be used for prophylaxis and are contra-indicated in ischaemic heart disease; previous myocardial infarction; coronary vasospasm (including Prinzmetal's angina); uncontrolled hypertension.

SIDE-EFFECTS. Side-effects of the 5HT₁ agonists include sensations of tingling, heat, heaviness, pressure, or tightness of any part of the body (including throat and chest—discontinue if intense, may be due to coronary vasoconstriction or to anaphylaxis; see also CSM advice under Sumatriptan); flushing, dizziness, feeling of weakness; fatigue; nausea and vomiting also reported.

Ergot alkaloids

The value of **ergotamine** for migraine is limited by difficulties in absorption and by its side-effects, particularly nausea, vomiting, abdominal pain, and *muscular cramps*; it is best avoided. The recommended doses of ergotamine preparations should **not** be exceeded and treatment should **not** be repeated at intervals of less than 4 days.

To avoid habituation the frequency of administration of ergotamine should be limited to **no more than** twice a month. It should **never** be prescribed prophylactically but in the management of cluster headache a low dose (e.g. ergotamine 1 mg at night for 6 nights in 7) is occasionally given daily for 1 to 2 weeks [unlicensed indication].

A nasal spray containing **dihydroergotamine mesilate** has been introduced recently.

Anti-emetics

Anti-emetics (section 4.6), such as **metoclopramide** or **domperidone**, or phenothiazine and antihistamine anti-emetics, relieve the nausea associated with migraine attacks. Anti-emetics may be given by intramuscular injection or rectally if vomiting is a problem. Metoclopramide and domperidone have the added advantage of promoting gastric emptying and normal peristalsis; a single dose should be given at the onset of symptoms. Oral analgesic preparations containing metoclopramide or domperidone are a convenient alternative (**important:** for warnings relating to extrapyramidal effects of metoclopramide particularly in children and young adults, see p. 201).

Other drugs for migraine

Isometheptene mucate (in combination with paracetamol) is licensed for the treatment of acute attacks of migraine; other effective treatments are however available now.

ANALGESICS

■ Aspirin
Section 4.7.1

■ Paracetamol
Section 4.7.1

■ With anti-emetics

Domperamol® (Servier) P͟o͟M͟
Tablets, f/c, paracetamol 500 mg, domperidone (as maleate) 10 mg, net price 16-tab pack = £7.00. Label: 17, 30
Dose: 2 tablets at onset of attack then up to every 4 hours; max. 8 tablets daily; CHILD not recommended

Migraleve® (Pfizer Consumer) ◣
Tablets, all f/c, *pink tablets*, buclizine hydrochloride 6.25 mg, paracetamol 500 mg, codeine phosphate 8 mg; *yellow tablets*, paracetamol 500 mg, codeine phosphate 8 mg. Net price 48-tab *Migraleve* P͟o͟M͟ (32 pink + 16 yellow) = £5.10; 48 pink (*Migraleve Pink*) = £5.56; 48 yellow (*Migraleve Yellow*) = £4.70. Label: 2 (*Migraleve Pink*), 17, 30
Dose: 2 pink tablets at onset of attack, or if it is imminent, then 2 yellow tablets every 4 hours if necessary; max. in 24 hours 2 pink and 6 yellow; CHILD under 10 years, only under close medical supervision; 10–14 years, half adult dose

Paramax® (Sanofi-Synthelabo) P͟o͟M͟
Tablets, scored, paracetamol 500 mg, metoclopramide hydrochloride 5 mg. Net price 42-tab pack = £7.00. Label: 17, 30
Sachets, effervescent powder, sugar-free, the contents of 1 sachet = 1 tablet; to be dissolved in ¼ tumblerful of liquid before administration. Net price 42-sachet pack = £9.10. Label: 13, 17, 30
Dose: (tablets or sachets): 2 at onset of attack then every 4 hours when necessary to max. of 6 in 24 hours; YOUNG ADULT 12–19 years, 1 at onset of attack then 1 every 4 hours when necessary to max. of 3 in 24 hours (max. dose of metoclopramide 500 micrograms/kg daily)
IMPORTANT. Metoclopramide can cause **severe extrapyramidal effects**, particularly in children and young adults (for further details, see p. 201)

◣ denotes preparations that are considered to be less suitable for prescribing (see p. vi)

DIHYDROERGOTAMINE MESILATE

Indications: treatment of acute migraine attacks

Cautions: see Ergotamine Tartrate; hepatic impairment (Appendix 2); **interactions:** Appendix 1 (Ergotamine)

Contra-indications: see Ergotamine Tartrate; pregnancy, breast-feeding (Appendix 5), concomitant use of parenteral dihydroergotamine, ergotamine, or sumatriptan

Side-effects: see Ergotamine Tartrate

Dose: *intranasally*, 1 mg (2 sprays, 1 in each nostril) as soon as possible after onset; further 1 mg (1 spray in each nostril) after 15 minutes if migraine persists; max. 2 mg (4 sprays) per attack Max. 2 mg (4 sprays) in 24 hours and 8 mg (16 sprays) in one week

CHILD under 16 years, not recommended

Migranal® (Novartis) ▼ PoM

Nasal spray, dihydroergotamine mesilate 500 micrograms/metered spray, net price 4-spray unit = £3.80. Label: 18, counselling, dosage

Note. Discard 8 hours after assembly

ERGOTAMINE TARTRATE

Indications: treatment of acute migraine attacks and migraine variants unresponsive to analgesics

Cautions: risk of peripheral vasospasm (see advice below); elderly; should not be used for migraine prophylaxis; **interactions:** Appendix 1 (ergotamine) and under Sumatriptan (Cautions), below

PERIPHERAL VASOSPASM. Warn patient to stop treatment immediately if numbness or tingling of extremities develops and to contact doctor.

Contra-indications: peripheral vascular disease, coronary heart disease, obliterative vascular disease and Raynaud's syndrome, hepatic and renal impairment, sepsis, severe or inadequately controlled hypertension, hyperthyroidism, pregnancy and breast-feeding, porphyria (section 9.8.2)

Side-effects: nausea, vomiting, vertigo, abdominal pain, diarrhoea, muscle cramps, and occasionally increased headache; precordial pain, myocardial ischaemia, rarely myocardial infarction; repeated high dosage may cause ergotism with gangrene and confusion; pleural and peritoneal fibrosis may occur with excessive use

Dose: see under preparations below

Cafergot® (Alliance) PoM

Tablets, ergotamine tartrate 1 mg, caffeine 100 mg. Net price 30-tab pack = £5.90. Label: 18, counselling, dosage

Dose: 1–2 tablets at onset; max. 4 tablets in 24 hours; not to be repeated at intervals of less than 4 days; max. 8 tablets in one week (but see also notes above); CHILD not recommended

Suppositories, ergotamine tartrate 2 mg, caffeine 100 mg. Net price 30 = £13.50. Label: 18, counselling, dosage

Dose: 1 suppository at onset; max. 2 in 24 hours; not to be repeated at intervals of less than 4 days; max. 4 suppositories in one week (but see also notes above); CHILD not recommended

Lingraine® (Sanofi-Synthelabo) PoM

Tablets (for sublingual use), green, ergotamine tartrate 2 mg. Net price 12 = £7.43. Label: 18, 26, counselling, dosage

Dose: 1 tablet at onset repeated after 30–60 minutes if necessary; max. 3 tablets in 24 hours and 6 tablets in one week (but see also notes above); CHILD not recommended

Migril® (CP) PoM

Tablets, scored, ergotamine tartrate 2 mg, cyclizine hydrochloride 50 mg, caffeine hydrate 100 mg. Net price 20 = £11.67. Label: 2, 18, counselling, dosage

Dose: 1 tablet at onset, followed after 30 minutes by ½–1 tablet, repeated every 30 minutes if necessary; max. 4 tablets per attack and 6 tablets in one week (but see also notes above); CHILD not recommended

> denotes preparations that are considered to be less suitable for prescribing (see p. vi)

ISOMETHEPTENE MUCATE

Indications: treatment of acute migraine attacks

Cautions: cardiovascular disease, hepatic and renal impairment, diabetes mellitus, hyperthyroidism; **interactions:** Appendix 1 (sympathomimetics)

Contra-indications: glaucoma, severe cardiac, hepatic and renal impairment, severe hypertension, pregnancy and breast-feeding; porphyria (section 9.8.2)

Side-effects: dizziness, circulatory disturbances, rashes, blood disorders also reported

¹**Midrid**® (Shire) PoM

Capsules, red, isometheptene mucate 65 mg, paracetamol 325 mg. Net price 100-cap pack = £13.12. Label: 30, counselling, dosage

Dose: migraine, 2 capsules at onset of attack, followed by 1 capsule every hour if necessary; max. 5 capsules in 12 hours; CHILD not recommended

1. A pack containing 15 capsules may be sold to the public

NARATRIPTAN

Indications: treatment of acute migraine attacks

Cautions: see above; renal impairment; **interactions:** Appendix 1 (5HT₁ agonists)

DRIVING. Drowsiness may affect performance of skilled tasks (e.g. driving)

Contra-indications: see above; peripheral vascular disease

Side-effects: see above, bradycardia or tachycardia; visual disturbances

Dose: 2.5 mg as soon as possible after onset; if migraine recurs after initial response, dose may be repeated after 4 hours (patient not responding should not take second dose for same attack); max. 5 mg in 24 hours

Naramig® (GlaxoWellcome) ▼ PoM

Tablets, f/c, green, naratriptan (as hydrochloride) 2.5 mg, net price 6-tab pack = £24.00, 12-tab pack = £48.00. Label: 3

RIZATRIPTAN

Indications: treatment of acute migraine attacks

Cautions: see above; renal impairment (Appendix 3); not to be taken until 24 hours after stopping an ergotamine-type preparation (ergotamine-type preparations not to be taken until 6 hours after rizatriptan); other **interactions:** Appendix 1 (5HT$_1$ agonists)

DRIVING. Drowsiness may affect performance of skilled tasks (e.g. driving)

Contra-indications: see above; previous cerebrovascular accident or transient ischaemic attack; peripheral vascular disease

Side-effects: see above; drowsiness, palpitation, tachycardia, dry mouth, diarrhoea, dyspepsia, thirst, pharyngeal discomfort, dyspnoea, headache, paraesthesia, decreased mental alertness, insomnia, tremor, ataxia, nervousness, vertigo, confusion, myalgia and muscle weakness, sweating, urticaria, pruritus, blurred vision; rarely syncope, hypertension

Dose: 10 mg as soon as possible after onset repeated after 2 hours if migraine recurs (patient not responding should not take second dose for same attack); max. 20 mg in 24 hours

CHILD under 18 years, not recommended

Note. Halve dose in patients taking propranolol and not to be taken within 2 hours of administration of propranolol

Maxalt® (MSD) ▼ PoM
Tablets, pink, rizatriptan (as benzoate) 5 mg, net price 6-tab pack = £26.74; 10 mg, 3-tab pack = £13.37, 6-tab pack = £26.74. Label: 3
Wafers (Maxalt® Melt), rizatriptan (as benzoate) 10 mg, net price 3-wafer pack = £13.37, 6-wafer pack = £26.74. Label: 3, counselling administration
COUNSELLING. *Maxalt® Melt* wafers should be placed on the tongue and allowed to dissolve
Excipients: include aspartame equivalent to phenylalanine 2.1 mg (section 9.4.1)

SUMATRIPTAN

Indications: treatment of acute migraine attacks; cluster headache (subcutaneous injection only)

Cautions: see above; renal impairment; should not be taken until 24 hours after stopping an ergotamine-containing preparation (ergotamine-containing preparations should not be taken until 6 hours after sumatriptan); other **interactions:** Appendix 1 (5HT$_1$ agonists)

DRIVING. Drowsiness may affect performance of skilled tasks (e.g. driving)

Contra-indications: see above

Side-effects: see above; drowsiness, transient increase in blood pressure, hypotension, bradycardia or tachycardia, altered liver function tests, seizures reported

CSM advice. Following reports of chest pain and tightness (coronary vasoconstriction) CSM has emphasised that sumatriptan should **not** be used in ischaemic heart disease or Prinzmetal's angina, and that use with ergotamine should be **avoided** (see also Cautions).

Dose: *by mouth,* 50 mg (some patients may require 100 mg) as soon as possible after onset (patient not responding should not take second dose for same attack); dose may be repeated if migraine recurs; max. 300 mg in 24 hours

By subcutaneous injection using auto-injector, 6 mg as soon as possible after onset (patients not responding should not take second dose for same attack); dose may be repeated once after not less than 1 hour if migraine recurs; max. 12 mg in 24 hours

IMPORTANT. **Not** for intravenous injection which may cause coronary vasospasm and angina

Intranasally, 20 mg (1 spray) into one nostril as soon as possible after onset (patient not responding should not take a second dose for same attack); dose may be repeated once after not less than two hours if migraine recurs; max. 40 mg in 24 hours

Imigran® (GlaxoWellcome) PoM
Tablets, f/c, sumatriptan (as succinate) 50 mg, net price 6-tab pack = £29.70, 12-tab pack = £56.43; 100 mg, 3-tab pack = £24.00, 6-tab pack = £48.00, 12-tab pack = £96.00. Label: 3, 10 patient information leaflet
Injection, sumatriptan (as succinate) 12 mg/mL (= 6 mg/0.5-mL syringe), net price, treatment pack (2 × 0.5-mL pre-filled syringes and auto-injector) = £41.14; refill pack (2 × 0.5-mL pre-filled syringes) = £39.14. Label: 3, 10 patient information leaflet
Nasal spray, sumatriptan 20 mg/0.1-mL unit-dose spray device, net price 2 unit-dose vials with applicator = £12.00, 6 unit-dose vials = £36.00. Label: 3, 10 patient information leaflet

TOLFENAMIC ACID

Indications: treatment of acute migraine attacks

Cautions: see section 10.1.1

Contra-indications: see section 10.1.1

Side-effects: see section 10.1.1; also dysuria (most commonly in men), tremor, euphoria, and fatigue reported

Dose: 200 mg at onset repeated once after 1–2 hours if necessary

Clotam® (Cortecs) PoM
Rapid Tablets, tolfenamic acid 200 mg. Net price 10-tab pack = £15.00

ZOLMITRIPTAN

Indications: treatment of acute migraine attacks

Cautions: see above; should not be taken within 12 hours of any other 5HT$_1$ agonist; **interactions:** Appendix 1 (5HT$_1$ agonists)

Contra-indications: see above; Wolff-Parkinson-White syndrome or arrhythmias associated with accessory cardiac conduction pathways

Side-effects: see above; drowsiness, transient increase in blood pressure; dry mouth, myalgia and muscle weakness, dysaesthesia reported

Dose: 2.5 mg as soon as possible after onset repeated after 2 hours if migraine persists or recurs (increase to 5 mg for subsequent attacks in patients not achieving satisfactory relief with 2.5-mg dose); max. 15 mg in 24 hours

Zomig® (Zeneca) ▼ PoM
Tablets, f/c, yellow, zolmitriptan 2.5 mg, net price 6-tab pack = £24.00, 12-tab pack = £48.00

4.7.4.2   Prophylaxis of migraine

Where migraine attacks are frequent, search should be made for provocative factors such as stress or diet (chocolate, cheese, alcohol, etc.). Benzodiazepines should be avoided because of the risk of dependence. In patients with more than one attack a month, one of four prophylactic agents may be tried: pizotifen, beta-blockers, tricyclic antidepressants (even when the patient is not obviously depressed), or sodium valproate. Long-term treatment with any of these prophylactic drugs is undesirable; the need for continuing therapy should be reviewed at intervals of about 6 months. Oral contraceptives may precipitate or worsen migraine; patients reporting a sharp increase in frequency of migraine or focal features should be recommended alternative contraceptive measures.

Pizotifen is an antihistamine and serotonin antagonist structurally related to the tricyclic antidepressants. It affords good prophylaxis but may cause weight gain. To avoid undue drowsiness treatment may be started at 500 micrograms at night and gradually increased to 3 mg; it is rarely necessary to exceed this dose.

The **beta-blockers** propranolol, metoprolol, nadolol, and timolol (section 2.4) are all effective. Propranolol is the most commonly used in an initial dose of 40 mg 2 to 3 times daily by mouth. Beta-blockers may also be given as a single daily dose of a long-acting preparation. The value of beta-blockers is limited by their contra-indications (section 2.4) and also by their interactions (see Appendix 1, beta-blockers).

Tricyclic antidepressants (section 4.3.1) [unlicensed] may usefully be prescribed in a dose, for example, of amitriptyline 10 mg at night, increasing to a maintenance dose of 50 to 75 mg at night.

Sodium valproate (section 4.8.1) [unlicensed] may be effective in a dose of 300 mg twice daily; it has been associated with severe hepatic and pancreatic toxicity, although these effects are rare.

There is some evidence that the **calcium-channel blockers** (section 2.6.2), e.g. verapamil and nifedipine may be useful in migraine prophylaxis.

Cyproheptadine (section 3.4.1), an antihistamine with serotonin-antagonist and calcium channel-blocking properties, may also be tried in refractory cases.

Clonidine (*Dixarit*®) is not recommended and may aggravate depression or produce insomnia. **Methysergide**, a semi-synthetic ergot alkaloid, has dangerous side-effects (retroperitoneal fibrosis and fibrosis of the heart valves and pleura); **important:** it should only be administered under hospital supervision.

PIZOTIFEN

Indications: prevention of vascular headache including classical migraine, common migraine, and cluster headache

Cautions: urinary retention; closed-angle glaucoma, renal impairment; pregnancy and breast-feeding; **interactions:** Appendix 1 (pizotifen)

DRIVING. Drowsiness may affect performance of skilled tasks (e.g. driving); effects of alcohol enhanced

Side-effects: antimuscarinic effects, drowsiness, increased appetite and weight gain; occasionally nausea, dizziness; CNS stimulation may occur in children

Dose: 1.5 mg at night *or* 500 micrograms 3 times daily (but see also notes above), adjusted according to response within the usual range 0.5–3 mg daily; max. single dose 3 mg, max. daily dose 4.5 mg; CHILD up to 1.5 mg daily in divided doses; max. single dose at night 1 mg

Pizotifen (Non-proprietary) PoM
Tablets, pizotifen (as hydrogen malate), 500 micrograms, net price 28-tab pack = £2.18; 1.5 mg, 28-tab pack = £7.78. Label: 2
Available from Cox, Norton

Sanomigran® (Novartis) PoM
Tablets, both ivory-yellow, s/c, pizotifen (as hydrogen malate), 500 micrograms, net price 60-tab pack = £2.57; 1.5 mg, 28-tab pack = £4.28. Label: 2
Elixir, pizotifen (as hydrogen malate) 250 micrograms/5 mL, net price 300 mL = £4.12. Label: 2

CLONIDINE HYDROCHLORIDE ▱

Indications: prevention of recurrent migraine (but see notes above), vascular headache, menopausal flushing; hypertension (section 2.5.2)

Cautions: depressive illness, concurrent antihypertensive therapy; porphyria (section 9.8.2); **interactions:** Appendix 1 (clonidine)

Side-effects: dry mouth, sedation, dizziness, nausea, nocturnal restlessness; occasionally rashes

Dose: 50 micrograms twice daily, increased after 2 weeks to 75 micrograms twice daily if necessary; CHILD not recommended

Dixarit® (Boehringer Ingelheim) PoM ▱
Tablets, blue, s/c, clonidine hydrochloride 25 micrograms. Net price 112-tab pack = £7.11
Catapres® PoM ▱ (hypertension), section 2.5.2

METHYSERGIDE ▱

Indications: prevention of severe recurrent migraine, cluster headache and other vascular headaches in patients who are refractory to other treatment and whose lives are seriously disrupted (**important:** hospital supervision only, see notes above); diarrhoea associated with carcinoid syndrome

Cautions: history of peptic ulceration; avoid abrupt withdrawal of treatment; after 6 months withdraw (gradually over 2 to 3 weeks) for reassessment for at least 1 month (see also notes above); **interactions:** Appendix 1 (ergotamine)

Contra-indications: renal, hepatic, pulmonary, and cardiovascular disease, severe hypertension, collagen disease, cellulitis, urinary-tract disorders, cachectic or septic conditions, pregnancy, breast-feeding

Side-effects: nausea, vomiting, heartburn, abdominal discomfort, drowsiness, and dizziness occur frequently in initial treatment; mental and behavioural disturbances, insomnia, oedema, weight gain, rashes, loss of scalp hair, cramps, arterial spasm (including coronary artery spasm with angina and possible myocardial infarction), paraesthesias of extremities, postural hypotension, and tachycardia also occur; retroperitoneal and other abnormal fibrotic reactions may occur on prolonged administration, requiring immediate withdrawal of treatment

Dose: initially 1 mg at bedtime, increased gradually over about 2 weeks to 1–2 mg 3 times daily with food (see notes above); CHILD not recommended

Diarrhoea associated with carcinoid syndrome, usual range, 12–20 mg daily (hospital supervision); CHILD not recommended

Deseril® (Alliance) [PoM] ▰▱

Tablets, s/c, methysergide (as maleate) 1 mg, net price 60-tab pack = £13.80. Label: 2, 21

> ▰▱ denotes preparations that are considered to be less suitable for prescribing (see p. vi)

4.8   Antiepileptics

4.8.1   Control of epilepsy
4.8.2   Drugs used in status epilepticus
4.8.3   Febrile convulsions

4.8.1   Control of epilepsy

The object of treatment is to prevent the occurrence of seizures by maintaining an effective plasma concentration of the drug. Careful adjustment of doses is necessary, starting with low doses and increasing gradually until seizures are controlled or there are overdose effects.

The frequency of administration is often determined by the plasma half-life, and should be kept as low as possible to encourage better patient compliance. Most antiepileptics, when used in average dosage, may be given twice daily. Phenobarbital and sometimes phenytoin, which have long half-lives, may often be given as a daily dose at bedtime. However, with large doses, some antiepileptics may need to be administered 3 times daily to avoid adverse effects associated with high peak plasma concentrations. Young children metabolise antiepileptics more rapidly than adults and therefore require more frequent doses and a higher amount per kilogram body-weight.

COMBINATION THERAPY. Therapy with two or more antiepileptic drugs concurrently should preferably only be used when monotherapy with several alternative drugs has proved ineffective. Combination therapy enhances toxicity and drug interactions may occur between antiepileptics (see below).

INTERACTIONS. Interactions between antiepileptics are complex and may enhance toxicity without a corresponding increase in antiepileptic effect. Interactions are usually caused by *hepatic enzyme induction* or *hepatic enzyme inhibition*; *displacement from protein binding sites* is not usually a problem. These interactions are highly variable and unpredictable. Plasma monitoring is therefore often advisable with combination therapy.

Interactions that occur between antiepileptics themselves are as follows:

Carbamazepine
often lowers plasma concentration of *clobazam, clonazepam, lamotrigine, phenytoin* (but may also raise phenytoin concentration), *tiagabine, topiramate, and valproate*
sometimes lowers plasma concentration of *ethosuximide, and primidone* (but tendency for corresponding increase in phenobarbital level)

Ethosuximide
sometimes raises plasma concentration of *phenytoin*

Lamotrigine
sometimes raises plasma concentration of *an active metabolite of carbamazepine*

Phenobarbital *or* Primidone
often lowers plasma concentration of *carbamazepine, clonazepam, lamotrigine, phenytoin* (but may also raise phenytoin concentration), *tiagabine, and valproate*
sometimes lowers plasma concentration of *ethosuximide*

Phenytoin
often lowers plasma concentration of *clonazepam, carbamazepine, lamotrigine, tiagabine, topiramate, and valproate*
often raises plasma concentration of *phenobarbital*
sometimes lowers plasma concentration of *ethosuximide, and primidone* (by increasing conversion to phenobarbital)

Topiramate
sometimes raises plasma concentration of *phenytoin*

Valproate
often raises plasma concentration of *an active metabolite of carbamazepine,* and of *lamotrigine, primidone, phenobarbital, and phenytoin* (but may also lower)
sometimes raises plasma concentration of *ethosuximide, and primidone* (and tendency for significant increase in phenobarbital level)

Vigabatrin
often lowers plasma concentration of *phenytoin*
sometimes lowers plasma concentration of *phenobarbital, and primidone*

For other important interactions see **Appendix 1**, and for FPA guidelines on enzyme-inducing antiepileptics and **oral contraceptives**, see section 7.3.1.

WITHDRAWAL. Abrupt withdrawal of antiepileptics, particularly the barbiturates and benzodiazepines, should be avoided, as this may precipitate severe rebound seizures. Reduction in dosage should be carried out in stages and, in the case of the barbiturates, the withdrawal process may take months. The changeover from one antiepileptic drug regimen to another should be made cautiously, withdrawing the first drug only when the new regimen has been largely established.

The decision to withdraw all antiepileptics from a seizure-free patient, and its timing, is often difficult and may depend on individual patient factors. Even in patients who have been seizure-free for several years, there is a significant risk of seizure recurrence on drug withdrawal.

In patients receiving several antiepileptic drugs, only one drug should be withdrawn at a time.

DRIVING. Patients suffering from epilepsy may drive a motor vehicle (but not a heavy goods or public service vehicle) provided that they have had a seizure-free period of one year or, if subject to attacks only while asleep, have established a three-year period of asleep attacks without awake attacks. Patients affected by drowsiness should not drive or operate machinery.

Guidance issued by the Drivers Medical Unit of the Driver and Vehicle Licensing Agency (DVLA) recommends that patients should be advised not to drive during withdrawal of antiepileptic drugs, or for six months afterwards.

PREGNANCY AND BREAST-FEEDING. During pregnancy, total plasma concentrations of anti-epileptics (particularly of phenytoin) may fall, particularly in the later stages but free plasma concentrations may remain the same (or even rise). There is an increased risk of teratogenicity associated with the use of antiepileptic drugs (reduced if treatment is limited to a single drug). In view of the increased risk of neural tube and other defects associated, in particular, with **carbamazepine**, **phenytoin** and **valproate** women taking antiepileptic drugs who *may become pregnant* should be **informed of the possible consequences**. Those who *wish to become pregnant* should be referred to an appropriate specialist for advice. Women who become pregnant should be **counselled** and offered **antenatal screening** (alpha-fetoprotein measurement and a second trimester ultrasound scan).

To counteract the risk of neural tube defects adequate folate supplements are advised for women before and during pregnancy; to prevent recurrence of neural tube defects, women should receive folic acid 5 mg daily (see section 9.1.2)—this dose may also be appropriate for women receiving established antiepileptic drugs.

In view of the risk of neonatal bleeding associated with carbamazepine, phenobarbital and phenytoin, prophylactic vitamin K_1 is recommended for the mother before delivery (as well as for the neonate).

Breast-feeding is acceptable with all antiepileptic drugs, taken in normal doses, with the possible exception of the barbiturates and ethosuximide, and also some of the more recently introduced ones, see Appendix 5.

Partial seizures with or without secondary generalisation

Carbamazepine, **sodium valproate** and **phenytoin** are the drugs of choice for secondary generalised tonic-clonic seizures and for partial (focal) seizures. Phenobarbital and primidone are also effective but are likely to be more sedating. Second-line drugs include clonazepam, clobazam, and acetazolamide. **Gabapentin**, **lamotrigine**, and **vigabatrin** are used where control is difficult to obtain and are effective in partial seizures with or without secondary generalisation. Partial epilepsy and secondarily generalised seizures are more difficult to control than tonic-clonic seizures as part of a syndrome of primary generalised epilepsy.

Generalised seizures

TONIC-CLONIC SEIZURES (GRAND MAL). The drugs of choice for tonic-clonic seizures are **carbamazepine**, **phenytoin**, and **sodium valproate**. For those patients who have tonic-clonic seizures as part of the syndrome of primary generalised epilepsy, **sodium valproate** is the drug of choice. **Phenobarbital** (phenobarbitone) and **primidone** are also effective but may be more sedating. There is evidence that **lamotrigine** is also effective.

ABSENCE SEIZURES (PETIT MAL). **Ethosuximide** and **sodium valproate** are the drugs of choice in simple absence seizures. Sodium valproate is also highly effective in treating the tonic-clonic seizures which may co-exist with absence seizures in primary generalised epilepsy.

MYOCLONIC SEIZURES. Myoclonic seizures (myoclonic jerks) occur in a variety of syndromes, and response to treatment varies considerably. **Sodium valproate** is the drug of choice and **clonazepam**, **ethosuximide**, or **lamotrigine** may be used. For reference to the adjunctive use of piracetam, see section 4.9.3.

ATYPICAL ABSENCE, ATONIC, AND TONIC SEIZURES. These seizure types are usually seen in childhood, in specific epileptic syndromes, or associated with cerebral damage or mental retardation. They may respond poorly to the traditional drugs. **Phenytoin**, **sodium valproate**, **lamotrigine**, **clonazepam**, **ethosuximide**, and **phenobarbital** may be tried. Second-line antiepileptic drugs that are occasionally helpful, include **acetazolamide** and **corticosteroids**.

Carbamazepine

Carbamazepine is a drug of choice for simple and complex partial seizures and for tonic-clonic seizures secondary to a focal discharge. It has a wider therapeutic index than phenytoin and the relationship between dose and plasma concentration is linear, but monitoring of plasma concentrations may be helpful in determining optimum dosage. It has generally fewer side-effects than phenytoin or the barbiturates, but reversible blurring of vision, dizziness, and unsteadiness are dose-related, and may be dose-limiting. These side-effects may be reduced by altering the timing of medication; use of modified release tablets also significantly lessens the incidence of dose-related side-effects. It is essential to initiate carbamazepine therapy at a low dose and build this up slowly with increments of 100–200 mg every two weeks.

CARBAMAZEPINE

Indications: partial and secondary generalised tonic-clonic seizures, some primary generalised seizures; trigeminal neuralgia; prophylaxis of bipolar disorder unresponsive to lithium

Cautions: hepatic or renal impairment; cardiac disease (see also Contra-indications), skin reactions (see also Side-effects), history of haematological reactions to other drugs; manufacturer recommends blood counts and hepatic and renal function tests (but evidence of practical value unsatisfactory); glaucoma; pregnancy (**important**: see p. 223 and Appendix 4 (neural tube screening)), breast-feeding (see p. 223); avoid sudden withdrawal; **interactions**: see p. 222 and Appendix 1 (carbamazepine)

BLOOD, HEPATIC or SKIN DISORDERS. Patients or their carers should be told how to recognise signs of blood, liver, or skin disorders, and advised to seek immediate medical attention if symptoms such as fever, sore throat, rash, mouth ulcers, bruising, or bleeding develop. Leucopenia which is severe, progressive or associated with clinical symptoms requires withdrawal (if necessary under cover of suitable alternative).

Contra-indications: AV conduction abnormalities (unless paced); history of bone marrow depression, porphyria (section 9.8.2)

Side-effects: nausea and vomiting, dizziness, drowsiness, headache, ataxia, confusion and agitation (elderly), visual disturbances (especially double vision and often associated with peak plasma concentrations); constipation or diarrhoea, anorexia; mild transient generalised erythematous rash may occur in a large number of patients (withdraw if worsens or is accompanied by other symptoms); leucopenia and other blood disorders (including thrombocytopenia, agranulocytosis and aplastic anaemia); other side-effects include cholestatic jaundice, hepatitis and acute renal failure, Stevens-Johnson syndrome, toxic epidermal necrolysis, alopecia, thromboembolism, arthralgia, fever, proteinuria, lymph node enlargement, cardiac conduction disturbances (sometimes arrhythmias), dyskinesias, paraesthesia, depression, impotence (and impaired fertility), gynaecomastia, galactorrhoea, aggression, activation of psychosis; photosensitivity, pulmonary hypersensitivity (with dyspnoea and pneumonitis), hyponatraemia, oedema, and disturbances of bone metabolism (with osteomalacia) also reported; suppositories may cause occasional rectal irritation

Dose: *by mouth*, epilepsy, initially, 100–200 mg 1–2 times daily, increased slowly (see notes above) to usual dose of 0.8–1.2 g daily in divided doses; in some cases 1.6–2 g daily may be needed; ELDERLY reduce initial dose; CHILD daily in divided doses, up to 1 year 100–200 mg, 1–5 years 200–400 mg, 5–10 years 400–600 mg, 10–15 years 0.6–1 g
Trigeminal neuralgia, initially 100 mg 1–2 times daily (but some patients may require higher initial dose), increased gradually according to response; usual dose 200 mg 3–4 times daily, up to 1.6 g daily in some patients
Prophylaxis of bipolar disorder unresponsive to lithium (see also section 4.2.3), initially 400 mg daily in divided doses increased until symptoms controlled; usual range 400–600 mg daily; max. 1.6 g daily

By rectum, as suppositories, see below

Note. Plasma concentration for optimum response 4–12 mg/litre (20–50 micromol/litre)

Carbamazepine (Non-proprietary) PoM
Tablets, carbamazepine 100 mg, net price 20 = 58p; 200 mg, 20 = £1.07; 400 mg, 20 = £2.11. Label: 3, 8, counselling, blood, hepatic or skin disorder symptoms (see above), driving (see notes above)
Available from APS, Cox, Generics, Hillcross, Norton (Epimaz®)
Note. Different preparations may vary in bioavailability; to avoid reduced effect or excessive side-effects, it may be prudent to avoid changing the formulation (see also notes above on how side-effects may be reduced)

Tegretol® (Novartis) PoM
Tablets, all scored, carbamazepine 100 mg, net price 84-tab pack = £2.43; 200 mg, 84-tab pack = £4.50; 400 mg, 56-tab pack = £5.90. Label: 3, 8, counselling, blood, hepatic or skin disorder symptoms (see above), driving (see notes above)
Chewtabs, orange, carbamazepine 100 mg, net price 56-tab pack = £2.95; 200 mg, 56-tab pack = £5.49. Label: 3, 8, 21, 24, counselling, blood, hepatic or skin disorder symptoms (see above), driving (see notes above)
Liquid, sugar-free, carbamazepine 100 mg/5 mL. Net price 300-mL pack = £5.72. Label: 3, 8, counselling, blood, hepatic or skin disorder symptoms (see above), driving (see notes above)
Suppositories, carbamazepine 125 mg, net price 5 = £7.50; 250 mg, 5 = £10.00. Label: 3, 8, counselling, blood, hepatic or skin disorder symptoms (see above), driving (see notes above)
Dose: epilepsy, for short-term use (max. 7 days) when oral therapy temporarily not possible; suppositories of 125 mg may be considered to be approximately equivalent in therapeutic effect to tablets of 100 mg but final adjustment should always depend on clinical response (plasma concentration monitoring recommended); max. by rectum 1 g daily in 4 divided doses

■ Modified release

Tegretol® Retard (Novartis) PoM
Tablets, m/r, both scored, carbamazepine 200 mg (beige-orange), net price 56-tab pack = £4.82; 400 mg (brown-orange), 56-tab pack = £9.48. Label: 3, 8, 25, counselling, blood, hepatic or skin disorder symptoms (see above), driving (see notes above)
Dose: epilepsy (ADULT and CHILD over 5 years), as above; trigeminal neuralgia, as above; total daily dose given in 2 divided doses

Teril® CR (Lagap) PoM
Tablets, m/r, scored, carbamazepine 200 mg, net price 100-tab pack = £8.22; 400 mg, 100-tab pack = £16.17. Label: 3, 8, 25, counselling, blood, hepatic or skin disorder symptoms (see above), driving (see notes above)
Dose: epilepsy (ADULT and CHILD over 5 years), as above; trigeminal neuralgia, as above; total daily dose given in 1–2 divided doses; bipolar disorder, as above

Timonil® retard (CP) PoM
Tablets, m/r, scored, carbamazepine 200 mg, net price 100-tab pack = £8.60; 400 mg, 100-tab pack = £16.92. Label: 3, 8, 25, counselling, blood, hepatic or skin disorder symptoms (see above), driving (see notes above)
Dose: epilepsy (ADULT and CHILD over 1 year), as above; bipolar disorder, as above; trigeminal neuralgia, as above; total daily dose given in 1–2 divided doses

Ethosuximide

Ethosuximide is the drug of choice in simple absence seizures; it may also be used in myoclonic seizures and in atypical absence, atonic, and tonic seizures.

ETHOSUXIMIDE

Indications: absence seizures

Cautions: see notes above; hepatic and renal impairment; manufacturer recommends blood counts and hepatic and renal function tests (but evidence of practical value unsatisfactory); pregnancy and breast-feeding (see notes above); avoid sudden withdrawal; porphyria (see section 9.8.2); **interactions:** Appendix 1 (ethosuximide)

BLOOD DISORDERS. Patients or their carers should be told how to recognise signs of blood disorders, and advised to seek immediate medical attention if symptoms such as fever, sore throat, mouth ulcers, bruising or bleeding develop

Side-effects: gastro-intestinal disturbances, weight loss, drowsiness, dizziness, ataxia, dyskinesia, hiccup, photophobia, headache, depression, and mild euphoria. Psychotic states, rashes, hepatic and renal changes (see Cautions), and haematological disorders such as agranulocytosis and aplastic anaemia occur rarely (blood counts required if signs or symptoms of infection); systemic lupus erythematosus and erythema multiforme (Stevens-Johnson syndrome) reported; other side-effects reported include gum hypertrophy, swelling of tongue, irritability, hyperactivity, sleep disturbances, night terrors, inability to concentrate, aggressiveness, increased libido, myopia, vaginal bleeding

Dose: ADULT and CHILD over 6 years initially, 500 mg daily, increased by 250 mg at intervals of 4–7 days to usual dose of 1–1.5 g daily; occasionally up to 2 g daily may be needed; CHILD up to 6 years initially 250 mg daily, increased gradually to usual dose of 20 mg/kg daily

Note. Plasma concentration for optimum response 40–100 mg/litre (300–700 micromol/litre)

Emeside® (LAB) PoM

Capsules, orange, ethosuximide 250 mg. Net price 112-cap pack = £11.15. Label: 8, counselling, blood disorders (see above), driving (see notes above)

Syrup, black currant, ethosuximide 250 mg/5 mL. Net price 200-mL pack = £6.00. Label: 8, counselling, blood disorders (see above), driving (see notes above)

Zarontin® (Parke-Davis) PoM

Capsules, yellow, ethosuximide 250 mg. Net price 56-cap pack = £4.51. Label: 8, counselling, blood disorders (see above), driving (see notes above)

Syrup, yellow, ethosuximide 250 mg/5 mL. Net price 200-mL pack = £3.73. Label: 8, counselling, blood disorders (see above), driving (see notes above)

Lamotrigine

Lamotrigine is an antiepileptic for partial seizures and primary and secondarily generalised tonic-clonic seizures. It is also used for myoclonic seizures and may be tried for atypical absence, atonic, and tonic seizures in the Lennox-Gastaut syndrome. Lamotrigine may rarely cause serious skin rash especially in children; dose recommendations should be adhered to closely.

Lamotrigine is used either as sole treatment or as an adjunct to treatment with other antiepileptic drugs. Valproate increases plasma-lamotrigine concentration whereas the enzyme inducing antiepileptics reduce it; care is therefore required in choosing the appropriate initial dose and subsequent titration. Where the potential for interaction is not known, treatment should be initiated with lower doses such as those used with valproate.

LAMOTRIGINE

Indications: monotherapy and adjunctive treatment of partial seizures and primary and secondarily generalised tonic-clonic seizures; seizures associated with Lennox-Gastaut syndrome

Cautions: closely monitor (including hepatic, renal and clotting parameters) and consider withdrawal if rash, fever, influenza-like symptoms, drowsiness, or worsening of seizure control develops (although causal relationship not established, lamotrigine given with other antiepileptics has been associated with rapidly progressive illness with status epilepticus, multi-organ dysfunction, disseminated intravascular coagulation and death); avoid abrupt withdrawal (taper off over 2 weeks or longer) unless serious skin reaction occurs; renal impairment; elderly; pregnancy and breast-feeding; monitor body-weight in children and review dose if necessary; **interactions:** see p. 222 and Appendix 1 (lamotrigine)

Contra-indications: hepatic impairment

Side-effects: commonly rashes (see also below)—fever, malaise, influenza-like symptoms, drowsiness and rarely hepatic dysfunction, lymphadenopathy, leucopenia, and thrombocytopenia reported in conjunction with rash; angioedema, and photosensitivity also reported; diplopia, blurred vision, conjunctivitis, dizziness, drowsiness, insomnia, headache, ataxia, tiredness, gastro-intestinal disturbances (including vomiting), irritability, aggression, tremor, agitation, confusion; headache, nausea, dizziness, diplopia and ataxia in patients also taking carbamazepine usually resolve when dose of either drug reduced

SKIN REACTIONS. Serious skin reactions including Stevens-Johnson syndrome and toxic epidermal necrolysis (rarely with fatalities) have developed in adults and especially in children; most rashes occur within 8 weeks of starting lamotrigine. The CSM has advised that factors associated with increased risk of serious skin reactions include concomitant use of valproate, initial lamotrigine dosing higher than recommended, and more rapid dose escalation than recommended.

COUNSELLING. Warn patients to see their doctor immediately if rash or influenza-like symptoms associated with hypersensitivity develop

Dose: IMPORTANT. Do not confuse the different combinations; see also notes above

Monotherapy, initially 25 mg daily for 14 days, increased to 50 mg daily for further 14 days, then increased by max. of 50–100 mg every 7–14 days; usual maintenance as monotherapy, 100–200 mg daily in 1–2 divided doses (up to 500 mg daily has been required)

Adjunctive therapy *with valproate*, initially 25 mg every other day for 14 days then 25 mg daily for further 14 days, thereafter increased by max. of 25–50 mg every 7–14 days; usual maintenance, 100–200 mg daily in 1–2 divided doses

Adjunctive therapy (with enzyme inducing drugs) *without valproate*, initially 50 mg daily for 14 days then 50 mg twice daily for further 14 days, thereafter increased by max. of 100 mg every 7–14 days; usual maintenance 200–400 mg daily in 2 divided doses (up to 700 mg daily has been required)

CHILD under 12 years, *monotherapy*, not recommended

CHILD 2–12 years, adjunctive therapy *with valproate*, initially 200 micrograms/kg daily for 14 days then 500 micrograms/kg daily for further 14 days (those weighing 12.5–25 kg may receive 5 mg on alternate days for first 14 days), thereafter increased by max. of 0.5–1 mg/kg every 7–14 days; usual maintenance 1–5 mg/kg daily in 1–2 divided doses

CHILD 2–12 years adjunctive therapy (with enzyme inducing drugs) *without valproate*, initially 2 mg/kg daily in 2 divided doses for 14 days then 5 mg/kg daily in 2 divided doses for further 14 days, thereafter increased by max. of 2–3 mg/kg every 7–14 days; usual maintenance 5–15 mg/kg daily in 2 divided doses

Lamictal® (GlaxoWellcome) ▼ PoM
Tablets, all yellow, lamotrigine 25 mg, net price 21-tab pack (*'Valproate Add-on therapy' Starter Pack*) = £7.49, 42-tab pack (*'Monotherapy' Starter Pack*) = £14.97, 56-tab pack = £19.97; 50 mg, 42-tab pack (*'Non-valproate Add-on therapy' Starter Pack*) = £25.46, 56-tab pack = £33.95; 100 mg, 56-tab pack = £58.57; 200 mg, 56-tab pack = £99.56. Label: 8, counselling, driving (see notes above)
Dispersible tablets, lamotrigine 5 mg (scored), net price 28-tab pack = £7.96; 25 mg, 56-tab pack = £19.97; 100 mg, 56-tab pack = £58.57. Label: 8, 13, counselling, driving (see notes above)

Phenobarbital and other barbiturates

Phenobarbital (phenobarbitone) is effective for tonic-clonic and partial seizures but may be sedative in adults and cause behavioural disturbances and hyperkinesia in children. It may be tried for atypical absence, atonic, and tonic seizures. Rebound seizures may be a problem on withdrawal. Monitoring plasma concentrations is less useful than with other drugs because tolerance occurs. **Methylphenobarbital** is largely converted to phenobarbital in the liver and has no advantages. **Primidone** is largely converted to phenobarbital

and this is probably responsible for its antiepileptic action. A small starting dose of primidone (125 mg) is essential, and the drug should be introduced over several weeks.

PHENOBARBITAL
(Phenobarbitone)
Indications: all forms of epilepsy except absence seizures; status epilepticus (section 4.8.2)
Cautions: elderly, debilitated, children, impaired renal or hepatic function, respiratory depression (avoid if severe), pregnancy and breast-feeding (see notes above); avoid sudden withdrawal; see also notes above; avoid in porphyria (see section 9.8.2); **interactions:** see p. 222 and Appendix 1 (barbiturates and primidone)
Side-effects: drowsiness, lethargy, mental depression, ataxia and allergic skin reactions; paradoxical excitement, restlessness and confusion in the elderly and hyperkinesia in children; megaloblastic anaemia (may be treated with folic acid); **overdosage:** see Emergency Treatment of Poisoning, p. 24
Dose: *by mouth*, 60–180 mg at night; CHILD 5–8 mg/kg daily
By intramuscular injection, 200 mg, repeated after 6 hours if necessary; CHILD 15 mg/kg
Status epilepticus, *by intravenous injection* (dilute injection 1 in 10 with water for injections), 10 mg/kg at a rate of not more than 100 mg/minute; max. 1 g
Note. For therapeutic purposes phenobarbital and phenobarbital sodium may be considered equivalent in effect. Plasma concentration for optimum response 15–40 mg/litre (60–180 micromol/litre)

[1]**Phenobarbital** (Non-proprietary) CD
Tablets, phenobarbital 15 mg, net price 20 = 7p; 30 mg, 20 = 11p; 60 mg, 20 = 19p. Label: 2, 8, counselling, driving (see notes above)
Elixir, phenobarbital 15 mg/5 mL in a suitable flavoured vehicle, containing alcohol 38%, net price 100 mL = 79p. Label: 2, 8, counselling, driving (see notes above)
Note. Some hospitals supply **alcohol-free** formulations of varying phenobarbital strengths
Injection, phenobarbital sodium 200 mg/mL in propylene glycol 90% and water for injections 10%, net price 1-mL amp = £1.33
Note. Must be diluted before intravenous administration (see under Dose)
Available from Concord (¹*Gardenal Sodium®* CD), Martindale; other strengths also available from Martindale.
1. See p. 7 for prescribing requirements for phenobarbital

METHYLPHENOBARBITAL
(Methylphenobarbitone)
Indications: see under Phenobarbital
Cautions: see under Phenobarbital; **interactions:** see p. 222 and Appendix 1 (barbiturates and primidone)
Side-effects: see under Phenobarbital
Dose: 100–600 mg daily

Prominal® (Sanofi-Synthelabo) CD
Tablets, methylphenobarbital 30 mg, net price 20 = 78p; 60 mg, 20 = £1.03; 200 mg, 20 = £2.20. Label: 2, 8, counselling, driving (see notes above)

PRIMIDONE

Indications: all forms of epilepsy except absence seizures; essential tremor (also section 4.9.3)

Cautions: see under Phenobarbital; **interactions:** see p. 222 and Appendix 1 (barbiturates and primidone)

Side-effects: see under Phenobarbital; drowsiness, ataxia, nausea, visual disturbances, and rashes, particularly at first, usually reversible on continued administration

Dose: epilepsy, initially, 125 mg daily at bedtime, increased by 125 mg every 3 days to 500 mg daily in 2 divided doses then increased by 250 mg every 3 days to a max. of 1.5 g daily in divided doses; CHILD under 2 years, 250–500 mg daily in 2 divided doses; 2–5 years, 500–750 mg daily in 2 divided doses; 6–9 years 0.75–1 g daily in 2 divided doses

Essential tremor, initially 50 mg daily (as suspension) increased gradually over 2–3 weeks according to response; max. 750 mg daily

Note. Monitor plasma concentrations of derived phenobarbital. Optimum range as for phenobarbital

Mysoline® (Zeneca) [PoM]

Tablets, scored, primidone 250 mg. Net price 100-tab pack = £1.77. Label: 2, 8, counselling, driving (see notes above)

Oral suspension, primidone 250 mg/5 mL. Net price 250-mL pack = £1.01. Label: 2, 8, counselling, driving (see notes above)

Phenytoin

Phenytoin is effective in tonic-clonic and partial seizures. It has a narrow therapeutic index and the relationship between dose and plasma concentration is non-linear; small dosage increases in some patients may produce large rises in plasma concentrations with acute toxic side-effects. Monitoring of plasma concentration greatly assists dosage adjustment. A few missed doses or a small change in drug absorption may result in a marked change in plasma concentration.

Phenytoin may cause coarse facies, acne, hirsutism, and gingival hyperplasia and so may be particularly undesirable in adolescent patients.

When only parenteral administration is possible, **fosphenytoin** (section 4.8.2), a pro-drug of phenytoin, may be convenient to give. Whereas phenytoin can be given intravenously only, fosphenytoin may also be given by intramuscular injection.

PHENYTOIN

Indications: all forms of epilepsy except absence seizures; trigeminal neuralgia if carbamazepine inappropriare (see also section 4.7.3)

Cautions: hepatic impairment (reduce dose), pregnancy (**important:** see notes above and Appendix 4), breast-feeding (see notes above); avoid sudden withdrawal; manufacturer recommends blood counts (but evidence of practical value unsatisfactory); avoid in porphyria (section 9.8.2); see also notes above; **interactions:** see p. 222 and Appendix 1 (phenytoin)

BLOOD OR SKIN DISORDERS. Patients or their carers should be told how to recognise signs of blood or skin disorders, and advised to seek immediate medical attention if symptoms such as fever, sore throat, rash, mouth ulcers, bruising, or bleeding develop. Leucopenia which is severe, progressive or associated with clinical symptoms requires withdrawal (if necessary under cover of suitable alternative)

Side-effects: nausea, vomiting, mental confusion, dizziness, headache, tremor, transient nervousness, insomnia occur commonly; rarely dyskinesias, peripheral neuropathy; ataxia, slurred speech, nystagmus and blurred vision are signs of overdosage; rashes (discontinue; if mild re-introduce cautiously but discontinue immediately if recurrence), coarse facies, acne and hirsutism, fever and hepatitis; lupus erythematosus, Stevens-Johnson syndrome, toxic epidermal necrolysis, polyarteritis nodosa; lymphadenopathy; gingival hypertrophy and tenderness; rarely haematological effects, including megaloblastic anaemia (may be treated with folic acid), leucopenia, thrombocytopenia, agranulocytosis, and aplastic anaemia; plasma-calcium concentration may be lowered (rickets and osteomalacia)

Dose: *by mouth*, initially 3–4 mg/kg daily *or* 150–300 mg daily (as a single dose *or* in 2 divided doses) increased gradually as necessary (with plasma-phenytoin concentration monitoring); usual dose 200–500 mg daily (exceptionally, higher doses may be used); CHILD initially 5 mg/kg daily in 2 divided doses, usual dose range 4–8 mg/kg daily (max. 300 mg)

By intravenous injection—section 4.8.2

Note. Plasma concentration for optimum response 10–20 mg/litre (40–80 micromol/litre)

COUNSELLING. Take preferably with or after food

Phenytoin (Non-proprietary) [PoM]

Capsules, phenytoin sodium 50 mg, net price 20 = 40p; 100 mg, 20 = 56p. Label: 8, counselling, administration, blood or skin disorder symptoms (see above), driving (see notes above)

Tablets, coated, phenytoin sodium 50 mg, net price 20 = 47p; 100 mg, 20 = 65p. Label: 8, counselling, administration, blood or skin disorder symptoms (see above), driving (see notes above)

Available from APS

Note. On the basis of single dose tests there are no clinically relevant differences in bioavailability between available phenytoin sodium tablets and capsules but there may be a pharmacokinetic basis for maintaining the same brand of phenytoin in some patients

Epanutin® (Parke-Davis) [PoM]

Capsules, phenytoin sodium 25 mg (white/purple), net price 20 = 39p; 50 mg (white/pink), 20 = 40p; 100 mg (white/orange), 20 = 56p; 300 mg (white/green), 20 = £1.69. Label: 8, counselling, administration, blood or skin disorder symptoms (see above), driving (see notes above)

Infatabs® (= chewable tablets), yellow, scored, phenytoin 50 mg. Net price 20 = £1.10. Label: 8, 24, counselling, blood or skin disorder symptoms (see above), driving (see notes above)

Note. Contain phenytoin 50 mg (as against phenytoin sodium) therefore care is needed on changing to capsules or tablets containing phenytoin sodium

Suspension, red, phenytoin 30 mg/5 mL. Net price 100 mL = 71p. Label: 8, counselling, administration, blood or skin disorder symptoms (see above), driving (see notes above)

Note. Suspension of phenytoin 90 mg in 15 mL may be considered to be approximately equivalent in therapeutic effect to capsules or tablets containing phenytoin sodium 100 mg, but nevertheless care is needed in making changes

Valproate

Sodium valproate is effective in controlling tonic-clonic seizures, particularly in primary generalised epilepsy. It is a drug of choice in primary generalised epilepsy, generalised absences and myoclonic seizures, and may be tried in atypical absence, atonic, and tonic seizures. Controlled trials in partial epilepsy suggest that it has similar efficacy to that of carbamazepine and phenytoin. Plasma-valproate concentrations are not a useful index of efficacy, therefore routine monitoring is unhelpful. The drug has widespread metabolic effects, and may have dose-related side-effects. There has been concern over severe hepatic or pancreatic toxicity, although these effects are rare.

SODIUM VALPROATE

Indications: all forms of epilepsy

Cautions: monitor liver function before therapy and during first 6 months especially in patients most at risk (see also below); ensure no undue potential for bleeding before starting and before major surgery; renal impairment (Appendix 3); pregnancy (**important** see notes above and Appendix 4 (neural tube screening)); breast-feeding; systemic lupus erythematosus; false-positive urine tests for ketones; avoid sudden withdrawal; see also notes above; **interactions:** see p. 222 and Appendix 1 (valproate)

LIVER TOXICITY. Liver dysfunction (including fatal hepatic failure) has occurred in association with valproate (especially in children under 3 years of age and those with metabolic or degenerative disorders, organic brain disease or severe seizure disorders associated with mental retardation) usually in the first 6 months of therapy and usually involving multiple antiepileptic therapy (monotherapy preferred). Raised liver enzymes are not uncommon during valproate treatment and are usually transient but patients should be reassessed clinically and liver function (including prothrombin time) monitored until return to normal—an abnormally prolonged prothrombin time (particularly in association with other relevant abnormalities) requires discontinuation of treatment. Any concomitant use of salicylates should be stopped.

BLOOD OR HEPATIC DISORDERS. Patients or their carers should be told how to recognise signs of blood or liver disorders, and advised to seek immediate medical attention if symptoms develop (advice is given on patient information leaflet).

Contra-indications: active liver disease, family history of severe hepatic dysfunction, porphyria (section 9.8.2)

Side-effects: gastric irritation, nausea, ataxia and tremor; hyperammonaemia, increased appetite and weight gain; transient hair loss (regrowth may be curly), oedema, thrombocytopenia, and inhibition of platelet aggregation; impaired hepatic function leading rarely to fatal hepatic failure (see also under Cautions—withdraw treat-ment immediately if vomiting, anorexia, jaundice, drowsiness, or loss of seizure control occurs); rashes; sedation reported (rarely lethargy and confusion associated with too high an initial dose) and also increased alertness (occasionally aggression, hyperactivity and behavioural disturbances); rarely pancreatitis (measure plasma amylase in acute abdominal pain), leucopenia, pancytopenia, red cell hypoplasia, fibrinogen reduction; irregular periods, amenorrhoea, gynaecomastia, hearing loss, Fanconi's syndrome, dementia, toxic epidermal necrolysis, Stevens-Johnson syndrome, and vasculitis also reported

Dose: *by mouth*, initially, 600 mg daily given in 2 divided doses, preferably after food, increasing by 200 mg/day at 3-day intervals to a max. of 2.5 g daily in divided doses, usual maintenance 1–2 g daily (20–30 mg/kg daily); CHILD up to 20 kg, initially 20 mg/kg daily in divided doses, may be increased provided plasma concentrations monitored (above 40 mg/kg daily also monitor clinical chemistry and haematological parameters); over 20 kg, initially 400 mg daily in divided doses increased until control (usually in range of 20–30 mg/kg daily); max. 35 mg/kg daily

By intravenous injection (over 3–5 minutes) or *by intravenous infusion*, continuation of valproate treatment when oral therapy not possible, same as current dose by oral route

Initiation of valproate therapy (when oral valproate not possible), *by intravenous injection* (over 3–5 minutes), 400–800 mg (up to 10 mg/kg) followed by *intravenous infusion* up to max. 2.5 g daily; CHILD, usually 20–30 mg/kg daily, may be increased provided plasma concentrations monitored (above 40 mg/kg daily also monitor clinical chemistry and haematological parameters)

Sodium Valproate (Non-proprietary) PoM

Tablets, e/c, sodium valproate 200 mg, net price 20 = £1.38; 500 mg, 20 = £3.27. Label: 5, 8, 25, counselling, blood or hepatic disorder symptoms (see above), driving (see notes above)

Available from Cox, CP (*Orlept*®), Hillcross, Norton

Oral solution, sodium valproate 200 mg/5 mL. Net price 100 mL = £1.96. Label: 8, counselling, blood or hepatic disorder symptoms (see above), driving (see notes above)

Available from APS, CP, (*Orlept*®, sugar-free), Hillcross, Norton (sugar-free)

Epilim® (Sanofi-Synthelabo) PoM

Tablets (crushable), scored, sodium valproate 100 mg. Net price 20 = 78p. Label: 8, counselling, blood or hepatic disorder symptoms (see above), driving (see notes above)

Note. Sodium valproate crushable tablets also available from Hillcross

Tablets, both e/c, lilac, sodium valproate 200 mg, net price 20 = £1.28; 500 mg, 20 = £3.21. Label: 5, 8, 25, counselling, blood or hepatic disorder symptoms (see above), driving (see notes above)

Liquid, red, sugar-free, sodium valproate 200 mg/5 mL. Net price 300-mL pack = £5.89. Label: 8, counselling, blood or hepatic disorder symptoms (see above), driving (see notes above)

Syrup, red, sodium valproate 200 mg/5 mL. Net price 300-mL pack = £5.89. Label: 8, counselling, blood or hepatic disorder symptoms (see above), driving (see notes above)

Epilim Chrono® (Sanofi-Synthelabo) PoM
Tablets, m/r, all lilac, sodium valproate 200 mg (as sodium valproate and valproic acid), net price 100-tab pack = £7.70; 300 mg, 100-tab pack = £11.55; 500 mg, 100-tab pack = £19.25. Label: 8, 25, counselling, blood or hepatic disorder symptoms (see above), driving (see notes above)
Dose: ADULT and CHILD over 20 kg, as above, total daily dose given in 1–2 divided doses

Epilim® Intravenous (Sanofi-Synthelabo) PoM
Injection, powder for reconstitution, sodium valproate. Net price 400-mg vial (with 4-mL amp water for injections) = £8.77

■ Valproic acid

Convulex® (Pharmacia & Upjohn) PoM
Capsules, e/c, valproic acid 150 mg, net price 100-cap pack = £3.68; 300 mg, 100-cap pack = £7.35; 500 mg, 100-cap pack = £12.25. Label: 8, 25, counselling, blood or hepatic disorder symptoms (see above), driving (see notes above)
Dose: ADULT and CHILD initially 15 mg/kg daily in 2–4 divided doses, gradually increasing in steps of 5–10 mg/kg up to 30 mg/kg daily
EQUIVALENCE TO SODIUM VALPROATE. Manufacturer advises that *Convulex®* has a 1:1 dose relationship with products containing sodium valproate, but nevertheless care is needed in making changes.

Vigabatrin

For partial epilepsy with or without secondary generalisation, **vigabatrin** is given in combination with other antiepileptic treatment; its use is restricted to patients in whom all other combinations are inadequate or are not tolerated. It can be used as sole therapy in the management of infantile spasms in West's syndrome.

About one-third of patients treated with vigabatrin have suffered visual field defects and **careful monitoring** for this side-effect is required. Vigabatrin has prominent behavioural side-effects in some patients.

VIGABATRIN

Indications: initiated and supervised by appropriate specialist, adjunctive treatment of partial seizures with or without secondary generalisation not satisfactorily controlled with other antiepileptics; monotherapy for management of infantile spasms (West's syndrome)
Cautions: renal impairment; elderly; closely monitor neurological function; avoid sudden withdrawal (taper off over 2–4 weeks); history of psychosis, depression or behavioural problems; pregnancy (see p. 223 and Appendix 4) and breast-feeding; **interactions:** see p. 222 and Appendix 1 (vigabatrin)
VISUAL FIELD DEFECTS. Vigabatrin is associated with visual field defects. The CSM has advised that onset of symptoms varies from 1 month to several years after starting. In most cases, visual field defects have persisted despite discontinuation. Product literature advises visual field testing before treatment and at 6-month intervals; a procedure for testing visual fields in those with a developmental age of less than 9 years is available from the manufacturers. Patients should be warned to report any new visual symptoms that develop and those with symptoms should be referred for an urgent ophthalmological opinion. Gradual withdrawal of vigabatrin should be considered.

Contra-indications: visual field defects
Side-effects: drowsiness (rarely marked sedation, stupor, and confusion with non-specific slow wave EEG), fatigue, visual field defects (see also under Cautions), dizziness, nervousness, irritability, excitation and agitation especially in children; depression, abnormal thinking, headache, nystagmus, ataxia, tremor, paraesthesia, impaired concentration; less commonly confusion, aggression, psychosis, mania, memory disturbance, visual disturbance (e.g. diplopia); also weight gain, oedema, gastro-intestinal disturbances, alopecia, rash; less commonly urticaria, occasional increase in seizure frequency (especially if myoclonic), decrease in liver enzymes, slight decrease in haemoglobin; photophobia and retinal disorders (e.g. peripheral retinal atrophy); optic neuritis, optic atrophy also reported
Dose: with current antiepileptic therapy, initially 1 g daily in single or 2 divided doses then increased according to response in steps of 500 mg at weekly intervals; usual range 2–3 g daily (max. 3 g daily); CHILD initially 40 mg/kg daily in single or 2 divided doses then adjusted according to body-weight 10–15 kg, 0.5–1 g daily; body-weight 15–30 kg, 1–1.5 g daily; body-weight 30–50 kg, 1.5–3 g daily; body-weight over 50 kg, 2–3 g daily
Infantile spasms (West's syndrome), *monotherapy*, 50 mg/kg daily, adjusted according to response over 7 days; up to 150 mg/kg daily used with good tolerability

Sabril® (Hoechst Marion Roussel) PoM
Tablets, f/c, scored, vigabatrin 500 mg, net price 100-tab pack = £44.85. Label: 3, 8, counselling, driving (see notes above)
Powder, sugar-free, vigabatrin 500 mg/sachet. Net price 50-sachet pack = £24.33. Label: 3, 8, 13, counselling, driving (see notes above)
Note. The contents of a sachet should be dissolved in water or a soft drink immediately before taking

Benzodiazepines

Clonazepam is occasionally used in tonic-clonic or partial seizures, but its sedative side-effects may be prominent. **Clobazam** may be used as adjunctive therapy in the treatment of epilepsy (section 4.1.2), but the effectiveness of these and other **benzodiazepines** may wane considerably after weeks or months of continuous therapy.

CLOBAZAM

Indications: adjunct in epilepsy; anxiety (short-term use)
Cautions: see under Diazepam (section 4.1.2)
Contra-indications: see under Diazepam (section 4.1.2)
Side-effects: see under Diazepam (section 4.1.2)
Dose: epilepsy, 20–30 mg daily; max. 60 mg daily; CHILD over 3 years, not more than half adult dose
Anxiety, 20–30 mg daily in divided doses or as a single dose at bedtime, increased in severe anxiety (in hospital patients) to a max. of 60 mg daily in divided doses; ELDERLY (or debilitated) 10–20 mg daily

¹ Clobazam (Non-proprietary) ᴺᴴˢ PoM

Tablets, clobazam 10 mg. Net price 30-tab pack = £9.98. Label: 2 *or* 19, 8, counselling, driving (see notes above)

1. ᴺᴴˢ except, for epilepsy and endorsed 'SLS'

Note. The brand name *Frisium*® ᴺᴴˢ (Hoechst Marion Roussel) is used for clobazam tablets

CLONAZEPAM

Indications: all forms of epilepsy; myoclonus; status epilepticus (section 4.8.2)

Cautions: see notes above; respiratory disease; hepatic and renal impairment; elderly and debilitated; pregnancy and breast-feeding (see notes above); avoid sudden withdrawal; porphyria (see section 9.8.2); **interactions:** see p. 222 and Appendix 1 (clonazepam)

DRIVING. Drowsiness may affect the performance of skilled tasks (e.g. driving); effects of alcohol enhanced

Contra-indications: respiratory depression; acute pulmonary insufficiency

Side-effects: drowsiness, fatigue, dizziness, muscle hypotonia, coordination disturbances; hypersalivation in infants, paradoxical aggression, irritability and mental changes; rarely, blood disorders, abnormal liver-function tests; **overdosage:** see Emergency Treatment of Poisoning, p. 24

Dose: 1 mg (elderly, 500 micrograms), initially at night for 4 nights, increased over 2–4 weeks to a usual maintenance dose of 4–8 mg daily in divided doses; CHILD up to 1 year 250 micrograms increased as above to 0.5–1 mg, 1–5 years 250 micrograms increased to 1–3 mg, 5–12 years 500 micrograms increased to 3–6 mg

Rivotril® (Roche) PoM

Tablets, both scored, clonazepam 500 micrograms (beige), net price 20 = 84p; 2 mg, 20 = £1.12. Label: 2, 8, counselling, driving (see notes above)

Injection, section 4.8.2

Other drugs

Acetazolamide (section 11.6), a carbonic anhydrase inhibitor, is a second-line drug for both tonic-clonic and partial seizures. It is occasionally helpful in atypical absence, atonic, and tonic seizures.

Piracetam (section 4.9.3) is used as adjunctive treatment for cortical myoclonus.

Gabapentin can be given as adjunctive therapy in partial epilepsy with or without secondary generalisation.

Topiramate can be given as adjunctive therapy in partial seizures with or without secondary generalisation.

Tiagabine is also used as adjunctive treatment for partial seizures, with or without secondary generalisation.

GABAPENTIN

Indications: adjunctive treatment of partial seizures with or without secondary generalisation not satisfactorily controlled with other antiepileptics

Cautions: avoid sudden withdrawal (taper off over at least 1 week); elderly (may need to reduce dose), renal impairment (Appendix 3), diabetes mellitus, false positive readings with some urinary protein tests; pregnancy (see p. 223 and Appendix 4) and breast-feeding (see p. 223 and Appendix 5); **interactions:** Appendix 1 (gabapentin)

Side-effects: somnolence, dizziness, ataxia, fatigue; also nystagmus, tremor, diplopia, amblyopia; pharyngitis, dysarthria, weight gain, dyspepsia, amnesia, nervousness, coughing, asthenia, paraesthesia, arthralgia, purpura, leucopenia; rhinitis, myalgia, headache, rarely pancreatitis, altered liver function tests, and Stevens-Johnson syndrome; nausea and vomiting reported

Dose: 300 mg on day 1, then 300 mg twice daily on day 2, then 300 mg 3 times daily (approx. every 8 hours) on day 3, then increased according to response in steps of 300 mg daily (in 3 divided doses) to max. 2.4 g daily, usual range 0.9–1.2 g daily; CHILD 6–12 years (specialist use only) 10 mg/kg on day 1, then 20 mg/kg on day 2, then 25–35 mg/kg daily (in 3 divided doses approx. every 8 hours), maintenance 900 mg daily (body-weight 26–36 kg) or 1.2 g daily (body-weight 37–50 kg)

Neurontin® (Parke-Davis) ▼ PoM

Capsules, gabapentin 100 mg (white), net price 100-cap pack = £22.86; 300 mg (yellow), 100-cap pack = £53.00; 400 mg (orange), 100-cap pack = £61.33. Label: 3, 5, 8, counselling, driving (see notes above)

TIAGABINE

Indications: adjunctive treatment for partial seizures with or without secondary generalisation not satisfactorily controlled with other antiepileptics

Cautions: liver impairment (Appendix 2)

DRIVING. May impair performance of skilled tasks (e.g. driving)

Side-effects: diarrhoea, dizziness, tiredness, nervousness, tremor, concentration difficulties, emotional lability, speech impairment; rarely, confusion, depression, drowsiness, psychosis; leucopenia reported

Dose: adjunctive therapy, with *enzyme-inducing* drugs, 5 mg twice daily for 1 week, then increased at weekly intervals in steps of 5–10 mg daily; usual maintenance dose 30–45 mg daily (doses above 30 mg given in 3 divided doses); in patients receiving *non-enzyme-inducing* drugs, initial maintenance dose should be 15–30 mg daily; CHILD under 12 years not recommended

Gabitril® (Sanofi-Synthelabo) ▼ PoM

Tablets, f/c, scored, tiagabine (as hydrochloride) 5 mg, net price 50-tab pack = £22.69, 100-tab pack = £45.37; 10 mg, 50-tab pack = £45.37, 100-tab pack = £90.74; 15 mg, 50-tab pack = £68.06, 100-tab pack = £136.11. Label: 21

TOPIRAMATE

Indications: adjunctive treatment of partial seizures with or without secondary generalisation not satisfactorily controlled with other antiepileptics; seizures associated with Lennox-Gastaut syndrome; primary generalised tonic-clonic seizures

Cautions: avoid abrupt withdrawal; ensure adequate hydration (especially if predisposition to nephrolithiasis); pregnancy (see notes above); hepatic impairment (Appendix 2); renal impairment (Appendix 3); **interactions:** see p. 222 and Appendix 1 (topiramate)

Contra-indications: breast-feeding

Side-effects: abdominal pain, nausea, anorexia, weight loss; impaired concentration and memory, confusion, impaired speech, emotional lability with mood disorders and depression, altered behaviour, ataxia, abnormal gait, paraesthesia, dizziness, drowsiness, fatigue, asthenia, visual disturbances, diplopia, nystagmus, taste disorder, also psychotic symptoms, aggression, cognitive problems, leucopenia

Dose: initially 50 mg daily for one week (lower dose may be used) *then* increased in steps of 50 mg daily at weekly intervals and taken in 2 divided doses; usual dose 200–400 mg daily in 2 divided doses; max. 800 mg daily; CHILD 2–16 years, initially 25 mg at night for one week then increased in steps of 1–3 mg/kg daily according to response at intervals of 1–2 weeks and taken in 2 divided doses; recommended dose range 5–9 mg/kg daily in 2 divided doses

Note. If patient cannot tolerate titration regimen recommended above then smaller steps or longer interval between steps may be used

Topamax® (Janssen-Cilag) PoM
Tablets, f/c, topiramate 25 mg, net price 60-tab pack = £22.02; 50 mg (light yellow), 60-tab pack = £36.17; 100 mg (yellow), 60-tab pack = £64.80; 200 mg (salmon), 60-tab pack £125.83. Label: 3, 8, counselling, driving (see notes above)
Sprinkle capsules, topiramate 15 mg, net price 60-cap pack = £16.88; 25 mg, 60-cap pack = £25.32. Label: 3, 8, counselling, administration, driving (see notes above)
COUNSELLING. Swallow whole or open capsule and sprinkle contents on soft food

4.8.2 Drugs used in status epilepticus

Major status epilepticus should be *treated initially* with intravenous **diazepam**, used with caution because of the risk of respiratory depression; in situations where facilities for resuscitation are not immediately available, *small doses* of diazepam can be given intravenously or the drug can be administered as a rectal solution. Absorption from intramuscular injection or from suppositories is too slow for treatment of status epilepticus. When diazepam is given intravenously there may be a high risk of venous thrombophlebitis which is minimised by using an emulsion (*Diazemuls®*). **Clonazepam** and **lorazepam** are also used; lorazepam has the advantage of a long duration of action.

To *prevent recurrence* **phenytoin sodium** may be given by slow intravenous injection, with ECG monitoring in a dose of 15 mg/kg at a rate of not more than 50 mg/minute (in adults) followed by the maintenance dosage. Intramuscular use of phenytoin is not recommended (absorption is slow and erratic).

Fosphenytoin, a pro-drug of phenytoin, can be given more rapidly and when given intravenously causes fewer reactions at the injection site. It can also be given intramuscularly, although absorption is too slow by this route for treatment of status epilepticus. Doses of fosphenytoin should be expressed in terms of phenytoin sodium.

Alternatively, **phenobarbital sodium** can be given by intravenous injection (section 4.8.1). Other drugs which can be tried include **clomethiazole** (chlormethiazole) given by intravenous infusion. Clomethiazole has a short half-life, and the rate of infusion can be titrated against the patient's clinical condition (see **cautions** below).

Paraldehyde also remains a valuable drug. Given rectally (or occasionally by deep intramuscular injection) it causes little respiratory depression and is therefore useful where facilities for resuscitation are poor.

If the above measures fail to control seizures, anaesthesia with **thiopental** or **a non-barbiturate anaesthetic** such as propofol, should be instituted with full intensive care support.

DIAZEPAM

Indications: status epilepticus; convulsions due to poisoning (see Emergency Treatment of Poisoning); other indications (section 4.1.2, section 10.2.2, and section 15.1.4.1)

Cautions: see section 4.1.2; when given intravenously facilities for reversing respiratory depression with mechanical ventilation must be at hand (but see also notes above)

SPECIAL CAUTIONS FOR INTRAVENOUS INFUSION. Intravenous infusion of diazepam is potentially hazardous (especially if prolonged), calling for close and constant observation and best carried out in specialist centres with intensive care facilities. Special cautions required on prolonged intravenous infusion are as for Clomethiazole, see below and p. 167

Contra-indications: see section 4.1.2

Side-effects: see section 4.1.2; hypotension and apnoea

Dose: *by intravenous injection*, 10–20 mg at a rate of 0.5 mL (2.5 mg) per 30 seconds, repeated if necessary after 30–60 minutes; may be followed by *intravenous infusion* to max. 3 mg/kg over 24 hours; CHILD 200–300 micrograms/kg *or* 1 mg per year of age

By rectum as rectal solution, ADULT and CHILD over 10 kg 500 micrograms/kg; ELDERLY 250 micrograms/kg

Diazepam (Non-proprietary) PoM
Injection (solution), diazepam 5 mg/mL. See Appendix 6. Net price 2-mL amp = 25p
Available from CP, Roche (*Valium®*)
Injection (emulsion), diazepam 5 mg/mL (0.5%). See Appendix 6. Net price 2-mL amp = 76p
Available from Dumex (*Diazemuls®*)

Rectal tubes (= rectal solution), diazepam 2 mg/mL, net price 1.25-mL (2.5-mg) tube = 94p, 2.5-mL (5-mg) tube = £1.27; 4 mg/mL, 2.5-mL (10-mg) tube = £1.62, 5-mL (20-mg) tube = £3.06

Available from CP (*Diazepam Rectubes®* 2.5 mg, 5 mg, 10 mg, 20 mg), Dumex (*Stesolid®* 5 mg, 10 mg), Lagap

■ Oral preparations, section 4.1.2

CLONAZEPAM

Indications: status epilepticus; other forms of epilepsy, and myoclonus (section 4.8.1)

Cautions: see section 4.8.1; facilities for reversing respiratory depression with mechanical ventilation must be at hand (but see also notes above)

SPECIAL CAUTIONS FOR INTRAVENOUS INFUSION. Intravenous infusion of clonazepam is potentially hazardous (especially if prolonged), calling for close and constant observation and best carried out in specialist centres with intensive care facilities. Special cautions required on prolonged intravenous infusion are as for Clomethiazole, see below and p. 167

Contra-indications: see section 4.8.1

Side-effects: see section 4.8.1; hypotension and apnoea

Dose: *by intravenous injection* into a large vein (over 30 seconds) *or by intravenous infusion*, 1 mg, repeated if necessary; CHILD all ages, 500 micrograms

Rivotril® (Roche) PoM

Injection, clonazepam 1 mg/mL in solvent, for dilution with 1 mL water for injections immediately before injection or as described in Appendix 6. Net price 1-mL amp (with 1 mL water for injections) = 68p

■ Oral preparations, section 4.8.1

CLOMETHIAZOLE

(Chlormethiazole)

Indications: status epilepticus; other indications (section 4.1.1, section 4.10, section 15.1.4.1); eclampsia, consult product literature

Cautions: see section 4.1.1 for general cautions; resuscitation facilities must be available; maintain clear airway (risk of mechanical obstruction in deep sedation); *rapid infusion* to be given only under direct medical supervision (risk of apnoea and hypotension—special care in those susceptible to cerebral or cardiac complications, e.g. the elderly); during *continuous infusion* sleep induced may lapse into deep unconsciousness and patient must be kept under close and constant observation; *prolonged infusion* may lead to accumulation and delay recovery, may also cause electrolyte imbalance (infusion contains only Na+ 32 mmol/litre and no other electrolytes); **interactions:** Appendix 1 (anxiolytics and hypnotics)

LENNOX-GASTAUT SYNDROME. Paradoxical worsening of epilepsy may occur in the Lennox-Gastaut syndrome

Contra-indications: acute pulmonary insufficiency

Side-effects: nasal congestion and irritation (with sneezing), conjunctival irritation, headache; localised thrombophlebitis, tachycardia and transient fall in blood pressure (apnoea and hypotension on rapid infusion, see Cautions); see also section 4.1.1

Dose: *by intravenous infusion*, as a 0.8% solution of clomethiazole edisilate, initially 5–15 mL (40–120 mg)/minute up to a max. total dose of 40–100 mL (320–800 mg); may then be continued if necessary at a reduced rate according to response (see notes above); usual rate 0.5–1 mL (4–8 mg)/minute

CHILD initially 0.01 mL (80 micrograms)/kg/minute, then dose increased every 2–4 hours if necessary until seizures controlled or drowsiness occurs; if no seizure for 2 days dose gradually reduced every 4–6 hours (if seizures recur dose increased to previous level)

IMPORTANT. See cautions for intravenous infusion under Cautions (above)

Heminevrin® (Astra) PoM

Intravenous infusion 0.8%, clomethiazole edisilate 8 mg/mL. Net price 500-mL bottle = £4.89

■ Oral preparations, section 4.1.1

FOSPHENYTOIN SODIUM

Note. Fosphenytoin is a pro-drug of phenytoin

Indications: status epilepticus; seizures associated with neurosurgery or head injury; when phenytoin by mouth not possible

Cautions: see Phenytoin Sodium; liver impairment (Appendix 2); renal impairment (Appendix 3); **interactions:** see p. 222 and Appendix 1 (phenytoin)

Contra-indications: see Phenytoin Sodium

Side-effects: see Phenytoin Sodium

Dose: expressed as **phenytoin sodium equivalent** (PE); fosphenytoin sodium 1.5 mg ≡ phenytoin sodium 1 mg

Status epilepticus, *by intravenous infusion* (at a rate of 100–150 mg(PE)/minute), initially 15 mg(PE)/kg then *by intramuscular injection* or *by intravenous infusion* (at a rate of 50–100 mg(PE)/minute), 4–5 mg(PE)/kg daily in 1–2 divided doses, dose adjusted according to response and trough plasma-phenytoin concentration

CHILD 5 years and over, *by intravenous infusion* (at a rate of 2–3 mg(PE)/kg/minute), initially 15 mg(PE)/kg then *by intravenous infusion* (at a rate of 1–2 mg(PE)/kg/minute), 4–5 mg(PE)/kg daily in 1–4 divided doses, dose adjusted according to response and trough plasma-phenytoin concentration

Prophylaxis or treatment of seizures associated with neurosurgery or head injury, *by intramuscular injection* or *by intravenous infusion* (at a rate of 50–100 mg(PE)/minute), initially 10–15 mg(PE)/kg then *by intramuscular injection* or *by intravenous infusion* (at a rate of 50–100 mg(PE)/minute), 4–5 mg(PE)/kg daily (in 1–2 divided doses), dose adjusted according to response and trough plasma-phenytoin concentration

CHILD 5 years and over, *by intravenous infusion* (at a rate of 1–2 mg(PE)/kg/minute), initially 10–15 mg(PE)/kg then 4–5 mg(PE)/kg daily in 1–4 divided doses, dose adjusted according to response and trough plasma-phenytoin concentration

Temporary substitution for oral phenytoin, *by intramuscular injection* or *by intravenous infusion* (at a rate of 50–100 mg(PE)/minute), same dose and dosing frequency as oral phenytoin therapy; CHILD 5 years and over, *by intravenous infusion* (at a rate of 1–2 mg(PE)/kg/minute), same dose and dosing frequency as oral phenytoin therapy ELDERLY consider 10–25% reduction in dose or infusion rate

---

Note. Prescriptions for fosphenytoin sodium should state the dose in terms of phenytoin sodium equivalent (PE)

Pro-Epanutin® (Parke-Davis) ▼ PoM

Injection concentrate, fosphenytoin sodium 75 mg/mL (equivalent to phenytoin sodium 50 mg/mL), net price 10-mL vial = £40.00

Electrolytes: phosphate 3.7 micromol/mg fosphenytoin sodium (phosphate 5.6 micromol/mg phenytoin sodium)

LORAZEPAM

Indications: status epilepticus; other indications, section 4.1.2

Cautions: see section 4.1.2; facilities for reversing respiratory depression with mechanical ventilation must be at hand

Contra-indications: see section 4.1.2

Side-effects: see section 4.1.2; hypotension and apnoea

Dose: *by intravenous injection* (into large vein), 4 mg; CHILD 2 mg

Preparations

Section 4.1.2

PARALDEHYDE

Indications: status epilepticus

Cautions: bronchopulmonary disease, hepatic impairment; pregnancy (Appendix 4) and breast-feeding (Appendix 5); avoid intramuscular injection near sciatic nerve (causes severe causalgia)

INTRAVENOUS INFUSION. Paraldehyde has been given by intravenous infusion (diluted in physiological saline) in specialist centres with intensive care facilities but this method of administration is no longer recommended

Contra-indications: gastric disorders; rectal administration in colitis

Side-effects: rashes; pain and sterile abscess after intramuscular injection; rectal irritation after enema

Dose: *by deep intramuscular injection*, as a single dose, 5–10 mL; usual max. 20 mL daily with not more than 5 mL at any one site; CHILD up to 3 months 0.5 mL, 3–6 months 1 mL, 6–12 months 1.5 mL, 1–2 years 2 mL, 3–5 years 3–4 mL, 6–12 years 5–6 mL

By intravenous infusion, formerly given in a dose of up to 4–5 mL diluted to a 4% solution with sodium chloride intravenous infusion 0.9%, but **no longer recommended**

By rectum, 5–10 mL, administered as a 10% enema in physiological saline (some centres mix paraldehyde with an equal volume of arachis (peanut) oil instead); CHILD as for intramuscular dose

Note. Do not use paraldehyde if it has a brownish colour or an odour of acetic acid. Avoid contact with rubber and plastics.

Paraldehyde (Non-proprietary) PoM

Injection, sterile paraldehyde, net price 5-mL amp = £8.26

Available from Faulding DBL

Note. May temporarily be unavailable

PHENYTOIN SODIUM

Indications: status epilepticus; seizures in neurosurgery; arrhythmias, but now obsolete (section 2.3.2)

Cautions: hypotension and heart failure; resuscitation facilities must be available; injection solutions alkaline (irritant to tissues); see also section 4.8.1; **interactions:** see p. 222 and Appendix 1 (phenytoin)

Contra-indications: sinus bradycardia, sino-atrial block, and second- and third-degree heart block; Stokes-Adams syndrome; porphyria (section 9.8.2)

Side-effects: intravenous injection may cause cardiovascular and CNS depression (particularly if injection too rapid) with arrhythmias, hypotension, and cardiovascular collapse; alterations in respiratory function (including respiratory arrest)

Dose: *by slow intravenous injection or infusion* (with blood pressure and ECG monitoring), status epilepticus, 15 mg/kg at a rate not exceeding 50 mg per minute, as a loading dose (see also notes above). Maintenance doses of about 100 mg should be given thereafter at intervals of every 6–8 hours, monitored by measurement of plasma concentrations; rate and dose reduced according to weight; CHILD 15 mg/kg as a loading dose (neonate 15–20 mg/kg at rate of 1–3 mg/kg/minute)

Ventricular arrhythmias (but use now obsolete), *by intravenous injection* via caval catheter, 3.5–5 mg/kg at a rate not exceeding 50 mg/minute, with blood pressure and ECG monitoring; repeat once if necessary

Note. Phenytoin is licensed for administration by intravenous infusion (at the same rate of administration as the injection—not exceeding 50 mg/minute, for further details of the infusion, see Appendix 6). To avoid local venous irritation each injection or infusion should be preceded and followed by an injection of sterile physiological saline through the same needle or catheter

By intramuscular injection, not recommended (see notes above)

Phenytoin (Non-proprietary) PoM

Injection, phenytoin sodium 50 mg/mL with propylene glycol 40% and alcohol 10% in water for injections, net price 5-mL amp = £3.40

Available from Antigen, Faulding DBL

Epanutin® Ready-Mixed Parenteral (Parke-Davis) PoM

Injection, phenytoin sodium 50 mg/mL with propylene glycol 40% and alcohol 10% in water for injections. Net price 5-mL amp = £4.07

Note. Phenytoin injection also available from Antigen, Faulding DBL

■ Oral preparations, section 4.8.1

Febrile convulsions

Brief febrile convulsions need only simple treatment such as tepid sponging or bathing, or antipyretic medication, e.g. **paracetamol** (section 4.7.1). *Prolonged febrile convulsions* (those lasting 15 minutes or longer), *recurrent convulsions*, or those occurring in a child at known risk must be treated more actively, as there is the possibility of resulting brain damage. **Diazepam** is the drug of choice given either by slow intravenous injection in a dose of 250 micrograms/kg (section 4.8.2) or preferably rectally in solution (section 4.8.2) in a dose of 500 micrograms/kg (max. 10 mg), repeated if necessary. The rectal route is preferred as satisfactory absorption is achieved within minutes and administration is much easier. Suppositories are not suitable because absorption is too slow.

Intermittent prophylaxis (i.e. the anticonvulsant administered at the onset of fever) is possible in only a small proportion of children. Again **diazepam** is the treatment of choice, orally or rectally.

The exact role of continuous prophylaxis in children at risk from prolonged or complex febrile convulsions is controversial. It is probably indicated in only a small proportion of children, including those whose first seizure occurred at under 14 months or who have pre-existing neurological abnormalities or who have had previous prolonged or focal convulsions. Thus long-term anticonvulsant prophylaxis is rarely indicated.

4.9 Drugs used in parkinsonism and related disorders

4.9.1   Dopaminergic drugs used in parkinsonism

4.9.2   Antimuscarinic drugs used in parkinsonism

4.9.3   Drugs used in essential tremor, chorea, tics, and related disorders

In idiopathic Parkinson's disease, progressive degeneration of pigment-containing cells of the substantia nigra leads to deficiency of the neurotransmitter dopamine. This, in turn, results in a neurohumoral imbalance in the basal ganglia, causing the characteristic signs and symptoms of the illness to appear. The pathogenesis of this process is still obscure and current drug therapy aims simply to correct the imbalance. Although this approach fails to prevent the progression of the disease, it greatly improves the quality and expectancy of life of most patients.

The patient should be advised at the outset of the limitations of treatment and possible side-effects. About 10 to 20% of patients are unresponsive to treatment.

ELDERLY. Antiparkinsonian drugs carry a special risk of inducing confusion in the elderly. It is particularly important to initiate treatment with low doses and to use small increments.

Dopaminergic drugs used in parkinsonism

Levodopa in combination with a **dopa-decarboxylase inhibitor** is the treatment of choice for patients disabled by idiopathic Parkinson's disease. It is least valuable in elderly patients and in those with long-standing disease who may not tolerate a dose large enough to overcome their deficit. It is also less valuable in patients with post-encephalitic disease who are particularly susceptible to the side-effects. Parkinsonism caused by generalised degenerative brain disease does not normally respond to levodopa. It should not be used for neuroleptic-induced parkinsonism.

Levodopa, the amino-acid precursor of dopamine, acts mainly by replenishing depleted striatal dopamine. It improves bradykinesia and rigidity more than tremor. It is administered in conjunction with an extracerebral dopa-decarboxylase inhibitor that prevents the peripheral degradation of levodopa to dopamine but, unlike levodopa, does not cross the blood-brain barrier. Effective brain concentrations of dopamine can thereby be achieved with lower doses of levodopa. At the same time the reduced peripheral formation of dopamine decreases peripheral side-effects such as nausea and vomiting and cardiovascular effects. There is also less delay in onset of therapeutic effect and a smoother clinical response. A disadvantage is an increased incidence of abnormal involuntary movements.

The extracerebral dopa-decarboxylase inhibitors used with levodopa are benserazide (in **co-beneldopa**) and carbidopa (in **co-careldopa**).

When co-careldopa 10/100 (10 mg of carbidopa for each 100 mg of levodopa) is used the dose of carbidopa may be insufficient to achieve full inhibition of extracerebral dopa-decarboxylase; co-careldopa 25/100 (25 mg of carbidopa for each 100 mg of levodopa) should then be used so that the daily dose of carbidopa is at least 75 mg.

Levodopa therapy should be initiated with low doses and gradually increased, by small increments, at intervals of 2 to 3 days. The final dose is usually a compromise between increased mobility and dose-limiting side-effects. Intervals between doses may be critical and should be chosen to suit the needs of the individual patient. Nausea and vomiting are rarely dose-limiting but doses should be taken after meals. Domperidone (section 4.6) may be useful in controlling vomiting. The most frequent dose-limiting side-effects of levodopa are involuntary movements and psychiatric complications. As the patient ages, the maintenance dose may need to be reduced.

During the first 6 to 18 months of levodopa therapy there may be a slow improvement in the response of the patient which is maintained for 1½ to 2 years; thereafter a slow decline may occur. Particularly troublesome is the 'on-off' effect the incidence of which increases as the treatment progresses. This is characterised by fluctuations in performance with normal performance during the 'on' period and weakness and akinesia lasting for 2 to 4 hours during the 'off' period.

'End-of-dose' deterioration may also occur where the duration of benefit after each dose becomes progressively shorter. Modified-release preparations may help with 'end-of-dose' deterioration or nocturnal immobility and rigidity.

Selegiline is a monoamine-oxidase-B inhibitor used in severe parkinsonism in conjunction with levodopa to reduce 'end-of-dose' deterioration. Early treatment with selegiline may delay the need for levodopa therapy but there is no convincing evidence that it delays disease progression. Selegiline given with levodopa may be associated with increased mortality in the longer term, but this remains to be confirmed. Selegiline need not necessarily be withdrawn from patients stabilised on treatment; sudden withdrawal of selegiline may exacerbate symptoms.

Entacapone has recently been introduced for use as an adjunct to co-beneldopa or co-careldopa for patients with Parkinson's disease who experience 'end-of-dose' deterioration and cannot be stabilised on these combinations.

The ergot derivatives, **bromocriptine, cabergoline, lisuride** (lysuride), and **pergolide** act by direct stimulation of surviving dopamine receptors. Although effective, they have no advantages over levodopa. They should be reserved for patients in whom levodopa alone is no longer adequate or who despite careful titration cannot tolerate levodopa. Ergot derivatives are sometimes useful in reducing 'off' periods and in ameliorating fluctuations in the later stage of Parkinson's disease. Their use is often limited by their side-effects and when used with levodopa, abnormal involuntary movements and confusional states are common; occasionally, ergot derivatives may cause neuropsychiatric effects and retroperitoneal fibrosis.

Ropinirole is a dopamine D_2 receptor agonist which improves the symptoms and signs in Parkinson's disease. Its side-effects are similar to those of bromocriptine. It is likely to be most useful as an adjunct to levodopa. Dopamine agonists such as ropinirole are often used as monotherapy, particularly in younger patients who are at risk of developing disabling dyskinesia with long-term levodopa therapy.

Pramipexole is a non-ergot dopamine D_2 and D_3 receptor agonist with antiparkinsonian activity. Side-effects are similar to those of other dopamine agonists. It is currently used as adjunctive therapy with levodopa.

Amantadine has modest antiparkinsonian effects. It improves mild bradykinetic disabilities as well as tremor and rigidity. Unfortunately only a small proportion of patients derive much benefit from this drug and tolerance to its effects occurs. However it has the advantage of being relatively free from side-effects.

Apomorphine is a potent stimulator of D_1 and D_2 receptors, which is sometimes helpful in stabilising patients experiencing unpredictable 'off' periods with levodopa treatment. It is essential to establish patients on domperidone for three days before starting apomorphine. Long-term specialist supervision is advisable throughout apomorphine treatment.

Tolcapone has been suspended following reports of serious hepatotoxicity associated with its use.

LEVODOPA

Indications: parkinsonism (but not drug-induced extrapyramidal symptoms), see notes above

Cautions: pulmonary disease, peptic ulceration, cardiovascular disease, diabetes mellitus, osteomalacia, open-angle glaucoma, skin melanoma, psychiatric illness (avoid if severe). In prolonged therapy, psychiatric, hepatic, haematological, renal, and cardiovascular surveillance is advisable. Warn patients who benefit from therapy to resume normal activities gradually; avoid abrupt withdrawal; pregnancy (toxicity in *animals*) and breast-feeding; **interactions:** Appendix 1 (levodopa)

Contra-indications: closed-angle glaucoma

Side-effects: anorexia, nausea and vomiting, insomnia, agitation, postural hypotension (rarely labile hypertension), dizziness, tachycardia, arrhythmias, reddish discoloration of urine and other body fluids, rarely hypersensitivity; abnormal involuntary movements and psychiatric symptoms which include hypomania and psychosis may be dose-limiting; depression, drowsiness, headache, flushing, sweating, gastro-intestinal bleeding, peripheral neuropathy, taste disturbance, pruritus, rash, and liver enzyme changes also reported; syndrome resembling neuroleptic malignant syndrome reported on withdrawal

Dose: initially 125–500 mg daily in divided doses after meals, increased according to response (but rarely used alone, see notes above)

Levodopa (Non-proprietary) PoM
Tablets, levodopa 500 mg. Net price 20 = £6.00. Label: 14, 21
Available from Cambridge

denotes preparations that are considered to be less suitable for prescribing (see p. vi)

CO-BENELDOPA

A mixture of benserazide hydrochloride and levodopa in mass proportions corresponding to 1 part of benserazide and 4 parts of levodopa

Indications: see under Levodopa and notes above

Cautions: see under Levodopa and notes above

Contra-indications: see under Levodopa

Side-effects: see under Levodopa and notes above

Dose: expressed as levodopa, initally 50 mg 3–4 times daily (100 mg 3 times daily in advanced disease), increased by 100 mg once or twice weekly according to response; usual maintenance dose 400–800 mg daily in divided doses after meals; ELDERLY initially 50 mg once or twice daily, increased by 50 mg every third or fourth day according to response

Note. When transferring patients from other levodopa preparations, it is recommended that the previous preparation should be discontinued 12 hours beforehand (although interval can be shorter); 3 capsules co-beneldopa 25/100 (*Madopar 125®*) should be substituted for 2 g levodopa; if transferring from another levodopa/dopa-decarboxylase inhibitor preparation, initial dose, expressed as levodopa, should be 50 mg 3–4 times daily

Madopar® (Roche) PoM
Capsules 62.5, blue/grey, co-beneldopa 12.5/50 (benserazide 12.5 mg (as hydrochloride), levo-dopa 50 mg). Net price 100-cap pack = £6.67. Label: 14, 21
Capsules 125, blue/pink, co-beneldopa 25/100 (benserazide 25 mg (as hydrochloride), levodopa 100 mg). Net price 100-cap pack = £9.29. Label: 14, 21
Capsules 250, blue/caramel, co-beneldopa 50/200 (benserazide 50 mg (as hydrochloride), levodopa 200 mg). Net price 100-cap pack = £15.84. Label: 14, 21
Dispersible tablets 62.5, scored, co-beneldopa 12.5/50 (benserazide 12.5 mg (as hydrochloride), levodopa 50 mg). Net price 100-tab pack = £7.92. Label: 14, 21, counselling, administration, see below
Dispersible tablets 125, scored, co-beneldopa 25/100 (benserazide 25 mg (as hydrochloride) levodopa 100 mg). Net price 100-tab pack = £14.04. Label: 14, 21, counselling, administration, see below
Note. The tablets may be dispersed in water or orange squash (not orange juice) or swallowed whole

Madopar® CR (Roche) PoM
Capsules 125, m/r, dark green/light blue, co-benel-dopa 25/100 (benserazide 25 mg (as hydro-chloride), levodopa 100 mg). Net price 100-cap pack = £17.16. Label: 5, 14, 25
Dose: Patients not receiving levodopa therapy, initially 1 capsule 3 times daily (max. initial dose 6 capsules daily) Fluctuations in response related to plasma-levodopa concentration or to timing of dose, initially 1 capsule substituted for every 100 mg of levodopa and given at same dosage frequency, subsequently increased every 2–3 days according to response; average increase of 50% needed over previous levodopa dose and titration may take up to 4 weeks
Supplementary dose of conventional *Madopar®* may be needed with first morning dose; if response still poor to total daily dose of *Madopar® CR* plus *Madopar®* corresponding to 1.2 g levodopa, consider alternative therapy

CO-CARELDOPA

A mixture of carbidopa and levodopa; the proportions are expressed in the form *x/y* where *x* and *y* are the strengths in milligrams of carbidopa and levodopa respectively
Indications: see under Levodopa and notes above
Cautions: see under Levodopa and notes above
Contra-indications: see under Levodopa
Side-effects: see under Levodopa and notes above
Dose: expressed as levodopa, initially 100 mg (with carbidopa 25 mg, as *Sinemet-Plus®*) 3 times daily, increased by 50–100 mg (with carbidopa 12.5–25 mg, as *Sinemet-62.5®* or *Sinemet-Plus®*) daily or on alternate days according to response, up to 800 mg (with carbidopa 200 mg) daily in divided doses
Note. Carbidopa 70–100 mg daily is necessary to achieve full inhibition of peripheral dopa-decarboxylase
Alternatively, initially 50–100 mg (with carbidopa 10–12.5 mg, as *Sinemet-62.5®* or *Sinemet-110®*) 3–4 times daily, increased by 50–100 mg daily or on alternate days according to response, up to 800 mg (with carbidopa 80–100 mg) daily in divided doses
Alternatively, initially 125 mg (with carbidopa 12.5 mg, as ½ tablet of *Sinemet-275®*) 1–2 times daily, increased by 125 mg (with carbidopa

12.5 mg) daily or on alternate days according to response
Note. When transferring patients from levodopa, 1 tablet co-careldopa 25/250 (*Sinemet-275®*) 3–4 times daily should be substituted for patients receiving more than 1.5 g levodopa daily; 1 tablet co-careldopa 25/100 (*Sinemet-Plus®*) 3–4 times daily should be substituted for patients receiving less than 1.5 g levodopa daily; levodopa should be discontinued 12 hours beforehand

Sinemet® (Du Pont) PoM
Sinemet-62.5® tablets, yellow, scored, co-carel-dopa 12.5/50 (carbidopa 12.5 mg (as mono-hydrate), levodopa 50 mg), net price 90-tab pack = £7.03. Label: 14, 21
Note. 2 tablets *Sinemet-62.5®* ≡ 1 tablet *Sinemet Plus®*; *Sinemet-62.5®* previously known as *Sinemet LS®*
Sinemet-110® tablets, blue, scored, co-careldopa 10/100 (carbidopa 10 mg (as monohydrate), levo-dopa 100 mg), net price 90-tab pack = £7.35. Label: 14, 21
Sinemet-Plus® tablets, yellow, scored, co-carel-dopa 25/100 (carbidopa 25 mg (as monohydrate), levodopa 100 mg), net price 90-tab pack = £10.81. Label: 14, 21
Note. The daily dose of carbidopa required to achieve full inhibition of extracerebral dopa-decarboxylase is 75 mg; co-careldopa 25/100 provides an adequate dose of carbidopa when low doses of levodopa are needed
Sinemet-275® tablets, blue, scored, co-careldopa 25/250 (carbidopa 25 mg (as monohydrate), levo-dopa 250 mg), net price 90-tab pack = £15.36. Label: 14, 21

■ Modified release

Half Sinemet® CR (Du Pont) PoM
Tablets, m/r, pink, co-careldopa 25/100 (carbidopa 25 mg (as monohydrate), levodopa 100 mg), net price 60-tab pack = £18.99. Label: 14, 25
Dose: for fine adjustment of *Sinemet® CR* dose (see below)

Sinemet® CR (Du Pont) PoM
Tablets, m/r, peach, co-careldopa 50/200 (carbi-dopa 50 mg (as monohydrate), levodopa 200 mg), net price 60-tab pack = £22.35. Label: 14, 25
Dose: initial treatment or fluctuations in response to conventional levodopa therapy, 1 *Sinemet® CR* tablet twice daily; both dose and interval then adjusted accord-ing to response at intervals of not less than 3 days; if transferring from existing levodopa therapy withdraw 8 hours beforehand; 1 tablet *Sinemet® CR* twice daily can be substituted for a daily dose of levodopa 300–400 mg in conventional *Sinemet®* tablets

AMANTADINE HYDROCHLORIDE

Indications: Parkinson's disease (but not drug-induced extrapyramidal symptoms); antiviral (section 5.3)
Cautions: hepatic, or renal impairment (Appendix 3), congestive heart disease (may exacerbate oedema), confused or hallucinatory states, eld-erly; avoid abrupt discontinuation in Parkinson's disease; **interactions:** Appendix 1 (amantadine)
DRIVING. May affect performance of skilled tasks (e.g. driving)
Contra-indications: epilepsy, history of gastric ulceration, severe renal impairment; pregnancy (toxicity in *animals*), breast-feeding
Side-effects: anorexia, nausea, nervousness, ina-bility to concentrate, insomnia, dizziness, con-

vulsions, hallucinations or feelings of detachment, blurred vision, gastro-intestinal disturbances, livedo reticularis and peripheral oedema; rarely leucopenia, rashes

Dose: 100 mg daily increased after one week to 100 mg twice daily, usually in conjunction with other treatment; some patients may require higher doses, max. 400 mg daily

ELDERLY 65 years and over, 100 mg daily

Symmetrel® (Alliance) [PoM]
Capsules, red-brown, amantadine hydrochloride 100 mg. Net price 56-cap pack = £15.35. Counselling, driving
Note. Also available as *Lysovir®* for the prophylaxis and treatment of influenza A
Syrup, amantadine hydrochloride 50 mg/5 mL. Net price 150-mL pack = £5.05. Counselling, driving

---

APOMORPHINE HYDROCHLORIDE

Indications: refractory motor fluctuations in Parkinson's disease ('off' episodes) inadequately controlled by levodopa or other dopaminergics (for capable and motivated patients under specialist supervision)

Cautions: tendency to nausea and vomiting; pulmonary, cardiovascular or endocrine disease, renal impairment; elderly and debilitated, history of postural hypotension (special care on initiation); hepatic, haemopoietic, renal, and cardiovascular monitoring; *on administration with levodopa* test initially and every 6 months for haemolytic anaemia (development calls for specialist haematological care with dose reduction and possible discontinuation); **interactions:** Appendix 1 (apomorphine)

Contra-indications: respiratory or CNS depression, hypersensitiviy to opioids; neuropsychiatric problems or dementia; not suitable if 'on' response to levodopa marred by severe dyskinesia, hypotonia or psychiatric effects; pregnancy and breast-feeding

Side-effects: nausea and vomiting (see below under Dose), dyskinesias during 'on' periods (may require discontinuation); postural instability and falls (impaired speech and balance may not improve), increasing cognitive impairment, and personality change during 'on' phase; confusion and hallucinations (if continued, specialist observation required with possible gradual dose reduction), sedation, postural hypotension; also euphoria, light-headedness, restlessness, tremors; haemolytic anaemia with levodopa (see Cautions) and rarely eosinophilia; local reactions common (include nodule formation and possible ulceration)—rotate injection sites, dilute with sodium chloride 0.9%, consider ultrasound, ensure no infection

Dose: *by subcutaneous injection*, usual range (after initiation as below) 3–30 mg daily in divided doses; subcutaneous infusion may be preferable in those requiring division of injections into more than 10 doses daily; max. single dose 10 mg; ADOLESCENT (under 18 years) and CHILD not recommended

By continuous subcutaneous infusion (those requiring division into more than 10 injections daily) initially 1 mg/hour daily increased according to response (not more often than every 4 hours) in max. steps of 500 micrograms/hour to max. 4 mg/hour (15–60 micrograms/kg/hour); change infusion site every 12 hours and give during waking hours only (24-hour infusions not advised unless severe night-time symptoms)—intermittent bolus boosts also usually needed (in those with severe dyskinesias only when absolutely necessary)

Total daily dose by either route (or combined routes) max. 100 mg

REQUIREMENTS FOR INITIATION. *Hospital admission* and at least 3 days of pretreatment with domperidone for nausea and vomiting, *after at least 3 days* withhold existing antiparkinsonian medication overnight to provoke 'off' episode, *determine* threshold dose, *re-establish* other antiparkinsonian drugs, *determine* effective apomorphine regimen, *teach* to administer by subcutaneous injection into lower abdomen or outer thigh at first sign of 'off' episode, *discharge* from hospital, *monitor* frequently and *adjust* dosage regimen as appropriate (domperidone may normally be withdrawn over several weeks or longer)—for full details of initiation requirements, consult product literature

Britaject® (Britannia) [PoM]
Injection, apomorphine hydrochloride 10 mg/mL, net price 2-mL amp = £7.95, 5-mL amp = £15.95; 3-mL pen injector = £21.00

BROMOCRIPTINE

Indications: parkinsonism (but not drug-induced extrapyramidal symptoms); endocrine disorders, section 6.7.1

Cautions: section 6.7.1
HYPOTENSIVE REACTIONS. Hypotensive reactions may be disturbing in some patients during the first few days of treatment and particular care should be exercised when driving or operating machinery; tolerance may be reduced by alcohol

Contra-indications: section 6.7.1

Side-effects: section 6.7.1

Dose: first week 1–1.25 mg at night, second week 2–2.5 mg at night, third week 2.5 mg twice daily, fourth week 2.5 mg 3 times daily then increasing by 2.5 mg every 3–14 days according to response to a usual range of 10–40 mg daily; taken with food

Preparations
Section 6.7.1

CABERGOLINE

Indications: adjunct to levodopa (with dopa-decarboxylase inhibitor) in Parkinson's disease; endocrine disorders (section 6.7.1)

Cautions: section 6.7.1
HYPOTENSIVE REACTIONS. Hypotensive reactions may be disturbing in some patients during the first few days of treatment and particular care should be exercised when driving or operating machinery; tolerance may be reduced by alcohol

Contra-indications: section 6.7.1

Side-effects: section 6.7.1

Dose: initially 1 mg daily, increased by increments of 0.5–1 mg at 7 or 14 day intervals; usual range 2–6 mg daily
Note. Concurrent dose of levodopa may be decreased gradually while dose of cabergoline is increased

Cabaser® (Pharmacia & Upjohn) ▼ PoM

Tablets, all scored, cabergoline 1 mg, net price 20-tab pack = £75.45; 2 mg, 20-tab pack = £75.45; 4 mg, 16-tab pack = £60.36. Label: 21, counselling, hypotensive reactions

Note. Dispense in original container (contains desiccant)

ENTACAPONE

Indications: adjunct to levodopa with dopa-decarboxylase inhibitor in Parkinson's disease and 'end-of-dose' motor fluctuations

Cautions: concurrent levodopa dose may need to be reduced by about 10–30%; **interactions:** Appendix 1 (entacapone)

Contra-indications: pregnancy and breast-feeding; hepatic impairment; phaeochromocytoma; history of neuroleptic malignant syndrome or non-traumatic rhabdomyolysis

Side-effects: nausea, vomiting, abdominal pain, constipation, diarrhoea, urine may be coloured reddish-brown, dry mouth, dyskinesias; dizziness; anaemia reported; rarely elevated liver enzymes

Dose: 200 mg with each dose of levodopa with dopa-decarboxylase inhibitor; max. 2 g daily

Comtess® (Orion) ▼ PoM

Tablets, f/c, brown/orange, entacapone 200 mg, net price 30-tab pack = £19.05, 100-tab pack = £63.50. Label: 14 (urine reddish-brown)

LISURIDE MALEATE

(Lysuride Maleate)

Indications: Parkinson's disease

Cautions: history of pituitary tumour; history of psychotic disturbance; pregnancy; porphyria (section 9.8.2); **interactions:** Appendix 1 (lysuride)

HYPOTENSIVE REACTIONS. Hypotensive reactions may be disturbing in some patients during the first few days of treatment and particular care should be exercised when driving or operating machinery

Contra-indications: severe disturbances of peripheral circulation; coronary insufficiency

Side-effects: see notes above; nausea and vomiting; dizziness; headache, lethargy, malaise, drowsiness, psychotic reactions (including hallucinations); occasionally severe hypotension, rashes; rarely abdominal pain and constipation; Raynaud's phenomenon reported

Dose: initially 200 micrograms at bedtime with food increased as necessary at weekly intervals to 200 micrograms twice daily (midday and bedtime) then to 200 micrograms 3 times daily (morning, midday, and bedtime); further increases made by adding 200 micrograms each week first to the bedtime dose, then to the midday dose and finally to the morning dose; max. 5 mg daily in 3 divided doses after food

Lisuride Maleate (Non-proprietary) PoM

Tablets, scored, lisuride maleate 200 micrograms. Net price 100-tab pack = £41.92. Label: 21, counselling, hypotensive reactions

Available from Cambridge

Note. The brand name *Revanil®* was formerly used for lisuride maleate tablets

PERGOLIDE

Indications: adjunct to levodopa in Parkinson's disease

Cautions: arrhythmias or underlying cardiac disease, history of confusion or hallucinations, dyskinesia (may cause or exacerbate), pregnancy, breast-feeding; increase dose gradually and avoid abrupt withdrawal; porphyria (section 9.8.2); **interactions:** Appendix 1 (pergolide)

HYPOTENSIVE REACTIONS. Hypotensive reactions may be disturbing in some patients during the first few days of treatment and particular care should be exercised when driving or operating machinery

Side-effects: see notes above; hallucinations, confusion, dizziness, dyskinesia, somnolence, abdominal pain, nausea, dyspepsia, diplopia, rhinitis, dyspnoea, pleuritis, pleural effusion, pleural fibrosis, pericarditis, pericardial effusion and retroperitoneal fibrosis, insomnia, constipation or diarrhoea, hypotension, syncope, tachycardia and atrial premature contractions, rash, fever reported; neuroleptic malignant syndrome also reported

Dose: 50 micrograms daily for 2 days, increased gradually by 100–150 micrograms every third day over next 12 days, usually given in 3 divided doses; further increases of 250 micrograms every third day; usual maintenance 3 mg daily (above 5 mg daily not evaluated); during pergolide titration levodopa dose may be reduced cautiously

Celance® (Lilly) PoM

Tablets, all scored, pergolide (as mesilate) 50 micrograms (ivory), net price 100-tab pack = £27.03; 250 micrograms (green), 100-tab pack = £40.77; 1 mg (pink), 100-tab pack = £147.15; 14-day starter pack of 75 × 50-microgram tablets with 6 × 250-microgram tablets = £22.49. Counselling, hypotensive reactions

PRAMIPEXOLE

Indications: adjunct to levodopa in advanced Parkinson's disease

Cautions: renal impairment (Appendix 3); psychotic disorders; ophthalmological testing recommended (risk of visual disorders); severe cardiovascular disease; pregnancy (Appendix 4); **interactions:** Appendix 1 (pramipexole)

HYPOTENSIVE REACTIONS. Hypotensive reactions may be disturbing in some patients during the first few days of treatment

DRIVING. Drowsiness (including sudden onset of sleep) may affect performance of skilled tasks; patients should **not** drive or undertake potentially dangerous activities

Contra-indications: breast-feeding (Appendix 5)

Side-effects: nausea, constipation, drowsiness (including sudden onset of sleep), hallucinations (mostly visual), dyskinesia during initial dose titration (more frequent in women—reduce levodopa dose)

Dose: initially, 264 micrograms daily in 3 divided doses, doubling the dose every 5–7 days to 1.08 mg daily in 3 divided doses; further increased if necessary by 540 micrograms daily at weekly intervals; max. 3.3 mg daily in 3 divided doses

Note. During pramipexole dose titration and maintenance, levodopa dose may be reduced

Important. Doses and strengths are stated in terms of pramipexole (base); equivalent strengths in terms of pramipexole dihydrochloride monohydrate (salt) are as follows: 88 micrograms base ≡ 125 micrograms salt; 180 micrograms base ≡ 250 micrograms salt; 700 micrograms base ≡ 1 mg salt

Mirapexin® (Pharmacia & Upjohn) ▼ PoM
Tablets, pramipexole (as hydrochloride)
88 micrograms, net price 30-tab pack = £7.96;
180 micrograms (scored), 30-tab pack = £15.92,
100-tab pack = £53.06; 700 micrograms (scored),
30-tab pack = £63.67, 100-tab pack = £212.24.
Counselling, hypotensive reactions, driving

ROPINIROLE

Indications: Parkinson's disease, either used alone
or as an adjunct to levodopa; see also notes above

Cautions: severe cardiovascular disease, major
psychotic disorders, avoid abrupt withdrawal;
interactions: Appendix 1 (ropinirole)

DRIVING. Drowsiness (including sudden onset of sleep)
may affect performance of skilled tasks; patients should
not drive or undertake potentially dangerous activities

Contra-indications: hepatic and severe renal
impairment; pregnancy and breast-feeding

Side-effects: nausea, drowsiness (including sudden onset of sleep), leg oedema, abdominal pain,
vomiting and syncope; dyskinesia, hallucinations
and confusion reported in adjunctive therapy;
occasionally severe hypotension and bradycardia

Dose: initially 750 micrograms daily in 3 divided
doses, increased by increments of
750 micrograms at weekly intervals to 3 mg daily;
further increased by increments of up to 3 mg at
weekly intervals according to response; usual
range 3–9 mg daily (but higher doses may be
required if used with levodopa); max. 24 mg daily

Note. When administered as adjunct to levodopa, concurrent dose of levodopa may be reduced by approx.
20%

Requip® (SmithKline Beecham) PoM
Tablets, f/c, ropinirole (as hydrochloride)
250 micrograms (white), net price 210-tab starter
pack = £43.12; 1 mg (green), 84-tab pack =
£46.20; 2 mg (pink), 84-tab pack = £92.40; 5 mg
(blue), 84-tab pack = £184.80. Label: 21, counselling, driving

SELEGILINE HYDROCHLORIDE

Indications: Parkinson's disease or symptomatic
parkinsonism (but not drug-induced extrapyramidal symptoms), used alone (in early disease) or
as adjunct to levodopa (but see notes above)

Cautions: gastric and duodenal ulceration (avoid
in active ulceration), uncontrolled hypertension,
arrhythmias, angina, psychosis, pregnancy and
breast-feeding, side-effects of levodopa may be
increased, concurrent levodopa dosage may need
to be reduced by 10–50%; **interactions:** Appendix 1 (selegiline)

Side-effects: constipation, diarrhoea, nausea and
vomiting, dry mouth, stomatitis, sore throat,
hypotension, depression, confusion, psychosis,
agitation, headache, tremor, dizziness, vertigo,
sleep disturbances; back pain, muscle cramps,
joint pain, difficulty in micturition, skin reactions
transient increase in liver enzymes reported

Dose: 10 mg in the morning, or 5 mg at breakfast
and midday; ELDERLY see below

ELDERLY. To avoid initial confusion and agitation, it may
be appropriate to start treatment with a dose of 2.5 mg
daily, particularly in the elderly

Selegiline Hydrochloride (Non-proprietary)
PoM
Tablets, selegiline hydrochloride 5 mg, net price
60-tab pack = £14.34; 10 mg, 30-tab pack =
£20.23
Available from Berk (*Stilline®*), Bioglan, Cox, Hillcross,
Lagap, Norton, Opus (*Centrapryl®*), Sanofi-Synthelabo

Eldepryl® (Orion) PoM
Tablets, both scored, selegiline hydrochloride
5 mg, net price 60-tab pack = £20.70; 10 mg, 30-
tab pack = £20.19
Oral liquid, selegiline hydrochloride 10 mg/5 mL,
net price 200-mL = £37.44

■ Oral lyophilisate

Zelapar® (Athena) PoM
Oral lyophilisates (= freeze-dried tablets), yellow,
selegiline hydrochloride 1.25 mg, net price 30-tab
pack = £55.50. Counselling, administration
Dose: initially 1.25 mg daily before breakfast
COUNSELLING. Tablets should be placed on the tongue
and allowed to dissolve. Advise patient not to drink,
rinse, or wash mouth out for 5 minutes after taking the
tablet
Excipients: include aspartame (section 9.4.1)
Note. Patients receiving 10 mg conventional selegiline
hydrochloride tablets can be switched to *Zelapar®*
1.25 mg

4.9.2 Antimuscarinic drugs used in parkinsonism

Antimuscarinic drugs (less correctly termed 'anticholinergics') are less effective than levodopa in
idiopathic Parkinson's disease although they may
supplement its action. Patients with mild symptoms, particularly where tremor predominates, may
be treated initially with antimuscarinic drugs (alone
or with selegiline, section 4.9.1), levodopa being
added or substituted as symptoms progress. They
have value in post-encephalitic parkinsonism.

Antimuscarinic drugs exert their antiparkinsonian
effect by correcting the relative central cholinergic
excess thought to occur in parkinsonism as a result
of dopamine deficiency. They reduce tremor and
rigidity but have little effect on bradykinesia. They
are useful in reducing sialorrhoea.

The antimuscarinic drugs also reduce the symptoms of drug-induced parkinsonism as seen, for
example, with antipsychotic drugs (section 4.2.1)
but there is no justification for giving them with
antipsychotics unless parkinsonian side-effects
occur. Tardive dyskinesia is not improved by the
antimuscarinic drugs and may be made worse.

No important differences exist between the many
synthetic antimuscarinic drugs available but some
patients appear to tolerate one better than another.
They may be taken before food if dry mouth is troublesome, or after food if gastro-intestinal symptoms
predominate. Those most commonly used are
orphenadrine and **trihexyphenidyl (benzhexol)**;
benzatropine and **procyclidine** are also used. Benzatropine is similar to trihexyphenidyl but is
excreted more slowly; changes in dose therefore
need to be carried out very gradually.

Procyclidine and benzatropine may be given
parenterally and are effective emergency treatment
for acute drug-induced dystonic reactions which
may be severe.

TRIHEXYPHENIDYL HYDROCHLORIDE/ BENZHEXOL HYDROCHLORIDE

Indications: parkinsonism; drug-induced extra-pyramidal symptoms (but not tardive dyskinesia, see notes above)

Cautions: cardiovascular disease, hepatic or renal impairment; elderly; avoid abrupt discontinuation of treatment; liable to abuse (may produce euphoric effect); **interactions:** Appendix 1 (anti-muscarinics)

DRIVING. May affect performance of skilled tasks (e.g. driving)

Contra-indications: untreated urinary retention, angle-closure glaucoma, gastro-intestinal obstruction

Side-effects: dry mouth, gastro-intestinal disturbances, dizziness, blurred vision; less commonly urinary retention, tachycardia, hypersensitivity, nervousness, and with high doses in susceptible patients, mental confusion, excitement, and psychiatric disturbances which may necessitate discontinuation of treatment

Dose: 1 mg daily, gradually increased; usual maintenance dose 5–15 mg daily in 3–4 divided doses; ELDERLY preferably lower end of range

Trihexyphenidyl/Benzhexol (Non-proprietary) PoM

Tablets, trihexyphenidyl hydrochloride 2 mg, net price 20 = 44p; 5 mg, 20 = 80p. Counselling, before or after food (see notes above), driving
Available from Genus

Broflex® (Alliance) PoM

Syrup, pink, trihexyphenidyl hydrochloride 5 mg/ 5 mL. Net price 200 mL = £6.36. Counselling, before or after food (see notes above), driving

BENZATROPINE MESILATE

Benztropine mesylate

Indications: see under Trihexyphenidyl Hydrochloride

Cautions: see under Trihexyphenidyl Hydrochloride

Contra-indications: see under Trihexyphenidyl Hydrochloride; avoid in children under 3 years

Side-effects: see under Trihexyphenidyl Hydrochloride, but causes sedation rather than stimulation

Dose: *by mouth,* 0.5–1 mg daily usually at bedtime, gradually increased; max. 6 mg daily; usual maintenance dose 1–4 mg daily in single or divided doses; ELDERLY preferably lower end of range
By intramuscular or intravenous injection, 1–2 mg, repeated if symptoms reappear; ELDERLY preferably lower end of range

Cogentin® (MSD) PoM

Tablets, scored, benzatropine mesilate 2 mg. Net price 20 = 29p. Label: 2
Injection, benzatropine mesilate 1 mg/mL. Net price 2-mL amp = 92p

BIPERIDEN

Indications: see under Trihexyphenidyl Hydrochloride

Cautions: see under Trihexyphenidyl Hydrochloride

Contra-indications: see under Trihexyphenidyl Hydrochloride

Side-effects: see under Trihexyphenidyl Hydrochloride, but may cause drowsiness; injection may cause hypotension

Dose: *by mouth,* biperiden hydrochloride 1 mg twice daily, gradually increased to 2 mg 3 times daily; usual maintenance dose 3–12 mg daily in divided doses; ELDERLY preferably lower end of range
By intramuscular or slow intravenous injection, biperiden lactate 2.5–5 mg up to 4 times daily; ELDERLY preferably lower end of range

Akineton® (Knoll) PoM

Tablets, scored, biperiden hydrochloride 2 mg. Net price 100-tab pack = £4.60. Label: 2
Injection, biperiden lactate 5 mg/mL. Net price 1-mL amp = 69p

ORPHENADRINE HYDROCHLORIDE

Indications: see under Trihexyphenidyl Hydrochloride

Cautions: see under Trihexyphenidyl Hydrochloride

Contra-indications: see under Trihexyphenidyl Hydrochloride; porphyria (section 9.8.2)

Side-effects: see under Trihexyphenidyl Hydrochloride, but more euphoric; may cause insomnia

Dose: 150 mg daily in divided doses, gradually increased; max. 400 mg daily; ELDERLY preferably lower end of range

Orphenadrine Hydrochloride (Non-proprietary) PoM

Oral solution, orphenadrine hydrochloride 50 mg/ 5 mL. Net price 200 mL = £7.25. Counselling, driving
Available from Rosemont (sugar-free)

Biorphen® (Alliance) PoM

Elixir, sugar-free, orphenadrine hydrochloride 25 mg/5 mL. Net price 200 mL = £7.25. Counselling, driving

Disipal® (Yamanouchi) PoM

Tablets, yellow, s/c, orphenadrine hydrochloride 50 mg. Net price 20 = 69p. Counselling, driving
Excipients: include tartrazine

PROCYCLIDINE HYDROCHLORIDE

Indications: see under Trihexyphenidyl Hydrochloride

Cautions: see under Trihexyphenidyl Hydrochloride

Contra-indications: see under Trihexyphenidyl Hydrochloride

Side-effects: see under Trihexyphenidyl Hydrochloride

Dose: *by mouth,* 2.5 mg 3 times daily, gradually increased if necessary; usual max. 30 mg daily (60 mg daily in exceptional circumstances); ELDERLY preferably lower end of range
Acute dystonia, *by intramuscular injection,* 5–10 mg repeated if necessary after 20 minutes; max. 20 mg daily; *by intravenous injection,* 5 mg (usually effective within 5 minutes); an occasional patient may need 10 mg or more and may require up to half an hour to obtain relief; ELDERLY preferably lower end of dose range

Procyclidine (Non-proprietary) [PoM]

Tablets, procyclidine hydrochloride 5 mg. Net price 20 = £1.07. Counselling, driving

Available from Cox, Opus (*Mucinil®*)

Arpicolin® (Rosemont) [PoM]

Syrup, sugar-free, procyclidine hydrochloride 2.5 mg/5 mL, net price 150 mL = £4.70; 5 mg/ 5 mL, 150 mL pack = £8.40. Counselling, driving

Kemadrin® (GlaxoWellcome) [PoM]

Tablets, scored, procyclidine hydrochloride 5 mg. Net price 20 = £1.17. Counselling, driving

Injection, procyclidine hydrochloride 5 mg/mL. Net price 2-mL amp = £1.49

4.9.3 Drugs used in essential tremor, chorea, tics, and related disorders

Tetrabenazine is mainly used to control movement disorders in Huntington's chorea and related disorders. It may act by depleting nerve endings of dopamine. It has useful action in only a proportion of patients and its use may be limited by the development of depression.

Haloperidol may be useful in improving motor tics and symptoms of Gilles de la Tourette syndrome and related choreas. **Pimozide** (see section 4.2.1 for CSM warning), **clonidine** (section 4.7.4.2) and **sulpiride** (section 4.2.1) are also used in Gilles de la Tourette syndrome. **Trihexyphenidyl (benzhexol)** (section 4.9.2) at high dosage may also improve some movement disorders; it is sometimes necessary to build the dose up over many weeks, to 20 to 30 mg daily or higher. **Chlorpromazine** and **haloperidol** are used to relieve intractable hiccup (section 4.2.1).

Propranolol or another beta-adrenoceptor blocking drug (section 2.4) may be useful in treating essential tremor or tremors associated with anxiety or thyrotoxicosis. Propranolol is given in a dosage of 40 mg 2 or 3 times daily, increased if necessary; 80 to 160 mg daily is usually required for maintenance.

Primidone (section 4.8.3) in some cases provides relief from benign essential tremor; the dose is increased slowly to reduce side-effects.

Piracetam is used as an adjunctive treatment for myoclonus of cortical origin.

Riluzole is used to extend life or the time to mechanical ventilation in patients with amyotrophic lateral sclerosis. Treatment should only be initiated by physicians experienced in treating motor neurone disease.

HALOPERIDOL

Indications: motor tics, adjunctive treatment in choreas and Gilles de la Tourette syndrome; other indications, section 4.2.1

Cautions: section 4.2.1

Contra-indications: section 4.2.1

Side-effects: section 4.2.1

Dose: *by mouth*, 0.5–1.5 mg 3 times daily adjusted according to the response; 10 mg daily or more may occasionally be necessary in Gilles de la Tourette syndrome; CHILD, Gilles de la Tourette syndrome up to 10 mg daily

Preparations
Section 4.2.1

PIRACETAM

Indications: adjunctive treatment of cortical myoclonus

Cautions: avoid abrupt withdrawal; elderly; renal impairment (avoid if severe)

Contra-indications: hepatic and severe renal impairment; pregnancy and breast-feeding

Side-effects: diarrhoea, weight gain; somnolence, insomnia, nervousness, depression; hyperkinesia; rash

Dose: initially 7.2 g daily in 2–3 divided doses, increased according to response by 4.8 g daily every 3–4 days to max. 20 g daily (subsequently, attempts should be made to reduce dose of concurrent therapy); CHILD under 16 years not recommended

ORAL SOLUTION. Follow the oral solution with a glass of water (or soft drink) to reduce bitter taste.

Nootropil® (UCB Pharma) ▼ [PoM]

Tablets, f/c, scored, piracetam 800 mg, net price 90-tab pack = £15.80; 1.2 g, 56-tab pack = £14.74. Label: 3

Oral solution, piracetam, 333.3 mg/mL, net price 300-mL pack = £21.93. Label: 3

RILUZOLE

Indications: to extend life or the time to mechanical ventilation for patients with amyotrophic lateral sclerosis, initiated by specialist physicians experienced in the management of motor neurone disease

Cautions: history of abnormal hepatic function (see product literature for details); **interactions:** Appendix 1 (riluzole)

BLOOD DISORDERS. Patients or their carers should be told how to recognise signs of neutropenia and advised to seek immediate medical attention if symptoms such as fever occur; white blood cell counts should be determined in febrile illness; neutropenia requires discontinuation of riluzole

DRIVING. Dizziness or vertigo may affect performance of skilled tasks (e.g. driving)

Contra-indications: hepatic and renal impairment; pregnancy and breast-feeding

Side-effects: nausea, vomiting, asthenia, tachycardia, somnolence, headache, dizziness, vertigo, abdominal pain, circumoral paraesthesia, alterations in liver function tests

Dose: 50 mg twice daily; CHILD not recommended

Rilutek® (Rhône-Poulenc Rorer) [PoM]

Tablets, f/c, riluzole 50 mg. Net price 56-tab pack = £286.00. Counselling, blood disorders, driving

TETRABENAZINE

Indications: movement disorders due to Huntington's chorea, hemiballismus, senile chorea, and related neurological conditions

Cautions: pregnancy; avoid in breast-feeding; **interactions:** Appendix 1 (tetrabenazine)

DRIVING. May affect performance of skilled tasks (e.g. driving)

Side-effects: drowsiness, gastro-intestinal disturbances, depression, extrapyramidal dysfunction, hypotension; rarely parkinsonism; neuroleptic malignant syndrome reported

Dose: initially 12.5 mg twice daily (elderly 12.5 mg daily) gradually increased to 12.5–25 mg 3 times daily; max. 200 mg daily

Tetrabenazine (Cambridge) [PoM]
Tablets, pale yellow-buff, scored, tetrabenazine 25 mg. Net price 112-tab pack = £100.00. Label: 2

Torsion dystonias and other involuntary movements

BOTULINUM A TOXIN-HAEMAGGLUTININ COMPLEX

Indications: dynamic equinus foot deformity due to spasticity in ambulant paediatric cerebral palsy patients over 2 years (only *Botox*® licensed); blepharospasm; hemifacial spasm; spasmodic torticollis (all specialist use only)

Cautions: potential for anaphylaxis; **interactions:** Appendix 1 (botulinum toxin)

SPECIFIC CAUTIONS WHEN TREATING BLEPHAROSPASM OR HEMIFACIAL SPASM. Avoid deep or misplaced injections—relevant anatomy (and any alterations due to previous surgery) must be understood before injecting; reduced blinking can lead to corneal exposure, persistent epithelial defect and corneal ulceration (especially in those with VIIth nerve disorders)—careful testing of corneal sensation in previously operated eyes, avoidance of injection in lower lid area to avoid ectropion and vigorous treatment of epithelial defect needed

SPECIFIC CAUTIONS WHEN TREATING TORTICOLLIS. Patients with defective neuromuscular transmission (risk of excessive muscle weakness)

COUNSELLING. All patients should be alerted to possible side-effects

Contra-indications: generalised disorders of muscle activity (e.g. myasthenia gravis); bleeding disorders; pregnancy and breast-feeding

Side-effects: increased electrophysiologic jitter in some distant muscles; misplaced injections may paralyse nearby muscle groups and excessive doses may paralyse distant muscles; rash; antibody formation (substantial deterioration in response); transient burning sensation after injection

SPECIFIC SIDE-EFFECTS WHEN TREATING PAEDIATRIC CEREBRAL PALSY. Leg pain, weakness; rarely leg cramps, fever, knee and ankle pain, lethargy

SPECIFIC SIDE-EFFECTS WHEN TREATING BLEPHAROSPASM OR HEMIFACIAL SPASM. Ptosis, lacrimation and irritation (including dry eye, lagophthalmos and photophobia); also ectropion, keratitis, diplopia and entropion; angle-closure glaucoma reported; bruising and ecchymosis in soft eyelid tissues minimised by applying gentle pressure at injection site immediately after injection

SPECIFIC SIDE-EFFECTS WHEN TREATING TORTICOLLIS. Dysphagia and pooling of saliva (occurs most frequently after injection into sternomastoid muscle); dry mouth, voice changes, weakness of neck muscles; generalised muscle weakness, malaise, nausea, diplopia and blurred vision; rarely respiratory difficulties (associated with high doses), drowsiness, numbness, stiffness, ptosis, headache, fever, influenza-like syndrome; CSM has warned of persistent dysphagia and sequelae (including death)—**important**, see also under Cautions

Dose: consult product literature (**important:** specific to **each individual preparation** and **not interchangeable**)

Botox® (Allergan) [PoM]
Injection, powder for reconstitution, botulinum A toxin-haemagglutinin complex, net price 100-unit vial = £128.93

Dysport® (Ipsen) [PoM]
Injection, powder for reconstitution, botulinum A toxin-haemagglutinin complex, net price 500-unit vial = £164.74

4.10   Drugs used in substance dependence

This section includes drugs used in alcohol dependence, cigarette smoking, and opioid dependence.

The health departments of the UK have produced a report, *Drug Misuse and Dependence* which contains guidelines on clinical management.

Drug Misuse and Dependence, London, The Stationery Office, 1999 can be obtained from:

The Publications Centre
PO Box 276, London SW8 5DT
Telephone orders (087) 0600 5522
Fax (087) 0600 5533

or from The Stationery Office bookshops and through all good booksellers.

It is **important** to be aware that *people who misuse drugs* may be at risk not only from the intrinsic toxicity of the drug itself but also from the practice of injecting preparations intended for administration by mouth. Excipients used in the production of oral dose forms are usually insoluble and may lead to *abscess formation at the site of injection*, or even to *necrosis and gangrene*; moreover, deposits in the heart or lungs may lead to *severe cardiac or pulmonary toxicity*. Additional hazards include *infection* following the use of a dirty needle or an unsterilised diluent.

Alcohol dependence

Disulfiram (*Antabuse*®) is used as an adjunct to the treatment of alcohol dependence. It gives rise to extremely unpleasant systemic reactions after the ingestion of even small amounts of alcohol because it leads to accumulation of acetaldehyde in the body. Reactions include flushing of the face, throbbing headache, palpitations, tachycardia, nausea, vomiting, and, with large doses of alcohol, arrhythmias, hypotension, and collapse. Even the small amounts of alcohol included in many oral medicines may be sufficient to precipitate a reaction (even toiletries containing alcohol should be avoided). It may be advisable for patients to carry a card warning of the danger of administration of alcohol.

Benzodiazepines (section 4.1) are used to attenuate withdrawal symptoms but they also have a dependence potential. To minimise the risk of dependence, administration should be for a limited period only (e.g. **chlordiazepoxide** 10–50 mg 4 times daily, gradually reducing over 7–14 days). Benzodiazepines should not be prescribed if the patient is likely to continue drinking alcohol.

Clomethiazole (chlormethiazole) (section 4.1.1) can be used in the management of withdrawal but again has a dependence potential and should not be prescribed if the patient is likely to continue drinking alcohol.

Acamprosate, in combination with counselling, may be helpful in maintaining abstinence in alcohol-dependent patients. It should be initiated as soon as possible *after* abstinence has been achieved and should be maintained if the patient relapses. Continued alcohol abuse, however, negates the therapeutic benefit of acamprosate.

ACAMPROSATE CALCIUM

Indications: maintenance of abstinence in alcohol dependence

Cautions: continued alcohol abuse (risk of treatment failure)

Contra-indications: renal and severe hepatic impairment; pregnancy and breast-feeding

Side-effects: diarrhoea, nausea, vomiting, abdominal pain, pruritus, occasionally maculopapular rash, rarely bullous skin reactions; fluctuation in libido

Dose: ADULT 18–65 years, 60 kg and over, 666 mg 3 times daily; less than 60 kg, 666 mg at breakfast, 333 mg at midday and 333 mg at night

TREATMENT COURSE. Treatment should be initiated as soon as possible after alcohol withdrawal period and maintained if patient relapses; recommended treatment period 1 year

Campral EC® (Lipha) PoM
Tablet, e/c, acamprosate calcium 333 mg. Net price 84-tab pack = £24.95. Label: 21, 25
Electrolytes: Ca²⁺ 0.8 mmol/tablet

DISULFIRAM

Indications: adjunct in the treatment of chronic alcohol dependence (under specialist supervision)

Cautions: ensure that alcohol not consumed for at least 24 hours before initiating treatment; see also notes above; alcohol challenge **not** recommended on routine basis (if considered essential—specialist units only with resuscitation facilities); hepatic or renal impairment, respiratory disease, diabetes mellitus, epilepsy; **interactions:** Appendix 1 (disulfiram)

ALCOHOL REACTION. Patients should be warned of unpredictable and occasionally severe nature of disulfiram-alcohol interactions. Reactions can occur within 10 minutes and last several hours (may require intensive supportive therapy—oxygen should be available). Patients should not ingest alcohol at all and should be warned of possible presence of alcohol in liquid medicines, remedies, tonics, foods and even in toiletries (alcohol should also be avoided for at least 1 week after stopping)

Contra-indications: cardiac failure, coronary artery disease, history of cerebrovascular accident, hypertension, psychosis, severe personality disorder, suicide risk, pregnancy, breast-feeding

Side-effects: initially drowsiness and fatigue; nausea, vomiting, halitosis, reduced libido; rarely psychotic reactions (depression, paranoia, schizophrenia, mania), allergic dermatitis, peripheral neuritis, hepatic cell damage

Dose: 800 mg as a single dose on first day, reducing over 5 days to 100–200 mg daily; should not be continued for longer than 6 months without review; CHILD not recommended

Antabuse® (Dumex) PoM
Tablets, scored, disulfiram 200 mg. Net price 50-tab pack = £18.38. Label: 2, counselling, alcohol reaction

Cigarette smoking

Nicotine chewing gum, patches, inhalation, sublingual tablets, or nasal spray may be used as an adjunct to counselling but are not generally available on the NHS.

Treatment with a nicotine replacement product should be continued for 10–12 weeks with gradual withdrawal over this period. If abstinence has not been achieved within 3 months, treatment should be reviewed.

NICOTINE PRODUCTS

Indications: adjunct to smoking cessation

Cautions: cardiovascular disease (avoid if severe); peripheral vascular disease; hyperthyroidism; diabetes mellitus; phaeochromocytoma, renal and hepatic impairment; history of gastritis and peptic ulcers; should not smoke or use nicotine replacement products in combination; *patches*, exercise may increase absorption and side-effects, skin disorders (patches should not be placed on broken skin); **interactions:** Appendix 1 (nicotine and tobacco)

DRIVING. The nasal spray should not be used when driving or operating machinery (sneezing or watering eyes could contribute to accident)

Contra-indications: severe cardiovascular disease (including severe arrhythmias or immediate post-myocardial infarction period); recent cerebrovascular accident (including transient ischaemic attacks); pregnancy and breast-feeding; *patches*, chronic generalised skin disease (patches should not be placed on broken skin); patches not for occasional smokers

Side-effects: nausea, dizziness, headache and cold and influenza-like symptoms, palpitations, dyspepsia and other gastro-intestinal disturbances, hiccups, insomnia, vivid dreams, myalgia; other side-effects reported include chest pain, blood pressure changes, anxiety and irritability, somnolence and impaired concentration, dysmenorrhoea; *with patches*, skin reactions (discontinue if severe)—vasculitis also reported; *with spray*, nasal irritation, nose bleeds, watering eyes, ear sensations; *with gum, sublingual tablets* or *inhalator*, aphthous ulceration (sometimes with swelling of tongue); *with spray, inhalator, sublingual* *tablets* or *gum*, throat irritation; *with inhalator,* cough, rhinitis, pharyngitis, stomatitis, sinusitis, dry mouth; *with sublingual tablets,* unpleasant taste

Dose: see under preparations, below
Note. Proprietary brands of nicotine products on sale to the public include *Boots Nicotine Gum* 2 mg, 4 mg and *Boots NRT Patch* 5 mg/16 hours, 10 mg/16 hours, 15 mg/16 hours

Nicorette® (Pharmacia & Upjohn)
Nicorette Microtab (sublingual), nicotine (as a cyclodextrin complex) 2 mg, net price starter pack of 2 × 15-tablet discs with dispenser = £3.57; refill pack of 7 × 15-tablet discs = £9.84. Label: 26
Dose: individuals smoking 20 cigarettes or less daily, *sublingually,* 2 mg each hour; for patients who fail to stop smoking or have significant withdrawal symptoms, consider increasing to 4 mg each hour
Individuals smoking more than 20 cigarettes daily, 4 mg each hour
Max. 80 mg daily; treatment should be continued for at least 3 months followed by a gradual reduction in dosage; max. period of treatment should not exceed 6 months
CHILD under 18 years not recommended

Nicorette chewing gum DHS, sugar-free, nicotine (as resin) 2 mg, net price pack of 15 = £1.71, pack of 30 = £3.25, pack of 105 = £8.89; 4 mg, net price pack of 15 = £2.11, pack of 30 = £3.99, pack of 105 = £10.83
Note. Also available in mint flavour
Dose: individuals smoking 20 cigarettes or fewer daily, initially one 2-mg piece chewed slowly for approx. 30 minutes, when urge to smoke occurs; individuals smoking more than 20 cigarettes daily or needing more than 15 pieces of 2-mg gum daily may need the 4-mg strength; max. 15 pieces of 4-mg strength daily; withdraw gradually after 3 months; CHILD under 18 years not recommended

Nicorette patches DHS, self-adhesive, all beige, nicotine, *'5 mg' patch* (releasing approx. 5 mg/16 hours), net price 7 = £7.20; *'10 mg' patch* (releasing approx. 10 mg/16 hours), 7 = £8.36; *'15 mg' patch* (releasing approx. 15 mg/16 hours), 7 = £9.07,
ADMINISTRATION: apply on waking to dry, non-hairy skin on hip, chest or upper arm, removing after approx. 16 hours, usually when retiring to bed; site next patch on different area (avoid using same area for several days); initially '15-mg' patch for 16 hours daily for 8 weeks then '10-mg' patch for 16 hours daily for 2 weeks then '5-mg' patch for 16 hours daily for 2 weeks; review treatment if abstinence not achieved in 3 months; CHILD not recommended

Nicorette nasal spray PoM DHS, nicotine 500 micrograms/metered spray. Net price 200-spray unit = £10.99
ADMINISTRATION: Apply 1 spray into each nostril as required to max. twice an hour for 16 hours daily (max. 64 sprays daily) for 8 weeks, then reduce gradually over next 4 weeks (reduce by half at end of first 2 weeks, stop altogether at end of next 2 weeks); max. treatment length 3 months; CHILD under 16 years not recommended

Nicorette inhalator (nicotine-impregnated plug for use in inhalator mouthpiece), nicotine 10 mg/cartridge. Net price 6-cartridge (starter) pack = £3.39, 42-cartridge (refill) pack = £11.37
ADMINISTRATION: Inhale when urge to smoke occurs; initially use between 6 and 12 cartridges daily for up to 8 weeks, then reduce number of cartridges used by half

over next 2 weeks and then stop altogether at end of further 2 weeks; review treatment if abstinence not achieved in 3 months; CHILD under 18 years not recommended

Nicotinell® (Novartis Consumer Health)
Chewing gum DHS, sugar-free, nicotine 2 mg, net price pack of 12 = £1.45, pack of 48 = £5.13, pack of 96 = £8.26; 4 mg, pack of 12 = £1.57, pack of 48 = £5.70, pack of 96 = £9.12
Note. Also available in fruit and mint flavours
Dose: initially one 2-mg piece chewed slowly for approx. 30 minutes, when urge to smoke occurs; max. 15 pieces daily; withdraw gradually after 3 months; CHILD under 18 years not recommended

Nicotinell mint lozenge, sugar-free, nicotine (as bitartrate) 1 mg, net price pack of 12 = £1.71, pack of 36 = £4.27, pack of 96 = £9.12. Label: 24
Excipients: include aspartame (section 9.4.1)
Dose: initially 1 lozenge every 1–2 hours, when urge to smoke occurs; max. 25 lozenges daily; withdraw gradually after 3 months; max. period of treatment should not usually exceed 6 months

TTS Patches DHS, self-adhesive, all yellowish-ochre, nicotine, *'10' patch* (releasing approx. 7 mg/24 hours), net price 7 = £9.12; *'20' patch* (releasing approx. 14 mg/24 hours), net price 2 = £2.57, 7 = £9.40; *'30' patch* (releasing approx. 21 mg/24 hours), net price 2 = £2.85, 7 = £9.97, 21 = £24.51
ADMINISTRATION: apply to dry, non-hairy skin on trunk or upper arm, removing after 24 hours and siting replacement patch on a different area (avoid using the same area for several days); individuals smoking 20 cigarettes daily or fewer, initially '20' patch daily; individuals smoking more than 20 cigarettes daily, initially '30' patch daily; withdraw gradually, reducing dose every 3–4 weeks; review treatment if abstinence not achieved in 3 months; CHILD under 18 years not recommended

NiQuitin CQ® (SmithKline Beecham Healthcare)
Patches, self-adhesive, pink/beige, nicotine *'7 mg' patch* (releasing approx. 7 mg/24 hours), net price 7 = £11.38; *'14 mg' patch* (releasing approx. 14 mg/24 hours), 7 = £11.38; *'21 mg' patch* (releasing approx. 21 mg/24 hours), 7 = £11.38, 14 = £20.50
ADMINISTRATION: apply on waking to dry, non-hairy skin site, removing after 24 hours and siting replacement patch on different area (avoid using same area for 7 days); individuals smoking 10 or more cigarettes daily, initially '21-mg' patch daily for 6 weeks then '14-mg' patch daily for 2 weeks then '7-mg' patch daily for 2 weeks; review treatment if abstinence not achieved in 10 weeks
Individuals smoking less than 10 cigarettes daily, initially '14-mg' patch daily for 6 weeks then '7-mg' patch daily for 2 weeks
CHILD not recommended
Note. Patients using the '21-mg' patch who experience excessive side-effects, which do not resolve within a few days, should change to '14-mg' patch for the remainder of the initial 6 weeks before switching to the '7-mg' patch for the final 2 weeks

Opioid dependence

Methadone, an opioid *agonist,* can be substituted for opioids such as diamorphine, preventing the onset of withdrawal symptoms; it is itself addictive and should only be prescribed for those who are physically dependent on opioids. It is administered in a single daily dose usually as methadone mixture 1 mg/mL. The dose is adjusted according to the degree of dependence with the aim of gradual reduction.

Buprenorphine is an opioid with both *agonist* and *antagonist* properties which, because of its abuse and dependence potential should be prescribed only for those who are already physically dependent on opioids. It can be used as substitution therapy for patients with moderate opioid dependence. In patients dependent on high doses of opioids, buprenorphine may precipitate withdrawal due to its partial antagonist properties; in these patients, the daily opioid dose should be reduced gradually before initiating therapy with buprenorphine.

Naltrexone, an opioid *antagonist*, blocks the action of opioids and precipitates withdrawal symptoms in opioid-dependent subjects. Since the euphoric action of opioid agonists is blocked by naltrexone it is given to former addicts as an aid to relapse prevention.

Lofexidine is used for the alleviation of symptoms in patients undergoing opioid withdrawal. Like clonidine it appears to act centrally to produce a reduction in sympathetic tone but reduction in blood pressure is less marked.

BUPRENORPHINE

Indications: adjunct in the treatment of opioid dependence; premedication, peri-operative analgesia, analgesia in other situations (section 4.7.2)

Cautions: see section 4.7.2 and notes above; effects only partially reversed by naloxone

Contra-indications: see section 4.7.2; breast-feeding (Appendix 5)

Side-effects: see section 4.7.2

Dose: *by sublingual administration*, initially, 0.8–4 mg as a single daily dose, adjusted according to response; max. 32 mg daily; withdraw gradually; CHILD under 16 years not recommended

Note. In those who have not undergone opioid withdrawal, buprenorphine should be administered at least 4 hours after last use of opioid or when signs of craving appear

For those receiving methadone, dose of methadone should be reduced to max. 30 mg daily before starting buprenorphine

Subutex® (Schering-Plough) ▼ CD

Tablets (sublingual), buprenorphine (as hydrochloride) 400 micrograms, net price 7-tab pack = £1.60; 2 mg, 7-tab pack = £6.72; 8 mg, 7-tab pack = £20.16. Label: 2, 26

LOFEXIDINE HYDROCHLORIDE

Indications: management of symptoms of opioid withdrawal

Cautions: severe coronary insufficiency, recent myocardial infarction, cerebrovascular disease, marked bradycardia (monitor pulse rate frequently); renal impairment; history of depression (on longer treatment); pregnancy and breast-feeding; withdraw gradually over 2–4 days (or longer) to minimise risk of rebound hypertension and associated symptoms; **interactions:** Appendix 1 (lofexidine)

Side-effects: drowsiness, dry mucous membranes (particularly dry mouth, throat and nose), hypotension, bradycardia, rebound hypertension on

withdrawal (see Cautions); sedation and coma in overdosage

Dose: initially, 200 micrograms twice daily, increased as necessary in steps of 200–400 micrograms daily to max. 2.4 mg daily; recommended duration of treatment 7–10 days if no opioid use (but longer may be required); withdraw gradually over 2–4 days or longer; CHILD not recommended

BritLofex® (Britannia) PoM

Tablets, peach, f/c, lofexidine hydrochloride 200 micrograms. Net price 60-tab pack = £77.95. Label: 2

METHADONE HYDROCHLORIDE

Indications: adjunct in treatment of opioid dependence, see notes above; analgesia (section 4.7.2); cough in terminal disease (section 3.9.1)

Cautions: section 4.7.2

Contra-indications: section 4.7.2

Side-effects: section 4.7.2; **overdosage:** see Emergency Treatment of Poisoning, p. 23

IMPORTANT: Methadone, even in low doses is a **special hazard** for children; non-dependent adults are also at risk; dependent adults are at risk if tolerance is incorrectly assessed during induction

INCOMPATIBILITY. Syrup preserved with hydroxybenzoate esters may be incompatible with methadone hydrochloride.

Dose: initially 10–20 mg daily, increased by 10–20 mg daily until no signs of withdrawal or intoxication; usual dose 40–60 mg daily; CHILD not recommended (see also important note above)

Methadone (Non-proprietary) CD

Mixture 1 mg/mL, methadone hydrochloride 1 mg/mL, net price 30 mL = 46p, 50 mL = 76p, 100 mL = £1.52, 500 mL = £7.59. Label: 2

Available from Generics (*Methex®*), Hillcross, Martindale (*Physeptone*, also as sugar-free), Rosemont (*Metharose®*, sugar-free), Thornton & Ross—taste and colour of different formulations may vary slightly

IMPORTANT. This preparation is 2½ times the strength of Methadone Linctus and is intended only for drug dependent persons for whom treatment may be ordered on form FP10HP(AD) or FP10(MDA), or in Scotland on forms HBP(A) or GP10. The title includes the strength and prescriptions should be written accordingly

Injection, section 4.7.2

Methadose® (Rosemont) CD

Oral concentrate, methadone hydrochloride 10 mg/mL (blue), net price 150 mL = £12.78; 20 mg/mL (brown), 200 mL = £34.07. Label: 2

Note. The final strength of the methadone mixture to be dispensed to the patient must be specified on the prescription

IMPORTANT. Care is required in prescribing and dispensing the **correct strength** since any confusion could lead to an overdose; this preparation should be dispensed only **after dilution** as appropriate with *Methadose® Diluent* (life of diluted solution 3 months) and is for drug dependent persons for whom treatment may be ordered on form FP10HP(AD) or FP10(MDA), or in Scotland on forms HBP(A)

NALTREXONE HYDROCHLORIDE

Indications: adjunct to prevent relapse in detoxified formerly opioid-dependent patients (who have remained opioid-free for at least 7–10 days)

Cautions: hepatic and renal impairment; liver function tests needed before and during treatment; test for opioid dependence with naloxone; avoid concomitant use of opioids but increased dose of opioid analgesic may be required for pain (monitor for opioid intoxication); pregnancy, breast-feeding

WARNING FOR PATIENTS. Patients need to be warned that an attempt to overcome the block could result in acute opioid intoxication

Contra-indications: patients currently dependent on opioids; acute hepatitis or liver failure

Side-effects: nausea, vomiting, abdominal pain; anxiety, nervousness, sleeping difficulty, headache, reduced energy; joint and muscle pain; less frequently, loss of appetite, diarrhoea, constipation, increased thirst; chest pain; increased sweating and lacrimation; increased energy, 'feeling down', irritability, dizziness, chills; delayed ejaculation, decreased potency; rash; occasionally, liver function abnormalities; reversible idiopathic thrombocytopenia reported

Dose: (initiate in specialist clinics only) 25 mg initially then 50 mg daily; the total weekly dose may be divided and given on 3 days of the week for improved compliance (e.g. 100 mg on Monday and Wednesday, and 150 mg on Friday); CHILD not recommended

Nalorex® (Du Pont) PoM
Tablets, yellow, f/c, scored, naltrexone hydrochloride 50 mg. Net price 28-tab pack = £42.51

4.11   Drugs for dementia

Acetylcholinesterase inhibiting drugs are used in the treatment of Alzheimer's disease, specifically for mild to moderate disease. The evidence to support the use of these drugs relates to their cognitive enhancement.

Treatment with acetylcholinesterase inhibitors should be initiated and supervised only by a specialist experienced in the management of dementia.

Benefit is assessed by repeating the cognitive assessment at around 3 months. Such assessment cannot demonstrate how the disease may have progressed in the absence of treatment but it can give a good guide to response. Up to half the patients given these drugs will show a slower rate of cognitive decline. The drug should be discontinued in those thought not to be responding. Many specialists repeat the cognitive assessment 4 to 6 weeks after discontinuation to assess deterioration; if significant deterioration occurs during this short period, consideration should be given to restarting therapy.

Donepezil is a reversible inhibitor of acetylcholinesterase that can be given once daily.

Rivastigmine is a reversible non-competitive inhibitor of acetylcholinesterase, which is given twice daily.

Donepezil and rivastigmine can cause unwanted dose-related cholinergic effects and should be started at a low dose and the dose increased according to response and tolerability.

DONEPEZIL HYDROCHLORIDE

Indications: mild to moderate dementia in Alzheimer's disease

Cautions: sick sinus syndrome or other supraventricular conduction abnormalities; patients at risk of developing peptic ulcers; asthma, obstructive airways disease; **interactions:** Appendix 1 (parasympathomimetics)

Contra-indications: pregnancy and breast-feeding

Side-effects: nausea, vomiting, diarrhoea, fatigue, insomnia, muscle cramps, less frequently headache, dizziness; rarely syncope, bradycardia, sino-atrial block and AV block; minor increase in plasma-creatine kinase concentration; anorexia, gastric and duodenal ulcers, gastro-intestinal haemorrhage, psychiatric disturbances and hepatitis reported, potential for bladder outflow obstruction, convulsions

Dose: 5 mg once daily at bedtime, increased if necessary after one month to 10 mg daily; max. 10 mg daily

Aricept® (Eisai, Pfizer) ▼ PoM
Tablets, f/c, donepezil hydrochloride 5 mg, net price 28-tab pack = £68.32; 10 mg (yellow), 28-tab pack = £95.76.

RIVASTIGMINE

Indications: mild to moderate dementia in Alzheimer's disease

Cautions: renal impairment, mild to moderate hepatic impairment (Appendix 2); sick sinus syndrome, conduction abnormalities; gastric or duodenal ulcers (and those at risk of developing ulcers); history of asthma or obstructive pulmonary disease; pregnancy (Appendix 4); monitor body-weight; **interactions:** Appendix 1 (parasympathomimetics)

Contra-indications: breast-feeding

Side-effects: asthenia, anorexia, weight loss, dizziness, nausea, vomiting, drowsiness, abdominal pain, agitation and confusion, depression, diarrhoea, dyspepsia, headache, insomnia, sweating, malaise, tremor; rarely angina pectoris, gastro-intestinal haemorrhage, syncope; potential for bladder outflow obstruction, convulsions

Note. Gastro-intestinal side-effects may occur more commonly in women

Dose: initially 1.5 mg twice daily, increased in steps of 1.5 mg twice daily at intervals of at least 2 weeks according to response and tolerance; usual range 3–6 mg twice daily; max. 6 mg twice daily

Exelon® (Novartis) ▼ PoM
Capsules, rivastigmine (as hydrogen tartrate) 1.5 mg (yellow), net price 28-cap pack = £31.50, 56-cap pack = £63.00; 3 mg (orange), 28-cap pack = £31.50, 56-cap pack = £63.00; 4.5 mg (red), 28-cap pack = £31.50, 56-cap pack = £63.00; 6 mg (red/orange), 28-cap pack = £31.50, 56-cap pack = £63.00. Label: 21, 25

5: Infections

Notifiable diseases

Doctors must notify the Proper Officer of the local authority (usually the consultant in communicable disease control) when attending a patient suspected of suffering from any of the diseases listed below; a form is available from the Proper Officer.

Anthrax	Mumps
Cholera	Ophthalmia neonatorum
Diphtheria	Paratyphoid fever
Dysentery (amoebic or bacillary)	Plague
Encephalitis, acute	Poliomyelitis, acute
Food poisoning	Rabies
Haemorrhagic fever (viral)	Relapsing fever
Hepatitis, viral	Rubella
Leprosy	Scarlet fever
Leptospirosis	Smallpox
Malaria	Tetanus
Measles	Tuberculosis
Meningitis	Typhoid fever
Meningococcal septi- caemia (without mening- itis)	Typhus
	Whooping cough
	Yellow fever

Note. It is good practice for doctors to also inform the consultant in communicable disease control of instances of other infections (e.g. psittacosis) where there could be a public health risk.

5.1   Antibacterial drugs

CHOICE OF A SUITABLE DRUG. Before selecting an antibiotic the clinician must first consider two factors—the patient and the known or likely causative organism. Factors related to the patient which must be considered include history of allergy, renal and hepatic function, resistance to infection (i.e. whether immunocompromised), ability to tolerate drugs by mouth, severity of illness, ethnic origin, age and, if female, whether pregnant, breast-feeding or taking an oral contraceptive.

The known or likely organism and its antibiotic sensitivity, in association with the above factors, will suggest one or more antibiotics, the final choice depending on the microbiological, pharmacological, and toxicological properties.

An example of a rational approach to the selection of an antibiotic is treatment of a urinary-tract infection in a patient complaining of nausea in early pregnancy. The organism is reported as being resistant to ampicillin but sensitive to nitrofurantoin (can cause nausea), gentamicin (can only be given by injection and best avoided in pregnancy), tetracycline (causes dental discoloration) and co-trimoxazole (folate antagonist therefore theoretical teratogenic risk), and cefalexin. The safest antibiotics in pregnancy are the penicillins and cephalosporins; therefore, cefalexin would be indicated for this patient.

The principles involved in selection of an antibiotic must allow for a number of variables including changing renal and hepatic function, increasing bacterial resistance, and new information on side-effects. Duration of therapy, dosage, and route of administration depend on site, type and severity of infection and response.

ANTIBIOTIC POLICIES. Many hospitals limit the antibiotics that may be used to achieve reasonable economy consistent with adequate cover, and to reduce the development of resistant organisms. A policy may indicate a range of drugs for general use, and permit other drugs only on the advice of the microbiologist or physician responsible for the control of infectious diseases.

BEFORE STARTING THERAPY. The following precepts should be considered before starting:
- Viral infections should not be treated with antibiotics;
- Samples should be taken for culture and sensitivity testing; **'blind'** antibiotic prescribing for unexplained pyrexia usually leads to further difficulty in establishing the diagnosis;
- Knowledge of **prevalent organisms** and their current sensitivity is of great help in choosing an antibiotic before bacteriological confirmation is available;
- The **dose** of an antibiotic will vary according to a number of factors including age, weight, renal function, and severity of infection. The prescribing of the so-called 'standard' dose in serious infections may result in failure of treatment or even death of the patient; therefore it is important to prescribe a dose appropriate to the condition. On the other hand, for an antibiotic with a narrow margin between the toxic and therapeutic dose (e.g. an aminoglycoside) it is also important to avoid an excessive dose and plasma concentration monitoring may be required;

- The **route** of administration of an antibiotic will often depend on the severity of the infection. Life-threatening infections require intravenous therapy. Whenever possible painful intramuscular injections should be avoided in children;
- **Duration** of therapy depends on the nature of the infection and the response to treatment. Courses should not be unduly prolonged as they are costly, encourage resistance and may lead to side-effects; in many cases a 5-day course is sufficient. However, in certain infections such as tuberculosis or chronic osteomyelitis it is necessary to continue treatment for relatively long periods. Conversely a single dose of an antibiotic may cure uncomplicated urinary-tract infections.

SUPERINFECTION. In general, broad-spectrum antibacterial drugs such as the cephalosporins are more likely to be associated with adverse reactions related to the selection of resistant organisms e.g. *fungal infections* or *antibiotic-associated colitis* (pseudomembranous colitis); other problems associated with superinfection include vaginitis and pruritus ani.

THERAPY. Suggested treatment is shown in table 1. When the pathogen has been isolated treatment may be changed to a more appropriate antibiotic if necessary. If no bacterium is cultured the antibiotic can be continued or stopped on clinical grounds. Infections for which prophylaxis is useful are listed in table 2.

Table I. Summary of antibacterial therapy

> If treating a patient suspected of suffering from a notifiable disease, the consultant in communicable disease control should be informed (see p. 247)

Gastro-intestinal system

Gastro-enteritis
Antibiotic not usually indicated
Frequently self-limiting and may not be bacterial
Campylobacter enteritis
Ciprofloxacin *or* erythromycin
Invasive salmonellosis
Ciprofloxacin *or* trimethoprim
Includes severe infections which may be invasive
Shigellosis
Ciprofloxacin *or* trimethoprim
Antibiotic not indicated for mild cases. Ciprofloxacin should be used for trimethoprim-resistant strains
Typhoid fever
Ciprofloxacin *or* cefotaxime *or* chloramphenicol
Infections from Indian subcontinent, Middle-East, and South-East Asia may be multiple-antibiotic-resistant and sensitivity results should be sought
Antibiotic-associated colitis (pseudomembranous colitis)
Oral metronidazole *or* oral vancomycin
Biliary-tract infection
A cephalosporin *or* gentamicin
Peritonitis
A cephalosporin (*or* gentamicin) + metronidazole (*or* clindamycin)

Peritoneal dialysis-associated peritonitis
Vancomycin[1] + gentamicin (*or* ceftazidime) added to dialysis fluid (*or* vancomycin added to dialysis fluid + oral ciprofloxacin)
Discontinue any antibiotic not required when sensitivity known; treat usually for 14 days or longer

Cardiovascular system

Endocarditis caused by streptococci (e.g. viridans streptococci)
Benzylpenicillin (*or* vancomycin[1] if penicillin-allergic) + low-dose gentamicin (i.e. 80 mg twice daily)
Treat for up to 4 weeks; stop after 2 weeks if organism fully sensitive to penicillin
Endocarditis caused by enterococci (e.g. *Enterococcus faecalis*)
Amoxicillin[2] (*or* vancomycin[1] if penicillin-allergic) + low-dose gentamicin (i.e. 80 mg twice daily)
Treat for 4 weeks; if gentamicin-resistant, substitute streptomycin for gentamicin and treat for at least 6 weeks
Endocarditis caused by staphylococci (including *Staph. aureus*, *Staph. epidermidis*)
Flucloxacillin (*or* benzylpenicillin if penicillin-sensitive *or* vancomycin if penicillin-allergic or if methicillin-resistant staphylococci) + gentamicin (*or* fusidic acid)
Treat for 4 weeks; stop gentamicin (or fusidic acid) after 1 week

Footnote—*see next page*

Respiratory system

Haemophilus influenzae epiglottitis
Cefotaxime *or* chloramphenicol
> Give intravenously

Exacerbations of chronic bronchitis
Amoxicillin[2] *or* tetracycline (*or* erythromycin[3])
> Some pneumococci and *Haemophilus influenzae* strains tetracycline-resistant; 15% *H. influenzae* strains amoxicillin-resistant

Uncomplicated community-acquired pneumonia
Amoxicillin[2] (*or* benzylpenicillin if previously healthy chest *or* erythromycin[3] if penicillin-allergic)
> Add flucloxacillin if staphylococcus suspected, e.g. in influenza or measles; add erythromycin[3] if atypical pneumonia suspected; pneumococci with decreased penicillin sensitivity being isolated but not yet common in UK

Severe community-acquired pneumonia of unknown aetiology
Erythromycin[3] + cefuroxime *or* cefotaxime
> Add flucloxacillin if staphylococcus suspected

Suspected atypical pneumonia
Erythromycin[3]
> Severe Legionella infections may require addition of rifampicin; tetracycline is an alternative for chlamydial and mycoplasma infections; treat for at least 10–14 days

Hospital-acquired pneumonia
A broad-spectrum cephalosporin (e.g. cefotaxime or ceftazidime) *or* an antipseudomonal penicillin + an aminoglycoside

Central nervous system

Meningitis: Initial 'blind' therapy
> If meningococcal disease suspected, general practitioners advised to give a single dose of benzylpenicillin before urgent transportation to hospital (see under Benzylpenicillin, section 5.1.1.1); cefotaxime (section 5.1.2) may be an alternative in penicillin allergy; chloramphenicol may be used if history of anaphylaxis due to penicillin

Meningitis caused by meningococci
Benzylpenicillin *or* cefotaxime
> Give rifampicin for 2 days before hospital discharge

Meningitis caused by pneumococci
Cefotaxime
> Substitute benzylpenicillin if organism penicillin-sensitive; if organism highly penicillin- and cephalosporin-resistant, add vancomycin

Meningitis caused by *Haemophilus influenzae*
Cefotaxime *or* chloramphenicol
> For *H. influenzae* type b give rifampicin for 4 days before hospital discharge

Meningitis caused by Listeria
Amoxicillin[2] + gentamicin

Urinary tract

Acute pyelonephritis or prostatitis
Trimethoprim *or* gentamicin *or* cephalosporin *or* a quinolone
> Treat prostatitis with trimethoprim or a quinolone for 4 weeks

'Lower' urinary-tract infection
Trimethoprim *or* amoxicillin[2] *or* nitrofurantoin *or* oral cephalosporin
> A short course (e.g. 3 days) is usually adequate for uncomplicated urinary-tract infections in women

Genital system

Syphilis
Procaine benzylpenicillin (*or* doxycycline *or* tetracycline *or* erythromycin if penicillin-allergic)
> Treat early syphilis for 14 days (10–14 days with procaine benzylpenicillin); treat late latent syphilis with procaine benzylpenicillin for 17–21 days (or with doxycycline for 28 days); contact tracing recommended

Gonorrhoea
Ciprofloxacin *or* ofloxacin (*or* for fully sensitive organisms amoxicillin[2] with probenecid)
> Single-dose treatment in uncomplicated infection; choice depends on locality where infection acquired—infection acquired abroad should be presumed to be penicillin-resistant; contact-tracing recommended; remember chlamydia; pharyngeal infection requires treatment with ciprofloxacin *or* ofloxacin

Uncomplicated genital chlamydial infection, non-gonococcal urethritis and non-specific genital infection
Doxycycline *or* azithromycin
> Treat with doxycycline for 7 days or with azithromycin 1 g as a single dose; alternatively treat with erythromycin 500 mg every 6 hours for 7 days; contact tracing recommended

Pelvic inflammatory disease
Metronidazole + doxycycline (*or* erythromycin)
> Treat for 14 days; severely ill patients may require initial treatment with doxycycline + a broad-spectrum parenteral cephalosporin (e.g. cefotaxime), then switching to oral treatment to complete 14 days' treatment; remember gonorrhoea

Blood

Septicaemia: Initial 'blind' therapy
Community-acquired septicaemia, aminoglycoside + a broad-spectrum penicillin *or* a broad-spectrum cephalosporin alone (e.g. cefotaxime)
Hospital-acquired septicaemia, aminoglycoside + a broad-spectrum antipseudomonal penicillin (*or* ceftazidime), *or* meropenem alone, *or* imipenem (with cilastatin as Primaxin®) alone
> Choice depends on local resistance patterns and clinical presentation; use aminoglycoside + broad-spectrum antipseudomonal penicillin if pseudomonas suspected; add metronidazole if anaerobic infection suspected; add flucloxacillin or vancomycin[1] if Gram-positive infection suspected

Meningococcal septicaemia
Benzylpenicillin *or* cefotaxime
> If meningococcal disease suspected, general practitioners advised to give a single dose of benzylpenicillin before urgent transportation to hospital (see under Benzylpenicillin, section 5.1.1.1); give rifampicin for 2 days before hospital discharge

Musculoskeletal system

Osteomyelitis and septic arthritis
Clindamycin alone *or* flucloxacillin + fusidic acid.
If *Haemophilus influenzae* give amoxicillin[2] *or* cefuroxime
> Under 5 years of age may be *H. influenzae*. Treat acute disease for at least 6 weeks and chronic infection for at least 12 weeks

Eye

Purulent conjunctivitis
Chloramphenicol *or* gentamicin eye-drops

---

1. Where vancomycin is suggested teicoplanin may be used.
2. Where amoxicillin is suggested ampicillin may be used.
3. Where erythromycin is suggested another macrolide (e.g. azithromycin or clarithromycin) may be used.

Ear, nose, and oropharynx

Dental infections

Phenoxymethylpenicillin (*or* amoxicillin[2]) *or* erythromycin *or* metronidazole

Tetracycline for chronic destructive forms of periodontal disease

Sinusitis

Amoxicillin[2] *or* doxycycline *or* erythromycin[3]

Treat for 3–10 days

Otitis externa

Flucloxacillin

Use ciprofloxacin (or an aminoglycoside) if pseudomonas suspected, see section 12.1.1

Otitis media

Amoxicillin[2] (*or* erythromycin[3] if penicillin-allergic)

Initial parenteral therapy (in severe infections) with benzylpenicillin, then oral therapy with phenoxymethylpenicillin; under 5 years of age may be *Haemophilus influenzae*; many infections are caused by viruses

Throat infections

Phenoxymethylpenicillin (*or* erythromycin[3] if penicillin-allergic) *or* oral cephalosporin

Most throat infections are caused by viruses and many do not require antibiotic therapy; restrict antibiotic prescribing for specific infections e.g. beta-haemolytic streptococcal pharyngitis (treat for at least 10 days); **avoid** amoxicillin if possibility of glandular fever, see section 5.1.1.3; initial parenteral therapy (in severe infection) with benzylpenicillin, then oral therapy with phenoxymethylpenicillin *or* amoxicillin[2]

Skin

Impetigo

Topical fusidic acid or mupirocin; oral flucloxacillin *or* erythromycin if widespread

Topical treatment for 7 days usually adequate; max. duration of topical treatment 10 days

Erysipelas

Phenoxymethylpenicillin

Cellulitis

Phenoxymethylpenicillin + flucloxacillin (*or* erythromycin alone if penicillin-allergic) *or* co-amoxiclav alone

Severe cellulitis may require parenteral benzylpenicillin + flucloxacillin or co-amoxiclav alone

Animal bites

Co-amoxiclav

Cleanse wound thoroughly; for tetanus prone wound, give human tetanus immunoglobulin (with adsorbed tetanus vaccine if necessary, according to immunisation history), see under Tetanus Vaccines, section 14.4

Acne—see section 13.6

---

1. Where vancomycin is suggested teicoplanin may be used.
2. Where amoxicillin is suggested ampicillin may be used.
3. Where erythromycin is suggested another macrolide (e.g. azithromycin or clarithromycin) may be used.

Table 2. Summary of antibacterial prophylaxis

Prevention of recurrence of rheumatic fever

Phenoxymethylpenicillin 250 mg twice daily *or* sulfadiazine 1 g daily (500 mg daily for patients under 30 kg)

Prevention of secondary case of meningococcal meningitis[1]

Rifampicin 600 mg every 12 hours for 2 days; CHILD 10 mg/kg (under 1 year, 5 mg/kg) every 12 hours for 2 days

or ciprofloxacin 500 mg as a single dose [not licensed for this indication]; CHILD obtain further advice[1]

or i/m ceftriaxone 250 mg as a single dose [not licensed for this indication]; CHILD under 12 years 125 mg

Prevention of secondary case of Haemophilus influenzae type b disease[1]

Rifampicin 600 mg once daily for 4 days (optimum regimen for adults); CHILD 1–3 months 10 mg/kg once daily for 4 days, over 3 months 20 mg/kg once daily for 4 days (max. 600 mg daily)

Prevention of secondary case of diphtheria in non-immune patient

Erythromycin 500 mg every 6 hours for 7–10 days; CHILD up to 2 years 125 mg every 6 hours, 2–8 years 250 mg every 6 hours

Prevention of pertussis

ADULT and CHILD erythromycin 50 mg/kg (max. 2 g) daily in 4 divided doses for 7–14 days

Note. Pertussis vaccine inappropriate for outbreak since 3 injections are required for protection

Prevention of pneumococcal infection in asplenia or in patients with sickle cell disease

Phenoxymethylpenicillin 500 mg every 12 hours; CHILD under 5 years 125 mg every 12 hours, 6–12 years 250 mg every 12 hours—if cover also needed for *H. influenzae* in CHILD give amoxicillin instead (under 5 years 125 mg every 12 hours, over 5 years 250 mg every 12 hours)

Note. Antibiotic prophylaxis is not fully reliable

Prevention of endocarditis[2] in patients with heart-valve lesion, septal defect, patent ductus, or prosthetic valve

Dental procedures[3] *under local or no anaesthesia,*

patients who have not received more than a single dose of a penicillin[4] in the previous month, including those with a prosthetic valve (but not those who have had endocarditis), oral amoxicillin 3 g 1 hour before procedure; CHILD under 5 years quarter adult dose; 5–10 years half adult dose

patients who are penicillin-allergic or have received more than a single dose of a penicillin[4] in the previous month, oral clindamycin[5] 600 mg 1 hour before procedure; CHILD under 5 years quarter adult dose; 5–10 years half-adult dose

patients who have had endocarditis, amoxicillin + gentamicin, as under general anaesthesia

Footnote—*see next page*

Dental procedures[3] *under general anaesthesia, no special risk* (including patients who have not received more than a single dose of a penicillin in the previous month),
either i/v amoxicillin 1 g at induction, then oral amoxicillin 500 mg 6 hours later; CHILD under 5 years quarter adult dose; 5–10 years half adult dose
or oral amoxicillin 3 g 4 hours before induction then oral amoxicillin 3 g as soon as possible after procedure; CHILD under 5 years quarter adult dose; 5–10 years half adult dose
or oral amoxicillin 3 g + oral probenecid 1 g 4 hours before procedure

special risk (patients with a prosthetic valve or who have had endocarditis), i/v amoxicillin 1 g + i/v gentamicin 120 mg at induction, then oral amoxicillin 500 mg 6 hours later; CHILD under 5 years amoxicillin quarter adult dose, gentamicin 2 mg/kg; 5–10 years amoxicillin half adult dose, gentamicin 2 mg/kg

patients who are penicillin-allergic or who have received more than a single dose of a penicillin in the previous month,
either i/v vancomycin 1 g over at least 100 minutes then i/v gentamicin 120 mg at induction or 15 minutes before procedure; CHILD under 10 years vancomycin 20 mg/kg, gentamicin 2 mg/kg
or i/v teicoplanin 400 mg + gentamicin 120 mg at induction or 15 minutes before procedure; CHILD under 14 years teicoplanin 6 mg/kg, gentamicin 2 mg/kg
or i/v clindamycin[5] 300 mg over at least 10 minutes at induction or 15 minutes before procedure then oral or i/v clindamycin 150 mg 6 hours later; CHILD under 5 years quarter adult dose; 5–10 years half adult dose

Upper respiratory-tract procedures, as for dental procedures; post-operative dose may be given parenterally if swallowing is painful

Genito-urinary procedures, as for *special risk* patients undergoing dental procedures under general anaesthesia except that clindamycin is not given, see above; if urine infected, prophylaxis should also cover infective organism

Obstetric, gynaecological and gastro-intestinal procedures (prophylaxis required for patients with prosthetic valves or those who have had endocarditis only), as for genito-urinary procedures

---

Joint prostheses and dental treatment

Advice of a Working Party of the British Society for Antimicrobial Chemotherapy is that patients with prosthetic joint implants (including total hip replacements) do not require antibiotic prophylaxis for dental treatment. The Working Party considers that it is unacceptable to expose patients to the adverse effects of antibiotics when there is no evidence that such prophylaxis is of any benefit, but that those who develop any intercurrent infection require prompt treatment with antibiotics to which the infecting organisms are sensitive.

The Working Party has commented that joint infections have rarely been shown to follow dental procedures and are even more rarely caused by oral streptococci.

Dermatological procedures

Advice of a Working Party of the British Society for Antimicrobial Chemotherapy is that patients who undergo dermatological procedures* do not require antibacterial prophylaxis against endocarditis.

* The British Association of Dermatologists Therapy Guidelines and Audit Subcommittee advise that such dermatological procedures include skin biopsies and excision of moles or of malignant lesions

---

Immunosuppression and indwelling intraperitoneal catheters

Advice of a Working Party of the British Society for Antimicrobial Chemotherapy is that patients who are immunosuppressed (including transplant patients) and patients with indwelling intraperitoneal catheters do not require antibiotic prophylaxis for dental treatment provided there is no other indication for prophylaxis.

The Working Party has commented that there is little evidence that dental treatment is followed by infection in immunosuppressed and immunodeficient patients nor is there evidence that dental treatment is followed by infection in patients with indwelling intraperitoneal catheters.

Prevention of **gas-gangrene** in high lower-limb amputations or following major trauma

Benzylpenicillin 300–600 mg every 6 hours for 5 days *or* if penicillin-allergic metronidazole 500 mg every 8 hours

---

1. For details of those who should receive chemoprophylaxis contact a consultant in communicable disease control (or a consultant in infectious diseases or the local public health laboratory). Unless there has been mouth to mouth contact, healthcare workers do not generally require chemoprophylaxis.

2. Advice on the prevention of endocarditis reflects the recommendations of a Working Party of the British Society for Antimicrobial Chemotherapy, *Lancet*, 1982, **2**, 1323–26; *idem*, 1986, **1**, 1267; *idem*, 1990, **335**, 88–9; *idem*, 1992, **339**, 1292–93; *idem*, 1997, **350**, 1100; also *J Antimicrob Chemother*, 1993; **31**, 437–8

3. Dental procedures that require antibiotic prophylaxis are, *extractions, scaling*, and *surgery involving gingival tissues*. Antibiotic prophylaxis for dental procedures may be supplemented with *chlorhexidine gluconate gel 1%* or *chlorhexidine gluconate mouthwash 0.2%*, used 5 minutes before procedure

4. For multistage procedures a max. of 2 single doses of a penicillin may be given in a month; alternative drugs should be used for further treatment and the penicillin should not be used again for 3–4 months

5. If **clindamycin** is used, periodontal or other multistage procedures should not be repeated at intervals of less than 2 weeks; clindamycin is not licensed for use in endocarditis prophylaxis

Prevention of **tuberculosis** in susceptible close contacts or those who have become tuberculin positive[1]

Isoniazid 300 mg daily for 6 months; CHILD 5–10 mg/kg daily (max. 300 mg daily) *or* isoniazid 300 mg daily + rifampicin 600 mg daily (450 mg if less than 50 kg) for 3 months; CHILD isoniazid 5–10 mg/kg daily (max. 300 mg daily) + rifampicin 10 mg/kg daily (max. 600 mg daily)

Prevention of infection in **abdominal surgery**

Operations on stomach or oesophagus for carcinoma, or cholecystectomy in patients with possibly infected bile

Single dose of gentamicin *or* a cephalosporin given within 2 hours before operation

Resections of colon and rectum for carcinoma, and resections in inflammatory bowel disease

Single dose of *either* gentamicin + metronidazole *or* cefuroxime + metronidazole given within 2 hours before operation

Hysterectomy

Cefuroxime i/v or i/m + metronidazole as suppository *or* single i/v dose

5.1.1   Penicillins

5.1.1.1	Benzylpenicillin and phenoxymethylpenicillin
5.1.1.2	Penicillinase-resistant penicillins
5.1.1.3	Broad-spectrum penicillins
5.1.1.4	Antipseudomonal penicillins

The penicillins are bactericidal and act by interfering with bacterial cell wall synthesis. They diffuse well into body tissues and fluids, but penetration into the cerebrospinal fluid is poor except when the meninges are inflamed. They are excreted in the urine in therapeutic concentrations. Probenecid (section 10.1.4) blocks the renal tubular excretion of the penicillins, producing higher and more prolonged plasma concentrations; it is not recommended in children under 2 years of age.

The most important side-effect of the penicillins is hypersensitivity which causes rashes and anaphylaxis, which can be fatal. Patients who are allergic to one penicillin will be allergic to all because the hypersensitivity is related to the basic penicillin structure. It should be borne in mind that very few 'penicillin-allergic' patients are at risk of anaphylaxis and therefore a penicillin should not be withheld unnecessarily for serious infections; appropriate resuscitation facilities should however be available.

A rare but serious toxic effect of the penicillins is encephalopathy due to cerebral irritation. This may result from excessively high doses or in patients with severe renal failure. The penicillins should **not** be given by intrathecal injection because they can cause encephalopathy which may be fatal.

Another problem relating to high doses of penicillin, or normal doses given to patients with renal failure, is the accumulation of electrolyte since most injectable penicillins contain either sodium or potassium.

Diarrhoea frequently occurs during oral penicillin therapy. It is most common with broad-spectrum penicillins, which can also cause antibiotic-associated colitis.

5.1.1.1   Benzylpenicillin and phenoxymethylpenicillin

Benzylpenicillin (Penicillin G) remains an important and useful antibiotic but is inactivated by bacterial beta-lactamases. It is effective for many streptococcal (including pneumococcal), gonococcal, and meningococcal infections and also for anthrax, diphtheria, gas-gangrene, leptospirosis, and treatment of Lyme disease in children. Pneumococci, meningococci, and gonococci which have decreased sensitivity to penicillin have been isolated; benzylpenicillin is no longer drug of first choice for pneumococcal meningitis. Although benzylpenicillin is effective in the treatment of tetanus, metronidazole (section 5.1.11) is preferred. Benzylpenicillin is inactivated by gastric acid and absorption from the gut is low; therefore it is best given by injection.

Procaine benzylpenicillin (procaine penicillin) is a sparingly soluble salt of benzylpenicillin. It is used in intramuscular depot preparations which provide therapeutic tissue concentrations for up to 24 hours. It is the preferred choice for the treatment of yaws and syphilis; neurosyphilis requires special consideration.

Phenoxymethylpenicillin (Penicillin V) has a similar antibacterial spectrum to benzylpenicillin, but is less active. It is gastric acid-stable, so is suitable for oral administration. It should not be used for serious infections because absorption can be unpredictable and plasma concentrations variable. It is indicated principally for respiratory-tract infections in children, for streptococcal tonsillitis, and for continuing treatment after one or more injections of benzylpenicillin when clinical response has begun. It should not be used for meningococcal or gonococcal infections. Phenoxymethylpenicillin is used for prophylaxis against streptococcal infections following rheumatic fever and against pneumococcal infections following splenectomy or in sickle cell disease.

BENZYLPENICILLIN
(Penicillin G)

Indications: throat infections, otitis media, streptococcal endocarditis, meningococcal meningitis, pneumonia (section 5.1, table 1); prophylaxis in limb amputation (section 5.1, table 2)

Cautions: history of allergy; renal impairment; **interactions:** Appendix 1 (penicillins)

Contra-indications: penicillin hypersensitivity

Side-effects: hypersensitivity reactions including urticaria, fever, joint pains, rashes, angioedema, anaphylaxis, serum sickness-like reactions, haemolytic anaemia and interstitial nephritis; neutropenia, thrombocytopenia, coagulation disorders and central nervous system toxicity including convulsions reported (especially with high doses or in severe renal impairment); paraesthesia with prolonged use; diarrhoea and antibiotic-associated colitis

---

1. The Joint Tuberculosis Committee recommends chemoprophylaxis for tuberculous infection in children under 16 years found at new immigrant or contact screening, tuberculin-positive children identified in BCG schools programme, neonates and children under 2 years in close contact with smear-positive tuberculosis, and adults with documented recent tuberculin conversion.

Dose: *by intramuscular or by slow intravenous injection or by infusion*, 1.2 g daily in 4 divided doses, increased if necessary to 2.4 g daily or more (see also below); PREMATURE INFANT and NEONATE, 50 mg/kg daily in 2 divided doses; INFANT 1–4 weeks, 75 mg/kg daily in 3 divided doses; CHILD 1 month–12 years, 100 mg/kg daily in 4 divided doses (higher doses may be required, see also below)

Bacterial endocarditis, *by slow intravenous injection or by infusion*, 7.2 g daily in 6 divided doses

Meningococcal meningitis, *by slow intravenous injection or by infusion*, 2.4 g every 4–6 hours; PREMATURE INFANT and NEONATE, 100 mg/kg daily in 2 divided doses; INFANT 1–4 weeks, 150 mg/kg daily in 3 divided doses; CHILD 1 month–12 years, 180–300 mg/kg daily in 4–6 divided doses

Important. If meningococcal disease is suspected general practitioners are advised to give a single injection of benzylpenicillin by intravenous injection (or by intramuscular injection) before transporting the patient urgently to hospital. Suitable doses are: ADULT 1.2 g; INFANT 300 mg; CHILD 1–9 years 600 mg, 10 years and over as for adult. In **penicillin allergy**, cefotaxime (section 5.1.2) may be an alternative; chloramphenicol may be used if there is a history of anaphylaxis to penicillins

By intrathecal injection, **not** recommended

Note. Benzylpenicillin doses in BNF may differ from those in product literature

Crystapen® (Britannia) [PoM]

Injection, powder for reconstitution, benzylpenicillin sodium (unbuffered), net price 600-mg vial = 44p, 2-vial 'GP pack' = 97p; 1.2-g vial = 88p
Electrolytes: Na⁺ 1.68 mmol/600-mg vial; 3.36 mmol/1.2-g vial

PHENOXYMETHYLPENICILLIN
(Penicillin V)

Indications: tonsillitis, otitis media, erysipelas; rheumatic fever and pneumococcal infection prophylaxis (section 5.1, table 2)

Cautions: see under Benzylpenicillin; **interactions:** Appendix 1 (penicillins)

Contra-indications: see under Benzylpenicillin

Side-effects: see under Benzylpenicillin

Dose: 500 mg every 6 hours increased to 750 mg every 6 hours in severe infections; CHILD, every 6 hours, up to 1 year 62.5 mg, 1–5 years 125 mg, 6–12 years 250 mg

Note. Phenoxymethylpenicillin doses in the BNF may differ from those in product literature

Phenoxymethylpenicillin (Non-proprietary)
[PoM]

Tablets, phenoxymethylpenicillin (as potassium salt) 250 mg, net price 28-tab pack = £2.04. Label: 9, 23
Available from APS (*Apsin®*), Berk, Cox, Generics, Kent (*Tenkicin®*)

Oral solution, phenoxymethylpenicillin (as potassium salt) for reconstitution with water, net price 125 mg/5 mL, 100 mL = £1.75; 250 mg/5 mL, 100 mL = £3.57. Label: 9, 23
Available from APS (*Apsin®*), Cox, Generics, Kent (*Tenkicin®*)

PROCAINE BENZYLPENICILLIN/ PROCAINE PENICILLIN

Indications: penicillin-sensitive infections
Cautions: see under Benzylpenicillin
Contra-indications: see under Benzylpenicillin; **not** for intravenous administration
Side-effects: see under Benzylpenicillin
Dose: see below

Bicillin® (Yamanouchi) [PoM]

Injection, powder for reconstitution, procaine benzylpenicillin 1.8 g, benzylpenicillin sodium 360 mg. Net price 6-mL multidose vial = £2.70
Electrolytes: Na⁺ 1 mmol/vial
Dose: when reconstituted with 4.6 mL water for injections, 1 mL (procaine benzylpenicillin 300 mg, benzylpenicillin sodium 60 mg) every 12–24 hours by intramuscular injection
Syphilis, by intramuscular injection, 2 mL daily for 10–14 days in early syphilis (for 17–21 days in late latent syphilis)
Note. Reconstitution with 4.6 mL water for injections produces 6 mL
Note. Doses in BNF may differ from those in product literature

5.1.1.2 Penicillinase-resistant penicillins

Most staphylococci are now resistant to benzylpenicillin because they produce penicillinases. **Flucloxacillin**, however, is not inactivated by these enzymes and is thus effective in infections caused by penicillin-resistant staphylococci, which is the sole indication for its use. Flucloxacillin is acid-stable and can, therefore, be given by mouth as well as by injection.

Flucloxacillin is well absorbed from the gut. For CSM warning on cholestatic jaundice see under Flucloxacillin.

Staphylococcus aureus strains resistant to methicillin [now discontinued] (methicillin-resistant *Staph. aureus*, MRSA) and to flucloxacillin have emerged in many hospitals; some of these organisms are sensitive only to vancomycin or teicoplanin (section 5.1.7). Other alternatives may include rifampicin and sodium fusidate; trimethoprim may be used for urinary-tract infections caused by some MRSA. The streptogramin antibiotics quinupristin and dalfopristin (section 5.1.7) are active against MRSA but the combination should be reserved for organisms resistant to other antibacterials. Treatment is guided by the sensitivity of the infecting strain.

FLUCLOXACILLIN

Indications: infections due to beta-lactamase-producing staphylococci including otitis externa; adjunct in pneumonia, impetigo, cellulitis and in staphylococcal endocarditis (section 5.1, table 1)

Cautions: see under Benzylpenicillin (section 5.1.1.1); porphyria (section 9.8.2)
CHOLESTATIC JAUNDICE. CSM has advised that cholestatic jaundice may occur up to several weeks after treatment with flucloxacillin has been stopped. Administration for more than 2 weeks and increasing age are risk factors

Contra-indications: see under Benzylpenicillin (section 5.1.1.1)

Side-effects: see under Benzylpenicillin (section 5.1.1.1); also hepatitis and cholestatic jaundice reported (see also CSM advice above)
Dose: *by mouth*, 250 mg every 6 hours, at least 30 minutes before food
By intramuscular injection, 250 mg every 6 hours
By slow intravenous injection or by infusion, 0.25–1 g every 6 hours
Doses may be doubled in severe infections
CHILD, any route, under 2 years quarter adult dose; 2–10 years half adult dose

Flucloxacillin (Non-proprietary) PoM
Capsules, flucloxacillin (as sodium salt) 250 mg, net price 20 = £1.84; 500 mg, 20 = £3.26. Label: 9, 23
Available from APS, Ashbourne (*Fluclomix*®), Berk (*Ladropen*®), Cox, Galen (*Galfloxin*®), Kent, Norton, Opus (*Zoxin*®)
Oral solution (= elixir or syrup), flucloxacillin (as sodium salt) for reconstitution with water, 125 mg/5 mL, net price 100 mL = £3.62. Label: 9, 23
Available from APS, Berk (*Ladropen*®), Cox, Kent, Norton
Injection, powder for reconstitution, flucloxacillin (as sodium salt). Net price 250-mg vial = £1.02; 500-mg vial = £2.04; 1-g vial = £4.08
Available from Berk (*Ladropen*®), CP

Floxapen® (SmithKline Beecham) PoM
Capsules, both black/caramel, flucloxacillin (as sodium salt) 250 mg, net price 28-cap pack = £6.79; 500 mg, 28-cap pack = £13.61. Label: 9, 23
Syrup, flucloxacillin (as magnesium salt) for reconstitution with water, 125 mg/5 mL, net price 100 mL = £3.49; 250 mg/5 mL, 100 mL = £6.97. Label: 9, 23
Injection, powder for reconstitution, flucloxacillin (as sodium salt). Net price 250-mg vial = 98p; 500-mg vial = £1.95; 1-g vial = £3.90
Electrolytes: Na⁺ 0.57 mmol/250-mg vial, 1.13 mmol/500-mg vial, 2.26 mmol/1-g vial

5.1.1.3   Broad-spectrum penicillins

Ampicillin is active against certain Gram-positive and Gram-negative organisms but is inactivated by penicillinases including those produced by *Staphylococcus aureus* and by common Gram-negative bacilli such as *Escherichia coli*. Almost all staphylococci, 50% of *E. coli* strains and 15% of *Haemophilus influenzae* strains are now resistant. The likelihood of resistance should therefore be considered before using ampicillin for the 'blind' treatment of infections; in particular, it should not be used for hospital patients without checking sensitivity.

Ampicillin is well excreted in the bile and urine. It is principally indicated for the treatment of exacerbations of chronic bronchitis and middle ear infections, both of which are usually due to *Streptococcus pneumoniae* and *H. influenzae*, and for urinary-tract infections (section 5.1.13) and gonorrhoea.

Ampicillin can be given by mouth but less than half the dose is absorbed, and absorption is further decreased by the presence of food in the gut.

Maculopapular rashes commonly occur with ampicillin (and amoxicillin) but are not usually related to true penicillin allergy. They almost always occur in patients with glandular fever; broad-spectrum penicillins should not therefore be used for 'blind' treatment of a sore throat. Rashes are also common in patients with chronic lymphatic leukaemia.

Amoxicillin (amoxycillin) is a derivative of ampicillin and has a similar antibacterial spectrum. It is better absorbed than ampicillin when given by mouth, producing higher plasma and tissue concentrations; unlike ampicillin, absorption is not affected by the presence of food in the stomach. Amoxicillin is used for endocarditis prophylaxis (section 5.1, table 2); it may also be used for the treatment of Lyme disease in children.

Co-amoxiclav consists of amoxicillin with the beta-lactamase inhibitor clavulanic acid. Clavulanic acid itself has no significant antibacterial activity but, by inactivating beta-lactamases, it makes the combination active against beta-lactamase-producing bacteria that are resistant to amoxicillin. These include resistant strains of *Staph. aureus*, *E. coli*, and *H. influenzae*, as well as many *Bacteroides* and *Klebsiella* spp. Co-amoxiclav should be reserved for infections likely, or known, to be caused by amoxicillin-resistant beta-lactamase-producing strains; for CSM warning on cholestatic jaundice see under Co-amoxiclav.

A combination of ampicillin with flucloxacillin (as co-fluampicil) is available.

AMOXICILLIN
(Amoxycillin)
Indications: see under Ampicillin; also endocarditis prophylaxis (section 5.1, table 2); adjunct in listerial meningitis (section 5.1, table 1); *Helicobacter pylori* eradication (section 1.3)
Cautions: see under Ampicillin
Contra-indications: see under Ampicillin
Side-effects: see under Ampicillin
Dose: *by mouth*, 250 mg every 8 hours, doubled in severe infections; CHILD up to 10 years, 125 mg every 8 hours, doubled in severe infections
Severe or recurrent purulent respiratory infection, 3 g every 12 hours
Short-course oral therapy
Dental abscess, 3 g repeated after 8 hours
Urinary-tract infections, 3 g repeated after 10–12 hours
Gonorrhoea, single dose of 2–3 g with probenecid 1 g
Otitis media, CHILD 3–10 years, 750 mg twice daily for 2 days
By intramuscular injection, 500 mg every 8 hours; CHILD, 50–100 mg/kg daily in divided doses
By intravenous injection or infusion, 500 mg every 8 hours increased to 1 g every 6 hours; CHILD, 50–100 mg/kg daily in divided doses

Amoxicillin (Non-proprietary) PoM
Capsules, amoxicillin (as trihydrate) 250 mg, net price 20 = £2.26; 500 mg, 20 = £2.21. Label: 9
Available from APS, Ashbourne (*Amix*®), Berk (*Almodan*®), Cox, DDSA, Eastern (*Amoram*®), Galen (*Galenamox*®), Hillcross, Kent, Norton, Ranbaxy (*Rimoxallin*®)
Oral suspension, amoxicillin (as trihydrate) for reconstitution with water, 125 mg/5 mL, net price 100 mL = £1.32; 250 mg/5 mL, 100 mL = £2.18. Label: 9
Note. Sugar-free versions are available and can be ordered by specifying 'sugar-free' on the prescription
Available from APS, Ashbourne (*Amix*®), Berk (*Almodan*®), Cox, Eastern (*Amoram*®), Galen (*Galenamox*®), Hillcross, Kent, Norton, Ranbaxy (*Rimoxallin*®)

Sachets, sugar-free, amoxicillin (as trihydrate) 3 g/
sachet, net price 2-sachet pack = £5.14, 14-sachet
pack = £33.76. Label: 9, 13
Available from Hillcross, Kent, Norton

Injection, powder for reconstitution, amoxicillin
(as sodium salt), net price 250-mg vial = 36p;
500-mg vial = 66p; 1-g vial = £1.31
Available from CP

Amoxil® (Bencard) PoM
Capsules, both maroon/gold, amoxicillin (as trihydrate), 250 mg, net price 21-cap pack = £3.86;
500 mg, 21-cap pack = £7.73. Label: 9
Syrup SF, both sugar-free, amoxicillin (as trihydrate) for reconstitution with water, 125 mg/5 mL,
net price 100 mL = £2.31; 250 mg/5 mL, 100 mL
= £4.62. Label: 9
Paediatric suspension, amoxicillin 125 mg (as trihydrate)/1.25 mL when reconstituted with water.
Net price 20 mL = £3.63. Label: 9, counselling,
use of pipette
Sachets SF, powder, sugar-free, amoxicillin (as trihydrate) 3 g/sachet, 2-sachet pack = £4.97. Label:
9, 13
Injection, powder for reconstitution, amoxicillin
(as sodium salt). Net price 250-mg vial = 34p;
500-mg vial = 63p; 1-g vial = £1.25
Electrolytes: Na+ 3.3 mmol/g

AMPICILLIN

Indications: urinary-tract infections, otitis media,
sinusitis, chronic bronchitis, invasive salmonellosis, gonorrhoea
Cautions: history of allergy; renal impairment;
erythematous rashes common in glandular fever,
chronic lymphatic leukaemia, and possibly HIV
infection (see notes above); **interactions:** Appendix 1 (penicillins)
Contra-indications: penicillin hypersensitivity
Side-effects: nausea, diarrhoea; rashes (discontinue
treatment); rarely, antibiotic-associated colitis; see
also under Benzylpenicillin (section 5.1.1.1)
Dose: *by mouth*, 0.25–1 g every 6 hours, at least 30
minutes before food
Gonorrhoea, 2–3 g as a single dose with probenecid 1 g
Urinary-tract infections, 500 mg every 8 hours
*By intramuscular injection or intravenous injection
or infusion*, 500 mg every 4–6 hours; higher doses
in meningitis
CHILD under 10 years, any route, half adult dose

Ampicillin (Non-proprietary) PoM
Capsules, ampicillin 250 mg, net price 20 = £1.25;
500 mg, 20 = £2.26. Label: 9, 23
Available from Cox, Kent, Norton, Ranbaxy (*Rimacil-
lin*®)
Oral suspension, ampicillin 125 mg/5 mL when
reconstituted with water, net price 100 mL =
£1.75; 250 mg/5 mL, 100 mL = £3.36. Label: 9, 23
Available from Cox, Kent, Norton, Ranbaxy (*Rimacil-
lin*®)

Penbritin® (SmithKline Beecham) PoM
Capsules, both black/red, ampicillin (as trihydrate)
250 mg, net price 28-cap pack = £2.26. Label: 9, 23
Injection, powder for reconstitution, ampicillin (as
sodium salt), net price 500-mg vial = 74p
Electrolytes: Na+ 1.47 mmol/500-mg vial

■ With flucloxacillin
See Co-fluampicil

CO-AMOXICLAV

A mixture of amoxicillin (as the trihydrate or as the sodium salt) and clavulanic acid (as potassium clavulanate);
the proportions are expressed in the form *x/y* where *x*
and *y* are the strengths in milligrams of amoxicillin and
clavulanic acid respectively

Indications: infections due to beta-lactamase-producing strains (where amoxicillin alone not
appropriate) including respiratory-tract infections, genito-urinary and abdominal infections,
cellulitis, animal bites, severe dental infection
with spreading cellulitis
Cautions: see under Ampicillin and notes above;
also caution in hepatic impairment (monitor
hepatic function), pregnancy
CHOLESTATIC JAUNDICE. CSM has advised that cholestatic jaundice has been identified as an adverse reaction
occuring either during, or shortly after, the use of co-
amoxiclav. An epidemiological study has shown that the
risk of acute liver toxicity was about 6 times greater with
co-amoxiclav than with amoxicillin. Cholestatic jaundice is more common in patients above the age of 65
years and in males; these reactions have only rarely been
reported in children. Jaundice is usually self-limiting
and very rarely fatal. The duration of treatment should
be appropriate to the indication and should not usually
exceed 14 days
Contra-indications: penicillin hypersensitivity,
history of co-amoxiclav-associated or penicillin-
associated jaundice or hepatic dysfunction
Side-effects: see under Ampicillin; hepatitis,
cholestatic jaundice (see above); erythema multiforme (including Stevens-Johnson syndrome),
toxic epidermal necrolysis, exfoliative dermatitis,
vasculitis reported; rarely prolongation of bleeding time, dizziness, headache, convulsions (particularly with high doses or in renal impairment);
superficial staining of teeth with suspension,
phlebitis at injection site
Dose: *by mouth*, expressed as amoxicillin, 250 mg
every 8 hours, dose doubled in severe infections;
CHILD see under preparations below (under 6
years *Augmentin®* '125/31 SF' suspension; 6–12
years *Augmentin®* '250/62 SF' suspension or for
short-term treatment with twice daily dosage in
CHILD 2 months–12 years *Augmentin-Duo®* 400/
57 suspension)
Severe dental infections (but not generally first-
line, see notes above), expressed as amoxicillin,
250 mg every 8 hours for 5 days
By intravenous injection over 3–4 minutes *or by
intravenous infusion*, expressed as amoxicillin,
1 g every 8 hours increased to 1 g every 6 hours in
more serious infections; INFANTS up to 3 months
25 mg/kg every 8 hours (every 12 hours in the
perinatal period and in premature infants); CHILD
3 months–12 years, 25 mg/kg every 8 hours
increased to 25 mg/kg every 6 hours in more serious infections
Surgical prophylaxis, expressed as amoxicillin,
1 g at induction; for high risk procedures (e.g.
colorectal surgery) a further 2–3 doses may be
given every 8 hours in first 24 hours (longer if
significantly increased risk of infection)

Augmentin® (SmithKline Beecham) PoM
Tablets 375 mg, f/c, co-amoxiclav 250/125 (amoxicillin 250 mg as trihydrate, clavulanic acid
125 mg as potassium salt), net price 21-tab pack =
£9.79. Label: 9

Tablets 625 mg, f/c, co-amoxiclav 500/125 (amoxicillin 500 mg as trihydrate, clavulanic acid 125 mg as potassium salt). Net price 21-tab pack = £15.73. Label: 9

Dispersible tablets, sugar-free, co-amoxiclav 250/125 (amoxicillin 250 mg as trihydrate, clavulanic acid 125 mg as potassium salt). Net price 21-tab pack = £10.99. Label: 9, 13

Suspension '125/31 SF', sugar-free, co-amoxiclav 125/31 (amoxicillin 125 mg as trihydrate, clavulanic acid 31 mg as potassium salt)/5 mL when reconstituted with water. Net price 100 mL = £4.57. Label: 9

Excipients: include aspartame 12.5 mg/5 mL (section 9.4.1)
Dose: CHILD 1–6 years (10–18 kg) 5 mL every 8 hours *or* INFANT and CHILD up to 6 years 0.8 mL/kg daily in 3 divided doses; in severe infections dose increased to 1.6 mL/kg daily in 3 divided doses

Suspension '250/62 SF', sugar-free, co-amoxiclav 250/62 (amoxicillin 250 mg as trihydrate, clavulanic acid 62 mg as potassium salt)/5 mL when reconstituted with water. Net price 100 mL = £6.42. Label: 9

Excipients: include aspartame 12.5 mg/5 mL (section 9.4.1)
Dose: CHILD 6–12 years (18–40 kg) 5 mL every 8 hours *or* 0.4 mL/kg daily in 3 divided doses; in severe infections dose increased to 0.8 mL/kg daily in 3 divided doses

Injection 600 mg, powder for reconstitution, co-amoxiclav 500/100 (amoxicillin 500 mg as sodium salt, clavulanic acid 100 mg as potassium salt). Net price per vial = £1.49

Electrolytes: Na⁺ 1.6 mmol, K⁺ 0.5 mmol/600-mg vial

Injection 1.2 g, powder for reconstitution, co-amoxiclav 1000/200 (amoxicillin 1 g as sodium salt, clavulanic acid 200 mg as potassium salt). Net price per vial = £2.97

Electrolytes: Na⁺ 3.1 mmol, K⁺ 1 mmol/1.2-g vial

Augmentin-Duo® (SmithKline Beecham) PoM

Suspension '400/57', sugar-free, co-amoxiclav 400/57 (amoxicillin 400 mg as trihydrate, clavulanic acid 57 mg as potassium salt)/5 mL when reconstituted with water. Net price 35 mL = £4.71, 70 mL = £6.61. Label: 9

Excipients: include aspartame 12.5 mg/5 mL (section 9.4.1)
Dose: CHILD 2 months–2 years 0.15 mL/kg twice daily, 2–6 years (13–21 kg) 2.5 mL twice daily, 7–12 years (22–40 kg) 5 mL twice daily, doubled in severe infections

CO-FLUAMPICIL

A mixture of equal parts by mass of flucloxacillin and ampicillin

Indications: mixed infections involving beta-lactamase-producing staphylococci

Cautions; Contra-indications; Side-effects: see under Ampicillin and Flucloxacillin

Dose: *by mouth*, co-fluampicil, 250/250 every 6 hours, dose doubled in severe infections; CHILD under 10 years half adult dose, dose doubled in severe infections

By intramuscular or slow intravenous injection or by intravenous infusion, co-fluampicil 250/250 every 6 hours, dose doubled in severe infections; CHILD under 2 years quarter adult dose, 2–10 years half adult dose, dose doubled in severe infections

Co-fluampicil (Non-proprietary) PoM

Capsules, co-fluampicil 250/250 (flucloxacillin 250 mg as sodium salt, ampicillin 250 mg as trihydrate). Net price 20 = £5.80. Label: 9, 22

Available from Cox, Generics (*Flu-Amp®*), Kent, Norton

Magnapen® (SmithKline Beecham) PoM

Capsules, black/turquoise, co-fluampicil 250/250 (flucloxacillin 250 mg as sodium salt, ampicillin 250 mg as trihydrate). Net price 20-cap pack = £6.15. Label: 9, 22

Syrup, co-fluampicil 125/125 (flucloxacillin 125 mg as magnesium salt, ampicillin 125 mg as trihydrate)/5 mL when reconstituted with water. Net price 100 mL = £4.99. Label: 9, 22

Injection 500 mg, powder for reconstitution, co-fluampicil 250/250 (flucloxacillin 250 mg as sodium salt, ampicillin 250 mg as sodium salt). Net price per vial = £1.33

Electrolytes: Na⁺ 1.3 mmol/vial

5.1.1.4   Antipseudomonal penicillins

The carboxypenicillin, **ticarcillin**, is principally indicated for serious infections caused by *Pseudomonas aeruginosa* although it also has activity against certain other Gram-negative bacilli including *Proteus* spp. and *Bacteroides fragilis*.

Ticarcillin is now available only in combination with clavulanic acid (section 5.1.1.3); the combination (*Timentin®*) is active against beta-lactamase-producing bacteria resistant to ticarcillin.

The ureidopenicillin, **piperacillin**, has a broad spectrum and it is more active than ticarcillin against *Ps. aeruginosa*.

Tazocin® (piperacillin with the beta-lactamase inhibitor tazobactam) is active against beta-lactamase-producing bacteria resistant to the ureidopenicillins; it has a spectrum of activity comparable to the carbapenems, imipenem and meropenem (section 5.1.2).

For pseudomonas septicaemias (especially in neutropenia or endocarditis) these antipseudomonal penicillins should be given with an aminoglycoside (e.g. gentamicin or netilmicin, section 5.1.4) since they have a synergistic effect. Penicillins and aminoglycosides must not, however, be mixed in the same syringe or infusion.

Owing to the sodium content of many of these antibiotics, high doses may lead to hypernatraemia.

PIPERACILLIN

Indications: infections due to *Pseudomonas aeruginosa*, see notes above; surgical prophylaxis

Cautions; Contra-indications; Side-effects: see under Benzylpenicillin (section 5.1.1.1); renal impairment (reduce dose; see Appendix 3); Stevens-Johnson syndrome reported rarely; leucopenia with prolonged use

Dose: *by deep intramuscular injection or by intravenous injection* over 3–5 minutes *or by intravenous infusion*, 100–150 mg/kg daily (in divided doses), increased to 200–300 mg/kg daily in severe infections, and to at least 16 g daily in life-threatening infections; single doses over 2 g intravenous route only; NEONATE *by intravenous injection* over 3–5 minutes *or by intravenous infusion*, aged up to 7 days *or over* 7 days but under 2 kg, 150 mg/kg daily in 3 divided doses; aged over 7 days and over 2 kg, 300 mg/kg daily in 3–4 divided doses; CHILD 1 month–12 years, 100–200 mg/kg daily in 3–4 divided doses, increased in severe infections to 200–300 mg/kg daily in 3–4 divided doses

Surgical prophylaxis, *by deep intramuscular injection or by intravenous injection* over 3–5 minutes *or by intravenous infusion*, 2 g just before surgery (or, in caesarean section, when umbilical cord clamped) followed by at least 2 doses of 2 g at 4 or 6 hour intervals within 24 hours of surgery

Acute gonorrhoea, *by deep intramuscular injection*, 2 g as a single dose

Pipril® (Lederle) PoM
Injection, powder for reconstitution, piperacillin (as sodium salt). Net price 1-g vial = £2.79; 2-g vial = £5.53
Infusion, powder for reconstitution, piperacillin 4 g (as sodium salt), with 50-mL bottle water for injections and transfer needle. Net price complete unit = £11.65
Electrolytes: Na⁺ 1.85 mmol/g

■ With tazobactam

Tazocin® (Lederle) PoM
Injection 2.25 g, powder for reconstitution, piperacillin 2 g (as sodium salt), tazobactam 250 mg (as sodium salt). Net price per vial = £7.24
Electrolytes: Na⁺ 4.69 mmol/2.25-g vial
Injection 4.5 g, powder for reconstitution, piperacillin 4 g (as sodium salt), tazobactam 500 mg (as sodium salt). Net price per vial = £13.16; infusion pack (4.5-g infusion bottle, 50-mL bottle water for injections and transfer needle) = £14.48
Electrolytes: Na⁺ 9.37 mmol/4.5-g vial
Dose: lower respiratory-tract, urinary-tract, intra-abdominal and skin infections, and septicaemia, ADULT and CHILD over 12 years, *by intravenous injection* over 3–5 minutes *or by intravenous infusion*, 2.25–4.5 g every 6–8 hours, usually 4.5 g every 8 hours; CHILD under 12 years, not yet recommended
Infections in neutropenic patients (in combination with an aminoglycoside), *by intravenous injection* over 3–5 minutes *or by intravenous infusion*, ADULT and CHILD over 50 kg, 4.5 g every 6 hours; CHILD less than 50 kg, 90 mg/kg every 6 hours

TICARCILLIN

Indications: infections due to *Pseudomonas* and *Proteus* spp, see notes above
Cautions; Contra-indications; Side-effects: see under Benzylpenicillin (section 5.1.1.1)
Dose: see under preparation

■ With clavulanic acid
Note. For a CSM warning on cholestatic jaundice possibly associated with clavulanic acid, see under Co-amoxiclav p. 255.

Timentin® (SmithKline Beecham) PoM
Injection 3.2 g, powder for reconstitution, ticarcillin 3 g (as sodium salt), clavulanic acid 200 mg (as potassium salt). Net price per vial = £6.08
Electrolytes: Na⁺ 16 mmol, K⁺ 1 mmol/3.2-g vial
Dose: by intravenous infusion, 3.2 g every 6–8 hours increased to every 4 hours in more severe infections; CHILD 80 mg/kg every 6–8 hours (every 12 hours in neonates)

5.1.1.5   Mecillinams

Pivmecillinam has significant activity against many Gram-negative bacteria including *Escherichia coli*, klebsiella, enterobacter and salmonellae. It is not active against *Pseudomonas aeruginosa* or enterococci. Pivmecillinam is hydrolysed to mecillinam, which is the active drug.

PIVMECILLINAM HYDROCHLORIDE

Indications: see under Dose below
Cautions: see under Benzylpenicillin (section 5.1.1.1); also liver and renal function tests required in long-term use; pregnancy; **interactions:** Appendix 1 (penicillins)
Contra-indications: see under Benzylpenicillin (section 5.1.1.1); also carnitine deficiency, oesophageal strictures, gastro-intestinal obstruction, infants under 3 months
Side-effects: see under Benzylpenicillin (section 5.1.1.1); nausea, vomiting, dyspepsia; also reduced serum and total body carnitine (especially with long-term or repeated use)
Dose: acute uncomplicated cystitis, ADULT and CHILD over 40 kg, initially 400 mg then 200 mg every 8 hours for 3 days
Chronic or recurrent bacteriuria, ADULT and CHILD over 40 kg, 400 mg every 6–8 hours
Urinary-tract infections, CHILD under 40 kg, 20–40 mg/kg daily in 3–4 divided doses
Salmonellosis, ADULT and CHILD over 40 kg, 1.2–2.4 g daily for 14 days (14–28 days for carriers); CHILD under 40 kg, 30–60 mg/kg daily in 3–4 divided doses
COUNSELLING. Tablets should be swallowed whole with plenty of fluid during meals while sitting or standing

Selexid® (Leo) PoM
Tablets, f/c, pivmecillinam hydrochloride 200 mg, net price 10-tab pack = £4.50. Label 9, 21, 27, counselling, posture (see Dose above)

5.1.2   Cephalosporins, cephamycins, and other beta-lactams

Antibiotics in this section include the **cephalosporins**, such as cefotaxime, ceftazidime, cefuroxime, cefalexin and cefradine, the **cephamycin**, cefoxitin, the **monobactam**, aztreonam, and the **carbapenems**, imipenem (a thienamycin derivative) and meropenem.

Cephalosporins and cephamycins

The cephalosporins are broad-spectrum antibiotics which are used for the treatment of septicaemia, pneumonia, meningitis, biliary-tract infections, peritonitis, and urinary-tract infections. All have a similar antibacterial spectrum although individual agents have differing activity against certain organisms. The pharmacology of the cephalosporins is similar to that of the penicillins, excretion being principally renal and blocked by probenecid. Cephalosporins penetrate the cerebrospinal fluid poorly unless the meninges are inflamed; cefotaxime is a suitable cephalosporin for infections of the CNS (e.g meningitis).

The principal side-effect of the cephalosporins is hypersensitivity and about 10% of penicillin-sensitive patients will also be allergic to the cephalosporins. Haemorrhage due to interference with blood clotting factors has been associated with several cephalosporins.

Cefradine (cephradine) and **cefazolin** (cephazolin) have generally been replaced by the newer cephalosporins mentioned below.

Cefuroxime and **cefamandole** (cephamandole) are 'second generation' cephalosporins and are less susceptible than the earlier cephalosporins to inactivation by beta-lactamases. They are, therefore, active against certain bacteria which are resistant to the other drugs and have greater activity against *Haemophilus influenzae* and *Neisseria gonorrhoeae*.

Cefotaxime, **ceftazidime** and **ceftriaxone** are 'third generation' cephalosporins with greater activity than the 'second generation' cephalosporins against certain Gram-negative bacteria. However, they are less active than cefuroxime and cefamandole against Gram-positive bacteria, most notably *Staphylococcus aureus*. Their broad antibacterial spectrum may encourage superinfection with resistant bacteria or fungi.

Ceftazidime has good activity against pseudomonas. It is also active against other Gram-negative bacteria.

Ceftriaxone has a longer half-life and therefore only needs once daily administration. Indications include serious infections such as septicaemia, pneumonia, and meningitis. The calcium salt of ceftriaxone forms a precipitate in the gall bladder which may rarely cause symptoms but these usually resolve when the antibiotic is stopped.

Cefpirome is indicated for urinary-tract, lower respiratory-tract and skin infections, bacteraemia, and infections associated with neutropenia.

Cefoxitin, a cephamycin antibiotic, is active against bowel flora including *Bacteroides fragilis* and because of this it has been recommended for abdominal sepsis such as peritonitis.

ORALLY ACTIVE CEPHALOSPORINS. The orally active 'first generation' cephalosporins, **cefalexin** (cephalexin), **cefradine**, and **cefadroxil** and the 'second generation' cephalosporins, **cefaclor** and **cefprozil**, have a similar antimicrobial spectrum. They are useful for urinary-tract infections which do not respond to other drugs or which occur in pregnancy, respiratory-tract infections, otitis media, sinusitis, and skin and soft-tissue infections. Cefaclor has good activity against *H. influenzae*, but it is associated with protracted skin reactions especially in children. Cefadroxil has a long duration of action and can be given twice daily; it has poor activity against *H. influenzae*. **Cefuroxime axetil**, an ester of the 'second generation' cephalosporin cefuroxime, has the same antibacterial spectrum as the parent compound.

Cefixime has a longer duration of action than the other cephalosporins that are active by mouth. It is presently only licensed for acute infections.

Cefpodoxime proxetil, is more active than the other oral cephalosporins against respiratory bacterial pathogens and it is licensed for upper and lower respiratory-tract infections.

CEFACLOR

Indications: infections due to sensitive Gram-positive and Gram-negative bacteria, but see notes above

Cautions: penicillin sensitivity; renal impairment (Appendix 3); pregnancy and breast-feeding (but appropriate to use); false positive urinary glucose (if tested for reducing substances) and false positive Coombs' test; **interactions:** Appendix 1 (cephalosporins)

Contra-indications: cephalosporin hypersensitivity; porphyria (section 9.8.2)

Side-effects: diarrhoea and rarely antibiotic-associated colitis (CSM has warned both more likely with higher doses), nausea and vomiting, abdominal discomfort, headache; allergic reactions including rashes, pruritus, urticaria, serum sickness-like reactions with rashes, fever and arthralgia, and anaphylaxis; erythema multiforme, toxic epidermal necrolysis reported; disturbances in liver enzymes, transient hepatitis and cholestatic jaundice; other side-effects reported include eosinophilia and blood disorders (including thrombocytopenia, leucopenia, agranulocytosis, aplastic anaemia and haemolytic anaemia); reversible interstitial nephritis, hyperactivity, nervousness, sleep disturbances, confusion, hypertonia, and dizziness

Dose: 250 mg every 8 hours, doubled for severe infections; max. 4 g daily; CHILD over 1 month, 20 mg/kg daily in 3 divided doses, doubled for severe infections, max. 1 g daily; *or* 1 month–1 year, 62.5 mg every 8 hours; 1–5 years, 125 mg; over 5 years, 250 mg; doses doubled for severe infections

Cefaclor (Non-proprietary) PoM
Capsules, cefaclor (as monohydrate) 250 mg, net price 21-cap pack = £6.80; 500 mg 21 = £22.74. Label: 9
Available from Cox, Galen (*Keftid*®), Hillcross, Kent
Suspension, cefaclor (as monohydrate) for reconstitution with water, 125 mg/5 mL, net price 100 mL = £5.07; 250 mg/5 mL, 100 mL = £8.86. Label: 9
Note. Sugar-free versions are available and can be ordered by specifying 'sugar-free' on the prescription
Available from Cox, Galen (*Keftid*®), Genus, Hillcross

Distaclor® (Dista) PoM
Capsules, cefaclor (as monohydrate) 500 mg (violet/grey), net price 20 = £21.66. Label: 9
Suspension, both pink, cefaclor (as monohydrate) for reconstitution with water, 125 mg/5 mL, net price 100 mL = £5.16; 250 mg/5 mL, 100 mL = £10.32. Label: 9

Distaclor MR® (Dista) PoM
Tablets, m/r, both blue, cefaclor (as monohydrate) 375 mg. Net price 14-tab pack = £6.93. Label: 9, 21, 25
Dose: 375 mg every 12 hours with food, dose doubled for pneumonia
Lower urinary-tract infections, 375 mg every 12 hours with food

CEFADROXIL

Indications: see under Cefaclor; see also notes above

Cautions; Contra-indications; Side-effects: see under Cefaclor

Dose: patients over 40 kg, 0.5–1 g twice daily; skin, soft tissue, and simple urinary-tract infections, 1 g daily; CHILD under 1 year, 25 mg/kg daily in divided doses; 1–6 years, 250 mg twice daily; over 6 years, 500 mg twice daily

Baxan® (Bristol-Myers) PoM
Capsules, cefadroxil (as monohydrate) 500 mg, net price 20 = £5.64. Label: 9
Suspension, cefadroxil (as monohydrate) for reconstitution with water, 125 mg/5 mL, net price 60 mL = £1.75; 250 mg/5 mL, 60 mL = £3.48; 500 mg/5 mL, 60 mL = £5.21. Label: 9

CEFALEXIN
(Cephalexin)
Indications: see under Cefaclor
Cautions; Contra-indications; Side-effects: see under Cefaclor
Dose: 250 mg every 6 hours *or* 500 mg every 8–12 hours increased to 1–1.5 g every 6–8 hours for severe infections; CHILD 25 mg/kg daily in divided doses, doubled for severe infections, max. 100 mg/kg daily; *or* under 1 year 125 mg every 12 hours, 1–5 years 125 mg every 8 hours, 6–12 years 250 mg every 8 hours
Prophylaxis of recurrent urinary-tract infection, ADULT 125 mg at night

Cefalexin (Non-proprietary) PoM
Capsules, cefalexin 250 mg, net price 28-cap pack = £3.56; 500 mg, 21-cap pack = £5.50. Label: 9
Available from APS, Cox, Hillcross, Kent (*Tenkorex®*), Ranbaxy
Tablets, cefalexin 250 mg, net price 20 = £2.36; 500 mg, 20 = £4.41. Label: 9
Available from APS, Berk (*Kiflone®*), Cox, Hillcross, Kent (*Tenkorex®*), Norton
Oral suspension, cefalexin for reconstitution with water, 125 mg/5 mL, net price 100 mL = £1.28; 250 mg/5 mL, 100 mL = £2.51. Label: 9
Available from APS, Cox, Hillcross, Kent (*Tenkorex®*)

Ceporex® (GlaxoWellcome) PoM
Capsules, both caramel/grey, cefalexin 250 mg, net price 28-cap pack = £4.47; 500 mg, 28-cap pack = £8.72. Label: 9
Tablets, all pink, f/c, cefalexin 250 mg, net price 28-tab pack = £4.47; 500 mg, 28-tab pack = £8.72; 1 g (scored), 14-tab pack = £8.72. Label: 9
Syrup, all orange, cefalexin for reconstitution with water, 125 mg/5 mL, net price 100 mL = £1.59; 250 mg/5 mL, 100 mL = £3.19; 500 mg/5 mL, 100 mL = £6.19. Label: 9

Keflex® (Lilly) PoM
Capsules, cefalexin 250 mg (green/white), net price 28-cap pack = £3.57; 500 mg (pale green/dark green), 21-cap pack = £5.23. Label: 9
Tablets, both peach, cefalexin 250 mg, net price 28-tab pack = £3.57; 500 mg (scored), 21-tab pack = £5.23. Label: 9
Suspension, cefalexin for reconstitution with water, 125 mg/5 mL (pink), net price 100 mL = £1.27; 250 mg/5 mL (orange), 100 mL = £2.55. Label: 9

CEFAMANDOLE
(Cephamandole)
Indications: see under Cefaclor; surgical prophylaxis
Cautions; Contra-indications; Side-effects: see under Cefaclor
Dose: *by deep intramuscular injection or by intravenous injection* over 3–5 minutes *or by intravenous infusion*, 0.5–2 g every 4–8 hours; CHILD over 1 month, 50–100 mg/kg daily in 3–6 divided doses increased to 150 mg/kg daily for severe infections
Surgical prophylaxis, *by intramuscular or intravenous injection*, 1–2 g 30–60 minutes before surgery followed by 1–2 g every 6 hours for 24–48 hours (up to 72 hours for implantation of prostheses)

Kefadol® (Dista) PoM
Injection, powder for reconstitution, cefamandole (as nafate) with sodium carbonate. Net price 1-g vial = £3.91
Electrolytes: Na+ 3.35 mmol/1-g vial

CEFAZOLIN
(Cephazolin)
Indications: see under Cefaclor; surgical prophylaxis
Cautions; Contra-indications; Side-effects: see under Cefaclor
Dose: *by intramuscular injection or intravenous injection or infusion*, 0.5–1 g every 6–12 hours; CHILD, 25–50 mg/kg daily (in divided doses), increased to 100 mg/kg daily in severe infections

Kefzol® (Lilly) PoM
Injection, powder for reconstitution, cefazolin (as sodium salt). Net price 500-mg vial = £2.45; 1-g vial = £4.63
Electrolytes: Na+ 2.1 mmol/g

CEFIXIME
Indications: see under Cefaclor and notes above
Cautions; Contra-indications; Side-effects: see under Cefaclor
Dose: ADULT and CHILD over 10 years, 200–400 mg daily in 1–2 divided doses; CHILD over 6 months 8 mg/kg daily in 1–2 divided doses *or* 6 months–1 year 75 mg daily; 1–4 years 100 mg daily; 5–10 years 200 mg daily

Suprax® (Rhône-Poulenc Rorer) PoM
Tablets, f/c, scored, cefixime 200 mg. Net price 7-tab pack = £12.03. Label: 9
Paediatric oral suspension, cefixime 100 mg/5 mL when reconstituted with water. Net price 37.5 mL (with double-ended spoon for measuring 3.75 mL or 5 mL since dilution not recommended) = £7.90; 75 mL = £14.18. Label: 9

CEFOTAXIME
Indications: see under Cefaclor; surgical prophylaxis; Haemophilus epiglottitis and meningitis (section 5.1 table 1); see also notes above
Cautions; Contra-indications; Side-effects: see under Cefaclor; rarely arrhythmias following rapid injection reported
Dose: *by intramuscular or intravenous injection or by intravenous infusion*, 1 g every 12 hours increased in severe infections (e.g. meningitis) to 8 g daily in 4 divided doses; higher doses (up to 12 g daily in 3–4 divided doses) may be required; NEONATE, 50 mg/kg daily in 2–4 divided doses increased to 150–200 mg/kg daily in severe infections; CHILD, 100–150 mg/kg daily in 2–4 divided doses increased up to 200 mg/kg daily in very severe infections
Gonorrhoea, 1 g as a single dose

Claforan® (Hoechst Marion Roussel) PoM
Injection, powder for reconstitution, cefotaxime (as sodium salt), net price 500-mg vial = £2.41; 1-g vial (with or without infusion connector) = £4.85; 2-g vial (with or without infusion connector) = £9.65
Electrolytes: Na+ 2.09 mmol/g

CEFOXITIN

Indications: see under Cefaclor; surgical prophylaxis; more active against Gram-negative bacteria

Cautions; Contra-indications; Side-effects: see under Cefaclor

Dose: *by deep intramuscular or by slow intravenous injection or by infusion*, 1–2 g every 6–8 hours, increased up to 12 g daily in divided doses for infections requiring higher doses; CHILD up to 1 week 20–40 mg/kg every 12 hours, 1–4 weeks 20–40 mg/kg every 8 hours, over 1 month 20–40 mg/kg every 6–8 hours, increased up to 200 mg/kg daily in divided doses (max. 12 g daily) in severe infections; intravenous route recommended for children

Uncomplicated urinary-tract infection, *by deep intramuscular injection*, 1 g every 12 hours for 10 days

Uncomplicated gonorrhoea, *by deep intramuscular injection*, 2 g as a single dose with probenecid 1 g by mouth

Surgical prophylaxis, *by deep intramuscular injection or by intravenous injection or infusion*, 2 g 30–60 minutes before surgery, dose repeated every 6 hours for usual max. 24 hours; CHILD 30–40 mg/kg 30–60 minutes before surgery, dose repeated every 6 hours for usual max. 24 hours (second and third doses every 8–12 hours in NEONATES); intravenous route recommended for children

Mefoxin® (MSD) ▒PoM▒

Injection, powder for reconstitution, cefoxitin (as sodium salt). Net price 1-g vial = £4.92; 2-g vial = £9.84

Electrolytes: Na⁺ 2.3 mmol/g

CEFPIROME

Indications: see under Cefaclor and notes above

Cautions; Contra-indications; Side-effects: see under Cefaclor; interference with creatinine assays using picrate method; taste disturbance shortly after injection reported

Dose: *by intravenous injection or infusion*, complicated upper and lower urinary-tract, skin and soft-tissue infections, 1 g every 12 hours increased to 2 g every 12 hours in very severe infections

Lower respiratory-tract infections, 1–2 g every 12 hours

Severe infections including bacteraemia and septicaemia and infections in neutropenic patients, 2 g every 12 hours

CHILD under 12 years not recommended

Cefrom® (Hoechst Marion Roussel) ▒PoM▒

Injection, powder for reconstitution, cefpirome (as sulphate), net price 1-g vial = £10.75; 2-g vial = £21.50

CEFPODOXIME

Indications: see under Dose

Cautions: see under Cefaclor

Contra-indications: see under Cefaclor

Side-effects: see under Cefaclor

Dose: upper respiratory-tract infections (but in pharyngitis and tonsillitis reserved for infections which are recurrent, chronic, or resistant to other antibiotics), 100 mg twice daily (200 mg twice daily in sinusitis)

Lower respiratory-tract infections (including bronchitis and pneumonia), 100–200 mg twice daily

Skin and soft tissue infections, 200 mg twice daily

Uncomplicated urinary-tract infections, 100 mg twice daily (200 mg twice daily in uncomplicated upper urinary-tract infections)

Uncomplicated gonorrhoea, 200 mg as a single dose

CHILD 15 days–6 months 4 mg/kg every 12 hours, 6 months–2 years 40 mg every 12 hours, 3–8 years 80 mg every 12 hours, over 9 years 100 mg every 12 hours

Orelox® (Hoechst Marion Roussel) ▒PoM▒

Tablets, f/c, cefpodoxime 100 mg (as proxetil), net price 10-tab pack = £9.26. Label: 5, 9, 21

Oral suspension, cefpodoxime (as proxetil) for reconstitution with water, 40 mg/5 mL, net price 50 mL = £6.50, 100 mL = £10.89. Label: 5, 9, 21

Excipients: include aspartame (section 9.4.1)

CEFPROZIL

Indications: see under Dose

Cautions: see under Cefaclor

Contra-indications: see under Cefaclor

Side-effects: see under Cefaclor

Dose: upper respiratory-tract infections and skin and soft tissue infections, 500 mg once daily usually for 10 days; CHILD 6 months–12 years, 20 mg/kg (max. 500 mg) once daily

Acute exacerbation of chronic bronchitis, 500 mg every 12 hours usually for 10 days

Otitis media, CHILD 6 months–12 years, 20 mg/kg (max. 500 mg) every 12 hours

Cefzil® (Bristol-Myers) ▼ ▒PoM▒

Tablets, cefprozil, 250 mg (orange), net price 20-tab pack = £14.95; 500 mg, 10-tab pack = £14.95. Label: 9

Suspension, cefprozil, 250 mg/5 mL when reconstituted with water, net price 100 mL = £15.22. Label: 9

Excipients: include aspartame equivalent to phenylalanine 28 mg/5 mL (section 9.4.1)

CEFRADINE

(Cephradine)

Indications: see under Cefaclor; surgical prophylaxis

Cautions; Contra-indications; Side-effects: see under Cefaclor

Dose: *by mouth*, 250–500 mg every 6 hours *or* 0.5–1 g every 12 hours; CHILD, 25–50 mg/kg daily in divided doses

By deep intramuscular injection or by intravenous injection over 3–5 minutes or by intravenous infusion, 0.5–1 g every 6 hours, increased to 8 g daily in severe infections; CHILD 50–100 mg/kg daily in 4 divided doses

Surgical prophylaxis, *by deep intramuscular injection or by intravenous injection over 3–5 minutes*, 1–2 g immediately prior to surgery

Cefradine (Non-proprietary) [PoM]
Capsules, cefradine 250 mg, net price 20-cap pack = £3.55; 500 mg, 20-cap pack = £7.00. Label: 9
Available from Galen (*Nicef®*), Norton

Velosef® (Squibb) [PoM]
Capsules, cefradine 250 mg (orange/blue), net price 20-cap pack = £3.55; 500 mg (blue), 20-cap pack = £7.00. Label: 9
Syrup, cefradine 250 mg/5 mL when reconstituted with water. Net price 100 mL = £4.22. Label: 9
Injection, powder for reconstitution, cefradine. Net price 500-mg vial = 99p; 1-g vial = £1.95

CEFTAZIDIME

Indications: see under Cefaclor; see also notes above
Cautions; Contra-indications; Side-effects: see under Cefaclor
Dose: *by deep intramuscular injection or intravenous injection or infusion*, 1 g every 8 hours *or* 2 g every 12 hours; 2 g every 8–12 hours in severe infections; single doses over 1 g intravenous route only; elderly usual max. 3 g daily; CHILD, up to 2 months 25–60 mg/kg daily in 2 divided doses, over 2 months 30–100 mg/kg daily in 2–3 divided doses; up to 150 mg/kg daily (max. 6 g daily) in 3 divided doses if immunocompromised or meningitis; intravenous route recommended for children
Urinary-tract and less serious infections, 0.5–1 g every 12 hours
Pseudomonal lung infection in cystic fibrosis, ADULT with normal renal function 100–150 mg/kg daily in 3 divided doses; CHILD up to 150 mg/kg daily (max. 6 g daily) in 3 divided doses; intravenous route recommended for children
Surgical prophylaxis, prostatic surgery, 1 g at induction of anaesthesia repeated if necessary when catheter removed

Fortum® (GlaxoWellcome) [PoM]
Injection, powder for reconstitution, ceftazidime (as pentahydrate), with sodium carbonate, net price 250-mg vial = £2.37, 500-mg vial = £4.73, 1-g vial = £9.45, 2-g vial (for injection and for infusion, both) = £18.91, 3-g vial (for injection or infusion) = £27.70; *Monovial*, 2 g (with transfer needle) = £18.91
Electrolytes: Na⁺ 2.3 mmol/g

Kefadim® (Lilly) [PoM]
Injection, powder for reconstitution, ceftazidime (as pentahydrate), with sodium carbonate, net price 500-mg vial = £4.95, 1-g vial = £9.90, 2-g vial (for injection and for infusion, both) = £19.80
Electrolytes: Na⁺ 2.3 mmol/g

CEFTRIAXONE

Indications: see under Cefaclor and notes above; surgical prophylaxis; prophylaxis of meningococcal meningitis [unlicensed indication] (section 5.1, table 2)
Cautions: see under Cefaclor; severe renal impairment (Appendix 3); hepatic impairment if accompanied by renal impairment (Appendix 2); premature neonates; may displace bilirubin from serum albumin, administer over 60 minutes in neonates (see also Contra-indications)
Contra-indications: see under Cefaclor; neonates with jaundice, hypoalbuminaemia, acidosis or impaired bilirubin binding

Side-effects: see under Cefaclor; calcium ceftriaxone precipitates in urine (particularly in very young, dehydrated or those who are immobilised) or in gall bladder—consider discontinuation if symptomatic; rarely prolongation of prothrombin time, pancreatitis
Dose: *by deep intramuscular injection, or by intravenous injection* over at least 2–4 minutes, *or by intravenous infusion*, 1 g daily; 2–4 g daily in severe infections; intramuscular doses over 1 g divided between more than one site
INFANT and CHILD 20–50 mg/kg daily; up to 80 mg/kg daily in severe infections; doses of 50 mg/kg and over by intravenous infusion only; NEONATES *by intravenous infusion* over 60 minutes, 20–50 mg/kg daily (max. 50 mg/kg daily)
Uncomplicated gonorrhoea, *by deep intramuscular injection*, 250 mg as a single dose
Surgical prophylaxis, *by deep intramuscular injection or by intravenous injection* over at least 2–4 minutes, 1 g as a single dose; colorectal surgery, *by deep intramuscular injection or by intravenous injection* over at least 2–4 minutes *or by intravenous infusion*, 2 g as a single dose; intramuscular doses over 1 g divided between more than one site

Rocephin® (Roche) [PoM]
Injection, powder for reconstitution, ceftriaxone (as sodium salt), net price 250-mg vial = £2.74; 1-g vial = £10.94; 2-g vial = £21.89
Electrolytes: Na⁺ 3.6 mmol/g

CEFUROXIME

Indications: see under Cefaclor; surgical prophylaxis; more active against *Haemophilus influenzae* and *Neisseria gonorrhoeae*
Cautions; Contra-indications; Side-effects: see under Cefaclor
Dose: *by mouth* (as cefuroxime axetil), 250 mg twice daily in most infections including mild to moderate lower respiratory-tract infections (e.g. bronchitis); doubled for more severe lower respiratory-tract infections or if pneumonia suspected
Urinary-tract infection, 125 mg twice daily, doubled in pyelonephritis
Gonorrhoea, 1 g as a single dose
CHILD over 3 months, 125 mg twice daily, if necessary doubled in child over 2 years with otitis media
By intramuscular injection or intravenous injection or infusion, 750 mg every 6–8 hours; 1.5 g every 6–8 hours in severe infections; single doses over 750 mg intravenous route only
CHILD usual dose 60 mg/kg daily (range 30–100 mg/kg daily) in 3–4 divided doses (2–3 divided doses in neonates)
Gonorrhoea, 1.5 g as a single dose by intramuscular injection (divided between 2 sites)
Surgical prophylaxis, 1.5 g by intravenous injection at induction; may be supplemented with 750 mg intramuscularly 8 and 16 hours later (abdominal, pelvic, and orthopaedic operations) *or* followed by 750 mg intramuscularly every 8 hours for further 24–48 hours (cardiac, pulmonary, oesophageal, and vascular operations)
Meningitis, 3 g intravenously every 8 hours; CHILD, 200–240 mg/kg daily (in 3–4 divided doses) reduced to 100 mg/kg daily after 3 days or on clinical improvement; NEONATE, 100 mg/kg daily reduced to 50 mg/kg daily

Zinacef® (GlaxoWellcome) PoM
Injection, powder for reconstitution, cefuroxime (as sodium salt). Net price 250-mg vial = 84p; 750-mg vial = £2.52; 1.5-g vial (for injection and for infusion) = £5.05
Electrolytes: Na⁺ 1.8 mmol/750-mg vial

Zinnat® (GlaxoWellcome) PoM
Tablets, both f/c, cefuroxime (as axetil) 125 mg, net price 14-tab pack = £4.73; 250 mg, 14-tab pack = £9.45. Label: 9, 21, 25
Suspension, cefuroxime (as axetil) 125 mg/5 mL when reconstituted with water, net price 70 mL = £5.40. Label: 9, 21
Sachets, cefuroxime (as axetil) 125 mg/sachet, net price 14-sachet pack = £5.40. Label: 9, 13, 21

Other beta-lactam antibiotics

Aztreonam is a monocyclic beta-lactam ('monobactam') antibiotic with an antibacterial spectrum limited to Gram-negative aerobic bacteria including *Pseudomonas aeruginosa*, *Neisseria meningitidis*, and *Haemophilus influenzae*; it should not be used alone for 'blind' treatment since it is not active against Gram-positive organisms. Aztreonam is also effective against *Neisseria gonorrhoeae* (but not against concurrent chlamydial infection). Side-effects are similar to those of the other beta-lactams although aztreonam may be less likely to cause hypersensitivity in penicillin-sensitive patients.

Imipenem, a carbapenem, has a broad spectrum of activity which includes many aerobic and anaerobic Gram-positive and Gram-negative bacteria. Imipenem is partially inactivated in the kidney by enzymatic activity and is therefore administered in combination with **cilastatin**, a specific enzyme inhibitor, which blocks its renal metabolism. Side-effects are similar to those of other beta-lactam antibiotics; neurotoxicity has been observed at very high dosage or in renal failure. **Meropenem** is similar to imipenem but is stable to the renal enzyme which inactivates imipenem and therefore can be given without cilastatin. Meropenem has less seizure-inducing potential and can be used to treat central nervous system infection.

AZTREONAM

Indications: Gram-negative infections including *Pseudomonas aeruginosa*, *Haemophilus influenzae*, and *Neisseria meningitidis*
Cautions: hypersensitivity to beta-lactam antibiotics; hepatic impairment; reduce dose in renal impairment; **interactions:** Appendix 1 (aztreonam)
Contra-indications: aztreonam hypersensitivity; pregnancy and breast-feeding
Side-effects: nausea, vomiting, diarrhoea, abdominal cramps; mouth ulcers, altered taste; jaundice and hepatitis; blood disorders (including thrombocytopenia and neutropenia); urticaria and rashes
Dose: *by deep intramuscular injection or by intravenous injection* over 3–5 minutes *or by intravenous infusion*, 1 g every 8 hours *or* 2 g every 12 hours; 2 g every 6–8 hours for severe infections (including systemic *Pseudomonas aeruginosa* and lung infections in cystic fibrosis); single doses over 1 g intravenous route only
CHILD over 1 week, *by intravenous injection or*

infusion*, 30 mg/kg every 6–8 hours increased in severe infections for child of 2 years or older to 50 mg/kg every 6–8 hours; max. 8 g daily
Urinary-tract infections, 0.5–1 g every 8–12 hours
Gonorrhoea/cystitis, *by intramuscular injection*, 1 g as a single dose

Azactam® (Squibb) PoM
Injection, powder for reconstitution, aztreonam. Net price 500-mg vial = £4.48; 1-g vial = £8.95; 2-g vial = £17.90

IMIPENEM WITH CILASTATIN

Indications: aerobic and anaerobic Gram-positive and Gram-negative infections; surgical prophylaxis; not indicated for CNS infections
Cautions: hypersensitivity to other beta-lactam antibiotics; renal impairment; CNS disorders (e.g. epilepsy); pregnancy; **interactions:** Appendix 1 (*Primaxin®*)
Contra-indications: hypersensitivity to imipenem or cilastatin; breast-feeding
Side-effects: nausea, vomiting, diarrhoea (antibiotic-associated colitis reported), taste disturbances; blood disorders, positive Coombs' test; allergic reactions (with rash, pruritus, urticaria, fever, anaphylactic reactions, rarely toxic epidermal necrolysis); myoclonic activity, convulsions, confusion and mental disturbances reported; slight increases in liver enzymes and bilirubin reported; increases in serum creatinine and blood urea; red coloration of urine in children reported; local reactions: erythema, pain and induration, and thrombophlebitis
Dose: *by deep intramuscular injection*, mild to moderate infections, in terms of imipenem, 500–750 mg every 12 hours; gonococcal urethritis or cervicitis, 500 mg as a single dose
By intravenous infusion, in terms of imipenem, 1–2 g daily (in 3–4 divided doses); less sensitive organisms, up to 50 mg/kg daily (to max. 4 g daily); CHILD 3 months and older, 60 mg/kg (up to max. of 2 g) daily in 4 divided doses
Surgical prophylaxis, *by intravenous infusion*, 1 g at induction of anaesthesia repeated after 3 hours, supplemented in high risk (e.g. colorectal) surgery by doses of 500 mg 8 and 16 hours after induction

Primaxin® (MSD) PoM
Intramuscular injection, powder for reconstitution, imipenem (as monohydrate) 500 mg with cilastatin (as sodium salt) 500 mg. Net price 15-mL vial = £15.00
Electrolytes: Na⁺ 1.47 mmol/vial
Intravenous infusion, powder for reconstitution, imipenem (as monohydrate) 500 mg with cilastatin (as sodium salt) 500 mg. Net price 120-mL vial = £15.00; *Monovial*, 20-mL vial (with transfer needle) = £15.00
Electrolytes: Na⁺ 1.72 mmol/vial

MEROPENEM

Indications: aerobic and anaerobic Gram-positive and Gram-negative infections
Cautions: hypersensitivity to penicillins, cephalosporins and other beta-lactam antibiotics; hepatic impairment (monitor liver function); renal impairment; pregnancy and breast-feeding
Contra-indications: hypersensitivity to meropenem

Side-effects: nausea, vomiting, diarrhoea (antibiotic-associated colitis reported), abdominal pain; disturbances in liver function tests; thrombocytopenia (reduction in partial thromboplastin time reported), positive Coombs' test, eosinophilia, neutropenia; headache, paraesthesia; rash, pruritus, urticaria; convulsions reported, local reactions including pain and thrombophlebitis at injection site

Dose: *by intravenous injection* over 5 minutes *or by intravenous infusion*, 500 mg every 8 hours, dose doubled in hospital-acquired pneumonia, peritonitis, septicaemia and infections in neutropenic patients; CHILD 3 months–12 years 10–20 mg/kg every 8 hours, over 50 kg body weight adult dose Meningitis, 2 g every 8 hours; CHILD 3 months–12 years 40 mg/kg every 8 hours, over 50 kg body weight adult dose
Exacerbations of chronic lower respiratory-tract infection in cystic fibrosis, up to 2 g every 8 hours; CHILD 4–18 years 25–40 mg/kg every 8 hours

Meronem® (Zeneca) [PoM]
Injection, powder for reconstitution, meropenem (as trihydrate), net price 250-mg vial = £9.55; 500-mg vial = £14.33; 1-g vial = £28.65
Intravenous infusion, powder for reconstitution, meropenem (as trihydrate), with 100-mL minibag sodium chloride 0.9%, net price 500-mg vial = £16.00; 1-g vial = £31.00
Electrolytes: Na⁺ 3.9 mmol/g

5.1.3 Tetracyclines

The tetracyclines are broad-spectrum antibiotics whose value has decreased owing to increasing bacterial resistance. They remain, however, the treatment of choice for infections caused by chlamydia (trachoma, psittacosis, salpingitis, urethritis, and lymphogranuloma venereum), rickettsia (including Q-fever), brucella (doxycycline with either streptomycin or rifampicin), and the spirochaete, *Borrelia burgdorferi* (Lyme disease). They are also used in respiratory and genital mycoplasma infections, in acne, in destructive (refractory) periodontal disease, in exacerbations of chronic bronchitis (because of their activity against *Haemophilus influenzae*), and for leptospirosis in penicillin hypersensitivity (as an alternative to erythromycin).

Microbiologically, there is little to choose between the various tetracyclines, the only exception being **minocycline** which has a broader spectrum; it is active against *Neisseria meningitidis* and has been used for meningococcal prophylaxis but is no longer recommended because of side-effects including dizziness and vertigo (see section 5.1, table 2 for current recommendations).

The tetracyclines are deposited in growing bone and teeth (being bound to calcium) causing staining and occasionally dental hypoplasia, and should **not** be given to children under 12 years or to pregnant or breast-feeding women. With the exception of **doxycycline** and **minocycline** the tetracyclines may exacerbate renal failure and should **not** be given to patients with kidney disease. Absorption of tetracyclines is decreased by milk (except doxycycline, lymecycline and minocycline), antacids, and calcium, iron and magnesium salts.

TETRACYCLINE

Indications: exacerbations of chronic bronchitis; brucellosis (see also notes above), chlamydia, mycoplasma, and rickettsia; acne vulgaris, rosacea (section 13.6)
Cautions: hepatic impairment; renal impairment (Appendix 3); **interactions:** Appendix 1 (tetracyclines)
Contra-indications: renal impairment (see Appendix 3), pregnancy and breast-feeding (see also Appendixes 4 and 5), children under 12 years of age, systemic lupus erythematosus
Side-effects: nausea, vomiting, diarrhoea, oesophageal irritation; erythema (discontinue treatment); headache and visual disturbances may indicate benign intracranial hypertension; hepatotoxicity, pancreatitis and antibiotic-associated colitis reported; rarely causes photosensitivity; see also notes above
Dose: *by mouth*, 250 mg every 6 hours, increased in severe infections to 500 mg every 6–8 hours
Acne, see section 13.6.2
Primary, secondary, or latent syphilis, 500 mg every 6 hours for 14–21 days
Non-gonococcal urethritis, 500 mg every 6 hours for 7–14 days (21 days if failure or relapse following the first course)
COUNSELLING. Tablets or capsules should be swallowed whole with plenty of fluid while sitting or standing

Tetracycline (Non-proprietary) [PoM]
Capsules, tetracycline hydrochloride 250 mg, net price 20 = 96p. Label: 7, 9, 23, counselling, posture, see above
Available from DDSA (*Economycin®*)
Tablets, coated, tetracycline hydrochloride 250 mg, net price 20 = 38p. Label: 7, 9, 23, counselling, posture, see above
Available from Cox, Hillcross, Kent, Norton
Achromycin® (Lederle) [PoM]
Capsules, orange, tetracycline hydrochloride 250 mg, net price 28-cap pack = £1.34. Label: 7, 9, 23, counselling, posture, see above

■ Compound preparations
Deteclo® (Lederle) [PoM]
Tablets, blue, f/c, tetracycline hydrochloride 115.4 mg, chlortetracycline hydrochloride 115.4 mg, demeclocycline hydrochloride 69.2 mg, net price 14 = £1.83. Label: 7, 9, 11, 23, counselling, posture, see above
Dose: 1 tablet every 12 hours; 3–4 tablets daily in more severe infections

DEMECLOCYCLINE HYDROCHLORIDE

Indications: see under Tetracycline; also inappropriate secretion of antidiuretic hormone, section 6.5.2
Cautions; Contra-indications; Side-effects: see under Tetracycline, but photosensitivity is more common; reversible nephrogenic diabetes insipidus reported
Dose: 150 mg every 6 hours *or* 300 mg every 12 hours

Ledermycin® (Lederle) [PoM]
Capsules, red, demeclocycline hydrochloride 150 mg. Net price 28 = £5.78. Label: 7, 9, 11, 23

DOXYCYCLINE

Indications: see under Tetracycline; brucellosis (with rifampicin); also chronic prostatitis and sinusitis; pelvic inflammatory disease (with metronidazole, section 5.1, table 1); malaria (section 5.4.1); acne, rosacea (section 13.6)

Cautions; Contra-indications; Side-effects: see under Tetracycline, but may be used in renal impairment; photosensitivity reported (avoid exposure to sunlight or sun lamps); avoid in porphyria (section 9.8.2)

Dose: 200 mg on first day, then 100 mg daily; severe infections (including refractory urinary-tract infections), 200 mg daily

Acne, see section 13.6.2

Early syphilis, 200 mg daily in 1–2 divided doses for 14 days; late latent syphilis 100–200 mg twice daily for 28 days (200 mg twice daily preferred)

Uncomplicated genital chlamydia, non-gonococcal urethritis, 100 mg twice daily for 7 days (14 days in pelvic inflammatory disease)

COUNSELLING. Capsules should be swallowed whole with plenty of fluid during meals while sitting or standing

Note. Doxycycline doses in BNF may differ from those in product literature

Doxycycline (Non-proprietary) PoM
Capsules, doxycycline (as hyclate) 50 mg, net price 28-cap pack = £7.30; 100 mg, 20 = £4.93. Label: 6, 9, 11, 27, counselling, posture, see above
Available from APS, Ashbourne (*Demix®*), Berk (*Cyclodox®*), Cox, Hillcross, Kent, Lagap (*Doxylar®*), Norton

Vibramycin® (Invicta) PoM
Capsules, doxycycline (as hyclate) 50 mg (green/ivory), net price 28-cap pack = £7.74, 56-cap pack (*Acne Pack*) = £17.80; 100 mg (green), 8-cap pack = £4.18. Label: 6, 9, 11, 27, counselling, posture, see above

Vibramycin-D® (Invicta) PoM
Dispersible tablets, off-white, doxycycline 100 mg. Net price 8-tab pack = £4.91. Label: 6, 9, 11, 13

LYMECYCLINE

Indications; Cautions; Contra-indications; Side-effects: see under Tetracycline

Dose: 408 mg every 12 hours, increased to 1.224–1.632 g daily in severe infections

Acne, 408 mg daily for at least 8 weeks

Tetralysal 300® (Galderma) PoM
Capsules, lymecycline 408 mg (≡tetracycline 300 mg). Net price 28-cap pack = £4.97. Label: 6, 9

MINOCYCLINE

Indications: see under Tetracycline; also meningococcal carrier state

Cautions; Contra-indications: see under Tetracycline, but may be used in renal impairment; if treatment continued for longer than 6 months, monitor for hepatotoxicity and for systemic lupus erythematosus—discontinue if these develop or if pre-existing systemic lupus erythematosus worsens

Side-effects: see under Tetracycline; also dizziness and vertigo (more common in women); severe exfoliative rashes, pigmentation (sometimes irreversible) discolouration of conjunctiva, tears and sweat, systemic lupus erythematosus and liver damage reported

Dose: 100 mg twice daily

Acne, see section 13.6.2

Gonorrhoea, initially 200 mg then 100 mg every 12 hours for at least 4 days in men; women may require longer treatment

Prophylaxis of asymptomatic meningococcal carrier state (but no longer recommended, see notes above), 100 mg twice daily for 5 days usually followed by rifampicin

Minocycline (Non-proprietary) PoM
Capsules, minocycline (as hydrochloride) 50 mg, net price 56-cap pack = £17.20; 100 mg, 28-cap pack = £14.74. Label: 6, 9
Available from Crookes (*Aknemin®*)
Tablets, minocycline (as hydrochloride) 50 mg, net price 28-tab pack = £7.65; 100 mg, 28-tab pack = £15.27. Label: 6, 9
Available from Ashbourne (*Blemix®*), Cox, CP, Hillcross, Kent, Lederle (*Minocin®*), Norton

Minocin MR® (Lederle) PoM
Capsules, m/r, orange/brown (enclosing yellow and orange pellets), minocycline (as hydrochloride) 100 mg. Net price 56-cap pack = £35.23. Label: 6, 25
Dose: acne, 1 capsule daily

OXYTETRACYCLINE

Indications; Cautions; Contra-indications; Side-effects: see under Tetracycline; avoid in porphyria (see section 9.8.2)

Dose: 250–500 mg every 6 hours

Acne, see section 13.6.2

Oxytetracycline (Non-proprietary) PoM
Tablets, coated, oxytetracycline dihydrate 250 mg, net price 20 = 70p. Label: 7, 9, 23
Available from APS, Ashbourne (*Oxytetramix®*), Cox, DDSA (*Oxymycin®*), Kent, Norton

Terramycin® (Pfizer) PoM
Tablets, yellow, s/c, oxytetracycline (as dihydrate) 250 mg, net price 28-tab pack = 96p. Label: 7, 9, 23

5.1.4   Aminoglycosides

These include amikacin, gentamicin, kanamycin, neomycin, netilmicin, streptomycin, and tobramycin. All are bactericidal and active against some Gram-positive and many Gram-negative organisms. Amikacin, gentamicin, and tobramycin are also active against *Pseudomonas aeruginosa*; streptomycin is active against *Mycobacterium tuberculosis* and is now almost entirely reserved for tuberculosis (section 5.1.9).

The aminoglycosides are not absorbed from the gut (although there is a risk of absorption in inflammatory bowel disease and liver failure) and must therefore be given by injection for systemic infections.

Excretion is principally via the kidney and accumulation occurs in renal impairment.

Most side-effects of this group of antibiotics are dose-related therefore care must be taken with dosage and whenever possible treatment should not exceed 7 days. The important side-effects are ototoxicity, and nephrotoxicity; they occur most commonly in the elderly and in patients with renal failure.

If there is impairment of renal function (or high pre-dose plasma concentrations) the interval between doses must be increased; if the renal impairment is severe the dose itself should be reduced as well.

Aminoglycosides may impair neuromuscular transmission and should not be given to patients with myasthenia gravis; large doses given during surgery have been responsible for a transient myasthenic syndrome in patients with normal neuromuscular function.

Aminoglycosides should not be given with potentially ototoxic diuretics (e.g. furosemide (frusemide)); if concurrent use is unavoidable administration of the aminoglycoside and of the diuretic should be separated by as long a period as practicable.

PLASMA CONCENTRATIONS. Plasma concentration monitoring avoids both excessive and subtherapeutic concentrations thus preventing toxicity and ensuring efficacy. In patients with normal renal function, aminoglycoside concentrations should be measured after 3 or 4 doses; patients with renal impairment may require early and more frequent measurement of aminoglycoside concentration.

Blood samples should be taken approximately 1 hour after intramuscular or intravenous administration ('peak' concentration) and also just before the next dose ('trough' concentration).

If possible plasma aminoglycoside concentrations should be measured in all patients and **must** be determined in infants, in the elderly, in obesity, and in cystic fibrosis, *or* if high doses are being given, *or* if there is renal impairment, *or* if treatment lasts longer than 7 days.

ONCE DAILY DOSAGE. Although aminoglycosides are generally given in 2–3 divided doses during the 24 hours, *once daily administration* is more convenient and is no more toxic than divided dose regimens (while ensuring adequate plasma concentrations) but **expert advice** about dosage and plasma concentrations should be obtained.

ENDOCARDITIS. Gentamicin is used in combination with other antibiotics for the treatment of bacterial endocarditis (Table 1, section 5.1). Plasma-gentamicin concentration should be determined twice each week (more often in renal impairment).

In *streptococcal* and *enterococcal endocarditis* gentamicin is given in a low dose of 80 mg twice daily, adjusted to achieve a one-hour ('peak') plasma-gentamicin concentration of 3–5 mg/litre and a pre-dose ('trough') concentration of less than 1 mg/litre. **Streptomycin** may be used as an alternative in gentamicin-resistant enterococcal endocarditis.

In *staphylococcal endocarditis*, gentamicin is given in conventional doses to achieve a one-hour ('peak') plasma-gentamicin concentration of 5–10 mg/litre and a pre-dose ('trough') concentration of less than 2 mg/litre.

Gentamicin is the most important of the aminoglycosides and is used widely for the treatment of serious infections. It is the aminoglycoside of choice in the UK. It has a broad spectrum but is inactive against anaerobes and has poor activity against haemolytic streptococci and pneumococci. When used for the 'blind' therapy of undiagnosed serious infections it is usually given in conjunction with a penicillin or metronidazole (or both). Gentamicin is used together with another antibiotic for the treatment of endocarditis (see above and Table 1, section 5.1).

The dose of gentamicin for most infections is up to 5 mg/kg daily given in divided doses every 8 hours (if renal function is normal); whenever possible treatment should not exceed 7 days. Higher doses are occasionally indicated for serious infections, especially in the neonate or the immunocompromised patient. Loading and maintenance doses may be calculated on the basis of the patient's weight and renal function (e.g. using a nomogram); adjustments are then made according to plasma gentamicin concentrations.

Amikacin is a derivative of kanamycin and has one important advantage over gentamicin in that it is more stable than gentamicin to enzyme inactivation. Amikacin is used in the treatment of serious infections caused by gentamicin-resistant Gram-negative bacilli.

Kanamycin has been superseded by other aminoglycosides. It is reserved for Gram-negative organisms resistant to other antibiotics; assays for kanamycin are not readily available.

Netilmicin has similar activity to gentamicin, but may cause less ototoxicity in those needing treatment for longer than 10 days. Netilmicin is active against a number of gentamicin-resistant Gram-negative bacilli but is less active against *Ps. aeruginosa* than gentamicin or tobramycin.

Tobramycin is similar to gentamicin. It is slightly more active against *Ps. aeruginosa* but shows less activity against certain other Gram-negative bacteria.

Neomycin is too toxic for parenteral administration and can only be used for infections of the skin or mucous membranes or to reduce the bacterial population of the colon prior to bowel surgery or in hepatic failure. Oral administration may lead to malabsorption. Small amounts of neomycin may be absorbed from the gut in patients with hepatic failure and, as these patients may also be uraemic, cumulation may occur with resultant ototoxicity.

PREGNANCY. Where possible, the aminoglycosides should be avoided in pregnancy as they cross the placenta and can cause fetal eighth nerve damage.

GENTAMICIN

Indications: septicaemia and neonatal sepsis; meningitis and other CNS infections; biliary-tract infection, acute pyelonephritis or prostatitis, endocarditis caused by viridans streptococci or *Enterococcus faecalis* (with a penicillin); pneumonia in hospital patients, adjunct in listerial meningitis (section 5.1, table 1)

Cautions: renal impairment, infants and elderly (adjust dose and monitor renal, auditory and vestibular function together with plasma gentamicin concentrations); avoid prolonged use; see also notes above; **interactions:** Appendix 1 (aminoglycosides)

Contra-indications: pregnancy, myasthenia gravis

Side-effects: vestibular and auditory damage, nephrotoxicity; rarely, hypomagnesaemia on prolonged therapy, antibiotic-associated colitis; also reported, nausea, vomiting, rash; see also notes above

Dose: *by intramuscular or by slow intravenous injection* over at least 3 minutes *or by intravenous infusion*, 2–5 mg/kg daily (in divided doses every 8 hours), see also notes above

CHILD up to 2 weeks, 3 mg/kg every 12 hours; 2 weeks–12 years, 2 mg/kg every 8 hours

By intrathecal injection, 1 mg daily (increased if necessary to 5 mg daily), with 2–4 mg/kg daily *by intramuscular injection* (in divided doses every 8 hours)

Endocarditis prophylaxis, section 5.1, table 2

Note. One-hour ('peak') concentration should not exceed 10 mg/litre; pre-dose ('trough') concentration should be less than 2 mg/litre

Gentamicin (Non-proprietary) PoM
Injection, gentamicin (as sulphate), net price 40 mg/mL, 1-mL amp = £1.40, 2-mL amp = £1.50, 2-mL vial = £1.54
Available from Faulding DBL

Cidomycin® (Hoechst Marion Roussel) PoM
Injection, gentamicin 40 mg (as sulphate)/mL. Net price 2-mL amp or vial = £1.55
Paediatric injection, gentamicin 10 mg (as sulphate)/mL. Net price 2-mL vial = 65p
Intrathecal injection, gentamicin 5 mg (as sulphate)/mL. Net price 1-mL amp = 77p

Genticin® (Roche) PoM
Injection, gentamicin 40 mg (as sulphate)/mL. Net price 2-mL amp = £1.58

Isotonic Gentamicin Injection (Baxter) PoM
Intravenous infusion, gentamicin 800 micrograms (as sulphate)/mL in sodium chloride intravenous infusion 0.9%. Net price 100-mL (80-mg) Viaflex® bag = £1.61
Electrolytes: Na+ 15.4 mmol/100-mL bag

AMIKACIN

Indications: serious Gram-negative infections resistant to gentamicin

Cautions; Contra-indications; Side-effects: see under Gentamicin

Dose: *by intramuscular or by slow intravenous injection or by infusion*, 15 mg/kg daily in 2 divided doses, see also notes above
Note. One-hour ('peak') concentration should not exceed 30 mg/litre; pre-dose ('trough') concentration should be less than 10 mg/litre

Amikacin (Non-proprietary) PoM
Injection, amikacin (as sulphate) 250 mg/mL. Net price 2-mL vial = £9.64
Electrolytes: Na+ 0.56 mmol/500-mg vial
Available from Faulding DBL

Amikin® (Bristol-Myers) PoM
Injection, amikacin (as sulphate) 250 mg/mL. Net price 2-mL vial = £10.14
Electrolytes: Na+ <0.5 mmol/vial
Paediatric injection, amikacin (as sulphate) 50 mg/mL. Net price 2-mL vial = £2.36
Electrolytes: Na+ <0.5 mmol/vial

KANAMYCIN ▱

Indications: superseded by other aminoglycosides (see notes above)

Cautions; Contra-indications; Side-effects: see under Gentamicin

Dose: *by intramuscular injection*, 250 mg every 6 hours *or* 500 mg every 12 hours, see also notes above

By intravenous infusion, 15–30 mg/kg daily in divided doses every 8–12 hours, see also notes above
Note. One-hour ('peak') concentration should not exceed 30 mg/litre; pre-dose ('trough') concentration should be less than 10 mg/litre

Kannasyn® (Sanofi-Synthelabo) PoM ▱
Powder (for preparing injections), kanamycin (as acid sulphate). Net price 1-g vial = £23.77

▱ denotes preparations that are considered to be less suitable for prescribing (see p. vi)

NEOMYCIN SULPHATE

Indications: bowel sterilisation prior to surgery, see also notes above

Cautions; Contra-indications; Side-effects: see under Gentamicin but too toxic for systemic use, see notes above; avoid in intestinal obstruction and in renal impairment

Dose: *by mouth*, bowel sterilisation, 1 g every 4 hours
Hepatic coma, up to 4 g daily in divided doses usually for max. 14 days

Nivemycin® (Sovereign) PoM
Tablets, neomycin sulphate 500 mg. Net price 20 = £3.44

NETILMICIN

Indications: serious Gram-negative infections resistant to gentamicin

Cautions; Contra-indications; Side-effects: see under Gentamicin

Dose: *by intramuscular injection or by intravenous injection* over 3–5 minutes *or by intravenous infusion*, 4–6 mg/kg daily, as a single daily dose or in divided doses every 8 or 12 hours; in severe infections, up to 7.5 mg/kg daily in divided doses every 8 hours (reduced as soon as clinically indicated, usually within 48 hours) NEONATE up to 1 week, 3 mg/kg every 12 hours; INFANT over 1 week, 2.5–3 mg/kg every 8 hours; CHILD 2–2.5 mg/kg every 8 hours

Urinary-tract infection, 150 mg as a single daily dose for 5 days

Gonorrhoea, 300 mg as a single dose
Note. For divided daily dose regimens, one-hour ('peak') concentration should not exceed 12 mg/litre; pre-dose ('trough') concentration should be less than 2 mg/litre

Netillin® (Schering-Plough) PoM

Injection, netilmicin (as sulphate) 10 mg/mL, net price 1.5-mL (15-mg) amp = £1.42; 50 mg/mL, 1-mL (50-mg) amp = £2.11; 100 mg/mL, 1-mL (100-mg) amp = £2.75; 1.5-mL (150-mg) amp = £3.92, 2-mL (200-mg) amp = £5.09

TOBRAMYCIN

Indications: see under Gentamicin and notes above

Cautions; Contra-indications; Side-effects: see under Gentamicin

Dose: *by intramuscular injection or by slow intravenous injection or by intravenous infusion*, 3 mg/kg daily in divided doses every 8 hours, see also notes above; in severe infections up to 5 mg/kg daily in divided doses every 6–8 hours (reduced to 3 mg/kg as soon as clinically indicated); NEONATE 2 mg/kg every 12 hours; CHILD over 1 week 2–2.5 mg/kg every 8 hours

Urinary-tract infection, *by intramuscular injection*, 2–3 mg/kg daily as a single dose

Note. One-hour ('peak') concentration should not exceed 10 mg/litre; pre-dose ('trough') concentration should be less than 2 mg/litre

Tobramycin (Non-proprietary) PoM

Injection, tobramycin (as sulphate) 40 mg/mL, net price 1-mL (40-mg) vial = £2.46, 2-mL (80-mg) vial = £3.77

Available from Faulding DBL, Cox

Nebcin® (Lilly) PoM

Injection, tobramycin (as sulphate) 10 mg/mL, net price 2-mL (20-mg) vial = £2.27; 40 mg/mL, 1-mL (40-mg) vial = £3.08, 2-mL (80-mg) vial = £5.52

5.1.5 Macrolides

Erythromycin has an antibacterial spectrum that is similar but not identical to that of penicillin; it is thus an alternative in penicillin-allergic patients.

Indications for erythromycin include respiratory infections, whooping cough, legionnaires' disease, and campylobacter enteritis. It has activity against gut anaerobes and has been used with neomycin for prophylaxis before bowel surgery. It is active against many penicillin-resistant staphylococci but some are now also resistant to erythromycin; it has poor activity against *Haemophilus influenzae*. Erythromycin is also active against chlamydia and mycoplasmas.

Erythromycin causes nausea, vomiting, and diarrhoea in some patients; in mild to moderate infections this can be avoided by giving a lower dose (250 mg 4 times daily) but if a more serious infection, such as Legionella pneumonia, is suspected higher doses are needed.

Azithromycin is a macrolide with slightly less activity than erythromycin against Gram-positive bacteria but enhanced activity against some Gram-negative organisms including *H. influenzae*. Plasma concentrations are very low but tissue concentrations are much higher. It has a long tissue half-life and once daily dosage is recommended.

Clarithromycin is an erythromycin derivative with slightly greater activity than the parent compound. Tissue concentrations are higher than with erythromycin. It is given twice daily.

Azithromycin and clarithromycin cause fewer gastro-intestinal side-effects than erythromycin.

Spiramycin is also a macrolide (section 5.4.7).

ERYTHROMYCIN

Indications: alternative to penicillin in hypersensitive patients; campylobacter enteritis, pneumonia, legionnaires' disease, syphilis, non-gonococcal urethritis, chronic prostatitis, diphtheria and whooping cough prophylaxis; acne vulgaris and rosacea (section 13.6)

Cautions: hepatic and renal impairment; prolongation of QT interval (ventricular tachycardia reported); porphyria (section 9.8.2); pregnancy (not known to be harmful) and breast-feeding (only small amounts in milk); **interactions:** Appendix 1 (erythromycin and other macrolides)

ARRHYTHMIAS. Avoid concomitant administration with cisapride, pimozide or terfenadine [other interactions, Appendix 1]

Contra-indications: estolate contra-indicated in liver disease

Side-effects: nausea, vomiting, abdominal discomfort, diarrhoea (antibiotic-associated colitis reported); urticaria, rashes and other allergic reactions; reversible hearing loss reported after large doses; cholestatic jaundice and cardiac effects (including chest pain and arrhythmias) also reported

Dose: *by mouth*, ADULT and CHILD over 8 years, 250–500 mg every 6 hours *or* 0.5–1 g every 12 hours (see notes above); up to 4 g daily in severe infections; CHILD up to 2 years 125 mg every 6 hours, 2–8 years 250 mg every 6 hours, doses doubled for severe infections

Early syphilis, 500 mg 4 times daily for 14 days

Non-gonococcal urethritis, 500 mg 4 times daily for 7 days

By intravenous infusion, ADULT and CHILD severe infections, 50 mg/kg daily by continuous infusion *or* in divided doses every 6 hours; mild infections (oral treatment not possible), 25 mg/kg daily

Erythromycin (Non-proprietary) PoM

Tablets, e/c, erythromycin 250 mg, net price 20 = £2.20. Label: 5, 9, 25

Available from Abbott, APS, Ashbourne (*Rommix®*), Cox, Kent, Norton

Erythromycin Ethyl Succinate (Non-proprietary) PoM

Oral suspension, erythromycin (as ethyl succinate) for reconstitution with water 125 mg/5 mL, net price 100 mL = £1.07; 250 mg/5 mL, 100 mL = £1.67; 500 mg/5 mL, 100 mL = £2.80. Label: 9

Note. Sugar-free versions are available and can be ordered by specifying 'sugar-free' on the prescription

Available from APS, Ashbourne (*Rommix®*), Cox, Hillcross, Kent, Norton, Rosemont (*Arpimycin®*)

Erythromycin Lactobionate (Non-proprietary) PoM

Intravenous infusion, powder for reconstitution, erythromycin (as lactobionate), net price 1-g vial = £9.90

Available from Abbott, Faulding DBL

Erymax® (Elan) PoM
Capsules, opaque orange/clear orange, enclosing orange and white e/c pellets, erythromycin 250 mg. Net price 30-cap pack = £5.80. Label: 5, 9, 25

Dose: 1 capsule every 6 hours *or* 2 capsules every 12 hours; acne, 1 capsule twice daily for 1 month then 1 capsule daily

Erythrocin® (Abbott) PoM
Tablets, both f/c, erythromycin (as stearate), 250 mg, net price 20 = £2.65; 500 mg, 20 = £5.46. Label: 9

Erythroped® (Abbott) PoM
Suspension SF, sugar-free, banana-flavoured, erythromycin (as ethyl succinate) for reconstitution with water, 125 mg/5 mL (*Suspension PI SF*), net price 140 mL = £2.89; 250 mg/5 mL, 140 mL = £5.63; 500 mg/5 mL (*Suspension SF Forte*), 140 mL = £9.99. Label: 9

Erythroped A® (Abbott) PoM
Tablets, yellow, f/c, erythromycin 500 mg (as ethyl succinate). Net price 28-tab pack = £9.26. Label: 9

Ilosone® (Dista) PoM
Capsules, ivory/red, erythromycin (as estolate) 250 mg, net price 20 = £6.26. Label: 9
Tablets, pink, erythromycin (as estolate) 500 mg, net price 24-tab pack = £7.48. Label: 9

Tiloryth® (Tillomed) PoM
Capsules, enclosing e/c microgranules, erythromycin 250 mg. Net price 30-cap pack = £6.08. Label 5, 9, 25

AZITHROMYCIN

Indications: respiratory-tract infections; otitis media; skin and soft-tissue infections; uncomplicated genital chlamydial infections

Cautions: see under Erythromycin; pregnancy and breast-feeding; **interactions:** Appendix 1 (erythromycin and other macrolides)

Contra-indications: hepatic impairment

Side-effects: see under Erythromycin; anorexia, dyspepsia, constipation; dizziness, headache, drowsiness; photosensitivity; hepatitis, interstitial nephritis, acute renal failure, asthenia, paraesthesia, convulsions and mild neutropenia reported; rarely tinnitus, hepatic necrosis, hepatic failure, Stevens-Johnson syndrome, toxic epidermal necrolysis and taste disturbances

Dose: 500 mg once daily for 3 days; CHILD over 6 months 10 mg/kg once daily for 3 days; *or* body-weight 15–25 kg, 200 mg once daily for 3 days; body-weight 26–35 kg, 300 mg once daily for 3 days; body-weight 36–45 kg, 400 mg once daily for 3 days
Genital chlamydial infections, 1 g as a single dose

Zithromax® (Pfizer) PoM
Capsules, azithromycin (as dihydrate) 250 mg, net price 4-cap pack = £8.95, 6-cap pack = £13.43. Label: 5, 9, 23
Tablets, f/c, azithromycin (as dihydrate) 500 mg, net price 3-tab pack = £10.99. Label: 5, 9
Oral suspension, cherry/banana-flavoured, azithromycin (as dihydrate) 200 mg/5 mL when reconstituted with water. Net price 15-mL pack = £5.08, 22.5-mL pack = £7.62, 30-mL pack = £13.80. Label: 5, 9

CLARITHROMYCIN

Indications: respiratory-tract infections, mild to moderate skin and soft tissue infections, otitis media; *Helicobacter pylori* eradication (section 1.3)

Cautions: see under Erythromycin; reduce dose in renal impairment; pregnancy and breast-feeding; **interactions:** Appendix 1 (erythromycin and other macrolides)
ARRHYTHMIAS. Avoid concomitant administration with cisapride, pimozide or terfenadine [other interactions, Appendix1]

Side-effects: see under Erythromycin; also reported, dyspepsia, headache, smell and taste disturbances, tooth and tongue discoloration, stomatitis, glossitis, arthralgia, myalgia, dizziness, vertigo, tinnitus, anxiety, insomnia, nightmares, confusion, psychosis, hypoglycaemia, cholestasis, jaundice, hepatitis, and Stevens-Johnson syndrome; on intravenous infusion, local tenderness, phlebitis

Dose: *by mouth*, 250 mg every 12 hours for 7 days, increased in severe infections to 500 mg every 12 hours for up to 14 days; CHILD body-weight under 8 kg, 7.5 mg/kg twice daily; 8–11 kg (1–2 years), 62.5 mg twice daily; 12–19 kg (3–6 years), 125 mg twice daily; 20–29 kg (7–9 years), 187.5 mg twice daily; 30–40 kg (10–12 years), 250 mg twice daily
By intravenous infusion into larger proximal vein, 500 mg twice daily; CHILD not recommended

Klaricid® (Abbott) PoM
Tablets, both yellow, f/c, clarithromycin 250 mg, net price 14-tab pack = £11.24; 500 mg, 14-tab pack = £22.49, 20-tab pack = £32.13. Label: 9
Paediatric suspension, clarithromycin for reconstitution with water 125 mg/5 mL, net price 70 mL = £6.00, 100 mL = £10.32; 250 mg/5 ml, 70ml = £12.00. Label: 9
Granules, clarithromycin 250 mg/sachet, net price 14-sachet pack = £12.00. Label: 9, 13
Intravenous infusion, powder for reconstitution, clarithromycin. Net price 500-mg vial = £12.14
Electrolyes: Na⁺ < 0.5 mmol/500-mg vial

Klaricid XL® (Abbott) PoM
Tablets, m/r, yellow, clarithromycin 500 mg, net price 7-tab pack = £10.68, 14-tab pack = £21.36. Label: 9, 21, 25
Dose: 500 mg once daily (doubled in severe infections) for 7–14 days

---

5.1.6 Clindamycin

Clindamycin has only a limited use because of serious side-effects. Its most serious toxic effect is antibiotic-associated colitis (section 1.5) which may be fatal and is most common in middle-aged and elderly women, especially following operation. Although it can occur with most antibiotics it is more frequently seen with clindamycin. Patients should therefore discontinue treatment immediately if diarrhoea develops.

Clindamycin is active against Gram-positive cocci, including penicillin-resistant staphylococci and also against many anaerobes, especially *Bacteroides fragilis*. It is well concentrated in bone and excreted in bile and urine.

Clindamycin is recommended for staphylococcal joint and bone infections such as osteomyelitis, and intra-abdominal sepsis. Clindamycin is also used for endocarditis prophylaxis (section 5.1, table 2).

CLINDAMYCIN

Indications: staphylococcal bone and joint infections, peritonitis; endocarditis prophylaxis [unlicensed indication], section 5.1, table 2

Cautions: discontinue immediately if diarrhoea or colitis develops; hepatic or renal impairment; monitor liver and renal function on prolonged therapy and in neonates and infants; pregnancy; breast-feeding (Appendix 5); avoid rapid intravenous administration; **interactions:** Appendix 1 (clindamycin)

Contra-indications: diarrhoeal states

Side-effects: diarrhoea (discontinue treatment), abdominal discomfort, nausea, vomiting, antibiotic-associated colitis; jaundice and altered liver function tests; neutropenia, eosinophilia, agranulocytosis and thrombocytopenia reported; rash, urticaria, erythema multiforme, exfoliative and vesiculobullous dermatitis reported; pain, induration, and abscess after intramuscular injection; thrombophlebitis after intravenous injection

Dose: *by mouth*, 150–300 mg every 6 hours; up to 450 mg every 6 hours in severe infections; CHILD, 3–6 mg/kg every 6 hours

COUNSELLING. Patients should discontinue immediately and contact doctor if diarrhoea develops; capsules should be swallowed with a glass of water.

By deep intramuscular injection or by intravenous infusion, 0.6–2.7 g daily (in 2–4 divided doses); life-threatening infection, up to 4.8 g daily; single doses above 600 mg by intravenous infusion only; single doses by intravenous infusion not to exceed 1.2 g

CHILD over 1 month, 15–40 mg/kg daily in 3–4 divided doses; severe infections, at least 300 mg daily regardless of weight

Dalacin C® (Pharmacia & Upjohn) [PoM]
Capsules, clindamycin (as hydrochloride) 75 mg (lavender), net price 24-cap pack = £5.93; 150 mg, (lavender/maroon), 24-cap pack = £10.92. Label: 9, 27, counselling, see above (diarrhoea)
Injection, clindamycin (as phosphate) 150 mg/mL. Net price 2-mL amp = £4.94; 4-mL amp = £9.83

5.1.7   **Some other antibiotics**

Antibacterials discussed in this section include chloramphenicol, fusidic acid, glycopeptide antibiotics (vancomycin and teicoplanin), the streptogramins (quinupristin and dalfopristin) and the polymyxin, colistin.

Chloramphenicol

Chloramphenicol is a potent broad-spectrum antibiotic; however, it is associated with serious haematological side-effects when given systemically and should therefore be reserved for the treatment of life-threatening infections, particularly those caused by *Haemophilus influenzae*, and also for typhoid fever.

Chloramphenicol eye drops (section 11.3.1) and chloramphenicol ear drops (section 12.1.1) are also available.

CHLORAMPHENICOL

Indications: see notes above

Cautions: avoid repeated courses and prolonged treatment; reduce doses in hepatic or renal impairment; blood counts required before and periodically during treatment; monitor plasma-chloramphenicol concentration in neonates (see below); **interactions:** Appendix 1 (chloramphenicol)

Contra-indications: pregnancy (see also Appendix 4), breast-feeding, porphyria (section 9.8.2)

Side-effects: blood disorders including reversible and irreversible aplastic anaemia (with reports of resulting leukaemia), peripheral neuritis, optic neuritis, erythema multiforme, nausea, vomiting, diarrhoea, stomatitis, glossitis; nocturnal haemoglobinuria reported; grey syndrome (abdominal distension, pallid cyanosis, circulatory collapse) may follow excessive doses in neonates with immature hepatic metabolism

Dose: *by mouth or by intravenous injection or infusion*, 50 mg/kg daily in 4 divided doses (exceptionally, can be doubled for severe infections such as septicaemia and meningitis, providing high doses reduced as soon as clinically indicated); CHILD, haemophilus epiglottitis and pyogenic meningitis, 50–100 mg/kg daily in divided doses (high dosages decreased as soon as clinically indicated); INFANTS under 2 weeks 25 mg/kg daily (in 4 divided doses), 2 weeks–1 year 50 mg/ kg daily (in 4 divided doses)

Note. Plasma concentration monitoring required in neonates and preferred in those under 4 years of age; recommended peak plasma concentration (measured approx. 1 hour after intravenous injection or infusion) 15–25 mg/litre; pre-dose ('trough') concentration should not exceed 15 mg/litre

Chloramphenicol (Non-proprietary) [PoM]
Capsules, chloramphenicol 250 mg. Net price 60 = £21.91
Available from Sussex

Kemicetine® (Pharmacia & Upjohn) [PoM]
Injection, powder for reconstitution, chloramphenicol (as sodium succinate). Net price 1-g vial = £1.15
Electrolytes: Na+ 3.14 mmol/g

Fusidic acid

Fusidic acid and its salts are narrow-spectrum antibiotics. The only indication for their use is in infections caused by penicillin-resistant staphylococci, especially osteomyelitis, as they are well concentrated in bone; they are also used for staphylococcal endocarditis (section 5.1, table 1). A second antistaphylococcal antibiotic is usually required to prevent emergence of resistance.

SODIUM FUSIDATE

Indications: see notes above

Cautions: liver-function tests required

Side-effects: nausea, vomiting, reversible jaundice, especially after high dosage or rapid infusion (withdraw therapy if persistent); rarely rashes, acute renal failure (usually with jaundice), blood disorders

Dose: see under Preparations, below

Fucidin® (Leo) [PoM]
Tablets, f/c, sodium fusidate 250 mg, net price 10-tab pack = £6.47. Label: 9
Dose: as sodium fusidate, 500 mg every 8 hours, doubled for severe infections
Skin infection, as sodium fusidate, 250 mg every 12 hours for 5–10 days
Suspension, off-white, fusidic acid 250 mg/5 mL. Net price 50 mL = £7.24. Label: 9, 21
Dose: as fusidic acid, ADULT 750 mg every 8 hours; CHILD up to 1 year 50 mg/kg daily (in 3 divided doses), 1–5 years 250 mg every 8 hours, 5–12 years 500 mg every 8 hours
Note. Fusidic acid is incompletely absorbed and doses recommended for suspension are proportionately higher than those for sodium fusidate tablets
Intravenous infusion, powder for reconstitution, sodium fusidate 500 mg (≡ fusidic acid 480 mg), with buffer. Net price per vial (with diluent) = £7.78
Electrolytes: Na+ 3.1 mmol/vial when reconstituted with buffer
Dose: as sodium fusidate, by intravenous infusion, ADULT over 50 kg, 500 mg 3 times daily; ADULT under 50 kg and CHILD, 6–7 mg/kg 3 times daily

---

Vancomycin and teicoplanin

The glycopeptide antibiotics vancomycin and teicoplanin have bactericidal activity against aerobic and anaerobic Gram-positive bacteria.

Vancomycin is used by the intravenous route in the prophylaxis and treatment of endocarditis and other serious infections caused by Gram-positive cocci including multi-resistant staphylococci; however there are increasing reports of vancomycin-resistant enterococci. It has a relatively long duration of action and can therefore be given every 12 hours; plasma-vancomycin concentration should be monitored (especially in patients with renal impairment in whom the dose may need marked reduction). It is ototoxic and nephrotoxic. Vancomycin (added to dialysis fluid) is also used in the treatment of peritoneal dialysis-associated peritonitis [unlicensed route] (table 1 section 5.1). Vancomycin is **not effective** by mouth for systemic infections.

Vancomycin is effective in the treatment of antibiotic-associated colitis (pseudomembranous colitis, see also section 1.5) for which it is given by mouth; a dose of 125 mg every 6 hours for 7 to 10 days is considered to be adequate. Vancomycin should **not** be given by mouth for systemic infections since it is not significantly absorbed.

Teicoplanin is very similar to vancomycin but has a significantly longer duration of action allowing once daily administration. Unlike vancomycin, teicoplanin can be given by intramuscular as well as by intravenous injection.

VANCOMYCIN

Indications: see notes above

Cautions: avoid rapid infusion (risk of anaphylactoid reactions, see Side-effects); rotate infusion sites; renal impairment; elderly; avoid if history of deafness; blood counts, urinalysis and renal function tests required in all patients; monitor auditory function and plasma-vancomycin concentration in elderly or if renal impairment; pregnancy and breast-feeding; systemic absorption may follow oral administration especially in inflammatory bowel disorders or following multiple doses; **interactions:** Appendix 1 (vancomycin)

Side-effects: after parenteral administration: nephrotoxicity including renal failure and interstitial nephritis; ototoxicity (discontinue if tinnitus occurs); blood disorders including neutropenia (usually after 1 week or cumulative dose of 25 g), rarely agranulocytosis and thrombocytopenia; nausea; chills, fever; eosinophilia, anaphylaxis, rashes (including exfoliative dermatitis, Stevens-Johnson syndrome and vasculitis); phlebitis (irritant to tissue); on rapid infusion, severe hypotension (including shock and cardiac arrest), wheezing, dyspnoea, urticaria, pruritus, flushing of the upper body ('red man' syndrome), pain and muscle spasm of back and chest

Dose: *by mouth*, antibiotic-associated colitis, 125 mg every 6 hours for 7–10 days, see notes above; CHILD 5 mg/kg every 6 hours, over 5 years, half adult dose
Note. Oral paediatric dose is lower than that on product literature but is adequate
By intravenous infusion, 500 mg over at least 60 minutes every 6 hours *or* 1 g over at least 100 minutes every 12 hours; NEONATE up to 1 week, 15 mg/kg initially then 10 mg/kg every 12 hours; INFANT 1–4 weeks, 15 mg/kg initially then 10 mg/kg every 8 hours; CHILD over 1 month, 10 mg/kg every 6 hours
Endocarditis prophylaxis, section 5.1, table 2
Note. Plasma concentration monitoring required; peak plasma concentration (measured 2 hours after intravenous infusion) should not exceed 30 mg/litre; pre-dose ('trough') concentration should not exceed 10 mg/litre

Vancomycin (Non-proprietary) [PoM]
Capsules, vancomycin (as hydrochloride) 125 mg, net price 28-cap pack = £66.23; 250 mg, 28-cap pack = £132.47. Label: 9
Available from Dumex
Injection, powder for reconstitution, vancomycin (as hydrochloride), for use as an infusion, net price 500-mg vial = £7.88; 1-g vial = £15.85
Note. Can be used to prepare solution for oral administration
Available from Antigen, Dumex, Faulding DBL

Vancocin® (Lilly) [PoM]
Matrigel capsules, vancomycin (as hydrochloride) 125 mg (blue/peach), net price 20-cap pack = £63.08; 250 mg (blue/grey), 20-cap pack = £126.16. Label: 9
Injection, powder for reconstitution, vancomycin (as hydrochloride), for use as an infusion, net price 500-mg vial = £8.66; 1-g vial = £17.32
Note. Can be used to prepare solution for oral administration

TEICOPLANIN

Indications: potentially serious Gram-positive infections including endocarditis, dialysis-associated peritonitis, and serious infections due to *Staphylococcus aureus*; prophylaxis in endocarditis [unlicensed indication] and in orthopaedic surgery at risk of infection with Gram-positive organisms

Cautions: vancomycin sensitivity; blood counts and liver and kidney function tests required; in renal impairment (Appendix 3)— monitor renal and auditory function on prolonged administration or if other nephrotoxic or neurotoxic drugs given; pregnancy (Appendix 4) and breast-feeding

Side-effects: nausea, vomiting, diarrhoea; rash, pruritus, fever, bronchospasm, rigors, urticaria, angioedema, anaphylaxis; dizziness, headache; blood disorders including eosinophilia, leucopenia, neutropenia, and thrombocytopenia; disturbances in liver enzymes, transient increase of serum creatinine, renal failure; tinnitus, mild hearing loss, and vestibular disorders also reported; rarely exfoliative dermatitis, Stevens-Johnson syndrome, toxic epidermal necrolysis; local reactions include erythema, pain, thrombophlebitis, injection site abscess and rarely flushing with infusion

Dose: *by intramuscular injection or by intravenous injection or infusion*, initially 400 mg (for severe infections, *by intravenous injection or infusion*, initially 400 mg every 12 hours for 3 doses), then 200 mg daily (400 mg daily for severe infections); higher doses may be required in patients of over 85 kg and in severe burns or endocarditis (consult product literature)

CHILD over 2 months *by intravenous injection or infusion*, initially 10 mg/kg every 12 hours for 3 doses, subsequently 6 mg/kg daily (severe infections or in neutropenia, 10 mg/kg daily); subsequent doses can be given *by intramuscular injection* (but intravenous administration preferred in children); NEONATE *by intravenous infusion*, initially a single dose of 16 mg/kg, subsequently 8 mg/kg daily

Orthopaedic surgery prophylaxis, *by intravenous injection*, 400 mg at induction of anaesthesia

Endocarditis prophylaxis [unlicensed indication], section 5.1, table 2

Targocid® (Hoechst Marion Roussel) [PoM]
Injection, powder for reconstitution, teicoplanin, net price 200-mg vial (with diluent) = £18.90; 400-mg vial (with diluent) = £38.30
Electrolytes: Na⁺ < 0.5 mmol/200- and 400-mg vial

Quinupristin and dalfopristin

A combination of the streptogramin antibiotics, **quinupristin** and **dalfopristin** (as *Synercid®*) has recently been licensed for infections due to Gram-positive bacteria. The combination should be reserved for treating infections which have failed to respond to other antibiotics (e.g. methicillin-resistant *Staphylococcus aureus*, MRSA) or for patients who cannot be treated with other antibiotics. Quinupristin and dalfopristin are not active against *Enterococcus faecalis* and they need to be given in combination with other antibiotics for mixed infections which also involve Gram-negative organisms.

QUINUPRISTIN WITH DALFOPRISTIN

A mixture of quinupristin and dalfopristin (both as mesilate salts) in the proportions 3 parts to 7 parts

Indications: serious Gram-positive infections where no alternative antibacterial is suitable including hospital-acquired pneumonia, skin and soft-tissue infections, infections due to vancomycin-resistant *Enterococcus faecium*

Cautions: hepatic impairment (Appendix 2); renal impairment (Appendix 3); pregnancy (Appendix 4); breast-feeding (Appendix 5); **interactions**: Appendix 1 (Quinupristin/Dalfopristin)

Side-effects: nausea, vomiting, diarrhoea, headache, arthralgia, myalgia, asthenia, rash, pruritus; injection site reactions on peripheral venous administration; less frequently oral candidiasis, stomatitis, constipation, abdominal pain, antibiotic-associated colitis, peripheral oedema, hypotension, chest pain, dyspnoea, insomnia, anxiety, confusion, dizziness, paraesthesia, hypertonia, hepatitis, jaundice, pancreatitis, gout; also reported, raised bilirubin and liver enzymes, anaemia, thrombocytopenia, leucopenia, eosinophilia, increased urea and creatinine, electrolyte disturbances

Dose: expressed as a combination of quinupristin and dalfopristin (in a ratio of 3:7)

ADULT over 18 years, *by intravenous infusion* preferably into central vein, 7.5 mg/kg every 8 hours for 10 days in hospital-acquired pneumonia; duration of treatment in *E. faecium* infection depends on site of infection

Skin and soft-tissue infections, 7.5 mg/kg every 12 hours (every 8 hours when due to macrolide-resistant *Staphylococcus aureus* or pending sensitivity test results for MRSA) for 7 days

Synercid® (Rhône-Poulenc Rorer) ▼ [PoM]
Intravenous infusion, powder for reconstitution, quinupristin (as mesilate) 150 mg, dalfopristin (as mesilate) 350 mg, net price 500-mg vial = £37.00

Polymyxins

The polymyxin antibiotic, **colistin**, is active against Gram-negative organisms, including *Pseudomonas aeruginosa*. It is **not** absorbed by mouth and thus needs to be given by injection to obtain a systemic effect; however, it is toxic and has few, if any, indications for systemic use.

Colistin is used by mouth in bowel sterilisation regimens in neutropenic patients (usually with nystatin); it is **not** recommended for gastro-intestinal infections. It is also given by inhalation of a nebulised solution as an adjunct to standard antibiotic therapy.

Both colistin and polymyxin B are included in some preparations for topical application.

COLISTIN

Indications: see notes above

Cautions: renal impairment; porphyria (section 9.8.2); **interactions:** Appendix 1 (colistin)

Contra-indications: myasthenia gravis; pregnancy; breast-feeding

Side-effects: perioral and peripheral paraesthesia, vertigo, muscle weakness, apnoea, nephrotoxicity; rarely vasomotor instability, slurred speech, visual disturbance, confusion and psychosis; neurotoxicity reported with excessive doses; bronchospasm on inhalation

Dose: *by mouth,* bowel sterilisation, 1.5–3 million units every 8 hours

By intramuscular injection or intravenous injection or infusion, 2 million units every 8 hours (but see notes above)

By inhalation of nebulised solution, patients over 40 kg, 1 million units every 12 hours; patients under 40 kg, 500 000 units every 12 hours

Note. Colistin doses in BNF may differ from those in product literature

Colomycin® (Pharmax) [PoM]
Tablets, scored, colistin sulphate 1.5 million units. Net price 50 = £62.18
Syrup, colistin sulphate 250 000 units/5 mL when reconstituted with water. Net price 80 mL = £3.71
Injection, powder for reconstitution, colistimethate sodium (colistin sulphomethate sodium). Net price 500 000-unit vial = £1.22; 1 million-unit vial = £1.79
Electrolytes: (before reconstitution) Na+ < 0.5 mmol/500 000- and 1 million-unit vial

5.1.8   Sulphonamides and trimethoprim

The importance of the sulphonamides has decreased as a result of increasing bacterial resistance and their replacement by antibiotics which are generally more active and less toxic.

Sulfamethoxazole (sulphamethoxazole) and trimethoprim are used in combination (as **co-trimoxazole**) because of their synergistic activity, but see below for important CSM recommendations limiting the use of this combination.

CSM recommendations. Co-trimoxazole should be limited to the role of drug of choice in *Pneumocystis carinii* pneumonia; it is also indicated for *toxoplasmosis* and *nocardiasis.* It should now only be considered for use in *acute exacerbations of chronic bronchitis* and *infections of the urinary tract* when there is good bacteriological evidence of sensitivity to co-trimoxazole and good reason to prefer this combination to a single antibiotic; similarly it should only be used in *acute otitis media in children* when there is good reason to prefer it. Review of the safety of co-trimoxazole using spontaneous adverse drug reaction data has indicated that the profile of reported adverse reactions with trimethoprim is similar to that with co-trimoxazole; *blood and generalised skin disorders* are the most serious reactions with both drugs and predominantly have been reported to occur in **elderly patients.** A recent large post-marketing study has demonstrated that such reactions are very rare with co-trimoxazole; the study did not distinguish between co-trimoxazole and trimethoprim with respect to *serious hepatic, renal, blood or skin disorders.*

Trimethoprim can be used alone for urinary- and respiratory-tract infections and for prostatitis, shigellosis, and invasive salmonella infections.

Side-effects of the sulphonamides include rashes, Stevens-Johnson syndrome, renal failure (especially with the less soluble preparations), and blood dyscrasias, notably bone marrow depression and agranulocytosis.

The **longer-acting sulphonamide**, sulfametopyrazine (sulfalene) which is highly bound to plasma proteins, has the advantage of requiring less frequent administration, but toxic effects due to accumulation are more likely to occur.

For *topical preparations* of sulphonamides used in the treatment of burns see section 13.10.1.1.

CO-TRIMOXAZOLE

A mixture of trimethoprim and sulfamethoxazole in the proportions of 1 part to 5 parts

Indications: see CSM recommendations above

Cautions: hepatic and renal impairment; maintain adequate fluid intake; avoid in blood disorders (unless under specialist supervision); monitor blood counts on prolonged treatment; discontinue immediately if blood disorders or rash develop; elderly (see CSM recommendations above); asthma; G6PD deficiency (see section 9.1.5); pregnancy (see Appendix 4) and breast-feeding; avoid in infants under 6 weeks (except for treatment or prophylaxis of pneumocystis pneumonia); **interactions:** Appendix 1 (co-trimoxazole)

Contra-indications: hepatic or renal failure; porphyria (see section 9.8.2)

Side-effects: nausea, vomiting; rash (including Stevens-Johnson syndrome, toxic epidermal necrolysis, photosensitivity)—discontinue immediately; blood disorders (including neutropenia, thrombocytopenia, rarely agranulocytosis and purpura)—discontinue immediately; rarely, allergic reactions, diarrhoea, glossitis, stomatitis, anorexia, arthralgia, myalgia; also reported, liver damage including jaundice and hepatic necrosis, pancreatitis, antibiotic-associated colitis, eosinophilia, cough and shortness of breath, pulmonary infiltrates, aseptic meningitis, headache, depression, convulsions, ataxia, tinnitus, megaloblastic anaemia due to trimethoprim, electrolyte disturbances, crystalluria, renal disorders including interstitial nephritis

Dose: *by mouth,* 960 mg every 12 hours, increased to 1.44 g in severe infections; 480 mg every 12 hours if treated for more than 14 days; CHILD, every 12 hours, 6 weeks–5 months, 120 mg; 6 months–5 years, 240 mg; 6–12 years, 480 mg

By intravenous infusion, 960 mg every 12 hours increased to 1.44 g every 12 hours in severe infections; CHILD 36 mg/kg daily in 2 divided doses increased to 54 mg/kg daily in severe infections

Treatment of *Pneumocystis carinii* infections (undertaken where facilities for appropriate monitoring available—consult microbiologist and product literature), *by mouth or by intravenous infusion,* 120 mg/kg daily in 2–4 divided doses for 14 days

Note. 480 mg of co-trimoxazole consists of sulfamethoxazole 400 mg and trimethoprim 80 mg

Co-trimoxazole (Non-proprietary) [PoM]
Tablets, co-trimoxazole 480 mg, net price 20 = £2.67; 960 mg, 20 = £1.79. Label: 9
Available from Ashbourne (*Comixco®*), Cox, DDSA (*Fectrim®, Fectrim® Forte*), Hillcross, Kent, Norton
Paediatric oral suspension, co-trimoxazole 240 mg/5 mL, net price 100 mL = £1.12. Label: 9
Available from Ashbourne (*Comixco®*), Norton, Rosemont (*Chemotrim®*)

Oral suspension, co-trimoxazole 480 mg/5 mL.
Net price 100 mL = £3.50. Label: 9
Available from Kent
Strong sterile solution, co-trimoxazole 96 mg/mL.
For dilution and use as an intravenous infusion.
Net price 5-mL amp = £1.58, 10-mL amp = £3.06
Available from Faulding DBL

Septrin® (GlaxoWellcome) PoM
Tablets, co-trimoxazole 480 mg. Net price 20 =
£3.34. Label: 9
Dispersible tablets, orange, sugar-free, co-trimox-
azole 480 mg. Net price 20 = £3.55. Label: 9, 13
Forte tablets, scored, co-trimoxazole 960 mg. Net
price 20 = £5.05. Label: 9
Adult suspension, co-trimoxazole 480 mg/5 mL.
Net price 100 mL = £4.74. Label: 9
Paediatric suspension, sugar-free, co-trimoxazole
240 mg/5 mL. Net price 100 mL = £2.63. Label: 9
Intravenous infusion, co-trimoxazole 96 mg/mL. To
be diluted before use. Net price 5-mL amp = £1.59

SULFADIAZINE
(Sulphadiazine)

Indications: prevention of rheumatic fever recurrence, toxoplasmosis [unlicensed]—see section
5.4.7
Cautions; Contra-indications; Side-effects:
see under Co-trimoxazole; avoid in severe renal
impairment
Dose: prevention of rheumatic fever, *by mouth*, 1 g
daily (500 mg daily for patients less than 30kg)

Sulfadiazine (Non-proprietary) PoM
Tablets, sulfadiazine 500 mg, net price 56-tab pack
= £17.60. Label: 9, 27
Available from CP
Injection, sulfadiazine (as sodium salt) 250 mg/
mL, net price 4-mL amp = £4.97
Available from Concord

SULFAMETOPYRAZINE ◣
(Sulfalene)

Indications: urinary-tract infections, chronic
bronchitis
Cautions; Contra-indications; Side-effects:
see under Co-trimoxazole
Dose: 2 g once weekly

Kelfizine W® (Pharmacia & Upjohn) PoM ◣
Tablets, sulfametopyrazine 2 g, net price 5-tab
pack = £6.38. Label: 9, 13

> ◣ denotes preparations that are considered to
> be less suitable for prescribing (see p. vi)

TRIMETHOPRIM

Indications: urinary-tract infections, acute and
chronic bronchitis
Cautions: renal impairment, pregnancy (Appendix
4), breast-feeding (Appendix 5), predisposition to
folate deficiency, manufacturer recommends
blood counts on long-term therapy (but evidence
of practical value unsatisfactory); neonates (specialist supervision required); porphyria (section
9.8.2); **interactions:** Appendix 1 (trimethoprim)
BLOOD DISORDERS. On long-term treatment, patients
and their carers should be told how to recognise signs of
blood disorders and advised to seek immediate medical
attention if symptoms such as fever, sore throat, rash,
mouth ulcers, purpura, bruising or bleeding develop

Contra-indications: severe renal impairment,
blood dyscrasias
Side-effects: gastro-intestinal disturbances including nausea and vomiting, pruritus, rashes, depression of haematopoiesis; rarely erythema
multiforme, toxic epidermal necrolysis; aseptic
meningitis reported
Dose: *by mouth*, acute infections, 200 mg every 12
hours; CHILD, twice daily, 6 weeks–5 months
25 mg, 6 months–5 years 50 mg, 6–12 years
100 mg
Chronic infections and prophylaxis, 100 mg at
night; CHILD 1–2 mg/kg at night
By slow intravenous injection or infusion, 150–
250 mg every 12 hours; CHILD under 12 years, 6–
9 mg/kg daily in 2–3 divided doses

Trimethoprim (Non-proprietary) PoM
Tablets, trimethoprim 100 mg, net price 20 = 42p;
200 mg, 20 = 75p. Label: 9
Available from APS, Berk (*Trimopan®*), Cox, Kent, Norton

Monotrim® (Solvay) PoM
Tablets, both scored, trimethoprim 100 mg, net
price 20 = 97p; 200 mg, 20 = £1.75. Label: 9
Suspension, sugar-free, trimethoprim 50 mg/5 mL.
Net price 100 mL = £1.77. Label: 9
Injection, trimethoprim (as lactate) 20 mg/mL. Net
price 5-mL amp = £1.11

Trimopan® (Berk) PoM
Suspension, sugar-free, trimethoprim 50 mg/5 mL.
Net price 100 mL = £1.77. Label: 9

5.1.9   Antituberculous drugs

Tuberculosis is treated in two phases—an *initial
phase* using at least three drugs and a *continuation
phase* using two drugs in fully sensitive cases.
Treatment requires specialised knowledge, particularly where the disease involves resistant organisms
or non-respiratory organs.

The regimens given below are based on the Joint
Tuberculosis Committee of the British Thoracic
Society guidelines for the treatment of tuberculosis
in the UK; variations occur in other countries.

INITIAL PHASE. The concurrent use of at least
three drugs during the initial phase is designed to
reduce the bacterial population as rapidly as possible and to prevent the emergence of drug-resistant
bacteria. Treatment of choice for the initial phase is
the daily use of isoniazid, rifampicin, pyrazinamide
and ethambutol; ethambutol can be omitted from
the regimen if the risk of resistance to isoniazid is
low (e.g. those who have not been treated previously for tuberculosis, those who are not immunosuppressed, and those who have not been in contact
with organisms likely to be drug resistant). Streptomycin is rarely used in the UK although it may be
used in the initial phase of treatment if resistance to
isoniazid has been established before therapy is
commenced. The initial phase drugs should be continued for 2 months. Where a positive culture for *M.
tuberculosis* has been obtained, but susceptibility
results are not available after 2 months, treatment
with pyrazinamide (and ethambutol if appropriate)
should be continued until full susceptibility is confirmed, even if this is for longer than 2 months.

CONTINUATION PHASE. After the initial phase, treatment is continued for a further 4 months with isoniazid and rifampicin; longer treatment is necessary for meningitis and for resistant organisms.

Recommended dosage for standard unsupervised 6-month regimen
Isoniazid (initial and continuation phases)
ADULT 300 mg daily; CHILD 5–10 mg/kg (max. 300 mg) daily
Rifampicin (initial and continuation phases)
ADULT under 50 kg 450 mg daily, 50 kg and over 600 mg daily; CHILD 10 mg/kg daily
Pyrazinamide (initial phase only)
ADULT under 50 kg 1.5 g daily, 50 kg and over 2 g daily; CHILD 35 mg/kg daily
[1]**Ethambutol** (initial phase only)
ADULT and CHILD 15 mg/kg daily
1. Ethambutol may be omitted from the regimen if the risk of isoniazid resistance is low

PREGNANCY AND BREAST-FEEDING. The standard regimen (above) may be used during pregnancy and breast-feeding. Streptomycin should not be given in pregnancy.

CHILDREN. Children are given isoniazid, rifampicin, and pyrazinamide for the first 2 months followed by isoniazid and rifampicin during the next 4 months. Ethambutol should be included in the first 2 months in children with a high risk of resistant infection (see Initial Phase, above). However, care is needed in young children because of the difficulty in testing eyesight and in obtaining reports of visual symptoms (see below).

SUPERVISED TREATMENT. Treatment needs to be fully supervised (directly observed therapy, DOT) in patients who cannot be relied upon to comply with the treatment regimen. These patients are given isoniazid, rifampicin, pyrazinamide and ethambutol (or streptomycin) 3 times a week under supervision for the first 2 months followed by isoniazid and rifampicin 3 times a week for a further 4 months.

Recommended dosage for intermittent supervised 6-month treatment
Isoniazid (initial and continuation phases)
ADULT and CHILD 15 mg/kg 3 times a week
Rifampicin (initial and continuation phases)
ADULT 600–900 mg 3 times a week; CHILD 15 mg/kg 3 times a week
Pyrazinamide (initial phase only)
ADULT under 50 kg 2 g 3 times a week, 50 kg and over 2.5 g 3 times a week; CHILD 50 mg/kg 3 times a week
[1]**Ethambutol** (initial phase only)
ADULT and CHILD 30 mg/kg 3 times a week
1. Ethambutol may be omitted from the regimen if the risk of isoniazid resistance is low

IMMUNOCOMPROMISED PATIENTS. Immunocompromised patients may develop tuberculosis owing to reactivation of previously latent disease or to new infection. Multi-resistant *Mycobacterium tuberculosis* may be present or the infection may be caused by other mycobacteria e.g. *M. avium* complex in which case specialist advice is needed. Culture should always be carried out and the type of organism and its sensitivity confirmed. Confirmed *M. tuberculosis* infection sensitive to first-line drugs should be treated with a standard 6-month regimen; after completion of treatment, patients should be closely monitored. Specialist advice should be sought about treatment of or chemoprophylaxis against tuberculosis in a HIV-positive individual; care is required in choosing the regimen and in avoiding potentially hazardous interactions.

MONITORING. Since isoniazid, rifampicin and pyrazinamide are associated with liver toxicity (see Appendix 2), *hepatic function* should be checked before treatment with these drugs. Those with pre-existing liver disease should have frequent checks particularly in the first 2 months. If there is no evidence of liver disease (and pre-treatment liver function is normal), further checks are only necessary if the patient develops fever, malaise, vomiting, jaundice or unexplained deterioration during treatment. In view of the need to comply fully with antituberculous treatment on the one hand and to guard against serious liver damage on the other, patients and their carers should be informed carefully how to recognise signs of liver disorders and advised to discontinue treatment and seek **immediate** medical attention should symptoms of liver disease occur.

Renal function should be checked before treatment with antituberculous drugs and appropriate dosage adjustments made. Streptomycin or ethambutol should preferably be avoided in patients with renal impairment, but if used, the dose should be reduced and the plasma-drug concentration monitored.

Visual acuity should be tested before ethambutol is used (see below).

> Major causes of treatment failure are incorrect prescribing by the physician and inadequate compliance by the patient. Avoid both excessive and inadequate dosage. Treatment should be supervised by a specialist physician.

Isoniazid is cheap and highly effective. Like rifampicin it should always be included in any antituberculous regimen unless there is a specific contra-indication. Its only common side-effect is peripheral neuropathy which is more likely to occur where there are pre-existing risk factors such as diabetes, alcoholism, chronic renal failure, malnutrition and HIV infection. In these circumstances pyridoxine 10 mg daily should be given prophylactically from the start of treatment. Other side-effects such as hepatitis (important: see Monitoring above) and psychosis are rare.

Rifampicin, a rifamycin, is a key component of any antituberculous regimen. Like isoniazid it should always be included unless there is a specific contra-indication.

During the first two months of rifampicin administration transient disturbance of liver function with elevated serum transaminases is common but generally does not require interruption of treatment. Occasionally more serious liver toxicity requires a change of treatment particularly in those with pre-existing liver disease (important: see Monitoring above).

On intermittent treatment six toxicity syndromes have been recognised—influenza-like, abdominal, and respiratory symptoms, shock, renal failure, and thrombocytopenic purpura—and can occur in 20 to 30% of patients.

Rifampicin induces hepatic enzymes which accelerate the metabolism of several drugs including oestrogens, corticosteroids, phenytoin, sulphonylureas, and anticoagulants; **interactions:** Appendix 1 (rifamycins). **Important:** the effectiveness of oral contraceptives is reduced and alternative family planning advice should be offered (section 7.3.1).

Rifabutin, a newly introduced rifamycin, is indicated for *prophylaxis* against *M. avium* complex infections in patients with a low CD4 count; it is also licensed for the *treatment* of non-tuberculous mycobacterial disease and pulmonary tuberculosis. As with rifampicin it induces hepatic enzymes and the effectiveness of oral contraceptives is reduced requiring alternative family planning methods.

Pyrazinamide is a bactericidal drug only active against intracellular dividing forms of *Mycobacterium tuberculosis*; it exerts its main effect only in the first two or three months. It is particularly useful in tuberculous meningitis because of good meningeal penetration. It is not active against *M. bovis*. Serious liver toxicity may occasionally occur (important: see Monitoring above).

Ethambutol is included in a treatment regimen if isoniazid resistance is suspected; it can be omitted if the risk of resistance is low.

Side-effects of ethambutol are largely confined to visual disturbances in the form of loss of acuity, colour blindness, and restriction of visual fields. These toxic effects are more common where excessive dosage is used or if the patient's renal function is impaired. The earliest features of ocular toxicity are subjective and patients should be advised to discontinue therapy immediately if they develop deterioration in vision and promptly seek further advice. Early discontinuation of the drug is almost always followed by recovery of eyesight. Patients who cannot understand warnings about visual side-effects should, if possible, be given an alternative drug. In particular, ethambutol should be used with caution in children until they are at least 5 years old and capable of reporting symptomatic visual changes accurately.

Visual acuity should be tested by Snellen chart before treatment with ethambutol.

Streptomycin is now rarely used in the UK except for resistant organisms. It is given intramuscularly in a dose of 15 mg/kg (max. 1 g) daily; the dose is reduced in those under 50 kg, those over 40 years or those with renal impairment. Plasma-drug concentration should be measured in patients with impaired renal function in whom streptomycin must be used with great care. Side-effects increase after a cumulative dose of 100 g, which should only be exceeded in exceptional circumstances.

Drug-resistant tuberculosis should be treated by a specialist physician with experience in such cases, and where appropriate facilities for infection-control exist. Second-line drugs available for infections caused by resistant organisms, or when first-line drugs cause unacceptable side-effects, include capreomycin, cycloserine, newer macrolides (e.g. azithromycin and clarithromycin), quinolones (e.g. ciprofloxacin and ofloxacin) and protionamide (prothionamide) (no longer on UK market). Advice on the availability of second-line antituberculous drugs can be obtained from Regional Drug Information Services.

CAPREOMYCIN

Indications: in combination with other drugs, tuberculosis resistant to first-line drugs

Cautions: renal, hepatic, or auditory impairment; monitor renal, hepatic, auditory, and vestibular function and electrolytes; pregnancy (teratogenic in *animals*) and breast-feeding; **interactions:** Appendix 1 (capreomycin)

Side-effects: hypersensitivity reactions including urticaria and rashes; leucocytosis or leucopenia, rarely thrombocytopenia; changes in liver function tests; nephrotoxicity, electrolyte disturbances; hearing loss with tinnitus and vertigo; neuromuscular block after large doses, pain and induration at injection site

Dose: *by deep intramuscular injection*, 1 g daily (not more than 20 mg/kg) for 2–4 months, then 1 g 2–3 times each week

Capastat® (Dista) PoM
Injection, powder for reconstitution, capreomycin sulphate 1 million units (≡ capreomycin approx. 1 g). Net price per vial = £16.47

CYCLOSERINE

Indications: in combination with other drugs, tuberculosis resistant to first-line drugs

Cautions: reduce dose in renal impairment (avoid if severe); monitor haematological, renal, and hepatic function; pregnancy and breast-feeding; **interactions:** Appendix 1 (cycloserine)

Contra-indications: severe renal impairment, epilepsy, depression, severe anxiety, psychotic states, alcohol dependence, porphyria (section 9.8.2)

Side-effects: mainly neurological, including headache, dizziness, vertigo, drowsiness, tremor, convulsions, confusion, psychosis, depression (discontinue or reduce dose if symptoms of CNS toxicity); rashes, allergic dermatitis (discontinue or reduce dose); megaloblastic anaemia; changes in liver function tests; heart failure at high doses reported

Dose: initially 250 mg every 12 hours for 2 weeks increased according to blood concentration and response to max. 500 mg every 12 hours; CHILD initially 10 mg/kg daily adjusted according to blood concentration and response

Note. Blood concentration monitoring required especially in renal impairment or if dose exceeds 500 mg daily or if signs of toxicity; blood concentration should not exceed 30 mg/litre

Cycloserine (Lilly) PoM
Capsules, red/grey cycloserine 250 mg, net price 100-cap pack = £220.69. Label: 2, 8

ETHAMBUTOL HYDROCHLORIDE

Indications: tuberculosis, in combination with other drugs

Cautions: reduce dose in renal impairment and monitor plasma-ethambutol concentration; elderly; pregnancy; warn patients to report visual changes—see notes above

Contra-indications: young children (see notes), optic neuritis, poor vision

Side-effects: optic neuritis, red/green colour blindness, peripheral neuritis, rarely rash, pruritus, urticaria, thrombocytopenia
Dose: see notes above
Note. One-hour ('peak') concentration should be 4–6 mg/litre (20–30 micromol/litre); pre-dose ('trough') concentration should be less than 1 mg/litre (5 micromol/litre)

Ethambutol (Non-proprietary) PoM
Tablets, ethambutol hydrochloride 100 mg (yellow), net price 100-tab pack = £11.85; 400 mg (grey), 100-tab pack = £43.96. Label: 8
Available from Genus

ISONIAZID

Indications: tuberculosis, in combination with other drugs; prophylaxis—section 5.1, table 2
Cautions: hepatic impairment (monitor hepatic function, see also below); renal impairment; slow acetylator status (increased risk of side-effects); epilepsy; history of psychosis; alcoholism; pregnancy and breast-feeding; porphyria (section 9.8.2); **interactions:** Appendix 1 (isoniazid)
HEPATIC DISORDERS. Patients or their carers should be told how to recognise signs of liver disorder, and advised to discontinue treatment and seek immediate medical attention if symptoms such as persistent nausea, vomiting, malaise or jaundice develop
Contra-indications: drug-induced liver disease
Side-effects: nausea, vomiting; peripheral neuritis with high doses (pyridoxine prophylaxis, see notes above), optic neuritis, convulsions, psychotic episodes; hypersensitivity reactions including fever, erythema multiforme, purpura; agranulocytosis; hepatitis (especially over age of 35); systemic lupus erythematosus-like syndrome, pellagra, hyperglycaemia, and gynaecomastia reported
Dose: *by mouth or by intramuscular or intravenous injection*, see notes above

Isoniazid (Non-proprietary) PoM
Tablets, isoniazid 50 mg, net price 20 = £3.01; 100 mg, 20 = 83p. Label: 8, 22
Available from Norton
Elixir (BPC), isoniazid 50 mg, citric acid monohydrate 12.5 mg, sodium citrate 60 mg, concentrated anise water 0.05 mL, compound tartrazine solution 0.05 mL, glycerol 1 mL, double-strength chloroform water 2 mL, water to 5 mL. Label: 8, 22
'Special order' [unlicensed] product; contact Martindale, Rosemont, or regional hospital manufacturing unit
Injection, isoniazid 25 mg/mL, net price 2-mL amp = £6.77
Available from Cambridge

PYRAZINAMIDE

Indications: tuberculosis in combination with other drugs
Cautions: hepatic impairment (monitor hepatic function, see also below); renal impairment; diabetes; gout; **interactions:** Appendix 1 (pyrazinamide)
HEPATIC DISORDERS. Patients or their carers should be told how to recognise signs of liver disorder, and advised to discontinue treatment and seek immediate medical attention if symptoms such as persistent nausea, vomiting, malaise or jaundice develop

Contra-indications: liver damage, porphyria (section 9.8.2)
Side-effects: hepatotoxicity including fever, anorexia, hepatomegaly, jaundice, liver failure; nausea, vomiting, arthralgia, sideroblastic anaemia, urticaria
Dose: see notes above

Zinamide® (MSD) PoM
Tablets, scored, pyrazinamide 500 mg. Net price 20 = £1.44. Label: 8

RIFABUTIN

Indications: see under Dose
Cautions: see under Rifampicin; renal impairment (Appendix 3); porphyria (section 9.8.2)
Side-effects: nausea, vomiting; leucopenia, thrombocytopenia, anaemia, rarely haemolysis; raised liver enzymes, jaundice, rarely hepatitis; uveitis following high doses or administration with drugs which raise plasma concentration—see also **interactions:** Appendix 1 (rifamycins); arthralgia, myalgia, influenza-like syndrome, dyspnoea; also hypersensitivity reactions including fever, rash, eosinophilia, bronchospasm, shock; urine, saliva and other body secretions coloured orange-red; asymptomatic corneal opacities reported with long-term use
Dose: prophylaxis of *Mycobacterium avium* complex infections in immunosuppressed patients with low CD4 count (see product literature), 300 mg daily as a single dose
Treatment of non-tuberculous mycobacterial disease, in combination with other drugs, 450–600 mg daily as a single dose for up to 6 months after cultures negative
Treatment of pulmonary tuberculosis, in combination with other drugs, 150–450 mg daily as a single dose for at least 6 months
CHILD not recommended

Mycobutin® (Pharmacia & Upjohn) PoM
Capsules, red-brown, rifabutin 150 mg. Net price 30-cap pack = £78.59. Label: 8, 14, counselling, lenses, see under Rifampicin

RIFAMPICIN

Indications: see under Dose
Cautions: reduce dose in hepatic impairment (see Appendix 2; liver function tests and blood counts in hepatic disorders and on prolonged therapy, see also below); renal impairment (if above 600 mg daily); pregnancy and breast-feeding (see notes above and Appendixes 4 and 5); porphyria (section 9.8.2); **important:** advise patients on oral contraceptives to use additional means (see also section 7.3.1); discolours soft contact lenses; see also notes above; **interactions:** Appendix 1 (rifamycins)
Note. If treatment interrupted re-introduce with low dosage and increase gradually; discontinue permanently if serious side-effects develop
HEPATIC DISORDERS. Patients or their carers should be told how to recognise signs of liver disorder, and advised to discontinue treatment and seek immediate medical attention if symptoms such as persistent nausea, vomiting, malaise or jaundice develop
Contra-indications: jaundice

Side-effects: gastro-intestinal symptoms including anorexia, nausea, vomiting, diarrhoea (antibiotic-associated colitis reported); those occurring mainly on intermittent therapy include influenza-like symptoms (with chills, fever, dizziness, bone pain), respiratory symptoms (including shortness of breath), collapse and shock, haemolytic anaemia, acute renal failure, and thrombocytopenic purpura; alterations of liver function, jaundice; flushing, urticaria, and rashes; other side-effects reported include oedema, muscular weakness and myopathy, leucopenia, eosinophilia, menstrual disturbances; urine, saliva, and other body secretions coloured orange-red; thrombophlebitis reported if infusion used for prolonged period

Dose: brucellosis, legionnaires' disease and serious staphylococcal infections, in combination with other drugs, *by mouth or by intravenous infusion*, 0.6–1.2 g daily (in 2–4 divided doses)

Tuberculosis, in combination with other drugs, see notes above

Leprosy, section 5.1.10

Prophylaxis of meningococcal meningitis and *Haemophilus influenzae* (type b) infection, section 5.1, table 2

Rifampicin (Non-proprietary) PoM
Capsules, rifampicin 150 mg, net price 20 = £3.71; 300 mg, 20 = £7.41. Label: 8, 14, 22, counselling, see lenses above
Available from Generics

Rifadin® (Hoechst Marion Roussel) PoM
Capsules, rifampicin 150 mg (blue/red), net price 20 = £3.73; 300 mg (red), 20 = £7.45. Label: 8, 14, 22, counselling, see lenses above
Syrup, red, rifampicin 100 mg/5 mL. Net price 120 mL = £3.62. Label: 8, 14, 22, counselling, see lenses above
Intravenous infusion, powder for reconstitution, rifampicin. Net price 600-mg vial (with solvent) = £7.80
Electrolytes: Na+ <0.5 mmol/vial

Rimactane® (Novartis) PoM
Capsules, rifampicin 150 mg (red), net price 56-tab pack = £11.39; 300 mg (red/brown), 56-tab pack = £22.77. Label: 8, 14, 22, counselling, see lenses above
Syrup, red, rifampicin 100 mg/5 mL. Net price 100 mL = £3.06. Label: 8, 14, 22, counselling, see lenses above
Intravenous infusion, powder for reconstitution, rifampicin (as sodium salt). Net price 300-mg vial (with diluent) = £8.01
Electrolytes: Na+ <0.5 mmol/vial
Note. Owing to risk of contact sensitisation care must be taken to avoid contact during preparation and infusion

■ Combined preparations

Rifater® (Hoechst Marion Roussel) PoM
Tablets, pink-beige, s/c, rifampicin 120 mg, isoniazid 50 mg, pyrazinamide 300 mg. Net price 20 = £4.29. Label: 8, 14, 22, counselling, see lenses above
Dose: initial treatment of pulmonary tuberculosis, patients up to 40 kg 3 tablets daily preferably before breakfast, 40–49 kg 4 tablets daily, 50–64 kg 5 tablets daily, 65 kg or more, 6 tablets daily; not suitable for use in children

Rifinah 150® (Hoechst Marion Roussel) PoM
Tablets, pink, s/c, rifampicin 150 mg, isoniazid 100 mg, net price 84-tab pack = £16.18, 100-tab pack = £19.26. Label: 8, 14, 22, counselling, see lenses above
Dose: ADULT under 50 kg, 3 tablets daily, preferably before breakfast

Rifinah 300® (Hoechst Marion Roussel) PoM
Tablets, orange, s/c, rifampicin 300 mg, isoniazid 150 mg, net price 56-tab pack = £21.38, 100-tab pack = £38.19. Label: 8, 14, 22, counselling, see lenses above
Dose: ADULT 50 kg and over, 2 tablets daily, preferably before breakfast

Rimactazid 150® (Novartis) PoM
Tablets, pink, s/c, rifampicin 150 mg, isoniazid 100 mg, net price 84-tab pack = £16.42. Label: 8, 14, 22, counselling, see lenses above
Excipients: include gluten
Dose: ADULT under 50 kg, 3 tablets daily, preferably before breakfast

Rimactazid 300® (Novartis) PoM
Tablets, orange, s/c, rifampicin 300 mg, isoniazid 150 mg, net price 56-tab pack = £21.71. Label: 8, 14, 22, counselling, see lenses above
Excipients: include gluten
Dose: ADULT 50 kg and over, 2 tablets daily, preferably before breakfast

STREPTOMYCIN

Indications: tuberculosis, in combination with other drugs; adjunct to doxycycline in brucellosis

Cautions; Contra-indications; Side-effects: see under Aminoglycosides, section 5.1.4; also hypersensitivity reactions, paraesthesia of mouth

Dose: *by deep intramuscular injection*, tuberculosis, see notes above; brucellosis, expert advice essential
Note. One-hour ('peak') concentration should be 15–40 mg/litre; pre-dose ('trough') concentration should be less than 5 mg/litre (less than 1 mg/litre in renal impairment or in those over 50 years)

Streptomycin Sulphate (Medeva) PoM
Injection, powder for reconstitution, streptomycin (as sulphate), net price 1-g vial = £5.62

5.1.10 Antileprotic drugs

Advice from a member of the Panel of Leprosy Opinion is essential for the treatment of leprosy (Hansen's disease). Details of the Panel can be obtained from the Department of Health telephone (020) 7972 4480.

The World Health Organization has made recommendations to overcome the problem of dapsone resistance and to prevent the emergence of resistance to other antileprotic drugs. Drugs recommended are **dapsone**, **rifampicin** (section 5.1.9), and **clofazimine**. Other drugs with significant activity against *Mycobacterium leprae* include ofloxacin, minocycline and clarithromycin, but none of these are as active as rifampicin; at present they should be reserved as second-line drugs for leprosy.

A three-drug regimen is recommended for *multibacillary leprosy* (lepromatous, borderline-lepromatous, and borderline leprosy) and a two-drug regimen for *paucibacillary leprosy* (borderlinetuberculoid, tuberculoid, and indeterminate). The following regimens are widely used throughout the world (with minor local variations):

Multibacillary leprosy (3-drug regimen)

Rifampicin	600 mg once-monthly, supervised (450 mg for adults weighing less than 35 kg)
Dapsone	100 mg daily, self-administered (50 mg daily or 1–2 mg/kg daily for adults weighing less than 35 kg)
Clofazimine	300 mg once-monthly, supervised, *and* 50 mg daily (or 100 mg on alternate days), self-administered

Multibacillary leprosy should be treated for at least 2 years. Treatment should be continued unchanged during both type I (reversal) or type II (erythema nodosum leprosum) reactions. During reversal reactions neuritic pain or weakness can herald the rapid onset of permanent nerve damage. Treatment with prednisolone (initially 40–60 mg daily) should be instituted at once. Mild type II reactions may respond to aspirin or chloroquine. Severe type II reactions may require corticosteroids; thalidomide [unlicensed] is also useful in men and post-menopausal women who have become corticosteroid dependent, but it should be used under **specialist supervision** and it should **never** be used in women of child-bearing potential (significant teratogenic risk—for CSM guidance on prescribing, see *Current Problems in Pharmacovigilance* 1994; **20**, 8). Increased doses of clofazimine 100 mg 3 times daily for the first month with subsequent reductions, are also useful but may take 4–6 weeks to attain full effect.

Paucibacillary leprosy (2-drug regimen)

Rifampicin	600 mg once-monthly, supervised (450 mg for those weighing less than 35 kg)
Dapsone	100 mg daily, self-administered (50 mg daily or 1–2 mg/kg daily for adults weighing less than 35 kg)

Paucibacillary leprosy should be treated for 6 months. If treatment is interrupted the regimen should be recommenced where it was left off to complete the full course.

Neither the multibacillary nor the paucibacillary antileprosy regimen is sufficient to treat tuberculosis.

DAPSONE

Indications: leprosy, dermatitis herpetiformis

Cautions: cardiac or pulmonary disease; anaemia (treat severe anaemia before starting); G6PD-deficiency (including breast-feeding of affected children, section 9.1.5); pregnancy; avoid in porphyria (section 9.8.2); **interactions:** Appendix 1 (dapsone)

BLOOD DISORDERS. On long-term treatment, patients and their carers should be told how to recognise signs of blood disorders and advised to seek immediate medical attention if symptoms such as fever, sore throat, rash, mouth ulcers, purpura, bruising or bleeding develop

Side-effects: (dose-related and uncommon at doses used for leprosy), haemolysis, methaemoglobinaemia, neuropathy, allergic dermatitis (rarely including toxic epidermal necrolysis and Stevens-Johnson syndrome), anorexia, nausea,

vomiting, headache, insomnia, psychosis, hepatitis, agranulocytosis; dapsone syndrome (rash with fever and eosinophilia)—discontinue immediately (may progress to exfoliative dermatitis, hepatitis, hypoalbuminaemia, psychosis and death)

Dose: leprosy, 1–2 mg/kg daily, see notes above
Dermatitis herpetiformis, see specialist literature

Dapsone (Non-proprietary) [PoM]
Tablets, dapsone 50 mg, net price 28-tab pack = £1.98; 100 mg, 28-tab pack = £2.83. Label: 8
Available from Cox

CLOFAZIMINE

Indications: leprosy

Cautions: hepatic and renal impairment; pregnancy and breast-feeding; may discolour soft contact lenses; avoid if persistent abdominal pain and diarrhoea

Side-effects: nausea, vomiting (hospitalise if persistent), abdominal pain; headache, tiredness; brownish-black discoloration of lesions and skin including areas exposed to light; reversible hair discoloration; dry skin; red discoloration of faeces, urine and other body fluids; also rash, pruritus, photosensitivity, acne-like eruptions, anorexia, eosinophilic enteropathy, bowel obstruction, dry eyes, dimmed vision, macular and subepithelial corneal pigmentation; elevation of blood sugar, weight loss, splenic infarction lymphadenopathy

Dose: leprosy, see notes above
Lepromatous lepra reactions, dosage increased to 300 mg daily for max. of 3 months

Lamprene® (Alliance) [PoM]
Capsules, brown, clofazimine 100 mg, net price 100-cap pack = £23.50. Label: 8, 14, 21

5.1.11   Metronidazole and tinidazole

Metronidazole is an antimicrobial drug with high activity against anaerobic bacteria and protozoa; indications include trichomonal vaginitis (section 5.4.3), bacterial vaginosis (notably *Gardnerella vaginalis* infections), and *Entamoeba histolytica* and *Giardia lamblia* infections (section 5.4.2). It is also used for surgical and gynaecological sepsis in which its activity against colonic anaerobes, especially *Bacteroides fragilis*, is important. Metronidazole is also effective in the treatment of antibiotic-associated colitis (pseudomembranous colitis, see also section 1.5) in a dose of 400 mg by mouth 3 times daily. Metronidazole by the rectal route is an effective alternative to the intravenous route when oral administration is not possible. Intravenous metronidazole is used for the treatment of established cases of tetanus; diazepam (section 10.2.2) and tetanus immunoglobulin (section 14.5) are also used.

Topical metronidazole (section 13.10.1.2) reduces the odour produced by anaerobic bacteria in fungating tumours; it is also used in the management of rosacea (section 13.6).

Tinidazole is similar to metronidazole but has a longer duration of action.

METRONIDAZOLE

Indications: anaerobic infections (including dental), see under Dose below; protozoal infections (section 5.4.2); *Helicobacter pylori* eradication (section 1.3); skin (section 13.10.1.2)

Cautions: disulfiram-like reaction with alcohol, hepatic impairment and hepatic encephalopathy (Appendix 2); pregnancy and breast-feeding (Appendixes 4 and 5); clinical and laboratory monitoring advised if treatment exceeds 10 days; **interactions:** Appendix 1 (metronidazole)

Side-effects: nausea, vomiting, unpleasant taste, furred tongue, and gastro-intestinal disturbances; rashes; rarely drowsiness, headache, dizziness, ataxia, darkening of urine, erythema multiforme, pruritus, urticaria, angioedema, and anaphylaxis; also reported abnormal liver function tests, hepatitis, jaundice, thrombocytopenia, aplastic anaemia, myalgia, arthralgia; on prolonged or intensive therapy peripheral neuropathy, transient epileptiform seizures, and leucopenia

Dose: anaerobic infections (usually treated for 7 days), *by mouth, either* 800 mg initially then 400 mg every 8 hours *or* 500 mg every 8 hours, CHILD, 7.5 mg/kg every 8 hours; *by rectum*, 1 g every 8 hours for 3 days, then 1 g every 12 hours, CHILD, every 8 hours for 3 days, then every 12 hours, up to 1 year 125 mg, 1–5 years 250 mg, 5–10 years 500 mg, over 10 years, adult dose; *by intravenous infusion*, 500 mg every 8 hours; CHILD, 7.5 mg/kg every 8 hours

Leg ulcers and pressure sores, *by mouth*, 400 mg every 8 hours for 7 days

Bacterial vaginosis, *by mouth*, 400–500 mg twice daily for 5–7 days *or* 2 g as a single dose

Acute ulcerative gingivitis, *by mouth*, 200–250 mg every 8 hours for 3 days; CHILD 1–3 years 50 mg every 8 hours for 3 days; 3–7 years 100 mg every 12 hours; 7–10 years 100 mg every 8 hours

Acute dental infections, *by mouth*, 200 mg every 8 hours for 3–7 days

Surgical prophylaxis, *by mouth*, 400 mg every 8 hours started 24 hours before surgery, then continued postoperatively *by intravenous infusion* or *by rectum* (see below) until oral administration can be resumed; CHILD 7.5 mg/kg every 8 hours
By rectum, 1 g every 8 hours; CHILD 5–10 years 500 mg every 8 hours
By intravenous infusion, 500 mg shortly before surgery then every 8 hours until oral administration can be started; CHILD, 7.5 mg/kg every 8 hours

Metronidazole (Non-proprietary) [PoM]
Tablets, metronidazole 200 mg, net price 20 = £2.03; 400 mg, 20 = £4.75. Label: 4, 9, 21, 25, 27
Available from APS, Cox, DDSA (*Vaginyl®*), Hillcross, Kent, Norton, Rosemont
Tablets, metronidazole 500 mg, net price 21-tab pack = £3.50. Label: 4, 9, 21, 25, 27
Available from Dumex
Suspension, metronidazole (as benzoate) 200 mg/ 5 mL. Net price 100 mL = £7.20. Label: 4, 9, 23
Available from Hillcross, Rosemont
Intravenous infusion, metronidazole 5 mg/mL. Net price 20-mL amp = £1.70, 100-mL container = £3.83
Available from Braun, Faulding DBL, Phoenix

Flagyl® (Hawgreen) [PoM]
Tablets, both f/c, ivory, metronidazole 200 mg, net price 21-tab pack = £3.89; 400 mg, 14-tab pack = £5.50. Label: 4, 9, 21, 25, 27
Intravenous infusion, metronidazole 5 mg/mL. Net price 100-mL Viaflex® bag = £3.41
Electrolytes: Na⁺ 13.6 mmol/100-mL bag
Suppositories, metronidazole 500 mg, net price 10 = £13.17; 1 g, 10 = £20.00. Label: 4, 9

Flagyl S® (Hawgreen) [PoM]
Suspension, metronidazole (as benzoate) 200 mg/ 5 mL. Net price 100 mL = £6.96. Label: 4, 9, 23

Metrolyl® (Lagap) [PoM]
Intravenous infusion, metronidazole 5 mg/mL, net price 100-mL Steriflex® bag = £1.22
Electrolytes: Na⁺ 14.53 mmol/100-mL bag
Suppositories, metronidazole 500 mg, net price 10 = £13.27; 1 g, 10 = £19.76. Label: 4, 9

■ With antifungal

Flagyl Compak® (Hawgreen) [PoM]
Treatment pack, tablets, off-white, f/c, metronidazole 400 mg, with pessaries, yellow, nystatin 100 000 units. Net price 14 tablets and 14 pessaries (with applicator) = £9.49
Dose: for mixed trichomonal and candidal infections, 1 tablet twice daily for 7 days and 1 pessary inserted twice daily for 7 days *or* 1 pessary at night for 14 nights

TINIDAZOLE

Indications: anaerobic infections, see under Dose below; protozoal infections (section 5.4.2); *Helicobacter pylori* eradication (section 1.3)

Cautions; Side-effects: see under Metronidazole; pregnancy (manufacturer advises avoidance in first trimester)

Dose: anaerobic infections *by mouth*, 2 g initially, followed by 1 g daily *or* 500 mg twice daily, usually for 5–6 days
Bacterial vaginosis and acute ulcerative gingivitis, a single 2-g dose
Abdominal surgery prophylaxis, a single 2-g dose approximately 12 hours before surgery

Fasigyn® (Pfizer) [PoM]
Tablets, f/c, tinidazole 500 mg. Net price 20-tab pack = £11.50. Label: 4, 9, 21, 25

5.1.12 Quinolones

Nalidixic acid, cinoxacin, and **norfloxacin** are effective in uncomplicated urinary-tract infections.

Ciprofloxacin is active against both Gram-positive and Gram-negative bacteria. It is particularly active against Gram-negative bacteria, including salmonella, shigella, campylobacter, neisseria, and pseudomonas. Ciprofloxacin has only moderate activity against Gram-positive bacteria such as *Streptococcus pneumoniae* and *Enterococcus faecalis*; it is not the drug of first choice for pneumococcal pneumonia. It is active against chlamydia and some mycobacteria. Most anaerobic organisms are not susceptible. Uses for ciprofloxacin include infections of the respiratory tract (but not for pneumococcal pneumonia) and of the urinary tract, and of the gastro-intestinal system (including typhoid fever), and gonorrhoea and septicaemia caused by sensitive organisms.

Ofloxacin is used for urinary-tract infections, lower respiratory-tract infections, gonorrhoea, and non-gonococcal urethritis and cervicitis.

Levofloxacin is a recently introduced quinolone that is active against Gram-positive and Gram-negative organisms. It has greater activity against pneumococci than ciprofloxacin.

Although, ciprofloxacin, levofloxacin and ofloxacin are licensed for skin and soft-tissue infections, many staphylococci are resistant to the quinolones and their use should be avoided in methicillin-resistant *Staphylococcus aureus* (MRSA) infections.

CAUTIONS. Quinolones should be used with caution in patients with a history of epilepsy or conditions that predispose to seizures, in G6PD deficiency (section 9.1.5), in pregnancy, during breast-feeding, and in children or adolescents (arthropathy has developed in weight-bearing joints in young *animals*—see below). Exposure to excessive sunlight should be avoided (discontinue if photosensitivity occurs). The CSM has warned that quinolones may induce **convulsions** in patients with or without a history of convulsions; taking NSAIDs at the same time may also induce them. Other **interactions**: Appendix 1 (quinolones).

USE IN CHILDREN. Quinolones cause arthropathy in the weight-bearing joints of immature *animals* and are therefore generally not recommended in children and growing adolescents. However, the significance of this effect in humans is uncertain and in some specific circumstances short-term use of a quinolone in children may be justified. Nalidixic acid is used for urinary-tract infections in children over 3 months of age and ciprofloxacin is licensed for pseudomonal infections in cystic fibrosis for children above 5 years of age.

> **CSM advice (tendon damage)**
> At the first sign of pain or inflammation, patients taking quinolones should discontinue the treatment and rest the affected limb until tendon symptoms have resolved.

SIDE-EFFECTS. Side-effects of the quinolones include nausea, vomiting, dyspepsia, abdominal pain, diarrhoea (rarely antibiotic-associated colitis), headache, dizziness, sleep disorders, rash (rarely Stevens-Johnson syndrome and toxic epidermal necrolysis), and pruritus. Less frequent side-effects include anorexia, transient disturbances in liver enzymes and bilirubin, increase in blood urea and creatinine; drowsiness, restlessness, depression, confusion, hallucinations, convulsions, paraesthesia; photosensitivity, hypersensitivity reactions including fever, urticaria, angioedema, arthralgia, myalgia, and anaphylaxis; blood disorders (including eosinophilia, leucopenia, thrombocytopenia); disturbances in vision, taste, hearing and smell. Also isolated reports of tendon inflammation and damage (especially in the elderly and in those taking corticosteroids, see also CSM advice above). Side-effects that have been reported to the CSM also include haemolytic anaemia, renal impairment, and hepatic dysfunction. The drug should be **discontinued** if psychiatric, neurological or hypersensitivity reactions (including severe rash) occur.

CINOXACIN

Indications: urinary-tract infections
Cautions: see notes above; renal impairment (avoid if moderate or severe—Appendix 3); **interactions:** Appendix 1 (quinolones)
DRIVING. May impair performance of skilled tasks (e.g. driving)

Side-effects: see notes above; also reported, perineal burning, tinnitus, photophobia
Dose: 500 mg every 12 hours; prophylaxis, 500 mg at night

Cinobac® (Lilly) PoM
Capsules, green/orange, cinoxacin 500 mg. Net price 14-cap pack = £10.41. Label: 6, 9, counselling, driving

CIPROFLOXACIN

Indications: see notes above and under Dose
Cautions: see notes above; renal impairment (Appendix 3); avoid excessive alkalinity of urine and ensure adequate fluid intake (risk of crystalluria); **interactions:** Appendix 1 (quinolones)
DRIVING. May impair performance of skilled tasks (e.g. driving); effects enhanced by alcohol
Side-effects: see notes above; also reported flatulence, dysphagia, tremor, altered prothrombin concentration, jaundice and hepatitis with necrosis, renal failure, nephritis, vasculitis, erythema nodosum, petechiae, haemorrhagic bullae, tinnitus, tenosynovitis and tachycardia; pain and phlebitis at injection site
Dose: *by mouth*, respiratory-tract infections, 250–750 mg twice daily
Urinary-tract infections, 250–500 mg twice daily (100 mg twice daily for 3 days in acute uncomplicated cystitis in women)
Gonorrhoea, 500 mg as a single dose
Pseudomonal lower respiratory-tract infection in cystic fibrosis, 750 mg twice daily; CHILD 5–17 years (see Cautions above), up to 20 mg/kg twice daily (max. 1.5 g daily)
Most other infections, 500–750 mg twice daily
Surgical prophylaxis, 750 mg 60–90 minutes before procedure
Prophylaxis of meningococcal meningitis [not licensed], section 5.1, table 2
By intravenous infusion (over 30–60 minutes; 400 mg over 60 minutes), 200–400 mg twice daily
Pseudomonal lower respiratory-tract infection in cystic fibrosis, 400 mg twice daily; CHILD 5–17 years (see Cautions above), up to 10 mg/kg 3 times daily (max. 1.2 g daily)
Urinary-tract infections, 100 mg twice daily
Gonorrhoea, 100 mg as a single dose
CHILD not recommended (see Cautions above) but where benefit outweighs risk, *by mouth*, 10–30 mg/kg daily in 2 divided doses *or by intravenous infusion*, 8–16 mg/kg daily in 2 divided doses

Ciproxin® (Bayer) PoM
Tablets, all f/c, ciprofloxacin (as hydrochloride) 100 mg, net price 6-tab pack = £2.80; 250 mg (scored), 10-tab pack = £7.50, 20-tab pack = £15.00; 500 mg (scored), 10-tab pack = £14.20, 20-tab pack = £28.40; 750 mg, 10-tab pack = £20.00. Label: 6, 9, 25, counselling, driving
Suspension, strawberry-flavoured, ciprofloxacin for reconstitution with diluent provided, 250 mg/5 mL, net price 100 mL = £15.00. Label: 6, 9, 25, counselling, driving
Intravenous infusion, ciprofloxacin (as lactate) 2 mg/mL, in sodium chloride 0.9%, net price 50-mL bottle = £8.65
Electrolytes: Na⁺ 15.4 mmol/100-mL bottle

Intravenous infusion (*Flexibag*), ciprofloxacin (as lactate) 2 mg/mL, in glucose 5%, net price 100-mL infusion bag = £16.89, 200-mL infusion bag = £25.70

LEVOFLOXACIN

Indications: see under Dose
Cautions: see notes above; renal impairment (Appendix 3); **interactions:** Appendix 1 (quinolones)
DRIVING. May impair performance of skilled tasks (e.g. driving)
Side-effects: see notes above; asthenia; rarely tremor, anxiety, tachycardia, hypotension, hypoglycaemia, hepatitis, interstitial nephritis, pneumonitis, rhabdomyolysis; local reactions and transient hypotension reported with infusion
Dose: *by mouth*, acute sinusitis, 500 mg daily for 10–14 days
Exacerbation of chronic bronchitis, 250–500 mg daily for 7–10 days
Community-acquired pneumonia, 500 mg once or twice daily for 7–14 days
Complicated urinary-tract infections, 250 mg daily for 7–10 days
Skin and soft tissue infections, 250 mg daily *or* 500 mg once or twice daily for 7–14 days
By intravenous infusion (over at least 60 minutes for 500 mg), community-acquired pneumonia, 500 mg once or twice daily
Complicated urinary-tract infections, 250 mg daily, increased in severe infections
Skin and soft tissue infections, 500 mg twice daily

Tavanic® (Hoechst Marion Roussel) ▼ PoM
Tablets, f/c, scored, levofloxacin 250 mg, net price 5-tab pack = £7.77, 10-tab pack = £15.54; 500 mg, 5-tab pack = £13.90, 10-tab pack = £27.80. Label: 6, 9, 25, counselling, driving
Intravenous infusion, levofloxacin 5 mg/mL, net price 100-mL bottle = £28.39

NALIDIXIC ACID

Indications: urinary-tract infections
Cautions: see notes above; avoid in porphyria (section 9.8.2); liver disease; renal impairment (Appendix 3); false positive urinary glucose (if tested for reducing substances); monitor blood counts, renal and liver function if treatment exceeds 2 weeks; **interactions:** Appendix 1 (quinolones)
Side-effects: see notes above; also reported toxic psychosis, weakness, increased intracranial pressure, cranial nerve palsy, cholestasis, metabolic acidosis
Dose: 1 g every 6 hours for 7 days, reduced in chronic infections to 500 mg every 6 hours; CHILD over 3 months max. 50 mg/kg daily in divided doses; reduced in prolonged therapy to 30 mg/kg daily

Mictral® (Sanofi-Synthelabo) PoM
Granules, effervescent, nalidixic acid 660 mg, sodium citrate (as sodium citrate and citric acid) 4.1 g/sachet (Na+ 41 mmol/sachet). Net price 9-sachet pack = £5.48. Label: 9, 11, 13
Dose: 1 sachet in water 3 times daily for 3 days

Negram® (Sanofi-Synthelabo) PoM
Tablets, beige, nalidixic acid 500 mg. Net price 56-tab pack = £12.83. Label: 9, 11, 23

Suspension, pink, sugar-free, nalidixic acid 300 mg/5 mL. Net price 150 mL = £12.85. Label: 9, 11, 23

Uriben® (Rosemont) PoM
Suspension, pink, nalidixic acid 300 mg/5 mL, net price 150 mL = £16.18. Label: 9, 11

NORFLOXACIN

Indications: see under Dose
Cautions: see notes above; severe renal impairment (Appendix 3); **interactions:** Appendix 1 (quinolones)
DRIVING. May impair performance of skilled tasks (e.g. driving)
Side-effects: see notes above; also reported euphoria, anxiety, tinnitus, exfoliative dermatitis, hepatitis, interstitial nephritis, pancreatitis, vasculitis
Dose: urinary-tract infections, 400 mg twice daily for 7–10 days (for 3 days in uncomplicated lower urinary-tract infections)
Chronic relapsing urinary-tract infections, 400 mg twice daily for up to 12 weeks; may be reduced to 400 mg once daily if adequate suppression within first 4 weeks

Utinor® (MSD) PoM
Tablets, scored, norfloxacin 400 mg. Net price 6-tab pack = £2.88, 14-tab pack = £6.72. Label: 6, 9, counselling, driving

OFLOXACIN

Indications: see under Dose
Cautions: see notes above; hepatic and renal impairment (Appendixes 2 and 3); history of psychiatric illness; **interactions:** Appendix 1 (quinolones)
DRIVING. May affect performance of skilled tasks (e.g. driving); effects enhanced by alcohol
Side-effects: see notes above; also reported, tachycardia, transient hypotension, vasculitic reactions, anxiety, unsteady gait and tremor, hypaesthesia, neuropathy, extrapyramidal symptoms, psychotic reactions (discontinue treatment—see notes above); very rarely changes in blood sugar; isolated cases of pneumonitis, cholestatic jaundice, hepatitis, interstitial nephritis; on intravenous infusion, hypotension and local reactions (including thrombophlebitis)
Dose: *by mouth*, urinary-tract infections, 200–400 mg daily preferably in the morning, increased if necessary in upper urinary-tract infections to 400 mg twice daily
Lower respiratory-tract infections, 400 mg daily preferably in the morning, increased if necessary to 400 mg twice daily
Skin and soft-tissue infections, 400 mg twice daily
Uncomplicated gonorrhoea, 400 mg as a single dose
Non-gonococcal urethritis and cervicitis, 400 mg daily in single or divided doses
By intravenous infusion (over at least 30 minutes for each 200 mg), complicated urinary-tract infection, 200 mg daily
Lower respiratory-tract infection, 200 mg twice daily
Septicaemia, 200 mg twice daily
Skin and soft-tissue infections, 400 mg twice daily
Severe or complicated infections, dose may be increased to 400 mg twice daily

Tarivid® (Hoechst Marion Roussel) PoM

Tablets, f/c, scored, ofloxacin 200 mg, net price 10-tab pack = £10.26, 20-tab pack = £20.50; 400 mg (yellow), 5-tab pack = £10.24, 10-tab pack = £20.43. Label: 6, 9, 11, counselling, driving

Intravenous infusion, ofloxacin (as hydrochloride) 2 mg/mL, net price 50-mL bottle = £15.41; 100-mL bottle = £22.01 (both hosp. only)

5.1.13   Urinary-tract infections

Urinary-tract infection is more common in women than in men; when it occurs in men there is frequently an underlying abnormality of the renal tract. Recurrent episodes of infection are an indication for radiological investigation especially in children in whom untreated pyelonephritis may lead to permanent kidney damage.

Escherichia coli is the most common cause of urinary-tract infection. Less common causes include Proteus and Klebsiella spp. *Pseudomonas aeruginosa* infections are almost invariably associated with functional or anatomical abnormalities of the renal tract. *Staphylococcus epidermidis* and *Enterococcus faecalis* infection may complicate catheterisation or instrumentation. Whenever possible a specimen of urine should be collected for culture and sensitivity testing before starting antibiotic therapy.

Uncomplicated lower urinary-tract infections often respond to ampicillin, nalidixic acid, nitrofurantoin, or trimethoprim given for 5–7 days (3 days may be adequate for infections in women); those caused by fully sensitive bacteria respond to two 3-g doses of amoxicillin (section 5.1.1.3). Bacterial resistance, however, especially to ampicillin (to which approximately 50% of *E. coli* are now resistant), has increased the importance of urine culture prior to therapy. Alternatives for resistant organisms include co-amoxiclav (amoxicillin with clavulanic acid), an oral cephalosporin, or a quinolone. Methenamine (hexamine) should **not** be used because it is only bacteriostatic, requires an acidic urine, and frequently causes side-effects.

Long-term low dose therapy may be required in selected patients to prevent *recurrence of infection*; indications include frequent relapses and significant kidney damage. Trimethoprim, nitrofurantoin and cefalexin have been recommended for long-term therapy.

Acute pyelonephritis can be associated with septicaemia and is best treated initially by injection of a broad-spectrum antibiotic such as cefuroxime, some quinolones, or gentamicin especially if the patient is severely ill.

Prostatitis can be difficult to cure and requires treatment for several weeks with an antibiotic which penetrates prostatic tissue such as trimethoprim, erythromycin, or some quinolones.

Where infection is localised and associated with an indwelling *catheter* a bladder instillation is often effective (section 7.4.4).

Patients with *heart-valve lesions* undergoing instrumentation of the urinary tract should be given a parenteral antibiotic to prevent bacteraemia and endocarditis (section 5.1, table 2).

Urinary-tract infection in *pregnancy* may be asymptomatic and requires prompt treatment to prevent progression to acute pyelonephritis. Penicillins and cephalosporins can be given in pregnancy but trimethoprim, sulphonamides, quinolones, and tetracyclines should be avoided.

In *renal failure* antibiotics normally excreted by the kidney accumulate with resultant toxicity unless the dose is reduced. This applies especially to the aminoglycosides which should be used with great caution; tetracyclines, hexamine, and nitrofurantoin should be avoided altogether.

NITROFURANTOIN

Indications: urinary-tract infections

Cautions: anaemia; diabetes mellitus; electrolyte imbalance; vitamin B and folate deficiency; pulmonary disease; hepatic impairment; monitor lung and liver function on long-term therapy, especially in the elderly; susceptibility to peripheral neuropathy; false positive urinary glucose (if tested for reducing substances); urine may be coloured yellow or brown; **interactions:** Appendix 1 (nitrofurantoin)

Contra-indications: impaired renal function, infants less than 3 months old, G6PD deficiency (including pregnancy at term, and breast-feeding of affected infants, see section 9.1.5 and Appendixes 4 and 5), porphyria (section 9.8.2)

Side-effects: anorexia, nausea, vomiting, and diarrhoea; acute and chronic pulmonary reactions (may be associated with lupus erythematosus-like syndrome); peripheral neuropathy; also reported, angioedema, urticaria, rash and pruritus; rarely, cholestatic jaundice, hepatitis, exfoliative dermatitis, erythema multiforme, pancreatitis, arthralgia, blood disorders (including agranulocytosis, thrombocytopenia, and aplastic anaemia), benign intracranial hypertension, and transient alopecia

Dose: acute uncomplicated infection, 50 mg every 6 hours with food for 7 days; CHILD over 3 months, 3 mg/kg daily in 4 divided doses

Severe chronic recurrent infection, 100 mg every 6 hours with food for 7 days (dose reduced or discontinued if severe nausea)

Prophylaxis (but see Cautions), 50–100 mg at night; CHILD over 3 months, 1 mg/kg at night

Nitrofurantoin (Non-proprietary) PoM

Tablets, nitrofurantoin 50 mg and 100 mg. Label: 9, 14, 21

Available from Biorex, Cox, Kent

Furadantin® (Goldshield) PoM

Tablets, all yellow, scored, nitrofurantoin 50 mg, net price 20 = £1.96; 100 mg, 20 = £3.62. Label: 9, 14, 21

Macrobid® (Goldshield) PoM

Capsules, m/r, blue/yellow, nitrofurantoin 100 mg (as nitrofurantoin macrocrystals and nitrofurantoin monohydrate). Net price 14-cap pack = £4.89. Label: 9, 14, 21, 25

Dose: uncomplicated urinary-tract infection, 1 capsule twice daily with food

Genito-urinary surgical prophylaxis, 1 capsule twice daily on day of procedure and for 3 days after

Macrodantin® (Goldshield) [PoM]
Capsules, nitrofurantoin 50 mg (yellow/white), net
price 30-cap pack = £3.05; 100 mg (yellow), 20 =
£3.84. Label: 9, 14, 21

METHENAMINE HIPPURATE ◤

(Hexamine hippurate)
Indications: prophylaxis and long-term treatment
of recurrent urinary-tract infections
Cautions: pregnancy; avoid concurrent adminis-
tration with sulphonamides (risk of crystalluria)
or urinary alkalinising agents; **interactions:**
Appendix 1 (hexamine)
Contra-indications: severe renal impairment,
dehydration, metabolic acidosis
Side-effects: gastro-intestinal disturbances,
bladder irritation, rash
Dose: 1 g every 12 hours (may be increased in
patients with catheters to 1 g every 8 hours);
CHILD 6–12 years 500 mg every 12 hours

Hiprex® (3M) ◤
Tablets, scored, methenamine hippurate 1 g. Net
price 60-tab pack = £7.07. Label: 9

> ◤ denotes preparations that are considered to
> be less suitable for prescribing (see p. vi)

5.2 Antifungal drugs

Treatment of fungal infections

The systemic treatment of common fungal infections is outlined below; specialist treatment is
required in most forms of systemic or disseminated
fungal infections. For local treatment of fungal
infections, see section 7.2.2 (genital), section 7.4.4
(bladder), section 11.3.2 (eye), section 12.1.1 (ear),
section 12.3.2 (oropharynx), and section 13.10.2
(skin).

ASPERGILLOSIS. Aspergillosis most commonly
affects the respiratory tract although, in severely
immunocompromised patients, invasive forms can
affect the sinuses, heart, brain, and skin. **Amphotericin** by intravenous infusion is the drug of choice
but response can be variable; liposomal amphotericin or oral **itraconazole** are alternatives in
patients in whom initial treatment has failed.

CANDIDIASIS. Many superficial candidal infections are treated locally including infections of the
vagina (section 7.2.2) and of the skin (section
13.10.2).
Oropharyngeal candidiasis generally responds to
topical therapy (section 12.3.2); an imidazole or triazole antifungal is given by mouth for unresponsive
infections. Fluconazole is effective and is reliably
absorbed.
For *deep and disseminated candidiasis*, **amphotericin** by intravenous infusion is used alone or with
flucytosine by intravenous infusion; an alternative
is **fluconazole** given alone, particularly in AIDS
patients (in whom flucytosine is best avoided
because of its bone marrow toxicity).

CRYPTOCOCCOSIS. Cryptococcosis is uncommon but infection in the immunocompromised,
especially in AIDS patients, can be life-threatening;
cryptococcal meningitis is the most common form
of fungal meningitis. The treatment of choice is
amphotericin by intravenous infusion with or
without **flucytosine** by intravenous infusion. **Fluconazole** given alone intravenously is an alternative; it is also used by mouth in AIDS patients who
have had cryptococcal meningitis, for lifelong
prophylaxis against relapse.

HISTOPLASMOSIS. Histoplasmosis is rare in tem-
perate climates; it can be life-threatening, particularly in HIV-infected persons. **Itraconazole** by
mouth or **ketoconazole** by mouth can be used for
the treatment of immunocompetent patients with
indolent non-meningeal infection including chronic
pulmonary histoplasmosis. **Amphotericin** by intravenous infusion is preferred in patients with fulminant or severe infections.

SKIN AND NAIL INFECTIONS. Mild localised
fungal infections of the skin (including tinea corporis, tinea cruris, and tinea pedis) respond to topical therapy (section 13.10.2). Systemic therapy is
appropriate if topical therapy fails, if many areas
are affected, or if the site of infection is difficult to
treat such as in infections of the nails (onychomycosis) and of the scalp (tinea capitis).
Griseofulvin was used extensively in tinea of
various sites but has now largely been replaced by
newer antifungals. Oral imidazole or triazole antifungals (particularly **itraconazole**) and **terbinafine** are used more commonly because they have a
broader spectrum of activity and require a shorter
duration of treatment.
Pityriasis versicolor may be treated with **itraconazole** by mouth if topical therapy is ineffective; **fluconazole** by mouth is an alternative.
Terbinafine and **itraconazole** have largely
replaced griseofulvin for the systemic treatment of
onychomycosis, particularly of the toenail; terbinafine is considered to be the drug of choice. Itraconazole can be administered as intermittent 'pulse'
therapy.

IMMUNOCOMPROMISED PATIENTS. Immunocompromised patients are at particular risk of
fungal infections and may receive antifungal drugs
prophylactically; oral imidazole or triazole antifungals are the drugs of choice. Fluconazole is more
reliably absorbed than itraconazole and ketoconazole; fluconazole is considered to be less toxic
than ketoconazole on long-term use.

Drugs used in fungal infections

POLYENE ANTIFUNGALS. The polyene antifungals include amphotericin and nystatin; neither drug
is absorbed when given by mouth. They are used
for oral, oropharyngeal, and perioral infections by
local application in the mouth (section 12.3.2).
Amphotericin by intravenous infusion is used for
the treatment of systemic fungal infections and is
active against most fungi and yeasts. It is highly
protein bound and penetrates poorly into body fluids and tissues. When given parenterally amphot-

ericin is toxic and side-effects are common. Lipid formulations of amphotericin (*Abelcet®*, *AmBisome®*, and *Amphocil®*) are significantly less toxic and are recommended when the conventional formulation of amphotericin is contra-indicated because of toxicity, especially nephrotoxicity; lipid formulations are more expensive.

Nystatin is used principally for *Candida albicans* infections of the skin and mucous membranes, including oesophageal and intestinal candidiasis.

IMIDAZOLE ANTIFUNGALS.Clotrimazole, econazole, fenticonazole, isoconazole, sulconazole, and tioconazole are used for the local treatment of vaginal candidiasis (section 7.2.2) and for dermatophyte infections (section 13.10.2).

Ketoconazole is better absorbed by mouth than other imidazoles. It has been associated with fatal hepatotoxicity; the CSM has advised that prescribers should weigh the potential benefits of ketoconazole treatment against the risk of liver damage and should carefully monitor patients both clinically and biochemically. It should not be used for superficial fungal infections.

Miconazole can be used locally for oral infections; it is also effective in intestinal infections. Systemic absorption may follow use of miconazole oral gel and may result in significant drug interactions.

TRIAZOLE ANTIFUNGALS. **Fluconazole** is very well absorbed after oral administration. It also achieves good penetration into the cerebrospinal fluid to treat fungal meningitis.

Itraconazole is active against a wide range of dermatophytes. It requires an acid environment in the stomach for optimal absorption.

Itraconazole has been associated with liver damage and should not be given to patients with a history of liver disease; fluconazole is less frequently associated with hepatotoxicity.

OTHER ANTIFUNGALS. **Flucytosine** is often used with amphotericin in a synergistic combination. Bone marrow depression can occur which limits its use, particularly in AIDS patients; weekly blood counts are necessary during prolonged therapy. Resistance to flucytosine can develop during therapy and sensitivity testing is essential before and during treatment.

Griseofulvin is effective for widespread or intractable dermatophyte infections but has been superseded by newer antifungals, particularly for nail infections. It is usually well tolerated and is licensed for use in children. Duration of therapy is dependent on the site of the infection and may be required for a number of months.

Terbinafine is the drug of choice for fungal nail infections and is also used for ringworm infections where oral treatment is considered appropriate.

AMPHOTERICIN

(Amphotericin B)

Indications: See under Dose

Cautions: when given parenterally, toxicity common (close supervision necessary and test dose required); renal impairment (Appendix 3); hepatic and renal-function tests, blood counts,

and plasma electrolyte monitoring required; corticosteroids (avoid except to control reactions); pregnancy and breast-feeding; avoid rapid infusion (risk of arrhythmias); **interactions:** Appendix 1 (amphotericin)

ANAPHYLAXIS. The CSM has advised that anaphylaxis occurs rarely with any intravenous amphotericin product and a test dose is advisable before the first infusion; the patient should be carefully observed for about 30 minutes after the test dose. Prophylactic antipyretics or hydrocortisone should only be used in patients who have previously experienced acute adverse reactions (in whom continued treatment with amphotericin is essential)

Side-effects: when given parenterally, anorexia, nausea and vomiting, diarrhoea, epigastric pain; febrile reactions, headache, muscle and joint pain; anaemia; disturbances in renal function (including hypokalaemia and hypomagnesaemia) and renal toxicity; also cardiovascular toxicity (including arrhythmias), blood disorders, neurological disorders (including hearing loss, diplopia, convulsions, peripheral neuropathy), abnormal liver function (discontinue treatment), rash, anaphylactoid reactions (see Anaphylaxis, above); pain and thrombophlebitis at injection site

Dose: *by mouth*, intestinal candidiasis, 100–200 mg every 6 hours; INFANT and CHILD, 100 mg 4 times daily

Prophylaxis NEONATE 100 mg once daily

Oral and perioral infections, see section 12.3.2

By intravenous infusion, see under preparations, below

Fungilin® (Squibb) PoM

Tablets, yellow, scored, amphotericin 100 mg, net price 56-tab pack = £8.32. Label: 9

Suspension, yellow, sugar-free, amphotericin 100 mg/mL, net price 12 mL = £2.31. Label: 9, counselling, use of pipette

Fungizone® (Squibb) PoM

Intravenous infusion, powder for reconstitution, amphotericin (as sodium deoxycholate complex). Net price 50-mg vial = £3.70

Electrolytes: Na$^+$ <0.5 mmol/vial

Dose: by intravenous infusion, systemic fungal infections, initial test dose of 1 mg over 20–30 minutes then 250 micrograms/kg daily, gradually increased if tolerated to 1 mg/kg daily; max. (severe infection) 1.5 mg/kg daily or on alternate days

Note. Prolonged treatment usually necessary; if interrupted for longer than 7 days recommence at 250 micrograms/kg daily and increase gradually

■ Lipid formulations

Abelcet® (Wyeth) PoM

Intravenous infusion, amphotericin 5 mg/mL as lipid complex with L-α-dimyristoylphosphatidylcholine and L-α-dimyristoylphosphatidylglycerol. Net price 10-mL vial = £50.00, 20-mL vial = £86.00 (hosp. only)

Dose: severe invasive candidiasis; severe systemic fungal infections in patients not responding to conventional amphotericin or to other antifungal drugs or where toxicity or renal impairment precludes conventional amphotericin, including invasive aspergillosis, cryptococcal meningitis and disseminated cryptococcosis in HIV patients, by intravenous infusion, ADULT and CHILD, initial test dose 1 mg over 15 minutes then 5 mg/kg daily for at least 14 days

AmBisome® (NeXstar) PoM

Intravenous infusion, powder for reconstitution, amphotericin 50 mg encapsulated in liposomes. Net price 50-mg vial = £145.00

Electrolytes: Na⁺ <0.5 mmol/vial

Dose: severe systemic or deep mycoses where toxicity (particularly nephrotoxicity) precludes use of conventional amphotericin, by intravenous infusion, ADULT and CHILD initial test dose 1 mg over 10 minutes then 1 mg/kg daily as a single dose increased gradually if necessary to 3 mg/kg daily as a single dose

Infections in febrile neutropenic patients unresponsive to broad-spectrum antibiotics, ADULT and CHILD, initial test dose 1 mg over 10 minutes then 3 mg/kg daily as a single dose until afebrile for 3 consecutive days; max. period of treatment 42 days

Visceral leishmaniasis, see section 5.4.5 and product literature

Amphocil® (Zeneca) PoM

Intravenous infusion, powder for reconstitution, amphotericin as a complex with sodium cholesteryl sulphate. Net price 50-mg vial = £104.10, 100-mg vial = £190.05

Electrolytes: Na⁺ <0.5 mmol/vial

Dose: severe systemic or deep mycoses where toxicity or renal failure preclude use of conventional amphotericin, by intravenous infusion, ADULT and CHILD initial test dose 2 mg over 10 minutes then 1 mg/kg daily as a single dose increased gradually if necessary to 3–4 mg/kg daily as a single dose

---

FLUCONAZOLE

Indications: see under Dose

Cautions: renal impairment (Appendix 3); pregnancy (Appendix 4) and breast-feeding (Appendix 5); raised liver enzymes (review need for treatment if raised significantly, risk of hepatic necrosis); **interactions:** Appendix 1 (antifungals, imidazole and triazole)

ARRHYTHMIAS. Avoid concomitant administration with cisapride or terfenadine; [other interactions, Appendix 1]

Side-effects: nausea, abdominal discomfort, diarrhoea, and flatulence; occasionally abnormalities of liver enzymes; headache; rarely rash (discontinue treatment or monitor closely if infection invasive or systemic); angioedema, anaphylaxis, bullous lesions, toxic epidermal necrolysis, and Stevens-Johnson syndrome reported; severe cutaneous reactions in AIDS patients also reported

Dose: vaginal candidiasis and candidal balanitis, *by mouth*, a single dose of 150 mg

Mucosal candidiasis (except genital), *by mouth*, 50 mg daily (100 mg daily in unusually difficult infections) given for 7–14 days in oropharyngeal candidiasis (max. 14 days except in severely immunocompromised patients); for 14 days in atrophic oral candidiasis associated with dentures; for 14–30 days in other mucosal infections (e.g. oesophagitis, candiduria, non-invasive bronchopulmonary infections); CHILD *by mouth or by intravenous infusion*, 3–6 mg/kg on first day then 3 mg/kg daily (every 72 hours in NEONATE up to 2 weeks old, every 48 hours in neonate 2–4 weeks old)

Tinea pedis, corporis, cruris, pityriasis versicolor, and dermal candidiasis, *by mouth*, 50 mg daily for 2–4 weeks (for up to 6 weeks in tinea pedis); max. duration of treatment 6 weeks

Invasive candidal infections (including candidaemia and disseminated candidiasis) and cryptococcal infections (including meningitis), *by mouth or intravenous infusion*, 400 mg initially then 200 mg daily, increased if necessary to 400 mg daily; treatment continued according to response (at least 6–8 weeks for cryptococcal meningitis); CHILD 6–12 mg/kg daily (every 72 hours in NEONATE up to 2 weeks old, every 48 hours in NEONATE 2–4 weeks old); max. 400 mg daily

Prevention of relapse of cryptococcal meningitis in AIDS patients after completion of primary therapy, *by mouth or by intravenous infusion*, 100–200 mg daily

Prevention of fungal infections in immunocompromised patients following cytotoxic chemotherapy or radiotherapy, *by mouth or by intravenous infusion*, 50–400 mg daily adjusted according to risk; 400 mg daily if high risk of systemic infections e.g. following bone-marrow transplantation; commence treatment before anticipated onset of neutropenia and continue for 7 days after neutrophil count in desirable range; CHILD according to extent and duration of neutropenia, 3–12 mg/kg daily (every 72 hours in NEONATE up to 2 weeks old, every 48 hours in NEONATE 2–4 weeks old); max. 400 mg daily

Diflucan® (Pfizer)

¹ *Capsules* PoM, fluconazole 50 mg (blue/white), net price 7-cap pack = £16.61; 150 mg (blue), single-capsule pack = £7.12; 200 mg (purple/white), 7-cap pack = £66.42. Label: 50 and 200 mg, 9

1. Can be sold to the public for vaginal candidiasis in women aged 16–60 years, in a container or packaging containing not more than 150 mg and labelled to show a max. dose of 150 mg; a proprietary brand (*Diflucan® One*) containing a single 150-mg capsule is on sale to the public

Oral suspension PoM, fluconazole for reconstitution with water, 50 mg/5 mL, net price 35 mL = £16.61; 200 mg/5 mL, 35 mL = £66.42. Label: 9

Intravenous infusion PoM, fluconazole 2 mg/mL in sodium chloride intravenous infusion 0.9%, net price 25-mL bottle = £7.32; 100-mL bottle = £29.28

Electrolytes: Na⁺ 15 mmol/100-mL bottle

FLUCYTOSINE

Indications: systemic yeast and fungal infections; adjunct to amphotericin (or fluconazole) in cryptococcal meningitis, adjunct to amphotericin in severe systemic candidiasis and in other severe or long-standing infections

Cautions: renal impairment (Appendix 3); elderly; blood disorders; liver- and kidney-function tests and blood counts required (weekly in renal impairment or blood disorders); pregnancy, breast-feeding

Side-effects: nausea, vomiting, diarrhoea, rashes; less frequently confusion, hallucinations, convulsions, headache, sedation, vertigo, alterations in liver function tests (hepatitis and hepatic necrosis reported); blood disorders including thrombocytopenia, leucopenia, and aplastic anaemia reported

Dose: *by intravenous infusion* over 20–40 minutes, ADULT and CHILD, 200 mg/kg daily in 4 divided doses usually for not more than 7 days; extremely sensitive organisms, 100–150 mg/kg daily may be sufficient; treat for at least 4 months in cryptococcal meningitis

Note. For plasma concentration monitoring blood should be taken shortly before starting the next infusion; plasma concentration for optimum response 25–50 mg/litre (200–400 micromol/litre)—should not be allowed to exceed 80 mg/litre (620 micromol/litre)

Ancotil® (ICN) [PoM]

Intravenous infusion, flucytosine 10 mg/mL. Net price 250-mL infusion bottle = £35.69 (hosp. only)

Electrolytes: Na⁺ 34.5 mmol/250-mL bottle

Note. Flucytosine tablets may be available on a named-patient basis from Bell and Croyden; the brand name *Alcobon®* was used formerly for flucytosine infusion

GRISEOFULVIN

Indications: dermatophyte infections of the skin, scalp, hair and nails where topical therapy has failed or is inappropriate

Cautions: rarely aggravation or precipitation of systemic lupus erythematosus; breast-feeding; **interactions:** Appendix 1 (griseofulvin)

DRIVING. May impair performance of skilled tasks (e.g. driving); effects of alcohol enhanced

Contra-indications: severe liver disease, lupus erythematosus and related conditions, porphyria (section 9.8.2); pregnancy (**avoid** pregnancy **during** and for **1 month after** treatment; men should not father children within 6 months of treatment)

Side-effects: headache, nausea, vomiting, rashes, photosensitivity; dizziness, fatigue, agranulocytosis and leucopenia reported; lupus erythematosus, erythema multiforme, toxic epidermal necrolysis, peripheral neuropathy, confusion and impaired co-ordination also reported

Dose: 500 mg daily, in divided doses or as a single dose, in severe infection dose may be doubled, reducing when response occurs; CHILD, 10 mg/kg daily in divided doses or as a single dose

Fulcin® (Zeneca) [PoM]

Tablets, griseofulvin 125 mg (scored), net price 20 = 61p; 500 mg (f/c), 20 = £2.29. Label: 9, 21, counselling, driving

Oral suspension, brown, griseofulvin 125 mg/5 mL. Net price 100 mL = £1.10. Label: 9, 21, counselling, driving

Grisovin® (GlaxoWellcome) [PoM]

Tablets, both f/c, griseofulvin 125 mg, net price 20 = 47p; 500 mg, 20 = £1.75. Label: 9, 21, counselling, driving

ITRACONAZOLE

Indications: see under Dose

Cautions: liver disease (Appendix 2); liver function tests required if history of liver disease or if treatment exceeds 1 month or if anorexia, nausea, vomiting, fatigue, abdominal pain or dark urine develop (discontinue if test abnormal); renal impairment (bioavailability may be reduced); absorption reduced in AIDS and neutropenia (monitor plasma-itraconazole concentration and increase dose if necessary); discontinue treatment if peripheral neuropathy; pregnancy (Appendix 4)

and breast-feeding; **interactions:** Appendix 1 (antifungals, imidazole and triazole)

ARRHYTHMIAS. Avoid concomitant administration with cisapride or terfenadine [other interactions, Appendix 1]

Side-effects: nausea, abdominal pain, dyspepsia, constipation (vomiting and diarrhoea with oral liquid), headache, dizziness, raised liver enzymes, menstrual disorders; allergic reactions (including pruritus, rash, urticaria and angioedema), hepatitis and cholestatic jaundice (especially if treatment exceeds 1 month), peripheral neuropathy (discontinue treatment), and Stevens-Johnson syndrome reported; on prolonged use hypokalaemia, oedema and hair loss reported

Dose: oropharyngeal candidiasis, 100 mg daily (200 mg daily in AIDS or neutropenia) for 15 days; see also under *Sporanox®* oral liquid below

Vulvovaginal candidiasis, 200 mg twice daily for 1 day

Pityriasis versicolor, 200 mg daily for 7 days

Tinea corporis and tinea cruris, *either* 100 mg daily for 15 days *or* 200 mg daily for 7 days

Tinea pedis and tinea manuum, *either* 100 mg daily for 30 days *or* 200 mg twice daily for 7 days

Onychomycosis, *either* 200 mg daily for 3 months *or* course ('pulse') of 200 mg twice daily for 7 days, subsequent courses repeated after 21-day interval; fingernails 2 courses, toenails 3 courses

Histoplasmosis, 200 mg 1–2 times daily

Systemic infections (aspergillosis, candidiasis and cryptococcosis including cryptococcal meningitis) where other antifungal drugs inappropriate or ineffective, 200 mg once daily (candidiasis 100–200 mg once daily) increased in invasive or disseminated disease and in cryptococcal meningitis to 200 mg twice daily

Maintenance in AIDS patients to prevent relapse of underlying fungal infection and prophylaxis in neutropenia when standard therapy inappropriate, 200 mg once daily, increased to 200 mg twice daily if low plasma-itraconazole concentration (see Cautions)

CHILD and ELDERLY not recommended

Sporanox® (Janssen-Cilag) [PoM]

Capsules, blue/pink, enclosing coated beads, itraconazole 100 mg, net price 4-cap pack = £5.72; 15-cap pack = £21.45; 28-cap pack (*Sporanox®-Pulse*) = £40.04; 60-cap pack = £85.80. Label: 5, 9, 21, 25

Oral liquid, sugar-free, itraconazole 10 mg/mL, net price 150 mL (with 10-mL measuring cup) = £52.28. Label: 9, counselling, administration

Dose: oral or oesophageal candidiasis in HIV-positive or other immunocompromised patients, 20 mL (2 measuring cups) daily in 1–2 divided doses for 1 week (continue for another week if no response)

Fluconazole-resistant oral or oesophageal candidiasis, 20–40 mL (2–4 measuring cups) daily in 1–2 divided doses for 2 weeks (continue for another 2 weeks if no response)

COUNSELLING. Do not take with food; swish around mouth and swallow, do not rinse afterwards

KETOCONAZOLE

Indications: systemic mycoses, serious chronic resistant mucocutaneous candidiasis, serious resistant gastro-intestinal mycoses, chronic resistant vaginal candidiasis, resistant dermatophyte infections of skin or finger nails (not toe nails); prophylaxis of mycoses in immunosuppressed patients

Cautions: monitor liver function clinically and biochemically—for treatment lasting longer than 14 days perform liver function tests before starting, 14 days after starting, then at monthly intervals (for details consult product literature)—for CSM advice see p. 284; avoid in porphyria (section 9.8.2); **interactions:** Appendix 1 (antifungals, imidazole and triazole)
ARRHYTHMIAS. Avoid concomitant administration with cisapride or terfenadine [other interactions, Appendix 1]
Contra-indications: hepatic impairment; pregnancy (Appendix 4) and breast-feeding
Side-effects: nausea, vomiting, abdominal pain; headache; rashes, urticaria, pruritus; rarely angioedema, thrombocytopenia, paraesthesia, photophobia, dizziness, alopecia, gynaecomastia and oligospermia; fatal liver damage—see also under Cautions, risk of developing hepatitis greater if given for longer than 14 days
Dose: 200 mg once daily with food, usually for 14 days; if response inadequate after 14 days continue until at least 1 week after symptoms have cleared and cultures negative; max. 400 mg (ELDERLY 200 mg) daily
CHILD 3 mg/kg daily
Chronic resistant vaginal candidiasis, 400 mg once daily with food for 5 days
Prophylaxis and maintenance treatment in immunosuppressed patients, 200 mg daily

Nizoral® (Janssen-Cilag) PoM
Tablets, scored, ketoconazole 200 mg. Net price 30-tab pack = £15.69. Label: 5, 9, 21

MICONAZOLE

Indications: see under Dose
Cautions: pregnancy and breast-feeding; avoid in porphyria (section 9.8.2); **interactions:** Appendix 1 (antifungals, imidazole and triazole)
ARRHYTHMIAS. Avoid concomitant administration with cisapride or terfenadine [other interactions, Appendix 1]
Contra-indications: hepatic impairment
Side-effects: nausea and vomiting, diarrhoea (usually on long-term treatment); rarely allergic reactions; isolated reports of hepatitis
Dose: prevention and treatment of oral and intestinal fungal infections, 5–10 mL in the mouth after food 4 times daily; retain near lesions before swallowing; CHILD under 2 years, 2.5 mL twice daily, 2–6 years, 5 mL twice daily, over 6 years, 5 mL 4 times daily
Localised lesions, smear on affected area with clean finger

¹ **Daktarin®** (Janssen-Cilag) PoM
Oral gel, sugar-free, orange-flavoured, miconazole 24 mg/mL. Net price 15-g tube = £2.27, 80-g tube = £5.00. Label: 9, counselling advised, hold in mouth, after food
1. 15-g tube can be sold to public

NYSTATIN

Indications: candidiasis; vaginal infection (section 7.2.2); oral infection (section 12.3.2); skin infection (section 13.10.2)
Side-effects: nausea, vomiting, diarrhoea at high doses; oral irritation and sensitisation; rash (including urticaria) and rarely Stevens-Johnson syndrome reported

Dose: *by mouth*, intestinal candidiasis 500 000 units every 6 hours, doubled in severe infections; CHILD 100 000 units 4 times daily
Prophylaxis, 1 million units once daily; NEONATE 100 000 units once daily

Nystatin (Non-proprietary) PoM
Oral suspension, nystatin 100 000 units/mL. Net price 30 mL = £2.20. Label: 9, counselling use of pipette
Available from Hillcross, Kent, Rosemont (sugar-free, *Nystamont®*)

Nystan® (Squibb) PoM
Tablets, brown, s/c, nystatin 500 000 units, net price 56-tab pack = £4.70. Label: 9
Suspension, yellow, nystatin 100 000 units/mL, net price 30 mL with pipette = £2.05. Label: 9, counselling, use of pipette

TERBINAFINE

Indications: dermatophyte infections of the nails, ringworm infections (including tinea pedis, cruris, and corporis) where oral therapy appropriate (due to site, severity or extent)
Cautions: hepatic and renal impairment (Appendixes 2 and 3); pregnancy, breast-feeding (Appendix 5); **interactions:** Appendix 1 (terbinafine)
Side-effects: abdominal discomfort, anorexia, nausea, diarrhoea; headache; rash and urticaria occasionally with arthralgia or myalgia; serious skin reactions including Stevens-Johnson syndrome and toxic epidermal necrolysis reported (discontinue treatment if progressive skin rash); taste disturbance, photosensitivity, and rarely liver toxicity (discontinue treatment) including jaundice, cholestasis and hepatitis also reported
Dose: 250 mg daily usually for 2–6 weeks in tinea pedis, 2–4 weeks in tinea cruris, 4 weeks in tinea corporis, 6 weeks–3 months in nail infections (occasionally longer in toenail infections); CHILD not recommended

Lamisil® (Novartis) PoM
Tablets, off-white, scored, terbinafine 250 mg (as hydrochloride), net price 14-tab pack = £23.16, 28-tab pack = £44.66. Label: 9

5.3 Antiviral drugs

The specific therapy of virus infections is generally unsatisfactory and treatment is, therefore, primarily symptomatic. Fortunately, the majority of infections resolve spontaneously in the immunocompetent. This section includes notes on herpes simplex and varicella-zoster, human immunodeficiency virus, cytomegalovirus, respiratory syncytial virus, viral hepatitis and influenza.

Herpes simplex and varicella–zoster

Aciclovir is active against herpes viruses but does not eradicate them. It is effective only if started at the onset of infection. Uses of aciclovir include the systemic treatment of varicella–zoster (chickenpox–shingles) and the systemic and topical treatment of herpes simplex infections of the skin and mucous membranes (including initial and recurrent genital herpes); it is also used topically in the eye. It can be life-saving in herpes simplex and varicella–zoster infections in the immunocompromised, and is also used for prevention of recurrence and for herpes simplex prophylaxis in the immunocompromised. Aciclovir may also be given by mouth to immunocompetent adults and older adolescents with chickenpox; it is not generally indicated for immunocompetent children in whom the disease is milder. See also section 11.3.3 (eye) and section 13.10.3 (skin, including herpes labialis).

Famciclovir, a prodrug of penciclovir, is similar to aciclovir and it is recommended for herpes zoster and initial and recurrent genital herpes. Penciclovir itself is used as a cream for herpes simplex labialis (section 13.10.3). **Valaciclovir** is an ester of aciclovir which is licensed for herpes zoster and for herpes simplex infections of the skin and mucous membranes (including initial and recurrent genital herpes).

Idoxuridine (section 13.10.3) is also only effective if started at the onset of infection; it is too toxic for systemic use. It has been used topically in the treatment of herpes simplex lesions of the skin and external genitalia with variable results; it has also been used topically in the treatment of zoster, but evidence of its value is dubious.

Inosine pranobex has been used by mouth for herpes simplex infections; its effectiveness has not been established.

ACICLOVIR
(Acyclovir)

Indications: herpes simplex and varicella–zoster (see also under Dose)

Cautions: maintain adequate hydration (especially with infusion or high doses); renal impairment (Appendix 3); pregnancy and breast-feeding; **interactions:** Appendix 1 (aciclovir and famciclovir)

Side-effects: rashes; gastro-intestinal disturbances; rises in bilirubin and liver enzymes, increases in blood urea and creatinine, decreases in haematological indices, headache, neurological reactions (including dizziness), fatigue; on intravenous infusion, severe local inflammation (sometimes leading to ulceration), also confusion, hallucinations, agitation, tremors, somnolence, psychosis, convulsions and coma

Dose: *by mouth,*
Herpes simplex, treatment, 200 mg (400 mg in the immunocompromised or if absorption impaired) 5 times daily, usually for 5 days; CHILD under 2 years, half adult dose, over 2 years, adult dose
Herpes simplex, prevention of recurrence, 200 mg 4 times daily *or* 400 mg twice daily possibly reduced to 200 mg 2 or 3 times daily and interrupted every 6–12 months
Herpes simplex, prophylaxis in the immunocompromised, 200–400 mg 4 times daily; CHILD under 2 years, half adult dose, over 2 years, adult dose
Varicella and herpes zoster, treatment, 800 mg 5 times daily for 7 days; CHILD, varicella, 20 mg/kg (max. 800 mg) 4 times daily for 5 days *or* under 2 years 200 mg 4 times daily, 2–5 years 400 mg 4 times daily, over 6 years 800 mg 4 times daily

By intravenous infusion, treatment of herpes simplex in the immunocompromised, severe initial genital herpes, and varicella–zoster, 5 mg/kg every 8 hours usually for 5 days, doubled to 10 mg/kg every 8 hours in varicella–zoster in the immunocompromised and in simplex encephalitis (usually given for 10 days in encephalitis); prophylaxis of herpes simplex in the immunocompromised, 5 mg/kg every 8 hours
NEONATE up to 3 months, herpes simplex, 10 mg/kg every 8 hours usually for 10 days; CHILD 3 months–12 years, herpes simplex or varicella–zoster, 250 mg/m^2 every 8 hours usually for 5 days, doubled to 500 mg/m^2 every 8 hours for varicella–zoster in the immunocompromised and in simplex encephalitis (usually given for 10 days in encephalitis)
By topical application, see sections 13.10.3 (skin) and 11.3.3 (eye)

Aciclovir (Non-proprietary) ▣PoM▣
Tablets, aciclovir 200 mg, net price 25-tab pack = £10.72; 400 mg, 56-tab pack = £34.40; 800 mg, 35-tab pack = £93.12. Label:9
Available from Cox, CP, Opus (*Virovir®*), Sovereign, Zurich
Dispersible tablets, aciclovir 200 mg, net price 25-tab pack = £21.62; 400 mg, 56-tab pack = £77.32; 800 mg, 35-tab pack = £75.35. Label: 9
Available from Genus, Hillcross, Norton, Pharmacia & Upjohn, Ranbaxy
Intravenous infusion, powder for reconstitution, aciclovir (as sodium salt). Net price 250-mg vial = £9.14; 500-mg vial = £17.59
Electrolytes: Na$^+$ 1.1 mmol/250-mg vial
Available from Genus, Zurich
Intravenous infusion, aciclovir (as sodium salt), 25 mg/mL, net price 10-mL (250-mg) vial = £10.37; 20-mL (500-mg) vial = £19.21; 40-mL (1-g) vial = £40.44
Electrolytes: Na$^+$ 1.16 mmol/250-mg vial
Available from Faulding DBL

Zovirax® (GlaxoWellcome) ▣PoM▣
Tablets, all dispersible, aciclovir 200 mg (blue), net price 25-tab pack = £20.22; 400 mg (pink), 56-tab pack = £74.17; 800 mg (scored, *Shingles Treatment Pack*), 35-tab pack = £75.11. Label: 9
Suspension, both off-white, sugar-free, aciclovir 200 mg/5 mL (banana-flavoured), net price 125 mL = £28.89; 400 mg/5 mL (*Chickenpox Treatment*, orange-flavoured) 50 mL = £16.14. Label: 9
Intravenous infusion, powder for reconstitution, aciclovir (as sodium salt). Net price 250-mg vial = £10.91; 500-mg vial = £20.22
Electrolytes: Na$^+$ 1.1 mmol/250-mg vial

FAMCICLOVIR

Note. Famciclovir is a pro-drug of penciclovir

Indications: treatment of herpes zoster, acute genital herpes simplex and suppression of recurrent genital herpes

Cautions: renal impairment (Appendix 3); pregnancy and breast-feeding; **interactions:** Appendix 1 (aciclovir and famciclovir)

Side-effects: nausea, vomiting; headache; rarely dizziness, confusion, hallucinations, rash; abdominal pain and fever have been reported in immunocompromised patients

Dose: herpes zoster, 250 mg 3 times daily for 7 days *or* 750 mg once daily for 7 days (in immuno-compromised, 500 mg 3 times daily for 10 days)
Genital herpes, first episode, 250 mg 3 times daily for 5 days; recurrent infection, 125 mg twice daily for 5 days (in immunocompromised, all episodes, 500 mg twice daily for 7 days)
Genital herpes, suppression, 250 mg twice daily (in HIV patients, 500 mg twice daily) interrupted every 6–12 months
CHILD not recommended

Famvir® (SmithKline Beecham) PoM
Tablets, all f/c, famciclovir 125 mg, net price 10-tab pack = £28.12; 250 mg, 15-tab pack = £84.35, 21-tab pack = £118.08; 56-tab pack = £314.90; 500 mg, 14-tab pack = £157.47, 30-tab pack = £337.34, 56-tab pack = £629.89; 750 mg, 7-tab pack = £112.72. Label: 9

INOSINE PRANOBEX

Indications: see under Dose
Cautions: avoid in renal impairment; history of gout or hyperuricaemia
Side-effects: reversible increase in serum and urinary uric acid
Dose: mucocutaneous herpes simplex, 1 g 4 times daily for 7–14 days
Adjunctive treatment of genital warts, 1 g 3 times daily for 14–28 days

Imunovir® (Ardern) PoM
Tablets, inosine pranobex 500 mg. Net price 100 = £39.50. Label: 9

denotes preparations that are considered to be less suitable for prescribing (see p. vi)

VALACICLOVIR

Note. Valaciclovir is a pro-drug of aciclovir
Indications: treatment of herpes zoster; treatment of initial and suppression of recurrent herpes sim-plex infections of skin and mucous membranes including initial and recurrent genital herpes
Cautions: renal impairment (Appendix 3); pregnancy and breast-feeding; **interactions:** Appendix 1 (aciclovir and famciclovir)
Side-effects: nausea, vomiting, diarrhoea, abdo-minal pain, headache, rash; neurological reactions including dizziness, confusion, hallucinations, and drowsiness reported
Dose: herpes zoster, 1 g 3 times daily for 7 days
Herpes simplex, first episode, 500 mg twice daily for 5 days (up to 10 days if severe); recurrent infection, 500 mg twice daily for 5 days
Herpes simplex, suppression, 500 mg daily in 1–2 divided doses (in immunocompromised, 500 mg twice daily)
CHILD not recommended

Valtrex® (GlaxoWellcome) PoM
Tablets, f/c, valaciclovir (as hydrochloride) 500 mg, net price 10-tab (*HS Treatment*) pack = £23.50, 42-tab (*Shingles Treatment*) pack = £98.50. Label: 9

Human immunodeficiency virus

There is no cure for infection caused by the human immunodeficiency virus (HIV) but there are a number of drugs which slow the progression of HIV infection.

PRINCIPLES OF TREATMENT. Drugs for HIV infection are potentially toxic and expensive; treat-ment should be undertaken only by those experi-enced in their use. Advice on the management of HIV infection is subject to rapid change.

Treatment is aimed at reducing the plasma viral load as much as possible and for as long as possi-ble; it should be started before the immune system is irreversibly damaged. The need for early drug treatment should, however, be balanced against the development of toxicity. The development of drug resistance is reduced by using a combination of drugs; such combinations should have synergistic or additive activity while ensuring that their toxicity is not additive. Testing for resistance to antiviral drugs particularly in therapeutic failure should be considered.

INITIATION OF TREATMENT. The optimum time for initiation of antiviral treatment will depend on the CD4 cell count, the plasma viral load, and clini-cal symptoms. Initiating treatment with a combina-tion of 3 drugs (including 2 nucleoside reverse transcriptase inhibitors with *either* a protease inhib-itor *or* a non-nucleoside reverse transcriptase inhib-itor) is recommended, particularly in patients with high plasma viral loads; initiating treatment with a combination of 2 nucleoside reverse transcriptase inhibitors (without another antiretroviral drug) should be considered only in exceptional circum-stances.

SWITCHING THERAPY. Deterioration of the con-dition (including clinical and virological changes) may require either switching therapy or adding another antiviral drug. The choice of an alternative regimen depends on factors such as the response to previous treatment, tolerance and the possibility of cross-resistance.

PREGNANCY AND BREAST-FEEDING. Treatment of HIV infection in pregnancy aims to reduce the risk of toxicity to the fetus (although the teratogenic potential of most antiretroviral drugs is unknown), to minimise the viral load and disease progression in the mother, and to prevent transmission of infec-tion to the neonate. **All treatment options require careful assessment by a specialist.** Zidovudine monotherapy reduces transmission of infection to the neonate. Combination antiretroviral therapy is used where indicated.

Breast-feeding by HIV-positive mothers may cause HIV infection in the infant and should be avoided.

POST-EXPOSURE PROPHYLAXIS. Treatment with antiviral drugs may be appropriate following occupa-tional exposure to HIV-contaminated material. Immediate expert advice should be sought in such cases; national guidelines on post-exposure prophy-laxis for healthcare workers have been developed (by the Chief Medical Officer's Expert Advisory Group on AIDS) and local ones may also be available.

DRUGS USED FOR HIV INFECTION. **Zidovudine**, a nucleoside reverse transcriptase inhibitor (or 'nucleoside analogue'), was the first anti-HIV drug to be introduced; it penetrates the blood-brain barrier and may be useful in preventing the AIDS dementia complex. Other nucleoside reverse transcriptase inhibitors include **abacavir**, **didanosine**, **lamivudine**, **stavudine**, and **zalcitabine**.

The protease inhibitors, **indinavir**, **nelfinavir**, **ritonavir** and **saquinavir** have been introduced recently. Indinavir, nelfinavir, ritonavir and possibly saquinavir inhibit the cytochrome P450 enzyme system and therefore have a potential for significant drug interactions. Protease inhibitors are associated with lipodystrophy and metabolic effects (see below).

The non-nucleoside reverse transcriptase inhibitors **efavirenz** and **nevirapine** have been introduced recently; they may interact with a number of drugs metabolised in the liver. Efavirenz and nevirapine are associated with a high incidence of rash (including Stevens-Johnson syndrome).

LIPODYSTROPHY AND METABOLIC EFFECTS The MCA has advised that combination antiretroviral therapy, including regimens containing a protease inhibitor, is associated with redistribution of body fat in some patients (e.g. decreased fat under the skin, increased abdominal fat, 'buffalo humps' and breast enlargement). Protease inhibitors are also associated with metabolic abnormalities such as hyperlipidaemia, insulin resistance, and hyperglycaemia. Clinical examination should include an evaluation of fat distribution; measurement of serum lipids and blood glucose should be considered.

Nucleoside reverse transcriptase inhibitors

ABACAVIR

Indications: HIV infection in combination with other antiretroviral drugs

Cautions: hepatic impairment (see below and Appendix 2); renal impairment (Appendix 3)

HYPERSENSITIVITY REACTION. Life-threatening hypersensitivity reactions reported—characterised by fever or rash with other symptoms including nausea, vomiting, diarrhoea, abdominal pain, lethargy, malaise, respiratory symptoms, musculoskeletal symptoms, headache, paraesthesia, oedema, mucous membrane lesions, lymphadenopathy, hypotension, renal failure and anaphylaxis; symptoms usually appear in first 6 weeks of treatment, but may occur at any time; monitor for symptoms every 2 weeks for first 2 months of treatment; discontinue immediately if symptoms of hypersensitivity develop and do not rechallenge; care needed with concomitant use of other drugs which cause skin toxicity. Patients should be told the importance of regular dosing (intermittent therapy may increase sensitisation), how to recognise signs of hypersensitivity, and advised to seek immediate medical attention if symptoms develop

HEPATIC DISEASE. Potentially life-threatening lactic acidosis and severe hepatomegaly with steatosis reported therefore caution in liver disease, liver enzyme abnormalities, or risk factors for liver disease (particularly in obese women); suspend or discontinue if deterioration in liver function tests, hepatic steatosis, progressive hepatomegaly or unexplained lactic acidosis

Contra-indications: pregnancy (Appendix 4); breast-feeding

Side-effects: hypersensitivity reactions (see above), nausea, vomiting, diarrhoea, anorexia lethargy, fatigue, fever, headache, lactic acidosis (see above)

Dose: 300 mg every 12 hours; CHILD safety and efficacy not established

Ziagen® (GlaxoWellcome) ▼ PoM
Tablets, yellow, f/c, abacavir (as sulphate) 300 mg, net price 60-tab pack = £238.50
Oral solution, sugar-free, banana and strawberry-flavoured, abacavir (as sulphate) 20 mg/ml, net price 240-mL = £63.60.

DIDANOSINE
(ddI, DDI)

Indications: HIV infection in combination with other antiretroviral drugs

Cautions: history of pancreatitis (extreme caution, see also below); peripheral neuropathy or hyperuricaemia (see under Side-effects); history of liver disease (see below); hepatic and renal impairment (see Appendixes 2 and 3); pregnancy; dilated retinal examinations recommended (especially in children) every 6 months, or if visual changes occur; **interactions:** Appendix 1 (didanosine)

PANCREATITIS. If symptoms of pancreatitis develop or if serum amylase or lipase is raised (even if asymptomatic) suspend treatment until diagnosis of pancreatitis excluded; on return to normal values re-initiate treatment only if essential (using low dose increased gradually if appropriate). Whenever possible avoid concomitant treatment with other drugs known to cause pancreatic toxicity (e.g. intravenous pentamidine isetionate); monitor closely if concomitant therapy unavoidable. Since significant elevations of triglycerides cause pancreatitis monitor closely if elevated

HEPATIC DISEASE. Potentially life-threatening lactic acidosis and severe hepatomegaly with steatosis reported therefore caution in liver disease, liver enzyme abnormalities, or risk factors for liver disease (particularly in obese women); suspend or discontinue if deterioration in liver function tests, hepatic steatosis, progressive hepatomegaly or unexplained lactic acidosis

Contra-indications: breast-feeding

Side-effects: pancreatitis (see also under Cautions); peripheral neuropathy especially in advanced HIV infection—suspend (reduced dose may be tolerated when symptoms resolve); hyperuricaemia (suspend treatment if significant elevation); diarrhoea (occasionally serious); also reported, nausea, vomiting, dry mouth, asthenia, headache, hypersensitivity reactions, retinal and optic nerve changes (especially in children), diabetes mellitus, raised liver function tests (see also under Cautions) liver failure

Dose: ADULT under 60 kg 250 mg daily in 1–2 divided doses, 60 kg and over 400 mg daily in 1–2 divided doses; CHILD over 3 months, 240 mg/m² daily (180 mg/m² daily in combination with zidovudine) in 1–2 divided doses

Videx® (Bristol-Myers) PoM
Tablets, both with calcium and magnesium antacids, didanosine 25 mg, net price 60-tab pack = £28.60; 100 mg, 60-tab pack = £88.00; 150 mg,

60-tab pack = £132.00. Label: 23, counselling, administration, see below

Excipients: include aspartame equivalent to phenylalanine 36.5 mg per tablet (section 9.4.1)

Note. Antacids in formulation may affect absorption of other drugs—see **interactions:** Appendix 1 (antacids and adsorbents)

COUNSELLING. To ensure sufficient antacid, each dose to be taken as 2 tablets (CHILD under 1 year 1 tablet) chewed thoroughly, crushed or dispersed in water; clear apple juice may be added for flavouring

LAMIVUDINE
(3TC)

Indications: see preparations below

Cautions: renal impairment (Appendix 3), hepatic disease (see below); pregnancy (Appendix 4); **interactions:** Appendix 1 (lamivudine)

HEPATIC DISEASE. Potentially life-threatening lactic acidosis and severe hepatomegaly with steatosis reported therefore caution in liver disease, liver enzyme abnormalities, or risk factors for liver disease; suspend or discontinue if deterioration in liver function tests, hepatic steatosis, progressive hepatomegaly or unexplained lactic acidosis. Recurrent hepatitis in patients with chronic hepatitis B may occur on discontinuation of lamivudine. When treating chronic hepatitis B with lamivudine, monitor liver function tests at least every 3 months and serological markers of hepatitis B every 6 months, more frequently in patients with advanced liver disease or following transplantation (monitoring to continue after discontinuation)—consult product literature

Contra-indications: breast-feeding

Side-effects: nausea, vomiting, diarrhoea, abdominal pain; cough; headache, insomnia; malaise, fever, rash, alopecia, musculoskeletal pain; nasal symptoms; peripheral neuropathy reported; rarely pancreatitis (discontinue); neutropenia and anaemia (in combination with zidovudine); thrombocytopenia; lactic acidosis; raised liver enzymes and serum amylase reported

Dose: see preparations below

Epivir® (GlaxoWellcome) ▼ PoM

Tablets, f/c, lamivudine 150 mg, net price 60-tab pack = £163.59

Oral solution, banana and strawberry-flavoured, lamivudine 50 mg/5 mL, net price 240-mL pack = £44.53

Excipients: include sucrose 1 g/5 mL

Dose: HIV infection in combination with other antiretroviral drugs, 150 mg every 12 hours; CHILD 3 months–12 years, 4 mg/kg every 12 hours; max. 300 mg daily

Zeffix® (GlaxoWellcome) ▼ PoM

Tablets, brown, f/c, lamivudine 100 mg, net price 28-tab pack = £76.34

Oral solution, banana and strawberry-flavoured, lamivudine 25 mg/5 mL, net price 240-mL pack = £22.27

Excipients: include sucrose 1 g/5 mL

Dose: chronic hepatitis B infection (with evidence of viral replication and decompensated liver disease or histologically documented active liver inflammation or fibrosis), ADULT over 16 years, 100 mg daily; patients receiving lamivudine for concomitant HIV infection should continue to receive lamivudine in a dose appropriate for HIV infection

■ With zidovudine
See under Zidovudine

STAVUDINE
(d4T)

Indications: progressive or advanced HIV infection, see notes above

Cautions: history of peripheral neuropathy (see below); history of pancreatitis or concomitant use with other drugs associated with pancreatitis; renal impairment (see Appendix 3); pregnancy; monitor liver enzymes (reduce dose if significant elevation); **interactions:** Appendix 1 (stavudine)

PERIPHERAL NEUROPATHY. Suspend if peripheral neuropathy develops—characterised by persistent numbness, tingling or pain in feet or hands; if symptoms resolve satisfactorily on withdrawal, resume treatment at half previous dose

LIVER ENZYMES. If liver enzymes raised significantly, manage as for peripheral neuropathy, above

Contra-indications: breast-feeding

Side-effects: peripheral neuropathy (dose-related, see above); pancreatitis; nausea, vomiting, diarrhoea, constipation, anorexia, abdominal discomfort; chest pain; dyspnoea; headache, dizziness, insomnia, mood changes; asthenia, musculoskeletal pain; influenza-like symptoms, rash and other allergic reactions; lymphadenopathy; neoplasms; elevated liver enzymes (see above) and serum amylase; neutropenia, thrombocytopenia

Dose: ADULT under 60 kg, 30 mg every 12 hours preferably at least 1 hour before food; 60 kg and over, 40 mg every 12 hours; CHILD over 3 months, under 30 kg, 1 mg/kg every 12 hours; 30 kg and over, adult dose

Zerit® (Bristol-Myers) ▼ PoM

Capsules, stavudine 15 mg (yellow/red), net price 56-cap pack = £153.87; 20 mg (brown), 56-cap pack = £159.19; 30 mg (light orange/dark orange), 56-cap pack = £166.94; 40 mg (dark orange), 56-cap pack = £171.98 (all hosp. only)

Oral solution, cherry-flavoured, stavudine for reconstitution with water, 1 mg/mL, net price 200 mL = £24.35

ZALCITABINE
(ddC, DDC)

Indications: HIV infection in combination with other antiretroviral drugs

Cautions: patients at risk of developing peripheral neuropathy (see below); pancreatitis (see also below)—monitor serum amylase in those with history of elevated serum amylase, pancreatitis, alcohol abuse, or receiving parenteral nutrition; cardiomyopathy, history of congestive cardiac failure; hepatotoxicity (see below); pregnancy (women of childbearing age should use effective contraception during treatment); renal impairment (Appendix 3); **interactions:** Appendix 1 (zalcitabine)

PERIPHERAL NEUROPATHY. Discontinue immediately if peripheral neuropathy develops—characterised by numbness and burning dysaesthesia possibly followed by sharp shooting pains or severe continuous burning and potentially irreversible pain; extreme caution and close monitoring required in those at risk of peripheral neuropathy (especially those with low CD4 cell count for whom risk is greater and those receiving another drug known to cause peripheral neuropathy)

PANCREATITIS. Discontinue permanently if clinical pancreatitis develops; suspend if raised serum amylase associated with dysglycaemia, rising triglyceride, decreasing serum calcium or other signs of impending pancreatitis until pancreatitis excluded; suspend if treatment required with another drug known to cause pancreatic toxicity (e.g. intravenous pentamidine isetionate); caution and close monitoring if history of pancreatitis (or of elevated serum amylase) or if at risk of pancreatitis

HEPATIC DISEASE. Potentially life-threatening lactic acidosis and severe hepatomegaly with steatosis reported therefore caution in liver disease, liver enzyme abnormalities, or history of alcohol abuse or hepatitis; suspend or discontinue if deterioration in liver function tests, hepatic steatosis, progressive hepatomegaly or unexplained lactic acidosis

Contra-indications: peripheral neuropathy (see also above); breast-feeding

Side-effects: peripheral neuropathy (discontinue immediately, see also above); oral ulcers, nausea, vomiting, dysphagia, anorexia, diarrhoea, abdominal pain, constipation; pharyngitis; headache, dizziness; myalgia, arthralgia; rash, pruritus, sweating, weight loss, fatigue, fever, rigors, chest pain, anaemia, leucopenia, neutropenia, thrombocytopenia, disorders of liver function; less frequently pancreatitis (see also above), oesophageal ulcers (suspend treatment if no response to treatment for specific organisms); rectal ulcers, jaundice and hepatocellular damage (see also under Cautions); other less frequent side-effects include taste, hearing and visual disturbances, tachycardia, cardiomyopathy, congestive heart failure, dyspnoea, seizures, tremor, movement disorders, mood changes, sleep disturbances, alopecia, hyperuricaemia and renal disorders

Dose: 750 micrograms every 8 hours; CHILD under 13 years safety and efficacy not established

---

Hivid® (Roche) ▼ PoM

Tablets, both f/c, zalcitabine 375 micrograms (beige), net price 100-tab pack = £99.51; 750 micrograms (grey), 100-tab pack = £151.57

ZIDOVUDINE

(Azidothymidine, AZT)

Note. The abbreviation AZT which has sometimes been used for zidovudine has also been used for another drug

Indications: HIV infection in combination with other antiretroviral drugs; monotherapy for prevention of maternal-fetal HIV transmission (by treating pregnant women and their newborn infants)

Cautions: haematological toxicity (blood tests at least every 2 weeks for first 3 months then at least once a month, early disease with good bone marrow reserves may require less frequent tests e.g. every 1–3 months); vitamin B_{12} deficiency (increased risk of neutropenia); reduce dose or interrupt treatment according to product literature if anaemia or myelosuppression; renal impairment (Appendix 3); hepatic impairment (see below and Appendix 2); risk of lactic acidosis, (see below); elderly; pregnancy; **interactions:** Appendix 1 (zidovudine)

HEPATIC DISEASE. Potentially life threatening lactic acidosis and severe hepatomegaly with steatosis reported therefore caution in liver disease, liver enzyme abnormalities, or risk factors for liver disease (particularly in obese women), suspend or discontinue if deterioration in liver function tests, hepatic steatosis, progressive hepatomegaly or unexplained lactic acidosis

Contra-indications: abnormally low neutrophil counts or haemoglobin values (consult product literature); neonates with hyperbilirubinaemia requiring treatment other than phototherapy, or with raised transaminase (consult product literature); breast-feeding

Side-effects: anaemia (may require transfusion), neutropenia, and leucopenia (all more frequent with high dose and advanced disease); also include, nausea and vomiting, anorexia, abdominal pain, dyspepsia, diarrhoea, flatulence, headache, rash, fever, myalgia, paraesthesia, neuropathy, dizziness, somnolence, insomnia, malaise, and asthenia; also reported, anxiety, depression, loss of mental acuity, convulsions (and other cerebral effects), myopathy, pigmentation of nail, skin and oral mucosa, pancytopenia (with bone marrow hypoplasia and rarely thrombocytopenia), liver disorders including fatty change and raised bilirubin and liver enzymes (see also under Cautions), dyspnoea, cough, urinary frequency, taste disturbance, chest pain, influenza-like symptoms, gynaecomastia, pancreatitis

Dose: *by mouth*, 500–600 mg daily in 2–3 divided doses (at least 1 g daily for treatment or prevention of HIV-associated neurological dysfunction); CHILD over 3 months 360–480 mg/m² daily in 3–4 divided doses; max. 200 mg every 6 hours; (at least 180 mg/m² every 6 hours for treatment or prevention of HIV-associated neurological dysfunction)

Prevention of maternal-fetal HIV transmission, women over 14 weeks gestation, *by mouth*, 100 mg 5 times daily until beginning of labour *then* during labour and delivery, *by intravenous infusion* initially 2 mg/kg over 1 hour *then* 1 mg/kg/hour until umbilical cord clamped (for planned caesarean section, start intravenous infusion 4 hours before operation); newborn INFANT starting within 12 hours of birth, *by mouth*, 2 mg/kg every 6 hours continued until 6 weeks old (or if unable to take by mouth, *by intravenous infusion* over 30 minutes, 1.5 mg/kg every 6 hours)

Patients temporarily unable to take zidovudine by mouth, *by intravenous infusion* over 1 hour, 1–2 mg/kg every 4 hours (approximating to 1.5–3 mg/kg every 4 hours by mouth) usually for not more than 2 weeks; CHILD 80–160 mg/m² every 6 hours (120 mg/m² every 6 hours approximates to 180 mg/m² every 6 hours by mouth)

Retrovir® (GlaxoWellcome) PoM

Capsules, zidovudine 100 mg (white/blue band), net price 100 = £119.33; 250 mg (blue/white/dark blue band), 40-cap pack = £119.33

Tablets, zidovudine 300 mg, net price 60 = £214.76

Syrup, sugar-free, strawberry-flavoured, zidovudine 50 mg/5 mL, net price 200-mL pack with 10-mL oral syringe = £23.87

Injection, zidovudine 10 mg/mL. For dilution and use as an intravenous infusion. Net price 20-mL vial = £11.98

■ With lamivudine

For cautions, contra-indications, and side-effects of lamivudine, see Lamivudine

Combivir® (GlaxoWellcome) ▼ PoM

Tablets, f/c, zidovudine 300 mg, lamivudine 150 mg, net price 60-tab pack = £342.58

Dose: 1 tablet twice daily

Protease inhibitors

INDINAVIR

Indications: HIV infection in combination with nucleoside reverse transcriptase inhibitors

Cautions: hepatic impairment (Appendix 2); ensure adequate hydration to reduce risk of nephrolithiasis; diabetes; haemophilia (possible increased bleeding); pregnancy; metabolism of many drugs inhibited if administered concomitantly, **interactions:** Appendix 1 (indinavir)

Contra-indications: breast-feeding

Side-effects: nausea, vomiting, diarrhoea, abdominal discomfort, dry mouth, taste disturbances; headache, dizziness, insomnia; myalgia, asthenia, paraesthesia; rash (including Stevens-Johnson syndrome), pruritus, dry skin, hyperpigmentation, alopecia; nephrolithiasis (may require interruption or discontinuation), dysuria, haematuria, crystalluria, proteinuria; elevated liver enzymes and bilirubin, hepatitis; blood disorders including neutropenia, haemolytic anaemia; lipodystrophy and metabolic effects, see notes above

Dose: 800 mg every 8 hours (600 mg every 8 hours if receiving concurrent ketoconazole *or* in hepatic impairment), CHILD safety and efficacy not established

Crixivan® (MSD) ▼ PoM

Capsules, indinavir (as sulphate), 200 mg net price 360-cap pack = £217.81; 400 mg 180-cap pack = £217.81. Counselling, administration

COUNSELLING. Administer 1 hour before or 2 hours after a meal; may be administered with a low-fat, light meal; in combination with didanosine, allow 1 hour between each drug (antacids in didanosine tablets reduce absorption of indinavir)

Note. Containers include desiccant canisters

NELFINAVIR

Indications: progressive or advanced HIV infection, in combination with nucleoside reverse transcriptase inhibitors

Cautions: hepatic and renal impairment; diabetes; haemophilia (possible increased bleeding); pregnancy; **interactions:** Appendix 1 (nelfinavir)

Contra-indications: breast-feeding

Side-effects: diarrhoea, nausea, flatulence; rash; reports of elevated creatine kinase, hepatitis, neutropenia, lipodystrophy and metabolic effects, see notes above

Dose: 750 mg 3 times daily; CHILD 2–13 years, initially 25–30 mg/kg 3 times daily, under 2 years safety and efficacy not established

Viracept® (Roche) ▼ PoM

Tablets, nelfinavir (as mesilate) 250 mg. Net price 270-tab pack = £289.23. Label: 21

Oral powder, nelfinavir (as mesilate) 50 mg/g. Net price 144 g (with 1-g scoop) = £30.88. Label: 21, counselling, administration

Excipients: include aspartame (section 9.4.1)

COUNSELLING. Powder may be mixed with water, milk, formula feeds or pudding; it should **not** be mixed with acidic foods or juices due to taste

RITONAVIR

Indications: progressive or advanced HIV infection in combination with nucleoside reverse transcriptase inhibitors

Cautions: hepatic impairment; diabetes; haemophilia (possible increased bleeding); pregnancy; metabolism of many drugs inhibited and toxicity increased if administered concomitantly, **interactions:** Appendix 1 (ritonavir)

PANCREATITIS. Signs and symptoms suggestive of pancreatitis (including raised serum amylase and lipase) should be evaluated—discontinue if pancreatitis diagnosed

Contra-indications: severe hepatic impairment; breast-feeding

Side-effects: nausea, vomiting, diarrhoea (may impair absorption—close monitoring required), abdominal pain, taste disturbances, dyspepsia, anorexia, throat irritation; vasodilatation; headache, circumoral and peripheral paraesthesia, hyperaesthesia, dizziness, sleep disturbances, asthenia, rash, leucopenia; raised liver enzymes, bilirubin, and uric acid; occasionally flatulence, eructation, dry mouth and ulceration, cough, anxiety, fever, pain, myalgia, weight loss, decreased thyroxine, sweating, pruritus, electrolyte disturbances, anaemia, neutropenia, increased prothrombin time; pancreatitis (see also under Cautions); lipodystrophy and metabolic effects, see notes above

Dose: 600 mg every 12 hours; CHILD over 2 years initially 250 mg/m² every 12 hours, increased by 50 mg/m² at intervals of 2–3 days to 350 mg/m² every 12 hours (max. 600 mg every 12 hours)

Norvir® (Abbott) ▼ PoM

Capsules, ritonavir 100 mg, net price 336-cap pack = £377.39. Label 21

Excipients: include alcohol 12%

Oral solution, sugar-free, ritonavir 400 mg/5 mL, net price 5 × 90-mL packs (with measuring cup) = £403.20. Label: 21, counselling, administration

COUNSELLING. Oral solution contains 43% alcohol; bitter taste can be masked by mixing with chocolate milk; do not mix with water, measuring cup must be dry

SAQUINAVIR

Indications: see preparations below

Cautions: hepatic impairment (Appendix 2); renal impairment (Appendix 3); diabetes; haemophilia (possible increased bleeding); pregnancy; **interactions:** Appendix 1 (saquinavir)

Contra-indications: severe hepatic impairment, breast-feeding

Side-effects: diarrhoea, buccal and mucosal ulceration, abdominal discomfort, nausea, vomiting; headache, peripheral neuropathy, paraesthesia, dizziness, musculoskeletal pain, asthenia; fever, pruritus, rash and other skin eruptions, rarely Stevens-Johnson syndrome; other rare side-effects include thrombocytopenia and other blood disorders, seizures, liver damage, pancreatitis and nephrolithiasis; reports of elevated creatine kinase, raised liver enzymes and neutropenia when used in combination therapy; lipodystrophy and metabolic effects, see notes above

Dose: see preparations below

Note. To avoid confusion between the different formulations of saquinavir, prescribers should specify the brand to be dispensed

Fortovase® (Roche) ▼ PoM

Capsules (gel-filled), beige, saquinavir 200 mg, net price 180-cap pack = £99.33. Label: 21

Dose: HIV infection in combination with other antiretroviral drugs, 1.2 g every 8 hours (within 2 hours after a meal); CHILD under 16 years, safety and efficacy not established

Invirase® (Roche) ▼ PoM

Capsules, brown/green, saquinavir (as mesilate) 200 mg, net price 270-cap pack = £289.23. Label: 21

Dose: HIV infection in combination with nucleoside reverse transcriptase inhibitors, 600 mg every 8 hours (within 2 hours after a meal); CHILD under 16 years, safety and efficacy not established

Non-nucleoside reverse transcriptase inhibitors

EFAVIRENZ

Indications: HIV infection in combination with other antiretroviral drugs

Cautions: hepatic impairment (avoid if severe; Appendix 2); severe renal impairment; pregnancy; elderly; **interactions:** Appendix 1 (efavirenz)

RASH. Rash, usually occurring in the first 2 weeks, is the most severe side-effect; discontinue if severe rash with blistering, desquamation, mucosal involvement or fever; if rash mild or moderate may continue without interruption—rash usually resolves within 1 month

Contra-indications: breast-feeding

Side-effects: rash including Stevens-Johnson syndrome (see also above); dizziness, headache, insomnia, somnolence, abnormal dreams, fatigue, impaired concentration, depression, psychosis (administration at bedtime especially in the first 2–4 weeks reduces CNS effects); nausea; raised plasma triglycerides and cholesterol, elevated liver enzymes (especially if seropositive for hepatitis B or C); diarrhoea, pancreatitis reported

Dose: 600 mg once daily; CHILD over 3 years, body-weight 13–14 kg, 200 mg once daily; body-weight 15–19 kg, 250 mg once daily; body-weight 20–24 kg, 300 mg once daily; body-weight 25–32.5 kg, 350 mg once daily; body-weight 32.5–39 kg, 400 mg once daily; body-weight 40 kg and over, adult dose

Sustiva (Du Pont) ▼ PoM

Capsules, efavirenz 50 mg (yellow/white), net price 30-cap pack = £19.60; 100 mg (white), 30-cap pack = £39.15; 200 mg (yellow), 90-cap pack = £224.09

NEVIRAPINE

Indications: progressive or advanced HIV infection, in combination with at least two other antiretroviral drugs

Cautions: hepatic impairment (see below and Appendix 2); renal impairment; pregnancy; **interactions:** Appendix 1 (nevirapine)

HEPATIC DISEASE. Potentially life threatening hepatotoxicity including fatal fulminant hepatitis reported; monitor liver function before treatment and for at least 6 months during treatment; suspend if moderate or severe abnormalities in liver function tests; discontinue permanently if moderate or severe abnormalities recur

Note. If treatment interrupted for more than 7 days reintroduce with 200 mg daily (CHILD 4 mg/kg daily) and increase dose cautiously

RASH. Rash, usually occurring in first 6 weeks, is most common side-effect; incidence reduced if introduced at low dose and dose increased gradually; discontinue permanently if severe rash or if rash accompanied by fever, pruritus, blistering, oral lesions, conjunctivitis, swelling, muscle or joint aches, general malaise or clinically significant liver function test abnormality; if rash mild or moderate may continue without interruption but dose should not be increased until rash resolves

Contra-indications: breast-feeding

Side-effects: rash including Stevens-Johnson syndrome and rarely, toxic epidermal necrolysis (see also above); hepatitis or jaundice reported (see also Cautions); nausea, vomiting, abdominal pain, diarrhoea, headache, drowsiness, fatigue, fever; myalgia; also reported hypersensitivity reactions (including anaphylaxis, angioedema, urticaria), eosinophilia, leucopenia, renal dysfunction

Dose: 200 mg daily for first 14 days then (if no rash present) 200 mg twice daily; CHILD 2 months–8 years, 4 mg/kg daily for first 14 days then (if no rash present) 7 mg/kg twice daily (max. 400 mg daily); 8–16 years, 4 mg/kg daily for first 14 days then (if no rash present) 4 mg/kg twice daily (max. 400 mg daily)

Viramune® (Boehringer Ingelheim) ▼ PoM

Tablets, nevirapine 200 mg, net price 60-tab pack = £168.00

Suspension, nevirapine 50 mg/5 mL, net price 240-mL pack = £50.40

Cytomegalovirus (CMV)

Ganciclovir is related to aciclovir but is more active against cytomegalovirus; it is also much more toxic than aciclovir and should therefore only be prescribed when the potential benefit outweighs the risks. Ganciclovir is administered by intravenous infusion; slow-release ocular implants (*Vitrasert®*, available from Bausch & Lomb) may also be inserted surgically to treat immediate sight-threatening CMV retinitis but they do not protect against systemic infection or infection in the other eye. Capsules are available for *maintenance treatment* of CMV retinitis in AIDS patients following intravenous therapy if the condition is stable. Ganciclovir causes profound myelosuppression when given with zidovudine; the two should not normally be given together particularly during initial ganciclovir therapy.

Foscarnet is also active against cytomegalovirus; it is toxic and can cause renal impairment.

Cidofovir is a DNA polymerase chain inhibitor which is given for CMV retinitis in AIDS patients when ganciclovir and foscarnet are contra-indicated; it is given in combination with probenecid. It is nephrotoxic.

CIDOFOVIR

Indications: cytomegalovirus retinitis in AIDS patients for whom other drugs are inappropriate

Cautions: monitor renal function (serum creatinine and urinary protein) and neutrophil count within 24 hours before each dose; co-treatment with probenecid and prior hydration with intravenous fluids necessary to minimise potential nephrotoxicity (see below); diabetes mellitus (increased risk of ocular hypotony)

NEPHROTOXICITY. Do not initiate treatment in renal impairment (assess creatinine clearance and proteinuria—consult product literature); discontinue treatment and hydrate with intravenous fluids if deterioration of renal function occurs—consult product literature

OCULAR DISORDERS. Regular ophthalmological examinations recommended; iritis and uveitis have been reported which may respond to a topical corticosteroid with or without a cycloplegic drug—discontinue cidofovir if no response to topical corticosteroid or if condition worsens, or if iritis or uveitis recurs after successful treatment

Contra-indications: renal impairment (creatinine clearance 55 mL/minute or less); concomitant administration of potentially nephrotoxic drugs (discontinue potentially nephrotoxic drugs at least 7 days before starting cidofovir); pregnancy (avoid pregnancy during and for 1 month after treatment, men should not father a child during or within 3 months of treatment), breast-feeding

Side-effects: dose-dependent nephrotoxicity (see Cautions above); neutropenia, fever, asthenia, alopecia, nausea, vomiting, decreased intra-ocular pressure, iritis, uveitis (see Cautions above); for side-effects related to probenecid see section 10.1.4

Dose: *by intravenous infusion* over 1 hour, initial (induction) treatment, 5 mg/kg once weekly for 2 weeks (give probenecid and intravenous fluids with each dose, see below); CHILD not recommended

Maintenance treatment, beginning 2 weeks after completion of induction, *by intravenous infusion* over 1 hour, 5 mg/kg once every 2 weeks (give probenecid and intravenous fluids with each dose, see below)

PROBENECID CO-TREATMENT, *by mouth* (preferably after food), probenecid 2 g 3 hours before cidofovir infusion followed by probenecid 1 g at 2 hours and 1 g at 8 hours after the end of cidofovir infusion (total probenecid 4 g); for cautions, contra-indications and side-effects of probenecid see section 10.1.4

PRIOR HYDRATION, sodium chloride 0.9%, *by intravenous infusion*, 1 litre over 1 hour immediately before cidofovir infusion (if tolerated an additional 1 litre may be given over 1–3 hours, starting at the same time as the cidofovir infusion or immediately afterwards

Vistide® (Pharmacia & Upjohn) ▼ PoM
Intravenous infusion, cidofovir 75 mg/mL, net price 5-mL vial = £570.00
CAUTION IN HANDLING. Wear gloves and safety glasses and prepare infusion in a laminar flow biological safety cabinet; if solution comes into contact with skin or mucosa immediately wash with water

GANCICLOVIR

Indications: life-threatening or sight-threatening cytomegalovirus infections in immunocompromised patients only; prevention of cytomegalovirus disease during immunosuppressive therapy following organ transplantation

Cautions: close monitoring of blood counts (consult product literature); history of cytopenia; low platelet count; concomitant use of myelosuppressants or drugs which inhibit rapid cell replication; potential carcinogen and teratogen; renal impairment (consult product literature); ensure adequate hydration during administration; vesicant—infuse into vein with adequate flow preferably via a plastic cannula; limited experience in children (possible risk of long-term carcinogenic or reproductive toxicity—not for neonatal or congenital cytomegalovirus disease); **interactions:** see notes above and Appendix 1 (ganciclovir)

Contra-indications: pregnancy (includes effective contraception during treatment and barrier contraception for men during and for 90 days after treatment); breast-feeding (until 72 hours after last dose); hypersensitivity to ganciclovir or aciclovir; abnormally low neutrophil or platelet counts (see product literature)

Side-effects: most frequent, leucopenia and thrombocytopenia; less frequent, anaemia, pancytopenia, fever, rash, abnormal liver function tests; also chills, oedema, infections, malaise; nausea, vomiting, mouth ulcers, dyspepsia, dysphagia, diarrhoea, anorexia, gastro-intestinal haemorrhage, abdominal pain; chest pain, arrhythmias, hypertension, hypotension, deep thrombophlebitis, migraine, vasodilation; dyspnoea; psychosis, confusion, mood disturbances, nervousness, dry mouth, drowsiness, dizziness, abnormal gait, ataxia, paraesthesia, tremor, headache, coma; eosinophilia; decrease in blood glucose; haematuria, raised serum creatinine and blood urea nitrogen; breast pain, urinary frequency, urinary-tract infection, aspermatogenesis; myasthenia, myalgia; disturbances in taste and vision, eye pain, deafness; retinal detachment in AIDS patients with retinitis; alopecia, acne, sweating, rash, pruritus, urticaria; local inflammation, pain and phlebitis at injection site

Dose: *by intravenous infusion*, initial (induction) treatment, 5 mg/kg every 12 hours for 14–21 days for treatment or for 7–14 days for prevention; maintenance (for patients at risk of relapse of retinitis) 6 mg/kg daily on 5 days per week *or* 5 mg/kg daily every day; if retinitis progresses initial induction treatment may be repeated

Maintenance treatment in AIDS patients where retinitis stable (following at least 3 weeks of intravenous ganciclovir), *by mouth*, 1 g 3 times daily with food *or* 500 mg 6 times daily with food

Cymevene® (Roche) PoM
Capsules, green, ganciclovir 250 mg, net price 84-cap pack = £253.70. Label: 21

Intravenous infusion, powder for reconstitution, ganciclovir (as sodium salt). Net price 500-mg vial = £33.98

Electrolytes: Na⁺ 2 mmol/500-mg vial

CAUTION IN HANDLING. Wear gloves and safety glasses when reconstituting; if solution contacts skin or mucosa immediately wash with soap and water

FOSCARNET SODIUM

Indications: cytomegalovirus retinitis in AIDS patients; mucocutaneous herpes simplex virus infections unresponsive to aciclovir in immunocompromised patients

Cautions: renal impairment (reduce dose or avoid if severe); monitor electrolytes, particularly calcium and magnesium; monitor serum creatinine every second day during induction and every week during maintenance; ensure adequate hydration; avoid rapid infusion

Contra-indications: pregnancy, breast-feeding

Side-effects: nausea, vomiting, diarrhoea (occasionally constipation and dyspepsia), abdominal pain, anorexia; changes in blood pressure and ECG; headache, fatigue, mood disturbances (including psychosis), asthenia, paraesthesia, convulsions, tremor, dizziness, and other neurological disorders; rash; impairment of renal function including acute renal failure; hypocalcaemia (sometimes symptomatic) and other electrolyte disturbances; abnormal liver function tests; decreased haemoglobin concentration, leucopenia, granulocytopenia, thrombocytopenia; thrombophlebitis if given undiluted by peripheral vein; genital irritation and ulceration (due to high concentrations excreted in urine); isolated reports of pancreatitis

Dose: CMV retinitis induction, *by intravenous infusion*, 60 mg/kg every 8 hours for 2–3 weeks then maintenance, 60 mg/kg daily, increased to 90–120 mg/kg if tolerated; if retinitis progresses on maintenance dose, repeat induction regimen
Mucocutaneous herpes simplex infection, *by intravenous infusion*, 40 mg/kg every 8 hours for 2–3 weeks or until lesions heal

Foscavir® (Astra) [PoM]
Intravenous infusion, foscarnet sodium hexahydrate 24 mg/mL, net price 250-mL bottle = £31.35, 500-mL bottle = £52.24

Viral hepatitis

The management of uncomplicated acute viral hepatitis is largely symptomatic. Hepatitis B and hepatitis C viruses are major causes of chronic hepatitis.

CHRONIC HEPATITIS B. **Interferon alfa** (section 8.2.4) is used in the treatment of chronic hepatitis B but its use is limited by a response rate of less than 50%, and relapse is frequent. If no improvement occurs after 3–4 months of treatment, interferon alfa should be discontinued. Interferon alfa is contra-indicated in patients with decompensated liver disease and in those receiving immunosuppressant treatment (or who have received it recently).

Lamivudine (see p. 291) has been licensed recently for the treatment of chronic hepatitis B. Unlike interferon alfa, lamivudine can be used in patients with decompensated liver disease. Treatment should be continued if there is no loss of efficacy and until adequate seroconversion is achieved (consult product literature); it is continued long-term in decompensated liver disease. Hepatitis B viruses with reduced susceptibility to lamivudine have emerged following

extended therapy. In patients with HIV infection not requiring anti-retroviral therapy, the use of lamivudine alone for chronic hepatitis B may give rise to lamivudine-resistant HIV.

CHRONIC HEPATITIS C. **Tribavirin** (*Rebetol®*, see p. 297) can be used in combination with **interferon alfa-2b** (section 8.2.4) for the treatment of chronic hepatitis C; tribavirin monotherapy is ineffective. The combination should usually be continued for 24 weeks but in some cases it may be necessary to extend treatment by a further 24 weeks (consult product literature).

Monotherapy with interferon alfa has also been used in the treatment of hepatitis C but it is less effective and relapse is more common.

Influenza

Amantadine may be used for prophylaxis during an outbreak of influenza A **only** in:

- unimmunised patients in 'at risk' groups (see under Influenza vaccine, section 14.4), for 2 weeks while the vaccine takes effect

- patients in 'at risk' groups for whom immunisation is contra-indicated, for the duration of the outbreak

- health care workers and other key personnel (to prevent disruption of service), during an epidemic

The Joint Committee on Vaccination and Immunisation has advised that amantadine should not be used for both prophylaxis and treatment of influenza in the same household (risk of resistance). Amantadine has also been used by mouth for herpes zoster, but its effectiveness has not been established.

Zanamivir is licensed for the treatment of influenza A or B within 48 hours after the onset of symptoms. In otherwise healthy individuals it reduces the duration of symptoms by about 1 day. There is currently little information about the benefit of zanamivir in preventing complications in high-risk patients (such as the elderly, the immunosuppressed and those with cardiovascular disease, asthma, or chronic obstructive pulmonary disease); in these patients immunisation with influenza vaccine is recommended (section 14.4).

AMANTADINE HYDROCHLORIDE

Indications: see under Dose; parkinsonism (section 4.9.1)

Cautions; Contra-indications; Side-effects: see section 4.9.1

Dose: herpes zoster (but see notes above), 100 mg twice daily for 14 days, if necessary extended for a further 14 days for post-herpetic pain
Influenza A (see also notes above), ADULT and CHILD over 10 years, treatment, 100 mg daily for 4–5 days; prophylaxis, 100 mg daily usually for 6 weeks *or* with influenza vaccination for 2–3 weeks after vaccination
ELDERLY 100 mg daily

Preparations
Section 4.9.1

ZANAMIVIR

Indications: treatment of influenza A or B within 48 hours after onset of symptoms when influenza is endemic in the community

Cautions: elderly; asthma and chronic pulmonary disease (risk of bronchospasm—fast acting bronchodilator should be available); immunocompromised patients, uncontrolled chronic illness; other inhaled drugs should be administered before zanamivir; pregnancy (Appendix 4)

Contra-indications: breast-feeding

Side-effects: gastro-intestinal disturbances; reported rarely, bronchospasm, respiratory impairment, and rash

Dose: *by inhalation of powder*, 10 mg twice daily for 5 days, CHILD under 12 years not recommended

Relenza® (GlaxoWellcome) ▼ PoM
Dry powder for inhalation, disks containing 4 blisters of zanamivir 5 mg/blister, net price 5 disks with *Diskhaler®* device = £24.00
NICE advice. The National Institute for Clinical Excellence has advised that zanamivir should not be prescribed during the 1999-2000 influenza season. New guidance will be offered for the 2000–2001 influenza season following further appraisal

Respiratory syncytial virus

Tribavirin inhibits a wide range of DNA and RNA viruses. It is given by inhalation for the treatment of severe bronchiolitis caused by the respiratory syncytial virus (RSV) in infants, especially when they have other serious diseases. Tribavirin is given by mouth with interferon alfa-2b for the treatment of chronic hepatitis C infection (see Viral Hepatitis, p. 296). It is also effective in Lassa fever.

Palivizumab is a monoclonal antibody indicated for the prevention of respiratory syncytial virus infection in infants at high risk of infection. It is licensed for monthly use during the RSV season; the first dose should be administered before the start of the RSV season.

PALIVIZUMAB

Indications: prevention of serious lower respiratory-tract infection caused by respiratory syncytial virus (RSV) requiring hospitalisation in children born at 35 weeks gestation or less and who are less than 6 months old at onset of RSV season, or in children less than 2 years old who have received treatment for bronchopulmonary dysplasia within the last 6 months

Cautions: moderate to severe acute infection or febrile illness; congenital heart disease; thrombocytopenia; facilities for cardiopulmonary resuscitation must be at hand

Contra-indications: hypersensitivity to humanised monoclonal antibodies

Side-effects: fever, injection site reactions, nervousness; less frequently diarrhoea, vomiting, rhinitis, cough, wheeze, pain, rash, leucopenia, abnormal liver function tests

Dose: *by intramuscular injection* (preferably in anterolateral thigh), 15 mg/kg once a month during season of RSV risk; injection volume over 1 mL should be given as a divided dose

Synagis® (Abbott) ▼ PoM
Injection, powder for reconstitution, palivizumab, net price 50-mg vial = £424.00; 100-mg vial = £706.00

TRIBAVIRIN

(Ribavirin)

Indications: severe respiratory syncytial virus bronchiolitis in infants and children; in combination with interferon alfa-2b for chronic hepatitis C not previously treated in patients without liver decompensation and who have fibrosis or high inflammatory activity or for relapse following previous response to interferon alfa

Cautions:

SPECIFIC CAUTIONS FOR INHALED TREATMENT. Maintain standard supportive respiratory and fluid management therapy; monitor electrolytes closely; monitor equipment for precipitation; pregnant women (and those planning pregnancy) should avoid exposure to aerosol

SPECIFIC CAUTIONS FOR ORAL TREATMENT. Exclude pregnancy before treatment; effective contraception essential during treatment and for 4 months after treatment in women and for 7 months after treatment in men; routine monthly pregnancy tests recommended; condoms must be used if partner of male patient is pregnant (tribavirin excreted in semen); cardiac disease (assessment including ECG recommended before and during treatment—discontinue if deterioration occurs); gout; determine full blood count, platelets, electrolytes, serum creatinine, liver function tests and uric acid before starting treatment and then on weeks 2 and 4 of treatment, then as indicated clinically—adjust dose if adverse reactions or laboratory abnormalities develop (consult product literature)

Contra-indications: pregnancy (**important teratogenic risk**: see Cautions and Appendix 4); breast-feeding

SPECIFIC CONTRA-INDICATIONS FOR ORAL TREATMENT. Severe cardiac disease, including unstable or uncontrolled cardiac disease in previous 6 months; haemoglobinopathies; severe debilitating medical conditions; renal impairment (Appendix 3); severe hepatic dysfunction or decompensated cirrhosis (Appendix 2); autoimmune disease (including autoimmune hepatitis); history of severe psychiatric condition; uncontrolled thyroid disease

Side-effects:

SPECIFIC SIDE-EFFECTS FOR INHALED TREATMENT. Worsening respiration, bacterial pneumonia, and pneumothorax reported; rarely non-specific anaemia and haemolysis

SPECIFIC SIDE-EFFECTS FOR ORAL TREATMENT. Haemolytic anaemia, reticulocytosis; also reported (in combination with interferon alfa-2b) nausea, vomiting, anorexia, abdominal pain, diarrhoea; chest pain; dyspnoea, rhinitis, pharyngitis; sleep disturbances, irritability, anxiety, depression, dizziness, myalgia, arthralgia, paraesthesia, influenza-like symptoms, headache; thyroid disorders, hyperuricaemia; rash, pruritus, alopecia, dry skin, taste disturbance, blurred vision; leucopenia, thrombocytopenia

Dose: Bronchiolitis, *by aerosol inhalation or nebulisation* (via small particle aerosol generator) of solution containing 20 mg/mL for 12–18 hours for at least 3 days; max. 7 days
Chronic hepatitis C, *by mouth*, ADULT over 18 years, 75 kg or less, 400 mg in the morning and 600 mg in the evening, over 75 kg 600 mg in the morning and 600 mg in the evening

Rebetol® (Schering-Plough) ▼ PoM
Capsules, tribavirin 200 mg, net price 84-cap pack = £296.40, 140-cap pack = £494.00, 168-cap pack = £592.80. Label 21

Virazole® (ICN) [PoM]

Inhalation, tribavirin 6 g for reconstitution with 300 mL water for injections. Net price 3 × 6-g vials = £349.00

Note. The brand name *Virazid®* was used formerly for tribavirin inhalation

5.4 Antiprotozoal drugs

5.4.1	Antimalarials
5.4.2	Amoebicides
5.4.3	Trichomonacides
5.4.4	Antigiardial drugs
5.4.5	Leishmaniacides
5.4.6	Trypanocides
5.4.7	Drugs for toxoplasmosis
5.4.8	Drugs for pneumocystis pneumonia

Advice on specific problems available from:

Malaria Reference
Laboratory	
Birmingham	(020) 7927 2437 (prophylaxis only)
	0121-766 6611
Glasgow	0141-300 1130
Liverpool	0151-708 9393
London	(020) 7387 4411 (treatment)
	(020) 8388 9600 (travel prophylaxis)
	(020) 8200 6868 extn 3421 (travel prophylaxis)
Oxford	(01865) 225217

Recorded advice
for Travellers   0891 600350
(49p/minute standard rate, 39p/minute cheap rate)

5.4.1 Antimalarials

Recommendations on the prophylaxis and treatment of malaria reflect guidelines agreed by UK malaria specialists.

The centres listed above should be consulted for advice on special problems.

Treatment of malaria

If the infective species is **not known**, or if the infection is **mixed**, initial treatment should be with quinine or mefloquine or *Malarone®* (or rarely with halofantrine) as for *falciparum malaria*.

Falciparum malaria (treatment)

Falciparum malaria (malignant malaria) is caused by *Plasmodium falciparum*. In most parts of the world *P. falciparum* is now resistant to chloroquine which should not therefore be given for treatment[1].

Quinine, **mefloquine**, *Malarone®* (proguanil with atovaquone) or **halofantrine** can be given *by mouth* if the patient can swallow tablets and there are no serious manifestations (e.g. impaired consciousness); quinine should be given *by intravenous infusion* (see below) if the patient is seriously ill or unable to take tablets. Specialist advice should be sought in difficult cases since other drugs such as **artesunate** (given intravenously) and **artemether** (given intramuscularly) may be available for 'named-patient use'.

Oral. The adult dosage regimen for **quinine** *by mouth* is:

600 mg (of quinine salt[2]) every 8 hours for 7 days *and* (if quinine resistance known or suspected) *followed by*
either **Fansidar®** 3 tablets as a single dose
or (if *Fansidar®*-resistant) **doxycycline** 200 mg daily for at least 7 days.

Alternatively **mefloquine**, *Malarone®* (or **halofantrine** but now rarely used—see warnings on p. 303) may be given instead of quinine but resistance has been reported in several countries. It is not necessary to give *Fansidar®* or doxycycline after mefloquine, *Malarone®*, or halofantrine treatment. The adult dosage regimen for **mefloquine** *by mouth* is:

20–25 mg/kg (of mefloquine base) as a single dose (up to maximum 1.5 g) *or preferably* as 2–3 divided doses 6–8 hours apart.

Malarone® (atovaquone and proguanil hydrochloride) has been introduced recently; the adult dose *by mouth* is:

4 tablets once daily for 3 days.

Halofantrine is now rarely used (see warnings on p. 303); the adult dosage regimen *by mouth* is:

1.5 g of halofantrine hydrochloride divided into 3 doses of 500 mg given at intervals of 6 hours (on an empty stomach); this course should be repeated after an interval of 1 week.

Parenteral. If the patient is seriously ill, **quinine** should be given *by intravenous infusion*. The adult dosage regimen for quinine *by infusion* is:

loading dose[3] of 20 mg/kg[4] (up to maximum 1.4 g) of quinine salt[2] infused over 4 hours *then after 8–12 hours* maintenance dose of 10 mg/kg[5] (up to maximum 700 mg) of quinine salt[2] infused over 4 hours every 8–12 hours (until patient can swallow tablets to complete the 7-day course) *followed by* either *Fansidar®* or doxycycline as above. Alternatively, after at least 2–3 days' treatment with a parenteral quinine salt, treatment may be completed with mefloquine by mouth started at least 12 hours after parenteral quinine salt has been administered.

CHILDREN.
Oral. **Quinine** is well tolerated by children although the salts are bitter. The dosage regimen for quinine *by mouth* for children is:

10 mg/kg (of quinine salt[2]) every 8 hours for 7 days *then* (if quinine resistance known or suspected) *Fansidar®* as a single dose: up to 4 years ½ tablet, 5–6 years 1 tablet, 7–9 years 1½ tablets, 10–14 years 2 tablets.

Alternatively **mefloquine** or *Malarone®* (or **halofantrine** but now rarely used—see warnings on p. 303) may be given instead of quinine; it is not necessary to give *Fansidar®* after mefloquine or halofantrine treatment. The dosage regimen for mefloquine *by mouth* for children is calculated on a mg/kg basis as for adults (see above). The dosage regimen for *Malarone®* *by mouth* for children over 40 kg is the same as for adults (see above); the dosage regimen for *Malarone®* for smaller children is reduced as follows:

weight under 11 kg, no suitable dose form
weight 11–20 kg, 1 tablet daily for 3 days
weight 21–30 kg, 2 tablets daily for 3 days
weight 31–40 kg, 3 tablets daily for 3 days.

Footnotes—*see next page*

The dosage regimen for halofantrine *by mouth* (**important:** see warnings on p. 303) for children over 37 kg is the same as for adults (see above); the dosage regimen for halofantrine for smaller children is reduced as follows:

    weight under 23 kg, no suitable dose form;
    weight 23–31 kg, 250 mg every 6 hours for 3 doses;
    weight 32–37 kg, 375 mg every 6 hours for 3 doses.

This course of halofantrine should be repeated after an interval of 1 week.

Parenteral. The dosage regimen for quinine *by intravenous infusion* for children is calculated on a mg/kg basis as for adults (see above).

PREGNANCY. Falciparum malaria is particularly dangerous in pregnancy, especially in the last trimester. The adult treatment doses of oral and intravenous quinine given above (including the loading dose) can safely be given to pregnant women. Halofantrine is contra-indicated in pregnancy and doxycycline should be avoided (causes dental discoloration); *Fansidar*® and mefloquine are also best avoided until more information is available.

Benign malarias (treatment)

Benign malaria is usually caused by *Plasmodium vivax* and less commonly by *P. ovale* and *P. malariae.* **Chloroquine**[6] is the drug of choice for the treatment of benign malarias (but chloroquine-resistant *P. vivax* infection has been reported from New Guinea and some adjacent islands).

The adult dosage regimen for **chloroquine** *by mouth* is:

    initial dose of 600 mg (of base) *then*
    a single dose of 300 mg after 6 to 8 hours *then*
    a single dose of 300 mg daily for 2 days
    (approximate total cumulative dose of 25 mg/kg of base)

Chloroquine alone is adequate for *P. malariae* infections but in the case of *P. vivax* and *P. ovale,* a *radical cure* (to destroy parasites in the liver and thus prevent relapses) is required. This is achieved with **primaquine**[7] in an adult dosage of 15 mg daily for 14 to 21 days given after the chloroquine; a 21-day (or even longer) course may be needed for Chesson-type strains of *P. vivax* from south-east Asia and western Pacific.

CHILDREN. The dosage regimen of chloroquine for benign malaria in children is:

    initial dose of 10 mg/kg (of base) *then*
    a single dose of 5 mg/kg after 6–8 hours *then*
    a single dose of 5 mg/kg daily for 2 days

For a *radical cure* children are then given primaquine[7] in a dose of 250 micrograms/kg daily.

PREGNANCY. The adult treatment doses of chloroquine can be given for benign malaria. In the case of *P. vivax* or *P. ovale,* however, the radical cure with primaquine should be **postponed** until the pregnancy is over; instead chloroquine should be continued at a dose of 600 mg each week during the pregnancy.

Prophylaxis against malaria

The recommendations on prophylaxis reflect guidelines agreed by UK malaria specialists; the advice is aimed at residents of the UK who travel to endemic areas. The choice of drug (see next page) takes account of:

    risk of exposure to malaria;
    extent of drug resistance;
    efficacy of the recommended drugs;
    side-effects of the drugs;
    patient-related criteria (e.g. age, pregnancy, renal or hepatic impairment).

PROTECTION AGAINST BITES. **Prophylaxis is relative and not absolute**, and breakthrough can occur with any of the drugs recommended. Personal protection against being bitten is very important. Mosquito nets impregnated with permethrin provide the most effective barrier protection against insects; coils, mats and vaporised insecticides are also useful. Diethyltoluamide (DEET) in lotions, sprays or roll-on formulations is safe and effective when applied to the skin but the protective effect only lasts for a few hours. Long sleeves and trousers worn after dusk also provide protection.

---

1. For chloroquine-sensitive strains of falciparum malaria chloroquine is effective *by mouth* in the dosage schedule outlined under benign malarias but it should **not** be used unless there is an **unambiguous exposure history** in one of the few remaining areas of chloroquine sensitivity.
    If the patient with a *chloroquine-sensitive infection* is seriously ill, chloroquine is given *by continuous intravenous infusion*. The dosage (for adults and children) is chloroquine 10 mg/kg (of base) infused over 8 hours, followed by three 8-hour infusions of 5 mg/kg (of base) each. *Oral therapy* is started as soon as possible to complete the course; the total cumulative dose for the course should be 25 mg/kg of base.

2. Valid for quinine hydrochloride, dihydrochloride, and sulphate; not valid for quinine bisulphate which contains a correspondingly smaller amount of quinine.

3. In intensive care units the loading dose can alternatively be given as quinine salt[2] 7 mg/kg infused over 30 minutes followed immediately by 10 mg/kg over 4 hours then (after 8 hours) maintenance dose as described.

4. **Important:** the loading dose of 20 mg/kg should **not** be used if the patient has received quinine (or quinidine) or mefloquine during the previous 24 hours—**for additional warnings** relating to halofantrine, see p. 303

5. Maintenance dose should be reduced to 5–7 mg/kg of salt if parenteral treatment is required for more than 48 hours.

6. Mefloquine is also active in benign malarias (but is not required since chloroquine is usually effective); as with chloroquine a radical cure is required for *P. vivax* and *P. ovale* infections; halofantrine is active against *P. vivax* but is not generally used.

7. Before starting primaquine blood should be tested for glucose-6-phosphate dehydrogenase (G6PD) activity since the drug can cause haemolysis in G6PD-deficient patients. In G6PD deficiency primaquine, in a dose for adults of 30 mg once a week (children 500–750 micrograms/kg once a week) for 8 weeks, has been found useful and without undue harmful effects.

LENGTH OF PROPHYLAXIS. In order to determine tolerance and to establish habit, prophylaxis should be started one week (preferably 2–3 weeks in the case of mefloquine) before travel into an endemic area (or if not possible at earliest opportunity up to 1 or 2 days before travel); it should be continued for **at least 4 weeks after leaving**.

In those requiring long-term prophylaxis, chloroquine and proguanil may be used for periods of over 5 years. Mefloquine is licenced for up to 1 year (although it has been used for up to 2 years without undue problems). Specialist advice should be sought for long-term prophylaxis and especially for travel to areas where chloroquine, proguanil or mefloquine are inappropriate.

RETURN FROM MALARIAL REGION. It is important to be aware that **any illness** that occurs within 1 year and **especially within 3 months of return might be malaria** even if all recommended precautions against malaria were taken. Travellers should be **warned** of this and told that if they develop any illness **particularly within 3 months** of their return they should go **immediately** to a doctor and specifically mention their exposure to malaria.

CHILDREN. The following prophylactic doses are based on guidelines agreed by UK malaria experts and may differ from advice in data sheets. If in doubt telephone centres listed on p. 298.

| Age | Weight (kg) | Percentage of adult dose | |
		Chloroquine Proguanil	Maloprim®
0–5 weeks		12.5%	—
6 weeks–11 months		25%	—
1–5 years	10–19	50%	25%
6–11 years	20–39	75%	50%
12 years	40	adult dose	adult dose

Note. Weight is a better guide than age for children over 6 months old. Specialist advice should be obtained for use of *Maloprim®* in children under 1 year of age.
For children's doses of mefloquine see p. 304.
Prophylaxis is required in **breast-fed infants**; although antimalarials are excreted in milk, the amounts are too variable to give reliable protection.

EPILEPSY. Both chloroquine and mefloquine are unsuitable for malaria prophylaxis in subjects with a history of epilepsy. In areas *without chloroquine resistance* proguanil 200 mg daily alone is recommended; in areas *with chloroquine resistance* doxycycline may be considered [unlicensed indication, specialist advice needed] but its metabolism may be influenced by antiepileptics (see **interactions:** Appendix 1 (tetracyclines)). *Maloprim®* may be another alternative; it should be supplemented with folic acid (5 mg daily) in those taking phenytoin or phenobarbital.

RENAL IMPAIRMENT. Avoidance (or dosage reduction) of proguanil is recommended since it is excreted by the kidneys. Chloroquine is only partially excreted by the kidneys and reduction of the dose for prophylaxis is not required except in severe impairment. Mefloquine is considered to be appropriate to use in renal impairment and does not require dosage reduction. Doxycycline is also considered to be appropriate [unlicensed indication, specialist advice needed].

PREGNANCY. Travel to malarious areas should be avoided during pregnancy; if travel is unavoidable, effective prophylaxis must be used. Chloroquine and proguanil may be given in usual doses in areas where *P. falciparum* strains are sensitive; in the case of proguanil, folic acid 5 mg daily should be given. Although the manufacturer advises that mefloquine should be avoided in the first trimester (see p. 304), studies of mefloquine in pregnancy (including use in the first trimester) have revealed no evidence of harm; it may therefore be considered for travel to chloroquine-resistant areas. *Maloprim®* is contraindicated in the first trimester; folate supplements should be given if *Maloprim®* is prescribed in the second and third trimester. The centres listed on p. 298 should be consulted for advice on prophylaxis in resistant areas.

Specific recommendations

Where a journey requires two regimens, the regimen for the higher risk area should be used for the whole journey. Those travelling to remote or little-visited areas may require expert advice.

> Risk may vary in different parts of a country—check under all risk levels

> WARNING. Settled immigrants (or long-term visitors) to the UK may be unaware that they will have **lost some of their immunity** and also that the areas where they previously lived **may now be malarious**

North Africa and the Middle East

VERY LOW RISK. Risk *very low* in Abu Dhabi, Algeria, tourist areas of Egypt, Libya, Morocco, Tunisia, most tourist areas of Turkey:

> no prophylaxis recommended but consider malaria if fever presents

LOW RISK. Risk *low* in southern border areas of Azerbaijan, Egypt (El Fayoum only, June–October), rural north Iraq (May–November), north border of Syria (May–October), Turkey (plain around Adana, Side, south-east Anatolia, March–November), south border areas of Tajikistan:

preferably

> chloroquine 300 mg (as base) once weekly

or

(if chloroquine not appropriate)

> proguanil hydrochloride 200 mg once daily

RISK. Risk *present* and *chloroquine resistance present* in Afghanistan (below 2000 m, May–November), Iran (March–November), Oman, Saudi Arabia (except Northern, Eastern and Central Provinces, Asir plateau, and western border cities where very little risk), northern rural United Arab Emirates, Yemen:

both

chloroquine 300 mg (as base) once weekly

and

proguanil hydrochloride 200 mg once daily

Sub-Saharan Africa

VERY HIGH RISK. Risk *very high* (or *locally very high*) and *chloroquine resistance very widespread* in Angola, Benin, Burkina Faso, Burundi, Cameroon, Central African Republic, Chad, Comoros, Congo, Democratic Republic of the Congo (formely Zaïre), Djibouti, Equatorial Guinea, Eritrea, Ethiopia, Gabon, Gambia[1], Ghana, Guinea, Guinea-Bissau, Ivory Coast, Kenya[1], Liberia, Madagascar, Malawi, Mali, Mozambique, Niger, Nigeria, Principe, Rwanda, São Tomé, Senegal, Sierra Leone, Somalia, Sudan, Swaziland, Tanzania[1], Togo, Uganda, Zambia, Zimbabwe (Zambezi valley, see also below):

preferably

mefloquine 250 mg once weekly

or
(if mefloquine not appropriate)
both

| chloroquine 300 mg (as base) once weekly |
| **and** |
| proguanil hydrochloride 200 mg once daily |

1. Visitors for periods of 2 weeks or less to tourist resorts of Gambia (between January and May), of coastal Kenya and of coastal Tanzania can take chloroquine plus proguanil; however, mefloquine provides better protection and is recommended for longer visits, higher exposure risk (e.g. backpacking, staying in rural areas, safaris) and for Gambia between June and December

RISK. Risk *present* (in *parts of country*) and *some chloroquine resistance* in northern half of Botswana (November–June), Mauritania (all year in southern half; July–October in northern half), northern third of Namibia (November–June), north-east part of South Africa (low altitude areas of north and eastern Transvaal and eastern Natal to 100 kilometres north of Durban), areas below 1200 m in Zimbabwe (November–June; all year in Zambezi valley *where mefloquine preferable*):

preferably

both
chloroquine 300 mg (as base) once weekly
and
proguanil hydrochloride 200 mg once daily

or
(if chloroquine plus proguanil not appropriate)

mefloquine 250 mg once weekly

Note. In Zimbabwe and neighbouring countries, *Maloprim®* (also known as *Deltaprim®*) prophylaxis is used by local residents (sometimes with chloroquine).

No prophylaxis recommended for Cape Verde and non-rural areas of Mauritius (but consider malaria if fever presents); *chloroquine prophylaxis* appropriate for rural areas of **Mauritius**

South Asia

HIGH RISK. Risk *high* and *chloroquine resistance high* in Bangladesh (only in Chittagong Hill Tracts):

preferably

mefloquine 250 mg once weekly

or
(if mefloquine not appropriate)

both
chloroquine 300 mg (as base) once weekly
and
proguanil hydrochloride 200 mg once daily

VARIABLE RISK. Risk *variable* and *chloroquine resistance usually moderate* in Bangladesh (except in Chittagong Hill Tracts, see above; no risk in Dhaka city), southern districts of Bhutan, India (no risk in mountain states of north), Nepal (below 1300 m; no risk in Kathmandu), Pakistan (below 2000 m), Sri Lanka (no risk in and just south of Colombo):

both
chloroquine 300 mg (as base) once weekly
and
proguanil hydrochloride 200 mg once daily

South-East Asia

VERY LOW RISK. Risk *very low* in Bali, Brunei, main tourist areas of China (but *substantial risk* in Yunnan and Hainan, see below; *chloroquine prophylaxis* appropriate for other remote areas), Hong Kong, Malaysia (but *variable risk* in Sabah, and in deep forests, see below), Sarawak (but *variable risk* in deep forests, see below), Singapore (no risk), Thailand (Bangkok, main tourist centres and rural areas not near borders—**important:** regional risk exists, see under Low but significant risk, below):

no prophylaxis recommended but consider malaria if fever presents

VARIABLE RISK. Risk *variable* and *some chloroquine resistance* in Indonesia (very low risk in Bali and cities but *substantial risk* in Irian Jaya, see below), rural Philippines below 600 m (no risk in Cebu, Leyte, Bohol, Catanduanes), deep forests of peninsular Malaysia and Sarawak, Sabah:

both
chloroquine 300 mg (as base) once weekly
and
proguanil hydrochloride 200 mg once daily

SUBSTANTIAL RISK. Risk *substantial* and *drug resistance common* in Cambodia (**important:** specialist advice needed for western provinces, see below), China (Yunnan and Hainan; *chloroquine prophylaxis* appropriate for other remote areas), Irian Jaya, Laos, Myanmar (formerly Burma), Vietnam (no risk in cities, Red River delta area, coastal plain north of Nha Trang):

mefloquine 250 mg once weekly

LOW BUT SIGNIFICANT RISK. Risk *low but significant* because *mefloquine resistance present* in western provinces of Cambodia, borders of Thailand with Cambodia and Myanmar, and Ko Chang:

> doxycycline 100 mg once daily [unlicensed indication—specialist advice needed and not for longer than 3 months]

Oceania

RISK. Risk *high* and *chloroquine resistance high* in Papua New Guinea (below 1800 m), Solomon Islands, Vanuatu:

preferably

> doxycycline 100 mg once daily [unlicensed]

or

> mefloquine 250 mg once weekly

Latin America and Caribbean

VARIABLE TO LOW RISK. Risk *variable to low* in Argentina (small area in north-west only), rural Belize (except Belize district), rural Costa Rica (below 500 m), Dominican Republic, El Salvador, Guatemala (below 1500 m), Haiti, Honduras, some rural areas of Mexico (not regularly visited by tourists), Nicaragua, Panama (west of Panama Canal but *variable to high risk* east of Panama Canal, see below), rural Paraguay (October–May):

preferably

> chloroquine 300 mg (as base) once weekly

or
(if chloroquine not appropriate)

> proguanil hydrochloride 200 mg once daily

VARIABLE TO HIGH RISK. Risk *variable to high* and *chloroquine resistance present* in rural areas of Bolivia (below 2500 m), Ecuador (below 1500 m), Panama (east of Panama Canal), rural areas of Peru (below 1500 m), rural areas of Venezuela (except on coast, Caracas free of malaria):

preferably

> **both**
> chloroquine 300 mg (as base) once weekly
> **and**
> proguanil hydrochloride 200 mg once daily

or
(if chloroquine plus proguanil not appropriate)

> mefloquine 250 mg once weekly

Note. Prophylaxis with *Maloprim®* (in a dose of 1 tablet once weekly) plus chloroquine (in a dose of 300 mg as base once weekly) is also an alternative

HIGH RISK. Risk *high* and *marked chloroquine resistance* in Bolivia (Amazon basin area), Brazil (throughout 'Legal Amazon' area which includes the Amazon basin region, Mato Grosso and Maranhao only; elsewhere *very low risk*—no prophylaxis), Colombia (most areas below 800 m), French Guiana, all interior regions of Guyana, Surinam

(except Paramaribo and coast), Venezuela (Amazon basin area):

preferably

> mefloquine 250 mg once weekly

or
(if mefloquine not appropriate)

> **both**
> chloroquine 300 mg (as base) once weekly
> **and**
> proguanil hydrochloride 200 mg once daily

STANDBY TREATMENT. Adults travelling for prolonged periods to areas of chloroquine-resistance who are unlikely to have easy access to medical care should carry a standby treatment course. Self-medication should be **avoided** if medical help is accessible; prophylaxis should be continued during and after the attack.

In order to avoid excessive self-medication, the traveller should be provided with **written instructions** that urgent medical attention should be sought if fever (38°C or more) develops 7 days (or more) after arriving in a malarious area and that self treatment is indicated if medical help is not immediately available or the condition is worsening.

In view of the continuing emergence of resistant strains and of the different regimens required for different areas expert advice should be sought on the best treatment course for an individual traveller.

Chloroquine

Chloroquine is used for the *prophylaxis of malaria* in areas of the world where the *risk of chloroquine resistant falciparum malaria is still low*. It is also used with proguanil when chloroquine resistant falciparum malaria is present although this regimen may not be that of first choice (see specific recommendations by country, pp. 300-302). Chloroquine is also combined with *Maloprim®* in some areas.

Chloroquine is **no longer recommended** for the *treatment of falciparum malaria* owing to widespread resistance, nor is it recommended if the infective species is *not known* or if the infection is *mixed*; in these cases treatment should be with quinine, mefloquine or rarely halofantrine (for details, see pp. 298-99). It is still recommended for the *treatment of benign malarias* (for details, see p. 299).

CHLOROQUINE

Indications: chemoprophylaxis and treatment of malaria, see notes above; rheumatoid arthritis and lupus erythematosus (section 10.1.3)

Cautions: hepatic impairment, renal impairment (see notes above), pregnancy (but for malaria benefit outweighs risk, see Appendix 4, Antimalarials), may exacerbate psoriasis, neurological disorders (avoid for prophylaxis if history of epilepsy, see notes above), may aggravate myasthenia gravis, severe gastro-intestinal disorders, G6PD deficiency (see section 9.1.5); ophthalmic examination and long-term therapy; see under Chloroquine, section 10.1.3; avoid concurrent therapy with hepatotoxic drugs and with halofantrine (see CSM advice under Halofantrine)—other **interactions**: Appendix 1 (chloroquine)

Side-effects: gastro-intestinal disturbances, headache; also convulsions, visual disturbances, depigmentation or loss of hair, skin reactions (rashes, pruritus); rarely, bone-marrow suppression; other side-effects (not usually associated with malaria prophylaxis or treatment), see under Chloroquine, section 10.1.3; very toxic in **overdosage**—immediate advice from poisons centres essential (see also p. 23)

Dose: see notes above

COUNSELLING. Warn travellers about **importance** of avoiding mosquito bites, **importance** of taking prophylaxis regularly, and **importance** of immediate visit to doctor if ill within 1 year and **especially** within 3 months of return. For details, see notes above

*Avloclor® (Zeneca) PoM
Tablets, scored, chloroquine phosphate 250 mg (≡ chloroquine base 155 mg). Net price 20-tab pack = £1.11. Label: 5, counselling, prophylaxis, see above
* Can be sold to the public provided it is licensed and labelled for the prophylaxis of malaria

Nivaquine® (Rhône-Poulenc Rorer)
* *Tablets* PoM, f/c, yellow, chloroquine sulphate 200 mg (≡ chloroquine base 150 mg), net price 28-tab pack = £1.34. Label: 5, counselling, prophylaxis, see above
* *Syrup* PoM, golden, chloroquine sulphate 68 mg/5 mL (≡ chloroquine base 50 mg/5 mL), net price 100 mL = £2.82. Label: 5, counselling, prophylaxis, see above
* Can be sold to the public provided it is licensed and labelled for the prophylaxis of malaria

Injection PoM, chloroquine sulphate 54.5 mg/mL (≡ chloroquine base 40 mg/mL), net price 5-mL amp = 76p

■ With proguanil
For cautions and side-effects of proguanil see Proguanil; for dose see notes above

Paludrine/Avloclor® (Zeneca)
Travel Pack, 14 tablets of chloroquine phosphate 250 mg (≡ chloroquine base 155 mg) and 98 tablets of proguanil hydrochloride 100 mg, net price 112-tab pack = £8.79. Label 5, 21, counselling, prophylaxis, see above
Available as a generic from Boots

Halofantrine

Halofantrine is not suitable for the *prophylaxis of malaria*.

Halofantrine is licensed for the *treatment of falciparum malaria* but is now rarely used—see warnings below (for details on the treatment of falciparum malaria, see p. 298-99). It should not be used for the *treatment of benign malarias*, as chloroquine is usually effective. It should not be used where mefloquine has been used for prophylaxis (see Cautions below).

HALOFANTRINE HYDROCHLORIDE

Indications: treatment of uncomplicated chloroquine-resistant falciparum malaria or of chloroquine-resistant vivax malaria, but see notes above

Cautions: no experience of use in cerebral or complicated malaria; cardiac disease (see below);

interactions: see below and Appendix 1 (halofantrine)

ARRHYTHMIAS. Halofantrine prolongs QT interval and has a potential for inducing hazardous arrhythmias in susceptible individuals, especially if dose excessive or if taken with food (which enhances absorption). It should **not** be used for standby treatment. Recommendations of the **CSM** are that halofantrine:
should **not** be taken with meals;
should **not** be taken with other drugs which may induce arrhythmias (e.g. *chloroquine, mefloquine, quinine, tricyclic antidepressants, antipsychotics, certain antiarrhythmics,* and *antihistamines such as terfenadine*);
should **not** be taken with drugs causing electrolyte disturbances;
should **not** be administered to those with known prolongation of the QT interval;
should **not** be administered to those with any form of cardiac disease associated with QT interval prolongation or ventricular arrhythmias (e.g. coronary heart disease, cardiomyopathy, and congenital heart disease)

Contra-indications: cardiac disorders including family history of congenital QT interval prolongation (**important:** see also above); other conditions associated with prolonged QT interval (e.g. hypokalaemia, hypomagnesaemia or other electrolyte disorders, thiamine deficiency); unexpected syncopal attacks; pregnancy and breast-feeding (avoid during treatment)

Side-effects: diarrhoea, abdominal pain, nausea, vomiting; transient elevation of serum transaminases; pruritus, rash, intravascular haemolysis, and hypersensitivity reactions also reported; **important**: ventricular arrhythmias (see also above)

Dose: see notes above

Halfan® (SK&F) PoM
Tablets, scored, halofantrine hydrochloride 250 mg. Net price 12-tab pack = £13.96. Label: 23

Mefloquine

Mefloquine is used for the *prophylaxis of malaria* in areas of the world where there is a *high risk of chloroquine-resistant falciparum malaria* (for details, see specific recommendations by country, pp. 300-302).

Mefloquine is used for the *treatment of falciparum malaria* or if the infective species is *not known* or if the infection is *mixed* (for details, see pp. 298-99). It is also effective for the *treatment of benign malarias*, but is not required as chloroquine is usually effective. Mefloquine should not be used for treatment if it has been used for prophylaxis.

CSM recommendation. The CSM has advised that:

• Patients should be informed about adverse reactions associated with mefloquine and, if they occur, advised to seek medical advice on alternative antimalarials before the next dose is due

• When possible mefloquine prophylaxis should be started 2–3 weeks before travel to enable any adverse reactions to be identified before departure

• Mefloquine is contra-indicated in patients with a history of neuropsychiatric disease including convulsions and depression

• The patient information leaflet, which describes adverse reactions should always be provided when dispensing mefloquine

MEFLOQUINE

Indications: chemoprophylaxis of malaria, treatment of uncomplicated falciparum malaria and chloroquine-resistant vivax malaria, see notes above

Cautions: exclude pregnancy before starting chemoprophylaxis (see also under Contra-indications); avoid for chemoprophylaxis in severe hepatic impairment; cardiac conduction disorders; epilepsy (avoid for prophylaxis); not recommended in infants under 3 months (5 kg); halofantrine must not be given with or after mefloquine (danger of fatal arrhythmias—see also under Halofantrine); other **interactions:** Appendix 1 (mefloquine)

DRIVING. Dizziness or a disturbed sense of balance may affect performance of skilled tasks (e.g. driving); effects may persist for up to 3 weeks

Contra-indications: chemoprophylaxis in first trimester of pregnancy (teratogenic in *animals*, manufacturer advises **avoid** pregnancy **during** and for **3 months after** but see notes under Prophylaxis against malaria), breast-feeding, and history of neuropsychiatric disorders, including depression, or convulsions; hypersensitivity to quinine

Side-effects: nausea, vomiting, diarrhoea, abdominal pain; dizziness, loss of balance, headache, sleep disorders (insomnia, drowsiness, abnormal dreams); also neuropsychiatric reactions (including sensory and motor neuropathies, tremor, ataxia, anxiety, depression, panic attacks, agitation, hallucinations, overt psychosis, convulsions), tinnitus and vestibular disorders, visual disturbances, circulatory disorders (hypotension and hypertension), tachycardia, bradycardia, cardiac conduction disorders, muscle weakness, myalgia, arthralgia, rash, urticaria, pruritus, alopecia, disturbances in liver function tests, asthenia, malaise, fatigue, fever, loss of appetite, leucopenia or leucocytosis, thrombocytopenia; rarely Stevens-Johnson syndrome, AV block and encephalopathy

Dose: chemoprophylaxis, starting 1–3 weeks before departure (see p. 299) and continued for 4 weeks after leaving malarious area, ADULT and CHILD over 45 kg 250 mg each week; CHILD 5–19 kg (3 months–5 years) quarter adult dose, 20–30 kg (6–8 years) half adult dose, 31–45 kg (9–14 years) three-quarters adult dose

LONG-TERM CHEMOPROPHYLAXIS. Mefloquine prophylaxis can be taken for up to 1 year

Treatment, see notes above

COUNSELLING. See CSM recommendation in notes above. Also warn travellers about **importance** of avoiding mosquito bites, **importance** of taking prophylaxis regularly, and **importance** of immediate visit to doctor if ill within 1 year and **especially** within 3 months of return. For details, see notes above

[1] **Lariam®** (Roche) PoM

Tablets, scored, mefloquine (as hydrochloride) 250 mg. Net price 8-tab pack = £14.53. Label: 21, 25, 27, counselling, driving, prophylaxis, see above

1. Prescriptions may be referred to Health Authorities to investigate circumstances under which written since prescriptions for chemoprophylaxis of malaria may not be reimbursable

Primaquine

Primaquine is used to eliminate the liver stages of *P. vivax or P. ovale following chloroquine treatment* (for details, see p. 299).

PRIMAQUINE

Indications: adjunct in the treatment of *Plasmodium vivax* and *P. ovale* malaria (eradication of liver stages)

Cautions: G6PD deficiency (see notes above); systemic diseases associated with granulocytopenia (e.g. rheumatoid arthritis, lupus erythematosus); pregnancy and breast-feeding; **interactions:** Appendix 1 (primaquine)

Side-effects: nausea, vomiting, abdominal pain; less commonly methaemoglobinaemia, haemolytic anaemia especially in G6PD deficiency

Dose: see notes above

Primaquine (Non-proprietary)

Tablets, primaquine (as phosphate) 7.5 mg

Available from Durbin [unlicensed—special order]

Proguanil

Proguanil is used (usually *with chloroquine*, but occasionally *alone*) for the *prophylaxis of malaria*, (for details, see specific recommendations by country, see pp. 300-302).

Proguanil used alone is not suitable for the *treatment of malaria*; a combination of atovaquone and proguanil is, however, licensed for the treatment of acute uncomplicated falciparum malaria.

PROGUANIL HYDROCHLORIDE

Indications: chemoprophylaxis of malaria

Cautions: renal impairment (see notes under Prophylaxis against malaria and Appendix 3); pregnancy (folate supplements needed); **interactions:** Appendix 1 (proguanil)

Side-effects: mild gastric intolerance and diarrhoea; occasionally mouth ulcers and stomatitis; skin reactions and hair loss reported

Dose: see notes above

COUNSELLING. Warn travellers about **importance** of avoiding mosquito bites, **importance** of taking prophylaxis regularly, and **importance** of immediate visit to doctor if ill within 1 year and **especially** within 3 months of return. For details, see notes above

Paludrine® (Zeneca)

Tablets, scored, proguanil hydrochloride 100 mg. Net price 98-tab pack = £7.43. Label: 21, counselling, prophylaxis, see above

■ With chloroquine

See under Chloroquine

PROGUANIL HYDROCHLORIDE WITH ATOVAQUONE

Indications: treatment of acute uncomplicated falciparum malaria, particularly where resistance to other antimalarial drugs is suspected

Cautions: acute renal failure, diarrhoea or vomiting (reduced absorption of atovaquone), pregnancy; avoid breast-feeding; efficacy not evaluated in cerebral or complicated malaria (including hyperparasitaemia, pulmonary oedema or renal failure); **interactions:** see Appendix 1 (proguanil, atovaquone)

Side-effects: nausea, vomiting, diarrhoea, abdominal pain, anorexia; headache, cough, occasionally elevated liver enzymes

Dose: see under preparation

Malarone® (GlaxoWellcome) ▼ PoM
Tablets, pink, f/c, proguanil hydrochloride 100 mg, atovaquone 250 mg. Net price 12-tab pack = £22.92. Label: 21
Dose: ADULT and CHILD over 40 kg, 4 tablets once daily for 3 days; CHILD 11–20 kg 1 tablet daily for 3 days; 21–30 kg 2 tablets once daily for 3 days; 31–40 kg 3 tablets once daily for 3 days

Pyrimethamine

Pyrimethamine should not be used alone, but is used with sulfadoxine (in *Fansidar®*) and with dapsone (in *Maloprim®*).

Fansidar® is not recommended for the *prophylaxis of malaria*, but it is used in the treatment of *falciparum malaria* and can be used *with (or following) quinine*.

Maloprim® is used with *chloroquine* for the *prophylaxis of malaria* in certain areas where there is a *high risk of chloroquine-resistant falciparum malaria* (for details see specific recommendations by country, see pp. 300-302). *Maloprim®* is not suitable for the *treatment of malaria*.

PYRIMETHAMINE

Indications: malaria (but used only in combined preparations incorporating dapsone or sulfadoxine); toxoplasmosis [not licensed]—section 5.4.7

Cautions: hepatic or renal impairment, folate supplements in pregnancy, breast-feeding, blood counts required with prolonged treatment; **interactions:** Appendix 1 (pyrimethamine)

Side-effects: depression of haematopoiesis with high doses, rashes, insomnia

Dose: malaria, no dose stated because not recommended
Toxoplasmosis, section 5.4.7

Daraprim® (GlaxoWellcome) PoM ▰
Tablets, scored, pyrimethamine 25 mg. Net price 30-tab pack = £2.12

▰ denotes preparations that are considered to be less suitable for prescribing (see p. vi)

PYRIMETHAMINE WITH SULFADOXINE

Indications: adjunct to quinine in treatment of *Plasmodium falciparum* malaria (see notes above); **not** recommended for prophylaxis

Cautions; Contra-indications; Side-effects: see under Pyrimethamine and under Co-trimoxazole (section 5.1.8); contra-indicated in sulphonamide allergy; pregnancy and breast-feeding (see

Appendixes 4 and 5); severe side-effects on long-term use therefore not recommended for prophylaxis; pulmonary infiltrates (e.g. eosinophilic or allergic alveolitis) reported—discontinue if cough or shortness of breath

Dose: treatment, see notes above
Prophylaxis, not recommended by UK malaria experts

Fansidar® (Roche) PoM
Tablets, scored, pyrimethamine 25 mg, sulfadoxine 500 mg. Net price 3-tab pack = 80p

PYRIMETHAMINE WITH DAPSONE

Indications: prophylaxis of *Plasmodium falciparum* malaria (limited use, see notes above)

Cautions; Contra-indications; Side-effects: see under Pyrimethamine and under Dapsone (section 5.1.10); contra-indicated in sulphonamide allergy; caution in G6PD deficiency (section 9.1.5); pregnancy (see notes under Prophylaxis against Malaria and Appendix 4) and breast-feeding (Appendix 5); side-effects including methaemoglobinaemia, thrombocytopenia, mononucleosis-like syndrome, psychosis, jaundice, pneumonia with eosinophilic pulmonary infiltration, and on prolonged treatment hypoalbuminaemia reported

Dose: malaria prophylaxis, see notes above
COUNSELLING. Warn travellers about **importance** of avoiding mosquito bites, **importance** of taking prophylaxis regularly, and **importance** of immediate visit to doctor if ill within 1 year and **especially** within 3 months of return. For details, see notes above

Maloprim® (GlaxoWellcome) PoM
Tablets, scored, pyrimethamine 12.5 mg, dapsone 100 mg. Net price 30-tab pack = £2.64. Counselling, prophylaxis, see above

Quinine

Quinine is not suitable for the *prophylaxis of malaria*.

Quinine is used for the *treatment of falciparum malaria* or if the infective species is *not known* or if the infection is *mixed* (for details see pp. 298-99).

QUININE

Indications: falciparum malaria; nocturnal leg cramps, see section 10.2.2

Cautions: atrial fibrillation, conduction defects, heart block, pregnancy (but appropriate for treatment of malaria); monitor blood glucose concentration during parenteral treatment; G6PD deficiency (see section 9.1.5); avoid concurrent administration with halofantrine (see CSM advice under Halofantrine), other **interactions:** Appendix 1 (quinine)

Contra-indications: haemoglobinuria, optic neuritis

Side-effects: cinchonism, including tinnitus, headache, hot and flushed skin, nausea, abdominal pain, rashes, visual disturbances (including temporary blindness), confusion; hypersensitivity reactions including angioedema, blood disorders (including thrombocytopenia and intravascular coagulation), and acute renal failure; hypoglycaemia (especially after parenteral administration); cardiovascular effects (see Cautions); very toxic in **overdosage**—immediate advice from poisons centres essential (see also p. 23)

Dose: see notes above

Note. Quinine (anhydrous base) 100 mg ≡ quinine bisulphate   169 mg ≡ quinine   dihydrochloride 122 mg ≡ quinine hydrochloride 122 mg ≡ quinine sulphate 121 mg. Quinine bisulphate 300-mg tablets are available but provide less quinine than 300 mg of the dihydrochloride, hydrochloride, or sulphate

Quinine Sulphate (Non-proprietary) PoM
Tablets, coated, quinine sulphate 200 mg, net price 20 = 81p; 300 mg, 20 = 86p
Available from APS, Cox, CP, Hillcross, Kent

Quinine Dihydrochloride (Non-proprietary) PoM
Injection, quinine dihydrochloride 300 mg/mL. For dilution and use as an infusion. 1- and 2-mL amps
Available from Martindale (special order) or from specialist centres (see p. 298)
Note. Intravenous injection of quinine is so hazardous that it has been superseded by infusion

Tetracyclines

Doxycycline (section 5.1.3) is used for the *prophylaxis of malaria* [unlicensed indication—specialist advice needed] in areas of *widespread mefloquine and chloroquine resistance* and also as a second-line drug for those who are unable to take chloroquine or mefloquine (for details, see specific recommendations by country, pp. 300-302).

Doxycycline is also used as an *adjunct to quinine in the treatment of falciparum malaria* (for details see p. 298).

5.4.2   Amoebicides

Metronidazole is the drug of choice for *acute invasive amoebic dysentery* since it is very effective against vegetative forms of *Entamoeba histolytica* in ulcers; it is given in an adult dose of 800 mg three times daily for 5 days. **Tinidazole** is also effective. Metronidazole and tinidazole are also active against amoebae which may have migrated to the liver. Treatment with metronidazole (or tinidazole) is followed by a 10-day course of diloxanide furoate.

Diloxanide furoate is the drug of choice for asymptomatic patients with *E. histolytica* cysts in the faeces; metronidazole and tinidazole are relatively ineffective. Diloxanide furoate is relatively free from toxic effects and the usual course is of 10 days, given alone for chronic infections or following metronidazole or tinidazole treatment.

For *amoebic abscesses* of the liver **metronidazole** is effective in doses of 400 mg 3 times daily for 5–10 days; tinidazole is an alternative. The course may be repeated after 2 weeks if necessary. Aspiration of the abscess is indicated where it is suspected that it may rupture or where there is no improvement after 72 hours of metronidazole; the aspiration may need to be repeated. Aspiration aids penetration of metronidazole and, for abscesses with more than 100 mL of pus, if carried out in conjunction with drug therapy, may reduce the period of disability.

Diloxanide furoate is not effective against hepatic amoebiasis, but a 10-day course should be given at the completion of metronidazole or tinidazole treatment to destroy any amoebae in the gut.

DILOXANIDE FUROATE

Indications: see notes above; chronic amoebiasis and as adjunct to metronidazole or tinidazole in acute amoebiasis

Contra-indications: pregnancy (Appendix 4), breast-feeding (Appendix 5)

Side-effects: flatulence, vomiting, urticaria, pruritus

Dose: 500 mg every 8 hours for 10 days; CHILD over 25 kg, 20 mg/kg daily in 3 divided doses for 10 days
See also notes above

Furamide® (Sovereign) PoM
Tablets, scored, diloxanide furoate 500 mg, net price 15-tab pack = £1.92. Label: 9

METRONIDAZOLE

Indications: see under Dose below; anaerobic infections, section 5.1.11

Cautions; Side-effects: section 5.1.11

Dose: *by mouth*, invasive intestinal amoebiasis, 800 mg every 8 hours for 5 days; CHILD 1–3 years 200 mg every 8 hours; 3–7 years 200 mg every 6 hours; 7–10 years 400 mg every 8 hours
Extra-intestinal amoebiasis (including liver abscess) and symptomless amoebic cyst passers, 400–800 mg every 8 hours for 5–10 days; CHILD 1–3 years 100–200 mg every 8 hours; 3–7 years 100–200 mg every 6 hours; 7–10 years 200–400 mg every 8 hours
Urogenital trichomoniasis, 200 mg every 8 hours for 7 days *or* 400–500 mg every 12 hours for 5–7 days, *or* 2 g as a single dose; CHILD 1–3 years 50 mg every 8 hours for 7 days; 3–7 years 100 mg every 12 hours; 7–10 years 100 mg every 8 hours
Giardiasis, 2 g daily for 3 days *or* 500 mg twice daily for 7–10 days; CHILD 1–3 years 500 mg daily for 3 days; 3–7 years 600–800 mg daily; 7–10 years 1 g daily

Preparations
Section 5.1.11

TINIDAZOLE

Indications: see under Dose below; anaerobic infections, section 5.1.11

Cautions; Side-effects: section 5.1.11

Dose: intestinal amoebiasis, 2 g daily for 2–3 days; CHILD 50–60 mg/kg daily for 3 days
Amoebic involvement of liver, 1.5–2 g daily for 3–6 days; CHILD 50–60 mg/kg daily for 5 days
Urogenital trichomoniasis and giardiasis, single 2-g dose; CHILD single dose of 50–75 mg/kg (repeated once if necessary)

Preparations
Section 5.1.11

5.4.3   Trichomonacides

Metronidazole (section 5.4.2) is the treatment of choice for *Trichomonas vaginalis* infection.

If metronidazole is ineffective, **tinidazole** may be tried; it is usually given as a single 2-g dose, with food. A further 2-g dose may be given if there is no clinical improvement.

Alcohol should be avoided during treatment with both metronidazole and tinidazole.

5.4.4 Antigiardial drugs

Metronidazole (section 5.4.2) is the treatment of choice for *Giardia lamblia* infections, given by mouth in a dosage of 2 g daily for 3 days or 400 mg every 8 hours for 5 days.

Alternative treatments are **tinidazole** (section 5.4.2) 2 g as a single dose or **mepacrine hydrochloride** 100 mg every 8 hours for 5–7 days.

MEPACRINE HYDROCHLORIDE

Indications: giardiasis; discoid lupus erythematosus—section 10.1.3

Cautions: hepatic impairment, elderly, history of psychosis; avoid in psoriasis; **interactions:** Appendix 1 (mepacrine)

Side-effects: gastro-intestinal disturbances; dizziness, headache; with large doses nausea, vomiting and occasionally transient acute toxic psychosis and CNS stimulation; on prolonged treatment yellow discoloration of skin and urine, chronic dermatoses (including severe exfoliative dermatitis), hepatitis, aplastic anaemia; also reported blue/black discoloration of palate and nails and corneal deposits with visual disturbances

Dose: giardiasis, 100 mg every 8 hours for 5–7 days; CHILD 2 mg/kg every 8 hours

Mepacrine Hydrochloride

Tablets, mepacrine hydrochloride 100 mg. Label: 4, 9, 14, 21

Available from BCM Specials [unlicensed—special order]

5.4.5 Leishmaniacides

Cutaneous leishmaniasis frequently heals spontaneously but if skin lesions are extensive or unsightly, treatment is indicated, as it is in visceral leishmaniasis (kala-azar).

Sodium stibogluconate, an organic pentavalent antimony compound, is the treatment of choice for visceral leishmaniasis. The dose is 20 mg/kg daily (max. 850 mg) for at least 20 days by intramuscular or intravenous injection; the dosage varies with different geographical regions and expert advice should be obtained. Skin lesions are treated for 10 days.

Amphotericin is used with or after an antimony compound for visceral leishmaniasis unresponsive to the antimonial alone; side-effects may be reduced by using liposomal amphotericin (*AmBisome®*—section 5.2) at a dose of 1–3 mg/kg daily for 10–21 days to a cumulative dose of 21–30 mg/kg. Other lipid formulations of amphotericin (*Abelcet®* and *Amphocil®*) are also likely to be effective but less information is available.

Pentamidine isetionate (pentamidine isethionate) (section 5.4.8) has been used in antimony-resistant visceral leishmaniasis, but although the initial response is often good, the relapse rate is high; it is associated with serious side-effects. Other treatments include paromomycin (available on named-patient basis from IDIS).

SODIUM STIBOGLUCONATE

Indications: leishmaniasis

Cautions: hepatic impairment; pregnancy; intravenous injections must be given slowly over 5 minutes (to reduce risk of local thrombosis) and stopped if coughing or substernal pain; mucocutaneous disease (see below); heart disease (withdraw if conduction disturbances occur); treat intercurrent infection (e.g. pneumonia)

MUCOCUTANEOUS DISEASE. Successful treatment of mucocutaneous leishmaniasis may induce severe inflammation around the lesions (may be life-threatening if pharyngeal or tracheal involvement)—may require corticosteroid

Contra-indications: significant renal impairment; breast-feeding

Side-effects: anorexia, nausea, vomiting, abdominal pain; ECG changes; headache, lethargy, myalgia; raised liver enzymes; coughing and substernal pain (see Cautions); rarely anaphylaxis; also reported, fever, sweating, flushing, vertigo, bleeding from nose or gum, jaundice, rash; pain and thrombosis on intravenous administration, intramuscular injection also painful

Dose: see notes above

Pentostam® (GlaxoWellcome) [PoM]

Injection, sodium stibogluconate equivalent to pentavalent antimony 100 mg/mL. Net price 100-mL bottle = £64.94

5.4.6 Trypanocides

The prophylaxis and treatment of trypanosomiasis is difficult and differs according to the strain of organism. Expert advice should therefore be obtained.

5.4.7 Drugs for toxoplasmosis

Most infections caused by *Toxoplasma gondii* are self-limiting, and treatment is not necessary. Exceptions are patients with eye involvement (toxoplasma choroidoretinitis), and those who are immunosuppressed. Toxoplasmic encephalitis is a common complication of AIDS. The treatment of choice is a combination of pyrimethamine and sulfadiazine (sulphadiazine), given for several weeks (expert advice **essential**). Pyrimethamine is a folate antagonist, and adverse reactions to this combination are relatively common (folinic acid supplements and weekly blood counts needed). Alternative regimens use combinations of pyrimethamine with clindamycin or clarithromycin or azithromycin. Long-term secondary prophylaxis is required after treatment of toxoplasmosis in AIDS.

If toxoplasmosis is acquired in pregnancy, transplacental infection may lead to severe disease in the fetus. Spiramycin (available on named-patient basis from IDIS) may reduce the risk of transmission of maternal infection to the fetus.

5.4.8 Drugs for pneumocystis pneumonia

Pneumonia caused by *Pneumocystis carinii* occurs in immunosuppressed or severely debilitated patients. It is the commonest cause of pneumonia in AIDS.

Co-trimoxazole (section 5.1.8) in high dosage is the drug of choice for the treatment of pneumocystis pneumonia.

Pentamidine isetionate (pentamidine isethionate) is an alternative to co-trimoxazole and is particularly indicated for patients with a history of adverse reactions to, or who have not responded to, co-trimoxazole. Pentamidine isetionate is a potentially toxic drug that can cause severe hypotension during or immediately after administration; it should only be administered by those experienced in its use. Pentamidine isetionate is given by intravenous infusion but can also be administered by inhalation which reduces side-effects (although systemic absorption may still occur).

In moderate to severe infections associated with HIV infection, prednisolone 50–80 mg daily is given for 5 days (alternatively, hydrocortisone may be given parenterally); the role of corticosteroids in pneumocystic infections in the absence of HIV infection is not clear.

Intermittent *prophylactic inhalation* of pentamidine isetionate may prevent relapse but co-trimoxazole is easier to administer and just as effective (in a dose of 960 mg twice daily) for prophylaxis.

Atovaquone has recently become available for the treatment of mild to moderate Pneumocystis pneumonia in patients who are intolerant of co-trimoxazole.

Trimetrexate is an alternative in AIDS patients who are intolerant of co-trimoxazole and pentamidine isetionate or who do not respond to these drugs. Trimetrexate is a potent dihydrofolate reductase inhibitor and must be given with calcium folinate.

ATOVAQUONE

Indications: treatment of mild to moderate *Pneumocystis carinii* pneumonia in patients intolerant of co-trimoxazole

Cautions: initial diarrhoea and difficulty in taking with food may reduce absorption (and require alternative therapy); other causes of pulmonary disease should be sought and treated; elderly; hepatic and renal impairment; pregnancy; avoid breast-feeding; **interactions:** Appendix 1 (atovaquone)

Side-effects: diarrhoea, nausea, vomiting; headache, insomnia; rash, fever; elevated liver enzymes and amylase; anaemia, neutropenia; hyponatraemia

Dose: 750 mg twice daily with food (particularly high fat) for 21 days; CHILD not recommended

Wellvone® (GlaxoWellcome) [PoM]
Suspension, sugar-free, fruit-flavoured, atovaquone 750 mg/5 mL. Net price 210 mL = £360.18. Label: 21

■ With proguanil hydrochloride
See section 5.4.1

PENTAMIDINE ISETIONATE

Indications: see under Dose (should only be given by specialists)

Cautions: risk of severe hypotension following administration (establish baseline blood pressure and administer with patient lying down; monitor blood pressure closely during administration, and at regular intervals, until treatment concluded); hepatic and renal impairment; hypertension or hypotension; hyperglycaemia or hypoglycaemia; leucopenia, thrombocytopenia, or anaemia; pregnancy and breast-feeding; carry out laboratory monitoring according to product literature; care required to protect personnel during handling and administration

Side-effects: severe reactions, sometimes fatal, due to hypotension, hypoglycaemia, pancreatitis, and arrhythmias; also leucopenia, thrombocytopenia, acute renal failure, hypocalcaemia; also reported: azotaemia, abnormal liver-function tests, anaemia, hyperkalaemia, nausea and vomiting, dizziness, syncope, flushing, hyperglycaemia, rash, and taste disturbances; Stevens-Johnson syndrome reported; on inhalation, bronchoconstriction (may be prevented by prior use of bronchodilators), cough, shortness of breath, and wheezing; discomfort, pain, induration, abscess formation, and muscle necrosis at injection site

Dose: *Pneumocystis carinii* pneumonia, *by intravenous infusion*, 4 mg/kg daily for at least 14 days (reduced according to product literature in renal impairment)

By inhalation of nebulised solution (using suitable equipment—consult product literature) 600 mg pentamidine isetionate daily for 3 weeks; secondary prevention, 300 mg every 4 weeks *or* 150 mg every 2 weeks

Visceral leishmaniasis (kala-azar, section 5.4.5), *by deep intramuscular injection*, 3–4 mg/kg on alternate days to max. total of 10 injections; course may be repeated if necessary

Cutaneous leishmaniasis, *by deep intramuscular injection*, 3–4 mg/kg once or twice weekly until condition resolves (but see also section 5.4.5)

Trypanosomiasis, *by deep intramuscular injection or intravenous infusion*, 4 mg/kg daily or on alternate days to total of 7–10 injections

Note. Direct bolus intravenous injection should be avoided whenever possible and **never** given rapidly; intramuscular injections should be deep and preferably given into the buttock

Pentacarinat® (JHC) [PoM]
Injection, powder for reconstitution, pentamidine isetionate. Net price 300-mg vial = £32.74
Nebuliser solution, pentamidine isetionate. Net price 300-mg bottle = £34.57
CAUTION IN HANDLING. Pentamidine isetionate is toxic and personnel should be adequately protected during handling and administration—consult product literature

---

TRIMETREXATE

Indications: treatment of moderate to severe *Pneumocystis carinii* pneumonia in AIDS patients intolerant of, or refractory to, standard therapy or for whom standard therapy is contra-indicated (specialist use only)

Cautions: administer calcium folinate during treatment and for 72 hours after last dose (to avoid potentially serious or life-threatening bone-marrow suppression, oral and gastro-intestinal ulceration, and renal and hepatic dysfunction); suspend myelosupressive drugs (e.g. zidovudine) to administer therapeutic doses of trimetrexate; hepatic and renal impairment; **interactions:** Appendix 1 (trimetrexate)

MONITORING. Monitor at least twice weekly full blood count, renal and hepatic function; interrupt treatment if significant change in renal or hepatic function (see product literature); adjust dose of trimetrexate and calcium folinate if significant haematological toxicity (see product literature)

Contra-indications: pregnancy (following administration to woman or man, avoid conception for **at least 6 months** after treatment), breast-feeding

Side-effects: blood disorders including thrombocytopenia, granulocytopenia and anaemia (dose modification may be necessary, see also monitoring, above); vomiting, diarrhoea, oral and gastrointestinal mucosal ulceration (discontinue if interfering with eating and drinking); fever (discontinue if uncontrolled by antipyretics); confusion, rarely seizures; disturbances in liver enzymes; disturbances in plasma calcium, potassium and magnesium reported; rash, anaphylaxis very rarely reported; rarely local irritation at injection site

Dose: by intravenous infusion, 45 mg/m^2 daily for 21 days together with calcium folinate by mouth or by intravenous injection (over 5–10 minutes), 20 mg/m^2 every 6 hours for 24 days

Note. Calcium folinate must not be given with trimetrexate in the same intravenous line (administer either before or after trimetrexate infusion)

Neutrexin® (Ipsen) ▼ PoM
Injection, powder for reconstitution, trimetrexate (as glucuronate). Net price 25-mg vial = £33.86

5.5   Anthelmintics

5.5.1   Drugs for threadworms
5.5.2   Ascaricides
5.5.3   Drugs for tapeworm infections
5.5.4   Drugs for hookworms
5.5.5   Schistosomicides
5.5.6   Filaricides
5.5.7   Drugs for cutaneous larva migrans
5.5.8   Drugs for strongyloidiasis

Advice on prophylaxis and treatment of helminth infections is available from:

Birmingham   0121-766 6611
Glasgow   0141-300 1130
Liverpool   0151-708 9393
London   (020) 7387 4411 (treatment)

5.5.1   Drugs for threadworms
(pinworms, Enterobius vermicularis)

Anthelmintics are effective in threadworm infections, but their use needs to be combined with hygienic measures to break the cycle of auto-infection. All members of the family require treatment.

Adult threadworms do not live for longer than 6 weeks and for development of fresh worms, ova must be swallowed and exposed to the action of digestive juices in the upper intestinal tract. Direct multiplication of worms does not take place in the large bowel. Adult female worms lay ova on the perianal skin which causes pruritus; scratching the area then leads to ova being transmitted on fingers to the mouth, often via food eaten with unwashed hands. Washing hands and scrubbing nails before each meal and after each visit to the toilet is essential. A bath taken immediately after rising will remove ova laid during the night.

Mebendazole is the drug of choice for patients of all ages over 2 years. It is given as a single dose; as reinfection is very common, a second dose may be given after 2–3 weeks.

Piperazine salts are preferably given daily for 7 days (followed by a second course if necessary 7 days later); single-dose preparations are also available.

MEBENDAZOLE

Indications: threadworm, roundworm, whipworm, and hookworm infections

Cautions: pregnancy (toxicity in rats), breast-feeding; **interactions:** Appendix 1 (mebendazole)

Note. The package insert in the Vermox® pack includes the statement that it is not suitable for women known to be pregnant or children under 2 years

Side-effects: rarely abdominal pain, diarrhoea; hypersensitivity reactions (including exanthema, rash, urticaria, and angioedema) reported

Dose: threadworms, ADULT and CHILD over 2 years, 100 mg as a single dose; if reinfection occurs second dose may be needed after 2–3 weeks; CHILD under 2 years, not yet recommended

Whipworms, ADULT and CHILD over 2 years, 100 mg twice daily for 3 days; CHILD under 2 years, not yet recommended

Roundworms—section 5.5.2

Hookworms—section 5.5.4

¹ Mebendazole (Non-proprietary) PoM
Tablets, chewable, mebendazole 100 mg
1. Can be sold to the public if supplied for oral use in the treatment of enterobiasis in adults and children over 2 years provided its container or package is labelled to show a max. single dose of 100 mg and it is supplied in a container or package containing not more than 800 mg; proprietary brands on sale to the public include Boots Threadworm Treatment®, Ovex® and Pripsen® Mebendazole.

Vermox® (Janssen-Cilag) PoM
Tablets, orange, scored, chewable, mebendazole 100 mg. Net price 6-tab pack = £1.53
Suspension, mebendazole 100 mg/5 mL. Net price 30 mL = £1.77

PIPERAZINE

Indications: threadworm and roundworm infections

Cautions: renal impairment (avoid if severe), liver disease, neurological disease; epilepsy, pregnancy (see also Appendix 4—packs on sale to the general public carry a warning to avoid in epilepsy and pregnancy)

Side-effects: nausea, vomiting, colic, diarrhoea, allergic reactions including urticaria, bronchospasm, and rare reports of Stevens-Johnson syndrome and angioedema; rarely dizziness, mus-

cular incoordination ('worm wobble'); drowsiness, confusion and clonic contractions in patients with neurological or renal abnormalities
Dose: see under Preparations, below

Piperazine Citrate (Non-proprietary)
Elixir, piperazine hydrate 750 mg/5 mL (as citrate)
Available from, SSL (*Pripsen® Worm Elixir*)
Dose: threadworms, 15 mL once daily for 7 days; CHILD under 2 years (on doctor's advice only) 0.3–0.5 mL/kg once daily for 7 days, 2–3 years 5 mL once daily for 7 days, 4–6 years 7.5 mL once daily for 7 days, 7–12 years 10 mL once daily for 7 days; repeat course after 1 week if necessary
Roundworms, 30 mL as a single dose; CHILD under 1 year (on doctor's advice only) 0.8 mL/kg as a single dose, 1–3 years 10 mL as a single dose, 4–5 years 15 mL as a single dose, 6–8 years 20 mL as a single dose, 9–12 years 25 mL as a single dose; repeat dose after 2 weeks

Pripsen® (SSL)
Oral powder, piperazine phosphate 4 g and sennosides 15.3 mg/sachet. Net price two-dose sachet pack = £1.25. Label: 13
Dose: threadworms, stirred into a small glass of milk or water and drunk immediately, ADULT and CHILD over 6 years, 1 sachet, repeated after 14 days; INFANT 3 months–1 year (on doctor's advice only), 1 level 2.5- mL spoonful, repeated after 14 days; CHILD 1–6 years, 1 level 5- mL spoonful, repeated after 14 days
Roundworms, first dose as for threadworms; repeat at monthly intervals for up to 3 months if reinfection risk

5.5.2   Ascaricides
(common roundworm infections)

Levamisole (available on named-patient basis from IDIS) is very effective against *Ascaris lumbricoides* and is generally considered to be the drug of choice. It is very well tolerated; mild nausea or vomiting has been reported in about 1% of treated patients; it is given as a single dose of 120–150 mg in adults.

Mebendazole (section 5.5.1) is also active against ascaris; the usual dose is 100 mg twice daily for 3 days. **Piperazine** may be given in a single adult dose equivalent to 4–4.5 g of piperazine hydrate see Piperazine, above.

5.5.3   Drugs for tapeworm infections

Taenicides

Niclosamide is the most widely used drug for tapeworm infections and side-effects are limited to occasional gastro-intestinal upset, lightheadedness, and pruritus; it is not effective against larval worms. Fears of developing cysticercosis in *Taenia solium* infections have proved unfounded. All the same, it is wise to anticipate this possibility by using an anti-emetic on wakening.

Praziquantel (available on named-patient basis from Bayer (*Biltricide®*) and from Merck (*Cysticide®*)) is as effective as niclosamide and is given as a single dose of 10–20 mg/kg after a light breakfast (a single dose of 25 mg/kg for *Hymenolepis nana*).

NICLOSAMIDE

Indications: tapeworm infections—see notes above and under Dose
Side-effects: nausea, retching, abdominal pain; lightheadedness; pruritus

Dose: *Taenia solium*, ADULT and CHILD over 6 years 2 g as a single dose after a light breakfast followed by a purgative after 2 hours; CHILD under 2 years 500 mg, 2–6 years 1 g
T. saginata and *Diphyllobothrium latum*, as for *T. solium* but half the dose may be taken after breakfast and the remainder 1 hour later followed by a purgative 2 hours after last dose
Hymenolepis nana, ADULT and CHILD over 6 years 2 g as a single dose on first day then 1 g daily for 6 days; CHILD under 2 years 500 mg on first day then 250 mg daily for 6 days, 2–6 years 1 g on first day then 500 mg daily for 6 days
COUNSELLING. Tablets should be chewed thoroughly (or crushed) before washing down with water

Yomesan® (Bayer)
Tablets, yellow, chewable, niclosamide 500 mg. Net price 4-tab pack = £1.41. Label: 4, 24, counselling, administration

Hydatid disease

Cysts caused by *Echinococcus granulosus* grow slowly and asymptomatic patients do not always require treatment. Surgical treatment remains the method of choice in many situations. **Albendazole** is used in conjunction with surgery to reduce the risk of recurrence or as primary treatment in inoperable cases. Alveolar echinococcosis due to *E. multilocularis* is usually fatal if untreated. Surgical removal with albendazole cover is the treatment of choice, but where effective surgery is impossible, repeated cycles of albendazole (for a year or more) may help. Careful monitoring of liver function is particularly important during drug treatment.

ALBENDAZOLE

Indications: adjunct to surgery in hydatid cysts caused by *Echinococcus granulosus* or *E. multilocularis*, or primary treatment if surgery not possible; strongyloidiasis (section 5.5.8)
Cautions: blood counts and liver function tests before treatment and twice during each cycle; breast-feeding; exclude pregnancy before starting treatment (non-hormonal contraception during and for 1 month after treatment)
Contra-indications: pregnancy (see also Cautions)
Side-effects: gastro-intestinal disturbances, headache, dizziness, changes in liver enzymes; rarely reversible alopecia; rash, fever, blood disorders including leucopenia and pancytopenia reported; allergic shock if cyst leakage; convulsions and meningism in cerebral disease
Dose: *E. granulosus*, ADULT over 60 kg, medical treatment, 800 mg daily in divided doses for 28 days followed by 14 tablet-free days; up to 3 cycles of treatment may be given
Adjunct in surgical treatment, *pre-surgery*, 800 mg daily in divided doses for 28 days followed by 14 tablet-free days, repeat cycle once before surgery; *post-surgery* (if viable cysts after pre-surgery treatment, or if no pre-surgery treatment, or if only short pre-surgery course), 800 mg daily in divided doses for 28 days followed by 14 tablet-free days, repeat cycle once
E. multilocularis, ADULT over 60 kg, 800 mg daily in divided doses for 28 days followed by 14 tablet-free days; prolonged treatment may be required, see notes above

Eskazole® (SmithKline Beecham) PoM
Tablets, orange, scored, chewable, albendazole
400 mg. Net price 60-tab pack = £72.00. Label: 9

5.5.4 Drugs for hookworms
(ancylostomiasis, necatoriasis)

Hookworms live in the upper small intestine and
draw blood from the point of their attachment to
their host. An iron-deficiency anaemia may thereby
be produced and, if present, effective treatment of
the infection requires not only expulsion of the
worms but treatment of the anaemia.

Mebendazole (section 5.5.1) has a useful broad-
spectrum activity, and is effective against hookworms;
the usual dose is 100 mg twice daily for 3 days.

5.5.5 Schistosomicides
(bilharziasis)

Adult *Schistosoma haematobium* worms live in the
genito-urinary veins and adult *S. mansoni* in those
of the colon and mesentery. *S. japonicum* is more
widely distributed in veins of the alimentary tract
and portal system.

Praziquantel (available on named-patient basis
from Bayer (*Biltricide®*) and from Merck (*Cysti-
cide®*)) is effective against all human schistosomes.
The dose is 40 mg/kg in 2 divided doses 4–6 hours
apart on one day (60 mg/kg in 3 divided doses on
one day for *S. japonicum* infections). No serious
toxic effects have been reported. Of all the available
schistosomicides, it has the most attractive combination of effectiveness, broad-spectrum activity,
and low toxicity.

Hycanthone, lucanthone, niridazole, oxamniquine,
and sodium stibocaptate have now been superseded.

5.5.6 Filaricides

Diethylcarbamazine (*Hetrazan®*, Lederle) is effective against microfilariae and adults of *Loa loa*,
Wuchereria bancrofti, and *Brugia malayi*. To minimise reactions treatment is commenced with a dose
of diethylcarbamazine citrate 1 mg/kg on the first
day and increased gradually over 3 days to 6 mg/kg
daily in divided doses; this dosage is maintained for
21 days and usually gives a radical cure for these
infections. Close medical supervision is necessary
particularly in the early phase of treatment.

In heavy infections there may be a febrile reaction, and in heavy *Loa loa* infection there is a small
risk of encephalopathy. In such cases treatment
must be given under careful in-patient supervision
and stopped at the first sign of cerebral involvement
(and specialist advice sought).

Ivermectin (*Mectizan®*, MSD, available on
named-patient basis) is very effective in *onchocerciasis* and it is now the drug of choice. A single
dose of 150 micrograms/kg by mouth produces a
prolonged reduction in microfilarial levels. Retreatment at intervals of 6 to 12 months depending on
symptoms must be given until the adult worms die
out. Reactions are usually slight and most commonly take the form of temporary aggravation of
itching and rash. Diethylcarbamazine or suramin
should no longer be used for onchocerciasis
because of their toxicity.

5.5.7 Drugs for cutaneous larva migrans
(creeping eruption)

Dog and cat hookworm larvae may enter human
skin where they produce slowly extending itching
tracks usually on the foot. Single tracks can be
treated with topical tiabendazole (no commercial
preparation available). Multiple infections respond
to **ivermectin** (*Mectizan®*, MSD, available on
named-patient basis), **albendazole** [unlicensed
indication] or **tiabendazole** (thiabendazole) (section 5.5.8) by mouth.

5.5.8 Drugs for strongyloidiasis

Adult *Strongyloides stercoralis* live in the gut and
produce larvae which penetrate the gut wall and
invade the tissues, setting up a cycle of auto-infection. **Tiabendazole** (thiabendazole) is the drug of
choice for adults (but side-effects are much more
marked in the elderly); it is given at a dosage of
25 mg/kg (max. 1.5 g) every 12 hours for 3 days.
Albendazole (section 5.5.3) is an alternative [unli-
censed] with fewer side-effects; it is given in a dose
of 400 mg twice daily for 3 days, repeated after 3
weeks if necessary. **Ivermectin** (*Mectizan®*, MSD,
available on named-patient basis) in a dose of
200 micrograms/kg daily for 2 days may be the
most effective drug for chronic *Strongyloides* infection.

TIABENDAZOLE
(Thiabendazole)

Indications: strongyloidiasis, cutaneous and
visceral larva migrans, dracontiasis, symptoms of
trichinosis; secondary treatment for threadworm
when mixed with above infestations; adjunct in
hookworm, whipworm, or roundworm (but not
suitable for mixed infections involving roundworms—risk of migration); not for prophylactic
use

Cautions: hepatic or renal impairment; elderly;
discontinue if hypersensitivity reactions occur;
correct anaemia, dehydration or malnutrition
preferably before treatment; **interactions**:
Appendix 1 (tiabendazole)

DRIVING. May impair performance of skilled tasks (e.g.
driving)

Contra-indications: pregnancy (teratogenesis in
animal studies) and breast-feeding

Side-effects: include anorexia, nausea, vomiting,
dizziness, diarrhoea, headache, pruritus, drowsiness; hypersensitivity reactions including fever,
chills, angioedema, rashes, erythema multiforme
and Stevens-Johnson syndrome; rarely tinnitus,
collapse, parenchymal liver damage (may be
severe and irreversible), visual disorders

Dose: see notes above

Mintezol® (MSD) PoM
Tablets, orange, chewable, tiabendazole 500 mg.
Net price 6-tab pack = 62p. Label: 3, 21, 24

6: Endocrine system

6.1   Drugs used in diabetes

Diabetes mellitus occurs because of a lack of insulin or resistance to its action. Diabetes is clinically defined by measurement of fasting or random blood-glucose concentration (and occasionally by glucose tolerance test). There are two principal classes of diabetes (and many subtypes not listed here):

TYPE 1 DIABETES. Type 1 diabetes, also referred to as insulin-dependent diabetes mellitus (IDDM), is due to a deficiency of insulin following autoimmune destruction of pancreatic beta cells. Patients with type 1 diabetes require administration of insulin.

TYPE 2 DIABETES. Type 2 diabetes, also referred to as non-insulin dependent diabetes (NIDDM), is due to reduced secretion of insulin or to peripheral resistance to the action of insulin. Although patients may be controlled on diet alone, many require administration of oral antidiabetic drugs or insulin to maintain satisfactory control.

Treatment should be aimed at alleviating symptoms and minimising the risk of long-term complications by appropriate control of diabetes. Other risk factors for cardiovascular disease (smoking, hypertension, obesity and hyperlipidaemia) should be addressed.

PREVENTION OF DIABETIC COMPLICATIONS. Optimal glycaemic control in both type 1 diabetes and type 2 diabetes, in the long term, reduces the risk of microvascular complications including retinopathy, development of albuminuria and to some extent neuropathy.

A measure of the total glycated (or glycosylated) haemoglobin (HbA_1) or a specific fraction (HbA_{1c}) provides a good indication of long-term glycaemic control. The ideal HbA_{1c} level is around 7% although this cannot always be achieved, and for those on insulin there are significantly increased risks of severe hypoglycaemia. Tight control of blood pressure in hypertensive patients with type 2 diabetes reduces mortality significantly and protects visual acuity (by reducing considerably the risks of maculopathy and retinal photocoagulation) (see also section 2.5).

6.1.1 Insulins

6.1.1.1	Short-acting insulins
6.1.1.2	Intermediate- and long-acting insulins
6.1.1.3	Hypodermic equipment

Insulin plays a key role in the regulation of carbohydrate, fat, and protein metabolism. It is a polypeptide hormone of complex structure. There are differences in the amino-acid sequence of animal insulins, human insulins and the human insulin analogues. Insulin may be extracted from pork pancreas and purified by crystallisation; it may also be extracted from beef pancreas, but beef insulins are now rarely used. Human sequence insulin may be produced semisynthetically by enzymatic modification of porcine insulin (emp) or biosynthetically by recombinant DNA technology using Escherichia coli (crb, prb, or pyr).

All insulin preparations are to a greater or lesser extent immunogenic in man but immunological resistance to insulin action is uncommon. Preparations of human sequence insulin should theoretically be less immunogenic, but no real advantage has been shown in trials.

Insulin is inactivated by gastro-intestinal enzymes, and must therefore be given by injection; the subcutaneous route is ideal in most circumstances. It is usually injected into the upper arms, thighs, buttocks, or abdomen; there may be increased absorption from a limb site if the limb is used in strenuous exercise following the injection. Generally subcutaneous insulin injections cause few problems; fat hypertrophy does however occur but can be minimised by rotating the injection sites. Local allergic reactions are now scarcely seen.

Insulin is needed by all patients, regardless of age, presenting with ketoacidosis, and most of those with rapid onset of symptoms, weight loss, weakness and sometimes vomiting often associated with ketonuria. It is required by almost all children with diabetes. Insulin is also needed for type 2 diabetes when other methods have failed to achieve good control, and temporarily in the presence of intercurrent illness or perioperatively. Pregnant women with type 2 diabetes should be treated with insulin when diet alone fails. The majority of those who are obese can be managed by dietary changes or, if diet alone fails to achieve adequate control, by also administering oral hypoglycaemic drugs.

MANAGEMENT OF DIABETES WITH INSULIN. The aim of treatment is to achieve the best possible control of plasma glucose concentration without making the patient obsessional and to avoid disabling hypoglycaemia; close co-operation is needed between the patient and the medical team since good control reduces the incidence of complications. Mixtures of insulin preparations may be required and appropriate combinations have to be determined for the individual patient. For patients with acute-onset diabetes, treatment should be started with soluble insulin given 3 times daily with medium-acting insulin at bedtime. For those less severely ill, treatment is usually started with a mixture of premixed short- and medium-acting insulins (most commonly in a proportion of 30% soluble insulin and 70% isophane insulin) given twice daily; 8 units twice daily is a suitable initial dose for most ambulant patients. The proportion of the short-acting soluble component can be increased in those with excessive post-prandial hyperglycaemia.

The dose of insulin is adjusted on an individual basis, by gradually increasing the dose but avoiding troublesome hypoglycaemic reactions.

There are 3 main types of insulin preparations:

- those of **short** duration which have a relatively rapid onset of action, namely soluble insulin, insulin lispro and insulin aspart;
- those with an **intermediate** action, e.g. isophane insulin and insulin zinc suspension; and
- those whose action is slower in onset and lasts for **long** periods, e.g. crystalline insulin zinc suspension

The duration of action of a particular type of insulin varies considerably from one patient to another, and needs to be assessed individually.

Examples of recommended insulin regimens

- Short-acting insulin mixed with intermediate-acting insulin: twice daily (before meals)
- Short-acting insulin mixed with intermediate-acting insulin: before breakfast
  Short-acting insulin: before evening meal
  Intermediate-acting insulin: at bedtime
- Short-acting insulin: three times daily (before breakfast, midday and evening meal)
  Intermediate-acting insulin: at bedtime
- Intermediate-acting insulin with or without short-acting insulin: once daily either before breakfast or at bedtime suffices for some patients with type 2 diabetes who need insulin

Insulin requirements may be increased by infection, stress, accidental or surgical trauma, puberty and, during the second and third trimesters of pregnancy. Requirements may be decreased in patients with renal or hepatic impairment and in those with some endocrine disorders (e.g. Addison's disease, hypopituitrism) or coeliac disease. In pregnancy insulin requirements should be assessed frequently by an experienced diabetes physician.

INSULIN ADMINISTRATION. Injection devices ('pens') (section 6.1.1.3) which hold the insulin in a cartridge and meter the required dose are convenient to use. The conventional syringe and needle is still the preferred method of insulin administration by many and is also required for insulins not available in cartridge form.

For intensive insulin regimens multiple injections (3 to 4 times daily) are usually recommended; soluble insulin can also be given by continuous subcutaneous infusion using an infusion pump. This delivers a continuous basal insulin infusion with preprandial boosts provided by patient-activated bolus doses. This technique has a limited place in the treatment of diabetes, and patients using it must be well motivated, reliable, able to monitor their own blood-glucose, and with access to expert advice at all times. Continuous subcutaneous insulin infusion is sometimes valuable for patients with serious problems from recurrent hypoglycaemia.

UNITS. The word 'unit' should not be abbreviated.

MONITORING. Many patients now monitor their own blood-glucose concentrations using blood glucose strips preferably with an electronic meter. Since blood-glucose concentrations vary substantially throughout the day, 'normoglycaemia' cannot always be achieved throughout a 24-hour period without causing damaging hypoglycaemia. It is therefore best to recommend that patients should maintain a blood-glucose concentration of between 4 and 10 mmol/litre for most of the time, while accepting that on occasions, for brief periods, it will be above these values; strenuous efforts should be made to prevent the blood-glucose concentration from falling below 4 mmol/litre. Patients should be advised to look for 'peaks' and 'troughs' of blood glucose, and to adjust their insulin dosage only once or twice weekly. Overall it is ideal to aim for an HbA_{1c} concentration of 7% or less (normal range 4–6%) or an HbA_1 of less than 8.8% (normal range 5–7.5%) although this is not always possible without causing disabling hypoglycaemia. Fructosamine can also be used for assessment of control; this is simpler and cheaper but the measurement of HbA_{1c} is generally a more reliable method.

The intake of energy and of simple and complex carbohydrates should be adequate to allow normal growth and development but obesity must be avoided. The carbohydrate intake needs to be regulated and should be distributed throughout the day. Fine control of plasma glucose can be achieved by moving portions of carbohydrate from one meal to another without altering the total intake.

HYPOGLYCAEMIA. Hypoglycaemia is a potential problem for all patients receiving insulin and careful instruction to the patient must be directed towards avoiding it.

Loss of warning of hypoglycaemia is common among insulin-treated patients and can be a serious hazard, especially for drivers and those in dangerous occupations. Very tight control of diabetes lowers the blood-glucose concentration needed to trigger hypoglycaemic symptoms; increase in the frequency of hypoglycaemic episodes reduces the warning symptoms experienced by the patient. Beta-blockers can also blunt hypoglycaemic awareness (and also delay recovery).

To restore the warning signs, episodes of hypoglycaemia must be reduced to a minimum; this involves appropriate adjustment of insulin type, dose and frequency together with suitable timing and quantity of meals and snacks.

Some patients have reported loss of hypoglycaemia warning after transfer to human insulin. If a patient believes that human insulin is responsible for the loss of warning it is reasonable to revert to animal insulin and to educate the patient about avoiding hypoglycaemia. Great care should be taken to specify whether a human or an animal preparation is required.

Few patients are now treated with beef insulins; when undertaking conversion from beef to human insulin, the total dose should be reduced by about 10% with careful monitoring for the first few days. When changing between pork and human sequence insulins, a dose change is not usually needed, but careful monitoring is still advised.

DRIVING. Drivers treated with insulin or oral antidiabetic drugs are required to notify the Driver and Vehicle Licensing Agency of their condition (as are drivers of heavy goods vehicles or public service vehicles whose diabetes is controlled by diet alone); the Agency's Drivers Medical Unit provides guidance on eligibility to drive.

Drivers need to be particularly careful to avoid hypoglycaemia (see also above) and should be warned of the problems. They should normally check their blood-glucose concentration before driving and, on long journeys, at intervals of approximately 2 hours and they should ensure that a supply of sugar is always available in the car. If hypoglycaemia occurs a car driver should switch off the ignition until recovery is complete, which may take up to 15 minutes or longer. Driving is not permitted when hypoglycaemic awareness has been lost.

DIABETES AND SURGERY. When an insulin-dependent diabetic patient requires surgery that is likely to require an intravenous infusion for longer than 12 hours the following regimen provides for intravenous administration of insulin (for an indefinite period).

- Give an injection of the patient's usual insulin on the night before the operation.
- Early on the day of the operation, start an intravenous infusion of glucose 5% or 10% containing potassium chloride 10 mmol/litre (provided that the patient is not hyperkalaemic) and run at a constant rate appropriate to the patient's fluid requirements (usually 125 mL per hour); make up a solution of soluble insulin 1 unit/mL in sodium chloride 0.9% and infuse intravenously using a syringe pump piggy-backed to the intravenous infusion.
- The rate of the insulin infusion should normally be:
  Blood glucose < 4 mmol/litre, give 0.5 units/hour
  Blood glucose 4–15 mmol/litre, give 2 units/hour
  Blood glucose 15–20 mmol/litre, give 4 units/hour
  Blood glucose > 20 mmol/litre, review.

In resistant cases (such as patients who are in shock or severely ill or those receiving corticosteroids or sympathomimetics) 2–4 times these rates or even more may be needed.

If a syringe pump is not available soluble insulin 16 units/litre should be added to the intravenous infusion of glucose 5 or 10% containing potassium chloride 10 mmol per litre (provided the patient is not hyperkalaemic) and the infusion run at the rate appropriate to the patient's fluid requirements (usually 125 mL per hour) with the insulin dose adjusted as follows:

  Blood glucose < 4 mmol/litre, give 8 units/litre
  Blood glucose 4–15 mmol/litre, give 16 units/litre
  Blood glucose 15–20 mmol/litre, give 32 units/litre
  Blood glucose > 20 mmol/litre, review.

The rate of intravenous infusion depends on the volume depletion, cardiac function, age, and other factors. Blood-glucose concentration should be measured pre-operatively and then hourly until stable, thereafter every 2 hours. The duration of action of intravenous insulin is only a few minutes and the infusion must not be stopped unless the patient becomes overtly hypoglycaemic (blood glucose < 3 mmol/litre) in which case it should be stopped for up to 30 minutes. The amount of potassium chloride required in the infusion needs to be assessed by regular measurement of plasma electrolytes. Sodium chloride 0.9% infusion should replace glucose 5% or 10% if the blood glucose is persistently above 15 mmol/litre.

Once the patient starts to eat and drink, give subcutaneous insulin before breakfast and stop intravenous insulin 30 minutes later; the dose may need to be 10–20% more than usual if the patient is still in bed or unwell. If the patient was not previously receiving insulin, an appropriate initial dose is 30–40 units daily in four divided doses using soluble insulin before meals and intermediate-acting insulin at bedtime and the dose adjusted from day to day. Patients with hyperglycaemia often relapse after conversion back to subcutaneous insulin calling for one of the following approaches:

- additional doses of soluble insulin at any of the four injection times (before meals or bedtime) *or*
- temporary addition of intravenous insulin infusion (while continuing the subcutaneous regimen) until blood-glucose concentration is satisfactory *or*
- complete reversion to the intravenous regimen (especially if the patient is unwell).

6.1.1.1   Short-acting insulins

Soluble Insulin is a short-acting form of insulin. For maintenance regimens it is usual to inject it 15 to 30 minutes before meals.

Soluble insulin is the only appropriate form of insulin for use in diabetic emergencies and at the time of surgery. It has the great advantage that it can be given intravenously and intramuscularly, as well as subcutaneously.

When injected subcutaneously, soluble insulin has a rapid onset of action (after 30 to 60 minutes), a peak action between 2 and 4 hours, and a duration of action of up to 8 hours. Human sequence preparations tend to have a more rapid onset and a shorter overall duration.

When injected intravenously, soluble insulin has a very short half-life of only about 5 minutes and its effect disappears within 30 minutes.

The recently introduced human insulin analogues, **insulin lispro** and **insulin aspart**, have a faster onset and shorter duration of action than soluble insulin; as a result, compared to soluble insulin, fasting and preprandial blood-glucose concentration is a little higher, postprandial blood-glucose concentration is a little lower, and hypoglycaemia occurs slightly less frequently. Subcutaneous injection of insulin lispro or of insulin aspart may prove convenient to those who wish to inject shortly before or, when necessary, shortly after a meal. They may also help those prone to pre-lunch hypoglycaemia and those who eat late in the evening and are prone to early nocturnal hypoglycaemia.

SOLUBLE INSULIN

(Insulin Injection; Neutral Insulin)
A sterile solution of insulin (i.e. bovine or porcine) or of human insulin; pH 6.6–8.0

Indications: diabetes mellitus; diabetic ketoacidosis (section 6.1.3)

Cautions: see notes above; reduce dose in renal impairment; **interactions:** Appendix 1 (antidiabetics)

Side-effects: see notes above; local reactions and fat hypertrophy at injection site; overdose causes hypoglycaemia

Dose: *by subcutaneous, intramuscular, or intravenous injection or intravenous infusion*, according to requirements
COUNSELLING. Show container to patient and confirm that patient is expecting the version dispensed

■ Highly purified animal

Hypurin® Bovine Neutral (CP) [PoM]
Injection, soluble insulin (bovine, highly purified) 100 units/mL. Net price 10-mL vial = £18.48; 5 × 1.5-mL cartridge = £13.86

Hypurin® Porcine Neutral (CP) [PoM]
Injection, soluble insulin (porcine, highly purified) 100 units/mL. Net price 10-mL vial = £16.80; 5 × 1.5-mL cartridge = £12.60

Pork Actrapid® (Novo Nordisk) [PoM]
Injection, soluble insulin (porcine, highly purified) 100 units/mL. Net price 10-mL vial = £6.58
Note. Not recommended for use in ambulatory insulin infusion pumps—may precipitate in catheter or needle

■ Human sequence

Human Actrapid® (Novo Nordisk) [PoM]
Injection, soluble insulin (human, pyr) 100 units/mL. Net price 10-mL vial = £7.10; *Penfill®* cartridge (for *NovoPen®* [DHS]) 5 × 1.5-mL = £9.87, 5 × 3-mL = £22.87; 5 × 3-mL *Actrapid®* prefilled disposable injection devices (range 2–78 units, allowing 2-unit dosage adjustment) = £25.28
Note. Not recommended for use in ambulatory insulin infusion pumps—may precipitate in catheter or needle

Human Velosulin® (Novo Nordisk) [PoM]
Injection, soluble insulin (human, emp) 100 units/mL. Net price 10-mL vial = £7.10

Humulin S® (Lilly) [PoM]
Injection, soluble insulin (human, prb) 100 units/mL. Net price 10-mL vial = £12.50; 5 × 1.5-mL cartridge (for *B-D Pen®* [DHS]) = £10.65; 5 × 3-mL cartridge (for *B-D Pen® 3 mL* or *HumaPen®* [DHS]) = £21.30; 5 × 3-mL *Humaject S®* prefilled disposable injection devices (range 2–96 units, allowing 2-unit dosage adjustment) = £26.33

■ Mixed preparations, see Biphasic Insulin and Biphasic Isophane Insulin (section 6.1.1.2)

INSULIN ASPART

(Recombinant human insulin analogue)
Indications: diabetes mellitus
Cautions: see under Soluble Insulin
Side-effects: see under Soluble Insulin
Dose: *by subcutaneous injection*, immediately before meals according to requirements
COUNSELLING. Show container to patient and confirm that patient is expecting the version dispensed

NovoRapid® (Novo Nordisk) ▼ [PoM]
Injection, insulin aspart (recombinant human insulin analogue) 100 units/mL, net price 10-mL vial = £15.71; *Penfill®* cartridge (for *NovoPen®* [DHS] devices) 5 × 3-mL = £26.78; 5 × 3-mL *NovoLet®* prefilled disposable injection devices (range 2–78 units, allowing 2-unit dosage adjustment) = £29.62

INSULIN LISPRO

(Recombinant human insulin analogue)
Indications: diabetes mellitus
Cautions: see under Soluble Insulin; children (use only if benefit likely compared to soluble insulin)
Side-effects: see under Soluble Insulin
Dose: *by subcutaneous injection or subcutaneous infusion*, according to requirements
COUNSELLING. Show container to patient and confirm that patient is expecting the version dispensed

Humalog® (Lilly) ▼ [PoM]
Injection, insulin lispro (recombinant human insulin analogue) 100 units/mL. Net price 10-mL vial = £15.71; 5 × 1.5-mL cartridge (for *B-D Pen®* [DHS]) = £13.39; 5 × 3-mL cartridge (for *B-D Pen® 3-mL* [DHS] or *HumaPen®* [DHS]) = £26.78

6.1.1.2 Intermediate- and long-acting insulins

When given by subcutaneous injection, intermediate- and long-acting insulins have an onset of action of approximately 1–2 hours, a maximal effect at 4–12 hours, and a duration of 16–35 hours. Some are given twice daily in conjunction with short-acting (soluble) insulin, and others are given once daily, particularly in elderly patients. They can be mixed with soluble insulin in the syringe, essentially retaining the properties of the two components, although there may be some blunting of the initial effect of the soluble insulin component (especially on mixing with protamine zinc insulin, see below).

Isophane insulin is a suspension of insulin with protamine which is of particular value for initiation of twice-daily insulin regimens. Patients usually mix isophane with soluble insulin but ready-mixed preparations may be appropriate (**biphasic isophane insulin** or **biphasic insulin lispro**).

Insulin zinc suspension (crystalline) has a more prolonged duration of action; it may be used independently or in **insulin zinc suspension** (30% amorphous, 70% crystalline).

Protamine zinc insulin is usually given once daily with short-acting (soluble) insulin. It has the drawback of binding with the soluble insulin when mixed in the same syringe, and is now rarely used.

INSULIN ZINC SUSPENSION

(Insulin Zinc Suspension (Mixed); I. Z. S.)
A sterile neutral suspension of bovine and/or porcine insulin or of human insulin in the form of a complex obtained by the addition of a suitable zinc salt; consists of rhombohedral crystals (10–40 microns) and of particles of no uniform shape (not exceeding 2 microns)

Indications: diabetes mellitus (long acting)

Cautions: see under Soluble Insulin (section 6.1.1.1)

Side-effects: see under Soluble Insulin (section 6.1.1.1)

Dose: *by subcutaneous injection*, according to requirements

COUNSELLING. Show container to patient and confirm that patient is expecting the version dispensed

■ Highly purified animal

Hypurin® Bovine Lente (CP) [PoM]
Injection, insulin zinc suspension (bovine, highly purified) 100 units/mL. Net price 10-mL vial = £18.48

Lentard MC® (Novo Nordisk) [PoM]
Injection, insulin zinc suspension (bovine and porcine, highly purified) 100 units/mL. Net price 10-mL vial = £5.78

■ Human sequence

Human Monotard® (Novo Nordisk) [PoM]
Injection, insulin zinc suspension (human, pyr) 100 units/mL. Net price 10-mL vial = £7.10

Humulin Lente® (Lilly) [PoM]
Injection, insulin zinc suspension (human, prb) 100 units/mL. Net price 10-mL vial = £12.50

INSULIN ZINC SUSPENSION (CRYSTALLINE)

(Cryst. I. Z. S.)
A sterile neutral suspension of bovine insulin or of human insulin in the form of a complex obtained by the addition of a suitable zinc salt; consists of rhombohedral crystals (10–40 microns)

Indications: diabetes mellitus (long acting)

Cautions: see under Soluble Insulin (section 6.1.1.1)

Side-effects: see under Soluble Insulin (section 6.1.1.1)

Dose: *by subcutaneous injection*, according to requirements

COUNSELLING. Show container to patient and confirm that patient is expecting the version dispensed

■ Human sequence

Human Ultratard® (Novo Nordisk) [PoM]
Injection, insulin zinc suspension, crystalline (human, pyr) 100 units/mL. Net price 10-mL vial = £7.10

Humulin Zn® (Lilly) [PoM]
Injection, insulin zinc suspension, crystalline (human, prb) 100 units/mL. Net price 10-mL vial = £12.50

ISOPHANE INSULIN

(Isophane Insulin Injection; Isophane Protamine Insulin Injection; Isophane Insulin (NPH))
A sterile suspension of bovine or porcine insulin or of human insulin in the form of a complex obtained by the addition of protamine sulphate or another suitable protamine

Indications: diabetes mellitus (intermediate acting)

Cautions: see under Soluble Insulin (section 6.1.1.1)

Side-effects: see under Soluble Insulin (section 6.1.1.1); protamine may cause allergic reactions

Dose: *by subcutaneous injection*, according to requirements

COUNSELLING. Show container to patient and confirm that patient is expecting the version dispensed

■ Highly purified animal

Hypurin® Bovine Isophane (CP) [PoM]
Injection, isophane insulin (bovine, highly purified) 100 units/mL. Net price 10-mL vial = £18.48; 5 × 1.5-mL cartridge = £13.86

Hypurin® Porcine Isophane (CP) [PoM]
Injection, isophane insulin (porcine, highly purified) 100 units/mL. Net price 10-mL vial = £16.80; 5 × 1.5-mL cartridge = £12.60

Pork Insulatard® (Novo Nordisk) [PoM]
Injection, isophane insulin (porcine, highly purified) 100 units/mL. Net price 10-mL vial = £6.58

■ Human sequence

Human Insulatard® ge (Novo Nordisk) [PoM]
Injection, isophane insulin (human, pyr) 100 units/mL. Net price 10-mL vial = £7.10; Penfill® cartridge (for Novopen® [NHS] devices) 5 × 1.5-mL = £9.87, 5 × 3-mL = £22.87; 5 × 3-mL prefilled disposable injection devices (range 2–78 units allowing 2-unit dosage adjustment) = £25.28

Humulin I® (Lilly) PoM
Injection, isophane insulin (human, prb) 100 units/
mL. Net price 10-mL vial = £12.50; 5 × 1.5-mL
cartridge (for *B-D Pen®* NHS) = £10.65; 5 × 3-
ml cartridge (for *B-D Pen®* 3 mL NHS or
HumaPen® NHS) = £21.30; 5 × 3-mL *Humaject
I®* prefilled disposable injection devices (range 2–
96 units, allowing 2-unit dosage adjustment) =
£26.33

■ Mixed preparations, see Biphasic Isophane
Insulin (below)

PROTAMINE ZINC INSULIN
(Protamine Zinc Insulin Injection)
A sterile suspension of insulin in the form of a complex
obtained by the addition of a suitable protamine and zinc
chloride; this preparation was included in BP 1980 but is
not included in BP 1988
Indications: diabetes mellitus (long acting)
Cautions: see under Soluble Insulin (section
6.1.1.1); see also notes above
Side-effects: see under Soluble Insulin (section
6.1.1.1); protamine may cause allergic reactions
Dose: *by subcutaneous injection*, according to
requirements
COUNSELLING. Show container to patient and confirm
that patient is expecting the version dispensed

Hypurin® Bovine Protamine Zinc (CP) PoM
Injection, protamine zinc insulin (bovine, highly
purified) 100 units/mL. Net price 10-mL vial =
£18.48

Biphasic insulins

BIPHASIC INSULIN LISPRO
Indications: diabetes mellitus (intermediate acting)
Cautions: see under Soluble Insulin (section
6.1.1.1)
Side-effects: see under Soluble Insulin (section
6.1.1.1); protamine may cause allergic reactions
Dose: *by subcutaneous injection*, according to
requirements
COUNSELLING. Show container to patient and confirm
that patient is expecting the version dispensed

Humalog® Mix25 (Lilly) ▼ PoM
Injection, biphasic insulin lispro (recombinant
human insulin analogue), 25% insulin lispro, 75%
insulin lispro protamine, 100 units/mL, net price
5 × 3-mL cartridge (for *B-D Pen®* 3 mL NHS or
Humapen® NHS) = £26.78; 5 × 3-mL prefilled
disposable injection devices = £29.62

BIPHASIC ISOPHANE INSULIN
(Biphasic Isophane Insulin Injection)
A sterile buffered suspension of either porcine or human
insulin complexed with protamine sulphate (or another
suitable protamine) in a solution of insulin of the same
species
Indications: diabetes mellitus (intermediate acting)
Cautions: see under Soluble Insulin (section
6.1.1.1)
Side-effects: see under Soluble Insulin (section
6.1.1.1); protamine may cause allergic reactions
Dose: *by subcutaneous injection*, according to
requirements
COUNSELLING. Show container to patient and confirm
that patient is expecting the version dispensed

■ Highly purified animal

**Hypurin® Porcine Biphasic Isophane 30/70
Mix** (CP) PoM
Injection, biphasic isophane insulin (porcine,
highly purified), 30% soluble, 70% isophane,
100 units/mL. Net price 10-mL vial = £16.80; 5 ×
1.5-ml cartridge = £12.60

Pork Mixtard 30® (Novo Nordisk) PoM
Injection, biphasic isophane insulin (porcine,
highly purified), 30% soluble, 70% isophane,
100 units/mL. Net price 10-mL vial = £6.58

■ Human sequence

Human Mixtard® 10 (Novo Nordisk) PoM
Injection, biphasic isophane insulin (human, pyr),
10% soluble, 90% isophane, 100 units/mL. Net
price *Penfill®* cartridge (for *Novopen®* NHS
devices) 5 × 1.5-mL = £9.87, 5 × 3-mL = £22.87;
5 × 3-mL prefilled disposable injection devices
(range 2–78 units, allowing 2-unit dosage adjustment) = £25.28

Human Mixtard® 20 (Novo Nordisk) PoM
Injection, biphasic isophane insulin (human, pyr),
20% soluble, 80% isophane, 100 units/mL. Net
price *Penfill®* cartridge (for *Novopen®* NHS
devices) 5 × 1.5-ml = £9.87, 5 × 3-mL = £22.87; 5
× 3-mL prefilled disposable injection devices
(range 2–78 units, allowing 2-unit dosage adjustment) = £25.28

Human Mixtard® 30 (Novo Nordisk) PoM
Injection, biphasic isophane insulin (human, pyr),
30% soluble, 70% isophane, 100 units/mL. Net
price *Penfill®* cartridge (for *Novopen®* NHS
devices) 5 × 1.5-mL = £9.87, 5 × 3-mL = £22.87;
5 × 3-mL prefilled disposable injection devices
(range 2–78 units, allowing 2-unit dosage adjustment) = £25.28

Human Mixtard® 30 ge (Novo Nordisk) PoM
Injection, biphasic isophane insulin (human, pyr),
30% soluble, 70% isophane, 100 units/mL. Net
price 10-mL vial = £7.10

Human Mixtard® 40 (Novo Nordisk) PoM
Injection, biphasic isophane insulin (human, pyr),
40% soluble, 60% isophane, 100 units/mL. Net
price *Penfill®* cartridge (for *Novopen®* NHS
devices) 5 × 1.5-mL = £9.87, 5 × 3-mL = £22.87;
5 × 3-mL prefilled disposable injection devices
(range 2–78 units, allowing 2-unit dosage adjustment) = £25.28

Human Mixtard® 50 (Novo Nordisk) PoM
Injection, biphasic isophane insulin (human, pyr),
50% soluble, 50% isophane, 100 units/mL. Net
price 10-mL vial = £7.10; *Penfill®* cartridge (for
Novopen® NHS devices) 5 × 1.5-mL = £9.87, 5
× 3-mL = £22.87; 5 × 3-mL prefilled disposable
injection devices (range 2–78 units, allowing 2-
unit dosage adjustment) = £25.28

Humulin M1® (Lilly) PoM
Injection, biphasic isophane insulin (human, prb),
10% soluble, 90% isophane, 100 units/mL. Net
price 10-mL vial = £12.50; 5 × 1.5-mL cartridge
(for *B-D Pen®* NHS) = £10.65; 5 × 3-mL cartridge (for *B-D Pen®* 3 mL NHS or
Humapen® NHS) = £21.30; 5 × 3-mL *Humaject
M1®* prefilled disposable injection devices (range
2–96 units, allowing 2-unit dosage adjustment) =
£26.33

Humulin M2® (Lilly) [PoM]

Injection, biphasic isophane insulin (human, prb), 20% soluble, 80% isophane, 100 units/mL. Net price 10-mL vial = £12.50; 5 × 1.5-mL cartridge (for *B-D Pen®* [NHS]) = £10.65; 5 × 3-mL cartridge (for *B-D Pen® 3 mL* [NHS] or *Humapen®* [NHS]) = £21.30; 5 × 3-mL *Humaject M2®* prefilled disposable injection devices (range 2–96 units, allowing 2-unit dosage adjustment) = £26.33

Humulin M3® (Lilly) [PoM]

Injection, biphasic isophane insulin (human, prb), 30% soluble, 70% isophane, 100 units/mL. Net price 10-mL vial = £12.50; 5 × 1.5-mL cartridge (for *B-D Pen®* [NHS]) = £10.65; 5 × 3-mL cartridge (for *B-D Pen® 3 mL* [NHS] or *Humapen®* [NHS]) = £21.30; 5 × 3-mL *Humaject M3®* prefilled disposable injection devices (range 2–96 units, allowing 2-unit dosage adjustment) = £26.33

Humulin M4® (Lilly) [PoM]

Injection, biphasic isophane insulin (human, prb), 40% soluble, 60% isophane, 100 units/mL. Net price 10-mL vial = £12.50; 5 × 1.5-mL cartridge (for *B-D Pen®* [NHS]) = £10.65; 5 × 3-mL cartridge (for *B-D Pen® 3 mL* [NHS] or *Humapen®* [NHS]) = £21.30; 5 × 3-mL *Humaject M4®* prefilled disposable injection devices (range 2–96 units, allowing 2-unit dosage adjustment) = £26.33

Humulin M5® (Lilly) [PoM]

Injection, biphasic isophane insulin (human, prb), 50% soluble, 50% isophane, 100 units/mL. Net price 10-mL vial = £12.50; 5 × 1.5-mL cartridge (for *B-D Pen®* [NHS]) = £10.65

6.1.1.3   Hypodermic equipment

Patients should be advised on the safe disposal of lancets, single-use syringes, and needles. Suitable arrangements for the safe disposal of contaminated waste must be made before these products are prescribed for patients who are carriers of infectious diseases.

■ Injection devices

Autopen® (Owen Mumford) [NHS]

Injection device, for use with Lilly and Novo Nordisk 1.5-mL insulin cartridges; allows adjustment of dosage in multiples of 1 unit, max. 16 units (single unit version); 2 units, max. 32 units (2-unit version). Net price (both) = £17.76

B-D Pen® (Becton Dickinson) [NHS]

Injection devices, for use with Lilly insulin cartridges; *B-D Pen®* (for 1.5-mL cartridges) allows adjustment of dosage in multiples of 1 unit, max. 30 units, net price = £23.86 (also available from clinics); *B-D Pen® 3 mL* (for 3-mL cartridges) allows adjustment of dosage in multiples of 1 unit, max. 69 units, net price = £28.00 (available only from clinics)

HumaPen® (Lilly) [NHS]

Injection device for use with *Humulin®* and *Humalog®* 3-mL cartridges; allows adjustment of dosage in multiples of 1 unit, max. 60 units (available free of charge from Lilly)

NovoPen® (Novo Nordisk) [NHS]

Injection devices, for use with *Penfill®* insulin cartridges; allows adjustment of dosage in multiples of 1 unit, max. 40 units (*NovoPen® 1.5 Classic* or *Fun*) *or* 1 unit, max. 70 units (*NovoPen® 3 Classic* or *Fun*). Available only from clinics

■ Lancets— sterile, single use

Type A (Drug Tariff). Cylindrical mount fluted longitudinally; compatible with *B-D Lancer®* [NHS] (Becton Dickinson), *Glucolet®* [NHS] (Bayer Diagnostics), *Monojector®* [NHS] (Kendall), *Penlet®* [NHS] II (Lifescan) and *Soft Touch®* [NHS] (Roche Diagnostics) finger-pricking devices

Available from Bayer (*Baylet®*, net price 100-lancet pack = £3.25; 200-lancet pack = £6.20), Becton Dickinson (*B-D Microfine®* +, net price 200-lancet pack = £6.13), Gainor Medical (*Cleanlet®* 25, net price 100-lancet pack = £3.19; 200-lancet pack = £6.08), Kendall (*Monolet®*, net price 100-lancet pack = £3.28; 200-lancet pack = £6.24; *Monolet Extra®*, net price 100-lancet pack = £3.28), Owen Mumford (*Unilet G® Superlite* net price 100-lancet pack = £3.17; 200-lancet pack = £6.01; *Unilet® Universal ComforTouch*, net price 100-lancet pack = £3.17; 200-lancet pack = £6.01)

Type B (Drug Tariff). Cylindrical mount with concentric ribs; compatible with *Autolet®* [NHS] (Owen Mumford) and *Glucolet®* [NHS] (Bayer Diagnostics) finger-pricking devices

Available from Bayer Diagnostics (*Ames®*, net price 100-lancet pack = £3.25; 200-lancet pack = £6.20), Gainor Medical (*Cleanlet® 25XL*, net price 100-lancet pack = £3.19; 200-lancet pack = £6.08), Owen Mumford (*Unilet® Superlite*, net price 100-lancet pack = £3.17; 200-lancet pack = £6.01; *Unilet® Universal ComferTouch*, net price 100-lancet pack = £3.17; 200-lancet pack = £6.01)

■ Needles

Hypodermic Needle , Sterile single use (Drug Tariff). For use with re-usable glass syringe, sizes 0.5 mm (25G), 0.45 mm (26G), 0.4 mm (27G). Net price 100-needle pack = £2.28

Available from Becton Dickinson (*Microlance®*), Kendall (*Monoject®*)

Needle Clipping (Chopping) Device (Drug Tariff). Consisting of a clipper to remove needle from its hub and container from which cut-off needles cannot be retrieved; designed to hold 1200 needles, not suitable for use with lancets. Net price = £1.12

Available from Becton Dickinson (*B-D Safe-clip®*)

■ Syringes

Hypodermic Syringe (Drug Tariff). Calibrated glass with Luer taper conical fitting, for use with U100 insulin. Net price 0.5 mL and 1 mL = £13.71

Available from Rand Rocket (*Abcare®*)

Pre-Set U100 Insulin Syringe (Drug Tariff). Calibrated glass with Luer taper conical fitting, supplied with dosage chart and strong box, for blind patients. Net price 1 mL = £20.87

Available from Rand Rocket

U100 Insulin Syringe with Needle (Drug Tariff). Disposable with fixed or separate needle for single use or single patient-use, colour coded orange, 0.45 mm (26G), 0.4 mm (27G), 0.36 mm (28G), 0.33 mm (29G). Net price 10 (with needle) , 0.3 mL = £1.24; 0.5 mL = £1.19; 1 mL = £1.20

Available from Becton Dickinson (*B-D Micro-Fine®* +, *Plastipak®*), Braun (*Omnikan®*), Codan (*Insupak®*), Kendall (*Monoject® Ultra*), Rand Rocket (*Clinipak®*)

6.1.2   Oral antidiabetic drugs

6.1.2.1   Sulphonylureas
6.1.2.2   Biguanides
6.1.2.3   Other antidiabetics

Oral antidiabetic drugs are used for non-insulin-dependent (type 2) diabetes; they should not be prescribed until patients have been shown not to respond adequately to at least three months' restriction of energy and carbohydrate intake and an increase in physical activity. They should be used to augment the effect of diet and exercise, and not to replace them.

6.1.2.1   Sulphonylureas

The sulphonylureas act mainly by augmenting insulin secretion and consequently are effective only when some residual pancreatic beta-cell activity is present; during long-term administration they also have an extrapancreatic action. All may cause hypoglycaemia but this is uncommon and usually indicates excessive dosage. Sulphonylurea-induced hypoglycaemia may persist for many hours and must always be treated in hospital.

Several sulphonylureas are available and choice is determined by side-effects and the duration of action as well as the patient's age and renal function. The long-acting sulphonylureas **chlorpropamide** and **glibenclamide** are associated with a greater risk of hypoglycaemia; for this reason they should be avoided in the elderly and shorter-acting alternatives, such as **gliclazide** or **tolbutamide**, should be used instead. Chlorpropamide also has more side-effects than the other sulphonylureas (see below) and therefore it is no longer recommended.

CAUTIONS AND CONTRA-INDICATIONS. Sulphonylureas can encourage weight gain and should be prescribed only if poor control and symptoms persist despite adequate attempts at dieting; metformin (section 6.1.2.2) should be considered in obese patients. Sulphonylureas should not be used during breast-feeding, and caution is needed in the elderly and those with hepatic and renal insufficiency because of the hazard of hypoglycaemia. The short-acting tolbutamide may be used in renal impairment, as may gliquidone and gliclazide which are principally metabolised and inactivated in the liver but careful monitoring of blood-glucose concentration is essential; care is required to choose the smallest possible dose that produces adequate control of blood glucose. Sulphonylureas should be avoided in porphyria (section 9.8.2).

Insulin therapy should be instituted temporarily during intercurrent illness (such as myocardial infarction, coma, infection, and trauma). Oral antidiabetic drugs should be omitted on the morning of surgery; insulin is often required because of the ensuing hyperglycaemia in these circumstances. Insulin therapy is also substituted during pregnancy (see also Appendix 4). Sulphonylureas are contra-indicated in the presence of ketoacidosis.

SIDE-EFFECTS. Side-effects of sulphonylureas are generally mild and infrequent and include gastro-intestinal disturbances and headache.

Chlorpropamide has appreciably more side-effects, mainly because of its very prolonged duration of action and the consequent hazard of hypoglycaemia. It may also cause facial flushing after drinking alcohol; this effect does not normally occur with other sulphonylureas. Chlorpropamide may also enhance antidiuretic hormone and very rarely cause hyponatraemia.

Sensitivity reactions (usually in first 6–8 weeks of therapy) include transient rashes, which rarely progress to erythema multiforme and exfoliative dermatitis, fever, and jaundice; photosensitivity has also rarely been reported with chlorpropamide. Blood disorders are rare too but include thrombocytopenia, agranulocytosis, and aplastic anaemia.

CHLORPROPAMIDE ◼

Indications: diabetes mellitus (for use in diabetes insipidus, see section 6.5.2)

Cautions: see notes above; **interactions:** Appendix 1 (antidiabetics)

Contra-indications: see notes above

Side-effects: see notes above

Dose: initially 250 mg daily (elderly patients 100–125 mg but avoid—see notes above), adjusted according to response; max. 500 mg daily; taken with breakfast

Chlorpropamide (Non-proprietary) [PoM] ◼
Tablets, chlorpropamide 100 mg, net price 20 = 36p; 250 mg, 20 = 43p. Label: 4
Available from APS, Regent, Sussex

> ◼ denotes preparations that are considered to be less suitable for prescribing (see p. vi)

GLIBENCLAMIDE

Indications: diabetes mellitus

Cautions: see notes above; **interactions:** Appendix 1 (antidiabetics)

Contra-indications: see notes above

Side-effects: see notes above

Dose: initially 5 mg daily (elderly patients 2.5 mg, but see also notes above), adjusted according to response; max. 15 mg daily; taken with breakfast

Glibenclamide (Non-proprietary) [PoM]
Tablets, glibenclamide 2.5 mg, net price 28-tab pack = £1.63; 5 mg, 20 = 75p
Available from APS, Ashbourne (*Diabetamide®*), Berk (*Calabren®*), Cox, CP, Generics, Hillcross, Kent (*Gliken®*), Norton

Daonil® (Hoechst Marion Roussel) [PoM]
Tablets, scored, glibenclamide 5 mg. Net price 28-tab pack = £2.63

Semi-Daonil® (Hoechst Marion Roussel) [PoM]
Tablets, scored, glibenclamide 2.5 mg. Net price 28-tab pack = £1.58

Euglucon® (Hoechst Marion Roussel) [PoM]
Tablets, glibenclamide 2.5 mg, net price 28-tab pack = £1.58; 5 mg (scored), 28-tab pack = £2.63

GLICLAZIDE

Indications: diabetes mellitus

Cautions: see notes above; **interactions:** Appendix 1 (antidiabetics)

Contra-indications: see notes above

Side-effects: see notes above

Dose: initially, 40–80 mg daily, adjusted according to response; up to 160 mg as a single dose, with breakfast; higher doses divided; max. 320 mg daily

Gliclazide (Non-proprietary) [PoM]
Tablets, scored, gliclazide 80 mg, net price 28-tab pack = £3.41, 60-tab pack = £7.67
Available from APS, Cox, Dominion, Generics (*DIAGLYK®*), Genus, Hillcross, Norton

Diamicron® (Servier) [PoM]
Tablets, scored, gliclazide 80 mg, net price 60-tab pack = £7.00

GLIMEPIRIDE

Indications: diabetes mellitus

Cautions: see notes above; regular hepatic and haematological monitoring; **interactions:** Appendix 1 (antidiabetics)

Contra-indications: see notes above; severe liver impairment (Appendix 2); severe renal impairment (Appendix 3); pregnancy (toxicity in *animal* studies; see also Appendix 4) and breast-feeding

Side-effects: see notes above; increase in liver enzymes and deterioration of liver function with cholestasis, icterus and hepatitis; severe hypersensitivity reactions and allergic vasculitis reported; decrease in plasma-sodium concentration

Dose: initially 1 mg daily, adjusted according to response in 1-mg steps at 1–2 week intervals; usual max. 4 mg daily (exceptionally, up to 6 mg daily may be used); taken shortly before or with first main meal

Note. If changing from other oral hypoglycaemic drugs, the strength and half-life of the previous drug must be taken into account and, if necessary, a washout period of a few days between drugs should be considered to minimise the risk of hypoglycaemia

Amaryl® (Hoechst Marion Roussel) ▼ PoM
Tablets, all scored, glimepiride 1 mg (pink), net price 30-tab pack = £4.90; 2 mg (green) 30-tab pack = £8.05; 3 mg (yellow) 30-tab pack = £12.15; 4 mg (blue) 30-tab pack = £16.10

GLIPIZIDE

Indications: diabetes mellitus

Cautions: see notes above; **interactions:** Appendix 1 (antidiabetics)

Contra-indications: see notes above

Side-effects: see notes above; dizziness, drowsiness

Dose: initially 2.5–5 mg daily, adjusted according to response; max. 20 mg daily; up to 15 mg may be given as a single dose before breakfast; higher doses divided

Glipizide (Non-proprietary) PoM
Tablets, glipizide 2.5 mg, net price 28-tab pack = £1.55; 5 mg, 56-tab pack = £4.07
Available from Cox, Hillcross, Norton

Glibenese® (Pfizer) PoM
Tablets, scored, glipizide 5 mg. Net price 56-tab pack = £3.63

Minodiab® (Pharmacia & Upjohn) PoM
Tablets, glipizide 2.5 mg, net price 28-tab pack = £1.48; 5 mg (scored), 28-tab pack = £1.58

GLIQUIDONE

Indications: diabetes mellitus

Cautions: see notes above; **interactions:** Appendix 1 (antidiabetics)

Contra-indications: see notes above

Side-effects: see notes above

Dose: initially 15 mg daily before breakfast, adjusted to 45–60 mg daily in 2 or 3 divided doses; max. single dose 60 mg, max. daily dose 180 mg

Glurenorm® (Sanofi-Synthelabo) PoM
Tablets, scored, gliquidone 30 mg. Net price 100-tab pack = £17.54

TOLAZAMIDE

Indications: diabetes mellitus

Cautions: see notes above; **interactions:** Appendix 1 (antidiabetics)

Contra-indications: see notes above

Side-effects: see notes above

Dose: initially 100–250 mg daily with breakfast adjusted according to response; max. 1 g daily; higher doses divided

Tolanase® (Pharmacia & Upjohn) PoM
Tablets, both scored, tolazamide 100 mg, net price 100-tab pack = £5.40; 250 mg, 100-tab pack = £11.74

TOLBUTAMIDE

Indications: diabetes mellitus

Cautions: see notes above; **interactions:** Appendix 1 (antidiabetics)

Contra-indications: see notes above

Side-effects: see notes above

Dose: 0.5–1.5 g (max. 2 g) daily in divided doses (see notes above)

Tolbutamide (Non-proprietary) PoM
Tablets, tolbutamide 500 mg. Net price 20 = 84p
Available from APS, Cox, CP, Hillcross, Sovereign

6.1.2.2   Biguanides

Metformin, the only available biguanide, has a different mode of action from the sulphonylureas, and is not interchangeable with them. It exerts its effect mainly by decreasing gluconeogenesis and by increasing peripheral utilisation of glucose; since it acts only in the presence of endogenous insulin it is effective only in diabetics with some residual functioning pancreatic islet cells.

Metformin is the drug of first choice in obese patients in whom strict dieting has failed to control diabetes. It is also used when diabetes is inadequately controlled with sulphonylurea treatment. When the combination of strict diet and metformin treatment fails other options which may be considered include:

- combining with acarbose (section 6.1.2.3), which may have a small beneficial effect, but flatulence can be a problem;
- combining with insulin (section 6.1.1) but weight gain and hypoglycaemia can be problems;
- combining with a sulphonylurea (section 6.1.2.1) (reports of increased hazard with this combination are at present unconfirmed).

Repaglinide (section 6.1.2.3) may be given with metformin if metformin alone does not control the diabetes adequately.

Insulin treatment is almost always required in medical and surgical emergencies; insulin should also be substituted before elective surgery (omit metformin on morning of surgery and give insulin if required).

Hypoglycaemia is not a problem with metformin; other advantages are the lower incidence of weight gain and lower plasma-insulin concentration. It does not exert a hypoglycaemic action in non-diabetic subjects unless given in overdose.

Gastro-intestinal side-effects are initially common with metformin, and may persist in some patients, particularly when very high doses such as 3 g daily are given.

Metformin may provoke lactic acidosis which is most likely to occur in patients with renal impairment; it should not be used in patients with even mild renal impairment. Metformin should also be avoided (or discontinued) in other situations which might predispose to lactic acidosis, e.g. severe dehydration, infection, shock, severe heart failure, myocardial infarction, hepatic impairment, alcohol dependency, use of x-ray contrast media, pregnancy and breast-feeding.

METFORMIN HYDROCHLORIDE

Indications: diabetes mellitus (see notes above)
Cautions: see notes above; **interactions:** Appendix 1 (antidiabetics)
Contra-indications: hepatic or renal impairment (withdraw if renal impairment suspected), predisposition to lactic acidosis, heart failure, severe infection or trauma, dehydration, alcohol dependence; pregnancy, breast-feeding
Side-effects: anorexia, nausea, vomiting, diarrhoea (usually transient), lactic acidosis (withdraw treatment), decreased vitamin-B_{12} absorption
Dose: 500 mg every 8 hours *or* 850 mg every 12 hours with or after food; max. 3 g daily in divided doses though most physicians limit this to 2 g daily (see notes above)

Metformin (Non-proprietary) PoM
Tablets, coated, metformin hydrochloride 500 mg, net price 20 = 51p; 850 mg, 56-tab pack = £2.15. Label: 21
Available from APS, Cox, CP, Hillcross, Norton, Opus (Glucamet®), Sovereign

Glucophage® (Lipha) PoM
Tablets, f/c, metformin hydrochloride 500 mg, net price 84-tab pack = £2.00; 850 mg, 56-tab pack = £2.22. Label: 21

6.1.2.3   Other antidiabetics

Acarbose, an inhibitor of intestinal alpha glucosidases, delays the digestion and absorption of starch and sucrose. It has a small but significant effect in lowering blood glucose and is used either on its own or as an adjunct to metformin or to sulphonylureas when they prove inadequate. Postprandial hyperglycaemia in insulin-dependent diabetes can be reduced by acarbose, but it has been little used for this purpose. Flatulence deters some from using acarbose although this side-effect tends to decrease with time.

Guar gum, if taken in adequate quantities, results in some reduction of postprandial plasma-glucose concentrations in diabetes mellitus, probably by retarding carbohydrate absorption. It is also used to relieve symptoms of the dumping syndrome.

Repaglinide stimulates insulin release. It has a rapid onset of action and short duration of activity and is administered shortly before a meal; the dose is omitted if the meal is missed. Repaglinide is indicated for non-insulin dependent diabetes which is inadequately controlled by diet and exercise; it can also be given with metformin if metformin alone does not control the diabetes adequately.

ACARBOSE

Indications: diabetes mellitus inadequately controlled by diet or by diet with oral hypoglycaemic agents
Cautions: monitor hepatic transaminase levels (higher doses); may enhance hypoglycaemic effects of insulin and sulphonylureas (hypoglycaemic episodes may be treated with oral glucose but not with sucrose); **interactions:** Appendix 1 (antidiabetics)
Contra-indications: pregnancy and breast-feeding; inflammatory bowel disease (e.g. ulcerative colitis, Crohn's disease), partial intestinal obstruction (or predisposition); hepatic impairment, severe renal impairment; hernia, history of abdominal surgery
Side-effects: flatulence, soft stools, diarrhoea (may need to reduce dose or withdraw), abdominal distention and pain; rarely abnormal liver function tests and skin reactions; jaundice and hepatitis reported
Note. Antacids not recommended for treating side-effects (unlikely to be beneficial)
Dose: 50 mg daily initially (to minimise side-effects) increased to 50 mg 3 times daily, then increased if necessary after 6–8 weeks to 100 mg 3 times daily; max. 200 mg 3 times daily; CHILD under 12 years not recommended
COUNSELLING. The tablets should either be chewed with first mouthful of food or swallowed whole with a little liquid immediately before food. In order to counteract possible hypoglycaemia, patients receiving insulin or a sulphonylurea as well as acarbose need to carry glucose (not sucrose—acarbose interferes with sucrose absorption)

Glucobay® (Bayer) PoM
Tablets, acarbose 50 mg, net price 90-tab pack = £9.68; 100 mg (scored). 90-tab pack = £12.51. Counselling, administration

GUAR GUM

Indications: see notes above
Cautions: maintain adequate fluid intake; **interactions:** Appendix 1 (guar gum)
COUNSELLING. Preparations that swell in contact with liquid should always be carefully swallowed with water and should not be taken immediately before going to bed.
Contra-indications: gastro-intestinal obstruction
Side-effects: flatulence, abdominal distension, intestinal obstruction

Guarem® (Rybar)
Granules, ivory, sugar-free, guar gum 5 g/sachet, net price 50 sachets = £8.70; 100 sachets = £15.67. Label: 13, counselling, administration
Dose: 5 g stirred into 200 mL fluid 3 times daily immediately before main meals (or sprinkled on food and eaten accompanied by 200 mL fluid)

REPAGLINIDE

Indications: diabetes mellitus (as monotherapy or in combination with metformin)
Cautions: substitute insulin during intercurrent illness (such as myocardial infarction, coma, infection, and trauma) and during surgery; renal

impairment (Appendix 3); **interactions:** Appendix 1 (repaglinide)

Contra-indications: diabetic ketoacidosis; severe renal or hepatic impairment; pregnancy (Appendix 4) and breast-feeding

Side-effects: abdominal pain, diarrhoea, constipation, nausea, vomiting; hypersensitivity reactions including rashes and urticaria; elevated liver enzymes

Dose: initially 500 micrograms within 30 minutes before main meals (1 mg if transferring from another oral hypoglycaemic), adjusted according to response at intervals of 1–2 weeks; up to 4 mg may be given as a single dose, max. 16 mg daily CHILD and ADOLESCENT under 18 years and ELDERLY over 75 years, not recommended

NovoNorm® (Novo Nordisk) ▼ PoM
Tablets, repaglinide 500 micrograms, net price 30-tab pack = £5.86, 90-tab pack = £17.57; 1 mg (yellow), 30-tab pack = £6.33, 90-tab pack = £18.98; 2 mg (red), 90-tab pack = £20.40

6.1.3   Diabetic ketoacidosis

Soluble insulin, the only form of insulin that may be given intravenously, is used in the management of diabetic ketoacidotic and hyperosmolar non-ketotic coma. It is preferable to use the type of soluble insulin that the patient has been using previously. It is necessary to achieve and to maintain an adequate plasma-insulin concentration until the metabolic disturbance is brought under control.

Insulin is best given by intravenous infusion, using an infusion pump, and diluted to 1 unit/mL (care in mixing, see Appendix 6). Adequate plasma-insulin concentration can usually be maintained with infusion rates of 6 units/hour for adults and 0.1 units/kg/hour for children. Blood glucose is expected to decrease by about 5 mmol/litre/hour; if the response is inadequate the infusion rate can be doubled or quadrupled. When the plasma glucose has fallen to 10 mmol/litre the infusion rate can be reduced to 3 units/hour for adults (about 0.02 units/kg/hour for children) and continued until the patient is ready to take food by mouth. The insulin infusion should not be stopped before subcutaneous insulin has been started.

No matter how large, a bolus intravenous injection of insulin can provide an adequate plasma concentration for a short time only; therefore if facilities for intravenous infusion are not available the insulin is given by *intramuscular injection.* An initial loading dose of 20 units intramuscularly is followed by 6 units intramuscularly every hour until the plasma-glucose concentration falls to 10 mmol/litre; intramuscular injections are then given every 2 hours. Although absorption of insulin is usually rapid after intramuscular injection, it may be impaired in the presence of hypotension and poor tissue perfusion; moreover insulin may accumulate during treatment and late hypoglycaemia should be watched for and treated appropriately.

Intravenous replacement of fluid and electrolytes (section 9.2.2) with **sodium chloride** intravenous infusion is an essential part of the management of ketoacidosis; **potassium chloride** is included in the infusion as appropriate to prevent the hypokalaemia induced by the insulin. **Sodium bicarbonate** infu-

sion (1.26% or 2.74%) is used only in cases of extreme acidosis and shock since the acid-base disturbance is normally corrected by the insulin. **Glucose** solution (5%) is infused once the blood glucose has decreased below 10 mmol/litre but insulin infusion must continue.

6.1.4   Treatment of hypoglycaemia

Initially glucose 10–20 g is given by mouth either in liquid form or as granulated sugar or sugar lumps. Glucose 10 g is available from 2 teaspoons sugar, 3 sugar lumps, *Hypostop*® *Gel* (glucose 10 g/23-g oral ampoule, available from Bio Diagnostics), milk 200 mL, and non-diet versions of *Lucozade*® *Sparkling Glucose Drink* 50–55 mL, *Coca-Cola*® 90 mL, *Ribena*® *Original* 15 mL (to be diluted). If necessary this may be repeated in 10–15 minutes.

If hypoglycaemia causes unconsciousness, 25–50 mL of **glucose intravenous infusion 50%** (section 9.2.2) should be given intravenously into a large vein through a large-gauge needle; care is required since this concentration is highly irritant especially if extravasation occurs. Glucose intravenous infusion 10% or 20% may be used but larger volumes are required.

Glucagon can be given as an alternative to parenteral glucose in hypoglycaemia. It is a polypeptide hormone produced by the alpha cells of the islets of Langerhans. Its action is to increase plasma-glucose concentration by mobilising glycogen stored in the liver. It can be injected by any route (intramuscular, subcutaneous, or intravenous) in a dose of 1 mg (1 unit) in circumstances when an intravenous injection of glucose would be difficult or impossible to administer. It may be issued to close relatives of insulin-treated patients for emergency use in hypoglycaemic attacks. It is often advisable to prescribe on an 'if necessary' basis to hospitalised insulin-treated patients, so that it may be given rapidly by the nurses during an hypoglycaemic emergency. If not effective in 10 minutes intravenous glucose should be given.

GLUCAGON

Indications: see notes above and under Dose

Cautions: see notes above, insulinoma, glucagonoma; ineffective in chronic hypoglycaemia, starvation, and adrenal insufficiency

Contra-indications: phaeochromocytoma

Side-effects: nausea, vomiting, diarrhoea, hypokalaemia, rarely hypersensitivity reactions

Dose: *by subcutaneous, intramuscular, or intravenous injection,* ADULT and CHILD over 25 kg, 1 unit; CHILD under 25 kg, 0.5 unit; if no response within 10 minutes intravenous glucose must be given
Diagnostic aid, consult product literature
Beta-blocker poisoning, see p. 23
Note. 1 unit of glucagon = 1 mg of glucagon or glucagon hydrochloride

GlucaGen® (Novo Nordisk) PoM
Injection, powder for reconstitution, glucagon (rys) as hydrochloride with lactose, net price 1-mg vial with prefilled syringe containing water for injection (*GlucaGen*® *Kit*) = £19.95

Chronic hypoglycaemia

Diazoxide, administered by mouth, is useful in the management of patients with chronic hypoglycaemia from excess endogenous insulin secretion, either from an islet cell tumour or islet cell hyperplasia. It has no place in the management of acute hypoglycaemia.

DIAZOXIDE

Indications: chronic intractable hypoglycaemia (for use in hypertensive crisis see section 2.5.1)

Cautions: ischaemic heart disease, pregnancy, labour, impaired renal function; haematological examinations and blood pressure monitoring required during prolonged treatment; growth, bone, and developmental checks in children; **interactions:** Appendix 1 (diazoxide)

Side-effects: anorexia, nausea, vomiting, hyperuricaemia, hypotension, oedema, tachycardia, arrhythmias, extrapyramidal effects; hypertrichosis on prolonged treatment

Dose: *by mouth*, ADULT and CHILD, initially 5 mg/ kg daily in 2–3 divided doses

Eudemine® (Medeva) [PoM]
Tablets, diazoxide 50 mg. Net price 20 = £7.68

6.1.5 Treatment of diabetic nephropathy and neuropathy

Diabetic nephropathy

Regular review of diabetic patients should include an annual test for urinary protein (using *Albustix®*). If this test is negative, the urine should be tested for microalbuminuria (the earliest sign of nephropathy). If reagent strip tests (*Micral-Test®* [NHS]) are used and prove positive, the result should be confirmed by a laboratory analysis of an overnight or 24-hour urine sample. All diabetic patients with nephropathy causing albuminuria and all insulin-dependent patients with establised microalbuminuria (at least 3 positive tests) should be treated with an ACE inhibitor (section 2.5.5.1) even if the blood pressure is normal; in any case, to minimise the risk of renal deterioration, blood pressure should be carefully controlled (section 2.5).

ACE inhibitors may potentiate the hypoglycaemic effect of insulin and oral antidiabetic drugs; this effect is more likely during the first weeks of combined treatment and in patients with renal impairment.

For the treatment of hypertension in diabetes, see section 2.5.

Diabetic neuropathy

Note. Several recommendations in this section involve non-licensed indications

Optimal diabetic control is beneficial for the management of *painful neuropathy*. Most patients should be treated with insulin, and relief can probably be accelerated by continuous insulin infusion. **Non-opioid analgesics** such as aspirin and paracetamol (section 4.7.1) are indicated for pain. Relief

may also be obtained with the **tricyclic antidepressants**, amitriptyline, imipramine, and nortriptyline (section 4.3.1) with or without a low dose of a **phenothiazine** (section 4.2). **Carbamazepine** (section 4.8.1) or mexiletine may be useful. **Capsaicin** applied topically as a cream (section 10.3.2) is now licenced for painful diabetic neuropathy and may have some effect, but it produces an intense burning sensation during the initial treatment period.

In *autonomic neuropathy* diabetic diarrhoea can often be aborted by 2 or 3 doses of **tetracycline** 250 mg (section 5.1.3). Otherwise **codeine phosphate** (section 1.4.2) is the best drug, but other antidiarrhoeal preparations can be tried. **Anti-emetics** or **cisapride** may control vomiting in gastroparesis. In the rare cases where they do not, erythromycin (especially when given intravenously) has been shown to be of benefit but further studies are needed. (**Important**: erythromycin and cisapride must not be given together—risk of dangerous arrhythmias).

In *neuropathic postural hypotension* an increased salt intake and the use of the **mineralocorticoid** fludrocortisone 100 to 400 micrograms daily (section 6.3.1) help by increasing plasma volume but uncomfortable oedema is a common side-effect. Fludrocortisone can also be combined with **flurbiprofen** (section 10.1.1) and **ephedrine hydrochloride** (section 3.1.1.2).

Gustatory sweating can be treated with **antimuscarinics** such as propantheline bromide (section 1.2); side-effects are common. In some patients with *neuropathic oedema*, **ephedrine hydrochloride** 30 to 60 mg 3 times daily offers impressive relief.

6.1.6 Diagnostic and monitoring agents for diabetes mellitus

Blood glucose monitoring

Blood glucose monitoring gives a direct measure of the glucose concentration at the time of the test and can detect hypoglycaemia as well as hyperglycaemia. Patients should be properly trained in the use of blood glucose monitoring systems and to take appropriate action on the results obtained. Inadequate understanding of the normal fluctuations in blood glucose may lead to confusion and inappropriate action. It is ideal for patients to observe the 'peaks' and 'troughs' of blood glucose over 24 hours and make adjustments of their insulin no more than once or twice weekly. Daily alterations to the insulin dose are highly undesirable (except during illness).

Blood glucose monitoring is best carried out by means of a meter. Visual colour comparison is often used but is much less satisfactory. Meters give a more precise reading and are useful for patients with poor eyesight or who are colour blind.

Note. In the UK blood-glucose concentration is expressed in mmol/litre and the British Diabetic Association advises that these units should be used for self-monitoring of blood glucose. In other European countries units of mg/100 mL (or mg/dL) are commonly used.

It is advisable to check that the meter is pre-set in the correct units.

■ Test strips

Biocare Glucose VT® (Biocare)
Reagent strips, for blood glucose monitoring, visual range (1.1–44.4 mmol/litre). Net price 50-strip pack = £8.50

BM-Accutest® (Roche Diagnostics)
Reagent strips, for blood glucose monitoring, range (1.1–33.3 mmol/litre), for use with *Accutrend®* [NHS] meters only. Net price 50-strip pack = £14.06

BM-Test 1–44® (Roche Diagnostics)
Reagent strips, for blood glucose monitoring, visual range (1–44 mmol/litre) meter range (0.5–27.7 mmol/litre), suitable for use with *Reflolux® S* [NHS]. Net price 50-strip pack = £14.81

Easistix® BG (Eastern)
Reagent strips, for blood glucose monitoring, visual range (0.5–28 mmol/litre). Net price 50-strip pack = £12.00

Esprit® Biosensor (Bayer Diagnostics)
Sensor discs, for blood glucose monitoring, range (0.6–33.3 mmol/L), for use with *Esprit®* [NHS] meter only. Net price 5 × 10-disc pack = £14.27

ExacTech® (MediSense)
Biosensor strips, for blood glucose monitoring, range (2.2–25 mmol/litre), for use with *ExacTech®* [NHS] meter only. Net price 50-strip pack = £13.96

Glucostix® (Bayer Diagnostics)
Reagent strips, for blood glucose monitoring, visual range (1–44 mmol/litre), meter range (2–22 mmol/litre), suitable for use with *Glucometer® GX* [NHS]. Net price 50-strip pack = £14.81

Glucotide® (Bayer Diagnostics)
Reagent strips, for blood glucose monitoring, range (0.6–33.3 mmol/litre), for use with *Glucometer® 4* [NHS] meter only. Net price 50-strip pack = £14.08

Glucotrend® (Roche Diagnostics)
Reagent strips, for blood glucose monitoring, range (0.6–33.3 mmol/litre), for use with *Glucotrend®* [NHS] and *Glucotrend® Premium* [NHS] meters only. Net price 50-strip pack = £14.51

Hypoguard® Supreme (Hypoguard)
Reagent strips, for blood glucose monitoring, range (2.2–27.7 mmol/litre), for use with *Hypoguard® Supreme Petit* [NHS] meter. Net price 50-strip pack = £12.95

MediSense G2® (MediSense)
Sensor strips, for blood glucose monitoring, range (1.1–33.3 mmol/litre) for use with *MediSense Card®* [NHS] or *MediSense Pen®* [NHS] meters only. Net price 50-strip pack = £13.42

Medi-Test® Glycaemie C (BHR)
Reagent strips, for blood glucose monitoring, visual range (1.1–44.4 mmol/litre), meter range (1.1–33.3 mmol/litre), suitable for use with *Glycotronic® C* [NHS] meter. Net price 50-strip pack = £13.21

One Touch® (LifeScan)
Reagent strips, for blood glucose monitoring, range (0–33.3 mmol/litre), for use with *One Touch® II*, *Profile* and *Basic* [NHS] meters only. Net price 50-strip pack = £14.11

■ Meters

Accutrend® (Roche Diagnostics) [NHS]
Meters for blood glucose monitoring for use with *BM-Accutest®* test strips. *Accutrend* = £34.00, *Accutrend Alpha* = £29.00

Esprit® (Bayer Diagnostics) [NHS]
Meter for blood glucose monitoring (for use with *Esprit® Biosensor* test sensor discs) = £17.49

ExacTech® (MediSense) [NHS]
Meters (Sensor) for blood glucose monitoring for use with *ExacTech®* test strips. *ExacTech Card* = £59.00, *ExacTech Card* starter pack = £69.00

Glucometer® (Bayer Diagnostics) [NHS]
Meters for blood glucose monitoring, *Glucometer 4* (for use with *Glucotide®* test strips) = £35.00; *Glucometer GX* (for use with *Glucostix®* test strips) = £29.00

Glucotrend® (Roche Diagnostics) [NHS]
Meters for blood glucose monitoring (for use with *Glucotrend®* test strips). *Glucotrend® Soft Test System* pack [NHS] = £29.00; *Glucotrend® Premium* meter only = £29.00; *Glucotrend® Premium* pack [NHS] = £49.00

Glycotronic® C (BHR) [NHS]
Meter for blood glucose monitoring (for use with *Medi-Test® Glycaemic C* test strips) = £40.00

Hypoguard® Supreme Petit (Hypoguard) [NHS]
Meter for blood glucose monitoring (for use with *Hypoguard® Supreme* test strips) = £19.49

MediSense® (MediSense) [NHS]
Meters (Sensor) for blood glucose monitoring for use with *MediSense G2®* test strips. *MediSense Card* = £35.00, *Medisense®* card starter pack = £45.00, *MediSense®* Pen = £35.00, *MediSense®* pen starter pack = £45.00

One Touch® (LifeScan) [NHS]
Meters for blood glucose monitoring for use with *One Touch®* test strips. *One Touch® Basic* system pack = £29.00, *One Touch® Profile* system pack = £49.00

Reflolux® S (Roche Diagnostics) [NHS]
Meter for blood glucose monitoring (for use with *BM-Test 1–44®* test strips) = £29.00

Urinalysis

Urine testing for glucose is useful in patients who find blood glucose monitoring difficult. Tests for glucose range from reagent strips specific to glucose to reagent tablets which detect all reducing sugars. Few patients still use *Clinitest®*; *Clinistix®* is suitable for screening purposes only. Tests for ketones by patients are rarely required unless they become unwell.

Microalbuminuria can be detected with *Micral-Test®* [NHS] but this should be followed by confirmation in the laboratory, since false positive results are common.

■ Glucose

Clinistix® (Bayer Diagnostics)
Reagent strips, for detection of glucose in urine. Net price 50-strip pack = £2.93

Clinitest® (Bayer Diagnostics)
Reagent tablets, for detection of glucose and other reducing substances in urine. Pocket set (test tube, dropper and 36 tablets), net price = £3.76, 36-tab pack = £1.87, 6-test tube pack = £2.10, 6-dropper pack = £2.10, test tube rack set [NHS] (6 tubes and 2 droppers) = £5.46

Diabur-Test 5000® (Roche Diagnostics)
Reagent strips, for detection of glucose in urine. Net price 50-strip pack = £2.41

Diastix® (Bayer Diagnostics)
Reagent strips, for detection of glucose in urine. Net price 50-strip pack = £2.49

Easistix® UG (Eastern)
Reagent strips, for detection of glucose in urine. Net price 50-strip pack = £1.99

Medi-Test® Glucose (BHR)
Reagent strips, for detection of glucose in urine. Net price 50-strip pack = £2.07

■ Ketones

Acetest® (Bayer Diagnostics)
Reagent tablets, for detection of ketones in urine. Net price 100-tab pack = £3.30

Ketostix® (Bayer Diagnostics)
Reagent strips, for detection of ketones in urine. Net price 50-strip pack = £2.64

Ketur Test® (Roche Diagnostics)
Reagent strips, for detection of ketones in urine. Net price 50-strip pack = £2.32

■ Protein

Albustix® (Bayer Diagnostics)

Reagent strips, for detection of protein in urine. Net price 50-strip pack = £3.62

Albym Test® (Roche Diagnostics)

Reagent strips, for detection of protein in urine. Net price 50-strip pack = £3.11

Medi-Test® Protein 2 (BHR)

Reagent strips, for detection of protein in urine. Net price 50-strip pack = £2.89

Other reagent strips available for urinalysis include *BM-Test-GP®* [NHS] (glucose and protein—Roche Diagnostics), *Ketodiastix®* [NHS] (glucose and ketones—Bayer Diagnostics), *Medi-Test Combi 2®* [NHS] (glucose and protein—BHR), *Micral-Test II®* [NHS] (albumin—Roche Diagnostics), *Microbumintest®* [NHS] (albumin—Bayer Diagnostics), *Uristix®* [NHS] (glucose and protein—Bayer Diagnostics)

Glucose tolerance test

The **glucose** tolerance test is now rarely needed for the diagnosis of diabetes when symptoms of hyperglycaemia are present, though it is still required to establish the presence of gestational diabetes. This generally involves giving anhydrous glucose 75 g (equivalent to Glucose BP 82.5 g) by mouth to the fasting patient, and measuring plasma-glucose concentrations at intervals.

The appropriate amount of glucose should be given with at least 300 mL fluid. Anhydrous glucose 75 g may alternatively be given as 116 mL *Hycal®* (SmithKline Beecham Healthcare) with extra fluid to administer a total volume of at least 300 mL.

6.2 Thyroid and antithyroid drugs

6.2.1   Thyroid hormones

6.2.2   Antithyroid drugs

6.2.1 Thyroid hormones

Thyroid hormones are used in hypothyroidism (myxoedema), and also in diffuse non-toxic goitre, Hashimoto's thyroiditis (lymphadenoid goitre), and thyroid carcinoma. Neonatal hypothyroidism requires prompt treatment for normal development.

Levothyroxine sodium (thyroxine sodium) is the treatment of choice for *maintenance* therapy. The initial dose should not exceed 100 micrograms daily, preferably before breakfast, or 25 to 50 micrograms in elderly patients or those with cardiac disease, increased by 25 to 50 micrograms at intervals of at least 4 weeks. The usual maintenance dose to relieve hypothyroidism is 100 to 200 micrograms daily which can be administered as a single dose.

In infants a daily dose of 10 micrograms/kg up to a maximum of 50 micrograms daily should be given; subsequent therapy should reach 100 micrograms daily by 5 years and 100–200 micrograms by 12 years, guided by clinical response, growth assessment, and measurements of plasma thyroxine and thyroid-stimulating hormone.

Liothyronine sodium has a similar action to levothyroxine but is more rapidly metabolised and has a more rapid effect; 20 micrograms is equivalent to 100 micrograms of levothyroxine. Its effects develop after a few hours and disappear within 24 to 48 hours of discontinuing treatment. It may be used in *severe hypothyroid states* when a rapid response is desired.

Liothyronine by intravenous injection is the treatment of choice in *hypothyroid coma.* Adjunctive therapy includes intravenous fluids, hydrocortisone, and antibiotics; assisted ventilation is often required.

LEVOTHYROXINE SODIUM/ THYROXINE SODIUM

Indications: hypothyroidism

Cautions: panhypopituitarism or predisposition to adrenal insufficiency from other causes (initiate corticosteroid therapy before starting levothyroxine), elderly, cardiovascular disorders (myocardial insufficiency or ECG evidence of myocardial infarction, see Initial Dosage below), long-standing hypothyroidism, diabetes insipidus, diabetes mellitus (dosage increase may be needed for antidiabetic drugs including insulin); pregnancy (Appendix 4) and breast-feeding (Appendix 5); **interactions:** Appendix 1 (levothyroxine)

INITIAL DOSAGE. A pre-therapy ECG is valuable as changes induced by hypothyroidism may be confused with evidence of ischaemia. If too rapid an increase of metabolism is produced (causing diarrhoea, nervousness, rapid pulse, insomnia, tremors and sometimes anginal pain where there is latent myocardial ischaemia), reduce dose or withhold for 1–2 days and start again at a lower dose

Contra-indications: thyrotoxicosis

Side-effects: usually at excessive dosage (see Initial Dosage above) include anginal pain, arrhythmias, palpitation, skeletal muscle cramps, tachycardia, diarrhoea, vomiting, tremors, restlessness, excitability, insomnia, headache, flushing, sweating, fever, heat intolerance, excessive loss of weight and muscular weakness

Dose: ADULT,   initially   50–100 micrograms (50 micrograms for those over 50 years) daily, preferably before breakfast, adjusted in steps of 50 micrograms every 3–4 weeks until normal metabolism   maintained   (usually   100–200 micrograms daily); where there is cardiac disease,   initially   25 micrograms   daily   *or* 50 micrograms on alternate days, adjusted in steps of 25 micrograms every 4 weeks; CHILD (see also notes   above),   congenital   hypothyroidism, 25 micrograms   daily   adjusted   in   steps   of 25 micrograms every 2–4 weeks until mild toxic symptoms then reduce dose slightly; juvenile myxoedema (child over 1 year), initially 2.5–5 micrograms/kg daily

Levothyroxine/Thyroxine (Non-proprietary)
[PoM]

Tablets, levothyroxine sodium 25 micrograms, net price 20 = 47p; 50 micrograms, 20 = 64p; 100 micrograms, 20 = £1.20

Various strengths available from APS, Cox, CP, Goldshield (including *Eltroxin®*), Hillcross, Kent, Norton

LIOTHYRONINE SODIUM
(L-Tri-iodothyronine sodium)
Indications: see notes above
Cautions: see under Levothyroxine Sodium
Contra-indications: see under Levothyroxine Sodium
Side-effects: see under Levothyroxine Sodium
Dose: *by mouth*, initially 20 micrograms daily gradually increased to 60 micrograms daily in 2–3 divided doses; elderly patients should receive smaller initial doses, gradually increased; CHILD, adult dose reduced in proportion to body-weight
By slow intravenous injection, hypothyroid coma, 5–20 micrograms repeated every 12 hours or more frequently (every 4 hours if necessary); alternatively 50 micrograms initially then 25 micrograms every 8 hours reducing to 25 micrograms twice daily

Tertroxin® (Goldshield) PoM
Tablets, scored, liothyronine sodium 20 micrograms. Net price 100-tab pack = £14.92
Triiodothyronine (Goldshield) PoM
Injection, powder for reconstitution, liothyronine sodium (with dextran). Net price 20-microgram amp = £37.92

6.2.2   Antithyroid drugs

Antithyroid drugs are used for hyperthyroidism either to prepare patients for thyroidectomy or for long-term management. In the UK carbimazole is the most commonly used drug. Propylthiouracil may be used in patients who suffer sensitivity reactions to carbimazole as sensitivity is not necessarily displayed to both drugs. Both drugs act primarily by interfering with the synthesis of thyroid hormones.

> **CSM warning (neutropenia and agranulocytosis)**
>
> Doctors are reminded of the importance of recognising bone marrow suppression induced by carbimazole and the need to stop treatment promptly.
>
> 1. Patient should be asked to report symptoms and signs suggestive of infection, especially sore throat.
>
> 2. A white blood cell count should be performed if there is any clinical evidence of infection.
>
> 3. Carbimazole should be stopped promptly if there is clinical or laboratory evidence of neutropenia.

Carbimazole is given in a daily dose of 20 to 60 mg and maintained at this dose until the patient becomes euthyroid, usually after 4 to 8 weeks; the dose may then be progressively reduced to a maintenance of between 5 and 15 mg daily; therapy is usually given for 18 months. Children may be given carbimazole in an initial dose of 250 micrograms/kg three times daily, adjusted according to response; treatment in children should be undertaken by a specialist. Rashes are common, and propylthiouracil may then be substituted. Pruritus and rashes can also be treated with antihistamines without discontinuing therapy, however patients should be advised to report any sore throat immediately because of the rare complication of agranulocytosis (see CSM warning, above).

Propylthiouracil is given in a dose of 300 to 600 mg daily in adults and this dose is maintained until the patient becomes euthyroid; the dose may then be gradually reduced to a maintenance dose of 50 to 150 mg daily.

Although antithyroid drugs have a short half-life they need only be given once daily because of their prolonged effect on the thyroid. Over-treatment with the rapid development of hypothyroidism is not uncommon and should be avoided particularly during pregnancy since it can cause fetal goitre.

A combination of carbimazole, 20 to 60 mg daily with levothyroxine, 50 to 150 micrograms daily, may be used in a *blocking-replacement regimen*; therapy is again usually given for 18 months. The blocking-replacement regimen is **not** suitable during pregnancy.

Before partial thyroidectomy **iodine** may be given for 10 to 14 days in addition to carbimazole or propylthiouracil to assist control and reduce vascularity of the thyroid. Iodine should not be used for long-term treatment since its antithyroid action tends to diminish.

Radioactive sodium iodide (^{131}I) solution is used increasingly for the treatment of thyrotoxicosis at all ages, particularly where medical therapy or compliance is a problem, in patients with cardiac disease, and in patients who relapse after thyroidectomy.

Propranolol is useful for rapid relief of thyrotoxic symptoms and may be used in conjunction with antithyroid drugs or as an adjunct to radioactive iodine. Beta-blockers are also useful in neonatal thyrotoxicosis and in supraventricular arrhythmias due to hyperthyroidism. Propranolol may be used in conjunction with iodine to prepare mildly thyrotoxic patients for surgery but it is still preferable to make the patient euthyroid with carbimazole before surgery. Laboratory tests of thyroid function are not altered by beta-blockers. Most experience in treating thyrotoxicosis has been gained with propranolol but **nadolol** is also used. For doses and preparations of beta-blockers see section 2.4.

Thyrotoxic crisis ('thyroid storm') requires emergency treatment with intravenous administration of fluids, propranolol (5 mg) and hydrocortisone (100 mg every 6 hours, as sodium succinate), as well as oral iodine solution and carbimazole or propylthiouracil which may need to be administered by nasogastric tube.

PREGNANCY AND BREAST-FEEDING. Radioactive iodine therapy is contra-indicated during pregnancy. Propylthiouracil and carbimazole can be given but the blocking-replacement regimen (see above) is **not** suitable. Both propylthiouracil and carbimazole cross the placenta and in high doses may cause fetal goitre and hypothyroidism—the lowest dose that will control the hyperthyroid state should be used (requirements in Graves' disease tend to fall during pregnancy). Rarely, carbimazole has been associated with aplasia cutis of the neonate.

Carbimazole and propylthiouracil appear in breast milk but this does not preclude breast-feeding as long as neonatal development is closely monitored and the lowest effective dose is used.

CARBIMAZOLE

Indications: hyperthyroidism

Cautions: liver disorders, pregnancy, breast-feeding (see notes)

Side-effects: nausea, mild gastrointestinal disturbances, headache, rashes and pruritus, arthralgia; rarely alopecia, agranulocytosis (see **CSM warning** above), jaundice

Dose: see notes above

COUNSELLING. Warn patient to tell doctor immediately if sore throat, mouth ulcers, bruising, fever, malaise, or non-specific illness develops

Neo-Mercazole® (Roche) PoM
Tablets, both pink, carbimazole 5 mg, net price 100-tab pack = £2.87; 20 mg, 100-tab pack = £10.65. Counselling, blood disorder symptoms

IODINE AND IODIDE

Indications: thyrotoxicosis (pre-operative)

Cautions: pregnancy, children; not for long-term treatment

Contra-indications: breast-feeding

Side-effects: hypersensitivity reactions including coryza-like symptoms, headache, lacrimation, conjunctivitis, pain in salivary glands, laryngitis, bronchitis, rashes; on prolonged treatment depression, insomnia, impotence; goitre in infants of mothers taking iodides

Aqueous Iodine Oral Solution (Lugol's Solution), iodine 5%, potassium iodide 10% in purified water, freshly boiled and cooled, total iodine 130 mg/mL. Net price 100 mL = £1.65. Label: 27
Dose: 0.1–0.3 mL 3 times daily well diluted with milk or water

PROPYLTHIOURACIL

Indications: hyperthyroidism

Cautions: see under Carbimazole; reduce dose in renal impairment (Appendix 3)

Side-effects: see under Carbimazole; urticaria, leucopenia; rarely cutaneous vasculitis, thrombocytopenia, aplastic anaemia, hepatitis, lupus erythematous-like syndromes

Dose: see notes above

Propylthiouracil (Non-proprietary) PoM
Tablets, propylthiouracil 50 mg. Net price 20 = £10.26
Available from CP, Hillcross, Norton

6.3   Corticosteroids

6.3.1   Replacement therapy
6.3.2   Glucocorticoid therapy

6.3.1   Replacement therapy

The adrenal cortex normally secretes hydrocortisone (cortisol) which has glucocorticoid activity and weak mineralocorticoid activity. It also secretes the mineralocorticoid aldosterone.

In deficiency states, physiological replacement is best achieved with a combination of **hydrocortisone** (section 6.3.2) and the mineralocorticoid

fludrocortisone; hydrocortisone alone does not usually provide sufficient mineralocorticoid activity for complete replacement.

In *Addison's disease* or following adrenalectomy, **hydrocortisone** 20 to 30 mg daily by mouth is usually required. This is given in 2 doses, the larger in the morning and the smaller in the evening, mimicking the normal diurnal rhythm of cortisol secretion. The optimum daily dose is determined on the basis of clinical response. Glucocorticoid therapy is supplemented by fludrocortisone 50 to 300 micrograms daily.

In *acute adrenocortical insufficiency*, **hydrocortisone** is given intravenously (preferably as sodium succinate) in doses of 100 mg every 6 to 8 hours in sodium chloride intravenous infusion 0.9%.

In *hypopituitarism* glucocorticoids should be given as in adrenocortical insufficiency, but since the production of aldosterone is also regulated by the renin-angiotensin system a mineralocorticoid is not usually required. Additional replacement therapy with levothyroxine (section 6.2.1) and sex hormones (section 6.4) should be given as indicated by the pattern of hormone deficiency.

Corticosteroid cover for *adrenalectomy*, for *hypophysectomy* or for operations on patients on long-term treatment with corticosteroids is determined logically from the knowledge that in a normal person major stress will not lead to the secretion of more than 300 mg of cortisol in 24 hours; once the stress is over, cortisol production rapidly returns to its usual level of approximately 20 mg per 24 hours. A simple way of mimicking this is to administer hydrocortisone. On the day of operation hydrocortisone 100 mg (usually as the sodium succinate) is given by intramuscular or intravenous injection with the premedication, and repeated every 8 hours. In the absence of complications, the dose can be halved every 24 hours until a normal maintenance dose of 20 to 30 mg per 24 hours is reached on the fifth postoperative day.

FLUDROCORTISONE ACETATE

Indications: mineralocorticoid replacement in adrenocortical insufficiency

Cautions: section 6.3.2

Contra-indications: section 6.3.2

Side-effects: section 6.3.2

Dose: adrenocortical insufficiency, 50–300 micrograms daily; CHILD 5 micrograms/kg daily

Florinef® (Squibb) PoM
Tablets, pink, scored, fludrocortisone acetate 100 micrograms. Net price 56-tab pack = £2.69.
Label: 10 steroid card

6.3.2   Glucocorticoid therapy

In comparing the relative potencies of corticosteroids in terms of their anti-inflammatory (glucocorticoid) effects it should be borne in mind that high glucocorticoid activity in itself is of no advantage unless it occurs in conjunction with relatively low mineralocorticoid activity so that the effect on water and electrolytes is not also increased. The mineralocorticoid activity of **fludrocortisone** (section 6.3.1) is so high that its anti-inflammatory activity is of no clinical relevance. The table below shows equivalent anti-inflammatory doses.

Equivalent Anti-inflammatory Doses of Corticosteroids

This table takes no account of mineralocorticoid effects, nor does it take account of variations in duration of action

Prednisolone 5 mg
≡ Betamethasone 750 micrograms
≡ Cortisone acetate 25 mg
≡ Deflazacort 6 mg
≡ Dexamethasone 750 micrograms
≡ Hydrocortisone 20 mg
≡ Methylprednisolone 4 mg
≡ Triamcinolone 4 mg

The relatively high mineralocorticoid activity of **cortisone** and **hydrocortisone**, and the resulting fluid retention, make them unsuitable for disease suppression on a long-term basis. However, they can be used for adrenal replacement therapy (section 6.3.1); hydrocortisone is preferred because cortisone requires conversion in the liver to hydrocortisone. Hydrocortisone is used on a short-term basis by intravenous injection for the emergency management of some conditions. The relatively moderate anti-inflammatory potency of hydrocortisone also makes it a useful topical corticosteroid for the management of inflammatory skin conditions because side-effects (both topical and systemic) are less marked (section 13.4); cortisone is not active topically.

Prednisolone has predominantly glucocorticoid activity and is the corticosteroid most commonly used by mouth for long-term disease suppression.

Betamethasone and **dexamethasone** have very high glucocorticoid activity in conjunction with insignificant mineralocorticoid activity. This makes them particularly suitable for high-dose therapy in conditions where water retention would be a disadvantage (e.g. cerebral oedema).

They also have a long duration of action and this, coupled with their lack of mineralocorticoid action makes them particularly suitable for conditions which require suppression of corticotropin (corticotrophin) secretion (e.g. congenital adrenal hyperplasia). Some esters of betamethasone and of **beclometasone** (beclomethasone) exert a considerably more marked topical effect (e.g. on the skin or the lungs) than when given by mouth; use is made of this to obtain topical effects without corresponding systemic activity (e.g. for skin applications and asthma inhalations).

Deflazacort is a newly introduced corticosteroid with high glucocorticoid activity; it is derived from prednisolone.

Disadvantages of corticosteroids

Overdosage or prolonged use may exaggerate some of the normal physiological actions of corticosteroids leading to mineralocorticoid and glucocorticoid side-effects.

Mineralocorticoid side-effects include hypertension, sodium and water retention and potassium loss. They are most marked with fludrocortisone, but are significant with cortisone, hydrocortisone, corticotropin, and tetracosactide (tetracosactrin). Mineralocorticoid actions are negligible with the high potency glucocorticoids, betamethasone and dexamethasone, and occur only slightly with methylprednisolone, prednisolone, and triamcinolone.

Glucocorticoid side-effects include diabetes and osteoporosis, which is a danger, particularly in the elderly, as it may result in osteoporotic fractures for example of the hip or vertebrae; in addition administration of high doses is associated with avascular necrosis of the femoral head. Mental disturbances may occur; a serious paranoid state or depression with risk of suicide may be induced, particularly in patients with a history of mental disorder. Euphoria is frequently observed. Muscle wasting (proximal myopathy) may also occur. Corticosteroid therapy is also weakly linked with peptic ulceration (the potential advantage of soluble or enteric-coated preparations to reduce the risk is speculative only).

High doses of corticosteroids may cause Cushing's syndrome, with moon face, striae, and acne; it is usually reversible on withdrawal of treatment, but this must always be gradually tapered to avoid symptoms of acute adrenal insufficiency (**important:** see also Adrenal Suppression p. 330).

In children, administration of corticosteroids may result in suppression of growth. For the effect of corticosteroids given in pregnancy see Pregnancy and breast-feeding, below.

Modification of tissue reactions may result in spread of infection; suppression of clinical signs may allow diseases such as septicaemia or tuberculosis to reach an advanced stage before being recognised—**important:** see also Infections p. 330.

Adrenal atrophy can persist for years after stopping prolonged corticosteroid therapy, therefore any illness or surgical emergency may require temporary reintroduction of corticosteroid therapy to compensate for lack of sufficient adrenocortical response. Anaesthetists **must** therefore know whether a patient is taking or has been taking corticosteroids to avoid a precipitous fall in blood pressure during anaesthesia or in the immediate postoperative period. Patients should therefore carry cards giving details of their dosage and possible complications.

Following concern about severe chickenpox associated with systemic corticosteroids, the CSM has issued a notice that **every** patient prescribed a *systemic* corticosteroid should receive the patient information leaflet supplied by the manufacturer.

Steroid treatment cards (see p. 329) should also be issued where appropriate.
Doctors and pharmacists can obtain supplies of the card from:
England and Wales
Department of Health, PO Box 777, London, SE1 6XH (Tel 0541 555 455)
Scotland
Banner Business Supplies, 20 South Gyle Crescent, Edinburgh, EH12 9EB (Tel 0131 479 3279)

For other references to the adverse effects of corticosteroids see section 11.4 (eye) and section 13.4 (skin).

STEROID TREATMENT CARD

I am a patient on STEROID treatment which must not be stopped suddenly

- If you have been taking this medicine for more than three weeks, the dose should be reduced gradually when you stop taking steroids unless your doctor says otherwise.

- Read the patient information leaflet given with the medicine.

- Always carry this card with you and show it to anyone who treats you (for example a doctor, nurse, pharmacist or dentist). For one year after you stop the treatment, you must mention that you have taken steroids.

- If you become ill, or if you come into contact with anyone who has an infectious disease, consult your doctor promptly. If you have never had chickenpox, you should avoid close contact with people who have chickenpox or shingles. If you do come into contact with chickenpox, see your doctor urgently.

- Make sure that the information on the card is kept up to date.

Clinical management

Dosage of corticosteroids varies widely in different diseases and in different patients. If the use of a corticosteroid can save or prolong life, as in exfoliative dermatitis, pemphigus, acute leukaemia or acute transplant rejection, high doses may need to be given, because the complications of therapy are likely to be less serious than the effects of the disease itself.

When long-term corticosteroid therapy is used in relatively benign chronic diseases such as rheumatoid arthritis the danger of treatment may become greater than the disabilities produced by the disease. To minimise side-effects the maintenance dose should be kept as low as possible (see also section 10.1.2.1).

When potentially less harmful measures are ineffective corticosteroids are used topically for the treatment of inflammatory conditions of the skin (section 13.4). Corticosteroids should be avoided or used only under specialist supervision in psoriasis (section 13.5).

Corticosteroids are used both topically (by rectum) and systemically (by mouth or intravenously) in the management of ulcerative colitis and Crohn's disease (section 1.5 and section 1.7.2).

Use can be made of the mineralocorticoid activity of fludrocortisone to treat postural hypotension in autonomic neuropathy (section 6.1.5).

Very high doses of corticosteroids have been given by intravenous injection in septic shock. However a recent study (using methylprednisolone sodium succinate) did not demonstrate efficacy and, moreover, suggested a higher mortality in some subsets of patients given the high-dose corticosteroid therapy.

Dexamethasone and betamethasone have little if any mineralocorticoid action and their long duration of action makes them particularly suitable for suppressing corticotropin secretion in congenital adrenal hyperplasia where the dose should be tailored to clinical response and by measurement of adrenal androgens and 17-hydroxyprogesterone. In common with all glucocorticoids their suppressive action on the hypothalamic-pituitary-adrenal axis is greatest and most prolonged when they are given at night. In most normal subjects a single dose of 1 mg of dexamethasone at night, depending on weight, is sufficient to inhibit corticotropin secretion for 24 hours. This is the basis of the 'overnight dexamethasone suppression test' for diagnosing Cushing's syndrome.

Betamethasone and dexamethasone are also appropriate for conditions where water retention would be a disadvantage, as for example in treating traumatic cerebral oedema with doses of 12 to 20 mg daily.

In acute hypersensitivity reactions such as angioedema of the upper respiratory tract and anaphylactic shock, corticosteroids are indicated as an adjunct to emergency treatment with adrenaline (epinephrine) (section 3.4.3). In such cases hydrocortisone (as sodium succinate) by intravenous injection in a dose of 100 to 300 mg may be required.

Corticosteroids are preferably used by inhalation in the management of asthma (section 3.2) but systemic therapy in association with bronchodilators is required for the emergency treatment of severe acute asthma (section 3.1.1).

Corticosteroids may also be useful in conditions such as rheumatic fever, chronic active hepatitis, and sarcoidosis; they may also lead to remissions of acquired haemolytic anaemia (section 9.1.3), and some cases of the nephrotic syndrome (particularly in children) and thrombocytopenic purpura (section 9.1.4).

Corticosteroids can improve the prognosis of serious conditions such as systemic lupus erythematosus, temporal arteritis, and polyarteritis nodosa; the effects of the disease process may be suppressed and symptoms relieved, but the underlying condition is not cured, although it may ultimately remit. It is usual to begin therapy in these conditions at fairly high dose, such as 40 to 60 mg prednisolone daily, and then to reduce the dose to the lowest commensurate with disease control.

For other references to the use of corticosteroids see Prescribing in palliative care, section 8.2.2 (immunosuppresion), section 11.4 (eye), section 12.1.1 (otitis externa), section 12.2.1 (allergic rhinitis), and section 12.3.1 (aphthous ulcers).

Pregnancy and breast-feeding

Following a review of the data on the safety of systemic corticosteroids used in pregnancy and breast-feeding the CSM has concluded:

- corticosteroids vary in their ability to cross the placenta; betamethasone and dexamethasone cross the placenta readily while 88% of prednisolone is inactivated as it crosses the placenta;
- there is no convincing evidence that systemic corticosteroids increase the incidence of congenital abnormalities such as cleft palate or lip;
- when administration is prolonged or repeated during pregnancy, systemic corticosteroids increase the risk of intra-uterine growth retardation; there is no evidence of intra-uterine growth retardation following short-term treatment (e.g. prophylactic treatment for neonatal respiratory distress syndrome);
- any adrenal suppression in the neonate following prenatal exposure usually resolves spontaneously after birth and is rarely clinically important;
- prednisolone appears in small amounts in breast milk but doses of up to 40 mg daily are unlikely to cause systemic effects in the infant; infants should be monitored for adrenal suppression if the mothers are taking a higher dose.

See also Appendix 4.

Administration

Whenever possible *local treatment* with creams, intra-articular injections, inhalations, eye-drops, or enemas should be used in preference to *systemic treatment*. The suppressive action of a corticosteroid on cortisol secretion is least when it is given in the morning, therefore in an attempt to reduce pituitary-adrenal suppression a corticosteroid (usually prednisolone) should normally be taken as a single dose in the morning. In an attempt to reduce pituitary-adrenal suppression further, the total dose for two days can sometimes be taken as a single dose on alternate days; alternate-day administration has not been very successful in the management of asthma (section 3.2). Pituitary-adrenal suppression can also be reduced by means of intermittent therapy with short courses. In some conditions it may be possible to reduce the dose of corticosteroid by adding a small dose of an immunosuppressive drug (section 8.2.1).

Withdrawal of corticosteroids

The CSM has recommended that *gradual* withdrawal of systemic corticosteroids should be considered in those whose disease is unlikely to relapse and have

- recently received repeated courses (particularly if taken for longer than 3 weeks)
- taken a short course within 1 year of stopping long-term therapy
- other possible causes of adrenal suppression
- received more than 40 mg daily prednisolone (or equivalent)
- been given repeat doses in the evening
- received more than 3 weeks' treatment

Systemic corticosteroids may be stopped abruptly in those whose disease is unlikely to relapse *and* have received treatment for 3 weeks or less *and* are not included in the patient groups described above.

During corticosteroid withdrawal the dose may be reduced rapidly down to physiological doses (equivalent to prednisolone 7.5 mg daily) and then reduced more slowly. Assessment of the disease may be needed during withdrawal to ensure that relapse does not occur.

PREDNISOLONE

Indications: suppression of inflammatory and allergic disorders; see also notes above; inflammatory bowel disease, section 1.5; asthma, section 3.2; immunosuppression, section 8.2.2; rheumatic disease, section 10.1.2

Cautions: adrenal suppression (see below), infection (see below), children and adolescents (growth retardation possibly irreversible), elderly (close supervision required particularly on long-term treatment); frequent monitoring required if history of tuberculosis (or X-ray changes), hypertension, recent myocardial infarction (rupture reported), congestive heart failure, liver failure, renal impairment, diabetes mellitus including family history, osteoporosis (post-menopausal women at special risk), glaucoma (including family history), severe affective disorders (particularly if history of steroid-induced psychosis), epilepsy, peptic ulcer, hypothyroidism, history of steroid myopathy; pregnancy and breast-feeding (see notes above); **interactions:** Appendix 1 (corticosteroids)

ADRENAL SUPPRESSION. During prolonged therapy *adrenal atrophy* may develop and persist for years after stopping. Abrupt withdrawal after a prolonged period may lead to adrenal insufficiency, hypotension or death; however in most asthma patients (who continue to receive other appropriate treatment, section 3.1), abrupt withdrawal after courses of up to 3 weeks has not resulted in adverse effects (see notes above on withdrawal). Withdrawal may also be associated with fever, myalgia, arthralgia, rhinitis, conjunctivitis, painful itchy skin nodules and weight loss.

Any significant intercurrent illness, trauma, or surgical procedure requires a temporary increase in dosage, or if already stopped, a temporary re-introduction of corticosteroid.

Patients should carry a Steroid Treatment Card giving clear guidance on precautions to minimise risk and providing details of prescriber, drug, dosage and duration of treatment.

INFECTIONS. Susceptibility and severity of infections may be increased and clinical presentation may be atypical. Serious infections e.g. *septicaemia* and *tuberculosis* may reach an advanced stage before being recognised. *Amoebiasis* or *strongyloidiasis* may be activated or exacerbated (exclude before initiating corticosteroid in those at risk or with suggestive symptoms). *Ocular infections* (fungal or viral) may also be exacerbated (see also section 11.4.1).

Chickenpox: unless they have had chickenpox, patients receiving oral or parenteral corticosteroids for purposes other than replacement should be regarded as being *at risk of severe chickenpox* (see Steroid Treatment Card). Manifestations of fulminant illness include pneumonia, hepatitis and disseminated intravascular coagulation; rash is not necessarily a prominent feature. Passive immunisation with varicella–zoster immunoglobulin (section 14.5) is needed by exposed non-immune patients receiving systemic corticosteroids or who have used them within the previous 3 months (preferably given within 3 days of exposure and not later than 10 days). Confirmed chickenpox warrants specialist care and urgent treatment. Corticosteroids should not be stopped (dosage may need to be increased). Currently there is no good evidence that topical, inhaled or rectal corticosteroids are associated with an increased risk of severe chickenpox.

Measles: Patients should be advised to take particular care to avoid exposure to measles and to seek medical advice without delay if exposure occurs; prophylaxis with intramuscular normal immunoglobulin (section 14.5) may be needed.

Contra-indications: systemic infection (unless specific antimicrobial therapy given); avoid live virus vaccines in those receiving immunosuppressive doses (serum antibody response diminished)

Side-effects: minimised by using lowest effective dose for minimum period possible; *gastro-intestinal effects* include dyspepsia, peptic ulceration (with perforation), abdominal distension, acute pancreatitis, oesophageal ulceration and candidiasis; *musculoskeletal effects* include proximal myopathy, osteoporosis, vertebral and long bone fractures, avascular osteonecrosis, tendon rupture; *endocrine effects* include adrenal suppression, menstrual irregularities and amenorrhoea, Cushing's syndrome (with high doses, usually reversible on withdrawal), hirsutism, weight gain, negative nitrogen and calcium balance, increased appetite; increased susceptibility to and severity of infection; *neuropsychiatric effects* include euphoria, psychological dependence, depression, insomnia, increased intracranial pressure with papilloedema in children (usually after withdrawal), psychosis and aggravation of schizophrenia, aggravation of epilepsy; *ophthalmic effects* include glaucoma, papilloedema, posterior subcapsular cataracts, corneal or scleral thinning and exacerbation of ophthalmic viral or fungal disease; *other side-effects* include impaired healing, skin atrophy, bruising, striae, telangiectasia, acne, myocardial rupture following recent myocardial infarction, fluid and electrolyte disturbance, leucocytosis, hypersensitivity reactions (including anaphylaxis), thromboembolism, nausea, malaise, hiccups

Dose: *by mouth,* initially, up to 10–20 mg daily (severe disease, up to 60 mg daily), preferably taken in the morning after breakfast; can often be reduced within a few days but may need to be continued for several weeks or months

Maintenance, usual range, 2.5–15 mg daily, but higher doses may be needed; cushingoid side-effects increasingly likely with doses above 7.5 mg daily

By intramuscular injection, prednisolone acetate, 25–100 mg once or twice weekly (for preparation see section 10.1.2.2)

Prednisolone (Non-proprietary) PoM
Tablets, prednisolone 1 mg, net price 28-tab pack = 58p; 5 mg, 28-tab pack = £1.04. Label: 10 steroid card, 21
Available from APS, Cox, CP, Hillcross, Norton, Hoechst Marion Roussel (Precortisyl®)
Tablets, both e/c, prednisolone 2.5 mg (brown), net price 30-tab pack = 26p; 5 mg (red), 30-tab pack = 43p. Label: 5, 10 steroid card, 25
Available from APS, Biorex, Cox, Norton (2.5 mg), Pfizer (Deltacortril Enteric®)
Injection, see section 10.1.2.2

Precortisyl Forte® (Hoechst Marion Roussel) PoM
Tablets, scored, prednisolone 25 mg. Net price 56-tab pack = £4.26. Label: 10 steroid card, 21

Prednesol® (Sovereign) PoM
Tablets, pink, scored, soluble, prednisolone 5 mg (as sodium phosphate). Net price 100-tab pack = £5.76. Label: 10 steroid card, 13, 21

BETAMETHASONE

Indications: suppression of inflammatory and allergic disorders; congenital adrenal hyperplasia; cerebral oedema; see also notes above; ear (section 12.1.1); eye (section 11.4.1); nose (section 12.2.1)

Cautions: see notes above and under Prednisolone

Contra-indications: see notes above and under Prednisolone

Side-effects: see notes above and under Prednisolone

Dose: *by mouth,* usual range 0.5–5 mg daily; see also Administration (above)

By intramuscular injection or slow intravenous injection or infusion, 4–20 mg, repeated up to 4 times in 24 hours; CHILD, *by slow intravenous injection,* up to 1 year 1 mg, 1–5 years 2 mg, 6–12 years 4 mg

Betnelan® (Medeva) PoM
Tablets, scored, betamethasone 500 micrograms. Net price 100-tab pack = £3.63. Label: 10 steroid card, 21

Betnesol® (Medeva) PoM
Tablets, pink, scored, soluble, betamethasone 500 micrograms (as sodium phosphate). Net price 100-tab pack = £3.20. Label: 10 steroid card, 13, 21
Injection, betamethasone 4 mg (as sodium phosphate)/mL. Net price 1-mL amp = 65p. Label: 10 steroid card

CORTISONE ACETATE ▰

Indications: see under Dose but now superseded, see also notes above

Cautions: see notes above and under Prednisolone

Contra-indications: see notes above and under Prednisolone

Side-effects: see notes above and under Prednisolone

Dose: *by mouth,* for replacement therapy, 25–37.5 mg daily in divided doses

Cortisyl® (Hoechst Marion Roussel) PoM ▰
Tablets, scored, cortisone acetate 25 mg. Net price 56-tab pack = £3.24. Label: 10 steroid card, 21

> ▰ denotes preparations that are considered to be less suitable for prescribing (see p. vi)

DEFLAZACORT

Indications: suppression of inflammatory and allergic disorders

Cautions: see notes above and under Prednisolone

Contra-indications: see notes above and under Prednisolone

Side-effects: see notes above and under Prednisolone

Dose: usual maintenance 3–18 mg daily (acute disorders, initially up to 120 mg daily); see also Administration (above)
CHILD 0.25–1.5 mg/kg daily (or on alternate days); see also Administration (above)

Calcort® (Shire) ▼ PoM
Tablets, deflazacort 1 mg, net price 100-tab pack = £8.00; 6 mg, 60-tab pack = £16.46; 30 mg, 30-tab pack = £22.80. Label: 5, 10 steroid card

DEXAMETHASONE

Indications: suppression of inflammatory and allergic disorders; shock; diagnosis of Cushing's disease, congenital adrenal hyperplasia; cerebral oedema; nausea and vomiting with chemotherapy (section 8.1); rheumatic disease (section 10.1.2); eye (section 11.4.1); see also notes above
Cautions: see notes above and under Prednisolone
Contra-indications: see notes above and under Prednisolone
Side-effects: see notes above and under Prednisolone; perineal irritation may follow intravenous administration of the phosphate ester
Dose: *by mouth*, usual range 0.5–10 mg daily; see also Administration (above)
By intramuscular injection or slow intravenous injection or infusion (as dexamethasone phosphate), initially 0.5–20 mg; CHILD 200–500 micrograms/kg daily
Cerebral oedema (as dexamethasone phosphate), *by intravenous injection*, 10 mg initially, then 4 mg *by intramuscular injection* every 6 hours as required for 2–10 days
Shock (as dexamethasone phosphate), *by intravenous injection or infusion*, 2–6 mg/kg, repeated if necessary after 2–6 hours (but see notes above)
Note. Dexamethasone 1 mg ≡ dexamethasone phosphate 1.2 mg ≡ dexamethasone sodium phosphate 1.3 mg

Dexamethasone (Non-proprietary) PoM
Tablets, dexamethasone 500 micrograms, net price 20 = 64p; 2 mg, 20 = £1.73. Label: 10 steroid card, 21
Available from Organon
Injection, dexamethasone phosphate (as dexamethasone sodium phosphate) 4 mg/mL, net price 1-mL amp = £1.00, 2-mL vial = £1.98; 24 mg/mL, 5-mL vial = £16.66. Label: 10 steroid card
Available from Faulding DBL
Injection, dexamethasone sodium phosphate 5 mg/mL, net price 1-mL amp = 83p, 2-mL vial = £1.27. Label: 10 steroid card
Available from Organon

Decadron® (MSD) PoM
Tablets, scored, dexamethasone 500 micrograms, net price 30-tab pack = 96p. Label: 10 steroid card, 21
Injection, dexamethasone phosphate (as dexamethasone sodium phosphate) 4 mg/mL, net price 2-mL vial = £1.76. Label: 10 steroid card

HYDROCORTISONE

Indications: adrenocortical insufficiency (section 6.3.1); shock; see also notes above; hypersensitivity reactions e.g. anaphylactic shock and angio-edema (section 3.4.5); inflammatory bowel disease (section 1.5); haemorrhoids (section 1.7.2); rheumatic disease (section 10.1.2); eye (section 11.4.1); skin (section 13.4)
Cautions: see notes above and under Prednisolone
Contra-indications: see notes above and under Prednisolone

Side-effects: see notes above and under Prednisolone; perineal irritation may follow intravenous administration of the phosphate ester
Dose: *by mouth*, replacement therapy, 20–30 mg daily in divided doses—see section 6.3.1; CHILD 10–30 mg
By intramuscular injection or slow intravenous injection or infusion, 100–500 mg, 3–4 times in 24 hours or as required; CHILD *by slow intravenous injection* up to 1 year 25 mg, 1–5 years 50 mg, 6–12 years 100 mg

Efcortesol® (Sovereign) PoM
Injection, hydrocortisone 100 mg (as sodium phosphate)/mL. Net price 1-mL amp = 75p; 5-mL amp = £3.40. Label: 10 steroid card
Note. Perineal irritation may follow intravenous injection of the phosphate ester

Hydrocortone® (MSD) PoM
Tablets, scored, hydrocortisone 10 mg, net price 30-tab pack = 70p; 20 mg, 30-tab pack = £1.07. Label: 10 steroid card, 21

Solu-Cortef® (Pharmacia & Upjohn) PoM
Injection, powder for reconstitution, hydrocortisone (as sodium succinate). Net price 100-mg vial = 92p, 100-mg vial with 2-mL amp water for injections = 97p. Label: 10 steroid card

METHYLPREDNISOLONE

Indications: suppression of inflammatory and allergic disorders; cerebral oedema; see also notes above; rheumatic disease (section 10.1.2); skin (section 13.4)
Cautions: see notes above and under Prednisolone; rapid intravenous administration of large doses associated with cardiovascular collapse
Contra-indications: see notes above and under Prednisolone
Side-effects: see notes above and under Prednisolone
Dose: *by mouth*, usual range 2–40 mg daily; see also Administration (above)
By intramuscular injection or slow intravenous injection or infusion, initially 10–500 mg; graft rejection, up to 1 g daily *by intravenous infusion* for up to 3 days

Medrone® (Pharmacia & Upjohn) PoM
Tablets, scored, methylprednisolone 2 mg (pink), net price 30-tab pack = £2.57; 4 mg, 30-tab pack = £4.93; 16 mg, 30-tab pack = £13.67; 100 mg (blue), 20-tab pack = £38.46. Label: 10 steroid card, 21

Solu-Medrone® (Pharmacia & Upjohn) PoM
Injection, powder for reconstitution, methylprednisolone (as sodium succinate) (all with solvent). Net price 40-mg vial = £1.26; 125-mg vial = £3.78; 500-mg vial = £7.64; 1-g vial = £13.77; 2-g vial = £26.15. Label: 10 steroid card

■ Intramuscular depot

Depo-Medrone® (Pharmacia & Upjohn) PoM
Injection (aqueous suspension), methylprednisolone acetate 40 mg/mL. Net price 1-mL vial = £2.61; 2-mL vial = £4.80; 3-mL vial = £6.79. Label: 10 steroid card
Dose: by deep intramuscular injection into gluteal muscle, 40–120 mg, a second injection may be given after 2–3 weeks if required

TRIAMCINOLONE

Indications: suppression of inflammatory and allergic disorders; see also notes above; rheumatic disease, section 10.1.2; mouth, section 12.3.1; skin, section 13.4

Cautions: see notes above and under Prednisolone; high dosage may cause proximal myopathy, avoid in chronic therapy

Contra-indications: see notes above and under Prednisolone

Side-effects: see notes above and under Prednisolone

Dose: *by deep intramuscular injection*, into gluteal muscle, 40 mg of acetonide for depot effect, repeated at intervals according to the patient's response; max. single dose 100 mg

Kenalog® (Squibb) PoM

Injection (aqueous suspension), triamcinolone acetonide 40 mg/mL. Net price 1-mL vial (intramuscular/intra-articular) = £1.70; 1-mL syringe (intramuscular only) = £2.11; 2-mL syringe (intramuscular only) = £3.66. Label: 10 steroid card

6.4   Sex hormones

Sex hormones are described under the following section headings:

6.4.1   Female sex hormones
6.4.2   Male sex hormones and antagonists
6.4.3   Anabolic steroids

6.4.1   Female sex hormones

6.4.1.1   Oestrogens and HRT
6.4.1.2   Progestogens

6.4.1.1   Oestrogens and HRT

Oestrogens are necessary for the development of female secondary sexual characteristics; they also stimulate myometrial hypertrophy with endometrial hyperplasia.

In terms of oestrogenic activity *natural oestrogens* (estradiol (oestradiol), estrone (oestrone), and estriol (oestriol)) have a more appropriate profile for hormone replacement therapy (HRT) than *synthetic oestrogens* (ethinylestradiol (ethinyloestradiol), mestranol, and diethylstilbestrol (stilboestrol)); the profile of *conjugated oestrogens* resembles that of natural oestrogens.

Oestrogen therapy is given cyclically or continuously for a number of gynaecological conditions. If long-term therapy is required a progestogen should be added to reduce the risk of cystic hyperplasia of the endometrium and possible transformation to cancer. This addition of a progestogen is not necessary if the patient has had a hysterectomy or in the case of tibolone.

Oestrogens are no longer used to *suppress lactation* because of their association with thromboembolism.

Hormone replacement therapy

Menopausal *vasomotor symptoms* and menopausal *vaginitis* are alleviated by administration of small doses of oestrogen. There is also good evidence that small doses of oestrogen given for several years starting in the perimenopausal period will diminish postmenopausal *osteoporosis* and some evidence that they will reduce the incidence of *stroke and myocardial infarction*. There is an increased risk of *endometrial cancer* (reduced by a progestogen) and, after some years of use, possibly an increased risk of *breast cancer* (see below).

Hormone replacement therapy (HRT) is indicated for menopausal women whose lives are inconvenienced by *vaginal atrophy* or *vasomotor instability*. Vaginal atrophy may respond to a short course of vaginal oestrogen preparation given for a few weeks and repeated if necessary. Systemic therapy is needed for vasomotor symptoms and should be given for at least a year; in a woman with a uterus a progestogen should be added to reduce the risk of endometrial cancer. HRT is also indicated for women with *early natural or surgical menopause (before age 45)*, since they are at high risk of osteoporosis; HRT should be given to the age of at least 50 and possibly for a further 10 years (for risk of breast cancer, see below).

Long-term HRT is almost certainly favourable in risk-benefit terms for menopausal women *without a uterus* because they do not require progestogen therapy; it should probably be continued for about 10 years (for risk of breast cancer, see below). The picture is less clear for menopausal women *with a uterus* because the need for administration of progestogen may blunt the protective effect of low-dose oestrogen against myocardial infarction and stroke; any effect of the progestogen (favourable or otherwise) on breast cancer is not yet known. Nevertheless, risk factors for osteoporosis should be borne in mind and, if there are several, consideration given to HRT. Risk factors include recent corticosteroid therapy or any disease predisposing to osteoporosis, family history, thinness, lack of exercise, alcoholism or smoking, and fracture of a hip or forearm before the age of 65; women of Afro-Caribbean origin appear to be less susceptible than those who are white or of Asian origin.

RISK OF BREAST CANCER. Following publication of an analysis of pooled original data, the CSM has advised that the increased risk of breast cancer is related to the duration of HRT use and that this excess risk disappears within about 5 years of stopping. Women who use HRT for a short time around the menopause have a very low excess risk. Breast cancers in HRT users were less likely to have spread beyond the breast than those in non-users.

About 45 in every 1000 women aged 50 years not using HRT will have breast cancer diagnosed over the next 20 years; in those using HRT for 5 years, this figure rises by 2 extra cases in 1000, in those using HRT for 10 years 6 extra cases in 1000 and in those using HRT for 15 years 12 extra cases in 1000.

The CSM's view is that these results do not provide a reason for women to stop their treatment but the results do emphasise the importance of breast awareness and regular mammograms.

RISK OF VENOUS THROMBOEMBOLISM. Recent studies show an increased risk of deep vein thrombosis and of pulmonary embolism in women currently taking HRT. The view of the CSM is that the new data do not change the overall positive balance between benefits and risks of treatment for most women. The CSM has advised that there is no need for *women without predisposing factors* for venous thromboembolism to stop taking HRT. In *women who have predisposing factors* (such as a personal or family history of deep vein thrombosis or pulmonary embolism, severe varicose veins, obesity, surgery, trauma or prolonged bed-rest) it may be prudent to review the need for HRT as in some cases the risks of HRT may be expected to exceed the benefits.

CHOICE. The choice of oestrogen for HRT is not straightforward and depends on an overall balance of indication, risk, and convenience. Oestrogen deficient vaginitis in a woman with a uterus can be treated for only a few weeks with an oestrogen, without addition of cyclical progestogen; this constraint includes vaginal preparations (section 7.2.1) since a significant amount is absorbed through the vaginal mucosa. Oestrogen therapy alone is suitable for long-term continuous therapy in a woman without a uterus. A woman with a uterus requires oestrogen with cyclical progestogen for the last 10 to 13 days of the cycle (or administration of a preparation which combines both oestrogenic and progestogenic activity). Oral preparations of oestrogen are subject to first-pass metabolism, therefore subcutaneous or transdermal administration reflects more closely endogenous hormone activity. In the case of subcutaneous implants, recurrence of vasomotor symptoms at supraphysiological plasma concentrations may occur; moreover, there is evidence of prolonged endometrial stimulation after discontinuation (calling for continued cyclical progestogen).

Provided that calcium intake is adequate calcium supplements (section 9.5.1) do not confer additional benefit on HRT.

CONTRACEPTION. HRT does **not** provide contraception and a woman is considered potentially fertile for *2 years after her last menstrual period* if she is *under 50 years*, and for *1 year* if she is *over 50 years*. A woman who is under 50 years and free of all risk factors for venous and arterial disease can use a low-oestrogen combined oral contraceptive pill (section 7.3.1) to provide both *relief of menopausal symptoms* and *contraception*; it is recommended that the oral contraceptive be stopped at 50 years of age since there are more suitable alternatives. If any potentially fertile woman needs to use HRT, *non-hormonal contraceptive measures* (such as condoms, or by this age, contraceptive foam, section 7.3.3) are necessary.

Although follicle-stimulating hormone measurements can be used as a guide to determine fertility, high measurements alone (particularly in women under the age of 50 years) do not necessarily preclude the possibility of pregnancy.

SURGERY. Surgery is a predisposing factor for venous thromboembolism and it may be prudent to review the need for HRT (see above). Oestrogenic activity may persist after discontinuation of estradiol implants (see above).

OESTROGENS FOR HRT

Note. Relates only to small amounts of oestrogens given for hormone replacement therapy

Indications: see notes above and under preparations

Cautions: prolonged exposure to unopposed oestrogens may increase risk of development of endometrial cancer (see notes above); migraine (or migraine-like headaches); history of breast nodules or fibrocystic disease—closely monitor breast status (risk of breast cancer, see notes above); pre-existing uterine fibroids may increase in size, symptoms of endometriosis may be exacerbated; predisposing factors to thromboembolism (see notes above); increased risk of gall bladder disease reported; porphyria (see section 9.8.2); **interactions:** Appendix 1 (oestrogens)

OTHER CONDITIONS. The product literature advises caution in other conditions including hypertension, cardiac or renal disease, diabetes, asthma, epilepsy, sickle-cell disease, melanoma, otosclerosis, multiple sclerosis and systemic lupus erythematosus. Evidence for caution in these conditions is unsatisfactory and many women with these conditions may stand to benefit from HRT.

Contra-indications: pregnancy; oestrogen-dependent cancer, active thrombophlebitis or thromboembolic disorders, liver disease (where liver function tests have failed to return to normal), Dubin-Johnson and Rotor syndromes (or monitor closely), undiagnosed vaginal bleeding, breast-feeding

Side-effects: nausea and vomiting, abdominal cramps and bloating, weight changes, breast enlargement and tenderness, premenstrual-like syndrome, sodium and fluid retention, changes in liver function, cholestatic jaundice, rashes and chloasma, changes in libido, depression, headache, migraine, dizziness, leg cramps (rule out venous thrombosis), contact lenses may irritate; transdermal delivery systems may cause contact sensitisation (possible severe hypersensitivity reaction on continued exposure), and headache has been reported on vigorous exercise

WITHDRAWAL BLEEDING. Cyclical HRT (where a progestogen is taken for 10–14 days of each 28-day oestrogen treatment cycle) usually results in a *regular withdrawal bleed* towards the end of the progestogen. The aim of continuous combined HRT (where a combination of oestrogen and progestogen is taken, usually in a single tablet, throughout each 28-day treatment cycle) is to avoid bleeding, but *irregular bleeding* may occur during the early treatment stages (if it continues endometrial abnormality should be excluded and consideration given to cyclical HRT instead)

Dose: see under preparations

COUNSELLING ON PATCHES. Patch should be removed after 3–4 days (or once a week in case of 7-day patch) and replaced with fresh patch on slightly different site; recommended sites: clean, dry, unbroken areas of skin on trunk below waistline; not to be applied on or near breasts or under waistband. If patch falls off in bath allow skin to cool before applying new patch

Women with uterus

The following preparations contain a **progestogen** as well as an **oestrogen** and are therefore suitable for a woman with an **intact uterus**; they are **not** suitable for use as (or with) hormonal contraceptives.

■ Conjugated oestrogens with progestogen

Premique® (Wyeth) PoM

Premique® tablets, s/c, blue, conjugated oestrogen (equine) 625 micrograms and medroxyprogesterone acetate 5 mg. Net price 3 × 28-tab pack = £22.62

Dose: menopausal symptoms and osteoporosis prophylaxis, in women with intact uterus, 1 tablet daily on a continuous basis, starting on day 1 of menstruation (or any time if cycles have ceased or are infrequent)

Note. Unsuitable for use in perimenopausal women or within 12 months of last menstrual period; may cause irregular bleeding in early stages of treatment—if bleeding continues exclude endometrial abnormality and consider changing to cyclical HRT, see below

Premique® Cycle Calendar pack, all s/c, 14 white tablets, conjugated oestrogens (equine) 625 micrograms; 14 green tablets, conjugated oestrogens (equine) 625 micrograms and medroxyprogesterone acetate 10 mg, net price 3 × 28-tab pack = £22.61

Dose: menopausal symptoms and osteoporosis prophylaxis, 1 white tablet daily for 14 days, starting on day 1 of menstruation (or at any time if cycles have ceased or are infrequent) then 1 green tablet daily for 14 days; subsequent courses are repeated without interval

Prempak-C® (Wyeth) PoM

Prempak C® 0.625 Calendar pack, s/c, 28 maroon tablets, conjugated oestrogens (equine) 625 micrograms; 12 light brown tablets, norgestrel 150 micrograms (≡ levonorgestrel 75 micrograms). Net price 3 × 40-tab pack = £14.73

Dose: menopausal symptoms and osteoporosis prophylaxis, in women with intact uterus, 1 maroon tablet daily on continuous basis, starting on day 1 of menstruation (or at any time if cycles are infrequent), and 1 brown tablet daily on days 17–28 of each 28-day treatment cycle; subsequent courses are repeated without interval

Prempak C® 1.25 Calendar pack, s/c, 28 yellow tablets, conjugated oestrogens (equine) 1.25 mg; 12 light brown tablets, norgestrel 150 micrograms (≡ levonorgestrel 75 micrograms). Net price 3 × 40-tab pack = £14.73

Dose: see under 0.625 Calendar pack, but taking 1 yellow tablet daily on continuous basis (instead of 1 maroon tablet) if symptoms not fully controlled with lower strength

■ Estradiol with progestogen

Climagest® (Novartis) PoM

Climagest® 1-mg tablets, 16 grey-blue, estradiol valerate 1 mg; 12 white, estradiol valerate 1 mg and norethisterone 1 mg. Net price 28-tab pack = £4.38; 3 × 28-tab pack = £12.75

Dose: menopausal symptoms, 1 grey-blue tablet daily for 16 days, starting on day 1 of menstruation (or at any time if cycles have ceased or are infrequent) then 1 white tablet for 12 days; subsequent courses are repeated without interval

Climagest® 2-mg tablets, 16 blue, estradiol valerate 2 mg; 12 yellow, estradiol valerate 2 mg and norethisterone 1 mg. Net price 28-tab pack = £4.38; 3 × 28-tab pack = £12.75

Dose: see *Climagest® 1-mg*, but starting with 1 blue tablet daily (instead of 1 grey-blue tablet) if symptoms not controlled with lower strength

Climesse® (Novartis) PoM

Tablets, pink, estradiol valerate 2 mg, norethisterone 700 micrograms. Net price 1 × 28-tab pack = £7.90; 3 × 28-tab pack = £23.70

Dose: menopausal symptoms and osteoporosis prophylaxis, in women with intact uterus, 1 tablet daily on a continuous basis

Note. Unsuitable for use in the perimenopause or within 12 months of the last menstrual period; may cause irregular bleeding in early stages of treatment—if bleeding continues exclude endometrial abnormality and consider changing to cyclical HRT

Cyclo-Progynova® (ASTA Medica) PoM

Cyclo-Progynova® 1-mg Tablets, all s/c, 11 beige, estradiol valerate 1 mg; 10 brown, estradiol valerate 1 mg and levonorgestrel 250 micrograms. Net price per pack = £3.34

Dose: menopausal symptoms, in women with intact uterus, 1 beige tablet daily for 11 days, starting on day 5 of menstruation (or at any time if cycles have ceased or are infrequent), then 1 brown tablet daily for 10 days, followed by a 7-day interval

Cyclo-Progynova® 2-mg Tablets, all s/c, 11 white, estradiol valerate 2 mg; 10 brown, estradiol valerate 2 mg and norgestrel 500 micrograms (≡ levonorgestrel 250 micrograms). Net price per pack = £3.34

Dose: menopausal symptoms and osteoporosis prophylaxis as *Cyclo-Progynova® 1-mg*, but starting with 1 white tablet daily for 11 days, then 1 brown tablet daily for 10 days, followed by a 7-day interval

Elleste-Duet® (Searle) PoM

Elleste-Duet® 1-mg tablets, 16 white, estradiol 1 mg; 12 green, estradiol 1 mg and norethisterone acetate 1 mg. Net price 3 × 28-tab pack = £9.72

Dose: menopausal symptoms, 1 white tablet daily for 16 days starting on day 1 of menstruation (or at any time if cycles have ceased or are infrequent), then 1 green tablet daily for 12 days; subsequent courses are repeated without interval

Elleste-Duet® 2-mg tablets, 16 orange, estradiol 2 mg; 12 grey, estradiol 2 mg, norethisterone acetate 1 mg. Net price 3 × 28-tab pack = £9.72

Dose: menopausal symptoms and osteoporosis prophylaxis, 1 orange tablet daily for 16 days, starting on day 1 of menstruation (or at any time if cycles have ceased or are infrequent) then 1 grey tablet daily for 12 days; subsequent courses are repeated without interval

Elleste-Duet Conti® tablets, grey, estradiol 2 mg, norethisterone acetate 1 mg. Net price 3 × 28–tab pack = £17.97.

Dose: menopausal symptoms, in women with intact uterus, 1 tablet daily on a continuous basis (if changing from cyclical HRT begin treatment at the end of scheduled bleed)

Note. Unsuitable for use in the perimenopause or within 12 months of the last menstrual period; may cause irregular bleeding in early stages of treatment—if bleeding continues exclude endometrial abnormality and consider changing to cyclical HRT

Estracombi® (Novartis) [PoM]

Combination pack, self-adhesive patches of *Estraderm TTS® 50* (releasing estradiol approx. 50 micrograms/24 hours) and of *Estragest TTS®* (releasing estradiol approx. 50 micrograms/24 hours and norethisterone acetate 250 micrograms/24 hours); net price 1-month pack (4 of each) = £11.14, 3-month pack (12 of each) = £33.42. Counselling, administration

Dose: menopausal symptoms and osteoporosis prophylaxis, in women with intact uterus, starting within 5 days of onset of menstruation (or any time if cycles have ceased or are infrequent), 1 *Estraderm TTS® 50* patch to be applied twice weekly for 2 weeks followed by 1 *Estragest TTS®* patch twice weekly for 2 weeks; subsequent courses are repeated without interval

Estrapak 50® (Novartis) [PoM]

Calendar pack, self-adhesive patches, releasing estradiol approx. 50 micrograms/24 hours, and tablets, red, norethisterone acetate 1 mg; net price 1-month pack (8 patches plus 12 tablets) = £9.48, 3-month pack (24 patches plus 36 tablets) = £28.44. Counselling, administration

Dose: menopausal symptoms and osteoporosis prophylaxis, in women with intact uterus, starting within 5 days of onset of menstruation (or at any time if cycles have ceased or are infrequent), apply 1 patch twice weekly on continuous basis, and take 1 tablet daily on days 15–26 of each 28-day treatment cycle

Evorel® (Janssen-Cilag) [PoM]

Evorel® Conti patches, self-adhesive, (releasing estradiol approx. 50 micrograms/24 hours and norethisterone acetate approx. 170 micrograms/24 hours), net price 8-patch pack = £12.90. Counselling, administration

Dose: menopausal symptoms and osteoporosis prophylaxis, in women with intact uterus, 1 patch to be applied twice weekly on a continuous basis

Evorel® Pak calendar pack, 8 self-adhesive patches (releasing estradiol approx. 50 micrograms/24 hours) and 12 tablets, norethisterone 1 mg, net price per pack = £8.45. Counselling, administration

Dose: menopausal symptoms and osteoporosis prophylaxis, in women with intact uterus, apply 1 patch twice weekly on a continuous basis (increased if necessary for menopausal symptoms to 2 patches twice weekly after first month) and take 1 tablet daily on days 15–26 of each 28-day treatment cycle

Evorel® Sequi combination pack, 4 self-adhesive patches of *Evorel® 50* (releasing estradiol approx. 50 micrograms/24 hours) and 4 self-adhesive patches of *Evorel® Conti* (releasing estradiol approx. 50 micrograms/24 hours and norethisterone acetate approx. 170 micrograms/24 hours), net price 8-patch pack = £11.00. Counselling, administration

Dose: menopausal symptoms and osteoporosis prophylaxis, in women with intact uterus, 1 *Evorel® 50* patch to be applied twice weekly for 2 weeks followed by 1 *Evorel® Conti* patch twice weekly for 2 weeks; subsequent courses are repeated without interval

Femapak® (Solvay) [PoM]

Femapak® 40 combination pack of 8 self-adhesive patches of *Fematrix® 40* (releasing estradiol approx. 40 micrograms/24 hours) and 14 tablets of *Duphaston®* (dydrogesterone 10 mg). Net price per pack = £8.45. Counselling, administration

Dose: see under *Femapak® 80*

Femapak® 80 combination pack of 8 self-adhesive patches of *Fematrix® 80* (releasing estradiol approx. 80 micrograms/24 hours) and 14 tablets of *Duphaston®* (dydrogesterone 10 mg). Net price per pack = £8.95. Counselling, administration

Dose: menopausal symptoms (and osteoporosis prophylaxis in case of *Femapak® 80* **only**), in women with intact uterus, starting within 5 days of onset of menstruation (or any time if cycles have ceased or are infrequent), apply 1 patch twice weekly on a continuous basis and take 1 tablet daily on days 15–28 of each 28-day treatment cycle; therapy should be initiated with *Femapak® 40* in those with menopausal symptoms, prolonged oestrogen deficiency or anticipated intolerance to higher strengths, subsequently adjusted to lowest effective dose

Femoston® (Solvay) [PoM]

Femoston® 1/10 tablets, both f/c, 14 white, estradiol 1 mg; 14 grey, estradiol 1 mg, dydrogesterone 10 mg. Net price 3 × 28-tab pack = £14.97

Dose: menopausal symptoms, in women with intact uterus, 1 white tablet daily for 14 days, starting within 5 days of onset of menstruation (or any time if cycles have ceased or are infrequent) then 1 grey tablet for 14 days; subsequent courses are repeated without interval

Femoston® 2/10 tablets, both f/c, 14 orange, estradiol 2 mg; 14 yellow, estradiol 2 mg, dydrogesterone 10 mg. Net price 3 × 28-tab pack = £14.97

Dose: menopausal symptoms and osteoporosis prophylaxis, in women with intact uterus, 1 orange tablet daily for 14 days, starting within 5 days of onset of menstruation (or any time if cycles have ceased or are infrequent) then 1 yellow tablet daily for 14 days; subsequent courses are repeated without interval; where therapy is required for control of menopausal symptoms alone, *Femoston® 1/10* is given initially and *Femoston® 2/10* substituted if symptom control is not achieved

Femoston® 2/20 tablets, both f/c, 14 orange, estradiol 2 mg; 14 blue, estradiol 2 mg, dydrogesterone 20 mg. Net price 3 × 28-tab pack = £22.44

Dose: see *Femoston® 2/10*, but taking 1 blue tablet (instead of 1 yellow tablet) if withdrawal bleed is early or endometrial biopsy shows inadequate progestational response

Femoston®-conti tablets, f/c, salmon, estradiol 1 mg, dydrogesterone 5 mg, net price 3 × 28-tab pack = £22.62

Dose: menopausal symptoms and osteoporosis prophylaxis, in women with intact uterus, 1 tablet daily on a continuous basis (if changing from cyclical HRT begin treatment the day after finishing oestrogen plus progestogen phase without a tablet-free interval)

Note. Unsuitable for use in the perimenopause or within 12 months of the last menstrual period; may cause irregular bleeding in early stages of treatment—if bleeding continues exclude endometrial abnormality and consider changing to cyclical HRT

Kliofem® (Novo Nordisk) [PoM]

Tablets, yellow, estradiol 2 mg, norethisterone acetate 1 mg. Net price 3 × 28-tab pack = £25.95

Dose: menopausal symptoms and osteoporosis prophylaxis, in women with intact uterus, 1 tablet daily on a continuous basis; start at end of scheduled bleed if changing from cyclical HRT

Note. Unsuitable for use in the perimenopause or within 12 months of the last menstrual period; may cause irregular bleeding in early stages of treatment—if bleeding continues, discontinue or change to cyclical HRT

Kliovance® (Novo Nordisk) [PoM]

Tablets, f/c, estradiol 1mg, norethisterone acetate 500 micrograms, net price 3 × 28-tab pack = £25.95

Dose: menopausal symptoms, in women with intact uterus, 1 tablet daily on a continuous basis; start at end of scheduled bleed if changing from cyclical HRT

Note. Unsuitable for use in the perimenopause or within 12 months of the last menstrual period; may cause irregular bleeding in the early stages of treatment—if bleeding continues discontinue and exclude endometrial abnormality

Nuvelle® (Schering Health) [PoM]

Nuvelle® tablets, all s/c, 16 white, estradiol valerate 2 mg; 12 pink, estradiol valerate 2 mg and levonorgestrel 75 micrograms. Net price 3 × 28-tab pack = £13.77

Dose: menopausal symptoms and osteoporosis prophylaxis, in women with intact uterus, 1 white tablet daily for 16 days, starting on day 5 of menstruation (or any time if cycles have ceased or are infrequent) then 1 pink tablet daily for 12 days; subsequent courses are repeated without interval

Nuvelle® *Continuous* tablets, f/c, pink, estradiol 2 mg, norethisterone acetate 1 mg, net price 3 x 28-tab pack = £18.02

Dose: menopausal symptoms and osteoporosis prophylaxis, in women with intact uterus, 1 tablet daily on a continuous basis; start at end of scheduled bleed if changing from cyclical HRT

Note. Unsuitable for use in the perimenopause or within 12 months of the last menstrual period; may cause irregular bleeding in early stages of treatment—if bleeding continues exclude endometrial abnormality, discontinue or change to cyclical HRT

Nuvelle® *TS*, combination pack of self-adhesive patches of *Nuvelle*® *TS Phase I* (releasing estradiol approx. 80 micrograms/24 hours) and of *Nuvelle*® *TS Phase II* (releasing estradiol approx. 50 micrograms/24 hours and levonorgestrel approx. 20 micrograms/24 hours); net price 1-month pack (4 of each) = £10.51. Counselling, administration

Dose: menopausal symptoms, in women with intact uterus, starting within 5 days of onset of menstruation (or any time if cycles have ceased or are infrequent) 1 *Phase I* patch to be applied twice weekly for 2 weeks followed by 1 *Phase II* patch twice weekly for 2 weeks; subsequent courses are repeated without interval

Tridestra® (Orion) [PoM]

Tablets, 70 white, estradiol valerate 2 mg; 14 blue, estradiol valerate 2 mg and medroxyprogesterone acetate 20 mg; 7 yellow, inactive. Net price 91-tab pack = £23.78

Dose: menopausal symptoms and osteoporosis prophylaxis, in women with intact uterus, 1 white tablet daily for 70 days, then 1 blue tablet daily for 14 days, then 1 yellow tablet daily for 7 days; subsequent courses are repeated without interval

Trisequens® (Novo Nordisk) [PoM]

Trisequens® tablets, 12 blue, estradiol 2 mg;10 white, estradiol 2 mg, norethisterone acetate 1 mg; 6 red, estradiol 1 mg, net price 3 × 28-tab pack = £14.40

Dose: menopausal symptoms and osteoporosis prophylaxis, in women with intact uterus, 1 blue tablet daily, starting on day 5 of menstruation (or at any time if cycles have ceased or are infrequent), then 1 tablet daily in sequence (without interruption)

Trisequens Forte® tablets, 12 yellow, estradiol 4 mg; 10 white, estradiol 4 mg, norethisterone acetate 1 mg; 6 red, estradiol 1 mg, net price 3 × 28-tab pack = £14.40

Dose: menopausal symptoms, see under *Trisequens*®, starting with 1 yellow tablet daily (instead of 1 blue tablet) if symptoms not fully controlled with lower strength

Women without uterus

The following preparations do **not** contain a **progestogen**; if the uterus is intact they need to be given with a progestogen in which case packs incorporating a suitable progestogen tablet are preferred (see above).

■ Conjugated oestrogens only

Premarin® (Wyeth) [PoM]

Tablets, all s/c, conjugated oestrogens (equine) 625 micrograms (maroon), net price 3 × 28-tab pack = £8.10; 1.25 mg (yellow), 3 × 28-tab pack = £10.99

Dose: menopausal symptoms and osteoporosis prophylaxis, (with progestogen for 12–14 days per cycle in women with intact uterus), 0.625–1.25 mg daily

Note. Premarin® tablets 2.5 mg (purple, net price 3 × 28-tab pack = £10.64) are still available, but no longer have a product licence for palliative care in breast cancer (and provide a higher dose than that having a product licence for osteoporosis prophylaxis)

■ Estradiol only

Estradiol Implants (Organon) [PoM]

Implant, estradiol 25 mg, net price each = £9.59; 50 mg, each = £19.16; 100 mg, each = £33.40

Dose: by implantation, oestrogen replacement, and osteoporosis prophylaxis (with cyclical progestogen on 10–13 days of each cycle in women with intact uterus, see notes above), 25–100 mg as required (usually every 4–8 months) according to oestrogen levels—check before each implant

Note. When removing implant for the last time from those with intact uterus, cyclical progesterone should be continued until cessation of withdrawal bleed

Climaval® (Novartis) [PoM]

Tablets, estradiol valerate 1 mg (grey-blue), net price 1 × 28-tab pack = £2.34, 3 × 28-tab pack = £7.02; 2 mg (blue), 1 × 28-tab pack = £2.34, 3 × 28-tab pack = £7.02

Dose: menopausal symptoms (if patient has had a hysterectomy), 1–2 mg daily

Dermestril® (Sanofi-Synthelabo) [PoM]

Patches, self-adhesive, estradiol, '25' patch (releasing approx. 25 micrograms/24 hours), net price 8-patch pack = £5.75; '50' patch (releasing approx. 50 micrograms/24 hours), 8-patch pack = £6.35; '100' patch (releasing approx. 100 micrograms/24 hours), 8-patch pack = £6.99. Counselling, administration

Dose: menopausal symptoms, 1 patch to be applied every 3–4 days on a continuous basis; (with cyclical progestogen on 10–12 days of each cycle in women with intact uterus); therapy should be initiated with '50' patch for first month, subsequently adjusted to lowest effective dose

Elleste-Solo® (Searle) PoM

Elleste-Solo® 1-mg tablets, estradiol 1 mg. Net price 3 × 28-tab pack = £5.34

Dose: menopausal symptoms, with cyclical progestogen on 12–14 days of each cycle in women with intact uterus, 1 mg daily starting on day 1 of menstruation (or at any time if cycles have ceased or are infrequent)

Elleste-Solo® 2-mg tablets, orange, estradiol 2 mg. Net price 3 × 28-tab pack = £5.34

Dose: menopausal symptoms not controlled with lower strength and osteoporosis prophylaxis, with cyclical progestogen on 12–14 days of each cycle in women with intact uterus, 2 mg daily starting on day 1 of menstruation (or at any time if cycles have ceased or are infrequent)

Elleste Solo® MX (Searle) PoM

Patches, self-adhesive, estradiol, *MX 40 patch* (releasing approx. 40 micrograms/24 hours), net price 8-patch pack = £5.19; *MX 80 patch* (releasing approx. 80 micrograms/24 hours), 8-patch pack = £5.99. Counselling, administration.

Dose: menopausal symptoms (and osteoporosis prophylaxis in case of *Elleste Solo MX 80®* **only**), 1 patch to be applied twice weekly on a continuous basis starting within 5 days of onset of menstruation (or at any time if cycles have ceased or are infrequent); with cyclical progestogen on 12–14 days of each cycle in women with intact uterus; therapy should be initiated with *MX 40* in those with menopausal symptoms, prolonged oestrogen deficiency or anticipated intolerance to higher strength, dosage may be increased if required, subsequently adjusted to lowest effective dose

Estraderm MX® (Novartis) PoM

Patches, self-adhesive, estradiol, *MX 25 patch* (releasing approx. 25 micrograms/24 hours), net price 8-patch pack = £5.20, 24-patch pack = £15.59; *MX 50 patch* (releasing approx. 50 micrograms/24 hours), 8-patch pack = £5.22, 24-patch pack = £15.65, 20-patch pack (hosp. only) = £13.04; *MX 75 patch* (releasing approx. 75 micrograms/24 hours), 8-patch pack = £6.08, 24-patch pack = £18.25; *MX 100 patch* (releasing approx. 100 micrograms/24 hours), 8-patch pack = £6.31, 24-patch pack = £18.94. Counselling, administration

Dose: menopausal symptoms (and osteoporosis prophylaxis in case of *Estraderm MX® 50* and *75* **only**), 1 patch to be applied twice weekly on a continuous basis, with cyclical progestogen on 12 days of each cycle in women with intact uterus; therapy should be initiated with *MX 50* for first month, subsequently adjusted to lowest effective dose

Estraderm TTS® (Novartis) PoM

Patches, self-adhesive, estradiol, *TTS 25 patch* (releasing approx. 25 micrograms/24 hours), net price, 8-patch pack = £6.21, 24-patch pack = £18.63; *TTS 50 patch* (releasing approx. 50 micrograms/24 hours), 8-patch pack = £6.23, 24-patch pack = £18.69; *TTS 100 patch* (releasing approx. 100 micrograms/24 hours), 8-patch pack = £7.52, 24-patch pack = £22.63, 20-patch pack (hosp. only) = £16.76 . Counselling, administration

Dose: menopausal symptoms (and osteoporosis prophylaxis in case of *Estraderm TTS® 50* **only**), 1 patch to be applied twice weekly on continuous basis, with cyclical progestogen on 12 days of each cycle in women with intact uterus; therapy should be initiated with *TTS 50* for first month, subsequently adjusted to lowest effective dose

Evorel® (Janssen-Cilag) PoM

Patches, self-adhesive, estradiol, *'25' patch* (releasing approx. 25 micrograms/24 hours), net price 8-patch pack = £5.87; *'50' patch* (releasing approx. 50 micrograms/24 hours), 8-patch pack = £6.48; *'75' patch* (releasing approx. 75 micrograms/24 hours), 8-patch pack = £6.87; *'100' patch* (releasing approx. 100 micrograms/24 hours), 8-patch pack = £7.13. Counselling, administration

Dose: menopausal symptoms and osteoporosis prophylaxis (except *Evorel® 25*), 1 patch to be applied twice weekly on a continuous basis, with cyclical progestogen on at least 12 days of each cycle in women with intact uterus; therapy should be initiated with *'50' patch* for first month, subsequently adjusted to lowest effective dose

Fematrix® (Solvay) PoM

Fematrix® 40 patch, self-adhesive, estradiol, *'40' patch* (releasing approx. 40 micrograms/24 hours). Net price 8-patch pack = £5.50. Counselling, administration

Dose: menopausal symptoms, 1 patch to be applied twice weekly on a continuous basis starting within 5 days of onset of menstruation (or at any time if cycles have ceased or are infrequent), with cyclical progestogen on 12–14 days of each cycle in women with intact uterus; *'80' patch* may be used if required (subsequently adjusted to lowest effective dose)

Fematrix® 80 patch, self-adhesive, estradiol (releasing approx. 80 micrograms/24 hours). Net price 8-patch pack = £6.00. Counselling, administration

Dose: menopausal symptoms and osteoporosis prophylaxis, as for *Fematrix® 40*; therapy should be initiated with *Fematrix® 40* in those with menopausal symptoms, prolonged oestrogen deficiency or anticipated intolerance to higher strength

FemSeven® (Merck) PoM

Patches, self-adhesive, estradiol, *'50' patch* (releasing approx. 50 micrograms/24 hours), net price 4-patch pack = £5.94, 12-patch pack = £17.04; *'75' patch* (releasing approx. 75 micrograms/24 hours), net price 4-patch pack = £6.55; *'100' patch* (releasing approx.100 micrograms/24 hours), net price 4-patch pack = £7.99. Counselling, administration

Dose: menopausal symptoms and osteoporosis prophylaxis, 1 patch to be applied once a week on a continuous basis, with cyclical progestogen on at least 10 days of each cycle in women with intact uterus; therapy should be initiated with *FemSeven® 50* patches for the first few months, subsequently adjusted according to response

Menorest® (Rhône-Poulenc Rorer) PoM

Patches, self-adhesive, estradiol, *'37.5' patch* (releasing approx. 37.5 micrograms/24 hours), net price 8-patch pack = £6.34; *'50' patch* (releasing approx. 50 micrograms/24 hours), 8-patch pack = £6.44; *'75' patch* (releasing approx. 75 micrograms/24 hours), 8-patch pack = £7.50. Counselling administration

Dose: menopausal symptoms and osteoporosis prophylaxis (except *Menorest® 37.5*), 1 patch to be applied every 3–4 days on a continuous basis, with cyclical progestogen on at least 12 days of each cycle in women with intact uterus; therapy should be initiated with *'50' patch* for first month, subsequently adjusted to lowest effective dose

Oestrogel® (Hoechst Marion Roussel) PoM

Gel, estradiol 0.06%, net price 64-dose pump pack = £7.95. Counselling, administration

Dose: menopausal symptoms and osteoporosis prophylaxis, 2 measures (estradiol 1.5 mg) once daily on a continuous basis to be applied over an area twice that of the template provided, starting within 5 days of menstruation (or anytime if cycles have ceased or are infrequent), with cyclical progestogen on 12 days of each cycle in women with intact uterus; for menopausal symptoms may be increased if necessary after 1 month to max. 4 measures daily

COUNSELLING. Apply gel to clean, dry, intact skin such as arms, shoulders or inner thighs and allow to dry for 5 minutes before covering with clothing. Not to be applied on or near breasts or on vulval region. Avoid skin contact with another person (particularly male) and avoid other skin products or washing the area for at least 1 hour after application

Progynova® (Schering Health) PoM

Tablets, both s/c, estradiol valerate 1 mg (beige), net price 3 × 28-tab pack = £7.02; 2 mg (blue), 3 × 28-tab pack = £7.02

Dose: menopausal symptoms, 1–2 mg daily on a continuous basis; osteoporosis prophylaxis, 2 mg daily on a continuous basis; with cyclical progestogen on 12 days of each cycle in women with intact uterus

Progynova® TS (Schering Health) PoM

Patches, self-adhesive, *Progynova®* TS (releasing estradiol approx. 50 micrograms/24 hours), net price 12-patch pack = £17.88; *Progynova® TS forte* (releasing estradiol approx. 100 micrograms/24 hours), 12-patch pack = £19.68. Counselling, administration

Dose: menopausal symptoms, 1 patch to be applied once a week on a continuous or cyclical basis (1 patch per week for three weeks followed by a 7-day patch-free interval), with cyclical progestogen on 12 days of each cycle in women with intact uterus; therapy should be initiated with *Progynova® TS* and subsequently adjusted to lowest effective dose

Sandrena® (Organon) PoM

Gel, estradiol (0.1%), 500 microgram/500 mg sachet, net price 28-sachet pack = £5.68, 1 mg/1 g sachet, 28-sachet pack = £6.54. Counselling, administration

Dose: menopausal symptoms, estradiol 1 mg (1 g gel) to be applied once daily over area 1–2 times size of hand; with cyclical progestogen on 10–12 days of each cycle in women with intact uterus; dose may be adjusted after 2–3 cycles to a usual dose of estradiol 0.5–1.5 mg (0.5–1.5 g gel) daily

COUNSELLING. Apply gel to intact areas of skin such as lower trunk or thighs, using right and left sides on alternate days. Wash hands after application. Not to be applied on the breasts or face and avoid contact with eyes. Allow area of application to dry for 5 minutes and do not wash area for at least 1 hour

Zumenon® (Solvay) PoM

Tablets, f/c, estradiol 1 mg, net price 84-tab pack = £7.65; 2 mg (orange), 84-tab pack = £7.65

Dose: menopausal symptoms, initially 1 mg daily starting on day 5 of menstruation (or any time if cycles have ceased or are infrequent) adjusted to 1–4 mg daily according to response; osteoporosis prophylaxis, 2 mg daily; with cyclical progestogen on 10–14 days of each cycle in women with intact uterus

■ Estradiol, estriol and estrone only

Hormonin® (Shire) PoM

Tablets, pink, estradiol 600 micrograms, estriol 270 micrograms, estrone 1.4 mg. Net price 90-tab pack = £7.08

Dose: menopausal symptoms and osteoporosis prophylaxis, 1–2 tablets daily, with cyclical progestogen on 12–14 days of each cycle in women with intact uterus

Note. Hormonin® tablets can be given continuously or cyclically (21 days out of 28)

■ Estriol only

Ovestin® (Organon) PoM

Tablets, scored, estriol 1 mg. Net price 30-tab pack = £4.20. Label: 25

Dose: genito-urinary symptoms associated with oestrogen-deficiency states, 0.5–3 mg daily, as single dose, for up to 1 month, then 0.5–1 mg daily until restoration of epithelial integrity (short-term use)

■ Estropipate only

Harmogen® (Pharmacia & Upjohn) PoM

Tablets, peach, scored, estropipate 1.5 mg. Net price 28-tab pack = £3.00

Dose: menopausal symptoms and osteoporosis prophylaxis, 1.5 mg daily on continuous basis (with cyclical progestogen on 10–13 days of each cycle in women with intact uterus); up to 3 mg daily (in single or divided doses) for vasomotor symptoms and menopausal vaginitis

Raloxifene

Raloxifene has been introduced recently for the prevention of vertebral fractures in postmenopausal women at increased risk of osteoporosis; it does not, however, reduce menopausal vasomotor symptoms.

RALOXIFENE HYDROCHLORIDE

Indications: prevention of vertebral fractures in postmenopausal women at increased risk of osteoporosis

Cautions: risk factors for venous thromboembolism (discontinue if prolonged immobilisation); **interactions:** Appendix 1 (raloxifene)

Contra-indications: history of venous thromboembolism, undiagnosed uterine bleeding, breast or endometrial cancer, hepatic impairment, cholestasis, severe renal impairment; pregnancy and breast-feeding

Side-effects: venous thromboembolism, thrombophlebitis, hot flushes, leg cramps, peripheral oedema

Dose: 60 mg once daily

Evista® (Lilly) ▼ PoM

Tablets, f/c, raloxifene hydrochloride 60 mg, net price 28-tab pack = £19.76; 84-tab pack = £59.28

Tibolone

Tibolone combines oestrogenic and progestogenic activity with weak androgenic activity. It is indicated for the treatment of vasomotor symptoms of the menopause and osteoporosis prophylaxis. Tibolone is given continuously, without cyclical progestogen.

TIBOLONE

Indications: vasomotor symptoms in oestrogen deficiency (including women being treated with gonadotrophin releasing hormone analogues), osteoporosis prophylaxis

Cautions: renal impairment, history of liver disease, epilepsy, migraine, diabetes mellitus, hypercholesterolaemia; withdraw if signs of thromboembolic disease, abnormal liver function tests or cholestatic jaundice; see also Note below; **interactions:** Appendix 1 (tibolone)

Contra-indications: hormone-dependent tumours, history of cardiovascular or cerebrovascular disease (e.g. thrombophlebitis, thromboembolism), uninvestigated vaginal bleeding, severe liver disease, pregnancy, breast-feeding

Side-effects: weight changes, oedema, dizziness, seborrhoeic dermatitis, vaginal bleeding, headache, abdominal pain, gastro-intestinal disturbances, increased facial hair; depression, arthralgia, myalgia, migraine, visual disturbances, liver-function changes, rash and pruritus also reported

Dose: 2.5 mg daily

Note. Unsuitable for use in the premenopause (unless being treated with gonadotrophin-releasing hormone analogue) and as (or with) an oral contraceptive; also unsuitable for use within 12 months of last menstrual period (may cause irregular bleeding); induce withdrawal bleed with progestogen if transferring from another form of HRT

Livial® (Organon) PoM

Tablets, tibolone 2.5 mg. Net price 28-tab pack = £13.05; 3 × 28-tab pack = £39.14

Ethinylestradiol

Ethinylestradiol (ethinyloestradiol) has been used as hormone replacement for menopausal symptoms in a dose of 10–20 micrograms daily. This has now been largely replaced by more appropriate forms of oestrogen.

Ethinylestradiol is occasionally used, under **specialist supervision**, for the management of *hereditary haemorrhagic telangiectasia* (but evidence of any beneficial effect is uncertain). Side-effects include nausea, fluid retention, and thrombosis. Impotence and gynaecomastia occur in men.

For use in breast cancer, see section 8.3.1.

ETHINYLESTRADIOL

(Ethinyloestradiol)

Indications: see notes above

Cautions: cardiovascular disease (sodium retention with oedema, thromboembolism), hepatic impairment (jaundice); see also under Combined Oral Contraceptives (section 7.3.1) and under Oestrogen for HRT (above)

Contra-indications: see under Combined Oral Contraceptives (section 7.3.1) and under Oestrogen for HRT (above)

Side-effects: feminising effects in men; see also under Combined Oral Contraceptives (section 7.3.1) and under Oestrogen for HRT (above)

Dose: see notes above

Ethinylestradiol (Non-proprietary) PoM

Tablets, ethinylestradiol 10 micrograms, net price 21-tab pack = £16.81; 50 micrograms, 21-tab pack = £22.70; 1 mg, 28-tab pack = £34.24

Available from Norton

6.4.1.2   Progestogens

There are two main groups of progestogen, *progesterone and its analogues* (dydrogesterone, hydroxyprogesterone, and medroxyprogesterone) and *testosterone analogues* (norethisterone and norgestrel). The newer progestogens (desogestrel, norgestimate, and gestodene) are all derivatives of norgestrel; levonorgestrel is the active isomer of norgestrel and has twice its potency. Progesterone and its analogues are less androgenic than the testosterone derivatives and neither progesterone nor dydrogesterone causes virilisation. Other synthetic derivatives are variably metabolised into testosterone and oestrogen; thus side-effects vary with the preparation and the dose.

Where *endometriosis* requires drug treatment, it may respond to a progestogen, e.g. norethisterone, administered on a continuous basis. Danazol, gestrinone, and gonadorelin analogues are also available (section 6.7.2).

Although oral progestogens have been used widely for *menorrhagia* they are relatively ineffective compared with tranexamic acid (section 2.11) or, particularly where dysmenorrhoea is also a factor, mefenamic acid (section 10.1.1); the levonorgestrel-releasing intra-uterine device (section 7.3.2.3) may be particularly useful for women also requiring contraception [currently licensed only as a contraceptive]. Oral progestogens have also been used for *severe dysmenorrhoea,* but where contraception is also required in younger women the best choice is a combined oral contraceptive (section 7.3.1).

Progestogens have also been advocated for the alleviation of *premenstrual symptoms,* but no convincing physiological basis for such treatment has been shown.

Progestogens have been used for the prevention of spontaneous abortion in women with a history of *recurrent miscarriage* (habitual abortion) but there is no evidence of benefit for this purpose and they are **not** recommended.

HORMONE REPLACEMENT THERAPY. In postmenopausal women receiving *long-term oestrogen therapy for hormone replacement,* a progestogen needs to be added to prevent cystic hyperplasia of the endometrium and possible transformation to cancer; it can be added on a cyclical or a continuous basis. Combined packs incorporating suitable progestogen tablets are available, see p. 335.

ORAL CONTRACEPTION. Desogestrel, etynodiol (ethynodiol), gestodene, levonorgestrel, norethisterone, and norgestimate are used in *combined oral contraceptives* and in *progestogen-only contraceptives* (section 7.3.1 and section 7.3.2).

CANCER. Progestogens also have a role in *neoplastic disease* (section 8.3.2).

DYDROGESTERONE

Indications: see under Dose and notes above

Cautions: see notes above and under Medroxyprogesterone Acetate

Contra-indications: see notes above and under Medroxyprogesterone Acetate

Side-effects: see notes above and under Medroxyprogesterone Acetate; breakthrough bleeding may occur (increase dose), also headache, dizziness and skin reactions reported

Dose: endometriosis, 10 mg 2–3 times daily from day 5 to 25 of cycle or continuously

Infertility, irregular cycles, 10 mg twice daily from day 11 to 25 for at least 6 cycles (but not recommended)

Habitual abortion, 10 mg twice daily from day 11 to 25 of cycle until conception, then continuously until week 20 of pregnancy and gradually reduced (but see notes above)

Dysfunctional uterine bleeding, 10 mg twice daily (together with an oestrogen) for 5–7 days to arrest bleeding; 10 mg twice daily (together with an oestrogen) from day 11 to 25 of cycle to prevent bleeding

Dysmenorrhoea (but see notes above), 10 mg twice daily from day 5 to 25 of cycle

Amenorrhoea, 10 mg twice daily from day 11 to 25 of cycle with oestrogen therapy from day 1 to 25 of cycle

Premenstrual syndrome, 10 mg twice daily from day 12 to 26 of cycle increased if necessary (but not recommended, see notes above)

Hormone replacement therapy, with continuous oestrogen therapy, see under *Duphaston® HRT* below

Duphaston® (Solvay) [PoM]
Tablets, scored, dydrogesterone 10 mg. Net price 60-tab pack = £4.49

Duphaston® HRT (Solvay) [PoM]
Tablets, scored, dydrogesterone 10 mg. Net price 42-tab pack = £3.14
  Dose: 10 mg daily on days 15–28 of each 28-day oestrogen HRT cycle, increased to 10 mg twice daily if withdrawal bleed is early or endometrial biopsy shows inadequate progestational response

HYDROXYPROGESTERONE CAPROATE

(Hydroxyprogesterone Hexanoate)

Indications: recurrent miscarriage but see notes above

Cautions: monitor pregnancy regularly; diabetes

Contra-indications: history of liver tumours; history of pemphigoid gestationis

Side-effects: see notes above; rarely local reactions at injection site; coughing, dyspnoea, circulatory irregularities; liver tumours reported rarely

Dose: *by slow intramuscular injection*, 250–500 mg weekly during first half of pregnancy

Proluton Depot® (Schering Health) [PoM]
Injection (oily), hydroxyprogesterone caproate 250 mg/mL. Net price 1-mL amp = £2.35; 2-mL amp = £3.69

MEDROXYPROGESTERONE ACETATE

Indications: see under Dose; contraception (section 7.3.2.2); malignant disease (section 8.3.2)

Cautions: diabetes, hypertension, cardiac or renal disease; **interactions:** Appendix 1 (progestogens)

Contra-indications: pregnancy, undiagnosed vaginal bleeding, hepatic impairment or active liver disease, severe arterial disease, breast or genital tract carcinoma; porphyria (section 9.8.2)

Side-effects: acne, urticaria, fluid retention, weight changes, gastro-intestinal disturbances, changes in libido, breast discomfort, premenstrual symptoms, irregular menstrual cycles; also depression, insomnia, somnolence, alopecia, hirsutism, anaphylactoid-like reaction; rarely jaundice

Dose: *by mouth*, 2.5–10 mg daily for 5–10 days beginning on day 16 to 21 of cycle, repeated for 2 cycles in dysfunctional uterine bleeding and 3 cycles in secondary amenorrhoea

Mild to moderate endometriosis, 10 mg 3 times daily for 90 consecutive days, beginning on day 1 of cycle

Provera® (Pharmacia & Upjohn) [PoM]
Tablets, all scored, medroxyprogesterone acetate 2.5 mg (orange), net price 30-tab pack = £1.84; 5 mg (blue), 10-tab pack = £1.23; 10 mg (white), 10-tab pack = £2.47, 90-tab pack = £22.16

■ Combined preparations
Section 6.4.1.1

NORETHISTERONE

Indications: see under Dose; HRT (section 6.4.1.1); contraception (section 7.3.1 and section 7.3.2); malignant disease (section 8.3.2)

Cautions: see under Medroxyprogesterone Acetate

Contra-indications: see under Medroxyprogesterone Acetate; history in pregnancy of idiopathic jaundice, severe pruritus or pemphigoid gestationis; pregnancy

Side-effects: see under Medroxyprogesterone Acetate but more virilising and greater incidence of liver disturbances and jaundice; exacerbation of epilepsy and migraine

Dose: endometriosis, 10–15 mg daily for 4–6 months or longer, starting on day 5 of cycle (if spotting occurs increase dose to 20–25 mg daily, reduced once bleeding has stopped)

Dysfunctional uterine bleeding, menorrhagia (but see notes above), 5 mg 3 times daily for 10 days to arrest bleeding; to prevent bleeding 5 mg twice daily from day 19 to 26

Dysmenorrhoea (but see notes above), 5 mg 3 times daily from day 5 to 24 for 3–4 cycles

Premenstrual syndrome, 5 mg 2–3 times daily from day 19 to 26 for several cycles (but not recommended, see notes above)

Postponement of menstruation, 5 mg 3 times daily starting 3 days before anticipated onset (menstruation occurs 2–3 days after stopping)

Progestogenic opposition of menopausal oestrogen HRT, see under *Micronor® HRT*, below

■ Tablets of 5 mg

Norethisterone (Non-proprietary) PoM
Tablets, norethisterone 5 mg, net price 30-tab pack
= £2.16; 100-tab pack = £7.20
Available from Cox, CP, Lagap

Primolut N® (Schering Health) PoM
Tablets, norethisterone 5 mg. Net price 30-tab pack
= £2.16

Utovlan® (Searle) PoM
Tablets, scored, norethisterone 5 mg, net price 30-
tab pack = £2.16, 90-tab pack = £6.48

■ Tablets of 1 mg for HRT

Micronor® HRT (Janssen-Cilag) PoM
Tablets, norethisterone 1 mg. Net price 3 × 12-tab
pack = £3.75
Dose: 1 tablet daily on days 15–26 of each 28-day oestrogen HRT cycle

■ Combined preparations
Section 6.4.1.1

PROGESTERONE

Indications: see under preparations
Cautions: history of depression; diabetes;
migraine; epilepsy; hypertension; cardiac disease;
hepatic impairment (avoid if severe), renal
impairment; breast-feeding; **interactions:**
Appendix 1 (progestogens)
Contra-indications: undiagnosed vaginal bleeding, missed or incomplete abortion, severe arterial
disease, mammary carcinoma; porphyria (section
9.8.2)
Side-effects: acne, urticaria, rashes, fluid retention, weight changes, gastro-intestinal disturbances, changes in libido, breast discomfort,
premenstrual symptoms, menstrual disturbances;
also chloasma, depression, pyrexia, insomnia,
somnolence, alopecia, hirsutism; rarely jaundice;
injection site reactions; pain, diarrhoea and flatulence can occur with rectal administration

Crinone® (Serono) PoM
Vaginal gel, progesterone 45 mg/application (4%),
net price 6 = £11.08; 90 mg/application (8%), 15
= £38.51
Dose: by vagina, progesterone deficiency, insert 1 applicatorful of 4% gel on alternate mornings from day 15 to
day 25 of cycle
Menopausal symptoms, insert 1 applicatorful of 4% gel
on alternate days for the last 12 days of oestrogen therapy in each cycle (section 6.4.1.1)
Infertility due to inadequate luteal phase, insert 1 applicatorful of 8% gel daily starting either after documented
ovulation or on day 18–21 of cycle
In vitro fertilisation, daily application of 8% gel, continued for 30 days after laboratory evidence of pregnancy

Cyclogest® (Shire) PoM ▭
Pessaries, progesterone 200 mg, net price 15 =
£5.22; 400 mg, 15 = £7.55
Dose: by vagina or rectum, premenstrual syndrome and
post-natal depression, 200 mg daily to 400 mg twice
daily; for premenstrual syndrome start on day 12–14 and
continue until onset of menstruation (but not recommended, see notes above); rectally if barrier methods of
contraception are used, in patients who have recently
given birth or in those who suffer from vaginal infection
or recurrent cystitis

Gestone® (Ferring) PoM
Injection, progesterone 25 mg/mL, net price 1-mL
amp = 34p; 50 mg/mL, 1-mL amp = 44p, 2-mL
amp = 58p
Dose: by deep intramuscular injection into buttock,
Dysfunctional uterine bleeding, 5–10 mg daily for 5–10
days until 2 days before expected onset of menstruation
Habitual abortion due to inadequate luteal phase (but see
notes above) or following *in vitro* fertilisation *or* gamete
intra-fallopian transfer, 25–100 mg 2–7 times a week
from day 15, or day of embryo *or* gamete transfer, until
8–16 weeks of pregnancy; max. 200 mg daily

6.4.2   Male sex hormones and antagonists

Androgens cause masculinisation; they may be
used as replacement therapy in castrated adults and
in those who are hypogonadal due to either pituitary
or testicular disease. In the normal male they inhibit
pituitary gonadotrophin secretion and depress spermatogenesis. Androgens also have an anabolic
action which led to the development of anabolic
steroids (section 6.4.3).

Androgens are useless as a treatment of impotence and impaired spermatogenesis unless there is
associated hypogonadism; they should not be given
until the hypogonadism has been properly investigated. Treatment should be under expert supervision.

When given to patients with hypopituitarism they
can lead to normal sexual development and potency
but not to fertility. If fertility is desired, the usual
treatment is with gonadotrophins or pulsatile
gonadotrophin-releasing hormone (section 6.5.1)
which will stimulate spermatogenesis as well as
androgen production.

Caution should be used when androgens or
chorionic gonadotrophin are used in treating boys
with delayed puberty since the fusion of epiphyses
is hastened and may result in short stature.

Intramuscular depot preparations of **testosterone
esters** are preferred for replacement therapy. Testosterone enantate or propionate or alternatively *Sus-
tanon®*, which consists of a mixture of testosterone
esters and has a longer duration of action, may be
used. Satisfactory replacement therapy can sometimes be obtained with 1 mL of *Sustanon 250®*,
given by intramuscular injection once a month,
although more frequent dose intervals are often
necessary. Implants of testosterone can be used for
hypogonadism; the implants are replaced every 4 to
5 months. Menopausal women are also sometimes
given implants of testosterone (in a dose of 50–
100 mg every 4–8 months) as an adjunct to hormone replacement therapy.

Of the orally active preparations, **testosterone
undecanoate** and **mesterolone** are available. Testosterone patches are now also available.

TESTOSTERONE AND ESTERS

Indications: see under preparations
Cautions: cardiac, renal, or hepatic impairment
(Appendix 2), elderly, ischaemic heart disease,
hypertension, epilepsy, migraine, skeletal metastases (risk of hypercalcaemia), undertake regular
examination of the prostate during treatment; pre-
pubertal boys (see notes above and under Side-
effects); **interactions:** Appendix 1 (testosterone)

Contra-indications: breast cancer in men, prostate cancer, history of primary liver tumours, hypercalcaemia, pregnancy, breast-feeding, nephrosis

Side-effects: prostate abnormalities and prostate cancer, headache, depression, gastro-intestinal bleeding, nausea, cholestatic jaundice, changes in libido, gynaecomastia, anxiety, asthenia, generalised paraesthesia, electrolyte disturbances including sodium retention with oedema and hypercalcaemia; increased bone growth; androgenic effects such as hirsuitism, male pattern baldness, seborrhoea, acne, excessive frequency and duration of penile erections, precocious sexual development and premature closure of epiphyses in pre-pubertal males, suppression of spermatogenesis in men and virilism in women; rarely liver tumours; *with patches*, local irritation and allergic reactions

■ Oral

Restandol® (Organon) PoM

Capsules, red-brown, testosterone undecanoate 40 mg in oily solution. Net price 28-cap pack = £8.30; 56-cap pack = £16.60. Label: 21, 25
Dose: androgen deficiency, 120–160 mg daily for 2–3 weeks; maintenance 40–120 mg daily

■ Intramuscular

Testosterone Enantate (Non-proprietary) PoM

Injection (oily), testosterone enantate 250 mg/mL. Net price 1-mL amp = £8.33
Available from Cambridge
The brand name *Primoteston Depot®* was formerly used for testosterone enantate injection
Dose: by slow intramuscular injection, hypogonadism, initially 250 mg every 2–3 weeks; maintenance 250 mg every 3–6 weeks
Breast cancer, 250 mg every 2–3 weeks

Sustanon 100® (Organon) PoM

Injection (oily), testosterone propionate 20 mg, testosterone phenylpropionate 40 mg, and testosterone isocaproate 40 mg/mL. Net price 1-mL amp = £1.17
Note. Contains arachis (peanut) oil
Dose: by deep intramuscular injection, androgen deficiency, 1 mL every 2 weeks

Sustanon 250® (Organon) PoM

Injection (oily), testosterone propionate 30 mg, testosterone phenylpropionate 60 mg, testosterone isocaproate 60 mg, and testosterone decanoate 100 mg/mL. Net price 1-mL amp = £2.74
Note. Contains arachis (peanut) oil
Dose: by deep intramuscular injection, androgen deficiency, 1 mL usually every 3 weeks

Virormone® (Ferring) PoM

Injection, testosterone propionate 50 mg/mL. Net price 2-mL amp = 46p
Dose: by intramuscular injection, androgen deficiency, 50 mg 2–3 times weekly
Delayed puberty, 50 mg weekly
Breast cancer, 100 mg 2–3 times weekly

■ Implant

Testosterone (Organon) PoM

Implant, testosterone 100 mg, net price = £7.40; 200 mg = £13.79
Dose: by implantation, male hypogonadism, 100–600 mg; 600 mg usually maintains plasma-testosterone concentration within the normal range for 4–5 months
Menopausal women, see notes above

■ Patch

Andropatch® (SmithKline Beecham) PoM

Patches, self-adhesive, releasing testosterone approx. 2.5 mg/24 hours, net price 60-patch pack = £52.80; releasing testosterone approx. 5 mg/24 hours, net price 30-patch pack = £52.80. Counselling, administration
Dose: androgen deficiency in men associated with primary or secondary hypogonadism, apply to clean, dry, unbroken skin on back, abdomen, upper arms or thighs, removing after 24 hours and siting replacement patch on a different area (with an interval of 7 days before using the same site); initially apply patches equivalent to testosterone 5 mg/24 hours (2.5 mg/24 hours in non-virilised patients) at night (approx. 10 p.m.), then adjust to 2.5 mg to 7.5 mg every 24 hours according to plasma-testosterone concentration (those with a body-weight over 130 kg may require 7.5 mg every 24 hours)

Testoderm® (Ferring) PoM

Scrotal patches, self-adhesive, releasing testosterone approx. 6 mg/24 hours, net price 30-patch pack = £53.70. Counselling, administration
Dose: testosterone deficiency, apply 1 patch to clean, dry, shaved scrotal skin in the morning, replace with fresh patch after 22–24 hours; measure plasma-testosterone concentration before and during treatment
Note. Not to be worn while swimming, or in the bath or shower; patches can be temporarily removed for up to 2 hours and then replaced

MESTEROLONE

Indications: see under Dose

Cautions: see under Testosterone and Esters

Contra-indications: see under Testosterone and Esters

Side-effects: see under Testosterone and Esters but spermatogenesis unimpaired

Dose: androgen deficiency and male infertility associated with hypogonadism, 25 mg 3–4 times daily for several months, reduced to 50–75 mg daily in divided doses for maintenance; CHILD not recommended

Pro-Viron® (Schering Health) PoM

Tablets, scored, mesterolone 25 mg. Net price 30-tab pack = £4.75

Anti-androgens

Cyproterone acetate is an anti-androgen used in the treatment of severe hypersexuality and sexual deviation in the male. It inhibits spermatogenesis and produces reversible infertility (but is not a male contraceptive); abnormal sperm forms are produced. Fully informed consent is recommended and an initial spermatogram. As hepatic tumours have been produced in *animal* studies, careful consideration should be given to the risk/benefit ratio before treatment. Cyproterone acetate is also used as an adjunct in prostatic cancer (section 8.3.4.2) and in the treatment of acne and hirsutism in women (section 13.6.2).

Finasteride is a specific inhibitor of the enzyme 5α-reductase which metabolises testosterone into the more potent androgen, dihydrotestosterone. This inhibition of testosterone metabolism leads to reduction in prostate size, with improvement in urinary flow rate and in obstructive symptoms. It is an alternative to alpha-blockers (section 7.4.1) particularly in men with a significantly enlarged prostate.

344 6.4.3 Anabolic steroids

CYPROTERONE ACETATE

Indications: see notes above; prostate cancer (section 8.3.4.2)

Cautions: ineffective for male hypersexuality in chronic alcoholism (relevance to prostate cancer not known); blood counts initially and throughout treatment; monitor hepatic function regularly (liver function tests should be performed before treatment, see also under Side-effects below); monitor adrenocortical function regularly; diabetes mellitus (see also Contra-indications)

DRIVING. Fatigue and lassitude may impair performance of skilled tasks (e.g. driving)

Contra-indications: (do not apply in prostate cancer) liver disease, severe diabetes (with vascular changes); sickle-cell anaemia, malignant or wasting disease, severe depression, history of thrombo-embolic disorders; youths under 18 years (may arrest bone maturation and testicular development)

Side-effects: fatigue and lassitude, breathlessness, weight changes, reduced sebum production (may clear acne), changes in hair pattern, gynaecomastia (rarely leading to galactorrhoea and benign breast nodules); rarely osteoporosis; inhibition of spermatogenesis (see notes above); hepatotoxicity reported (including jaundice, hepatitis and hepatic failure usually in men given 200–300 mg daily for prostatic cancer, see section 8.3.4.2 for details and warnings)

Dose: male hypersexuality, 50 mg twice daily after food

Androcur® (Schering Health) PoM
Tablets, scored, cyproterone acetate 50 mg. Net price 56-tab pack = £32.23. Label: 21
Note. Tablets containing cyproterone acetate 50 mg are also available from Cox, Generics, Hillcross

FINASTERIDE

Indications: benign prostatic hyperplasia

Cautions: obstructive uropathy, prostate cancer (may decrease markers such as prostate specific antigen); use of condoms recommended if sexual partner is pregnant or is likely to become pregnant (finasteride excreted in semen); women of child-bearing potential should avoid handling crushed or broken tablets

Side-effects: impotence, decreased libido, ejaculation disorders, breast tenderness and enlargement, hypersensitivity reactions (including lip swelling and rash)

Dose: 5 mg daily, review treatment after 6 months (may require several months treatment before benefit is obtained)

Proscar® (MSD) PoM
Tablets, blue, f/c, finasteride 5 mg. Net price 28-tab pack = £24.90

| 6.4.3 | **Anabolic steroids** |

All the anabolic steroids have some androgenic activity but they cause less virilisation than androgens in women. Their protein-building property led to the hope that they might be widely useful in medicine but this hope has not been realised. Their use

as body builders or tonics is quite unjustified; they are abused by some athletes.

Anabolic steroids have also been given for osteoporosis in women but are no longer advocated for this purpose.

Anabolic steroids are used in the treatment of some *aplastic anaemias* (section 9.1.3) and to reduce the itching of *chronic biliary obstruction* (see Prescribing in Palliative Care p. 14).

NANDROLONE

Indications: osteoporosis in postmenopausal women (but not recommended, see notes above); aplastic anaemia (section 9.1.3)

Cautions: cardiac and renal impairment, hepatic impairment (see Appendix 2), hypertension, diabetes mellitus, epilepsy, migraine; monitor skeletal maturation in young patients; skeletal metastases (risk of hypercalcaemia); **interactions:** Appendix 1 (anabolic steroids)

Contra-indications: severe hepatic impairment, prostate cancer, male breast cancer, pregnancy and breast-feeding, porphyria (section 9.8.2)

Side-effects: acne, sodium retention with oedema, virilisation with high doses including voice changes (sometimes irreversible), amenorrhoea, inhibition of spermatogenesis, premature epiphyseal closure; abnormal liver-function tests reported with high doses; liver tumours reported occasionally on prolonged treatment with anabolic steroids

Dose: see below

Deca-Durabolin® (Organon) PoM ▭
Injection (oily), nandrolone decanoate 25 mg/mL, net price 1-mL amp = £1.83; 50 mg/mL, 1-mL amp = £3.54
Note. Contains arachis (peanut) oil
Dose: by deep intramuscular injection, 50 mg every 3 weeks

STANOZOLOL

Indications: see under Dose

Cautions: cardiac or renal impairment; premature closure of epiphyses in children; peliosis hepatis and hepatic tumours reported on long-term treatment; breast cancer (possibility of hypercalcaemia); monitor liver function, haematocrit and haemoglobin; diabetes mellitus (possible dosage adjustments for oral hypoglycaemic drugs and avoid in insulin-dependent diabetes); **interactions:** Appendix 1 (anabolic steroids)

Contra-indications: pregnancy, breast-feeding, established liver disease (if history of jaundice—liver function tests before starting treatment); prostate cancer, insulin-dependent diabetes mellitus; not indicated for treatment of loss of appetite, unexplained weight loss, or failure to thrive in children; porphyria (section 9.8.2)

Side-effects: androgenic effects (generally mild and reversible on stopping treatment) include acne, hirsutism, amenorrhoea, sodium retention with oedema; voice change—usually at higher dosage (discontinue); menstrual irregularity, headache, muscle cramp, dyspepsia, rash, hair loss, euphoria, depression, increased haematocrit and haemoglobin; cholestatic jaundice and rarely peliosis hepatis and hepatic tumours also reported; changes in liver enzymes, in lipoproteins, and in thyroid hormones; also premature epiphyseal closure (on prolonged treatment)

Dose: *by mouth*, vascular manifestations of Behcet's disease, 10 mg daily

Hereditary angioedema, 2.5–10 mg daily to control attacks, reduced for maintenance (2.5 mg 3 times weekly may be sufficient); CHILD 1–6 years initially 2.5 mg daily, 6–12 years initially 2.5–5 mg daily, reduced for maintenance

Note. In hereditary angioedema restricted to well-established cases who have experienced serious attacks (and not for premenopausal women except in life-threatening situations)

Stromba® (Sanofi-Synthelabo) PoM
Tablets, scored, stanozolol 5 mg. Net price 56-tab pack = £26.26

6.5 Hypothalamic and pituitary hormones and anti-oestrogens

Hypothalamic and pituitary hormones are described under the following section headings:

6.5.1   Hypothalamic and anterior pituitary hormones and anti-oestrogens

6.5.2   Posterior pituitary hormones and antagonists

Use of preparations in these sections requires detailed prior investigation of the patient and *should be reserved for specialist centres.*

6.5.1 Hypothalamic and anterior pituitary hormones and anti-oestrogens

---

Anti-oestrogens

The anti-oestrogens **clomifene** (clomiphene) and **tamoxifen** (section 8.3.4.1) are used in the treatment of female infertility due to oligomenorrhoea or secondary amenorrhoea (e.g. associated with polycystic ovarian disease). They induce gonadotrophin release by occupying oestrogen receptors in the hypothalamus, thereby interfering with feedback mechanisms; chorionic gonadotrophin is sometimes used as an adjunct. Patients should be warned that there is a risk of multiple pregnancy (*rarely* more than twins).

CLOMIFENE CITRATE
(Clomiphene Citrate)

Indications: anovulatory infertility—see notes above

Cautions: see notes above; polycystic ovary syndrome (cysts may enlarge during treatment), ovarian hyperstimulation syndrome, uterine fibroids, ectopic pregnancy, incidence of multiple

births increased (consider ultrasound monitoring), visual symptoms (discontinue and initiate ophthalmological examination)

CSM Advice. The CSM has recommended that clomifene should not normally be used for longer than 6 cycles (possible increased risk of ovarian cancer in patients treated for longer than recommended).

Contra-indications: hepatic disease, ovarian cysts, hormone dependent tumours or abnormal uterine bleeding of undetermined cause, pregnancy (exclude before treatment)

Side-effects: visual disturbances (withdraw), ovarian hyperstimulation (withdraw), hot flushes, abdominal discomfort, occasionally nausea, vomiting, depression, insomnia, breast tenderness, headache, intermenstrual spotting, menorrhagia, endometriosis, convulsions, weight gain, rashes, dizziness, hair loss

Dose: 50 mg daily for 5 days, starting within about 5 days of onset of menstruation (preferably on 2nd day) or at any time (normally preceded by a progestogen-induced withdrawal bleed) if cycles have ceased; second course of 100 mg daily for 5 days may be given in absence of ovulation; most patients who are going to respond will do so in first course; 3 courses should constitute adequate therapeutic trial; long-term cyclical therapy not recommended—see CSM advice, above

Clomifene (Non-proprietary) PoM
Tablets, clomifene citrate 50 mg, net price 30-tab pack = £8.43
Available from Kent

Clomid® (Hoechst Marion Roussel) PoM
Tablets, yellow, scored, clomifene citrate 50 mg. Net price 30-tab pack = £11.27; 100-tab pack = £32.80

Serophene® (Serono) PoM
Tablets, scored, clomifene citrate 50 mg. Net price 10-tab pack = £4.12; 30-tab pack = £11.56; 100-tab pack = £33.64

Anterior pituitary hormones

Corticotrophins

Tetracosactide (tetracosactrin) an analogue of corticotropin (ACTH) is used to test adrenocortical function; corticotropin itself is no longer commercially available in the UK. Failure of the plasma cortisol concentration to rise after intramuscular administration indicates adrenocortical insufficiency.

Both corticotropin and tetracosactide were formerly used as alternatives to corticosteroids in conditions such as Crohn's disease or rheumatoid arthritis; their value was limited by the variable and unpredictable therapeutic response and by the waning of their effect with time.

TETRACOSACTIDE
(Tetracosactrin)

Indications: see notes above

Cautions: as for corticosteroids, section 6.3.2; **important**: risk of anaphylaxis (medical supervision; consult product literature)

Contra-indications: as for corticosteroids, section 6.3.2

Side-effects: as for corticosteroids, section 6.3.2

Synacthen® (Alliance) [PoM]
Injection, tetracosactide 250 micrograms (as acetate)/mL. Net price 1-mL amp = £3.00
Dose: diagnostic (30-minute test), *by intramuscular or intravenous injection*, 250 micrograms as a single dose

Synacthen Depot® (Alliance) [PoM]
Injection (aqueous suspension), tetracosactide 1 mg (as acetate)/mL, with zinc phosphate complex. Net price 1-mL amp = £4.29
Dose: diagnostic (5-hour test), *by intramuscular injection*, 1 mg as a single dose
Contra-indications: not for use in neonates owing to presence of benzyl alcohol as additive
Note. Formerly used therapeutically by intramuscular injection, in an initial dose of 1 mg daily (or every 12 hours in acute cases); reduced to 1 mg every 2–3 days, then 1 mg weekly (or 500 micrograms every 2–3 days) but value was limited (see notes above)

Gonadotrophins

Follicle-stimulating hormone (FSH) and luteinising hormone (LH) together (as in **human menopausal gonadotrophin**), follicle-stimulating hormone alone (as in **urofollitropin** (urofollitrophin) or **follitropin**), or chorionic gonadotrophin, are used in the treatment of infertility in women with proven hypopituitarism or who have not responded to clomifene, or in superovulation treatment for assisted conception (such as *in vitro* fertilisation).

The gonadotrophins are also occasionally used in the treatment of hypogonadotrophic hypogonadism and associated oligospermia. There is no justification for their use in primary gonadal failure.

Chorionic gonadotrophin has also been used in delayed puberty in the male to stimulate endogenous testosterone production, but has little advantage over testosterone (section 6.4.2).

CHORIONIC GONADOTROPHIN

(Human Chorionic Gonadotrophin; HCG)
A preparation of a glycoprotein fraction secreted by the placenta and obtained from the urine of pregnant women having the action of the pituitary luteinising hormone
Indications: see notes above
Cautions: cardiac or renal impairment, asthma, epilepsy, migraine; prepubertal boys (risk of premature epiphyseal closure or precocious puberty)
Side-effects: oedema (particularly in males—reduce dose), headache, tiredness, mood changes, gynaecomastia, local reactions; may aggravate ovarian hyperstimulation, multiple pregnancy
Contra-indications: androgen-dependant tumours
Dose: *by subcutaneous or intramuscular injection*, according to patient's response

Choragon® (Ferring) [PoM]
Injection, powder for reconstitution, chorionic gonadotrophin. Net price 5000-unit amp (with solvent) = £3.50. For intramuscular injection

Pregnyl® (Organon) [PoM]
Injection, powder for reconstitution, chorionic gonadotrophin. Net price 1500-unit amp = £2.37; 5000-unit amp = £3.52 (both with solvent). For subcutaneous or intramuscular injection

Profasi® (Serono) [PoM]
Injection, powder for reconstitution, chorionic gonadotrophin. Net price 2000-unit amp = £2.01; 5000-unit amp = 3.53; 10 000-unit amp = £7.06 (all with solvent). For subcutaneous or intramuscular injection

FOLLITROPIN ALFA and BETA

(Recombinant human follicle stimulating hormone)
Indications: see notes above
Cautions: see under Human Menopausal Gonadotrophins
Side-effects: see under Human Menopausal Gonadotrophins
Dose: *by subcutaneous or intramuscular injection*, according to patient's response

■ Follitropin alfa
Gonal-F® (Serono) [PoM]
Injection, powder for reconstitution, follitropin alfa. Net price 75-unit amp = £26.25; 150-unit amp = £52.50 (both with diluent)
Note. For subcutaneous injection

■ Follitropin beta
Puregon® (Organon) [PoM]
Injection, follitropin beta 100 units/mL, net price 0.5-mL (50-unit) vial = £20.15; 200 units/mL, 0.5-mL (100-unit) vial = £40.30; 300 units/mL, 0.5-mL (150-unit) vial = £54.43; 400 units/mL, 0.5-mL (200-unit) vial = £72.57
Note. For subcutaneous or intramuscular injection

HUMAN MENOPAUSAL GONADOTROPHINS

Purified extract of human post-menopausal urine containing follicle-stimulating hormone (FSH) and luteinising hormone (LH); the relative *in vivo* activity is designated as a ratio; the 1:1 ratio is also known as menotrophin
Indications: see notes above
Cautions: ovarian cysts, adrenal or thyroid disorders, hyperprolactinoma or pituitary tumour
Side-effects: ovarian hyperstimulation, multiple pregnancy; local reactions
Dose: *by deep intramuscular injection*, according to patient's response

Menogon® (Ferring) [PoM]
Injection, powder for reconstitution, menotrophin as follicle-stimulating hormone 75 units, luteinising hormone 75 units, net price per amp (with solvent) = £9.90

Pergonal® (Serono) [PoM]
Injection, powder for reconstitution, menotrophin as follicle-stimulating hormone 75 units, luteinising hormone 75 units. Net price per amp (with solvent) = £9.72

UROFOLLITROPIN

(Urofollitrophin)
Extract of the urine of postmenopausal women containing follicle-stimulating hormone
Indications: see notes above
Cautions: see under Human Menopausal Gonadotrophins
Side-effects: see under Human Menopausal Gonadotrophins
Dose: *by subcutaneous or intramuscular injection*, according to patient's response

Metrodin High Purity® (Serono) [PoM]
Injection, powder for reconstitution, urofollitropin as follicle-stimulating hormone, net price 75-unit amp = £18.62; 150-unit amp = £37.24 (both with solvent). For subcutaneous or intramuscular injection

Growth hormone

Growth hormone is used in the treatment of growth hormone deficiency (including short stature in Turner syndrome); only the human type is effective since growth hormone is species specific. Growth hormone of human origin (HGH; somatotrophin) has been replaced by a growth hormone of human sequence, **somatropin**, produced using recombinant DNA technology.

SOMATROPIN

(Synthetic Human Growth Hormone)

Indications: see under Dose

Cautions: diabetes mellitus (adjustment of antidiabetic therapy may be necessary), papilloedema (see under Side-effects), relative deficiencies of other pituitary hormones (notably hypothyroidism—periodic thyroid function tests recommended), history of malignant disease, disorders of the epiphysis of the hip (monitor for limping), resolved intracranial hypertension (monitor closely); breast-feeding; **interactions:** Appendix 1 (somatropin)

Contra-indications: evidence of tumour activity (complete antitumour therapy and ensure intracranial lesions inactive before starting); not to be used after renal transplantation in seriously ill patients or for growth promotion in children with closed epiphyses; pregnancy (interrupt treatment if pregnancy occurs)

Side-effects: headache, funduscopy for papilloedema recommended if severe or recurrent headache, visual problems, nausea and vomiting occur—if papilloedema confirmed consider benign intracranial hypertension (rare cases reported); fluid retention (peripheral oedema), arthralgia, myalgia, paraesthesia, antibody formation, hypothyroidism, reactions at injection site; leukaemia in children with growth hormone deficiency also reported

Dose: *by subcutaneous injection*, weekly dosage adjusted individually and given in 3, 6 or 7 divided doses (rotate injection sites to prevent lipoatrophy); alternatively *by intramuscular injection*, weekly dosage given in 3, 6 or 7 divided doses (but more painful)

Gonadal dysgenesis (Turner syndrome), 0.6–1 unit/kg weekly (18–30 units/m^2 body-surface area weekly) in divided doses given by subcutaneous injection

Insufficient secretion of growth hormone in children, 0.4–0.8 units/kg weekly (12–21 units/m^2 body-surface area weekly) in divided doses given by subcutaneous or intramuscular injection

Chronic renal insufficiency in children (renal function decreased to less than 50%), approx. 1 unit/kg weekly (28–30 units/m^2 body-surface area weekly) divided into daily subcutaneous injections, higher doses may be needed; adjustment may be required after 6 months

Adult growth hormone deficiency, initially 0.125 units/kg weekly (divided into daily subcutaneous injections) gradually increased if required to max. 0.25 units/kg weekly; use minimum effective dose (requirements may decrease with age)

Genotropin® (Pharmacia & Upjohn) PoM

Injection, two-compartment cartridge containing powder for reconstitution, somatropin (rbe) and diluent, net price 16-unit (5.3-mg) cartridge = £116.51, 36-unit (12-mg) cartridge = £262.15. For use with *Genotropin® Pen* NHS or *KabiPen®* NHS devices (available free of charge from clinics). For subcutaneous injection

KabiQuick injection, two-compartment single-dose syringe containing powder for reconstitution, somatropin (rbe) and diluent, net price 2-unit (0.7-mg) syringe = £15.28, 3-unit (1-mg) syringe = £22.92, 4-unit (1.3-mg) syringe = £30.56. For subcutaneous injection

KabiVial injection, two-compartment cartridge containing powder for reconstitution, somatropin (rbe) and diluent, net price 16-unit (5.3-mg) vial = £116.51. For subcutaneous injection

MiniQuick injection, two-compartment single-dose syringe containing powder for reconstitution, somatropin (rbe) and diluent, net price 0.6-unit (0.2-mg) syringe = £4.37, 1.2-unit (0.4-mg) syringe = £8.74, 1.8-unit (0.6-mg) syringe = £13.11, 2.4-unit (0.8-mg) syringe = £17.48, 3-unit (1-mg) syringe = £21.85. For subcutaneous injection

Humatrope® (Lilly) PoM

Injection, powder for reconstitution, somatropin (rbe), net price 4-unit (1.33-mg) vial (with diluent) = £30.50; 16-unit (5.33-mg) vial (with diluent) = £122.00; 18-unit (6-mg) cartridge = £137.25; 36-unit (12-mg) cartridge = £274.50; 72-unit (24-mg) cartridge = £549.00; all supplied with diluent. For subcutaneous or intramuscular injection; cartridges for subcutaneous injection

Norditropin® (Novo Nordisk) PoM

Injection, powder for reconstitution, somatropin (epr), net price 12-unit (4-mg) vial (with diluent) = £89.21. For subcutaneous injection (intramuscular route rarely used)

PenSet 12 injection, powder for reconstitution, somatropin (epr), net price 12-unit (4-mg) vial (with diluent in cartridge and needle) = £93.68. For use with *Nordiject®12* NHS device (available free of charge from clinics). For subcutaneous injection

PenSet 24 injection, powder for reconstitution, somatropin (epr), net price 24-unit (8-mg) vial (with diluent in cartridge and needle) = £187.35. For use with *Nordiject®24* NHS device (available free of charge from clinics). For subcutaneous injection

SimpleXx injection, somatropin (epr) 10 units (3.3 mg)/mL, net price 1.5-mL (15-unit, 5-mg) cartridge = £117.10; 20 units (6.7 mg)/mL, 1.5-mL (30-unit, 10-mg) cartridge = £234.20; 30 units (10 mg)/mL, 1.5-mL (45-unit, 15-mg) cartridge = £351.30. For use with appropriate *NordiPen®* NHS device (available free of charge from clinics). For subcutaneous injection

Saizen® (Serono) PoM

Injection, powder for reconstitution, somatropin (rmc), net price 4-unit (1.33-mg) vial (with diluent) = £30.50; 10-unit (3.33-mg) vial (with diluent) = £76.25. For subcutaneous or intramuscular injection

Easyject®, powder for reconstitution, somatropin (rmc), net price 24-unit (8-mg) vial (with diluent) = £183.00. For use with *Easyject®* NHS device (available free-of-charge from clinics). For subcutaneous injection

Zomacton® (Ferring) PoM

Injection, powder for reconstitution, somatropin (rbe), net price 12-unit (4-mg) vial (with diluent) = £83.28. For use with *ZomaJet®* 2 NHS needle-free device or with *Auto-Jector®* NHS (both available free of charge from clinics) or with needles and syringes. For subcutaneous injection

---

Hypothalamic hormones

Gonadorelin when injected intravenously in normal subjects leads to a rapid rise in plasma concentrations of both luteinising hormone (LH) and follicle-stimulating hormone (FSH). It has not proved to be very helpful, however, in distinguishing hypothalamic from pituitary lesions. **Gonadorelin analogues** are indicated in endometriosis and infertility (section 6.7.2) and in breast and prostate cancer (section 8.3.4).

Protirelin may be of value in difficult cases of hyperthyroidism but has been superseded largely by immunoassays. Failure of plasma thyrotrophin (TSH) concentration to rise after intravenous injection indicates excess circulating thyroid hormones. Impaired or absent responses also occur in some euthyroid patients with single adenoma, multinodular goitre, or endocrine exophthalmos; patients with hypopituitarism show a reduced or delayed rise.

Sermorelin, an analogue of growth hormone releasing hormone (somatorelin, GHRH), has recently been introduced as a diagnostic test for secretion of growth hormone.

GONADORELIN

(Gonadotrophin-releasing hormone; GnRH; LH–RH)
Indications: see preparations below
Cautions: pituitary adenoma
Side-effects: rarely, nausea, headache, abdominal pain, increased menstrual bleeding; rarely, hypersensitivity reaction on repeated administration of large doses; irritation at injection site
Dose: see under preparations

HRF® (Monmouth) PoM

Injection, powder for reconstitution, gonadorelin. Net price 100-microgram vial (with diluent) = £13.45 (hosp. only)
For assessment of pituitary function (adults), *by subcutaneous or intravenous injection*, 100 micrograms

---

PROTIRELIN

(Thyrotrophin-releasing hormone; TRH)
Indications: assessment of thyroid function and thyroid stimulating hormone reserve
Cautions: severe hypopituitarism, myocardial ischaemia, bronchial asthma and obstructive airways disease, pregnancy, breast-feeding (Appendix 5)
Side-effects: after rapid intravenous administration desire to micturate, flushing, dizziness, nausea, strange taste; transient increase in pulse rate and blood pressure; rarely bronchospasm
Dose: *by intravenous injection*, 200 micrograms; CHILD 1 microgram/kg

Protirelin (Non-proprietary) PoM

Injection, protirelin 100 micrograms/mL. Net price 2-mL amp = £7.89 (hosp. only)
Available from Cambridge
The brand name *TRH-Cambridge®* was formerly used for protirelin injection

---

SERMORELIN

Indications: see notes above
Cautions: epilepsy; discontinue growth hormone therapy 1–2 weeks before test; untreated hypothyroidism, antithyroid drugs; obesity, hyperglycaemia, elevated plasma fatty acids; avoid preparations which affect release of growth hormone (includes those affecting release of somatostatin, insulin or glucocorticoids and cyclo-oxygenase inhibitors such as aspirin and indometacin)
Contra-indications: pregnancy and breast-feeding
Side-effects: occasional facial flushing and pain at injection site
Dose: *by intravenous injection*, 1 microgram/kg in the morning after an overnight fast

Geref 50® (Serono) ▼ PoM

Injection, powder for reconstitution, sermorelin 50 micrograms (as acetate). Net price per amp (with solvent) = £52.53

| 6.5.2 | **Posterior pituitary hormones and antagonists** |

Posterior pituitary hormones

DIABETES INSIPIDUS. **Vasopressin** (antidiuretic hormone, ADH) is used in the treatment of *pituitary* ('cranial') *diabetes insipidus* as is its analogue **desmopressin.** Dosage is tailored to produce a slight diuresis every 24 hours to avoid water intoxication. Treatment may be required for a limited period only in diabetes insipidus following trauma or pituitary surgery.

Desmopressin has a longer duration of action than vasopressin; unlike vasopressin it has no vasoconstrictor effect. It is given by mouth or intranasally for maintenance therapy, and by injection in the postoperative period or in unconscious patients. Desmopressin is also used in the differential diagnosis of diabetes insipidus. Following a dose of 2 micrograms intramuscularly or 20 micrograms intranasally, restoration of the ability to concentrate urine after water deprivation confirms a diagnosis of cranial diabetes insipidus. Failure to respond occurs in nephrogenic diabetes insipidus.

In *nephrogenic* and *partial pituitary diabetes insipidus* benefit may be gained from the paradoxical antidiuretic effect of thiazides (section 2.2.1) e.g. chlortalidone 100 mg twice daily reduced to maintenance dose of 50 mg daily.

Chlorpropamide (section 6.1.2.1) is also useful in partial pituitary diabetes insipidus, and probably acts by sensitising the renal tubules to the action of remaining endogenous vasopressin; it is given in doses of up to 350 mg daily in adults and 200 mg daily in children, care being taken to avoid hypoglycaemia. Carbamazepine (section 4.8.1) is also sometimes useful (in a dose of 200 mg once or twice daily) [unlicensed]; its mode of action may be similar to that of chlorpropamide.

OTHER USES. Desmopressin injection is also used to boost factor VIII concentrations in mild to moderate haemophilia. For a comment on use of desmopressin in nocturnal enuresis see section 7.4.2.

Vasopressin infusion is used to control variceal bleeding in portal hypertension, prior to more definitive treatment and with variable results. Terlipressin, a derivative of vasopressin, is used similarly.

Oxytocin, another posterior pituitary hormone, is indicated in obstetrics (section 7.1.1).

VASOPRESSIN

Indications: pituitary diabetes insipidus; bleeding from oesophageal varices

Cautions: heart failure, hypertension, asthma, epilepsy, migraine or other conditions which might be aggravated by water retention; renal impairment (see also Contra-indications); pregnancy (Appendix 4); avoid fluid overload

Contra-indications: vascular disease (especially disease of coronary arteries) unless extreme caution, chronic nephritis (until reasonable blood nitrogen concentrations attained)

Side-effects: fluid retention, pallor, tremor, sweating, vertigo, headache, nausea, vomiting, belching, abdominal cramps, desire to defaecate, hypersensitivity reactions (including anaphylaxis), constriction of coronary arteries (may cause anginal attacks and myocardial ischaemia), peripheral ischaemia and rarely gangrene

Dose: *by subcutaneous or intramuscular injection,* diabetes insipidus, 5–20 units every four hours

By intravenous infusion, initial control of variceal bleeding, 20 units over 15 minutes

■ Synthetic vasopressin

Pitressin® (Goldshield) PoM

Injection, argipressin (synthetic vasopressin) 20 units/mL. Net price 1-mL amp = £14.29 (hosp. only)

DESMOPRESSIN

Indications: see under Dose

Cautions: see under Vasopressin; less pressor activity, but still considerable caution in renal impairment, in cardiovascular disease and in hypertension (not indicated for nocturnal enuresis or nocturia in these circumstances); elderly (avoid for nocturnal enuresis and nocturia in those over 65 years); also considerable caution in cystic fibrosis; in nocturia and nocturnal enuresis limit fluid intake to minimum and only to satisfy thirst for 8 hours after dose; in nocturia periodic blood pressure and weight checks needed to monitor for fluid overload; **interactions:** Appendix 1 (desmopressin)

HYPONATRAEMIC CONVULSIONS. The CSM has advised that patients being treated for primary nocturnal enuresis should be warned to avoid fluid overload (including during swimming) and to stop taking desmopressin during an episode of vomiting or diarrhoea (until fluid balance normal). The risk of hyponatraemic convulsions can also be minimised by keeping to the recommended starting doses and by avoiding concomitant use of drugs which increase secretion of vasopressin (e.g. tricyclic antidepressants)

Contra-indications: cardiac insufficiency and other conditions treated with diuretics

Side-effects: fluid retention, and hyponatraemia (in more serious cases with convulsions) on administration without restricting fluid intake; stomach pain, headache, nausea, and vomiting also reported; epistaxis, nasal congestion, rhinitis with nasal spray

Dose: *by mouth*

Diabetes insipidus, treatment, ADULT and CHILD initially 300 micrograms daily (in 3 divided doses); maintenance, 300–600 micrograms daily in 3 divided doses; range 0.2–1.2 mg daily

Primary nocturnal enuresis (if urine concentrating ability normal), ADULT (under 65 years) and CHILD over 5 years (preferably over 7 years) 200 micrograms at bedtime, only increased to 400 micrograms if lower dose not effective (**important:** see also Cautions); withdraw for at least 1 week for reassessment after 3 months

Postoperative polyuria/polydipsia, adjust dose according to urine osmolality

Intranasally

Diabetes insipidus, diagnosis, ADULT and CHILD 20 micrograms (limit fluid intake to 500 mL from 1 hour before to 8 hours after administration)

Diabetes insipidus, treatment, ADULT 10–40 micrograms daily (in 1–2 divided doses); CHILD 5–20 micrograms daily; infants may require lower doses

Primary nocturnal enuresis (if urine concentrating ability normal), ADULT (under 65 years) and CHILD over 5 years (preferably over 7 years) initially 20 micrograms at bedtime, only increased to 40 micrograms if lower dose not effective (**important:** see also Cautions); withdraw for at least 1 week for reassessment after 3 months

Nocturia associated with multiple sclerosis (when other treatments have failed), ADULT (under 65 years) 10–20 micrograms at bedtime (**important:** see also Cautions), dose not to be repeated within 24 hours

Renal function testing (empty bladder at time of administration and limit fluid intake to 500 mL from 1 hour before until 8 hours after administration), ADULT 40 micrograms; CHILD 1–15 years 20 micrograms, under 1 year 10 micrograms (restrict fluid intake to 50% at next 2 feeds to avoid fluid overload)

By injection

Diabetes insipidus, diagnosis (*subcutaneous or intramuscular*), ADULT and CHILD 2 micrograms (limit fluid intake to 500 mL from 1 hour before to 8 hours after administration)

Diabetes insipidus, treatment (*subcutaneous, intramuscular or intravenous*), ADULT 1–4 micrograms daily; CHILD 400 nanograms

Renal function testing (empty bladder at time of administration and limit fluid intake to 500 mL from 1 hour before until 8 hours after administration) (*subcutaneous or intramuscular*), ADULT and CHILD 2 micrograms; INFANT 400 nanograms (restrict fluid intake to 50% at next 2 feeds)

Mild to moderate haemophilia and von Willebrands disease, post lumbar puncture headache, fibrinolytic response testing, consult product literature

DDAVP® (Ferring) PoM
Tablets, both scored, desmopressin acetate
100 micrograms, net price 90-tab pack = £45.95;
200 micrograms, 90-tab pack = £91.90. Counselling, fluid intake, see above
Intranasal solution, desmopressin acetate
100 micrograms/mL. Net price 2.5-mL dropper
bottle and catheter = £9.50. Counselling, fluid
intake, see above
Injection, desmopressin acetate 4 micrograms/mL.
Net price 1-mL amp = £1.07

Desmotabs® (Ferring) PoM
Tablets, scored, desmopressin acetate
200 micrograms, net price 28-tab pack = £29.00.
Counselling, fluid intake, see above

Desmospray® (Ferring) PoM
Nasal spray, desmopressin acetate 10 micrograms/
metered spray. Net price 6-mL unit = £28.00.
Counselling, fluid intake, see above
Note. Children requiring dose of less than
10 micrograms should be given *DDAVP® intranasal
solution*

TERLIPRESSIN

Indications: bleeding from oesophageal varices
Cautions: see under Vasopressin
Contra-indications: see under Vasopressin
Side-effects: see under Vasopressin, but effects
milder
Dose: *by intravenous injection*, 2 mg followed by 1
or 2 mg every 4 to 6 hours until bleeding is controlled, for up to 72 hours

Glypressin® (Ferring) PoM
Injection, terlipressin, powder for reconstitution.
Net price 1-mg vial with 5 mL diluent = £19.00
(hosp. only)

Antidiuretic hormone antagonists

Demeclocycline (section 5.1.3) may be used in the
treatment of hyponatraemia resulting from inappropriate secretion of antidiuretic hormone. It is
thought to act by directly blocking the renal tubular
effect of antidiuretic hormone. Initially 0.9 to 1.2 g
is given daily in divided doses, reduced to 600–
900 mg daily for maintenance.

6.6　Drugs affecting bone metabolism

| 6.6.1 | Calcitonin |
| 6.6.2 | Bisphosphonates |

See also calcium (section 9.5.1.1), phosphorus (section 9.5.2), vitamin D (section 9.6.4), and oestrogens
in postmenopausal osteoporosis (section 6.4.1.1).

Osteoporosis

Osteoporosis occurs commonly in postmenopausal
women and in those taking long-term oral corticosteroids. Other risk factors for osteoporosis include
low body weight, cigarette smoking, excess alcohol
intake, lack of physical activity, family history of
osteoporosis, and early menopause.

> Those at risk of osteoporosis should maintain an
> adequate intake of **calcium and vitamin D** and
> any deficiency should be corrected by increasing dietary intake or taking supplements.

Elderly patients, especially those who are housebound or live in residential or nursing homes, are at
increased risk of calcium and vitamin D deficiency
and may benefit from supplements (section 9.5.1.1
and section 9.6.4). Reversible secondary causes of
osteoporosis such as hyperthyroidism, hyperparathyroidism, osteomalacia or hypogonadism should be
excluded before treatment for osteoporosis is initiated.

POSTMENOPAUSAL OSTEOPOROSIS. **Hormone
replacement therapy** (HRT, section 6.4.1.1) is recommended for *prophylaxis* of postmenopausal
osteoporosis but it needs to be continued for at least
5–10 years to be beneficial. **Etidronate** (section
6.6.2) or **calcitonin** (section 6.6.1) may be considered for those at high risk of osteoporosis for whom
HRT is unsuitable. **Raloxifene** (section 6.4.1.1) has
recently been introduced for the prevention of vertebral fractures in postmenopausal women.

HRT or a bisphosphonate (section 6.2.2) may be
used for the *treatment* of postmenopausal osteoporosis. The **bisphosphonates** etidronate and alendronate decrease the risk of vertebral fracture;
alendronate has also been shown to reduce non-vertebral fractures. If HRT and bisphosphonates are
unsuitable **calcitriol** (section 9.6.4) or **calcitonin**
may be considered. Calcitonin may also be useful
for pain relief for up to 3 months after a vertebral
fracture if other analgesics are ineffective.

CORTICOSTEROID-INDUCED OSTEOPOROSIS. To reduce the risk of osteoporosis doses of oral
corticosteroids should be as low as possible and
courses of treatment as short as possible. The greatest rate of bone loss occurs during the first 6–12
months of corticosteroid use and so early steps to
prevent the development of osteoporosis are important.

Patients taking the equivalent of prednisolone
7.5 mg or more each day for 3 months or longer
should be assessed and where necessary given prophylactic treatment; those aged over 65 years are at
greater risk. Patients taking oral corticosteroids who
have sustained a low-trauma fracture should receive
treatment for osteoporosis. The therapeutic options
for *prophylaxis* and *treatment* of corticosteroid-induced osteoporosis are the same:

* hormone replacement (HRT in women, testosterone in men) in those who are deficient;

* a bisphosphonate such as etidronate;

* calcitriol.

6.6.1　Calcitonin

Calcitonin is involved with parathyroid hormone in
the regulation of bone turnover and hence in the
maintenance of calcium balance and homoeostasis.
Calcitonin (salmon) (**salcatonin**, synthetic or
recombinant salmon calcitonin) is used to lower the
plasma-calcium concentration in some patients with
hypercalcaemia (notably when associated with
malignant disease). In the treatment of severe
Paget's disease of bone it is used mainly for relief of
pain but it is also effective in relieving some of the
neurological complications, for example deafness.

CALCITONIN (SALMON)/ SALCATONIN

Indications: see under Dose (all short term)

Cautions: history of allergy (skin test advised); renal impairment; heart failure; children—use for short periods only and monitor bone growth; pregnancy (Appendix 4), breast-feeding (Appendix 5)

Side-effects: nausea, vomiting, diarrhoea, flushing, dizziness, tingling of hands, unpleasant taste, rash; allergic reactions including anaphylaxis reported; inflammatory reactions at injection site

Dose: hypercalcaemia, *by subcutaneous or intramuscular injection*, range from 5–10 units/kg daily (in 1–2 divided doses) *to* 400 units every 6–8 hours adjusted according to clinical and biochemical response (no additional benefit with over 8 units/kg every 6 hours); *by slow intravenous infusion* (*Forcaltonin*® and *Miacalcic*® ampoules only), 5–10 units/kg over at least 6 hours

Paget's disease of bone, *by subcutaneous or intramuscular injection*, dose range 50 units 3 times weekly to 100 units daily, in single or divided doses

Bone pain in neoplastic disease, *by subcutaneous or intramuscular injection*, 200 units every 6 hours *or* 400 units every 12 hours for 48 hours; may be repeated at discretion of physician

Postmenopausal osteoporosis, *by subcutaneous or intramuscular injection*, 100 units daily with dietary calcium and vitamin D supplements (see section 9.5.1.1 and section 9.6.4)

Calsynar® (Rhône-Poulenc Rorer) [PoM]
Injection, calcitonin (salmon) 100 units/mL, net price 1-mL amp = £7.92; 200 units/mL, 2-mL vial = £28.47
For subcutaneous or intramuscular injection only

Forcaltonin® (Strakan) [PoM]
Injection, calcitonin (salmon) (recombinant) 100 units/mL, net price 1-mL amp = £3.56
For subcutaneous or intramuscular injection and for dilution and use as an intravenous infusion

Miacalcic® (Novartis) [PoM]
Injection, calcitonin (salmon) 50 units/mL, net price 1-mL amp = £3.56; 100 units/mL, 1-mL amp = £7.13; 200 units/mL, 2-mL vial = £25.62
For subcutaneous or intramuscular injection and for dilution and use as an intravenous infusion

---

6.6.2   Bisphosphonates

Bisphosphonates are used mainly in the treatment of *Paget's disease* of bone. They are adsorbed onto hydroxyapatite crystals, so slowing both their rate of growth and dissolution, and reduce the increased rate of bone turnover associated with the disease. They are also used in the treatment of *hypercalcaemia of malignancy* (section 9.5.1.2). Bisphosphonates may also have an important role in treating *osteoporosis in postmenopausal women*. Disodium etidronate (as *Didronel PMO*®) is also licensed for the prevention and treatment of corticosteroid-induced osteoporosis.

ALENDRONIC ACID

Indications: postmenopausal osteoporosis (treatment)

Cautions: upper gastro-intestinal disorders (dysphagia, symptomatic oesophageal disease, gastritis, duodenitis, or ulcers—see also under Contra-indications and Side-effects); renal impairment (manufacturer advises avoid if creatinine clearance is less than 35 mL/minute); correct disturbances of calcium and mineral metabolism (e.g. vitamin-D deficiency, hypocalcaemia) before starting; exclude other causes of osteoporosis; **interactions:** Appendix 1 (bisphosphonates)

Contra-indications: abnormalities of oesophagus and other factors which delay emptying (e.g. stricture or achalasia), hypocalcaemia, pregnancy and breast-feeding; inability to stand or sit upright for 30 minutes (see Counselling below)

Side-effects: oesophageal reactions (see below), abdominal pain and distension, diarrhoea or constipation, flatulence, musculoskeletal pain, headache; rarely rash, erythema, photosensitivity, uveitis, transient decrease in serum calcium and phosphate; nausea, vomiting, peptic ulceration and hypersensitivity reactions (including urticaria and angioedema) also reported

OESOPHAGEAL REACTIONS. Severe oesophageal reactions (oesophagitis, oesophageal ulcers, oesophageal stricture and oesophageal erosions) have been reported; patients should be advised to stop taking the tablets and to seek medical attention if they develop symptoms of oesophageal irritation such as dysphagia, new or worsening heartburn, pain on swallowing or retrosternal pain

Dose: 10 mg daily at least 30 minutes before breakfast

COUNSELLING. Swallow the tablets whole with a full glass of water on an empty stomach at least 30 minutes before breakfast (and any other oral medication); stand or sit upright for at least 30 minutes and do not lie down until after eating breakfast. Do not take the tablets at bedtime or before rising.

Fosamax® (MSD) ▼ [PoM]
Tablets, alendronic acid 10 mg (as alendronate sodium). Net price 28-tab pack = £25.69. Counselling, administration

---

DISODIUM ETIDRONATE

Indications: see under Dose

Cautions: reduce dose in mild renal impairment (avoid if moderate to severe); **interactions:** Appendix 1 (bisphosphonates)

Contra-indications: moderate to severe renal impairment; pregnancy and breast-feeding; not indicated for osteoporosis in presence of hypercalcaemia or hypercalciuria or for osteomalacia

Side-effects: nausea, diarrhoea or constipation, abdominal pain; asymptomatic hypocalcaemia; increased bone pain in Paget's disease, also increased risk of fractures with high doses in Paget's disease (discontinue if fractures occur); rarely skin reactions (including angioedema urticaria and pruritus), transient hyperphosphataemia, headache, paraesthesia, peripheral neuropathy reported; blood disorders (including leucopenia, agranulocytosis and pancytopenia) also reported

Dose: Paget's disease of bone, *by mouth,* 5 mg/kg as a single daily dose for up to 6 months; doses above 10 mg/kg daily for up to 3 months may be used with caution but doses above 20 mg/kg daily are not recommended; after interval of not less than 3 months may be repeated where evidence of reactivation—including biochemical indices (avoid premature retreatment)

MONITORING. Serum phosphate, serum alkaline phosphatase and (if possible) urinary hydroxyproline should be measured before starting and at intervals of 3 months—consult product literature for further details

Osteoporosis, see under *Didronel PMO®*

COUNSELLING. Avoid food for at least 2 hours before and after oral treatment, particularly calcium-containing products e.g. milk; also avoid iron and mineral supplements and antacids

Didronel® (Procter & Gamble Pharm.) PoM
Tablets, disodium etidronate 200 mg. Net price 60-tab pack = £43.88. Counselling, food and calcium (see above)

■ With calcium carbonate

For cautions and side-effects of calcium carbonate see section 9.5.1.1

Didronel PMO® (Procter & Gamble Pharm.) PoM
Tablets, 14 white, disodium etidronate 400 mg; 76 pink, effervescent, calcium carbonate 1.25 g (*Cacit®*). Net price per pack = £40.20. Label: 10 patient information leaflet, counselling, food and calcium (see above)

Dose: treatment of osteoporosis, prevention of bone loss in postmenopausal women (particularly if hormone replacement therapy inappropriate), and prevention and treatment of corticosteroid-induced osteoporosis, given in 90-day cycles, 1 *Didronel®* tablet daily for 14 days, then 1 *Cacit®* tablet daily for 76 days

DISODIUM PAMIDRONATE

Disodium pamidronate was formerly called aminohydroxypropylidenediphosphonate disodium (APD)

Indications: see under Dose

Cautions: renal impairment—monitor renal function in those with pre-existing renal disease or predisposition to renal impairment (e.g. in multiple myeloma or tumour-induced hypercalcaemia); cardiac disease (especially in elderly); previous thyroid surgery (risk of hypocalcaemia); monitor serum electrolytes, calcium and phosphate—possibility of convulsions due to electrolyte changes; avoid concurrent use with other bisphosphonates; **interactions:** Appendix 1 (bisphosphonates)

DRIVING. Patients should be warned against driving or operating machinery immediately after treatment (somnolence or dizziness may occur)

Contra-indications: pregnancy and breast-feeding

Side-effects: hypocalcaemia (rarely symptomatic), hypophosphataemia, transient rise in body temperature, fever and influenza-like symptoms (sometimes accompanied by malaise, rigors, fatigue and flushes); occasionally transient bone pain, arthralgia, myalgia, nausea, vomiting, headache, lymphocytopenia, hypomagnesaemia; rarely muscle cramps, anorexia, abdominal pain, diarrhoea, constipation, dyspepsia, agitation, con-

fusion, dizziness, insomnia, somnolence, lethargy, anaemia, leucopenia, hypotension or hypertension, rash, pruritus, hyperkalaemia or hypokalaemia, hypernatraemia; isolated cases of seizures, hallucinations, thrombocytopenia, haematuria, acute renal failure, deterioration of pre-existing renal disease, conjunctivitis and other ocular symptoms, abnormal liver function tests, reactivation of herpes simplex and zoster also reported; also local reactions at injection site

Dose: *by slow intravenous infusion* (via cannula in a relatively large vein), see also Appendix 6

Hypercalcaemia of malignancy, according to serum calcium concentration 15–60 mg in single infusion or in divided doses over 2–4 days; max. 90 mg per treatment course

Osteolytic lesions and bone pain in bone metastases associated with breast cancer or multiple myeloma, 90 mg every 4 weeks (or every 3 weeks to coincide with chemotherapy in breast cancer)

Paget's disease of bone, 30 mg once a week for 6 weeks (total dose 180 mg) *or* 30 mg in first week then 60 mg every other week (total dose 210 mg); max. total 360 mg (in divided doses of 60 mg) per treatment course; may be repeated every 6 months

CALCIUM AND VITAMIN D SUPPLEMENTS. Oral supplements are advised for those with Paget's disease at risk of calcium or vitamin D deficiency (e.g. through malabsorption or lack of exposure to sunlight) to minimise potential risk of hypocalcaemia

Aredia Dry Powder® (Novartis) PoM
Injection, powder for reconstitution, disodium pamidronate, for use as an infusion. Net price 15-mg vial = £27.27; 30-mg vial = £54.53; 90-mg vial = £155.80 (all with diluent). Counselling, driving, see above

SODIUM CLODRONATE

Indications: see under Dose

Cautions: monitor renal and hepatic function and white cell count; also monitor serum calcium and phosphate periodically; renal dysfunction reported in patients receiving concomitant NSAIDs; maintain adequate fluid intake during treatment; **interactions:** Appendix 1 (bisphosphonates)

Contra-indications: moderate to severe renal impairment; pregnancy and breast-feeding

Side-effects: nausea, diarrhoea; asymptomatic hypocalcaemia; skin reactions

Dose: osteolytic lesions, hypercalcaemia and bone pain associated with skeletal metastases in patients with breast cancer or multiple myeloma, *by mouth,* 1.6 g daily in single or 2 divided doses increased if necessary to a max. of 3.2 g daily

COUNSELLING. Avoid food for 1 hour before and after treatment, particularly calcium-containing products e.g. milk; also avoid iron and mineral supplements and antacids; maintain adequate fluid intake

Hypercalcaemia of malignancy, *by slow intravenous infusion,* 300 mg daily for max. 7–10 days *or* by single-dose infusion of 1.5 g

Bonefos® (Boehringer Ingelheim) PoM
Capsules, yellow, sodium clodronate 400 mg. Net price 30-cap pack = £43.54, 120-cap pack = £174.16. Counselling, food and calcium
Tablets, f/c, scored, sodium clodronate 800 mg. Net price 10-tab pack = £30.40; 60-tab pack = £182.39. Counselling, food and calcium
Concentrate (= intravenous solution), sodium clodronate 60 mg/mL, for dilution and use as infusion. Net price 5-mL amp = £13.78

Loron® (Roche) PoM
Loron® capsules, sodium clodronate 400 mg. Net price 30-cap pack = £43.54. Label: 10 patient information leaflet, counselling, food and calcium
Loron 520® tablets, f/c, scored, sodium clodronate 520 mg. Net price 10-tab pack = £29.03; 60-tab pack = £174.18. Label: 10 patient information leaflet, counselling, food and calcium
Dose: 2 tablets daily in single or two divided doses; may be increased to max. 4 tablets daily
Note. Due to greater bioavailability one *Loron 520*® tablet (520 mg) is equivalent to two *Loron*® capsules (2 × 400 mg)

Loron® for infusion (Roche) PoM
Intravenous solution, sodium clodronate 30 mg/mL, for dilution and use as infusion. Net price 10-mL amp = £13.78

TILUDRONIC ACID

Indications: Paget's disease of bone
Cautions: renal impairment (monitor renal function regularly, see under Contra-indications); correct disturbances of calcium metabolism (e.g. vitamin D deficiency, hypocalcaemia) before starting; avoid concomitant use of indometacin; **interactions:** Appendix 1 (bisphosphonates)
Contra-indications: severe renal impairment, juvenile Paget's disease, pregnancy and breast-feeding
Side-effects: stomach pain, nausea, diarrhoea; rarely asthenia, dizziness, headache and skin reactions
Dose: 400 mg daily as a single dose for 12 weeks; may be repeated if necessary after 6 months
COUNSELLING. Avoid food for 2 hours before and after treatment, particularly calcium-containing products e.g. milk; also avoid antacids

Skelid® (Sanofi-Synthelabo) PoM
Tablets, tiludronic acid (as tiludronate disodium) 200 mg. Net price 28-tab pack = £99.00. Counselling, food and calcium

---

6.7 **Other endocrine drugs**

This section includes:
6.7.1   Bromocriptine and other dopamine-receptor stimulants
6.7.2   Drugs affecting gonadotrophins
6.7.3   Metyrapone and trilostane

6.7.1 **Bromocriptine and other dopamine-receptor stimulants**

Bromocriptine is a stimulant of dopamine receptors in the brain; it also inhibits release of prolactin by the pituitary. Bromocriptine is used for the treat-

ment of galactorrhoea and cyclical benign breast disease, and for the treatment of prolactinomas (when it reduces both plasma prolactin concentration and tumour size). Bromocriptine also inhibits the release of growth hormone and is sometimes used in the treatment of acromegaly, but somatostatin analogues (such as octreotide, section 8.3.4.3) are more effective.

Cabergoline has actions and uses similar to those of bromocriptine, but its duration of action is longer. Its profile of side-effects appears to differ from that of bromocriptine, which means that patients intolerant of bromocriptine may be able to tolerate cabergoline (and *vice versa*).

Quinagolide has been introduced recently; its actions and uses are similar to those of bromocriptine, but its profile of side-effects differs slightly.

SUPPRESSION OF LACTATION. Although bromocriptine and cabergoline are licensed to suppress lactation, they are **not** recommended for routine suppression (or for the relief of symptoms of postpartum pain and engorgement) that can be adequately treated with simple analgesics and breast support. Quinagolide is not licensed for the suppression of lactation.

BROMOCRIPTINE

Indications: see notes above and under Dose; parkinsonism (section 4.9.1)
Cautions: specialist evaluation—monitor for pituitary enlargement, particularly during pregnancy, annual gynaecological assessment (postmenopausal, every 6 months), monitor for peptic ulceration in acromegalic patients; contraceptive advice if appropriate (oral contraceptives may increase prolactin concentration); caution in patients with history of serious mental disorders (especially psychotic disorders) or with cardiovascular disease or Raynaud's syndrome and monitor for retroperitoneal fibrosis; porphyria (section 9.8.2); **interactions:** Appendix 1 (bromocriptine and cabergoline)
HYPOTENSIVE REACTIONS. Hypotensive reactions may be disturbing in some patients during the first few days of treatment and particular care should be exercised when driving or operating machinery; tolerance may be reduced by alcohol
Contra-indications: hypersensitivity to bromocriptine or other ergot alkaloids; toxaemia of pregnancy and hypertension in postpartum women or in puerperium (see also below); advise women not to breast-feed if lactation prevention fails
POSTPARTUM OR PUERPERIUM. Should not be used postpartum or in puerperium in women with high blood pressure, coronary artery disease or symptoms (or history) of serious mental disorder; monitor blood pressure carefully (especially during first few days) in postpartum women. Very rarely hypertension, myocardial infarction, seizures or stroke (both sometimes preceded by severe headache) and mental disorders have been reported in postpartum women given bromocriptine for lactation suppression—caution with antihypertensive therapy and avoid other ergot alkaloids. Discontinue immediately if hypertension, unremitting headache or signs of CNS toxicity develop

Side-effects: nausea, vomiting, constipation, headache, dizziness, postural hypotension, drowsiness, vasospasm of fingers and toes particularly in patients with Raynaud's syndrome; *high doses,* confusion, psychomotor excitation, hallucinations, dyskinesia, dry mouth, leg cramps, pleural effusions (may necessitate withdrawal of treatment), retroperitoneal fibrosis reported (monitoring required)

Dose: prevention or suppression of lactation (but see notes above and under Contra-indications), 2.5 mg on day 1 (prevention) or daily for 2–3 days (suppression); then 2.5 mg twice daily for 14 days
Hypogonadism, galactorrhoea, infertility, initially 1–1.25 mg at bedtime, increased gradually; usual dose 7.5 mg daily in divided doses, increased if necessary to max. 30 mg daily, usual dose in infertility without hyperprolactinaemia, 2.5 mg twice daily
Cyclical benign breast disease and cyclical menstrual disorders (particularly breast pain), 1–1.25 mg at bedtime, increased gradually; usual dose 2.5 mg twice daily
Acromegaly, initially 1–1.25 mg at bedtime, increase gradually to 5 mg every 6 hours
Prolactinoma, initially 1–1.25 mg at bedtime; increased gradually to 5 mg every 6 hours (occasional patients may require up to 30 mg daily)
CHILD under 15, not recommended

Bromocriptine (Non-proprietary) PoM
Tablets, bromocriptine (as mesilate), 2.5 mg, net price 30-tab pack = £5.66. Label: 21, counselling, hypotensive reactions
Available from APS, Berk, Cox, Kent, Norton

Parlodel® (Novartis) PoM
Tablets, both scored, bromocriptine (as mesilate) 1 mg, net price 100-tab pack = £9.05; 2.5 mg, 30-tab pack = £5.28. Label: 21, counselling, hypotensive reactions
Capsules, bromocriptine (as mesilate) 5 mg (blue/white), net price 100-cap pack = £34.34; 10 mg (white), 100-cap pack = £63.53. Label: 21, counselling, hypotensive reactions

CABERGOLINE

Indications: see notes above and under Dose

Cautions: see under Bromocriptine; peptic ulcer, gastro-intestinal bleeding; severe hepatic impairment; fibrotic lung disease; monthly pregnancy tests during the amenorrhoeic period; advise non-hormonal contraception if pregnancy not desired (see also Contra-indications); **interactions:** Appendix 1 (bromocriptine and cabergoline)
HYPOTENSIVE REACTIONS. Hypotensive reactions may be disturbing in some patients during the first few days of treatment and particular care should be exercised when driving or operating machinary; tolerance may be reduced by alcohol

Contra-indications: see under Bromocriptine; exclude pregnancy before starting and avoid until at least 1 month after successful treatment (ovulatory cycles persist for 6 months)—discontinue if pregnancy occurs during treatment (specialist advice needed)

Side-effects: see under Bromocriptine (but profile of side-effects may differ, see notes above); dyspepsia, epigastric and abdominal pain, breast pain, palpitations, angina, epistaxis, peripheral oedema, hemianopia, asthenia, erythromelalgia, hot flushes, depression

Dose: prevention of lactation (but see notes above), during first day postpartum, 1 mg as a single dose; suppression of established lactation (but see notes above) 250 micrograms every 12 hours for 2 days
Hyperprolactinaemic disorders, 500 micrograms weekly (as a single dose *or* as 2 divided doses on separate days) increased at monthly intervals in steps of 500 micrograms until optimal therapeutic response (usually 1 mg weekly, range 0.25–2 mg weekly) with monthly monitoring of serum prolactin levels; reduce initial dose and increase more gradually if patient intolerant; over 1 mg weekly give as divided doses; up to 4.5 mg weekly has been used in hyperprolactinaemic patients
Parkinsonism, section 4.9.1
CHILD under 16 years, not recommended

Dostinex® (Pharmacia & Upjohn) ▼ PoM
Tablets, scored, cabergoline 500 micrograms. Net price 8-tab pack = £30.04. Label: 21, counselling, hypotensive reactions

QUINAGOLIDE

Indications: see notes above and under Dose

Cautions: see under Bromocriptine; advise non-hormonal contraception if pregnancy not desired; discontinue if pregnancy occurs during treatment (specialist advice needed); **interactions:** Appendix 1 (quinagolide)
HYPOTENSIVE REACTIONS. Hypotensive reactions may be disturbing in some patients during the first few days of treatment—monitor blood pressure for a few days after starting treatment and following dosage increases; particular care should be exercised when driving or operating machinery; tolerance may be reduced by alcohol

Contra-indications: see under Bromocriptine; hypersensitivity to quinagolide (but not ergot alkaloids)

Side-effects: see under Bromocriptine (but profile of side-effects may differ, see notes above); also syncope, anorexia, abdominal pain, diarrhoea, insomnia, oedema, flushing and nasal congestion

Dose: hyperprolactinaemia, 25 micrograms at bedtime for 3 days; increased at intervals of 3 days in steps of 25 micrograms to usual maintenance dose of 75–150 micrograms daily; for doses higher than 300 micrograms daily increase in steps of 75–150 micrograms at intervals of not less than 4 weeks
CHILD not recommended

Norprolac® (Novartis) PoM
Tablets, quinagolide (as hydrochloride) 75 micrograms (white), net price 30-tab pack = £57.00; 150 micrograms (white), 30-tab pack = £100.00; starter pack of 3 × 25-microgram tabs (pink) with 3 × 50-microgram tabs (blue) = £5.00. Label: 21, counselling, hypotensive reactions

6.7.2 Drugs affecting gonadotrophins

Danazol inhibits pituitary gonadotrophins; it combines androgenic activity with antioestrogenic and antiprogestogenic activity. It is used in the treatment of *endometriosis* and has also been used for *mammary dysplasia*, and *gynaecomastia* where other measures have proved unsatisfactory; it has been used for *menorrhagia* and other *menstrual disorders* but in view of its side-effects, treatment with other drugs may be preferable (section 6.4.1.2). It may also be effective in the long-term management of *hereditary angioedema* [unlicensed indication].

Gestrinone has general actions similar to those of danazol and is indicated for the treatment of endometriosis.

Cetrorelix is a luteinising hormone releasing hormone antagonist, which inhibits the release of gonadotrophins (luteinising hormone and follicle-stimulating hormone). It is used in the treatment of infertility by assisted reproductive techniques.

CETRORELIX

Indications: adjunct in the treatment of female infertility (under specialist supervision)

Contra-indications: pregnancy, breast-feeding, moderate renal impairment, moderate hepatic impairment

Side-effects: nausea, headache, injection site reactions

Dose: *by subcutaneous injection* into the lower abdominal wall,

either 250 micrograms in the morning, starting on day 5 or 6 of ovarian stimulation with gonadotrophins (*or* each evening starting on day 5 of ovarian stimulation); continue throughout administration of gonadotrophin including day of ovulation induction (*or* evening before ovulation induction)

or 3 mg on day 7 of ovarian stimulation with gonadotrophins; if ovulation induction not possible on day 5 after 3-mg dose, additional 250 micrograms once daily until day of ovulation induction

Cetrotide® (ASTA Medica) ▼ [PoM]
Injection, powder for reconstitution, cetrorelix (as acetate), net price 250-micrograms vial = £27.76; 3-mg vial = £194.29 (both with solvent)

DANAZOL

Indications: see notes above and under Dose

Cautions: cardiac, hepatic, or renal impairment (avoid if severe), elderly, polycythaemia, epilepsy, diabetes mellitus, hypertension, migraine, lipoprotein disorder, history of thrombosis or thromboembolic disease; withdraw if virilisation (may be irreversible on continued use); non-hormonal contraceptive methods should be used, if appropriate; **interactions:** Appendix 1 (danazol)

Contra-indications: pregnancy (Appendix 4), ensure that patients with amenorrhoea are not pregnant; breast-feeding; severe hepatic, renal or cardiac impairment; thromboembolic disease; undiagnosed genital bleeding; androgen-dependent tumours; porphyria (section 9.8.2)

Side-effects: nausea, dizziness, skin reactions including rashes, photosensitivity and exfoliative dermatitis, fever, backache, nervousness, mood changes, anxiety, changes in libido, vertigo, fatigue, epigastric and pleuritic pain, headache, weight gain; menstrual disturbances, vaginal dryness and irritation, flushing and reduction in breast size; musculo-skeletal spasm, joint pain and swelling, hair loss; androgenic effects including acne, oily skin, oedema, hirsutism, voice changes and rarely clitoral hypertrophy (see also Cautions); temporary alteration in lipoproteins and other metabolic changes, insulin resistance; thrombotic events; leucopenia, thrombocytopenia, eosinophilia, reversible erythrocytosis or polycythaemia reported; headache and visual disturbances may indicate benign intracranial hypertension; rarely cholestatic jaundice, pancreatitis, peliosis hepatis and benign hepatic adenomata

Dose: usually given in up to 4 divided doses; in women of child-bearing potential, treatment should start during menstruation, preferably on day 1

Endometriosis, 200–800 mg daily in up to 4 divided doses, adjusted to achieve amenorrhoea, usually for 6 months (up to 9 months in some cases)

Menorrhagia (but see notes above), 200 mg daily, usually for 3 months

Severe cyclical mastalgia, 100–400 mg daily usually for 3–6 months

Benign breast cysts, 300 mg daily usually for 3–6 months

Gynaecomastia, 400 mg daily in up to 4 divided doses for 6 months (adolescents 200 mg daily, increased to 400 mg daily if no response after 2 months)

For pre-operative thinning of endometrium, 400–800 mg daily in up to 4 divided doses for 3–6 weeks

Danazol (Non-proprietary) [PoM]
Capsules, danazol 100 mg, net price 20 = £5.07; 200 mg, 20 = £9.75
Available from APS, Cox, Generics, Hillcross, Kent, Norton, Sterwin

Danol® (Sanofi-Synthelabo) [PoM]
Capsules, danazol 100 mg (grey/white), net price 60-cap pack = £17.84; 200 mg (pink/white), 60-cap pack = £35.34

GESTRINONE

Indications: endometriosis

Cautions: cardiac and renal impairment; **interactions:** Appendix 1 (gestrinone)

Contra-indications: pregnancy (use non-hormonal method of contraception) and breast-feeding; severe cardiac, renal or hepatic impairment; metabolic or vascular disorders associated with previous sex hormone treatment

Side-effects: spotting; acne, oily skin, fluid retention, weight gain, hirsutism, voice change; liver enzyme disturbances; headache; gastro-intestinal disturbances; change in libido, flushing, decrease in breast size; nervousness, depression, change in appetite; muscle cramp

Dose: 2.5 mg twice weekly starting on first day of cycle with second dose 3 days later, repeated on same two days preferably at same time each week; duration of treatment usually 6 months

MISSED DOSES. One missed dose—2.5 mg as soon as possible and maintain original sequence; two or more missed doses—discontinue, re-start on first day of new cycle (following negative pregnancy test)

Dimetriose® (Florizel) PoM

Capsules, gestrinone 2.5 mg, net price 8-cap pack = £111.73

Gonadorelin analogues

Administration of **gonadorelin analogues** produces an initial phase of stimulation; continued administration is followed by down-regulation of gonadotrophin-releasing hormone receptors, thereby reducing the release of gonadotrophins (follicle stimulating hormone and luteinising hormone) which in turn leads to inhibition of androgen and oestrogen production.

Gonadorelin analogues are used in the treatment of endometriosis, infertility, anaemia due to uterine fibroids (together with iron supplementation), breast cancer (section 8.3.4.1), prostate cancer (section 8.3.4.2) and before intra-uterine surgery.

CAUTIONS. Non-hormonal, barrier methods of contraception should be used during entire treatment period with gonadorelin analogues; also use with caution in patients with metabolic bone disease because decrease in bone mineral density can occur.

CONTRA-INDICATIONS. Gonadorelin analogues are contra-indicated for use longer than 6 months (do not repeat), where there is undiagnosed vaginal bleeding, in pregnancy (exclude pregnancy—also give first injection during menstruation or shortly afterwards *or* use barrier contraception for 1 month beforehand) and in breast-feeding.

SIDE-EFFECTS. Side-effects of the gonadorelin analogues related to the inhibition of oestrogen production include menopausal-like symptoms (e.g. hot flushes, increased sweating, vaginal dryness, dyspareunia and loss of libido) and a decrease in trabecular bone density; these effects can be reduced by hormone replacement (e.g. with an oestrogen and a progestogen or with tibolone). Side-effects of gonadorelin analogues also include headache (rarely migraine) and hypersensitivity reactions including urticaria, pruritus, skin rashes, asthma and anaphylaxis; spray formulations can cause irritation of the nasal mucosa including nose bleeds; local reactions at injection site can occur; other side-effects also reported with some gonadorelin analogues include changes in breast size, arthralgia, visual disturbances, paraesthesia, changes in scalp and body hair, oedema of the face and extremities, weight changes, and mood changes including depression.

BUSERELIN

Indications: see under Dose; prostate cancer (section 8.3.4.2)

Cautions: see notes above; polycystic ovarian disease, depression, hypertension, diabetes

Contra-indications: see notes above; hormone-dependent tumours

Side-effects: see notes above; initially withdrawal bleeding and subsequently breakthrough bleeding, ovarian cysts (may require withdrawal), leucorrhoea; nausea, vomiting, constipation, diarrhoea; anxiety, memory and concentration disturbances, sleep disturbances, nervousness, dizziness, drowsiness; breast tenderness, lactation; abdominal pain; fatigue; increased thirst, changes in appetite, palpitations, worsening of hypertension; acne, dry skin, dry eyes; back and limb pain; altered liver function tests, altered blood lipids, leucopenia, thrombocytopenia; hearing disturbances; reduced glucose tolerance

Dose: endometriosis, *intranasally*, 300 micrograms (one 150-microgram spray in each nostril) 3 times daily (starting on days 1 or 2 of menstruation); max. duration of treatment 6 months (do not repeat)

Pituitary desensitisation before induction of ovulation by gonadotrophins for *in vitro* fertilisation (under specialist supervision), *by subcutaneous injection*, 200–500 micrograms daily given as a single injection (occasionally up to 500 micrograms twice daily may be needed) starting in early follicular phase (day 1) *or*, after exclusion of pregnancy, in midluteal phase (day 21) and continued until down-regulation achieved (usually about 1–3 weeks) then maintained during gonadotrophin administration (stopping gonadotrophin and buserelin on administration of chorionic gonadotrophin at appropriate stage of follicular development)

Intranasally, 150 micrograms (one spray in one nostril) 4 times daily during waking hours (occasionally up to 300 micrograms 4 times daily may be needed) starting in early follicular phase (day 1) *or*, after exclusion of pregnancy, in midluteal phase (day 21) and continued until down-regulation achieved (usually about 2–3 weeks) then maintained during gonadotrophin administration (stopping gonadotrophin and buserelin on administration of chorionic gonadotrophin at appropriate stage of follicular development)

COUNSELLING. Avoid use of nasal decongestants before and for at least 30 minutes after treatment

Suprecur® (Shire) PoM

Nasal spray, buserelin (as acetate) 150 micrograms/metered spray. Net price 2 × 100-dose pack (with metered dose pumps) = £75.43. Counselling, see above

Injection ▼, buserelin (as acetate) 1mg/mL. Net price 5.5-mL vial = £11.85.

GOSERELIN

Indications: see under Dose; prostate cancer (section 8.3.4.2); advanced breast cancer (section 8.3.4.1)

Cautions: see notes above; polycystic ovarian disease

Contra-indications: see notes above

Side-effects: see notes above; withdrawal bleeding, fibroid degeneration; ovarian cysts; transient changes in blood pressure

Dose: *by subcutaneous injection* into anterior abdominal wall, endometriosis, 3.6 mg every 28 days; max. duration of treatment 6 months (do not repeat); endometrial thinning before intra-uterine surgery, 3.6 mg (may be repeated after 28 days if uterus is large or to allow flexible surgical timing); before surgery in women who have anaemia due to uterine fibroids, 3.6 mg every 28 days (with supplementary iron); max. duration of treatment 3 months

Pituitary desensitisation before induction of ovulation by gonadotrophins for *in vitro* fertilisation (under specialist supervision), after exclusion of pregnancy, 3.6 mg to achieve pituitary down-regulation (usually 1–3 weeks) then gonadotrophin is administered (stopping gonadotrophin on administration of chorionic gonadotrophin at appropriate stage of follicular development)

Preparation
Section 8.3.4.2

LEUPRORELIN ACETATE

Indications: see under Dose; prostate cancer (section 8.3.4.2)

Cautions: see notes above; family history of osteoporosis; chronic use of other drugs which reduce bone density including alcohol and tobacco

Contra-indications: see notes above

Side-effects: see notes above; breast tenderness; nausea; sleep disturbances, dizziness, fatigue

Dose: *by subcutaneous or intramuscular injection*, endometriosis, 3.75 mg every 4 weeks, starting during the first 5 days of menstrual cycle; max. duration of treatment 6 months (do not repeat); endometrial thinning before intra-uterine surgery, 3.75 mg given 5–6 weeks before surgery starting between days 3 and 5 of menstrual cycle

Preparation
Section 8.3.4.2

NAFARELIN

Indications: see under Dose

Cautions: see notes above

Contra-indications: see notes above

Side-effects: see notes above; ovarian cysts (may require withdrawal); myalgia; acne; palpitations; altered liver function tests

Dose: women over 18 years, endometriosis, 200 micrograms twice daily as one spray in one nostril in the morning and one spray in the other nostril in the evening (starting on days 2–4 of menstruation), max. duration of treatment 6 months (do not repeat)

Pituitary desensitisation before induction of ovulation by gonadotrophins for *in vitro* fertilisation (under specialist supervision), 400 micrograms (one spray in each nostril) twice daily starting in early follicular phase (day 2) or, after exclusion of pregnancy, in midluteal phase (day 21) and continued until down-regulation achieved (usually

within 4 weeks) then maintained (usually for 8–12 days) during gonadotrophin administration (stopping gonadotrophin and nafarelin on administration of chorionic gonadotrophin at follicular maturity); discontinue if down-regulation not achieved within 12 weeks

COUNSELLING. Avoid use of nasal decongestants before and for at least 30 minutes after treatment; repeat dose if sneezing occurs during or immediately after administration

Synarel® (Searle) PoM
Nasal spray, nafarelin 200 micrograms (as acetate)/metered spray. Net price 30-dose unit = £30.74; 60-dose unit = £53.01. Label: 10 patient information leaflet, counselling, see above

---

TRIPTORELIN

Indications: see under dose; prostate cancer (section 8.3.4.2)

Cautions: see notes above

Contra-indications: see notes above

Side-effects: see notes above; myalgia; transient hypertension; asthenia

Dose: *by intramuscular injection*, endometriosis, 3 mg every 4 weeks starting during the first 5 days of menstrual cycle; max. duration of treatment 6 months (do not repeat)

Preparations
Section 8.3.4.2

Breast pain (mastalgia)

Once any serious underlying cause has been ruled out, most women will respond to reassurance and reduction in dietary fat; withdrawal of an oral contraceptive or of hormone replacement therapy may help resolve the pain.

Women whose symptoms persist for longer than 6 months may require drug treatment. Danazol is the most effective but may be unacceptable owing to its unpleasant side-effects (which occur in about one-third of patients). Bromocriptine (section 6.7.1) like danazol is associated with unpleasant side-effects. Gamolenic acid can be useful and, with its lack of antioestrogenic side-effects, may be preferred particularly in younger women who wish to continue taking an oral contraceptive; whereas bromocriptine and danazol act within 2 months, gamolenic acid may require 8–12 weeks to take effect.

Symptoms recur in about 50% of women within 2 years of withdrawal of therapy but may be less severe.

GAMOLENIC ACID

Indications: symptom relief of cyclical and non-cyclical mastalgia; atopic eczema (section 13.5.1)

Cautions: history of epilepsy, concomitant treatment with epileptogenic drugs e.g. phenothiazines; pregnancy

Side-effects: occasional nausea, indigestion, headache; rarely hypersensitivity reactions including rash, urticaria, pruritus and abdominal pain

Dose: cyclical and non-cyclical mastalgia, 240–320 mg daily in 1–2 divided doses until response obtained then stopped or dose reduced (may take 8–12 weeks for response in some patients)

Efamast® (Searle) PoM
Efamast® 40 capsules, gamolenic acid 40 mg in evening primrose oil, net price 224-cap pack = £22.65
Excipients: include vitamin E
Efamast® 80 capsules, gamolenic acid 80 mg in evening primrose oil , net price 112-cap pack = £22.65
Excipients: include vitamin E

6.7.3   Metyrapone and trilostane

Metyrapone is a competitive inhibitor of 11β-hydroxylation in the adrenal cortex; the resulting inhibition of cortisol (and to a lesser extent aldosterone) production leads to an increase in ACTH production which, in turn, leads to increased synthesis and release of cortisol precursors. It may be used as a test of anterior pituitary function.

Although most types of *Cushing's syndrome* are treated surgically, that which occasionally accompanies carcinoma of the bronchus is not usually amenable to surgery. Metyrapone has been found helpful in controlling the symptoms of the disease; it is also used in other forms of Cushing's syndrome to prepare the patient for surgery. The dosages used are either low, and tailored to cortisol production, or high, in which case corticosteroid replacement therapy is also needed.

Trilostane reversibly inhibits 3β-hydroxysteroid dehydrogenase/delta 5-4 isomerase in the adrenal cortex; the resulting inhibition of the synthesis of mineralocorticoids and glucocorticoids may be useful in *Cushing's syndrome* and *primary hyperaldosteronism*. Trilostane appears to be less effective than metyrapone for Cushing's syndrome (where it is tailored to corticosteroid production). It also has a minor role in post-menopausal breast cancer that has relapsed following initial oestrogen antagonist therapy (corticosteroid replacement therapy is also required).

See also aminoglutethimide (section 8.3.4)

METYRAPONE

Indications: see notes above and under Dose (specialist supervision in hospital)

Cautions: gross hypopituitarism (risk of precipitating acute adrenal failure); hypertension on long-term administration; hypothyroidism or hepatic impairment (delayed response); many drugs interfere with diagnostic estimation of steroids
DRIVING. Drowsiness may affect the performance of skilled tasks (e.g. driving)

Contra-indications: adrenocortical insufficiency (see Cautions); pregnancy, breast-feeding

Side-effects: occasional nausea, vomiting, dizziness, headache, hypotension, sedation; rarely abdominal pain, allergic skin reactions, hypoadrenalism, hirsutism

Dose: differential diagnosis of ACTH-dependent Cushing's syndrome, 750 mg every 4 hours for 6 doses; CHILD 15 mg/kg (minimum 250 mg) every 4 hours for 6 doses
Management of Cushing's syndrome, range 0.25–6 g daily, tailored to cortisol production; see notes above

Resistant oedema due to increased aldosterone secretion in cirrhosis, nephrosis, and congestive heart failure (with glucocorticoid replacement therapy) 3 g daily in divided doses

Metopirone® (Alliance) PoM
Capsules, metyrapone 250 mg. Net price 100-tab pack = £42.50. Label: 21, counselling, driving

TRILOSTANE

Indications: see notes above and under Dose (specialist supervision)

Cautions: breast cancer (concurrent corticosteroid replacement therapy needed, see under Dose), adrenal cortical hyperfunction (tailored to cortisol and electrolytes, concurrent corticosteroid therapy may be needed, see under Dose); hepatic and renal impairment; **interactions:** Appendix 1 (trilostane)

Contra-indications: pregnancy (use non-hormonal method of contraception) and breast-feeding; children

Side-effects: flushing, tingling and swelling of mouth, rhinorrhoea, nausea, vomiting, diarrhoea, and rashes reported; rarely granulocytopenia

Dose: adrenal cortical hyperfunction, 240 mg daily in divided doses for at least 3 days then tailored according to response with regular monitoring of plasma electrolytes and circulating corticosteroids (both mineralocorticoid and glucocorticoid replacement therapy may be needed); usual dose: 120–480 mg daily (may be increased to 960 mg)
Postmenopausal breast cancer (with glucocorticoid replacement therapy) following relapse to initial oestrogen receptor antagonist therapy, initially 240 mg daily increased every 3 days in steps of 240 mg to a maintenance dose of 960 mg daily (720 mg daily if not tolerated)

Modrenal® (Wanskerne) PoM
Capsules, trilostane 60 mg (pink/black), net price 100-cap pack = £49.50;120 mg (pink/yellow), 100-cap pack = £98.50. Label: 21

7: Obstetrics, gynaecology, and urinary-tract disorders

For hormonal therapy of gynaecological disorders see section 6.4.1, section 6.5.1 and section 6.7.2.

7.1 Drugs used in obstetrics

Because of the complexity of dosage regimens in obstetrics, in all cases **detailed specialist literature** should be consulted.

7.1.1 Prostaglandins and oxytocics

Prostaglandins and oxytocics are used to induce abortion or induce or augment labour and to minimise blood loss from the placental site. They include oxytocin, ergometrine, and the prostaglandins. All induce uterine contractions with varying degrees of pain according to the strength of contractions induced.

INDUCTION OF ABORTION. **Gemeprost**, administered vaginally as pessaries is the preferred prostaglandin for the medical induction of late therapeutic abortion. Gemeprost ripens and softens the cervix before surgical abortion, particularly in primigravida. The prostaglandin **misoprostol** is given by mouth or by vaginal administration to induce medical abortion [unlicensed indication]; intravaginal use ripens the cervix prior to surgical abortion [unlicensed indication]. Extra-amniotic **dinoprostone** is rarely used nowadays.

Pre-treatment with **mifepristone** can facilitate the process of medical abortion. It makes the uterus more sensitive to subsequent administration of a prostaglandin and, therefore, abortion occurs in a shorter time and with a lower dose of prostaglandin.

INDUCTION AND AUGMENTATION OF LABOUR. **Oxytocin** (*Syntocinon®*) is administered by slow intravenous infusion, using an infusion pump, to *induce or augment labour*, usually in conjunction with amniotomy. Uterine activity must be monitored carefully and hyperstimulation avoided. Large doses of oxytocin may result in excessive fluid retention.

Dinoprostone is available as vaginal tablets, pessaries and vaginal gels for the *induction of labour*. The intravenous solution and oral tablets are rarely used since tablets are less effective than vaginal preparations and both are associated with more side-effects.

Misoprostol is given orally or by vagina for the induction of labour [unlicensed indication].

PREVENTION AND TREATMENT OF HAEMORRHAGE. Bleeding due to *incomplete abortion* can be controlled with **ergometrine** and **oxytocin** (*Syntometrine®*) given intramuscularly, the dose being adjusted according to the patient's condition and blood loss. This is commonly used prior to surgical evacuation of the uterus, particularly when surgery is delayed. Oxytocin and ergometrine combined are more effective in early pregnancy than either drug alone.

For the routine management of the *third stage of labour* ergometrine 500 micrograms with oxytocin 5 units (*Syntometrine*® 1 mL) is given by intramuscular injection with or after delivery of the shoulders.

If ergometrine is inappropriate (e.g. in pre-eclampsia), oxytocin may be given by intramuscular injection with or after delivery of shoulder [unlicensed indication] instead of ergometrine with oxytocin.

For the prevention of postpartum haemorrhage in *high-risk cases*, intravenous injection of *either* ergometrine 125–250 micrograms alone *or* oxytocin 5–10 units is recommended, after delivery of the shoulders (repeated if necessary); alternatively intravenous infusion of oxytocin 10–20 units/500 mL can be given after delivery of the shoulders, particularly when the uterus is *atonic*. The use of **carboprost** now has an important role for severe events.

Provided causes such as infection or retained products of conception have been excluded, small secondary postpartum haemorrhage may be treated in domicillary practice with **ergometrine** by mouth in a dose of 500 micrograms three times daily for 3 days.

CARBOPROST

Indications: postpartum haemorrhage due to uterine atony in patients unresponsive to ergometrine and oxytocin

Cautions: history of glaucoma or raised intra-ocular pressure, asthma, hypertension, hypotension, anaemia, jaundice, diabetes, epilepsy; uterine scars; excessive dosage may cause uterine rupture

Contra-indications: acute pelvic inflammatory disease; cardiac, renal, pulmonary, or hepatic disease

Side-effects: nausea, vomiting and diarrhoea, hyperthermia and flushing, bronchospasm; less frequent effects include raised blood pressure, dyspnoea, and pulmonary oedema; chills, headache, diaphoresis, dizziness; cardiovascular collapse also reported; erythema and pain at injection site reported

Dose: *by deep intramuscular injection,* 250 micrograms repeated if necessary at intervals of 1½ hours (in severe cases the interval may be reduced but should not be less than 15 minutes); total dose should not exceed 2 mg (8 doses)

Hemabate® (Pharmacia & Upjohn) [PoM]
Injection, carboprost as trometamol salt (tromethamine salt) 250 micrograms/mL, net price 1-mL amp = £15.76 (hosp. only)

DINOPROSTONE

Indications: see notes above and under preparations below

Cautions: history of asthma, glaucoma and raised intra-ocular pressure; cardiac, hepatic or renal impairment; hypertension; history of epilepsy; monitor uterine activity and fetal status (particular care if history of uterine hypertony); uterine rupture; see also notes above; effect of oxytocin enhanced (care needed in monitoring uterine activity when used in sequence)—see also under *Propess*® and Appendix 1 (oxytocin)

Contra-indications: active cardiac, pulmonary, renal or hepatic disease; placenta praevia or unexplained vaginal bleeding during pregnancy, ruptured membranes, major cephalopelvic disproportion or fetal malpresentation, history of caesarean section or major uterine surgery, untreated pelvic infection, fetal distress, grand multiparas and multiple pregnancy, history of difficult or traumatic delivery; avoid extra-amniotic route in cervicitis or vaginitis

Side-effects: nausea, vomiting, diarrhoea; other side-effects include uterine hypertonus, severe uterine contractions, pulmonary or amniotic fluid embolism, abruptio placenta, fetal distress, maternal hypertension, bronchospasm, rapid cervical dilation, fever, backache; uterine hypercontractility with or without fetal bradycardia, low Apgar scores; cardiac arrest, uterine rupture, stillbirth or neonatal death also reported; vaginal symptoms (warmth, irritation, pain); after intravenous administration—flushing, shivering, headache, dizziness, temporary pyrexia and raised white blood cell count; also local tissue reaction and erythema after intravenous administration and possibility of infection after extra-amniotic administration

Dose: see under Preparations, below

IMPORTANT. Do not confuse dose of *Prostin E2*® vaginal **gel** with that of *Prostin E2*® vaginal **tablets**—not bioequivalent.

Propess® (Ferring) [PoM]
Pessaries (within retrieval system), releasing dinoprostone approx. 5 mg over 12 hours. Net price 1-pessary pack = £43.43
Dose: by vagina, cervical ripening and induction of labour at term, 1 pessary inserted high into posterior fornix; if cervical ripening insufficient, remove pessary 8–12 hours later and replace with a second pessary (which should also be removed not more than 12 hours later); max. 2 consecutive pessaries
IMPORTANT. Effect of oxytocin enhanced—particular care needed to monitor uterine activity when oxytocin used in sequence (remove pessary beforehand)

Prostin E2® (Pharmacia & Upjohn) [PoM]
Tablets ▰, dinoprostone 500 micrograms. Net price 10-tab pack = £14.26 (hosp. only)
Dose: by mouth, induction of labour, 500 micrograms, followed by 0.5–1 mg (max. 1.5 mg) at hourly intervals
Intravenous solution ▰, for dilution and use as an infusion, dinoprostone 1 mg/mL, net price 0.75-mL amp = £7.10; 10 mg/mL, 0.5-mL amp = £15.33 (both hosp. only; rarely used, consult product literature for dose and indications)
Extra-amniotic solution ▰, dinoprostone 10 mg/mL. Net price 0.5-mL amp (with diluent) = £16.05 (hosp. only; less commonly used nowadays, consult product literature for dose and indications)
Vaginal gel, dinoprostone 400 micrograms/mL, net price 2.5 mL (1 mg) = £13.87; 800 micrograms/mL, 2.5 mL (2 mg) = £15.28
Dose: by vagina, induction of labour, inserted high into posterior fornix (avoid administration into cervical canal), 1 mg (unfavourable primigravida 2 mg), followed after 6 hours by 1–2 mg if required; max. [gel] 3 mg (unfavourable primigravida 4 mg)
Vaginal tablets, dinoprostone 3 mg. Net price 8-vaginal tab pack = £62.11
Dose: by vagina, induction of labour, inserted high into posterior fornix, 3 mg, followed after 6–8 hours by 3 mg if labour is not established; max. 6 mg [vaginal tablets]
Note. Prostin E2 Vaginal Gel and *Vaginal Tablets* are **not** bioequivalent

ERGOMETRINE MALEATE

Indications: see notes above

Cautions: cardiac disease, hypertension, hepatic, and renal impairment, multiple pregnancy; porphyria (section 9.8.2)

Contra-indications: induction of labour, first and second stages of labour, vascular disease, severe cardiac disease, impaired pulmonary function, severe hepatic and renal impairment, sepsis, severe hypertension, eclampsia

Side-effects: nausea, vomiting, headache, dizziness, tinnitus, abdominal pain, chest pain, palpitation, dyspnoea, bradycardia, transient hypertension, vasoconstriction; stroke, myocardial infarction and pulmonary oedema also reported

Dose: see notes above

Ergometrine (Non-proprietary) PoM
Tablets, ergometrine maleate 500 micrograms, net price 21-tab pack = £24.98
Available from Norton
Injection, ergometrine maleate 500 micrograms/mL. Net price 1-mL amp = 30p
Available from Antigen, Phoenix

■ With oxytocin

Syntometrine® (Alliance) PoM
Injection, ergometrine maleate 500 micrograms, oxytocin 5 units/mL. Net price 1-mL amp = £1.38
Dose: by intramuscular injection, 1 mL; by intravenous injection, no longer recommended

GEMEPROST

Indications: see under Dose

Cautions: obstructive airways disease, cardiovascular insufficiency, raised intra-ocular pressure, cervicitis or vaginitis

IMPORTANT. For warnings relating to use of gemeprost in a patient undergoing termination with mifepristone, see under Mifepristone

Side-effects: vaginal bleeding and uterine pain; nausea, vomiting, or diarrhoea; headache, muscle weakness, dizziness, flushing, chills, backache, dyspnoea, chest pain, palpitations and mild pyrexia; uterine rupture reported (most commonly in multiparas or if history of uterine surgery or if given with intravenous oxytocics)

Dose: *by vagina* in pessaries, softening and dilation of the cervix to facilitate transcervical operative procedures in first trimester, inserted into posterior fornix, 1 mg 3 hours before surgery
Second trimester abortion, inserted into posterior fornix, 1 mg every 3 hours for max. of 5 administrations; second course may begin 24 hours after start of treatment (if treatment fails pregnancy should be terminated by another method)
Second trimester intra-uterine death, inserted into posterior fornix, 1 mg every 3 hours for max. of 5 administrations only; monitor for coagulopathy

Gemeprost (Farillon) PoM
Pessaries, gemeprost 1 mg. Net price 5-pessary pack = £161.94

OXYTOCIN

Indications: see under Dose and notes above

Cautions: particular caution needed when given for *induction or enhancement of labour* in presence of borderline cephalopelvic disproportion (avoid if significant), mild or moderate pregnancy-induced hypertension or cardiac disease, women over 35 years or with history of lower-uterine segment caesarean section (see also under Contra-indications below); if fetal death *in utero* or meconium-stained amniotic fluid avoid tumultuous labour (may cause amniotic fluid embolism); water intoxication and hyponatraemia—avoid large infusion volumes and restrict fluid intake by mouth (see also Appendix 6); effects enhanced by concomitant prostaglandins (very careful monitoring), caudal block anaesthesia (may enhance hypertensive effects of sympathomimetic vasopressors), see also **interactions:** Appendix 1 (oxytocin)

Contra-indications: hypertonic uterine contractions, mechanical obstruction to delivery, fetal distress; any condition where spontaneous labour or vaginal delivery inadvisable (e.g. significant cephalopelvic disproportion, malpresentation, placenta praevia, vasa praevia, placental abruption, cord presentation or prolapse, predisposition to uterine rupture as in multiple pregnancy, polyhydramnios, grand multiparity and presence of uterine scar from major surgery—including caesarean section); avoid prolonged administration in oxytocin-resistant uterine inertia, severe pre-eclamptic toxaemia or severe cardiovascular disease

Side-effects: uterine spasm (may occur at low doses), uterine hyperstimulation (usually with excessive doses—may cause fetal distress, asphyxia and death, or may lead to hypertonicity, tetanic contractions, soft-tissue damage or uterine rupture); water intoxication and hyponatraemia associated with high doses with large infusion volumes of electrolyte-free fluid (see also under Dose below); also nausea, vomiting, arrhythmias; rashes and anaphylactoid reactions (with dyspnoea, hypotension or shock) also reported; placental abruption and amniotic fluid embolism also reported on overdose

Dose: induction of labour for medical reasons or stimulation of labour in hypotonic uterine inertia, *by intravenous infusion,* 0.001–0.004 units/minute increased at intervals of not less than 20 minutes until labour pattern established similar to normal (usually less than 0.01 units/minute for pregnancy at term); max. recommended rate 0.02 units/minute (use solution containing 10 units/500 mL if higher rate required); do not use total of more than 5 units in any one day (may be repeated the following day starting again at 0.001–0.004 units/minute)

IMPORTANT. Careful monitoring of fetal heart rate and uterine motility essential to allow dose titration according to response (never give intravenous injection); discontinue immediately in uterine hyperactivity or fetal distress

Caesarean section, *by slow intravenous injection* immediately after delivery, 5 units

Prevention of postpartum haemorrhage, after delivery of placenta, *by slow intravenous injection,* 5 units (if infusion used for induction or enhancement of labour, increase rate during third stage and for next few hours)

Note. May be given in a dose of 10 units by intramuscular injection [unlicensed route] instead of oxytocin with ergometrine (*Syntometrine®*), see notes above

Treatment of postpartum haemorrhage, *by slow intravenous injection*, 5 units, followed in severe cases *by intravenous infusion* of 5–20 units in 500 mL of non-hydrating diluent (e.g. glucose 5% solution) at a rate sufficient to control uterine atony

IMPORTANT. Avoid rapid intravenous injection (may cause short-lasting drop in blood pressure); prolonged administration, see warning below

Incomplete, inevitable or missed abortion, *by slow intravenous injection*, 5 units followed if necessary *by intravenous infusion*, 0.02–0.04 units/minute or faster

IMPORTANT. Prolonged intravenous administration at high doses with large volume of fluid (as possible in inevitable or missed abortion or postpartum haemorrhage) may cause water intoxication with hyponatraemia. To avoid: use electrolyte-containing diluent (i.e. not glucose), increase oxytocin concentration to reduce fluid, restrict fluid intake by mouth; monitor fluid and electrolytes

Syntocinon® (Alliance) [PoM]
Injection, oxytocin, net price 5 units/mL, 1-mL amp = £1.23; 10 units/mL, 1-mL amp = £1.40

■ With ergometrine, see Syntometrine®, p. 361

7.1.1.1   Ductus arteriosus

Maintenance of patency

Alprostadil (prostaglandin E₁) is used to maintain patency of the ductus arteriosus in neonates with congenital heart defects, prior to corrective surgery in centres where intensive care is immediately available.

ALPROSTADIL

Indications: congenital heart defects in neonates prior to corrective surgery; erectile dysfunction (section 7.4.5)

Cautions: see notes above; history of haemorrhage, avoid in hyaline membrane disease, monitor arterial pressure

Side-effects: apnoea (particularly in infants under 2 kg), flushing, bradycardia, hypotension, tachycardia, cardiac arrest, oedema, diarrhoea, fever, convulsions, disseminated intravascular coagulation, hypokalaemia; cortical proliferation of long bones, weakening of the wall of the ductus arteriosus and pulmonary artery may follow prolonged use; gastric-outlet obstruction reported

Dose: *by intravenous infusion*, initially 50–100 nanograms/kg/minute, then decreased to lowest effective dose

Prostin VR® (Pharmacia & Upjohn) [PoM]
Intravenous solution, alprostadil 500 micrograms/mL in alcohol. For dilution and use as an infusion. Net price 1-mL amp = £59.84 (hosp. only)

Closure of ductus arteriosus

Indometacin (indomethacin) is used to close a patent ductus arteriosus in premature infants, probably by inhibiting prostaglandin synthesis.

INDOMETACIN

(Indomethacin)

Indications: patent ductus arteriosus in premature infants (under specialist supervision in neonatal intensive care unit); rheumatoid disease (section 10.1.1)

Cautions: may mask symptoms of infection; may reduce urine output by 50% or more (monitor carefully—see also under Anuria or Oliguria, below) and precipitate renal impairment especially if extracellular volume depleted, heart failure, sepsis, or hepatic impairment, or if receiving nephrotoxic drugs; may induce hyponatraemia; monitor renal function and electrolytes; inhibition of platelet aggregation (monitor for bleeding); **interactions:** Appendix 1 (NSAIDs)

ANURIA OR OLIGURIA. If anuria or marked oliguria (urinary output of 0.6 mL/kg/hour) at time of scheduled second or third dose, delay until renal function returns to normal

Contra-indications: untreated infection, bleeding (especially with active intracranial haemorrhage or gastro-intestinal bleeding); thrombocytopenia, coagulation defects, necrotising enterocolitis, renal impairment

Side-effects: include haemorrhagic, renal, gastro-intestinal, metabolic, and coagulation disorders; pulmonary hypertension, intracranial bleeding, fluid retention, and exacerbation of infection

Dose: *by intravenous injection*, over 20–30 minutes (using a suitable syringe driver), 3 doses at intervals of 12–24 hours (provided urine output remains adequate), age less than 48 hours, 200 micrograms/kg then 100 micrograms/kg then 100 micrograms/kg; age 2–7 days, 200 micrograms/kg then 200 micrograms/kg then 200 micrograms/kg; age over 7 days, 200 micrograms/kg then 250 micrograms/kg then 250 micrograms/kg; solution prepared with 1–2 mL sodium chloride 0.9% or water for injections (not glucose and no preservatives)

If ductus arteriosus reopens a second course of 3 injections may be given 48 hours after first course

Indocid PDA® (MSD) [PoM]
Injection, powder for reconstitution, indometacin (as sodium trihydrate). Net price 3 × 1-mg vials = £22.50 (hosp. only)

7.1.2   Mifepristone

MIFEPRISTONE

Indications: see under dose

Cautions: asthma, chronic obstructive pulmonary disease; cardiovascular disease or risk factors; prosthetic heart valve or history of infective endocarditis (prophylaxis recommended, see section 5.1 table 2); not recommended in hepatic or renal impairment; breast-feeding (Appendix 5); avoid aspirin and NSAIDs for at least 8–12 days after mifepristone; **interactions:** Appendix 1 (mifepristone)

Contra-indications: suspected ectopic pregnancy; chronic adrenal failure, long-term corticosteroid therapy, haemorrhagic disorders and anticoagulant therapy; smokers over 35 years of age when used in combination with gemeprost (smoking and alcohol must be avoided 2 days before and on the day of gemeprost administration); porphyria (section 9.8.2)

Side-effects: vaginal bleeding (sometimes severe) may occur between administration of mifepristone and surgery, and rarely abortion may occur before surgery; malaise, faintness, headache, nausea, vomiting, rashes; uterine pain after gemeprost (may be severe and require parenteral opioids); uterine and urinary-tract infections reported

Dose: therapeutic termination of intra-uterine pregnancy of up to 63 days gestation, *by mouth*, mifepristone 600 mg as a single dose in presence of doctor and observed for at least 2 hours, followed 36–48 hours later (unless abortion already complete) by gemeprost 1 mg *by vagina* and observed for at least 6 hours (or until bleeding or pain at acceptable level) with follow-up visit 8–12 days later to verify complete expulsion (if treatment fails essential that pregnancy be terminated by another method)

Softening and dilatation of cervix before mechanical cervical dilatation for termination of pregnancy, 36–48 hours before procedure, *by mouth*, mifepristone 600 mg as a single dose in presence of doctor

Termination of pregnancy of 13–20 weeks gestation (in combination with gemeprost), *by mouth*, mifepristone 600 mg as a single dose (presence of doctor and observed for at least 2 hours to ensure vomiting does not occur) followed 36–48 hours later by gemeprost 1 mg *by vagina* every 3 hours up to max. 5 mg; if abortion does not occur, 24 hours after start of treatment repeat course of gemeprost 1 mg *by vagina* up to max. 5 mg (if treatment fails pregnancy should be terminated by another method); follow-up visit after appropriate interval to assess vaginal bleeding recommended

Note. Careful monitoring essential for 6 hours after administration of gemeprost pessary (risk of profound hypotension)

Mifegyne® (Exelgyn) [PoM]
Tablets, yellow, mifepristone 200 mg. Net price 3-tab pack = £41.83 (supplied to NHS hospitals and premises approved under Abortion Act 1967).
Label: 10 patient information leaflet

7.1.3   Myometrial relaxants

Beta₂-adrenoceptor stimulants (beta₂-sympathomimetics) relax uterine muscle and are used in selected cases to inhibit *premature delivery.*

Beta₂-adrenoceptor stimulants are indicated for the inhibition of *uncomplicated* premature labour *between 24 and 33 weeks* of gestation and they may permit a delay in delivery of at least 48 hours; no statistically significant effect on perinatal mortality has as yet been observed. The greatest benefit is gained by using the delay to administer corticosteroid therapy (with care to avoid fluid overload) or to implement other measures known to improve perinatal health (including transfer to a unit with neonatal intensive care facility). Prolonged therapy should be avoided since risks to the mother (see under Ritodrine Hydrochloride, below) increase after 48 hours and furthermore, myometrial response is reduced; oral therapy following initial parenteral treatment is not therefore recommended.

Indometacin (indomethacin), a cyclo-oxygenase inhibitor, also inhibits labour [unlicensed indica-tion] and it may be useful in situations where a beta₂-adrenoceptor stimulant is not appropriate e.g. in cardiac disease; however, there are concerns about neonatal complications such as premature closure of ductus arteriosus.

RITODRINE HYDROCHLORIDE

Indications: uncomplicated premature labour (see notes above)

Cautions: suspected cardiac disease (physician experienced in cardiology to assess), hypertension, hyperthyroidism, hypokalaemia (special risk with potassium-depleting diuretics), diabetes mellitus (closely monitor blood glucose during intravenous treatment), mild to moderate pre-eclampsia (avoid if severe), monitor blood pressure and pulse rate (should not exceed 135–140 beats per minute) and avoid over-hydration (Appendix 6); **important:** closely monitor state of hydration (discontinue immediately and institute diuretic therapy if pulmonary oedema occurs); beta-blockers (effect antagonised—may be used to reverse increased tendency to uterine bleeding following caesarean section); drugs likely to enhance sympathomimetic side-effects or induce arrhythmias, see also **interactions**, Appendix 1 (sympathomimetics *and* sympathomimetics, beta₂)

Contra-indications: cardiac disease, eclampsia and severe pre-eclampsia, intra-uterine infection, intra-uterine fetal death, antepartum haemorrhage (requires immediate delivery), placenta praevia, cord compression; not for use in first or second trimesters

Side-effects: nausea, vomiting, flushing, sweating, tremor; hypokalaemia, tachycardia, palpitations, and hypotension (left lateral position throughout infusion to minimise risk), increased tendency to uterine bleeding (see Cautions); pulmonary oedema (see below and under Cautions); chest pain or tightness (with or without ECG changes) and arrhythmias reported; salivary gland enlargement also reported; on prolonged administration (several weeks) leucopenia and agranulocytosis reported; liver function abnormalities (including increased transaminases and hepatitis) reported

Dose: *by intravenous infusion* (**important:** minimum fluid volume, see below), premature labour, initially 50 micrograms/minute, gradually increased according to response by 50 micrograms/minute every 10 minutes to 150–350 micrograms/minute and continued for 12–48 hours after contractions have ceased (max. rate of 350 micrograms/minute should not be exceeded); or *by intramuscular injection*, 10 mg every 3–8 hours continued for 12–48 hours after contractions have ceased; then *by mouth* (but see notes above), 10 mg 30 minutes before termination of intravenous infusion, repeated every 2 hours for 24 hours, followed by 10–20 mg every 4–6 hours, max. oral dose 120 mg daily

IMPORTANT. Manufacturer states that although *fatal pulmonary oedema* associated with ritodrine infusion is almost certainly multifactorial in origin evidence suggests that **fluid overload** may be the most important single factor. The volume of infusion fluid should therefore be kept to a minimum; for further guidance see Appendix 6. For specific guidance on infusion rates to achieve the required dose, consult product literature

Yutopar® (Solvay) [PoM]
Tablets, yellow, scored, ritodrine hydrochloride
10 mg. Net price 90-tab pack = £19.80 �
Injection, ritodrine hydrochloride 10 mg/mL. Net
price 5-mL amp = £2.15

▰ denotes preparations that are considered to
be less suitable for prescribing (see p. vi)

SALBUTAMOL

Indications: uncomplicated premature labour (see
notes above); asthma (section 3.1.1)
Cautions: see under Ritodrine Hydrochloride
Contra-indications: see under Ritodrine Hydrochloride
Side-effects: see under Ritodrine Hydrochloride;
headache, rarely muscle cramps; hypersensitivity
reactions including bronchospasm, urticaria, and
angioedema reported
Dose: *by intravenous infusion,* initially
10 micrograms/minute, rate increased gradually
according to response at 10-minute intervals until
contractions diminish then increase rate slowly
until contractions cease (max. rate
45 micrograms/minute); maintain rate for 1 hour
after contractions have stopped, then gradually
reduce by 50% every 6 hours; then *by mouth* (but
see notes above), 4 mg every 6–8 hours

Preparations
Section 3.1.1.1

TERBUTALINE SULPHATE

Indications: uncomplicated premature labour (see
notes above); asthma (section 3.1.1)
Cautions: see under Ritodrine Hydrochloride
Contra-indications: see under Ritodrine Hydrochloride
Side-effects: see under Ritodrine Hydrochloride
Dose: *by intravenous infusion,* 5 micrograms/
minute for 20 minutes, increased every 20 minutes in steps of 2.5 micrograms/minute until contractions have ceased (more than 10 micrograms/
minute should **seldom** be given—20 micrograms/
minute should **not** be exceeded), continue for 1
hour then decrease every 20 minutes in steps of
2.5 micrograms/minute to lowest dose that maintains suppression, continue at this level for 12
hours then *by mouth* (but see notes above), 5 mg
every 8 hours for as long as is desirable to prolong pregnancy (or alternatively follow the *intravenous infusion* by *subcutaneous injection*
250 micrograms every 6 hours for a few days then
by mouth as above)

Preparations
Section 3.1.1.1

7.2   Treatment of vaginal and vulval conditions

7.2.1   Preparations for vaginal atrophy
7.2.2   Anti-infective drugs

Symptoms are primarily referable to the vulva, but
infections almost invariably involve the vagina
which should also be treated. Applications to the
vulva alone are likely to give only symptomatic
relief without cure.

Aqueous medicated douches may disturb normal
vaginal acidity and bacterial flora.
Topical anaesthetic agents give only symptomatic
relief and may cause sensitivity reactions. They are
indicated only in cases of pruritus where specific
local causes have been excluded.
Systemic drugs are required in the treatment of
infections such as gonorrhoea and syphilis (section
5.1).

7.2.1   Preparations for vaginal atrophy

Topical HRT

Application of cream containing an oestrogen may
be used on a short-term basis to improve the quality
of the vaginal epithelium in *menopausal atrophic
vaginitis*. It is **important** to bear in mind that topical oestrogens should be used in the **minimum
effective amount** to minimise absorption of the
oestrogen; if they are used on a long-term basis,
some require **oral progestogen** for 10–14 days of
each month to combat endometrial hyperplasia (for
details see under preparations below). Modified-
release vaginal tablets and an impregnated vaginal
ring are now also available.

Topical oestrogens are also used prior to vaginal
surgery in postmenopausal women for prolapse
when there is epithelial atrophy.

For a general comment on hormone replacement
therapy, including the role of topical oestrogens, see
section 6.4.1.1.

OESTROGENS, TOPICAL

Indications: see notes above
Cautions: see Oestrogens for HRT (section
6.4.1.1); interrupt treatment periodically to assess
need for continued treatment
Contra-indications: see Oestrogens for HRT
(section 6.4.1.1); pregnancy and breast-feeding
Side-effects: see Oestrogens for HRT (section
6.4.1.1); local irritation

Ortho® Dienoestrol (Janssen-Cilag) [PoM]
Cream, dienestrol 0.01%. Net price 78 g with
applicator = £2.61
Excipients: include arachis (peanut) oil
Condoms: damages latex condoms and diaphragms
Insert 1–2 applicatorfuls daily for 1–2 weeks, then
reduce to half the initial dose for 1–2 weeks; maintenance 1 applicatorful 1–3 times weekly if necessary;
attempts to reduce or discontinue should be made at 3–6
month intervals with re-examination

Ortho-Gynest® (Janssen-Cilag) [PoM]
Intravaginal cream, estriol 0.01%. Net price 80 g
with applicator = £2.72
Excipients: include arachis (peanut) oil
Condoms: damages latex condoms and diaphragms
Insert 1 applicatorful daily, preferably in evening;
reduced to 1 applicatorful twice a week; attempts to
reduce or discontinue should be made at 3–6 month
intervals with re-examination
Pessaries, estriol 500 micrograms. Net price 15
pessaries = £5.29
Excipients: include butylated hydroxytoluene
Condoms: damages latex condoms and diaphragms
Insert 1 pessary daily, preferably in the evening, until
improvement occurs; maintenance 1 pessary twice a
week; attempts to reduce or discontinue should be made
at 3–6 month intervals with re-examination

Ovestin® (Organon) [PoM]
Intravaginal cream, estriol 0.1%. Net price 15 g
with applicator = £4.98
Excipients: include polysorbates
Condoms: effect on latex condoms and diaphragms not yet known
Insert 1 applicator-dose daily for 2–3 weeks, then reduce
to twice a week (discontinue every 2–3 months for 4
weeks to assess need for further treatment); vaginal surgery, 1 applicator-dose daily for 2 weeks before surgery,
resuming 2 weeks after surgery

Premarin® (Wyeth) [PoM]
Vaginal cream, conjugated oestrogens (equine)
625 micrograms/g. Net price 42.5 g with calibrated applicator = £2.19
Excipients: include propylene glycol
Condoms: effect on latex condoms and diaphragms not yet known
Insert 1–2 g daily, starting on day 5 of cycle, for 3
weeks, followed by 1-week interval; if therapy long term
in women with intact uterus, oral progestogen for 10–14
days at end of each cycle essential

Tampovagan® (Co-Pharma) [PoM] ▰◣
Pessaries, diethylstilbestrol 500 micrograms, lactic acid 5%. Net price 10 pessaries = £8.95
Condoms: no evidence of damage to latex condoms and diaphragms
Insert 2 pessaries at night for 2–3 weeks (short-term
only, see notes above)

Vagifem® (Novo Nordisk) [PoM]
Vaginal tablets, f/c, m/r, estradiol 25 micrograms
in disposable applicators. Net price 15-applicator
pack = £14.62
Condoms: no evidence of damage to latex condoms and diaphragms
Insert 1 tablet daily for 2 weeks then reduce to 1 tablet
twice weekly; discontinue after 3 months to assess need
for further treatment

■ Vaginal ring
Note. For postmenopausal urogenital conditions—not
suitable for vasomotor symptoms or osteoporosis
prophylaxis

Estring® (Pharmacia & Upjohn) [PoM]
Vaginal ring, releasing estradiol approx.
7.5 micrograms/24 hours. Net price 1-ring pack =
£31.42. Label: 10 patient information leaflet
To be inserted into upper third of vagina and worn continuously; replace after 3 months; max. duration of continuous treatment 2 years

Non-hormonal preparations

Non-hormonal vaginal preparations include
Replens® [NHS] which has an acid pH and provides
a high moisture content for up to 3 days, and
Senselle® [NHS] which is a water-based lubricant.
See section 7.2.2 for the pH-modifying prepara-
tion *Aci-jel*®.

7.2.2 Anti-infective drugs

Effective specific treatments are available for the
common vaginal infections.

Fungal infections

Candidal vulvitis can be treated locally with cream
but is almost invariably associated with vaginal
infection which should also be treated. *Vaginal
candidiasis* is treated primarily with antifungal pessaries or cream inserted high into the vagina
(including during menstruation).

Imidazole drugs (clotrimazole, econazole, fenticonazole, isoconazole, and miconazole) are effective in short courses of 3 to 14 days according to the
preparation used; single dose preparations offer an
advantage when compliance is a problem. Vaginal
applications may be supplemented with antifungal
cream for vulvitis and to treat other superficial sites
of infection.

Nystatin is a well established treatment (but
stains clothing yellow). One or two pessaries are
inserted for 14 to 28 nights; they may be supplemented with cream for vulvitis and to treat other
superficial sites of infection.

Recurrence is common if the full course of treatment is not completed and is also particularly likely
if there are predisposing factors such as antibiotic
therapy, oral contraceptive use, pregnancy, or diabetes mellitus. Possible reservoirs of infection may
also lead to recontamination and should be treated.
These include other skin sites such as the digits, nail
beds, and umbilicus as well as the gastro-intestinal
tract and the bladder. The partner may also be the
source of re-infection and, if symptomatic, should
be treated with cream at the same time.

Oral treatment with fluconazole or itraconazole
(section 5.2) is also effective; oral ketoconazole has
been associated with fatal hepatotoxicity (see section 5.2 for CSM warning).

PREPARATIONS FOR VAGINAL AND VULVAL CANDIDIASIS
Side-effects: occasional local irritation

Clotrimazole (Non-proprietary)
Cream (topical), clotrimazole 1%, net price 20 g =
£1.45
Condoms: effect on latex condoms and diaphragms not yet known
Apply to anogenital area 2–3 times daily
Available from Generics, Genus
Pessary, clotrimazole 500 mg, net price 1 pessary
with applicator = £3.48
Insert 1 at night as a single dose
Available from Tillomed

Canesten® (Bayer Consumer Care)
Cream (topical), clotrimazole 1%. Net price 20 g =
£1.95; 50 g = £4.44
Condoms: damages latex condoms and diaphragms
Apply to anogenital area 2–3 times daily
Thrush Cream (topical) [NHS], clotrimazole 2%,
net price 20 g = £2.56
Excipients: include benzyl alcohol, polysorbates
Condoms: damages latex condoms and diaphragms
Apply to anogenital area 2–3 times daily
Vaginal cream (10% VC®), clotrimazole 10%. Net
price 5-g applicator pack = £3.48
Condoms: damages latex condoms and diaphragms
Insert 5 g at night as a single dose
Pessaries, clotrimazole 100 mg, net price 6 pessa-
ries with applicator = £3.62; 200 mg, 3 pessaries
with applicator = £3.62
Insert 200 mg for 3 nights *or* 100 mg for 6 nights
Condoms: damages latex condoms and diaphragms
Pessary , clotrimazole 500 mg. Net price 1 with
applicator = £3.48
Insert 1 at night as a single dose
Condoms: damages latex condoms and diaphragms
Combi, clotrimazole 500-mg pessary and cream
(topical) 1%. Net price 1 pessary and 20 g cream
= £4.50
Condoms: damages latex condoms and diaphragms

Ecostatin® (Squibb)

Cream (topical), econazole nitrate 1%. Net price 15 g = £1.49; 30 g = £2.75

Excipients: include butylated hydroxyanisole, fragrance
Condoms: damages latex condoms and diaphragms
Apply to anogenital area twice daily

¹ *Pessaries* PoM, econazole nitrate 150 mg. Net price 3 with applicator = £3.35

Condoms: damages latex condoms and diaphragms
Insert 1 pessary for 3 nights

¹ *Pessary (Ecostatin 1®)* PoM, econazole nitrate 150 mg, formulated for single-dose therapy. Net price 1 pessary with applicator = £3.35

Condoms: damages latex condoms and diaphragms
Insert 1 pessary at night as a single dose

¹ *Twinpack* PoM, econazole nitrate 150-mg pessaries and cream 1%. Net price 3 pessaries and 15 g cream = £4.35

Condoms: damages latex condoms and diaphragms

Flagyl Compak® PoM see section 5.1.11

¹ **Gyno-Daktarin®** (Janssen-Cilag) PoM

Intravaginal cream, miconazole nitrate 2%. Net price 78 g with applicators = £4.95

Excipients: include butylated hydroxyanisole
Condoms: damages latex condoms and diaphragms
Insert 5-g applicatorful once daily for 10–14 days or twice daily for 7 days; topical, apply to anogenital area twice daily

Pessaries, miconazole nitrate 100 mg. Net price 14 = £3.35

Condoms: damages latex condoms and diaphragms
Insert 1 pessary daily for 14 days or 1 pessary twice daily for 7 days

Combipack, miconazole nitrate 100-mg pessaries and cream (topical) 2%. Net price 14 pessaries and 15 g cream = £4.35

Condoms: damages latex condoms and diaphragms

Ovule (= vaginal capsule) (*Gyno-Daktarin 1®*), miconazole nitrate 1.2 g in a fatty basis. Net price 1 ovule (with finger stall) = £3.35

Excipients: include hydroxybenzoates (parabens)
Condoms: damages latex condoms and diaphragms
Insert 1 ovule at night as a single dose

Gyno-Pevaryl® (Janssen-Cilag)

Cream, econazole nitrate 1%. Net price 15 g = £1.50; 30 g = £3.45

Condoms: damages latex condoms and diaphragms
Insert 5-g applicatorful intravaginally and apply to vulva at night for at least 14 nights

Pessaries, econazole nitrate 150 mg. Net price 3 pessaries = £3.17

Condoms: damages latex condoms and diaphragms
Insert 1 pessary for 3 nights

Pessary (Gyno-Pevaryl 1®), econazole nitrate 150 mg, formulated for single-dose therapy. Net price 1 pessary with applicator = £3.37

Condoms: damages latex condoms and diaphragms
Insert 1 pessary at night as a single dose

Combipack, econazole nitrate 150-mg pessaries, econazole nitrate 1% cream. Net price 3 pessaries and 15 g cream = £4.35

Condoms: damages latex condoms and diaphragms

CP pack (Gyno-Pevaryl 1®), econazole nitrate 150-mg pessary, econazole nitrate 1% cream. Net price 1 pessary and 15 g cream = £4.35

Condoms: damages latex condoms and diaphragms

1. Can be sold to the public for the treatment of *vaginal candidiasis*. Unless packs labelled 'P' are available, those labelled 'PoM' can be sold providing the pharmacist *deletes* PoM from the pack and *substitutes* a capital **P** and provides *each purchaser* with a copy of the **patient information leaflet** supplied by the Professional Standards Directorate of the Royal Pharmaceutical Society of Great Britain.

Lomexin® (Dominion) PoM

Pessaries, fenticonazole nitrate 200 mg, net price 3 pessaries = £2.83; 600 mg, 1 pessary = £2.96

Excipients: include hydroxybenzoates (parabens)
Condoms: damages latex condoms and diaphragms
Insert 600 mg for 1 night or 200 mg for 3 nights

Masnoderm® (Dominion)

Cream, clotrimazole 1%. Net price 20 g = £1.47

Excipients: include benzyl alcohol, polysorbates
Condoms: damages latex condoms and diaphragms
Apply to anogenital area 2–3 times daily

Nizoral® (Janssen-Cilag) PoM

Cream (topical), ketoconazole 2%. Net price 30 g = £3.81

Excipients: include polysorbates, propylene glycol
Apply to anogenital area once or twice daily

Nystan® (Squibb) PoM

Cream and *Ointment*, see section 13.10.2

Vaginal cream, nystatin 100 000 units/4-g application. Net price 60 g with applicator = £2.77

Excipients: include benzyl alcohol, propylene glycol
Condoms: damages latex condoms and diaphragms
Insert 1–2 applicatorfuls at night for at least 14 nights

Pessaries, yellow, nystatin 100 000 units. Net price 28-pessary pack = £1.96

Condoms: no evidence of damage to latex condoms and diaphragms
Insert 1–2 pessaries at night for at least 14 nights

Pevaryl® (Janssen-Cilag)

Cream, econazole nitrate 1%. Net price 30 g = £2.65

Condoms: effect on latex condoms and diaphragms not yet known
Apply to anogenital area 2–3 times daily

¹ **Travogyn®** (Schering Health) PoM

Vaginal tablets (= pessaries), isoconazole nitrate 300 mg. Net price 2 = £3.37

Condoms: effect on latex condoms and diaphragms not yet known
Insert 2 pessaries as a single dose preferably at night

Other infections

Vaginal preparations intended to restore normal acidity (*Aci-Jel®*) may prevent recurrence of vaginal infections and permit the re-establishment of the normal vaginal flora.

Trichomonal infections commonly involve the lower urinary tract as well as the genital system and need systemic treatment with metronidazole or tinidazole (section 5.1.11).

Bacterial infections with Gram-negative organisms are particularly common in association with gynaecological operations and trauma. Metronidazole is effective against certain Gram-negative organisms, especially *Bacteroides* spp. and may be used prophylactically in gynaecological surgery.

Topical vaginal products containing povidone–iodine can be used to treat vaginitis due to candidal, trichomonal, non-specific or mixed infections; they are also used for the pre-operative preparation of the vagina. Clindamycin cream and metronidazole gel are also indicated for bacterial vaginosis; *Sultrin®* cream is licensed for the treatment of infections due to *Haemophilus vaginalis* only.

The antiviral drugs aciclovir, famciclovir and valaciclovir may be used in the treatment of genital infection due to *herpes simplex virus*, the HSV type 2 being a major cause of genital ulceration. They have a beneficial effect on virus shedding and healing, generally giving relief from pain and other symptoms. See section 5.3 for systemic preparations, and section 13.10.3 for topical preparations.

PREPARATIONS FOR OTHER VAGINAL INFECTIONS

Aci-Jel® (Janssen-Cilag)
Vaginal jelly, glacial acetic acid 0.94% in a buffered (pH 4) basis. Net price 85 g with applicator = £3.37
Excipients: include hydroxybenzoates (parabens), fragrance
Condoms: effect on latex condoms and diaphragms not yet known
Non-specific infections, insert 1 applicatorful once or twice daily to restore vaginal acidity

Betadine® (SSL)
Cautions: avoid in pregnancy (also if planned) and in breast-feeding; renal impairment (see Appendix 3); avoid regular use in thyroid disorders
Side-effects: rarely sensitivity; may interfere with thyroid function
Vaginal Cleansing Kit, solution, povidone-iodine 10%. Net price 250 mL with measuring bottle and applicator = £2.79
Condoms: effect on latex condoms and diaphragms not yet known
To be diluted and used once daily, preferably in the morning; may be used with Betadine® pessaries or vaginal gel
Pessaries, brown, povidone-iodine 200 mg. Net price 28 pessaries with applicator = £6.06
Condoms: effect on latex condoms and diaphragms not yet known
Vaginal gel, brown, povidone-iodine 10%. Net price 80 g with applicator = £2.79
Condoms: effect on latex condoms and diaphragms not yet known
Vaginal infections or pre-operatively, insert 1 moistened pessary night and morning for up to 14 days *or* use morning pessary with 5-g gel at night *or* morning douche with pessary (or 5-g gel) at night

Dalacin® (Pharmacia & Upjohn) [PoM]
Cream, clindamycin 2% (as phosphate). Net price 40-g pack with 7 applicators = £8.64
Excipients: include benzyl alcohol, polysorbates, propylene glycol
Condoms: damages latex condoms and diaphragms
Bacterial vaginosis, insert 5-g applicatorful at night for 3–7 nights

Sultrin® (Janssen-Cilag) [PoM] [▨]
Cautions: absorption of sulphonamides may produce systemic effects
Contra-indications: pregnancy; hypersensitivity to peanuts
Side-effects: sensitivity
Cream, sulfathiazole 3.42%, sulfacetamide 2.86%, sulphabenzamide 3.7%. Net price 80 g with applicator = £3.48
Excipients: include arachis (peanut) oil, hydroxybenzoates (parabens), propylene glycol, wool fat
Condoms: damages latex condoms and diaphragms
Bacterial vaginosis, insert 1 applicatorful of cream twice daily for 10 days, then once daily if necessary (but see also notes above)

Zidoval® (3M) [PoM]
Cautions: not recommended during menstruation; some absorption may occur, see section 5.1.11 for systemic effects
Side-effects: local effects including irritation, candidiasis, abnormal discharge, increased pelvic pressure
Vaginal gel, metronidazole 0.75%. Net price 40-g pack with 5 applicators = £4.63
Excipients: include hydroxybenzoates (parabens), propylene glycol
Bacterial vaginosis, insert 5-g applicatorful at night for 5 nights

[▨] denotes preparations that are considered to be less suitable for prescribing (see p. vi)

7.3   Contraceptives

The criteria by which contraceptive methods should be judged are effectiveness, acceptability, and freedom from side-effects.

Hormonal contraception is the most effective method of fertility control, short of sterilisation, but has unwanted major and minor side-effects, especially for certain groups of women.

Intra-uterine devices have a high use-effectiveness but may produce undesirable side-effects, especially menorrhagia, or be otherwise unsuitable in a significant proportion of women; their use is generally inadvisable in nulliparous women because of the increased risk of pelvic sepsis and infertility.

Barrier methods alone (condoms, diaphragms, and caps) are less effective but can be very reliable for well-motivated couples if used in conjunction with a **spermicide**. Occasionally sensitivity reactions occur. The female condom (*Femidom®*) is now also available; it is prelubricated but does not contain a spermicide.

7.3.1   Combined oral contraceptives

Oral contraceptives containing an oestrogen and a progestogen are the most effective preparations for general use. Their advantages include:
reliability;
avoidance of dysmenorrhoea;
less iron-deficiency anaemia;
avoidance of pre-menstrual tension;
less benign breast disease;
protection against endometrial and ovarian cancer;
protection against pelvic inflammatory disease.

CHOICE. The oestrogen content ranges from 20 to 50 micrograms and generally a preparation with the lowest oestrogen and progestogen content which gives good cycle control and minimal side-effects in the individual woman is chosen.

- *Low strength preparations* (containing ethinylestradiol (ethinyloestradiol) 20 micrograms) are particularly appropriate for obese or older women provided a combined oral contraceptive is otherwise suitable. It is recommended that the combined oral contraceptive is not continued beyond 50 years of age since there exist more suitable alternatives.
- *Standard strength preparations* (containing ethinylestradiol 30 or 35 micrograms or in 30/40 microgram *phased* preparations) are appropriate for standard use—but see Risk of Venous Thromboembolism below. Phased preparations are more complex to take, but provide better cycle control than the equivalent 'monophasic' levonorgestrel or norethisterone formulations.
- *High strength preparations* (containing either ethinylestradiol 50 micrograms or mestranol 50 micrograms) provide greater contraceptive security but increase the possibility of side-effects. These are used mainly in circumstances of reduced bioavailability (e.g. during long-term use of enzyme-inducing antiepileptics, see FPA advice under Interactions below).

The progestogens desogestrel, gestodene and nor-gestimate in combination with ethinylestradiol have been reported to have less adverse effects on lipids than etynodiol, levonorgestrel and norethisterone in combination with ethinylestradiol. Desogestrel and gestodene may be considered for women who experience side-effects (such as acne, headache, depression, weight gain, breast symptoms and breakthrough bleeding) with other progestogens. However, women should be advised that desogestrel and gestodene have also been associated with an increased risk of *venous thromboembolism*.

RISK OF VENOUS THROMBOEMBOLISM. There is an increased risk of venous thromboembolic disease in users of oral contraceptives but this risk is considerably smaller than that associated with pregnancy (about 60 cases of venous thromboembolic disease per 100 000 pregnancies). In all cases the risk of venous thromboembolism increases with age and in the presence of other risk factors for venous thromboembolism (e.g. obesity).

The incidence of venous thromboembolism in healthy, non-pregnant women who are not taking an oral contraceptive is about 5 cases per 100 000 women per year. For those using combined oral contraceptives containing second generation progestogens e.g. levonorgestrel, this incidence is about 15 per 100 000 women per year of use. Some studies have reported a greater risk of venous thromboembolism in women using preparations containing the third generation progestogens desogestrel and gestodene; the incidence in these women is about 25 per 100 000 women per year of use.

The absolute risk of venous thromboembolism in women using combined oral contraceptives containing these third generation progestogens remains very small and well below the risk associated with pregnancy. Provided that women are informed of and accept the relative risks of venous thromboembolism, the choice of oral contraceptive is for the woman together with the prescriber jointly to decide in the light of her individual medical history and any contra-indications.

MISSED PILL. It is important to bear in mind that the critical time for loss of protection is when a pill is omitted at the *beginning* or *end* of a cycle (which lengthens the pill-free interval). The following advice is now recommended by family planning organisations:

'If you forget a pill, take it as soon as you remember, and the next one at your normal time. If you are 12 or more hours late with any pill (especially the first in the packet) the pill may not work. As soon as you remember, continue normal pill taking. However, you will not be protected for the next seven days and must either not have sex or use another method such as the sheath. If these seven days run beyond the end of your packet, start the next packet at once when you have finished the present one, i.e. do not have a gap between packets. This will mean you may not have a period until the end of two packets but this does you no harm. Nor does it matter if you see some bleeding on tablet-taking days. If you are using everyday (ED) pills—miss out the seven inactive pills. If you are not sure which these are, ask your doctor.'

DIARRHOEA AND VOMITING. Vomiting and severe diarrhoea can interfere with absorption and limit effectiveness. Additional precautions should

therefore be used during and for 7 days after recovery. If the vomiting and diarrhoea occurs during the last 7 tablets, the next pill-free interval should be omitted (in the case of ED tablets the inactive ones should be omitted).

INTERACTIONS. The effectiveness of both *combined* and *progestogen-only* oral contraceptives may be considerably reduced by interaction with drugs that induce hepatic enzyme activity (e.g. **carbamazepine, griseofulvin, modafinil, phenytoin, phenobarbital, primidone, topiramate,** and, above all, **the rifamycins (rifabutin and rifampicin)**).

Family Planning Association (FPA) advice relating to a *short-term course of an enzyme-inducing drug* (for rifampicin and rifabutin, see also below) is that additional contraceptive precautions should be taken whilst taking the enzyme-inducing drug and for at least 7 days after stopping it; if these 7 days run beyond the end of a packet the new packet should be started immediately without a break (in the case of ED tablets the inactive ones should be omitted). It should be noted that **rifampicin** and **rifabutin** are such potent enzyme-inducing drugs that even if a course lasts for less than 7 days the additional contraceptive precautions should be continued for at least 4 weeks after stopping.

FPA advice relating to a *long-term course of an enzyme-inducing drug* (for rifampicin and rifabutin, see also below) in a woman unable to use an alternative method of contraception is to take an oral contraceptive containing ethinylestradiol 50 micrograms or more; 'tricycling' with standard ('monophasic') tablets (i.e. taking 3 or 4 packets without a break followed by a short tablet-free interval of 4 days) is recommended. **Rifampicin** and **rifabutin** are such potent enzyme-inducing drugs that an alternative method of contraception (such as an IUD) is **always** recommended. Since the excretory function of the liver does not return to normal for several weeks after stopping an enzyme-inducing drug, FPA advice relating to *withdrawal* is that appropriate contraceptive measures are required for 4 to 8 weeks after stopping.

Some **broad-spectrum antibiotics** (e.g. ampicillin, doxycycline) may reduce the efficacy of *combined* oral contraceptives by impairing the bacterial flora responsible for recycling of ethinylestradiol from the large bowel. FPA advice is that additional contraceptive precautions should be taken whilst taking a *short course of a broad-spectrum antibiotic* and for 7 days after stopping. If these 7 days run beyond the end of a packet the next packet should be started immediately without a break (in the case of ED tablets the inactive ones should be omitted). If the antibiotic course *exceeds 3 weeks*, the bacterial flora develops antibiotic resistance and additional precautions become unnecessary; additional precautions are also unnecessary if a woman starting a *combined* oral contraceptive has been on a course of antibiotics for 3 weeks or more.

SURGERY. Oestrogen-containing oral contraceptives should preferably be discontinued (and adequate alternative contraceptive arrangements made) 4 weeks before major elective surgery and all surgery to the legs; they should normally be recommenced at the first menses occurring at least 2 weeks after full mobilisation. A depot injection of a progestogen-only contraceptive may be offered and the oestrogen-containing contraceptive restarted later—if preferred before the next injection would be due. When discontinuation of an oestrogen-containing contraceptive is not possible, e.g. after trauma or if a patient admitted for an elective procedure is still on an oestrogen-containing oral contraceptive, thromboprophylaxis (with heparin and graduated compression hosiery) is advised. These recommendations do not apply to minor surgery with short duration of anaesthesia, e.g. laparoscopic sterilisation or tooth extraction, or to women taking oestrogen-free hormonal contraceptives (whether by mouth or by injection).

REASON TO STOP IMMEDIATELY. Combined oral contraceptives should be stopped (pending investigation and treatment), if any of the following occur:

- Sudden severe chest pain (even if not radiating to left arm);
- Sudden breathlessness (or cough with blood-stained sputum);
- Severe pain in calf of one leg;
- Severe stomach pain;
- Serious neurological effects including unusual severe, prolonged headache especially if first time or getting progressively worse or sudden partial or complete loss of vision or sudden disturbance of hearing or other perceptual disorders or dysphasia or bad fainting attack or collapse or first unexplained epileptic seizure or weakness, motor disturbances, very marked numbness suddenly affecting one side or one part of body;
- Hepatitis, jaundice, liver enlargement;
- Severe depression;
- Blood pressure above systolic 160 mmHg and diastolic 100 mmHg;
- Detection of a risk factor see Cautions and Contra-indications under Combined Oral Contraceptives

COMBINED ORAL CONTRACEPTIVES

('COC')

Indications: contraception; menstrual symptoms (section 6.4.1.2)

Cautions: risk factors for venous thromboembolism (see below and also notes above); arterial disease and migraine, see below; hyperprolactinaemia (seek specialist advice); severe depression, sickle-cell disease, inflammatory bowel disease including Crohn's disease; **interactions:** see above and Appendix 1 (contraceptives, oral)

RISK FACTORS FOR VENOUS THROMBOEMBOLISM (see also notes above). Use with **caution** if any of following factors present but **avoid** if two or more factors present:

- *family history of venous thromboembolism* in first degree relative aged under 45 years (avoid contraceptive containing desogestrel or gestodene, or if known prothrombotic coagulation abnormality e.g. factor V Leiden or antiphospholipid antibodies (including lupus anticoagulant));
- *obesity*—body mass index above 30 kg/m^2 (avoid if body mass index above 39 kg/m^2);
- *long-term immobilisation* e.g. in a wheelchair (avoid if confined to bed or leg in plaster cast);
- *varicose veins* (avoid during sclerosing treatment or where definite history of thrombosis).

RISK FACTORS FOR ARTERIAL DISEASE. Use with **caution** if any of one following factors present but **avoid** if two or more factors present:

- *family history of arterial disease* in first degree relative aged under 45 years (avoid if atherogenic lipid profile);
- *diabetes mellitus* (avoid if diabetes complications present);
- *hypertension*—blood pressure above *systolic 140 mmHg* and *diastolic 90 mmHg* (avoid if blood pressure above *systolic 160 mmHg* and *diastolic 100 mmHg*);
- *smoking* (avoid if smoking 40 or more cigarettes daily);
- *age* over 35 years (avoid if over 50 years);
- *obesity* (avoid if body mass index above 39 kg/m^2);
- *migraine*—see below.

MIGRAINE. Subject should report any increase in headache frequency or onset of focal symptoms (discontinue immediately and refer urgently to neurology expert if focal neurological symptoms not typical of aura persist for more than 1 hour—see also Reason to stop immediately in notes above); **contra-indicated** in

- migraine with typical focal aura,
- severe migraine regularly lasting over 72 hours despite treatment,
- migraine treated with ergot derivatives;

use with **caution** in

- migraine without focal aura,
- migraine controlled with 5HT$_1$ agonist (section 4.7.4.1).

Contra-indications: pregnancy; personal history of venous or arterial thrombosis, severe or multiple risk factors for arterial disease or for venous thromboembolism (see above), heart disease associated with pulmonary hypertension or risk of embolus; migraine (see above), transient cerebral ischaemic attacks without headaches; liver disease including disorders of hepatic excretion (e.g. Dubin-Johnson or Rotor syndromes), infective hepatitis (until liver function returns to normal); systemic lupus erythematosus; porphyria (section 9.8.2); liver adenoma; gallstones; after evacuation of hydatidiform mole (until return to normal of urine and plasma gonadotrophin concentration); history of haemolytic uraemic syndrome or history during pregnancy of pruritus, cholestatic jaundice, chorea or deterioration of otosclerosis; pemphigoid gestationis; breast or genital-tract carcinoma; undiagnosed vaginal bleeding; breast-feeding (until weaning or for 6 months after birth)

Side-effects: nausea, vomiting, headache, breast tenderness, changes in body weight, fluid retention, thrombosis (more common when factor V Leiden present or in blood groups A, B, and AB; see also notes above), changes in libido, depression, chorea, skin reactions, chloasma, hypertension, contact lenses may irritate, impairment of liver function, hepatic tumours, reduced menstrual loss, 'spotting' in early cycles, absence of withdrawal bleeding; rarely photosensitivity

BREAST CANCER. There is a small increase in the risk of having breast cancer diagnosed in women taking the combined oral contraceptive pill; this relative risk may wholly or partly be due to an earlier diagnosis. In users of combined oral contraceptive pills the cancers are more likely to be localised to the breast. The most important risk factor appears to be the age at which the contraceptive is stopped rather than the duration of use; the risk disappears gradually during the 10 years after stopping and there is no excess risk by 10 years. The CSM has advised that a small increase in the risk of breast cancer should be weighed against the benefits and evidence of the protective effect against cancers of the ovary and endometrium

Dose: each tablet should be taken at approximately same time each day; if delayed by longer than 12 hours contraceptive protection may be lost

21-day combined (monophasic) preparations, 1 tablet daily for 21 days; subsequent courses repeated after a 7-day interval (during which withdrawal bleeding occurs); first course usually started on day 1 of cycle—if starting on day 4 of cycle or later additional precautions (barrier methods) necessary during first 7 days

Every day (ED) combined (monophasic) preparations, 1 *active* tablet starting on day 1 of cycle—if starting on day 4 of cycle or later additional precautions (barrier methods) necessary during first

7 days (14 days if course accidentally started with *inactive* tablets); withdrawal bleeding occurs when *inactive* tablets are being taken; subsequent courses repeated without interval

Biphasic and triphasic preparations, see under individual preparations below

CHANGING TO COMBINED PREPARATION CONTAINING DIFFERENT PROGESTOGEN.

> *21-day combined preparations:* continue current pack until last tablet and start first tablet of new brand the next day. If a 7-day break is taken before starting new brand, additional precautions (barrier methods) should be used during first 7 days of taking the new brand.
>
> *Every Day (ED) combined preparations:* start the new brand (first tablet a of *21-day preparation* or the first *active* tablet of an *ED preparation*) the day after taking the last *active* tablet of previous brand (omitting the *inactive* tablets). If not possible to avoid taking the *inactive* tablets of an *ED preparation*, additional precautions (barrier methods) necessary during first 14 days of taking the new brand

CHANGING FROM PROGESTOGEN-ONLY TABLET: start on day 1 of menstruation or any day if amenorrhoea present and pregnancy has been excluded

SECONDARY AMENORRHOEA (exclude pregnancy): start any day, additional precautions (barrier methods) necessary during first 7 days

AFTER CHILDBIRTH (*not* breast-feeding): start 3 weeks postpartum (increased risk of thrombosis if started earlier); later than 3 weeks postpartum additional precautions (barrier methods) necessary for first 7 days

Not recommended if woman breast-feeding—oral progestogen-only contraceptive preferred

AFTER ABORTION OR MISCARRIAGE: start same day

Low Strength

■ Ethinylestradiol with Norethisterone

Loestrin 20® (Parke-Davis) PoM
Tablets, norethisterone acetate 1 mg, ethinylestradiol 20 micrograms. Net price 3 × 21-tab pack = £2.58
Dose: 1 tablet daily for 21 days; subsequent courses repeated after 7-day tablet-free interval (during which withdrawal bleeding occurs); for 'starting routines' see under Dose above

■ Ethinylestradiol with Desogestrel
See Risk of venous thromboembolism in notes above before prescribing

Mercilon® (Organon) PoM
Tablets, desogestrel 150 micrograms, ethinylestradiol 20 micrograms. Net price 3 × 21-tab pack = £8.57
Dose: 1 tablet daily for 21 days; subsequent courses repeated after 7-day tablet-free interval (during which withdrawal bleeding occurs); for 'starting routines' see under Dose above

■ Ethinylestradiol with Gestodene
See Risk of venous thromboembolism in notes above before prescribing

Femodette® (Schering Health) PoM
Tablets, s/c, gestodene 75 micrograms, ethinylestradiol 20 micrograms, net price 3 × 21-tab pack = £7.50
Dose: 1 tablet daily for 21 days; subsequent courses repeated after 7-day tablet-free interval (during which withdrawal bleeding occurs); for 'starting routines' see under Dose above

---

Standard Strength

■ Ethinylestradiol with Levonorgestrel

Eugynon 30® (Schering Health) PoM
Tablets, levonorgestrel 250 micrograms, ethinylestradiol 30 micrograms. Net price 3 × 21-tab pack = £2.07
Dose: 1 tablet daily for 21 days; subsequent courses repeated after 7-day tablet-free interval (during which withdrawal bleeding occurs); for 'starting routines' see under Dose above

Logynon® (Schering Health) PoM
6 light brown tablets, ethinylestradiol 30 micrograms, levonorgestrel 50 micrograms;
5 white tablets, ethinylestradiol 40 micrograms, levonorgestrel 75 micrograms;
10 ochre tablets, ethinylestradiol 30 micrograms, levonorgestrel 125 micrograms.
Net price 3 × 21-tab pack = £3.27
Dose: 1 tablet daily for 21 days, starting with light brown tablet marked 1 on day 1 of cycle; repeat after 7-day tablet-free interval

Logynon ED® (Schering Health) PoM
6 light brown tablets, ethinylestradiol 30 micrograms, levonorgestrel 50 micrograms;
5 white tablets, ethinylestradiol 40 micrograms, levonorgestrel 75 micrograms;
10 ochre tablets, ethinylestradiol 30 micrograms, levonorgestrel 125 micrograms;
7 white, inactive tablets.
Net price 3 × 28-tab pack = £3.27
Dose: 1 tablet daily starting in red sector on day 1 of cycle; continue in sequence without interruption

Microgynon 30® (Schering Health) PoM
Tablets, s/c, levonorgestrel 150 micrograms, ethinylestradiol 30 micrograms. Net price 21-tab pack = 71p
Dose: 1 tablet daily for 21 days; subsequent courses repeated after 7-day tablet-free interval (during which withdrawal bleeding occurs); for 'starting routines' see under Dose above

Microgynon 30 ED® (Schering Health) PoM
Tablets, beige, levonorgestrel 150 micrograms, ethinylestradiol 30 micrograms, white inactive tablets. Net price 3 × 28-tab (7 are inactive) pack = £2.13
Dose: 1 tablet daily for 28 days (withdrawal bleeding occurs when inactive tablets being taken); subsequent courses repeated without interval; for 'starting routines' see under Dose above

Ovran 30® (Wyeth) PoM
Tablets, levonorgestrel 250 micrograms, ethinylestradiol 30 micrograms. Net price 21-tab pack = 63p
Dose: 1 tablet daily for 21 days; subsequent courses repeated after 7-day tablet-free interval (during which withdrawal bleeding occurs); for 'starting routines' see under Dose above

Ovranette® (Wyeth) PoM
Tablets, levonorgestrel 150 micrograms, ethinylestradiol 30 micrograms. Net price 3 × 21-tab pack = £2.05
Dose: 1 tablet daily for 21 days; subsequent courses repeated after 7-day tablet-free interval (during which withdrawal bleeding occurs); for 'starting routines' see under Dose above

Trinordiol® (Wyeth) [PoM]
6 light brown tablets, ethinylestradiol
  30 micrograms, levonorgestrel 50 micrograms;
5 white tablets, ethinylestradiol 40 micrograms,
  levonorgestrel 75 micrograms;
10 ochre tablets, ethinylestradiol 30 micrograms,
  levonorgestrel 125 micrograms.
Net price 3 × 21-tab pack = £3.61
  Dose: 1 tablet daily for 21 days, starting with light
  brown tablet marked 1 on day 1 of cycle; repeat after 7-
  day tablet-free interval

■ Ethinylestradiol with Norethisterone

BiNovum® (Janssen-Cilag) [PoM]
7 white tablets, ethinylestradiol 35 micrograms,
  norethisterone 500 micrograms;
14 peach tablets, ethinylestradiol 35 micrograms,
  norethisterone 1 mg.
Net price 3 × 21-tab pack = £2.24
  Dose: 1 tablet daily for 21 days, starting with white tablet on day 1 of cycle; repeat after 7-day tablet-free interval

Brevinor® (Searle) [PoM]
Tablets, blue, norethisterone 500 micrograms, ethinylestradiol 35 micrograms. Net price 3 × 21-tab
  pack = £1.67
  Dose: 1 tablet daily for 21 days; subsequent courses
  repeated after 7-day tablet-free interval (during which
  withdrawal bleeding occurs); for 'starting routines' see
  under Dose above

Loestrin 30® (Parke-Davis) [PoM]
Tablets, norethisterone acetate 1.5 mg, ethinylestradiol 30 micrograms. Net price 3 × 21-tab
  pack = £3.78
  Dose: 1 tablet daily for 21 days; subsequent courses
  repeated after 7-day tablet-free interval (during which
  withdrawal bleeding occurs); for 'starting routines' see
  under Dose above

Norimin® (Searle) [PoM]
Tablets, norethisterone 1 mg, ethinylestradiol
  35 micrograms. Net price 3 × 21-tab pack = £1.90
  Dose: 1 tablet daily for 21 days; subsequent courses
  repeated after 7-day tablet-free interval (during which
  withdrawal bleeding occurs); for 'starting routines' see
  under Dose above

Ovysmen® (Janssen-Cilag) [PoM]
Tablets, norethisterone 500 micrograms, ethinylestradiol 35 micrograms. Net price 3 × 21-tab
  pack = £1.70
  Dose: 1 tablet daily for 21 days; subsequent courses
  repeated after 7-day tablet-free interval (during which
  withdrawal bleeding occurs); for 'starting routines' see
  under Dose above

Synphase® (Searle) [PoM]
7 blue tablets, ethinylestradiol 35 micrograms,
  norethisterone 500 micrograms;
9 white tablets, ethinylestradiol 35 micrograms,
  norethisterone 1 mg;
5 blue tablets, ethinylestradiol 35 micrograms,
  norethisterone 500 micrograms.
Net price 21-tab pack = £1.08
  Dose: 1 tablet daily for 21 days, starting with blue tablet
  marked 1 on day 1 of cycle; repeat after 7-day tablet-free
  interval

TriNovum® (Janssen-Cilag) [PoM]
7 white tablets, ethinylestradiol 35 micrograms,
  norethisterone 500 micrograms;
7 light peach tablets, ethinylestradiol
  35 micrograms, norethisterone 750 micrograms;

7 peach tablets, ethinylestradiol 35 micrograms,
  norethisterone 1 mg.
Net price 3 × 21-tab pack = £3.11
  Dose: 1 tablet daily for 21 days, starting with white tablet on day 1 of cycle; repeat after 7-day tablet-free interval

■ Ethinylestradiol with Norgestimate

Cilest® (Janssen-Cilag) [PoM]
Tablets, blue, norgestimate 250 micrograms, ethinylestradiol 35 micrograms. Net price 3 × 21-tab
  pack = £6.42
  Dose: 1 tablet daily for 21 days; subsequent courses
  repeated after 7-day tablet-free interval (during which
  withdrawal bleeding occurs); for 'starting routines' see
  under Dose above

■ Ethinylestradiol with Desogestrel
See Risk of venous thromboembolism in notes
above before prescribing

Marvelon® (Organon) [PoM]
Tablets, desogestrel 150 micrograms, ethinylestradiol 30 micrograms. Net price 3 × 21-tab pack =
  £6.70
  Dose: 1 tablet daily for 21 days; subsequent courses
  repeated after 7-day tablet-free interval (during which
  withdrawal bleeding occurs); for 'starting routines' see
  under Dose above

■ Ethinylestradiol with Gestodene
See Risk of venous thromboembolism in notes
above before prescribing

Femodene® (Schering Health) [PoM]
Tablets, s/c, gestodene 75 micrograms, ethinylestradiol 30 micrograms. Net price 3 × 21-tab
  pack = £5.70
  Dose: 1 tablet daily for 21 days; subsequent courses
  repeated after 7-day tablet-free interval (during which
  withdrawal bleeding occurs); for 'starting routines' see
  under Dose above

Femodene® **ED** (Schering Health) [PoM]
Tablets, s/c, gestodene 75 micrograms, ethinylestradiol 30 micrograms. Net price 3 × 28-tab
  (7 are inactive) pack = £5.70
  Dose: 1 tablet daily for 28 days (withdrawal bleeding
  occurs when inactive tablets are being taken); subsequent courses repeated without interval; for 'starting
  routines' see under Dose above

Minulet® (Wyeth) [PoM]
Tablets, gestodene 75 micrograms, ethinylestradiol
  30 micrograms. Net price 3 × 21-tab pack = £5.70
  Dose: 1 tablet daily for 21 days; subsequent courses
  repeated after 7-day tablet-free interval (during which
  withdrawal bleeding occurs); for 'starting routines' see
  under Dose above

Triadene® (Schering Health) [PoM]
6 beige tablets, ethinylestradiol 30 micrograms,
  gestodene 50 micrograms;
5 dark brown tablets, ethinylestradiol
  40 micrograms, gestodene 70 micrograms;
10 white tablets, ethinylestradiol 30 micrograms,
  gestodene 100 micrograms.
Net price 3 × 21-tab pack = £7.95
  Dose: 1 tablet daily for 21 days, starting with beige tablet marked 'start' on day 1 of cycle; repeat after 7-day
  tablet-free interval

Tri-Minulet® (Wyeth) PoM
6 beige tablets, ethinylestradiol 30 micrograms,
gestodene 50 micrograms;
5 dark brown tablets, ethinylestradiol
40 micrograms, gestodene 70 micrograms;
10 white tablets, ethinylestradiol 30 micrograms,
gestodene 100 micrograms.
Net price 3 × 21-tab pack = £7.95
> *Dose:* 1 tablet daily for 21 days, starting with beige tab-
> let marked 1 on day 1 of the cycle; repeat after 7-day
> tablet-free interval

■ Ethinylestradiol with cyproterone acetate
See co-cyprindiol (section 13.6.2)

High Strength

■ Ethinylestradiol with Levonorgestrel
Ovran® (Wyeth) PoM
Tablets, levonorgestrel 250 micrograms, ethinylestradiol 50 micrograms. Net price 21-tab pack
= 41p
> *Dose:* 1 tablet daily for 21 days; subsequent courses
> repeated after 7-day tablet-free interval (during which
> withdrawal bleeding occurs); for 'starting routines' see
> under Dose above

■ Mestranol with Norethisterone
Norinyl-1® (Searle) PoM
Tablets, norethisterone 1 mg, mestranol
50 micrograms. Net price 3 × 21-tab pack = £1.83
> *Dose:* 1 tablet daily for 21 days; subsequent courses
> repeated after 7-day tablet-free interval (during which
> withdrawal bleeding occurs); for 'starting routines' see
> under Dose above

Emergency contraception

Hormonal methods
Two hormonal methods are available for emergency
contraception and involve the use of *either* levonorgestrel alone *or* the combined preparation containing ethinylestradiol (ethinyloestradiol) with
levonorgestrel. Both are effective if the first dose is
taken within 72 hours (3 days) of unprotected intercourse; taking the first dose as soon as possible
increases efficacy. Both methods are occasionally
used after 72 hours [unlicensed use] but there is no
clear proof of efficacy. Hormonal methods are however less effective than insertion of an intra-uterine
device (see below).
 Levonorgestrel is taken in a dose of
750 micrograms (*Levonelle-2®*) followed 12 hours
later by a further 750 micrograms; the levonor-
gestrel-only emergency contraceptive has fewer
side-effects than the combined hormonal emergency contraceptive. Levonorgestrel is not suitable
for women with current severe liver disease or
active acute porphyria.
 The combined hormonal (Yuzpe) method
involves taking 2 tablets, each containing **ethinylestradiol** (ethinyloestradiol) 50 micrograms and
levonorgestrel 250 micrograms, followed 12 hours
later by a further 2 tablets. The combined method is
not suitable for women with a history of thrombosis, active acute porphyria or for those with current

severe liver disease or focal migraine at the time of
presentation. Side-effects include nausea, vomiting,
headache, dizziness, breast discomfort, and menstrual irregularities. If vomiting occurs within 2
hours of taking the tablets, 2 replacement tablets
can be given with an anti-emetic (preferably not
metoclopramide which may cause extrapyramidal
effects in young women—domperidone may be
used).
 When prescribing either method of hormonal
emergency contraception the doctor should explain:

* that the next period may be early or late;
* that a barrier method of contraception needs to be
 used until the next period;
* the need to return promptly if any lower abdominal
 pain occurs (and also in 3 to 4 weeks if the subsequent menstrual bleed is abnormally light, heavy or
 brief, or is absent, or if she is otherwise concerned).

Pregnancy despite treatment: see Appendix 4
(contraceptives, oral)—doctor information leaflet
also available.

INTERACTIONS. The effectiveness of either hormonal method of emergency contraception is
reduced by enzyme-inducing drugs; the dose of
emergency contraception should be increased by
50%. There is no need to increase the dose for
emergency contraception if the patient is taking
antibiotics that are not enzyme inducers.

Levonelle®-2 (Schering Health) ▼ PoM
Tablets, levonorgestrel 750 micrograms, net price
2-tab pack = £5.00
> For post-coital contraception as an occasional emer-
> gency measure; should not be administered if menstrual
> bleeding overdue or if unprotected intercourse occurred
> more than 72 hours previously
> *Dose:* 1 tablet as soon as possible after coitus (up to 72
> hours) then 1 further tablet 12 hours later

Schering PC4® (Schering Health) PoM
Tablets, s/c, norgestrel 500 micrograms (≡ levonorgestrel 250 micrograms), ethinylestradiol
50 micrograms. Net price 4-tab pack = £1.60
> For post-coital contraception as an occasional emer-
> gency measure; should not be administered if menstrual
> bleeding overdue or if unprotected intercourse occurred
> more than 72 hours previously (but see notes above)
> *Dose:* 2 tablets as soon as possible after coitus (up to 72
> hours) then 2 further tablets 12 hours later
> *Note.* **Ovran®** also contains levonorgestrel
> 250 micrograms and ethinylestradiol 50 micrograms but
> is not licensed or packed for post-coital contraception

IUD

A copper intra-uterine contraceptive device (section
7.3.4) can be inserted up to 120 hours (5 days) after
unprotected intercourse; testing for sexually transmitted disease should be carried out and insertion of
the device should usually be covered by antibiotic
prophylaxis. If intercourse has occurred more than
5 days previously, the device can still be inserted up
to 5 days after the earliest likely calculated ovulation (i.e. within the minimum period before implantation). Insertion of an intra-uterine device is more
effective than the hormonal methods.

7.3.2 Progestogen-only contraceptives

- **7.3.2.1** Oral progestogen-only contraceptives
- **7.3.2.2** Parenteral progestogen-only contraceptives
- **7.3.2.3** Intra-uterine progestogen-only contraceptive

7.3.2.1 Oral progestogen-only contraceptives

Oral progestogen-only preparations may offer a suitable alternative when oestrogens are contra-indicated (including those patients with venous thrombosis or a past history or predisposition to venous thrombosis), but have a higher failure rate than combined preparations. They are suitable for older women, for heavy smokers, and for those with hypertension, valvular heart disease, diabetes mellitus, and migraine. Menstrual irregularities (oligomenorrhoea, menorrhagia) are more common but tend to resolve on long-term treatment.

INTERACTIONS. Effectiveness of oral progestogen-only preparations is not affected by broad-spectrum antibiotics but is reduced by enzyme-inducing drugs—see p. 368 and Appendix 1 (progestogens).

SURGERY. All progestogen-only contraceptives (including those given by injection) are suitable for use as an alternative to combined oral contraceptives before major elective surgery.

STARTING ROUTINE. 1 tablet daily, on a continuous basis, starting on 1st day of cycle and taken at the same time each day (if delayed by longer than 3 hours contraceptive protection may be lost). Additional contraceptive precautions are not necessary when initiating treatment.

Changing from a combined oral contraceptive: start on the day following completion of the combined oral contraceptive course without a break (or in the case of ED tablets omitting the inactive ones).

After childbirth: start any time after 3 weeks postpartum (increased risk of breakthrough bleeding if started earlier)—lactation is not affected.

MISSED PILL. The following advice is now recommended by family planning organisations:
'If you forget a pill, take it as soon as you remember and carry on with the next pill at the right time. If the pill was more than three hours overdue you are not protected. Continue normal pill-taking but you must also use another method, such as the sheath, for the next 7 days'.

DIARRHOEA AND VOMITING. Vomiting and severe diarrhoea can interfere with absorption and limit effectiveness. Additional precautions should be used during and for 7 days after recovery.

ORAL PROGESTOGEN-ONLY CONTRACEPTIVES

(Progestogen-only pill, 'POP')
Indications: contraception
Cautions: heart disease, sex-steroid dependent cancer, past ectopic pregnancy, malabsorption syndromes, functional ovarian cysts, active liver disease, recurrent cholestatic jaundice, history of jaundice in pregnancy; **interactions:** p. 368 and Appendix 1 (progestogens)
OTHER CONDITIONS. The product literature advises caution in patients with history of thromboembolism, hypertension, diabetes and migraine; evidence for caution in these conditions is unsatisfactory
Contra-indications: pregnancy, undiagnosed vaginal bleeding; severe arterial disease; liver adenoma, porphyria (section 9.8.2); after evacuation of hydatidiform mole (until return to normal of urine and plasma gonadotrophin values)
Side-effects: menstrual irregularities (see also notes above); nausea, vomiting, headache, dizziness, breast discomfort, depression, skin disorders, disturbance of appetite, weight changes, changes in libido
BREAST CANCER. There is a small increase in the risk of having breast cancer diagnosed in women using, or who have recently used, a progestogen-only contraceptive pill; this relative risk may wholly or partly be due to an earlier diagnosis. The most important risk factor appears to be the age at which the contraceptive is stopped rather than the duration of use; the risk disappears gradually during the 10 years after stopping and there is no excess risk by 10 years. The CSM has advised that a small increase in the risk of breast cancer should be weighed against the benefits
Dose: 1 tablet daily at same time each day, starting on day 1 of cycle then continuously; if administration delayed for 3 hours or more it should be regarded as a 'missed pill', see notes above

Femulen® (Searle) ▣PoM▣
Tablets, etynodiol diacetate 500 micrograms. Net price 3 × 28-tab pack = £2.76
Micronor® (Janssen-Cilag) ▣PoM▣
Tablets, norethisterone 350 micrograms. Net price 3 × 28-tab pack = £1.89
Microval® (Wyeth) ▣PoM▣
Tablets, levonorgestrel 30 micrograms. Net price 35-tab pack = 90p
Neogest® (Schering Health) ▣PoM▣
Tablets, brown, s/c, norgestrel 75 micrograms (≡ levonorgestrel 37.5 micrograms). Net price 35-tab pack = 82p
Norgeston® (Schering Health) ▣PoM▣
Tablets, s/c, levonorgestrel 30 micrograms. Net price 35-tab pack = 82p
Noriday® (Searle) ▣PoM▣
Tablets, norethisterone 350 micrograms. Net price 3 × 28-tab pack = £1.75

7.3.2.2 Parenteral progestogen-only contraceptives

Medroxyprogesterone acetate (*Depo-Provera®*) is a long-acting progestogen given by intramuscular injection; it is as effective as the combined oral preparations but because of its prolonged action should never be given without *full counselling backed by the manufacturer's approved leaflet*. It may be used as a short-term or long-term contraceptive for women who have been appropriately counselled concerning the likelihood of menstrual disturbance and the potential for a delay in return to full fertility. Delayed return of fertility and irregular cycles may occur after discontinuation of treatment but there is no evidence of permanent infertility. Heavy bleeding has been reported in patients given medroxyprogesterone acetate in the immediate puerperium (the first dose is best delayed until 5 to 6 weeks postpartum). If the woman is not breast-feeding, the first injection may be given within 5 days postpartum (she should be warned that the risk of heavy or prolonged bleeding may be increased). Reduction in bone mineral density has also been reported. **Norethisterone enantate** (*Noristerat®*) is a long-acting progestogen given as an oily injection which provides contraception for 8 weeks to provide short-term interim contraception e.g. before vasectomy becomes effective. The **cautions** and **contra-indications** of oral progestogen-only contraceptives apply except that since the injection also reliably inhibits ovulation, it protects against ectopic pregnancy and functional ovarian cysts.

An **etonogestrel-releasing implant** (*Implanon®*), consisting of a single flexible rod, is also available; the rod is inserted subdermally into the lower surface of the upper arm and is effective for up to 3 years. In overweight women, the implant may not provide effective contraception during the third year and earlier replacement should be considered in such patients. Local reactions such as bruising and itching may occur at the insertion site. The **cautions**, **contra-indications** and **side-effects** of oral preparations apply; the contraceptive .effect of *Implanon®* is reversible on removal of the implant. *The doctor or nurse administering (or removing) the system should be fully trained in the technique and should provide full counselling backed by the manufacturer's approved leaflet.*

The **levonorgestrel-releasing implant system** (*Norplant®*, Hoechst Marion Roussel) has recently been discontinued, but some women may have the system in place until 2004. Unlike the injectable progestogen-only contraceptive method, the effects of *Norplant®* are almost immediately reversible on removal of the implants. *The doctor removing the system should be fully trained in the technique.*

INTERACTIONS. Effectiveness of parenteral progestogen-only contraceptives is not affected by broad-spectrum antibiotics. However, effectiveness may be reduced by enzyme-inducing drugs; another method of contraception may be used additionally or, more usually in long-term users, the interval between injections of medroxyprogesterone acetate should be reduced from 12 weeks to 10 weeks—see p. 368 and Appendix 1 (progestogens)

PARENTERAL PROGESTOGEN-ONLY CONTRACEPTIVES

Indications: contraception, see also notes above and under preparations (roles vary according to preparation)

Cautions: see notes above and under preparations; possible risk of breast cancer, see oral progestogen-only contraceptives (section 7.3.2.1); history during pregnancy of pruritis or of deterioration of otosclerosis, disturbances of lipid metabolism; **interactions:** see notes above, p. 368 and Appendix 1 (progestogens)

COUNSELLING. Full counselling backed by *manufacturer's approved leaflet* required before administration

Contra-indications: see notes above

Side-effects: see notes above

Dose: see under preparations

■ Injectable preparations

Depo-Provera® (Pharmacia & Upjohn) PoM

Injection (aqueous suspension), medroxyprogesterone acetate 150 mg/mL, net price 1-mL pre-filled syringe = £4.55. Counselling, see patient information leaflet

Dose: by deep intramuscular injection, 150 mg within first 5 days of cycle or within first 5 days after parturition (delay until 6 weeks after parturition if breast-feeding); for long-term contraception, repeated every 12 weeks (if interval greater than 12 weeks and 5 days, exclude pregnancy before next injection and advise patient to use additional contraceptive measures (e.g. barrier) for 14 days after the injection)

Note. The 150 mg/mL strength is also available in 3.3-mL vial for use in cancer as *Depo-Provera Oncology®* (section 8.3.2)

Noristerat® (Schering Health) PoM

Injection (oily), norethisterone enantate 200 mg/mL. Net price 1-mL amp = £3.00. Counselling, see patient information leaflet

Dose: by deep intramuscular injection given very slowly *into gluteal muscle*, short-term contraception, 200 mg within first 5 days of cycle or immediately after parturition (duration 8 weeks); may be repeated once after 8 weeks (withhold breast-feeding for neonates with severe or persistent jaundice requiring medical treatment)

■ Implants

Implanon® (Organon) ▼ PoM

Implant, containing etonogestrel 68 mg in each flexible rod, net price = £90.00. Counselling, see patient information leaflet

Dose: by subdermal implantation, no previous hormonal contraceptive, 1 implant inserted during first 5 days of cycle; parturition or abortion in second trimester, 1 implant inserted between days 21–28 after delivery or abortion (if inserted after 28 days additional precautions necessary for next 7 days); abortion in first trimester, 1 implant inserted immediately; changing from an oral contraceptive, consult product literature; remove within 3 years of insertion

7.3.2.3 Intra-uterine progestogen-only contraceptive

Levonorgestrel is released directly into the uterine cavity from an intra-uterine system (*Mirena®*). Effects are therefore mainly local and hormonal including prevention of proliferation of the endometrium, sperm-impeding changes to the utero-cervical fluid, and suppression of ovulation in some women (in some cycles); the physical presence of the system in the uterus may also make a minor contribution to the overall contraceptive effect. Return of fertility after removal is rapid and appears to be complete. Advantages over copper intra-uterine devices are that there may be an improvement in any dysmenorrhoea and a reduction in blood loss; there is also evidence that the frequency of pelvic inflammatory disease may be reduced (particularly in the youngest age groups who are most at risk). Generally the **cautions** and **contra-indications** are as for standard intra-uterine devices (section 7.3.4) but the risk of ectopic pregnancy is considerably reduced and pre-existing heavy menses and anaemia may be alleviated. Moreover, since the progestogen is released close to the site of the main contraceptive action (on cervical mucus and endometrium) progestogenic side-effects and interactions are less likely to be a problem—in particular, enzyme-inducing drugs are unlikely to have much influence on the contraceptive effect. Initially changes in the pattern and duration of menstrual bleeding (spotting or prolonged bleeding) are common and full counselling (backed by patient information leaflet) should be undertaken before insertion. Improvement usually occurs a few months after insertion and bleeding may often become scanty or absent; this may therefore be a method of choice for women who have excessively heavy menses. Functional ovarian cysts (usually asymptomatic) may occur and usually resolve spontaneously (ultrasound monitoring recommended).

INTRA-UTERINE PROGESTOGEN-ONLY CONTRACEPTIVE

Indications: contraception

Cautions; Contra-indications; Side-effects: see notes above; in case of pregnancy—remove system (teratogenicity cannot be excluded); not suitable for emergency contraception; **interactions:** see notes above and Appendix 1 (progestogens)

Mirena® (Schering Health) PoM
Intra-uterine system, T-shaped plastic frame (impregnated with barium sulphate and with threads attached to base) with polydimethylsiloxane reservoir releasing levonorgestrel 20 micrograms/24 hours. Net price = £89.25. Counselling, see patient information leaflet
Insert into uterine cavity within 7 days of onset of menstruation (anytime if replacement) or immediately after first-trimester termination by curettage; postpartum insertions should be delayed until 6 weeks after delivery; effective for 5 years

7.3.3 Spermicidal contraceptives

Spermicidal contraceptives are useful additional safeguards but do **not** give adequate protection if used alone except where fertility is already significantly diminished (section 6.4.1.1); they are suitable for use with barrier methods. They have two components: a spermicide and a vehicle which itself may have some inhibiting effect on sperm activity.

CSM Advice. Products such as petroleum jelly (vaseline), baby oil and oil-based vaginal and rectal preparations are likely to damage condoms and contraceptive diaphragms made from latex rubber, and may render them less effective as a barrier method of contraception and as a protection from sexually transmitted diseases (including AIDS).

Condoms: no evidence of harm to latex condoms and diaphragms with the products listed below

Delfen® (Janssen-Cilag)
Foam, nonoxinol '9' 12.5%, pressurised aerosol unit in a water-miscible basis. Net price 20 g (with applicator) = £4.65
Excipients: include hydroxybenzoates (parabens), propylene glycol, fragrance

Duragel® (LRC)
Gel, nonoxinol '9' 2% in a water-soluble basis. Net price 100-g tube = £3.28
Excipients: include propylene glycol

Gynol II® (Janssen-Cilag)
Jelly, nonoxinol '9' 2% in a water-soluble basis. Net price 81 g = £2.61; applicator = 75p
Excipients: include hydroxybenzoates (parabens), propylene glycol, sorbic acid

Ortho-Creme® (Janssen-Cilag)
Cream, nonoxinol '9' 2% in a water-miscible basis. Net price 70 g = £2.44; applicator = 75p
Excipients: include hydroxybenzoates (parabens), propylene glycol, sorbic acid, fragrance

Orthoforms® (Janssen-Cilag)
Pessaries, nonoxinol '9' 5% in a water-soluble basis. Net price 15 pessaries = £2.40

7.3.4 Contraceptive devices

Intra-uterine devices

The intra-uterine device (IUD) is suitable for older parous women and as a second-line contraceptive in young nulliparous women who should be carefully selected because of their increased background risk of pelvic inflammatory disease. Inert intra-uterine devices are no longer on the UK market but may still be worn by some women.

Smaller devices have been introduced to minimise side-effects; these consist of a plastic carrier wound with copper wire or fitted with copper bands; some also have a central core of silver to prevent fragmentation of the copper. Family planning organisations now recommend that the replacement time for these devices should be 5 years; any copper intra-uterine device licensed currently in the UK, which is fitted in a woman over the age of 40, may remain in the uterus until menopause. The intra-uterine device *Gyne-T 380®* (Janssen-Cilag) is no longer available, but some women may have the device in place until 2009.

The timing and technique of fitting an intra-uterine device are critical for its subsequent performance and call for proper training and experience. Devices should not be fitted during the heavy days of the period; they are best fitted after the end of menstruation and before the calculated time of implantation. The main excess risk of infection occurs in the first 20 days after insertion and is believed to be related to existing carriage of a sexually transmitted disease, therefore pre-screening (at least for chlamydia) should ideally be performed. The woman should be advised to attend *as an emergency* if she experiences sustained pain during the next 20 days.

An intra-uterine device should not be removed in mid-cycle unless an additional contraceptive was used for the previous 7 days. If removal is essential (e.g. to treat severe pelvic infection) post-coital contraception should be considered.

If an intra-uterine device fails and the woman wishes to continue to full-term the device should be removed in the first trimester if possible.

INTRA-UTERINE CONTRACEPTIVE DEVICES

Indications: see notes above

Cautions: anaemia, heavy menses (progestogen intra-uterine system might be preferable, section 7.3.2.3), endometriosis, severe primary dysmenorrhoea, history of pelvic inflammatory disease, history of ectopic pregnancy or tubal surgery, diabetes, fertility problems, nulliparity and young age, severely scarred uterus (including after endometrial resection) or severe cervical stenosis, valvular heart disease (antibiotic cover needed—section 5.1 table 2)—avoid if prosthetic valve or history of infective endocarditis; HIV infection or immunosuppressive therapy (risk of infection—avoid if marked immunosuppression); joint and other prostheses (increased risk of infection); epilepsy; increased risk of expulsion if inserted before uterine involution; gynaecological examination before insertion, 6 weeks after (or sooner if there is a problem), then after 6 months, then yearly; anticoagulant therapy (avoid if possible); remove if pregnancy occurs; if pregnancy occurs, increased likelihood that it may be ectopic

Contra-indications: pregnancy, severe anaemia, recent sexually transmitted infection (if not fully investigated and treated), unexplained uterine bleeding, distorted or small uterine cavity, genital malignancy, active trophoblastic disease, pelvic inflammatory disease, established or marked immunosuppression; *copper devices:* copper allergy, Wilson's disease, medical diathermy

Side-effects: uterine or cervical perforation, displacement, expulsion; pelvic infection may be exacerbated, heavy menses, dysmenorrhoea, allergy; *on insertion:* pain (alleviated by NSAID such as ibuprofen 30 minutes before insertion) and bleeding, occasionally, epileptic seizure, vasovagal attack

Multiload® Cu250 (Organon) PoM

Intra-uterine device, copper wire, surface area approx. 250 mm² wound on vertical stem of plastic carrier, 3.5 cm length, with 2 down-curving flexible arms, monofilament thread attached to base of vertical stem; preloaded in inserter. Net price = £7.01

For uterine length 6–9 cm; replacement every 3 years (but see notes above)

Multiload® Cu250 Short (Organon) PoM

Intra-uterine device, as above, with vertical stem length 2.4 cm. Net price = £7.01

For uterine length 5–7 cm; replacement every 3 years (but see notes above)

Multiload® Cu375 (Organon) PoM

Intra-uterine device, as above, with copper surface area approx. 375 mm² and vertical stem length 3.5 cm. Net price = £9.08

For uterine length 6–9 cm; replacement every 5 years (see notes above)

Nova-T® (Schering Health) PoM

Intra-uterine device, copper wire with silver core, surface area approx. 200 mm² wound on vertical stem of T-shaped plastic carrier, impregnated with barium sulphate for radio-opacity, threads attached to base of vertical stem. Net price = £10.27

For uterine length over 6.5 cm; replacement every 5 years (see notes above)

Other contraceptive devices

■ Contraceptive caps

Type A contraceptive pessary
Opaque rubber, sizes 1 to 5 (55–75 mm rising in steps of 5 mm), net price = £6.62
Available from Lamberts (*Dumas Vault Cap®*)

Type B contraceptive pessary
Opaque rubber, sizes 22 to 31 mm (rising in steps of 3 mm), net price = £7.71
Available from Lamberts (*Prentif Cavity Rim Cervical Cap®*)

Type C contraceptive pessary
Opaque rubber, sizes 1 to 3 (42, 48 and 54 mm), net price = £6.62
Available from Lamberts (*Vimule Cap®*)

■ Contraceptive diaphragms

Type A Diaphragm with flat metal spring
Transparent rubber with flat metal spring, sizes 55–95 mm (rising in steps of 5 mm), net price = £5.49
Available from Lamberts (*Reflexions®*)

Type B Diaphragm with coiled metal rim
Opaque rubber with coiled metal rim, sizes 55–100 mm (rising in steps of 5 mm), net price = £5.74
Available from Janssen-Cilag (*Ortho®*)

Type C Arcing Spring Diaphragm
Opaque rubber with arcing spring, sizes 55–95 mm (rising in steps of 5 mm), net price = £6.53
Available from Janssen-Cilag (*All-Flex®*)

■ Fertility thermometer

Fertility (Ovulation) Thermometer (Zeal)
Mercury in glass thermometer, range 35 to 39°C (graduated in 0.1°C). Net price = £1.65
For monitoring ovulation for the fertility awareness method of contraception

7.4 Drugs for genito-urinary disorders

7.4.1	Drugs for urinary retention
7.4.2	Drugs for urinary frequency, enuresis, and incontinence
7.4.3	Drugs used in urological pain
7.4.4	Bladder instillations and urological surgery
7.4.5	Drugs for impotence

For drugs used in the treatment of urinary-tract infections see section 5.1.13.

7.4.1 Drugs for urinary retention

Acute retention is painful and is treated by catheterisation.

Chronic retention is painless and often long-standing. Catheterisation is unnecessary unless there is deterioration of renal function. After the cause has initially been established and treated, drugs may be required to increase detrusor muscle tone.

Benign prostatic hyperplasia is treated either surgically or medically with alpha-blockers (see below) or with the anti-androgen finasteride (section 6.4.2).

Alpha-blockers

The selective alpha-blockers, **alfuzosin**, **doxazosin**, **indoramin**, **prazosin**, **tamsulosin** and **terazosin** relax smooth muscle in benign prostatic hyperplasia producing an increase in urinary flow-rate and an improvement in obstructive symptoms. Side-effects of selective alpha-blockers include sedation, dizziness and hypotension (notably postural hypotension, particularly after the first dose); other side-effects associated with this group of drugs include drowsiness, weakness and lack of energy, depression, headache, dry mouth, nausea, urinary frequency and incontinence, and tachycardia and palpitations. They should be avoided in patients with a history of orthostatic hypotension and micturition syncope; special care (and reduced dosage) is needed when initiating them in the elderly, and in renal and possibly hepatic impairment. Since selective alpha-blockers are also antihypertensive, patients receiving antihypertensive treatment require reduced dosage and specialist supervision (as do those with cardiac disorders). **Interactions:** see Appendix 1 (alpha-blockers).

DRIVING. Selective alpha-blockers may cause drowsiness and so affect ability to drive or operate machinery.

ALFUZOSIN HYDROCHLORIDE

Indications: see notes above
Cautions: see notes above
Contra-indications: see notes above; severe liver impairment
Side-effects: see notes above
Dose: 2.5 mg 3 times daily, max.10 mg daily; ELDERLY initially 2.5 mg twice daily
FIRST DOSE EFFECT. First dose may cause collapse due to hypotensive effect (therefore should be taken on retiring to bed). Patient should be warned to lie down if symptoms such as dizziness, fatigue or sweating develop, and to remain lying down until they abate completely

Xatral® (Sanofi-Synthelabo) PoM
Tablets, f/c, alfuzosin hydrochloride 2.5 mg. Net price 60-tab pack = £19.00; 90-tab pack = £25.00. Label: 3, counselling, see dose above

■ Modified release
Xatral® SR (Sanofi-Synthelabo) PoM
Tablets, m/r, yellow, f/c, alfuzosin hydrochloride 5 mg. Net price 60-tab pack = £23.80. Label: 3, 25, counselling, see dose above
Dose: 5 mg twice daily; ELDERLY initially 5 mg in the evening

DOXAZOSIN

Indications: see notes above and section 2.5.4
Cautions: see notes above and section 2.5.4
Contra-indications: see notes above and section 2.5.4
Side-effects: see notes above and section 2.5.4
Dose: initially 1 mg daily; increased if necessary at intervals of 1–2 weeks to max. 8 mg daily; usual maintenance 2–4 mg daily

Cardura® (Invicta) PoM
Tablets, doxazosin (as mesilate) 1 mg, net price 28-tab pack = £10.56; 2 mg, 28-tab pack = £14.08; 4 mg, 28-tab pack = £17.60

INDORAMIN

Indications: see notes above and section 2.5.4
Cautions: see notes above and section 2.5.4
Contra-indications: see notes above and section 2.5.4
Side-effects: see notes above and section 2.5.4
Dose: 20 mg twice daily; increased if necessary by 20 mg every 2 weeks to max. 100 mg daily in divided doses; ELDERLY, 20 mg at night may be adequate

Doralese® (Bencard) PoM
Tablets, yellow, f/c, indoramin 20 mg, net price 60-tab pack = £12.30. Label: 2

PRAZOSIN HYDROCHLORIDE

Indications: see notes above and section 2.5.4
Cautions: see notes above and section 2.5.4
Contra-indications: see notes above and section 2.5.4
Side-effects: see notes above and section 2.5.4
Dose: initially 500 micrograms twice daily for 3–7 days, subsequently adjusted according to response; usual maintenance (and max.) 2 mg twice daily; ELDERLY initiate with lowest possible dose
FIRST DOSE EFFECT. First dose may cause collapse due to hypotensive effect (therefore should be taken on retiring to bed). Patient should be warned to lie down if symptoms such as dizziness, fatigue or sweating develop, and to remain lying down until they abate completely

Hypovase® (Invicta) PoM
Tablets, prazosin hydrochloride 500 micrograms, net price 56-tab pack = £2.09; 1 mg (orange, scored), 56-tab pack = £2.69; 2 mg (scored), 56-tab pack = £3.66; starter pack of 8 × 500-microgram tabs with 32 × 1-mg tabs = £2.52. Label: 3, counselling, see dose above

TAMSULOSIN HYDROCHLORIDE

Indications: see notes above
Cautions: see notes above
Contra-indications: see notes above; severe liver impairment
Side-effects: see notes above
Dose: 400 micrograms daily after breakfast

Flomax® MR (Yamanouchi) ▼ PoM
Capsules, m/r, tamsulosin hydrochloride 400 micrograms. Net price 30-cap pack = £23.90. Label: 25

TERAZOSIN

Indications: see notes above and section 2.5.4
Cautions: see notes above and section 2.5.4
Contra-indications: see notes above and section 2.5.4
Side-effects: see notes above and section 2.5.4
Dose: initially 1 mg at bedtime; dose may be doubled at weekly intervals according to response, to max. 10 mg once daily; usual maintenance 5–10 mg daily
FIRST DOSE EFFECT. First dose may cause collapse due to hypotensive effect (therefore should be taken on retiring to bed). Patient should be warned to lie down if symptoms such as dizziness, fatigue or sweating develop, and to remain lying down until they abate completely

Hytrin BPH® (Abbott) [PoM]

Tablets, terazosin (as hydrochloride) 2 mg (yellow), net price 28-tab pack = £8.07; 5 mg (tan), 28-tab pack = £13.07; 10 mg (blue), 28-tab pack = £26.59; starter pack of 7 × 1-mg tab with 14 × 2-mg tab and 7 × 5-mg tab = £10.97. Label: 3, counselling, see dose above

Parasympathomimetics

Parasympathomimetics produce the effects of parasympathetic nerve stimulation; they possess the muscarinic rather than the nicotinic effects of acetylcholine and improve voiding efficiency by increasing detrusor muscle contraction. In the absence of obstruction to the bladder outlet they have a limited role in the relief of urinary retention. Generalised parasympathomimetic side-effects such as sweating, bradycardia, and intestinal colic may occur, particularly in the elderly.

Carbachol and **bethanechol** are choline esters that have been used in postoperative urinary retention. Bethanechol has a more selective action on the bladder than carbachol but the use of both has now been superseded by catheterisation.

Distigmine inhibits the breakdown of acetylcholine. It may help patients with an upper motor neurone neurogenic bladder.

BETHANECHOL CHLORIDE [▨]

Indications: urinary retention, but see notes above

Contra-indications: intestinal or urinary obstruction or where increased muscular activity of urinary or gastro-intestinal tract harmful; asthma, bradycardia, hyperthyroidism, recent myocardial infarction, epilepsy, hypotension, parkinsonism, vagotonia, peptic ulceration, pregnancy; **interactions**: Appendix 1 (parasympathomimetics)

Side-effects: parasympathomimetic effects such as nausea, vomiting, sweating, blurred vision, bradycardia, and intestinal colic

Dose: 10–25 mg 3–4 times daily half an hour before food

Myotonine® (Glenwood) [PoM] [▨]

Tablets, both scored, bethanechol chloride 10 mg, net price 20 = 90p; 25 mg, 20 = £1.15. Label: 22

CARBACHOL [▨]

Indications: urinary retention, but see notes above

Contra-indications: see under Bethanechol Chloride

Side-effects: see under Bethanechol Chloride but side-effects more acute

Dose: *by mouth*, 2 mg 3 times daily half an hour before food

By subcutaneous injection (acute symptoms, postoperative urinary retention) 250 micrograms, repeated twice if necessary at 30-minute intervals

Note. Inadvertent intravenous administration of carbachol is **extremely hazardous** and calls for emergency treatment with atropine

Carbachol (Non-proprietary) [PoM] [▨]

Tablets, carbachol 2 mg. Net price 20 = £5.45. Label: 22

Available from Norton

Injection, carbachol 250 micrograms/mL

DISTIGMINE BROMIDE

Indications: urinary retention (see notes above); myasthenia gravis, (section 10.2.1)

Cautions: asthma, bradycardia, hyperthyroidism, recent myocardial infarction, epilepsy, hypotension, parkinsonism, vagotonia, peptic ulceration, pregnancy; **interactions:** Appendix 1 (parasympathomimetics)

Contra-indications: intestinal or urinary obstruction or where increased muscular activity of urinary or gastro-intestinal tract harmful

Side-effects: see under Bethanechol Chloride, but action slower therefore side-effects less acute; see also Neostigmine (section 10.2.1)

Dose: 5 mg daily or on alternate days, half an hour before breakfast

Ubretid® (Rhône-Poulenc Rorer) [PoM]

Tablets, scored, distigmine bromide 5 mg. Net price 30-tab pack = £31.26. Label: 22

[▨] denotes preparations that are considered to be less suitable for prescribing (see p. vi)

7.4.2   Drugs for urinary frequency, enuresis, and incontinence

Urinary incontinence

Antimuscarinic drugs such as **oxybutynin** and **flavoxate** are used to treat *urinary frequency*; they increase bladder capacity by diminishing unstable detrusor contractions. Both drugs may cause dry mouth and blurred vision and may precipitate glaucoma. Oxybutynin has a high level of side-effects which limits its use; the dosage needs to be carefully assessed, particularly in the elderly. Flavoxate has less marked side-effects but is also less effective. **Tolterodine** and **propiverine** are also antimuscarinic drugs which have been introduced recently for urinary frequency, urgency and incontinence. **Propantheline** was formerly widely used in urinary incontinence but had a low response rate with a high incidence of side-effects; it is now used mainly for adult enuresis. The need for continuing antimuscarinic drug therapy should be reviewed after 6 months. The **tricyclic antidepressants** imipramine, amitriptyline, and nortriptyline (section 4.3.1) are sometimes effective in the management of the unstable bladder.

Conservative methods of managing stress and urge incontinence, such as pelvic floor exercises and behavourial therapy, are effective alternatives.

Purified bovine collagen implant (*Contigen®*, Bard) is indicated for *urinary incontinence* caused by intrinsic sphincter deficiency (poor or non-functioning bladder outlet mechanism). The implant should only be used by surgeons or physicians familiar with the use of a cystoscope and trained in the technique for injection of the implant.

FLAVOXATE HYDROCHLORIDE

Indications: urinary frequency and incontinence, dysuria, urgency; bladder spasms due to catheterisation

Cautions: see under Oxybutynin Hydrochloride (antimuscarinic effect considerably less marked)

Contra-indications: see under Oxybutynin Hydrochloride

Side-effects: antimuscarinic side-effects (see Atropine Sulphate, section 1.2); see also notes above

Dose: 200 mg 3 times daily; CHILD under 12 years not recommended

Urispas 200® (Shire) ▣PoM▣
Tablets, s/c, flavoxate hydrochloride 200 mg, net price 90-tab pack = £11.87

OXYBUTYNIN HYDROCHLORIDE

Indications: urinary frequency, urgency and incontinence, neurogenic bladder instability and nocturnal enuresis

Cautions: frail elderly; hepatic and renal impairment; neuropathy; hyperthyroidism; cardiac disease where increase in heart rate undesirable; prostatic hypertrophy; hiatus hernia with reflux oesophagitis; pregnancy and breast-feeding; porphyria (section 9.8.2); **interactions:** Appendix 1 (antimuscarinics)

Contra-indications: intestinal obstruction or atony, severe ulcerative colitis or toxic megacolon; significant bladder outflow obstruction; glaucoma; myasthenia gravis

Side-effects: include dry mouth, constipation, blurred vision, nausea, abdominal discomfort, facial flushing (more marked in children), difficulty in micturition (less commonly urinary retention); also headache, dizziness, drowsiness, dry skin, rash, angioedema, photosensitivity, diarrhoea, arrhythmia, restlessness, disorientation, hallucination (children at higher risk of excitatory effects); convulsions; see also notes above

Dose: 5 mg 2–3 times daily increased if necessary to max. 5 mg 4 times daily

ELDERLY 2.5–3 mg twice daily initially, increased to 5 mg twice daily according to response and tolerance

CHILD over 5 years, neurogenic bladder instability, 2.5–3 mg twice daily increased to 5 mg twice daily (max. 5 mg 3 times daily); nocturnal enuresis (preferably over 7 years, see notes below), 2.5–3 mg twice daily increased to 5 mg 2–3 times daily (last dose before bedtime)

Oxybutynin Hydrochloride (Non-proprietary) ▣PoM▣
Tablets, oxybutynin hydrochloride 2.5 mg, net price 56-tab pack = £5.72, 84-tab pack = £10.91; 3 mg, 56-tab pack = £9.15; 5 mg, 56-tab pack = £14.22, 84-tab pack = £20.77. Label: 3
Available from APS, Ashbourne (*Promictuline®*), Berk (*Contimin®*), Cox, Dominion, Generics, Genus, Lagap, Norton, Pharmacia & Upjohn, Sterwin

Cystrin® (Sanofi-Synthelabo) ▣PoM▣
Tablets, oxybutynin hydrochloride 3 mg, net price 56-tab pack = £9.15; 5 mg (scored), 84-tab pack = £22.88. Label: 3

Ditropan® (Sanofi-Synthelabo) ▣PoM▣
Tablets, both blue, scored, oxybutynin hydrochloride 2.5 mg, net price 21-tab pack = £2.93, 84-tab pack = £9.80; 5 mg, 21-tab pack = £5.72, 84-tab pack = £19.05. Label: 3
Elixir, oxybutynin hydrochloride 2.5 mg/5 mL. Net price 150-mL pack = £4.78. Label: 3.

PROPANTHELINE BROMIDE

Indications: adult enuresis, see notes above

Cautions: see under Oxybutynin Hydrochloride

Contra-indications: see under Oxybutynin Hydrochloride

Side-effects: antimuscarinic side-effects (see Atropine Sulphate, section 1.2); see also notes above

Dose: 15–30 mg 2–3 times daily one hour before meals

Preparations
Section 1.2

PROPIVERINE HYDROCHLORIDE

Indications: urinary frequency, urgency and incontinence; neurogenic bladder instability

Cautions: frail elderly; neuropathy; hyperthyroidism; cardiac disease; prostatic hypertrophy; hiatus hernia with reflux oesophagitis; **interactions:** Appendix 1 (antimuscarinics)

Contra-indications: intestinal obstruction or atony, severe ulcerative colitis or toxic megacolon; significant bladder outflow obstruction; glaucoma; myasthenia gravis; liver impairment; severe renal impairment; pregnancy (Appendix 4) and breast-feeding (Appendix 5)

Side-effects: dry mouth, blurred vision; less commonly gastro-intestinal disturbances, hypotension, drowsiness, difficulty in micturition, tiredness; rarely tachycardia, irritability, restlessness, hot flushes, rash

Dose: 15 mg 2–3 times daily increased if necessary to max. 15 mg 4 times daily

ELDERLY initially 15 mg twice daily, increased if necessary to 15 mg 3 times daily

CHILD not recommended

Detrunorm® (Schering-Plough) ▼ ▣PoM▣
Tablets, pink, s/c, propiverine hydrochloride 15 mg, net price 28-tab pack = £15.28, 56-tab pack = £30.56. Label: 3

TOLTERODINE TARTRATE

Indications: urinary frequency, urgency and incontinence

Cautions: significant bladder outflow obstruction; gastro-intestinal obstruction; hiatus hernia; neuropathy; liver impairment (Appendix 2); renal impairment; **interactions:** Appendix 1 (antimuscarinics)

Contra-indications: urinary retention; uncontrolled angle-closure glaucoma; myasthenia gravis; severe ulcerative colitis or toxic megacolon

Side-effects: dry mouth, dyspepsia, constipation, abdominal pain, flatulence, vomiting; headache; dry skin; dry eyes; drowsiness, nervousness; paraesthesia; less commonly blurred vision, chest pain; rarely urinary retention, confusion

Dose: 2 mg twice daily; reduce to 1mg twice daily if necessary to minimise side-effects; review after 6 months

CHILD not recommended

Detrusitol® (Pharmacia & Upjohn) ▼ PoM
Tablets, f/c, tolterodine tartrate 1 mg, net price 56-tab pack = £27.50; 2mg, 56-tab pack = £30.56

Nocturnal enuresis

Nocturnal enuresis is a normal occurrence in young children but persists in as many as 5% by 10 years of age. In the absence of urinary-tract infection simple measures such as *bladder training* or the use of an *alarm system* may be successful. Drug therapy is not usually appropriate for children under 7 years of age and should be reserved for when alternative measures have failed preferably on a short-term basis to cover periods away from home. The possible side-effects of the various drugs should be borne in mind when they are prescribed.

Desmopressin (section 6.5.2), an analogue of vasopressin, is used for nocturnal enuresis; particular care is needed to avoid fluid overload and treatment should not be continued for longer than 3 months without stopping for a week for full re-assessment.

Tricyclics (section 4.3.1) such as **amitriptyline**, **imipramine**, and less often **nortriptyline** are also used but behaviour disturbances may occur and relapse is common after withdrawal. Treatment should not normally exceed 3 months unless a full physical examination is given and the child is fully re-assessed; toxicity following overdosage with tricyclics is of particular concern.

7.4.3   Drugs used in urological pain

The acute pain of *ureteric colic* may be relieved with **pethidine** (section 4.7.2). **Diclofenac** by injection or as suppositories (section 10.1.1) is also effective and compares favourably with pethidine; other non-steroidal anti-inflammatory drugs are occasionally given by injection.

Lidocaine (lignocaine) gel is a useful topical application in *urethral pain* or to relieve the discomfort of catheterisation (section 15.2).

Alkalinisation of urine

Alkalinisation of urine may be undertaken with **potassium citrate**. The alkalinising action may relieve the discomfort of *cystitis* caused by lower urinary tract infections. **Sodium bicarbonate** is used as a urinary alkalinising agent in some metabolic and renal disorders (section 9.2.1.3).

POTASSIUM CITRATE
Indications: relief of discomfort in mild urinary-tract infections; alkalinisation of urine
Cautions: renal impairment, cardiac disease; elderly; **interactions:** Appendix 1 (potassium salts)
Side-effects: hyperkalaemia on prolonged high dosage, mild diuresis

Potassium Citrate Mixture BP
(Potassium Citrate Oral Solution)
Oral solution, potassium citrate 30%, citric acid monohydrate 5% in a suitable vehicle with a lemon flavour. Extemporaneous preparations should be recently prepared according to the following formula: potassium citrate 3 g, citric acid

monohydrate 500 mg, syrup 2.5 mL, quillaia tincture 0.1 mL, lemon spirit 0.05 mL, double-strength chloroform water 3 mL, water to 10 mL. Contains about 28 mmol K⁺/10 mL. Label: 27
Dose: 10 mL 3 times daily well diluted with water
Note. Concentrates for preparation of Potassium Citrate Mixture BP are available from Hillcross
Proprietary brands of potassium citrate on sale to the public for the relief of discomfort in mild urinary-tract infections include *Cystopurin®* (Roche Consumer Health) and *Effercitrate®* (Typharm)

SODIUM BICARBONATE
Indications: relief of discomfort in mild urinary-tract infections; alkalinisation of urine
Cautions: see section 1.1.2; elderly
Side-effects: see section 1.1.2
Dose: 3 g in water every 2 hours until urinary pH exceeds 7; maintenance of alkaline urine 5–10 g daily

Preparations
Section 9.2.1.3

SODIUM CITRATE
Indications: relief of discomfort in mild urinary-tract infections
Cautions: renal impairment, cardiac disease, hypertension, pregnancy, patients on a sodium-restricted diet; elderly
Side-effects: mild diuresis

Note. Proprietary brands of Sodium Citrate on sale to the public for the relief of discomfort in mild urinary-tract infections include *Boots Cystitis Relief Sachets* and *Tablets*, *Canesten® Oasis* (Bayer), *Cymalon®* (SSL), *Cystemme®* (Abbott), and *Cystoleve®* (SSL)

Acidification of urine

Acidification of urine has been undertaken with **ascorbic acid** but it is not always reliable. Large doses may cause gastro-intestinal disturbances including diarrhoea; renal stones have also been reported in patients with hyperoxaluria.

For pH-modifying solutions for the maintenance of indwelling urinary catheters, see section 7.4.4.

ASCORBIC ACID ▨
Indications: acidification of urine but see notes above; prevention and treatment of scurvy (section 9.6.3)
Dose: *by mouth*, 4 g daily in divided doses

Preparations
See section 9.6.3

Other preparations for urinary disorders

A terpene mixture (Rowatinex®) is claimed to be of benefit in *urolithiasis* for the expulsion of calculi.

Rowatinex® (Rowa) PoM ▨
Capsules, yellow, e/c, anethol 4 mg, borneol 10 mg, camphene 15 mg, cineole 3 mg, fenchone 4 mg, pinene 31 mg. Net price 50 = £7.35. Label: 25
Dose: 1–2 capsules 3–4 times daily before food; CHILD not recommended

▨ denotes preparations that are considered to be less suitable for prescribing (see p. vi)

7.4.4 Bladder instillations and urological surgery

BLADDER INFECTION. Various solutions are available as irrigations or washouts.

Aqueous **chlorhexidine** (section 13.11.2) may be used in the management of common infections of the bladder but it is ineffective against most *Pseudomonas* spp. Solutions containing chlorhexidine 1 in 5000 (0.02%) are used but they may irritate the mucosa and cause burning and haematuria (in which case they should be discontinued); sterile **sodium chloride solution 0.9%** (physiological saline) is usually adequate and is preferred as a mechanical irrigant.

Bladder irrigations of **amphotericin** 100 micrograms/mL (section 5.2) may be of value in mycotic infections.

DISSOLUTION OF BLOOD CLOTS. Clot retention is usually treated by irrigation with sterile **sodium chloride solution 0.9%** but sterile **sodium citrate solution for bladder irrigation 3%** may also be helpful. **Streptokinase-streptodornase** (*Varidase Topical®*, section 13.11.7) is an alternative.

LOCALLY ACTING CYTOTOXIC DRUGS. Bladder instillations of **doxorubicin** (section 8.1.2), **mitomycin** (section 8.1.2), and **thiotepa** (section 8.1.1) are used for recurrent superficial bladder tumours. Such instillations reduce systemic side-effects; adverse effects on the bladder (e.g. micturition disorders and reduction in bladder capacity) may occur.

Instillation of **epirubicin** (section 8.1.2) is used for treatment and prophylaxis of certain forms of superficial bladder cancer; instillation of **doxorubicin** (section 8.1.2) is also used for some papillary tumours.

INTERSTITIAL CYSTITIS. **Dimethyl sulfoxide** (dimethyl sulphoxide) may be used for symptomatic relief in patients with interstitial cystitis (Hunner's ulcer). 50 mL of a 50% solution (*Rimso-50®*—available on named-patient basis from Britannia) is instilled into the bladder, retained for 15 minutes, and voided by the patient. Treatment is repeated at intervals of 2 weeks. Bladder spasm and hypersensitivity reactions may occur and long-term use requires ophthalmic, renal, and hepatic assessment at intervals of 6 months.

SODIUM CITRATE

Indications: bladder washouts, see notes above

Sterile Sodium Citrate Solution for Bladder Irrigation, sodium citrate 3%, dilute hydrochloric acid 0.2%, in purified water, freshly boiled and cooled, and sterilised

Urological surgery

There is a high risk of fluid absorption from the irrigant used in endoscopic surgery within the urinary tract; if this occurs in excess, hypervolaemia, haemolysis, and renal failure may result. **Glycine** **irrigation solution 1.5%** is the irrigant of choice for transurethral resection of the prostate gland and bladder tumours; **sterile sodium chloride solution 0.9%** (physiological saline) is used for percutaneous renal surgery.

GLYCINE

Indications: bladder irrigation during urological surgery; see notes above
Cautions: see notes above
Side-effects: see notes above

Glycine Irrigation Solution (Non-proprietary)
Irrigation solution, glycine 1.5% in water for injections
Available from Baxter

Maintenance of indwelling urinary catheters

The deposition which occurs in catheterised patients is usually chiefly composed of phosphate and to minimise this the catheter (if latex) should be changed at least as often as every 6 weeks. If the catheter is to be left for longer periods a silicone catheter should be used together with the appropriate use of catheter maintenance solutions. Repeated blockage usually indicates that the catheter needs to be changed.

CATHETER PATENCY SOLUTIONS

Chlorhexidine 0.02%. Available from Braun (*Uro-Tainer Chlorhexidine®*, 100-mL sachet = £2.60), SSL (*Uriflex C®*, 100-mL sachet = £2.13)
Mandelic acid 1% Available from Braun (*Uro-Tainer Mandelic Acid®*, 100-mL sachet = £2.60)
Sodium chloride 0.9%. Available from Braun (*Uro-Tainer Sodium Chloride®*, 100-mL sachet = £2.45, *Uro-Tainer M®*, with integral drug additive port, 50- and 100-mL sachets = £2.90), SSL (*Uriflex S®*, 100-mL sachet = £2.00, *Uriflex SP®* with integral drug additive port, 100-mL sachet = £2.06)
Solution G, citric acid 3.23%, magnesium oxide 0.38%, sodium bicarbonate 0.7%, disodium edetate 0.01%. Available from Braun (*Uro-Tainer Suby G®*, 100-mL sachet = £2.60), SSL (*Uriflex G®*, 100-mL sachet = £2.13)
Solution R, citric acid 6%, gluconolactone 0.6%, magnesium carbonate 2.8%, disodium edetate 0.01%. Available from Braun (*Uro-Tainer Solution R®*, 100-mL sachet = £2.60), SSL (*Uriflex R®*, 100-mL sachet = £2.13)

7.4.5 Drugs for impotence

Reasons for failure to produce a satisfactory erection include *psychogenic, vascular, neurogenic,* and *endocrine abnormalities*; impotence can also be drug-induced. Intracavernosal injection or urethral application of vasoactive drugs under careful medical supervision is used for both diagnostic and therapeutic purposes.

Erectile disorders may also be treated with drugs given by mouth which increase the blood flow to the penis. Drugs should be used with caution if the penis is deformed (e.g. in angulation, cavernosal fibrosis, and Peyronie's disease).

Drug treatments for impotence may only be prescribed on the NHS under certain circumstances (see individual preparations). The Department of Health (England) has recommended that treatment should also be available from specialist services (commissioned by Health Authorities and Primary Care Groups, and operating under local agreement) when impotence is causing severe distress; specialist centres should use form FP10(HP) (or form HBP in Scotland) and endorse them 'SLS' if the treatment is to be dispensed in the community. The following criteria should be considered when assessing distress:

- significant disruption to normal social and occupational activities
- a marked effect on mood, behaviour, social and environmental awareness
- a marked effect on interpersonal relationships.

Alprostadil

Alprostadil (prostaglandin E_1) is given by intracavernosal injection or intraurethral application for the management of erectile dysfunction (after exclusion of treatable medical causes); it is also used as a diagnostic test.

ALPROSTADIL

Indications: erectile dysfunction (including aid to diagnosis); neonatal congenital heart defects (section 7.1.1.1)

Cautions: priapism—patients should be instructed to report any erection lasting 4 hours or longer—for recommendations, see below; anatomical deformations of penis (painful erection more likely)—follow up regularly to detect signs of penile fibrosis (consider discontinuation if angulation, cavernosal fibrosis or Peyronie's disease develop); **interactions:** Appendix 1 (alprostadil)

Contra-indications: predisposition to prolonged erection (as in sickle cell anaemia, multiple myeloma or leukaemia); not for use with other agents for erectile dysfunction, in patients with penile implants or when sexual activity medically inadvisable; urethral application also contra-indicated in urethral stricture, severe hypospadia, severe curvature, balanitis, urethritis

Side-effects: penile pain, priapism (see below and under Cautions); reactions at injection site include haematoma, haemosiderin deposits, ecchymosis, penile rash, penile oedema, penile fibrosis, haemorrhage, inflammation, swelling; other local reactions include balanitis, urethral burning, urethral bleeding, penile warmth, numbness, penile or urinary-tract infection, irritation, sensitivity, phimosis, pruritus, erythema, venous leak, abnormal ejaculation; systemic effects reported include testicular pain and swelling, scrotal disorders, changes in micturition (including haematuria), nausea, dry mouth, fainting, hypotension (very rarely circulatory collapse) or hypertension, rapid pulse, vasodilatation, chest pain, supraventricular extrasystole, peripheral vascular disorder, dizziness, weakness, localised pain (buttocks, legs, genital, perineal, abdominal),

headache, pelvic pain, back pain, influenza-like syndrome, swelling of the leg veins

PRIAPISM. If priapism should occur treatment should not be delayed more than 6 hours and is as follows:

Initial therapy by penile aspiration—using aseptic technique a 19–21 gauge butterfly needle inserted into the corpus cavernosum and 20–50 mL of blood aspirated; if necessary the procedure may be repeated on the opposite side.

If aspiration unsuccessful, *cautious* intracavernosal injection of a sympathomimetic with action on alpha-adrenergic receptors, continuously monitoring blood pressure and pulse (*extreme caution:* coronary heart disease, hypertension, cerebral ischaemia or if taking antidepressant) as follows:

- intracavernosal injections of phenylephrine 100–200 micrograms (0.5–1 mL of a 200 microgram/mL solution) every 5–10 minutes; max. total dose 1 mg [unlicensed indication] [*important:* if suitable strength of phenylephrine injection not available may be specially prepared by diluting 0.1 mL of the phenylephrine 1% (10 mg/mL) injection to 5 mL with sodium chloride 0.9%];
alternatively
- intracavernosal injections of adrenaline 10–20 micrograms (0.5–1mL of a 20 microgram/mL solution) every 5–10 minutes; max. total dose 100 micrograms [*important:* if suitable strength of adrenaline not available may be specially prepared by diluting 0.1 mL of the adrenaline 1 in 1000 (1mg/mL) injection to 5 mL with sodium chloride 0.9%];
alternatively
- intracavernosal injection of metaraminol (*caution: has been associated with fatal hypertensive crises*); metaraminol 1 mg (0.1 mL of 10 mg/mL metaraminol injection) is diluted to 50 mL with sodium chloride injection 0.9% and given carefully by slow injection into the corpora in 5-mL injections every 15 minutes [unlicensed indication].

If necessary the sympathomimetic injections can be followed by further aspiration of blood through the same butterfly needle.

If sympathomimetics unsuccessful, urgent surgical referral for management (possibly including shunt procedure).

Dose: see under preparations below

■ Intracavernosal injection

¹**Caverject®** (Pharmacia & Upjohn) [NHS] [PoM]

Injection, powder for reconstitution, alprostadil, net price 5-microgram vial = £6.44; 10-microgram vial = £7.35; 20-microgram vial = £9.50; 40-microgram vial = £17.98 (all with diluent-filled syringe, needles and swabs)

Dose: by direct intracavernosal injection, erectile dysfunction, first dose 2.5 micrograms, second dose 5 micrograms (if some response to first dose) *or* 7.5 micrograms (if no response to first dose), increasing in steps of 5–10 micrograms to obtain dose suitable for producing erection not lasting more than 1 hour (neurological dysfunction, first dose 1.25 micrograms, second dose 2.5 micrograms, third dose 5 micrograms, increasing in steps of 5 micrograms to obtain suitable dose); if no response to dose then next higher dose can be given within 1 hour, if there is a response the next dose should not be given for at least 24 hours; usual range 5–20 micrograms; max. 60 micrograms (max. frequency of injection not more than once daily and not more than 3 times in any 1 week)

Note. The first dose must be given by medically trained personnel; self-administration may only be undertaken after proper training

Aid to diagnosis, 20 micrograms as a single dose (where evidence of neurological dysfunction, initially 5 micrograms and max. 10 micrograms)—consult product literature for details

1. See footnote 1 on p. 383

¹**Viridal®** (Schwarz) NHS PoM

Injection, powder for reconstitution, alprostadil. Net price 5-microgram vial = £6.44; 10-microgram vial = £7.35; 20-microgram vial = £9.50 (all with diluent-filled syringe)

Viridal Duo® Starter Pack (hosp. only), contents as for *Continuation Pack* below plus *Duoject* applicator, 10-microgram starter pack = £21.65, 20-microgram starter pack = £26.39, 40-microgram starter pack = £32.08; *Viridal Duo® Continuation Pack*, 2 double-chamber cartridges (containing alprostadil and diluent), 2 needles, swabs, 10-microgram continuation pack = £16.18, 20-microgram continuation pack = £20.91, 40-microgram continuation pack = £26.61; *Duoject®* applicator available free of charge from Schwarz

Dose: by direct intracavernosal injection, erectile dysfunction, initially 5 micrograms (2.5 micrograms in primary psychogenic or neurogenic erectile dysfunction) increasing in steps of 2.5–5 micrograms to obtain dose suitable for producing erection not lasting more than 1 hour; usual range 10–20 micrograms; max. 40 micrograms (max. frequency of injection not more than once in any 1 day and not more than 2–3 times in any 1 week); erection lasting longer than 2 hours but less than 4 hours—retitrate dose

Note. The first dose must be given by medically trained personnel; self-administration may only be undertaken after proper training

■ Urethral application

COUNSELLING. If partner pregnant barrier contraception should be used

¹**MUSE®** (Astra) ▼ NHS PoM

Urethral application, alprostadil, net price 125-microgram single-use applicator = £9.14, 250-microgram single-use applicator = £9.95, 500-microgram single-use applicator = £9.95, 1-mg single-use applicator = £10.18 (all strengths also available in packs of 6 applicators)

Condoms: no evidence of harm to latex condoms and diaphragms

Dose: by direct urethral application, erectile dysfunction, initially 250 micrograms adjusted according to response (usual range 0.125–1 mg); max. 2 doses in 24 hours and 7 doses in 7 days)

Note. The first dose must be given by medically trained personnel; self-administration may only be undertaken after proper training

Aid to diagnosis, 500 micrograms as a single dose

Sildenafil

Sildenafil, has been introduced recently for the treatment of erectile dysfunction; it is given by mouth. Appropriate assessment should be carried out before prescribing sildenafil. Since sildenafil is administered systemically it has a potential for drug interactions; it should **not** be used in those receiving nitrates.

SILDENAFIL

Indications: erectile dysfunction

Cautions: cardiovascular disease; anatomical deformation of penis (e.g. angulation, cavernosal fibrosis, Peyronie's disease); predisposition to prolonged erection (as in sickle-cell anaemia, multiple myeloma, leukaemia); hepatic impairment (Appendix 2—avoid if severe); renal impairment (Appendix 3); not recommended for use in combination with other treatments for erectile dysfunction; **interactions:** Appendix 1 (sildenafil)

Contra-indications: treatment with nitrates; conditions in which sexual activity is inadvisable; manufacturer advises contra-indicated in recent stroke or myocardial infarction, blood pressure below 90/50 mmHg and hereditary degenerative retinal disorders

Side-effects: dyspepsia; headache, flushing, dizziness, visual disturbances and increased intra-ocular pressure, nasal congestion; priapism reported

Dose: initially 50 mg (ELDERLY 25 mg) approx. 1 hour before sexual activity, subsequent doses adjusted according to response to 25–100 mg as a single dose as needed; max. 1 dose in 24 hours (max. single dose 100 mg)

Note. Onset of effect may be delayed if taken with food

¹**Viagra®** (Pfizer) ▼ NHS PoM

Tablets, all blue, f/c, sildenafil (as citrate), 25 mg, net price 4-tab pack = £16.59, 8-tab pack = £33.19; 50 mg, 4-tab pack = £19.34, 8-tab pack = £38.67; 100 mg, 4-tab pack = £23.50, 8-tab pack = £46.99

Papaverine and phentolamine

Although not licensed the smooth muscle relaxant **papaverine** has also been given by intracavernosal injection for impotence. Patients with neurological or psychogenic impotence are more sensitive to the effect of papaverine than those with vascular abnormalities. **Phentolamine** is added if the response is inadequate [unlicensed indication].

Persistence of the erection for longer than 4 hours is an emergency, see advice under Alprostadil, above.

---

1. NHS except to treat erectile dysfunction in men who:
   - have diabetes, multiple sclerosis, Parkinson's disease, poliomyelitis, prostate cancer, severe pelvic injury, single gene neurological disease, spina bifida or spinal cord injury;
   - are receiving dialysis for renal failure;
   - have had radical pelvic surgery, prostatectomy, or kidney transplant;
   - were receiving *Caverject®, Erecnos®, MUSE®, Viagra®* or *Viridal®* for erectile dysfunction, at the expense of the NHS, on 14 September 1998;
   - are suffering severe distress as a result of impotence (prescribed by specialist centres only, see notes above);

   the prescription must be endorsed 'SLS'.

8: Malignant disease and immunosuppression

Malignant disease may be treated by surgery, radiotherapy, and chemotherapy. Certain tumours are highly sensitive to chemotherapy but many are not, and inappropriate drug administration in these circumstances can only increase morbidity or mortality.

8.1   Cytotoxic drugs

8.1.1   Alkylating drugs

8.1.2   Cytotoxic antibiotics

8.1.3   Antimetabolites

8.1.4   Vinca alkaloids and etoposide

8.1.5   Other antineoplastic drugs

The chemotherapy of cancer is complex and should be confined to specialists in oncology. Cytotoxic drugs have both anti-cancer activity and the potential for damage to normal tissue. Chemotherapy may be given with a curative intent or it may aim to prolong life or to palliate symptoms. In an increasing number of cases chemotherapy may be combined with radiotherapy or surgery or both as either neoadjuvant treatment (initial chemotherapy aimed at shrinking the primary tumour, thereby rendering local therapy less destructive or more effective) or as adjuvant treatment (which follows definitive treatment of the primary disease, when the risk of sub-clinical metastatic disease is known to be high). All chemotherapy drugs cause side-effects and a balance has to be struck between likely benefit and acceptable toxicity.

> **CRM guidelines on handling cytotoxic drugs :**
>
> 1. Trained personnel should reconstitute cytotoxics;
>
> 2. Reconstitution should be carried out in designated areas;
>
> 3. Protective clothing (including gloves) should be worn;
>
> 4. The eyes should be protected and means of first aid should be specified;
>
> 5. Pregnant staff should not handle cytotoxics;
>
> 6. Adequate care should be taken in the disposal of waste material, including syringes, containers, and absorbent material.

Cytotoxic drugs may be used either singly, or in combination. In the latter case, the initial letters of the approved or proprietary names of the drugs, identify the regimen used. Drug combinations are frequently more toxic than single drugs but may have the advantage in certain tumours of enhanced response, reduced development of drug resistance and increased survival. However for some tumours, single-agent chemotherapy remains the treatment of choice.

> Most cytotoxic drugs are teratogenic, and all may cause life-threatening toxicity; administration should, where possible, be confined to those experienced in their use.
>
> Because of the complexity of dosage regimens in the treatment of malignant disease, dose statements have been omitted from some of the drug entries in this chapter. *In all cases detailed specialist literature should be consulted.*
>
> Prescriptions should **not** be repeated except on the instructions of a specialist.

Cytotoxic drugs fall naturally into a number of classes, each with characteristic antitumour activity, sites of action, and toxicity. A knowledge of sites of metabolism and excretion is important because impaired drug handling as a result of disease is not uncommon and may result in enhanced toxicity.

Side-effects of cytotoxic drugs

Side-effects commonly encountered with cytotoxic drugs are discussed below whilst side-effects characteristic of a particular drug or class of drugs (e.g. neurotoxicity with vinca alkaloids) are described in the appropriate sections. Manufacturers' product literature should be consulted for full details of side-effects associated with individual drugs.

EXTRAVASATION OF INTRAVENOUS DRUGS. A number of cytotoxic drugs will cause severe local tissue necrosis if leakage into the extravascular compartment occurs. To reduce the risk of extravasation injury it is recommended that cytotoxic drugs are administered by appropriately trained staff. For information on the prevention and management of extravasation injury see section 10.3.

HYPERURICAEMIA. Hyperuricaemia, which can result in uric acid crystal formation in the urinary tract with associated renal dysfunction is a complication of the treatment of non-Hodgkin's lymphoma and leukaemia. Allopurinol (see section 10.1.4) should be started 24 hours before treating such tumours, and should be continued for 7 to 10 days (it is not required again unless further therapy is given for tumour relapse); patients should be adequately hydrated. The dose of mercaptopurine or azathioprine should be reduced if allopurinol needs to be given concomitantly (see Appendix 1).

NAUSEA AND VOMITING. Nausea and vomiting cause considerable distress to many patients who receive chemotherapy, and to a lesser extent abdominal radiotherapy, and may lead to refusal of further treatment. Symptoms may be acute (occurring within 24 hours of treatment), delayed (first occurring more than 24 hours after treatment) or anticipatory (occurring prior to subsequent doses). Delayed and anticipatory symptoms are more difficult to control than acute symptoms and require different management.

Patients vary in their susceptibility to drug-induced nausea and vomiting; those affected more often include women, patients under 50 years of age, anxious patients, and those who experience motion sickness. Susceptibility also increases with repeated exposure to the drug.

Drugs may be divided according to their emetogenic potential and some examples are given below, but the symptoms vary according to the dose, to other drugs administered and to individual susceptibility.

Mildly emetogenic treatment—fluorouracil, etoposide, methotrexate (less than $100 \, mg/m^2$), the vinca alkaloids, and abdominal radiotherapy.

Moderately emetogenic treatment—doxorubicin, intermediate and low doses of cyclophosphamide, mitoxantrone (mitozantrone), and high doses of methotrexate ($0.1–1.2 \, g/m^2$).

Highly emetogenic treatment—cisplatin, dacarbazine, and high doses of cyclophosphamide.

Prevention of acute symptoms. For patients at a low risk of emesis, pretreatment with oral phenothiazines (e.g. prochlorperazine) or with domperidone, continued for up to 24 hours after chemotherapy, is often effective (section 4.6). For patients at a higher risk dexamethasone (6–10 mg by mouth) alone or with lorazepam (1–2 mg by mouth) may be added prior to chemotherapy.

For patients at a high risk of emesis or when other therapies are ineffective, a specific ($5HT_3$) serotonin antagonist (section 4.6) is used, often with dexamethasone. The $5HT_3$ antagonists are highly effective in controlling early emesis and have largely replaced the use of high-dose intravenous metoclopramide (section 4.6).

Prevention of delayed symptoms. Dexamethasone is the drug of choice for the prevention of delayed symptoms; it is used alone or with metoclopramide or prochlorperazine. The $5HT_3$ antagonists may be less effective for delayed symptoms.

Prevention of anticipatory symptoms. Good symptom control is the best way to prevent anticipatory symptoms. The addition of lorazepam to antiemetic therapy is helpful because of its amnesic, sedative and anxiolytic effects.

BONE-MARROW SUPPRESSION. All cytotoxic drugs except vincristine and bleomycin cause bone-marrow depression. This commonly occurs 7 to 10 days after administration, but is delayed for certain drugs, such as carmustine, lomustine, and melphalan. Peripheral blood counts must be checked prior to each treatment, and doses should be reduced or therapy delayed if marrow recovery has not occurred. Fever occurring in a neutropenic patient (neutrophil count less than $0.8 \times 10^9/litre$) is an indication for immediate parenteral broad-spectrum antibiotic therapy (see section 5.1, table 1). Appropriate bacteriological investigations should be conducted as soon as possible.

It is now possible, in selected patients, to lessen both the duration and the severity of neutropenia by the use of parenterally administered bone marrow growth factors known as colony stimulating factors (section 9.1.6) or (in patients with ovarian carcinoma receiving cisplatin and cyclophosphamide) by the use of amifostine (see p. 386).

ALOPECIA. Reversible hair loss is a common complication, although it varies in degree between drugs and individual patients. No pharmacological methods of preventing this are available.

REPRODUCTIVE FUNCTION. Most cytotoxic drugs are teratogenic and should not be administered during pregnancy, especially during the first trimester.

Contraceptive advice should be offered where appropriate before cytotoxic therapy begins (and should cover the duration of contraception required after therapy has ended). Regimens that do not contain an alkylating drug may have less effect on fertility, but those with an alkylating drug carry the risk of causing permanent male sterility (there is no effect on potency). Pre-treatment counselling and consideration of sperm storage may be appropriate. Females are less severely affected, though the span of reproductive life may be shortened by the onset of a premature menopause. No increase in fetal abnormalities or abortion-rate has been recorded in patients who remain fertile after cytotoxic chemotherapy.

Drugs for cytotoxic-induced side-effects

Methotrexate-induced mucositis and myelosuppression

Folinic acid (given as calcium folinate) is used to counteract the folate-antagonist action of methotrexate and thus speed recovery from methotrexate-induced mucositis or myelosuppression. It is generally given 24 hours after the methotrexate, in a dose of 15 mg by mouth every 6 hours, for 2–8 doses (depending on the dose of methotrexate). It does not counteract the antibacterial activity of folate antagonists such as trimethoprim.

Folinic acid also interacts with fluorouracil; when the two are used together in metastatic colonic cancer a favourable effect has been demonstrated on response-rate.

The calcium salt of **levofolinic acid**, a single isomer of folinic acid, has been introduced recently for rescue therapy following methotrexate administration and for use with fluorouracil for colorectal cancer. The dose of calcium levofolinate is generally half that of calcium folinate.

CALCIUM FOLINATE

(Calcium leucovorin)
Indications: see notes above
Cautions: avoid simultaneous administration of methotrexate; as for Folic Acid (section 9.1.2) **not** indicated for pernicious anaemia or other megaloblastic anaemias where vitamin B_{12} deficient; pregnancy and breast-feeding; **interactions:** Appendix 1 (folic acid and folinic acid) IMPORTANT. Intrathecal injection **contra-indicated**
Side-effects: rarely, pyrexia after parenteral administration
Dose: expressed in terms of folinic acid
As an antidote to methotrexate (usually started 24 hours after the beginning of methotrexate infusion), in general up to 120 mg in divided doses over 12–24 hours *by intramuscular or intravenous injection or by intravenous infusion*, followed by 12–15 mg *intramuscularly or* 15 mg *by mouth* every 6 hours for the next 48–72 hours
Suspected methotrexate overdosage, immediate administration of folinic acid at a rate not exceeding 160 mg/minute in a dose equal to (or higher than) the dose of methotrexate
Adjunct to fluorouracil in colorectal cancer, consult product literature

Calcium Folinate (Non-proprietary) PoM
Tablets, scored, folinic acid (as calcium salt) 15 mg, net price 10-tab pack (Faulding DBL) = £37.85, (Hillcross) = £37.10, (Lederle) = £41.22; 30-tab pack (Pharmacia & Upjohn, *Refolinon*®) = £94.50
Injection, folinic acid (as calcium salt) 3 mg/mL, net price 1-mL amp (Faulding DBL) = £2.28, 10-mL amp (Pharmacia & Upjohn, *Refolinon*®) = £5.70
Injection, folinic acid (as calcium salt) 7.5 mg/mL, net price 2-mL amp (Faulding DBL) = £7.80
Injection, folinic acid (as calcium salt) 10 mg/mL, net price 5-mL vial (Faulding DBL) = £19.41, 10-mL vial (Faulding DBL) = £35.09, 30-mL vial (Faulding DBL) = £94.69, 35-mL vial (Lederle, *Lederfolin*®) = £90.98
Injection, powder for reconstitution, folinic acid (as calcium salt), net price 15-mg vial (Lederle) = £4.46; 30-mg vial (Lederle) = £8.36

CALCIUM LEVOFOLINATE

(Calcium levoleucovorin)
Indications: see notes above
Cautions: see Calcium Folinate
Side-effects: see Calcium Folinate
Dose: expressed in terms of levofolinic acid
As an antidote to methotrexate (usually started 24 hours after the beginning of methotrexate infusion), in general 7.5 mg, *by intramuscular injection, or by intravenous injection or by intravenous infusion* every 6 hours for 10 doses
Suspected methotrexate overdosage, immediate administration of levofolinic acid at a rate not exceeding 160 mg/minute in a dose which is at least 50% of the dose of methotrexate
Adjunct to fluorouracil in colorectal cancer, consult product literature

Isovorin® (Wyeth) ▼ PoM
Injection, levofolinic acid (as calcium salt) 10 mg/mL, net price 2.5-mL vial = £13.00, 5-mL vial = £26.00, 17.5-mL vial = £91.00

Platinum-induced neutropenic infection and nephrotoxicity

Amifostine is licensed for the reduction of risk of infection related to neutropenia in patients undergoing treatment with cisplatin and cyclophosphamide for advanced ovarian carcinoma and for the reduction of nephrotoxicity due to cisplatin. Amifostine has recently been licensed to protect against xerostomia during radiotherapy for head and neck cancer.

Other drugs for the reduction of risk of infection associated with neutropenia include granulocyte-colony stimulating factor and granulocyte macrophage-colony stimulating factor.

AMIFOSTINE

Indications: (specialist use only) see under dose
Cautions: ensure adequate hydration before treatment; infuse with patient supine and monitor arterial blood pressure (interrupt infusion if blood pressure decreases significantly, consult product literature); during chemotherapy interrupt antihypertensive therapy 24 hours before treatment

with amifostine and monitor closely, during radiotherapy monitor closely if concomitant antihypertensive therapy; monitor serum calcium in patients at risk of hypocalcaemia; not recommended in renal and hepatic impairment; pregnancy and breast-feeding; **interactions:** Appendix 1 (amifostine)

Side-effects: hypotension (reversed by infusion of physiological saline and postural management), nausea, vomiting, flushing, chills, dizziness, somnolence, hiccups, sneezing; rarely convulsions, clinical hypocalcaemia; allergic reactions

Dose: reduction of neutropenia-related risk of infection due to cyclophosphamide and cisplatin treatment in patients with advanced ovarian carcinoma, *by intravenous infusion* over 15 minutes, 910 mg/m^2 once daily started within 30 minutes before chemotherapy (reduced to 740 mg/m^2 for subsequent cycles if full dose could not be given first time due to hypotension lasting more than 5 minutes after interruption, see product literature)

Reduction of cumulative nephrotoxicity due to cisplatin in patients with advanced solid tumours of non-germ cell origin, consult product literature

Prevention of xerostomia during radiotherapy for head and neck cancer, *by intravenous infusion* over 3 minutes, 200 mg/m^2 once daily starting within 15–30 minutes before radiotherapy

CHILD and ELDERLY (over 70 years) not recommended

Ethyol® (Schering-Plough) [PoM]
Intravenous infusion, powder for reconstitution, amifostine, net price 375-mg vial = £108.00; 500-mg vial = £144.00

Urothelial toxicity

Haemorrhagic cystitis is a common manifestation of urothelial toxicity which occurs with cyclophosphamide and ifosfamide; it is caused by the metabolite acrolein. **Mesna** reacts specifically with this metabolite in the urinary tract, preventing toxicity. Mesna is used routinely (preferably by mouth) in patients receiving ifosfamide, and in patients receiving cyclophosphamide by the intravenous route at a high dose (e.g. more than 2 g) or in those who experienced urothelial toxicity when given cyclophosphamide previously.

MESNA

Indications: see notes above

Contra-indications: hypersensitivity to thiol-containing compounds

Side-effects: above max. therapeutic doses, nausea, vomiting (use intravenous route), colic, diarrhoea, fatigue, headache, limb and joint pains, depression, irritability, lack of energy, rash, hypotension and tachycardia; rarely hypersensitivity reactions (more common in patients with auto-immune disorders)

Dose: calculated according to oxazaphosphorine (cyclophosphamide or ifosfamide) treatment—for details consult product literature; when given *by mouth*, dose is given 2 hours *before* oxazaphosphorine treatment and repeated 2 and 6 hours *after* treatment; when given *by intravenous injection*, dose is given *with* oxazaphosphorine treatment and repeated 4 and 8 hours *after* treatment

Uromitexan® (ASTA Medica) [PoM]
Tablets, f/c, mesna 400 mg, net price 10-tab pack = £17.43; 600 mg, 10-tab pack = £22.63
Injection, mesna 100 mg/mL. Net price 4-mL amp = £1.61; 10-mL amp = £3.62
Note. For oral administration contents of ampoule are taken in a flavoured drink such as orange juice or cola which may be stored in a refrigerator for up to 24 hours in a sealed container

8.1.1 Alkylating drugs

Extensive experience is available with these drugs, which are among the most widely used in cancer chemotherapy. They act by damaging DNA, thus interfering with cell replication. In addition to the side-effects common to many cytotoxic drugs (section 8.1), there are two problems associated with prolonged usage. Firstly, gametogenesis is often severely affected (see above). Secondly, prolonged use of these drugs, particularly when combined with extensive irradiation, is associated with a marked increase in the incidence of acute non-lymphocytic leukaemia.

Cyclophosphamide is widely used in the treatment of chronic lymphocytic leukaemia, the lymphomas, and solid tumours. It is given by mouth or intravenously and is inactive until metabolised by the liver. A urinary metabolite of cyclophosphamide, acrolein, may cause haemorrhagic cystitis; this is a rare but very serious complication. An increased fluid intake, for 24–48 hours after intravenous injection, will help avoid this complication. When high-dose therapy (e.g. more than 2 g intravenously) is used or when the patient is considered to be at high risk of cystitis (e.g. previous pelvic irradiation) mesna (given initially intravenously then by mouth) will also help prevent this—see under Urothelial toxicity (section 8.1).

Ifosfamide is related to cyclophosphamide and is given intravenously; mesna (section 8.1) is routinely given with it to reduce urothelial toxicity.

Chlorambucil is commonly used to treat chronic lymphocytic leukaemia, the indolent non-Hodgkin's lymphomas, Hodgkin's disease, and ovarian cancer. It is given by mouth. Side-effects, apart from marrow suppression, are uncommon. However occasional patients develop severe widespread rashes which can progress to Stevens-Johnson syndrome or to toxic epidermal necrolysis. If a rash occurs further chlorambucil is contra-indicated and cyclophosphamide is substituted.

Melphalan is used to treat myeloma and occasionally solid tumours and lymphomas. It is usually given by mouth, but may also be given intravenously. Because bone marrow toxicity is delayed the drug is usually given at intervals of 4–6 weeks.

Busulfan (busulphan) is used almost exclusively to treat chronic myeloid leukaemia and is given by mouth. Frequent blood counts are necessary because excessive myelosuppression may result in irreversible bone-marrow aplasia. Hyperpigmentation of the skin is a common side-effect and, rarely, progressive pulmonary fibrosis may occur.

Lomustine is a lipid-soluble nitrosourea and is given by mouth. It is mainly used to treat Hodgkin's disease and certain solid tumours. Bone marrow toxicity is delayed, and the drug is therefore given at intervals of 4 to 6 weeks. Permanent bone marrow damage may occur with prolonged use. Nausea and vomiting are common and moderately severe.

Carmustine is given intravenously. It has similar activity and toxicity to lomustine and is most commonly given to patients with myeloma, lymphoma, and brain tumours. Cumulative renal damage and delayed pulmonary fibrosis may occur.

Chlormethine (mustine) is now much less commonly used. It is a very toxic drug which causes severe vomiting. The freshly prepared injection must be given into a fast-running intravenous infusion. Local extravasation causes severe tissue necrosis.

Estramustine is a combination of an oestrogen and chlormethine (mustine) used predominantly in prostate cancer. It is given by mouth and has both an antimitotic effect and (by reducing testosterone concentration) a hormonal effect.

Treosulfan is given by mouth or intravenously and is used to treat ovarian cancer. Skin pigmentation is a common side-effect and allergic alveolitis, pulmonary fibrosis and haemorrhagic cystitis occur rarely.

Thiotepa is usually used as an intracavitary drug for the treatment of malignant effusions or bladder cancer (section 7.4.4). It is also occasionally used to treat breast cancer, but requires parenteral administration.

Mitobronitol is occasionally used to treat chronic myeloid leukaemia; it is available on a named-patient basis only (as *Myelobromol*®, Sinclair).

BUSULFAN
(Busulphan)

Indications: chronic myeloid leukaemia
Cautions: see section 8.1 and notes above; avoid in porphyria (section 9.8.2)
Side-effects: see section 8.1 and notes above
Dose: induction of remission, 60 micrograms/kg to max. 4 mg daily; maintenance, 0.5–2 mg daily

Myleran® (GlaxoWellcome) PoM
Tablets, f/c, busulfan 2 mg, net price 25-tab pack = £5.08

CARMUSTINE

Indications: see notes above
Cautions: see section 8.1 and notes above
Side-effects: see section 8.1 and notes above; irritant to tissues

BiCNU® (Bristol-Myers) PoM
Injection, powder for reconstitution, carmustine. Net price 100-mg vial (with diluent) = £12.50

CHLORAMBUCIL

Indications: see notes above; immunosuppression (section 8.2.1)
Cautions: see section 8.1 and notes above; avoid in porphyria (section 9.8.2)
Side-effects: see section 8.1 and notes above
Dose: used alone, usually 100–200 micrograms/kg daily for 4–8 weeks

Leukeran® (GlaxoWellcome) PoM
Tablets, both yellow, chlorambucil 2 mg, net price 25-tab pack = £8.17; 5 mg, 25-tab pack = £12.45

CHLORMETHINE HYDROCHLORIDE/ MUSTINE HYDROCHLORIDE

Indications: Hodgkin's disease—see notes above
Cautions: see section 8.1 and notes above; caution in handling
Side-effects: see section 8.1 and notes above; irritant to tissues

Chlormethine Hydrochloride/Mustine Hydrochloride (Sovereign) PoM
Injection, powder for reconstitution, chlormethine hydrochloride, net price 10-mg vial = £39.98

CYCLOPHOSPHAMIDE

Indications: see notes above
Cautions: see section 8.1 and notes above; hepatic and renal impairment (Appendixes 2 and 3); avoid in porphyria (section 9.8.2); **interactions:** Appendix 1 (cyclophosphamide)
Side-effects: see section 8.1 and notes above

Cyclophosphamide (Pharmacia & Upjohn) PoM
Tablets, pink, s/c, cyclophosphamide (anhydrous) 50 mg. Net price 20 = £2.12. Label: 27
Injection, powder for reconstitution, cyclophosphamide. Net price 200-mg vial = £1.65; 500-mg vial = £2.88; 1-g vial = £5.04

Endoxana® (ASTA Medica) PoM
Tablets, s/c, cyclophosphamide 50 mg, net price 100-tab pack = £10.03. Label: 27
Injection, powder for reconstitution, cyclophosphamide. Net price 200-mg vial = £1.54; 500-mg vial = £2.68; 1-g vial = £4.68

ESTRAMUSTINE PHOSPHATE

Indications: prostate cancer
Cautions: see section 8.1; renal impairment
Contra-indications: peptic ulceration, severe liver disease (Appendix 2), cardiac disease
Side-effects: see section 8.1; also gynaecomastia, altered liver function, cardiovascular disorders (angina and rare reports of myocardial infarction)
Dose: 0.14–1.4 g daily in divided doses (usual initial dose 560 mg daily)
COUNSELLING. Each dose should be taken not less than 1 hour before or 2 hours after meals and should not be taken with dairy products

Estracyt® (Pharmacia & Upjohn) PoM
Capsules, estramustine phosphate 140 mg (as disodium salt). Net price 100-cap pack = £142.73. Label: 23, counselling, see above

IFOSFAMIDE

Indications: see notes above
Cautions: see section 8.1 and notes above; renal impairment (Appendix 3); **interactions:** Appendix 1 (cyclophosphamide and ifosfamide)
Contra-indications: hepatic impairment
Side-effects: see section 8.1 and notes above

Mitoxana® (ASTA Medica) PoM
Injection, powder for reconstitution, ifosfamide. Net price 1-g vial = £20.31; 2-g vial = £37.59 (hosp. only)

LOMUSTINE

Indications: see notes above
Cautions: see section 8.1 and notes above
Side-effects: see section 8.1 and notes above
Dose: used alone, 120–130 mg/m² body-surface every 6–8 weeks

Lomustine (Medac) [PoM]
Capsules, blue/clear, lomustine 40 mg. Net price 20-cap pack = £171.35
Note. The brand name *CCNU®* has been used for lomustine capsules

MELPHALAN

Indications: myelomatosis; see also notes above
Cautions: see section 8.1 and notes above; renal impairment (Appendix 3); **interactions:** Appendix 1 (melphalan)
Side-effects: see section 8.1 and notes above
Dose: *by mouth*,150–300 micrograms/kg daily for 4–6 days, repeated after 4–8 weeks

Alkeran® (GlaxoWellcome) [PoM]
Tablets, melphalan 2 mg, net price 25 = £11.20; 5 mg, 25 = £19.82
Injection, powder for reconstitution, melphalan 50 mg (as hydrochloride). Net price 50-mg vial (with solvent-diluent) = £26.99

THIOTEPA

Indications: see notes above and section 7.4.4
Cautions: see section 8.1; **interactions:** Appendix 1 (thiotepa)
Side-effects: see section 8.1

Thiotepa (Lederle) [PoM]
Injection, powder for reconstitution, thiotepa, net price 15-mg vial = £4.73

TREOSULFAN

Indications: see notes above
Cautions: see section 8.1
Side-effects: see section 8.1 and notes above
Dose: *by mouth*, courses of 1–2 g daily in 3–4 divided doses to provide total dose of 21–28 g over initial 8 weeks (with treatment-free intervals during this period—consult product literature)

Treosulfan (Medac) [PoM]
Capsules, treosulfan 250 mg. Net price 20 = £34.18. Label: 25
Injection, powder for reconstitution, treosulfan. Net price 1 g = £20.95; 5 g = £80.98 (both in infusion bottle with transfer needle)

8.1.2　Cytotoxic antibiotics

Drugs in this group are widely used. Many cytotoxic antibiotics act as radiomimetics and simultaneous use of radiotherapy should be **avoided** as it may result in markedly enhanced toxicity.

Aclarubicin, daunorubicin, doxorubicin, epirubicin and idarubicin are anthracycline antibiotics. Mitoxantrone (mitozantrone) is an anthracycline derivative.

Doxorubicin is one of the most successful and widely used antitumour drugs, and is used to treat the acute leukaemias, lymphomas, and a variety of solid tumours. It is given by fast running infusion, commonly at 21-day intervals. Local extravasation will cause severe tissue necrosis. Common toxic effects include nausea and vomiting, myelosuppression, alopecia, and mucositis. This drug is largely excreted by the biliary tract, and an elevated bilirubin concentration is an indication for reducing the dose. Supraventricular tachycardia related to drug administration is an uncommon complication. Higher cumulative doses are associated with development of a cardiomyopathy. It is customary to limit total cumulative doses to 450 mg/m² body-surface area as symptomatic and potentially fatal heart failure is increasingly common above this level. Patients with pre-existing cardiac disease, the elderly, and those who have received myocardial irradiation should be treated cautiously. Cardiac monitoring, for example by sequential radionuclide ejection fraction measurement, may assist in safely limiting total dosage. Evidence is available to suggest that weekly low-dose administration may be associated with less cardiac damage. Doxorubicin is also given by bladder instillation. A liposomal formulation for intravenous use has recently been licensed for Kaposi's sarcoma in AIDS patients.

Epirubicin is structurally related to doxorubicin and clinical trials suggest that it is as effective in the treatment of breast cancer. A maximum cumulative dose of 0.9–1 g/m² is recommended to help avoid cardiotoxicity. Like doxorubicin it is given intravenously and by bladder instillation.

Aclarubicin and **idarubicin** are anthracyclines with general properties similar to those of doxorubicin. They are both given intravenously. Idarubicin may also be given by mouth.

Daunorubicin also has general properties similar to those of doxorubicin. It should be given by intravenous infusion and is indicated for acute leukaemias. A liposomal formulation for intravenous use has recently been licensed for AIDS-related Kaposi's sarcoma.

Mitoxantrone (**mitozantrone**) is structurally related to doxorubicin; it is used in breast cancer. It is given intravenously and is well tolerated apart from myelosuppression and dose-related cardiotoxicity; cardiac examinations are recommended after a cumulative dose of 160 mg/m².

Bleomycin is given intravenously or intramuscularly to treat the lymphomas and certain solid tumours; it is given by the intracavitary route for malignant effusions. It causes little bone-marrow suppression but dermatological toxicity is common and increased pigmentation particularly affecting the flexures and subcutaneous sclerotic plaques may occur. Mucositis is also relatively common and an association with Raynaud's phenomenon is reported. Hypersensitivity reactions manifest by chills and fevers commonly occur a few hours after drug administration and may be prevented by simultaneous administration of a corticosteroid, for example hydrocortisone intravenously. The principal problem associated with the use of bleomycin is progressive pulmonary fibrosis. This is dose-related, occurring more commonly at cumulative doses greater than 300 000 units (see Bleomycin, below) and in the elderly. Basal lung crepitations or suspicious chest X-ray changes are an indication to stop therapy with this drug. Patients who have received extensive treatment with bleomycin (e.g. cumulative dose more than 100 000 units—see Bleomycin below) may be at risk of developing respiratory failure if a general anaesthetic is given with high inspired oxygen concentrations. Anaesthetists should be warned of this.

Dactinomycin is principally used to treat paediatric cancers; it is given intravenously. Its side-effects are similar to those of doxorubicin, except that cardiac toxicity is not a problem.

Mitomycin is given intravenously to treat upper gastro-intestinal and breast cancers and by bladder instillation for superficial bladder tumours. It causes delayed bone-marrow toxicity and therefore it is usually administered at 6-weekly intervals. Prolonged use may result in permanent bone-marrow damage. It may also cause lung fibrosis and renal damage.

ACLARUBICIN

Indications: acute non-lymphocytic leukaemia in patients who have relapsed or are resistant or refractory to first-line chemotherapy

Cautions: see section 8.1 and notes above; hepatic and renal impairment; irritant to tissues

Side-effects: see section 8.1 and notes above

Aclarubicin (Medac) [PoM]
Injection, powder for reconstitution, aclarubicin 20 mg (as hydrochloride). Net price 20-mg vial = £98.55
Note. The brand names *Aclacin®* and *Aclaplastin®* have been used for aclarubicin preparations

BLEOMYCIN

Indications: squamous cell carcinoma; see also notes above

Cautions: see section 8.1 and notes above; renal impairment (Appendix 3); caution in handling—irritant to tissues

Side-effects: see section 8.1 and notes above

Bleomycin (Non-proprietary) [PoM]
Injection, powder for reconstitution, bleomycin (as sulphate). Net price 15 000-unit amp = £16.29
Note. To conform to the European Pharmacopoeia ampoules previously labelled as containing '15 units' of bleomycin are now labelled as containing 15 000 units. The amount of bleomycin in the ampoule has not changed.
Available from Faulding DBL, Kyowa Hakko (*Bleo-Kyowa®*)

DACTINOMYCIN

(Actinomycin D)
Indications: see notes above
Cautions: see section 8.1 and notes above; caution in handling—irritant to tissues
Side-effects: see section 8.1 and notes above

Cosmegen Lyovac® (MSD) [PoM]
Injection, powder for reconstitution, dactinomycin, net price 500-microgram vial = £1.50

DAUNORUBICIN

Indications: see notes above
Cautions: see section 8.1 and notes above; caution in handling—irritant to tissues
Side-effects: see section 8.1 and notes above

Cerubidin® (Rhône-Poulenc Rorer) [PoM]
Injection, powder for reconstitution, daunorubicin (as hydrochloride). Net price 20-mg vial = £28.08

■ Lipid formulation
DaunoXome® (NeXstar) [PoM]
Concentrate for intravenous infusion, daunorubicin encapsulated in liposomes. For dilution before use. Net price 50-mg vial = £155.00
For advanced AIDS-related Kaposi's sarcoma

DOXORUBICIN HYDROCHLORIDE

Indications: see notes above and section 7.4.4
Cautions: see section 8.1 and notes above; hepatic impairment (Appendix 2); caution in handling—irritant to tissues; **interactions:** Appendix 1 (doxorubicin)
Side-effects: see section 8.1 and notes above

Doxorubicin Rapid Dissolution (Pharmacia & Upjohn) [PoM]
Injection, powder for reconstitution, doxorubicin hydrochloride, net price 10-mg vial = £18.72; 50-mg vial = £93.60
Note.This preparation has replaced *Adriamycin®*
Various strengths also available from Medac
Doxorubicin Solution for Injection (Pharmacia & Upjohn) [PoM]
Injection, doxorubicin hydrochloride 2 mg/mL, net price 5-ml vial = £20.60, 25-mL vial = £103.00
Various strengths and sizes also available from Faulding DBL

■ Lipid formulation
Caelyx® (Schering-Plough) ▼ [PoM]
Concentrate for intravenous infusion, doxorubicin hydrochloride 2 mg/mL encapsulated in liposomes. For dilution before use. Net price 10-mL vial = £457.00
For AIDS-related Kaposi's sarcoma in patients with low CD4 counts and extensive mucocutaneous or visceral disease

EPIRUBICIN HYDROCHLORIDE

Indications: see notes above and section 7.4.4
Cautions: see section 8.1 and notes above; hepatic impairment (Appendix 2); caution in handling—irritant to tissues
Side-effects: see section 8.1 and notes above

Pharmorubicin® Rapid Dissolution (Pharmacia & Upjohn) [PoM]
Injection, powder for reconstitution, epirubicin hydrochloride. Net price 10-mg vial = £16.09; 20-mg vial = £32.18; 50-mg vial = £80.45
Pharmorubicin® Solution for Injection (Pharmacia & Upjohn) [PoM]
Injection, epirubicin hydrochloride 2 mg/mL, net price 5-mL vial = £18.54, 25-mL vial = £92.70

IDARUBICIN HYDROCHLORIDE

Indications: advanced breast cancer after failure of first-line chemotherapy (not including anthracyclines); acute leukaemias—see notes above

Cautions: see section 8.1 and notes above; hepatic and renal impairment (Appendixes 2 and 3); caution in handling—irritant to tissues

Side-effects: see section 8.1 and notes above

Zavedos® (Pharmacia & Upjohn) PoM
Capsules, idarubicin hydrochloride, 5 mg (red), net price 1-cap pack = £27.50; 10 mg (red/white), 1-cap pack = £55.01; 25 mg (white), 1-cap pack = £137.52. Label: 25
Injection, powder for reconstitution, idarubicin hydrochloride, net price 5-mg vial = £69.52; 10-mg vial = £139.05

MITOMYCIN

Indications: see notes above and section 7.4.4
Cautions: see section 8.1 and notes above; caution in handling—irritant to tissues
Side-effects: see section 8.1 and notes above

Mitomycin (Non-proprietary) PoM
Injection, powder for reconstitution, mitomycin. Net price 10-mg vial = £22.67; 20-mg vial = £41.70
Available from Faulding DBL
Mitomycin C Kyowa® (Kyowa Hakko) PoM
Injection, powder for reconstitution, mitomycin. Net price 2-mg vial = £6.16; 10-mg vial = £20.28; 20-mg vial = £38.68 (hosp. only)

MITOXANTRONE/MITOZANTRONE

Indications: see notes above
Cautions: see section 8.1 and notes above; intrathecal administration not recommended
Side-effects: see section 8.1 and notes above

Novantrone® (Lederle) PoM
Intravenous infusion, mitoxantrone (as hydrochloride) 2 mg/mL, net price 10-mL vial = £150.43, 12.5-mL vial = £188.05, 15-mL vial = £225.60

8.1.3   Antimetabolites

Antimetabolites are incorporated into new nuclear material or combine irreversibly with vital cellular enzymes, preventing normal cellular division.

Methotrexate inhibits the enzyme dihydrofolate reductase, essential for the synthesis of purines and pyrimidines. It is given by mouth, intravenously, intramuscularly, or intrathecally.

Methotrexate is used as maintenance therapy for childhood acute lymphoblastic leukaemia. Other uses include choriocarcinoma, non-Hodgkin's lymphoma, and a number of solid tumours. Intrathecal methotrexate is used in the CNS prophylaxis of childhood acute lymphoblastic leukaemia, and as a therapy for established meningeal cancer or lymphoma.

Methotrexate causes myelosuppression, mucositis, and rarely pneumonitis. It is **contra-indicated** in significant renal impairment because it is excreted primarily by the kidney. It is also contra-indicated in patients with severe hepatic impairment. It should also be **avoided** if a significant

pleural effusion or ascites is present because it tends to accumulate at these sites, and its subsequent return to the circulation will be associated with myelosuppression. Systemic toxicity may occur following intrathecal administration and blood counts should be carefully monitored.

Folinic acid (section 8.1) following methotrexate administration helps to prevent methotrexate-induced mucositis or myelosuppression.

Cytarabine acts by interfering with pyrimidine synthesis. It is given subcutaneously, intravenously, or intrathecally. Its predominant use is in the induction of remission of acute myeloblastic leukaemia. It is a potent myelosuppressant and requires careful haematological monitoring.

Fludarabine is recommended for patients with B-cell chronic lymphocytic leukaemia (CLL) after initial treatment with an alkylating agent has failed; it is given intravenously daily for 5 days every 28 days. Fludarabine is generally well tolerated but does, however, cause myelosuppression which may be cumulative. CNS and pulmonary toxicity, visual disturbances, heart failure, and autoimmune haemolytic anaemia have been reported rarely.

Cladribine is an effective but potentially toxic drug given by intravenous infusion for the treatment of hairy cell leukaemia. It is also licensed for chronic lymphocytic leukaemia in patients who have failed to respond to standard regimens containing an alkylating agent; it is given by intravenous infusion. Myelosuppression may be severe and serious neurotoxicity has been reported rarely.

Gemcitabine is given intravenously for palliative treatment in patients with locally advanced or metastatic non-small cell lung and pancreatic cancer. It is generally well tolerated but may cause mild gastro-intestinal side-effects and rashes; renal impairment, pulmonary oedema and influenza-like symptoms have also been reported. Haemolytic uraemic syndrome has been reported rarely and gemcitabine should be discontinued if signs of microangiopathic haemolytic anaemia occur. Gemcitabine should not be used concurrently with radical radiotherapy.

Fluorouracil is usually given intravenously because absorption following oral administration is unpredictable. It is used to treat a number of solid tumours, including gastro-intestinal tract cancers and breast cancer. It is commonly used with folinic acid in advanced colorectal cancer. It may also be used topically for certain malignant and pre-malignant skin lesions. Toxicity is unusual, but may include myelosuppression, mucositis, and rarely a cerebellar syndrome.

Raltitrexed, a thymidylate synthase inhibitor, is given intravenously for palliation of metastatic colon cancer. It is probably of similar efficacy to fluorouracil. Raltitrexed is generally well tolerated, but can cause marked myelosuppression and gastro-intestinal side-effects.

Mercaptopurine is used almost exclusively as maintenance therapy for the acute leukaemias. Azathioprine, a derivative of mercaptopurine, is generally used as an immunosuppressant (section 8.2.1). The dose of both drugs should be reduced if the patient is receiving allopurinol since it interferes with their metabolism.

Tioguanine (thioguanine) is given by mouth to induce remission in acute myeloid leukaemia.

CLADRIBINE

Indications: see notes above
Cautions: see section 8.1 and notes above
Side-effects: see section 8.1 and notes above

Leustat® (Janssen-Cilag) PoM
Injection, cladribine 1 mg/mL. For dilution and use as an infusion, net price 10-mL vial = £182.29

CYTARABINE

Indications: acute leukaemias
Cautions: see section 8.1 and notes above
Side-effects: see section 8.1 and notes above

Cytarabine (Non-proprietary) PoM
Injection, cytarabine 20 mg/mL. Net price 5-mL vial = £3.84. For subcutaneous, intravenous, or intrathecal use
Injection, cytarabine 100 mg/mL. Net price 1-mL vial = £3.84; 5-mL vial = £19.00; 10-mL vial = £37.83; 20-mL vial = £71.88; 20-mL *Onco-vial®* = £79.10. **Not** for intrathecal use
All available from Faulding DBL
Cytosar® (Pharmacia & Upjohn) PoM
Injection, powder for reconstitution, cytarabine. Net price 100-mg vial = £2.87, 100-mg vial (with diluent) = £3.03; 500-mg vial = £14.28, 500-mg vial (with diluent) = £14.75. For intravenous injection or infusion and subcutaneous injection only; not recommended for intrathecal use

FLUDARABINE PHOSPHATE

Indications: see notes above
Cautions: see section 8.1 and notes above; renal impairment (Appendix 3) **interactions:** Appendix 1 (fludarabine)
Side-effects: see section 8.1 and notes above

Fludara® (Schering Health) PoM
Injection, powder for reconstitution, fludarabine phosphate. Net price 50-mg vial = £130.00

FLUOROURACIL

Indications: see notes above
Cautions: see section 8.1 and notes above; caution in handling—irritant to tissues; **interactions:** Appendix 1 (fluorouracil)
Side-effects: see section 8.1 and notes above
Dose: *by mouth*, maintenance 15 mg/kg weekly; max. in one day 1 g

Fluorouracil (Non-proprietary) PoM
Capsules, fluorouracil 250 mg.
Available from Cambridge on a named patient basis
Injection, fluorouracil (as sodium salt) 25 mg/mL, net price 10-mL vial = £3.20, 20-mL vial = £6.40, 100-mL vial = £32.00; 50 mg/mL, 10-mL vial = £6.40, 50-mL vial = £32.00, 100-mL vial = £64.00
Available from Faulding DBL
Efudix® (ICN) PoM
Cream, fluorouracil 5%. Net price 20 g = £18.27

GEMCITABINE

Indications: see notes above
Cautions: see section 8.1 and notes above
Side-effects: see section 8.1 and notes above

Gemzar® (Lilly) PoM
Injection, powder for reconstitution, gemcitabine (as hydrochloride), net price 200-mg vial = £32.55; 1-g vial = £162.76 (both hosp. only)

MERCAPTOPURINE

Indications: acute leukaemias
Cautions: see section 8.1 and notes above; renal impairment (Appendix 3); avoid in porphyria (section 9.8.2); **interactions:** Appendix 1 (mercaptopurine)
Side-effects: see section 8.1 and notes above
Dose: initially 2.5 mg/kg daily

Puri-Nethol® (GlaxoWellcome) PoM
Tablets, fawn, scored, mercaptopurine 50 mg. Net price 25 = £18.35

METHOTREXATE

Indications: see notes above and under Dose; rheumatoid arthritis (section 10.1.3); psoriasis (section 13.5.2)
Cautions: see section 8.1, notes above and section 13.5.2; hepatic and renal impairment (Appendixes 2 and 3); porphyria (section 9.8.2); **interactions:** Appendix 1 (methotrexate)
Side-effects: see section 8.1, notes above and section 13.5.2
Dose: *by mouth*, leukaemia in children (maintenance), 15 mg/m^2 weekly in combination with other drugs

Methotrexate (Non-proprietary) PoM
Tablets, yellow, methotrexate 2.5 mg. Net price 100 = £14.19. Counselling, NSAIDs, see section 13.5.2
Available from Faulding DBL, Lederle, Pharmacia & Upjohn (*Maxtrex®*)
Tablets, yellow, methotrexate 10 mg. Net price 100 (Faulding DBL) = £55.07; (Pharmacia & Upjohn, Maxtrex®) = £47.29. Counselling, NSAIDs, see section 13.5.2
Injection, methotrexate 2.5 mg (as sodium salt)/mL. Net price 2-mL vial (Faulding DBL) = £1.68
Injection, methotrexate 25 mg (as sodium salt)/mL. Net price 2-mL vial (Faulding DBL) = £4.58, (Lederle) = £2.62; 8-mL vial (Lederle) = £10.02; 20-mL vial (Faulding DBL) = £39.09, (Lederle) = £25.07; 40-mL vial (Lederle) = £44.57; 200-mL vial (Lederle) = £200.57
Injection, methotrexate 100 mg/mL (not for intrathecal use). Net price 10-mL vial (Faulding DBL) = £78.33; 50-mL vial (Faulding DBL) = £380.07

RALTITREXED

Indications: see notes above
Cautions: see section 8.1 and notes above; hepatic and renal impairment (Appendixes 2 and 3)
Side-effects: see section 8.1 and notes above

Tomudex® (Zeneca) PoM
Injection, powder for reconstitution, raltitrexed. Net price 2-mg vial = £116.00

TIOGUANINE

(Thioguanine)
Indications: acute leukaemias
Cautions: see section 8.1 and notes above; renal impairment (Appendix 3)

Side-effects: see section 8.1 and notes above
Dose: initially 2–2.5 mg/kg daily

Lanvis® (GlaxoWellcome) PoM
Tablets, yellow, scored, tioguanine 40 mg. Net price 25-tab pack = £44.39

8.1.4 Vinca alkaloids and etoposide

The vinca alkaloids, **vinblastine**, **vincristine**, and **vindesine**, are used to treat the acute leukaemias, lymphomas, and some solid tumours (e.g. breast and lung cancer). **Vinorelbine**, a semi-synthetic vinca alkaloid, has recently been introduced for advanced breast cancer (where anthracycline-containing regimens have failed) and for advanced non-small cell lung cancer.

Neurological toxicity, usually manifested as peripheral or autonomic neuropathy, is a feature of treatment with all vinca alkaloids and is a limiting side-effect of vincristine; it occurs less often with vindesine, vinblastine and vinorelbine. Patients with neurological toxicity commonly experience peripheral paraesthesia, loss of deep tendon reflexes, abdominal pain, and constipation. If symptoms of neurotoxicity are severe, doses should be reduced. Motor weakness can also occur, and increasing motor weakness calls for discontinuation of treatment with these drugs. Generally recovery of the nervous system is slow but complete.

Myelosuppression is the dose-limiting side-effect of vinblastine, vindesine and vinorelbine; vincristine causes negligible myelosuppression. The vinca alkaloids may cause reversible alopecia. They cause severe local irritation and care must be taken to avoid extravasation.

> Vinblastine, vincristine, vindesine and vinorelbine are for **intravenous administration only**. They are **not** for intrathecal administration because of severe neurotoxicity which is usually fatal.

Etoposide may be given orally or by slow intravenous infusion, the oral dose being double the intravenous dose. A preparation containing etoposide phosphate can be given by intravenous injection or infusion. Etoposide is usually given daily for 3–5 days and courses should not be repeated more frequently than at intervals of 21 days. It has particularly useful activity in small cell carcinoma of the bronchus, the lymphomas, and testicular cancer. Toxic effects include alopecia, myelosuppression, nausea, and vomiting.

ETOPOSIDE

Indications: see notes above
Cautions: see section 8.1 and notes above
Contra-indications: see section 8.1 and notes above; severe hepatic impairment
Side-effects: see section 8.1 and notes above; irritant to tissues

Etoposide (Non-proprietary) PoM
Concentrate for intravenous infusion, etoposide 20 mg/mL, net price 5-mL vial (Medac, *Eposin®*) = £13.50, 10-mL vial (APS) = £26.24, 25-mL vial (Medac, *Eposin®*) = £67.50

Etopophos® (Bristol-Myers) PoM
Injection, powder for reconstitution, etoposide (as phosphate), net price 100-mg vial = £29.87

Vepesid® (Bristol-Myers) PoM
Capsules, etoposide 50 mg, net price 20 = £113.95; 100 mg, 10-cap pack = £99.57 (hosp. only).
Label: 23
Concentrate for intravenous infusion, etoposide 20 mg/mL, net price 5-mL vial = £14.58 (hosp. only)

VINBLASTINE SULPHATE

Indications: see notes above
Cautions: see section 8.1 and notes above; hepatic impairment (Appendix 2); caution in handling
Contra-indications: see section 8.1 and notes above
IMPORTANT. Intrathecal injection **contra-indicated**
Side-effects: see section 8.1 and notes above; irritant to tissues

Vinblastine (Non-proprietary) PoM
Injection, vinblastine sulphate 1 mg/mL. Net price 10-mL vial = £13.09
Available from Faulding DBL

Velbe® (Lilly) PoM
Injection, powder for reconstitution, vinblastine sulphate. Net price 10-mg amp = £14.15

VINCRISTINE SULPHATE

Indications: see notes above
Cautions: see section 8.1 and notes above; hepatic impairment (Appendix 2); caution in handling; **interactions:** Appendix 1 (vincristine)
Contra-indications: see section 8.1 and notes above
IMPORTANT. Intrathecal injection **contra-indicated**
Side-effects: see section 8.1 and notes above; irritant to tissues

Vincristine (Non-proprietary) PoM
Injection, vincristine sulphate 1 mg/mL. Net price 1-mL vial = £10.92; 2-mL vial = £21.17; 5-mL vial = £44.16; 1-mL syringe = £13.27; 2-mL syringe = £20.55
Available from Faulding DBL

Oncovin® (Lilly) PoM
Injection, vincristine sulphate 1 mg/mL, net price 1-mL vial = £14.18; 2-mL vial = £28.05

VINDESINE SULPHATE

Indications: see notes above
Cautions: see section 8.1 and notes above; hepatic impairment (Appendix 2); caution in handling
Contra-indications: see section 8.1 and notes above
IMPORTANT. Intrathecal injection **contra-indicated**
Side-effects: see section 8.1 and notes above; irritant to tissues

Eldisine® (Lilly) PoM
Injection, powder for reconstitution, vindesine sulphate, net price 5-mg vial = £78.30 (hosp. only)

VINORELBINE

Indications: see notes above

Cautions: see section 8.1 and notes above; hepatic impairment (Appendix 2); caution in handling

Contra-indications: see section 8.1 and notes above

IMPORTANT. Intrathecal injection **contra-indicated**

Side-effects: see section 8.1 and notes above; irritant to tissues

Navelbine® (Fabre) PoM
Injection concentrate, vinorelbine (as tartrate) 10 mg/mL. Net price 1-mL vial = £31.25; 5-mL vial = £147.06

8.1.5 Other antineoplastic drugs

Amsacrine

Amsacrine has an action and toxic effects similar to those of doxorubicin (section 8.1.2) and is given *intravenously*. It is used in acute myeloid leukaemia. Side-effects include myelosuppression and mucositis; electrolytes should be monitored as fatal arrhythmias have occurred in association with hypokalaemia.

AMSACRINE

Indications: see notes above

Cautions: see section 8.1 and notes above; reduce dose in renal or hepatic impairment; also caution in handling—irritant to skin and tissues

Side-effects: see section 8.1 and notes above

Amsidine® (Goldshield) PoM
Concentrate for intravenous infusion, amsacrine 5 mg (as lactate)/mL, when reconstituted by mixing two solutions. Net price 1.5-mL (75-mg) amp with 13.5-mL diluent vial = £47.62 (hosp. only)
Note. Use glass apparatus for reconstitution

Altretamine

Altretamine has recently been introduced for the treatment of advanced ovarian cancer where other regimens have failed. It is given by mouth. Prophylactic anti-emetic treatment is recommended because nausea and vomiting are common and may not respond to symptomatic management. Peripheral and central neurotoxicity has been reported and regular neurological examination is therefore recommended. Altretamine should be discontinued if dose reduction fails to stabilise symptoms of neurological toxicity. Other side-effects include renal and hepatic toxicity, rash and pruritus.

ALTRETAMINE

Indications: see notes above

Cautions: see section 8.1 and notes above; hepatic and renal impairment (Appendixes 2 and 3); **interactions:** Appendix 1 (altretamine)

Contra-indications: see section 8.1 and notes above

Side-effects: see section 8.1 and notes above

Hexalen® (Ipsen) ▼ PoM
Capsules, altretamine 50 mg. Net price 60-cap pack = £142.77. Label: 21.

Crisantaspase

Crisantaspase is the enzyme asparaginase produced by *Erwinia chrysanthemi*. It is given *intramuscularly* or *subcutaneously* almost exclusively in acute lymphoblastic leukaemia. Facilities for the management of anaphylaxis should be available. Side-effects also include nausea, vomiting, CNS depression, and liver function and blood lipid changes; careful monitoring is therefore necessary and the urine is tested for glucose to exclude hyperglycaemia.

CRISANTASPASE

Indications: see notes above

Cautions: see section 8.1 and notes above

Side-effects: see section 8.1 and notes above

Erwinase® (Ipsen) PoM
Injection, powder for reconstitution, crisantaspase. Net price 10 000-unit vial = £39.94

Dacarbazine and temozolomide

Dacarbazine is used to treat metastatic melanoma and, in combination therapy, the soft tissue sarcomas. It is also a component of a commonly used combination for Hodgkin's disease (ABVD—doxorubicin [previously *Adriamycin®*], bleomycin, vinblastine, and dacarbazine). It is given *intravenously*. The predominant side-effects are myelosuppression and intense nausea and vomiting.

Temozolomide has been introduced recently for second-line treatment of malignant glioma.

DACARBAZINE

Indications: see notes above

Cautions: see section 8.1; hepatic and renal impairment (Appendixes 2 and 3); caution in handling

Side-effects: see section 8.1 and notes above; rarely liver necrosis due to hepatic vein thrombosis; irritant to skin and tissues

Dacarbazine (Non-proprietary) PoM
Injection, powder for reconstitution, dacarbazine (as citrate), net price 100-mg vial = £5.11 (Medac); 200-mg vial = £7.24 (Medac) or £7.50 (Faulding DBL); 500-mg vial = £16.50 (Medac); 1000-mg vial = £31.80 (Medac)
Available from Faulding DBL, Medac

DTIC-Dome® (Bayer) PoM
Injection, powder for reconstitution, dacarbazine. Net price 200-mg vial = £7.40

TEMOZOLOMIDE

Indications: see notes above

Cautions: see section 8.1; severe hepatic impairment and renal impairment; **interactions:** Appendix 1 (temozolomide)

Side-effects: see section 8.1

Temodal® (Schering-Plough) ▼ PoM
Capsules, temozolomide 5 mg, net price 5-cap
pack = £17.30, 20-cap pack = £69.20; 20 mg, 5-
cap pack = £69.20, 20-cap pack = £276.80;
100 mg, 5-cap pack = £346.00; 250 mg, 5-cap
pack = £865.00. Label: 22, 25

Hydroxycarbamide/Hydroxyurea

Hydroxycarbamide (**hydroxyurea**) is an orally
active drug used mainly in the treatment of chronic
myeloid leukaemia. It is occasionally used for polycythaemia (the usual treatment is venesection).
Myelosuppression, nausea, and skin reactions are
the most common toxic effects.

HYDROXYCARBAMIDE/
HYDROXYUREA
Indications: see notes above
Cautions: see section 8.1 and notes above
Side-effects: see section 8.1 and notes above
Dose: 20–30 mg/kg daily *or* 80 mg/kg every third
day

Hydrea® (Squibb) PoM
Capsules, pink/green, hydroxycarbamide 500 mg.
Net price 20 = £2.39

Pentostatin

Pentostatin is highly active in hairy cell leukaemia.
It is given *intravenously* on alternate weeks and is
capable of inducing prolonged complete remission.
It is potentially toxic, causing myelosuppression,
immunosuppression and a number of other side-
effects which may be severe. Its use is probably
best confined to specialist centres.

PENTOSTATIN
Indications: see notes above
Cautions: see section 8.1 and notes above; **inter-
actions:** Appendix 1 (pentostatin)
Side-effects: see section 8.1 and notes above

Nipent® (Lederle) PoM
Injection, powder for reconstitution, pentostatin.
Net price 10-mg vial = £774.00

Platinum compounds

Carboplatin, which has activity equivalent to that
of cisplatin in ovarian cancer, is given *intravenously*. It is also active in small cell lung cancer and
is under trial in a variety of other malignancies.
Carboplatin is better tolerated than cisplatin; nausea
and vomiting are reduced in severity and nephrotoxicity, neurotoxicity, and ototoxicity are much
less of a problem than with cisplatin. It is, however,
more myelosuppressive than cisplatin.
  Cisplatin has an alkylating action and is given
intravenously. It has useful antitumour activity in
certain solid tumours including ovarian cancer and
testicular teratoma. It is, however, a toxic drug.
Common problems include severe nausea and
vomiting, nephrotoxicity (pretreatment hydration
mandatory and renal function should be closely
monitored), myelotoxicity, ototoxicity (high tone

hearing loss and tinnitus), peripheral neuropathy,
optic neuritis, papilloedema, cerebral blindness, and
hypomagnesaemia. These toxic effects commonly
necessitate dose reduction or drug withdrawal. It is
preferable that treatment with this drug be supervised by specialists familiar with its use.
  Oxaliplatin is given *intravenously* for the treatment of metastatic colorectal cancer in combination
with fluorouracil and folinic acid. Neurotoxic side-
effects (including sensory peripheral neuropathy)
are dose limiting. Other side-effects include gastro-
intestinal disturbances, ototoxicity, and myelosuppression. Manufacturers advise renal function monitoring in moderate impairment.

CARBOPLATIN
Indications: see notes above
Cautions: see section 8.1 and notes above; renal
impairment (Appendix 3); **interactions:** Appen-
dix 1 (platinum compounds)
Side-effects: see section 8.1 and notes above

Carboplatin (Non-proprietary) PoM
Injection, carboplatin 10 mg/mL, net price 5-mL
vial = £22.86 (Faulding DBL), 15-mL vial =
£62.83 (APS) or £65.83 (Faulding DBL), 15-mL
Onco-vial®= £72.41 (Faulding DBL), 45-mL vial
= £187.61 (APS) or £197.48 (Faulding DBL), 45-
mL *Onco-vial*®= £217.23 (Faulding DBL), 60-
mL vial = £260.00 (Faulding DBL)
Available from APS, Faulding DBL
Paraplatin® (Bristol-Myers) PoM
Injection, carboplatin 10 mg/mL, net price 5-mL
vial = £22.86, 15-mL vial = £65.83, 45-mL vial =
£197.48

CISPLATIN
Indications: see notes above
Cautions: see section 8.1 and notes above; renal
impairment (Appendix 3); **interactions:** Appen-
dix 1 (platinum compounds)
Side-effects: see section 8.1 and notes above

Cisplatin (Non-proprietary) PoM
Injection, cisplatin 1 mg/mL. Net price 10-mL vial
= £5.85; 50-mL vial = £26.70 (APS) or £28.11
(Faulding DBL); 100-mL vial = £52.86 (APS) or
£55.64 (Faulding DBL)
Available from Faulding DBL, APS
Injection, powder for reconstitution, cisplatin. Net
price 10-mg vial = £4.89; 50-mg vial = £17.00
Available from Pharmacia & Upjohn

OXALIPLATIN
Indications: metastatic colorectal cancer in combination with fluorouracil and folinic acid
Cautions: see section 8.1 and notes above; renal
impairment (Appendix 3); **interactions:** Appendix 1 (platinum compounds)
Contra-indications: see section 8.1; peripheral
neuropathy with functional impairment
Side-effects: see section 8.1 and notes above

Eloxatin® (Sanofi-Synthelabo) ▼ PoM
Injection, powder for reconstitution, oxaliplatin,
net price 50-mg vial = £165.00, 100-mg vial =
£330.00

Procarbazine

Procarbazine is most often used in Hodgkin's disease, for example in MOPP (chlormethine (mustine), vincristine [*Oncovin*®], procarbazine, and prednisolone) chemotherapy. It is given *by mouth*. Toxic effects include nausea, myelosuppression, and a hypersensitivity rash preventing further use of this drug. It is a mild monoamine-oxidase inhibitor but dietary restriction is not considered necessary. Alcohol ingestion may cause a disulfiram-like reaction.

PROCARBAZINE

Indications: see notes above
Cautions: see section 8.1 and notes above; renal impairment (Appendix 3); **interactions:** Appendix 1 (procarbazine)
Side-effects: see section 8.1 and notes above
Dose: initially 50 mg daily, increased by 50 mg daily to 250–300 mg daily in divided doses; maintenance (on remission) 50–150 mg daily to cumulative total of at least 6 g

Procarbazine (Cambridge) PoM
Capsules, ivory, procarbazine 50 mg (as hydrochloride). Net price 50-cap pack = £37.44. Label: 4
Note. The brand name *Natulan*® was formerly used for procarbazine capsules

Razoxane

Razoxane has limited activity in the leukaemias, and is little used.

RAZOXANE

Indications: see notes above
Cautions: see section 8.1
Side-effects: see section 8.1
Dose: acute leukaemias, 150–500 mg/m^2 daily for 3–5 days

Razoxane (Cambridge) PoM
Tablets, scored, razoxane 125 mg. Net price 30-tab pack = £71.01

Taxanes

Paclitaxel is the first of a new group of drugs termed the taxanes. It is given by *intravenous infusion*. It is licensed for treatment of advanced ovarian cancer and for secondary treatment of breast and non-small cell lung cancer. There is increasing evidence that paclitaxel given with carboplatin or cisplatin is the treatment of choice for advanced ovarian cancer. Routine premedication with a corticosteroid, an antihistamine and a histamine H$_2$-receptor antagonist is recommended to prevent severe hypersensitivity reactions; hypersensitivity reactions may occur rarely despite premedication, although more commonly only bradycardia or asymptomatic hypotension occur.

Other side-effects of paclitaxel include myelosuppression, peripheral neuropathy, and cardiac conduction defects with arrhythmias (which are nearly always asymptomatic). It also causes alopecia and muscle pain; nausea and vomiting is mild to moderate.

Docetaxel is licensed for use in anthracycline-resistant breast cancer. Its side-effects are similar to those of paclitaxel but persistent fluid retention (commonly as leg oedema that worsens during treatment) can be resistant to treatment; hypersensitivity reactions also occur. Dexamethasone by mouth for 3 days, starting on the day before each course of docetaxel, is recommended for reducing fluid retention and hypersensitivity reactions. Caution is advised in hepatic impairment.

DOCETAXEL

Indications: advanced or metastatic breast cancer where adjuvant cytotoxic chemotherapy (including anthracycline) has failed
Cautions: see section 8.1 and notes above; **interactions:** Appendix 1 (docetaxel)
Side-effects: see section 8.1 and notes above

Taxotere® (Rhône-Poulenc Rorer) ▼ PoM
Concentrate for intravenous infusion, docetaxel 40 mg/mL. Net price 0.5-mL vial = £175.00, 2-mL vial = £575.00 (both with diluent). Hosp. only

PACLITAXEL

Indications: primary ovarian cancer (advanced or residual disease following laparotomy) in combination with cisplatin; metastatic ovarian cancer where standard platinum-containing therapy has failed; metastatic breast carcinoma where standard anthracycline-containing therapy has failed or is inappropriate; non-small cell lung cancer (in combination with cisplatin) when surgery or radiation therapy not appropriate
Cautions: see section 8.1 and notes above
Contra-indications: see section 8.1 and notes above; severe hepatic impairment
Side-effects: see section 8.1 and notes above

Taxol® (Bristol-Myers) ▼ PoM
Concentrate for intravenous infusion, paclitaxel 6 mg/mL, net price 5-mL vial = £124.79; 16.7-mL vial = £374.00 (hosp. only)
Note. Contains polyethoxylated castor oil which has been associated with anaphylaxis

Topoisomerase I inhibitors

Irinotecan and topotecan are recently introduced drugs which inhibit topoisomerase I, an enzyme involved in DNA replication.

Irinotecan is given by intravenous infusion in metastatic colorectal cancer in combination with fluorouracil and folinic acid or when treatment containing fluorouracil has failed.

Topotecan is given by intravenous infusion in metastatic ovarian cancer when first-line or subsequent therapy has failed.

In addition to dose-limiting myelosuppression, side-effects of irinotecan and topotecan include gastro-intestinal effects (delayed diarrhoea requiring prompt treatment may follow irinotecan treatment), asthenia, alopecia, and anorexia.

IRINOTECAN HYDROCHLORIDE

Indications: metastatic colorectal cancer in combination with fluorouracil and folinic acid or where treatment containing fluorouracil has failed

Cautions: see section 8.1 and notes above; raised plasma-bilirubin concentration (see under Contra-indications and Appendix 2)

Contra-indications: see section 8.1 and notes above, also chronic inflammatory bowel disease, bowel obstruction; plasma bilirubin concentration more than 1.5 times the upper limit of reference range; avoid conception for at least 3 months after cessation of treatment

Side-effects: see section 8.1 and notes above; also acute cholinergic syndrome (with early diarrhoea) and delayed diarrhoea (consult product literature)

Campto® (Rhône-Poulenc Rorer) PoM
Concentrate for intravenous infusion, irinotecan hydrochloride 20 mg/mL, net price 2-mL vial = £53.00; 5-mL vial = £130.00

TOPOTECAN

Indications: metastatic ovarian cancer where first-line or subsequent therapy has failed

Cautions: see section 8.1 and notes above

Contra-indications: see section 8.1 and notes above

Side-effects: see section 8.1 and notes above

Hycamtin® (SmithKline Beecham) ▼ PoM
Intravenous infusion, powder for reconstitution, topotecan (as hydrochloride), net price 4-mg vial = £312.50

Tretinoin

Tretinoin has recently been introduced for the induction of remission in acute promyelocytic leukaemia. It is used in previously untreated patients as well as in those who have relapsed after standard chemotherapy or who are refractory to it.

TRETINOIN

Note. Tretinoin is the acid form of vitamin A

Indications: see notes above; acne (section 13.6.1); photodamage (section 13.8.1)

Cautions: exclude pregnancy before starting treatment and avoid pregnancy during and for at least 1 month after treatment; monitor haematological profile, liver function and plasma lipids before and during treatment; increased risk of thromboembolism during first month of treatment; hepatic and renal impairment (Appendixes 2 and 3); **interactions:** Appendix 1 (retinoids)

Contra-indications: pregnancy (**important teratogenic risk:** see Cautions and Appendix 4) and breast-feeding

Side-effects: retinoic acid syndrome (fever, dyspnoea, acute respiratory distress, pulmonary infiltrates, pleural effusion, hyperleukocytosis, hypotension, oedema, weight gain, hepatic, renal and multi-organ failure) requires immediate treatment—consult product literature; gastro-intestinal disturbances, pancreatitis; arrhythmias, flushing, oedema; headache, benign intracranial hypertension (mainly in children), shivering, dizziness, confusion, anxiety, depression, insomnia, paraesthesia, visual and hearing disturbances; raised liver enzymes, serum creatinine and lipids; bone and chest pain, alopecia, rash, pruritus, sweating, dry skin, dryness of mucous membranes, cheilitis; thromboembolism reported

Vesanoid® (Roche) ▼ PoM
Capsules, yellow/brown, tretinoin 10 mg. Net price 100-cap pack = £183.36. Label: 21.

8.2 Drugs affecting the immune response

8.2.1	Antiproliferative immunosuppressants
8.2.2	Corticosteroids and other immunosuppressants
8.2.3	Rituximab
8.2.4	Interferons
8.2.5	Aldesleukin

Immunosuppressant therapy

Immunosuppressants are used to suppress rejection in organ transplant recipients and to treat a variety of chronic inflammatory and autoimmune diseases. Solid organ transplant patients are usually maintained on a corticosteroid combined with a calcineurin inhibitor (ciclosporin or tacrolimus), *or* with an antiproliferative drug (azathioprine or mycophenolate mofetil), *or* with both. Specialist management is required and other immunomodulators may be used to initiate treatment or to treat rejection.

IMPAIRED IMMUNE RESPONSIVENESS. Modification of tissue reactions caused by corticosteroids and other immunosuppressive drugs may result in the rapid *spread of infection*. Corticosteroids may suppress clinical signs of infection and allow diseases such as septicaemia or tuberculosis to reach an advanced stage before being recognised—**important:** for advice on measles and chickenpox (varicella) exposure, see Immunoglobulins (section 14.5). For general comments and warnings relating to corticosteroids and immunosuppressants see section 6.3.2 (under Prednisolone).

PREGNANCY. Transplant patients immunosuppressed with azathioprine should not discontinue it on becoming pregnant; there is no evidence that azathioprine is teratogenic. There is less experience of ciclosporin in pregnancy but it does not appear to be any more harmful than azathioprine. Any risk to the offspring of azathioprine-treated men is small. Tacrolimus and mycophenolate mofetil are contra-indicated by the manufacturers in pregnancy (Appendix 4).

8.2.1 Antiproliferative immunosuppressants

Azathioprine is widely used for transplant recipients and it is also used to treat a number of autoimmune conditions, usually when corticosteroid therapy alone provides inadequate control. It is metabolised to mercaptopurine, and doses should be reduced when allopurinol is given concurrently. The predominant toxic effect is myelosuppression, although hepatic toxicity is also well recognised.

Mycophenolate mofetil is metabolised to mycophenolic acid which has a more selective mode of action than azathioprine. It is licensed for the prophylaxis of acute rejection in renal or cardiac transplantation when used in combination with ciclosporin and corticosteroids. There is evidence that compared with similar regimens incorporating azathioprine, mycophenolate mofetil reduces the risk of acute rejection episodes; the risk of opportunistic infections (particularly due to tissue-invasive cytomegalovirus) and the occurrence of blood disorders such as leucopenia may be higher.

Cyclophosphamide and chlorambucil (section 8.1.1) are less commonly prescribed as immunosuppressants.

AZATHIOPRINE

Indications: see notes above

Cautions: monitor for toxicity throughout treatment; monitor full blood count weekly (more frequently with higher doses or if hepatic or renal impairment) for first 4 weeks (manufacturer advises weekly monitoring for 8 weeks but evidence of practical value unsatisfactory), thereafter reduce frequency of monitoring to at least every 3 months; hepatic impairment (Appendix 2); renal impairment (Appendix 3); reduce dose in elderly; pregnancy (see section 8.2)—treatment should not generally be initiated during pregnancy; **interactions:** Appendix 1 (azathioprine)

BONE MARROW SUPPRESSION. Patients should be warned to report immediately any signs or symptoms of bone marrow suppression e.g. inexplicable bruising or bleeding, infection

Contra-indications: hypersensitivity to azathioprine or mercaptopurine

Side-effects: hypersensitivity reactions (including malaise, dizziness, vomiting, diarrhoea, fever, rigors, myalgia, arthralgia, disturbed liver function, cholestatic jaundice, arrhythmias, rash, hypotension and interstitial nephritis—calling for immediate and permanent withdrawal); dose-related bone marrow suppression (see also Cautions); hair loss and increased susceptibility to infections and colitis in patients also receiving corticosteroids; nausea; rarely pancreatitis and pneumonitis

Dose: *by mouth, or* (if oral administration not possible—intravenous solution very irritant, see below) *by intravenous injection* over at least 1 minute (followed by 50 mL sodium chloride intravenous infusion), *or by intravenous infusion*, autoimmune conditions, 1–3 mg/kg daily, adjusted according to response (consider withdrawal if no improvement in 3 months)

Suppression of transplant rejection, initially up to 5 mg/kg then 1–4 mg/kg daily according to response

Note. Intravenous injection is alkaline and very irritant, intravenous route should therefore be used **only** if oral route not feasible, see also Appendix 6

Azathioprine (Non-proprietary) PoM
Tablets, azathioprine 25 mg, net price 20 = £6.65; 50 mg, 20 = £3.49. Label: 21
Available from APS, Ashbourne (*Immunoprin*®), Cox, Hillcross, Norton, Opus (*Oprisine*®), Penn (*Azamune*®)

Imuran® (GlaxoWellcome) PoM
Tablets, both f/c, azathioprine 25 mg (orange), net price 100-tab pack = £39.35; 50 mg (yellow), 100-tab pack = £65.61. Label: 21

Injection, powder for reconstitution, azathioprine (as sodium salt). Net price 50-mg vial = £16.54

MYCOPHENOLATE MOFETIL

Indications: prophylaxis of acute renal or cardiac transplant rejection (in combination with ciclosporin and corticosteroids) under specialist supervision

Cautions: full blood counts every week for 4 weeks then twice a month for 2 months then every month in the first year (possibly interrupt treatment if neutropenia develops); elderly (increased risk of infection, gastro-intestinal haemorrhage and pulmonary oedema); active serious gastro-intestinal disease (risk of haemorrhage, ulceration and perforation); delayed graft function; susceptibility to skin cancer (avoid exposure to strong sunlight); **interactions:** Appendix 1 (mycophenolate mofetil)

BONE MARROW SUPPRESSION. Patients should be warned to report immediately any signs or symptoms of bone marrow suppression e.g. infection and inexplicable bruising or bleeding

Contra-indications: pregnancy (exclude before starting and avoid for 6 weeks after discontinuation); breast-feeding

Side-effects: diarrhoea, vomiting, constipation, nausea, dyspepsia, abdominal pain; hypertension, oedema, chest pain; dyspnoea, cough, rhinitis; dizziness, insomnia, headache, tremor; infection (including cytomegalovirus viraemia, herpes simplex, candidiasis, aspergillosis, urinary-tract infection and pneumonia); leucopenia (see also Cautions), anaemia, thrombocytopenia, leucocytosis, polycythaemia; electrolyte disturbances, hyperglycaemia, hypercholesterolaemia; asthenia; renal damage, haematuria; acne; lymphoproliferative disease; less frequently, gastro-intestinal perforation, abnormal liver-function tests, hepatitis, gingivitis, mouth ulceration, haemorrhage, influenza-like syndrome, hypotension, arrhythmias, tachycardia, hypoglycaemia, weight gain; allergic reactions, benign neoplasm of skin and skin carcinoma reported

Dose: renal transplantation, *by mouth*, 1 g twice daily starting within 72 hours of transplantation *or by intravenous infusion*, 1 g twice daily starting within 24 hours of transplantation for up to max. 14 days (then transfer to oral therapy)

Cardiac transplantation, *by mouth*, 1.5 g twice daily starting within 5 days of transplantation

CellCept® (Roche) ▼ PoM
Capsules, blue/brown, mycophenolate mofetil 250 mg, net price 100-cap pack = £113.41. Label: 23

Tablets, lavender, mycophenolate mofetil 500 mg, net price 50-tab pack = £113.41. Label: 23

Intravenous infusion, powder for reconstitution, mycophenolate mofetil (as hydrochloride), net price 500-mg vial = £10.14

| 8.2.2 | **Corticosteroids and other immunosuppressants** |

Prednisolone (section 6.3.2) is widely used in oncology. It has a marked antitumour effect in acute lymphoblastic leukaemia, Hodgkin's disease, and the non-Hodgkin lymphomas. It is also active in hormone-sensitive breast cancer and may cause useful disease regression. Finally, it has a role in the palliation of symptomatic end-stage malignant disease when it may enhance appetite and produce a sense of well-being (see also Prescribing in Palliative Care).

The corticosteroids are also powerful immunosuppressants. They are used to prevent organ transplant rejection, and in high dose to treat rejection episodes.

Ciclosporin (cyclosporin), a calcineurin inhibitor, is a potent immunosuppressant which is virtually non-myelotoxic but markedly nephrotoxic. It has found particular use in the field of organ and tissue transplantation, for prevention of graft rejection following bone marrow, kidney, liver, pancreas, heart, and heart-lung transplantation, and for prophylaxis and treatment of graft-versus-host disease.

Tacrolimus is also a calcineurin inhibitor. Although not chemically related to ciclosporin it has a similar mode of action and side-effects, but the incidence of neurotoxicity and nephrotoxicity appears to be greater; cardiomyopathy has also been reported. Disturbance of glucose metabolism also appears to be significant; hypertrichosis appears to be less of a problem than with ciclosporin.

Basiliximab and **daclizumab** are monoclonal antibodies that prevent T-lymphocyte proliferation; they have recently been introduced for prophylaxis of acute rejection in allogenic renal transplantation. They are given with ciclosporin and corticosteroid immunosuppression regimens; their use should be confined to specialist centres.

BASILIXIMAB

Indications: see notes above

Contra-indications: pregnancy (Appendix 4) and breast-feeding

Side-effects: no specific side-effects reported with basiliximab; for side-effects of regimen see under cyclopsorin (below) and prednisolone (section 6.3.2)

Dose: *by intravenous infusion*, 20 mg within 2 hours before transplant surgery and a further 20 mg 4 days after surgery—withhold second dose if post-operative complications such as graft loss occur

Simulect® (Novartis) ▼ PoM
Injection, powder for reconstitution, basiliximab, net price 20-mg vial (with water for injections) = £770.00. For intravenous infusion

---

CICLOSPORIN

(Cyclosporin)

Indications: see notes above, and under Dose; atopic dermatitis and psoriasis (section 13.5.2); rheumatoid arthritis (section 10.1.3)

Cautions: monitor kidney function—dose dependent increase in serum creatinine and urea during first few weeks may necessitate dose reduction in transplant patients (exclude rejection if kidney transplant) or discontinuation in non-transplant patients; monitor liver function (dosage adjustment based on bilirubin and liver enzymes may be needed); monitor blood pressure—discontinue if hypertension develops that cannot be controlled by antihypertensives; hyperuricaemia; monitor serum potassium especially in marked renal dysfunction (and avoid high dietary potassium); measure blood lipids before treatment and thereafter as appropriate; pregnancy (see p. 397) and breast-feeding (Appendix 5); porphyria (section 9.8.2); apart from specialist use in transplant patients preferably avoid other immunosuppressants with the exception of corticosteroids (oversuppression may increase susceptibility to infection and lymphoma); **interactions:** Appendix 1 (ciclosporin)

ADDITIONAL CAUTIONS IN NEPHROTIC SYNDROME. *Contra-indicated* in uncontrolled hypertension, uncontrolled infections, and malignancy; reduce dose by 25–50% if serum creatinine more than 30% above baseline on more than one measurement; in renal impairment initially 2.5 mg/kg daily; in long-term management, perform renal biopsies at yearly intervals

ADDITIONAL CAUTIONS. Atopic Dermatitis and Psoriasis, section 13.5.2; Rheumatoid Arthritis, section 10.1.3

Side-effects: commonly dose-dependent increase in serum creatinine and urea during first few weeks (see also under Cautions), and less commonly renal structural changes on long-term administration; also hypertrichosis, tremor, hypertension (especially in heart transplant patients) hepatic dysfunction, fatigue, gingival hypertrophy, gastro-intestinal disturbances, and burning sensation in hands and feet (usually during first week); *occasionally* headache, rash (possibly allergic), mild anaemia, hyperkalaemia, hyperuricaemia, gout, hypomagnesaemia, hypercholesterolaemia, weight increase, oedema, pancreatitis, neuropathy, confusion, paraesthesia, convulsions, dysmenorrhoea or amenorrhoea; muscle weakness, cramps, myopathy, gynaecomastia (in patients receiving concomitant spironolactone), colitis also reported; thrombocytopenia (sometimes with haemolytic uraemic syndrome) also reported; incidence of malignancies and lymphoproliferative disorders similar to that with conventional immunosuppressive therapy

Dose: organ transplantation, used alone, 10–15 mg/ kg *by mouth* 4–12 hours before transplantation followed by 10–15 mg/kg daily for 1–2 weeks post-operatively then reduced to 2–6 mg/kg daily for maintenance (dose should be adjusted by monitoring blood concentrations and renal function); dose lower if given concomitantly with other immunosuppressant therapy (e.g. corticos-

teroids); if necessary one-third oral dose can be given *by intravenous infusion* over 2–6 hours
Bone-marrow transplantation, prevention and treatment of graft-versus-host disease, 3–5 mg/kg daily *by intravenous infusion* over 2–6 hours from day before transplantation to 2 weeks post-operatively (or 12.5–15 mg/kg daily *by mouth*) then 12.5 mg/kg daily *by mouth* for 3–6 months then tailed off (may take up to a year after transplantation)
Nephrotic syndrome, *by mouth*, 5 mg/kg daily in 2 divided doses; CHILD 6 mg/kg daily in 2 divided doses; maintenance treatment reduce to lowest effective dose according to proteinuria and serum creatinine measurements; discontinue after 3 months if no improvement in glomerulonephritis or glomerulosclerosis (after 6 months in membranous glomerulonephritis)

CONVERSION (between different brands of ciclosporin). Measure trough blood-ciclosporin concentration, serum creatinine and blood pressure then give same dose (mg for mg) of oral ciclosporin as the previous preparation; repeat measurements 4–7 days after conversion (further measurements may be needed in first 2 months, e.g. week 2 and week 4) and adjust dose accordingly; if temporary loss of efficacy acceptable, start with the lowest recommended dose and adjust according to response. Unlike oral *Sandimmun®* which may be taken either as a single daily dose (transplant recipients) or in 2 divided doses, *Neoral®* or *SangCya®* are always taken in 2 divided doses.

> Because of differences in bioavailability, the brand of ciclosporin to be dispensed should be specified by the prescriber

Neoral® (Novartis) [PoM]
Capsules, ciclosporin 10 mg (yellow/white), net price 30-cap pack = £8.22; 25 mg (blue/grey), 30-cap pack = £20.54; 50 mg (yellow/white), 30-cap pack = £40.22; 100 mg (blue/grey), 30-cap pack = £76.33. Counselling, administration
Oral solution, yellow, sugar-free, ciclosporin 100 mg/mL, net price 50 mL = £114.38. Counselling, administration
COUNSELLING. Total daily dose should be taken in 2 divided doses. Avoid grapefruit or grapefruit juice for 1 hour before dose.
Mix solution with orange juice (or squash) or apple juice (to improve taste) or with water immediately before taking (and rinse with more to ensure total dose). Do not mix with grapefruit juice. Keep medicine measure away from other liquids (including water)

Sandimmun® (Novartis) [PoM]
[1]*Capsules*, ciclosporin 25 mg (pale pink), 30-cap pack; 50 mg (yellow), 30-cap pack; 100 mg (dusky pink), 30-cap pack. Counselling, administration
[1]*Oral solution*, oily, yellow, sugar-free, ciclosporin 100 mg/mL, 50 mL. Counselling, administration
COUNSELLING. Total daily dose may be taken as a single dose (transplant recipients) or in 2 divided doses. Avoid grapefruit or grapefruit juice for 1 hour before dose
To mask taste, mix solution with cold milk, cold chocolate drink, cola, or orange juice immediately before taking (and rinse with more to ensure total dose). Do not mix with grapefruit juice. Do not use plastic cup. Keep medicine measure away from other liquids (including water)
1. *Sandimmun®* capsules and oral solution available only on named-patient basis for patients who cannot be transferred to other brands of oral ciclosporin

Concentrate for intravenous infusion (oily), ciclosporin 50 mg/mL. To be diluted before use. Net price 1-mL amp = £1.77; 5-mL amp = £8.38
Note. Contains polyethoxylated castor oil which has been associated with anaphylaxis—observe for at least 30 minutes after starting infusion and at frequent intervals thereafter

SangCya® (Sangstat) [PoM]
Oral solution, sugar-free, ciclosporin 100 mg/mL, net price 50 mL = £94.36. Counselling, administration
COUNSELLING. Total daily dose should be taken in 2 divided doses. Avoid grapefruit or grapefruit juice for 1 hour before dose.
To mask taste, mix solution with cold milk, cold chocolate drink, cola or orange juice immediately before taking (and rinse with more to ensure total dose). Do not mix with grapefruit juice. Keep medicine measure away from other liquids (including water)

DACLIZUMAB
Indications: see notes above
Contra-indications: pregnancy and breast-feeding
Side-effects: no specific side-effects reported with daclizumab; for side-effects of regimen see under Ciclosporin (above) and Prednisolone (section 6.3.2)
Dose: *by intravenous infusion*, 1 mg/kg within the 24-hour period before transplantation, then 1 mg/kg every 14 days for a total of 5 doses

Zenapax® (Roche) ▼ [PoM]
Concentrate for intravenous infusion, daclizumab 5 mg/mL, net price 5-mL = £245.23

TACROLIMUS
Indications: primary immunosuppression in liver and kidney allograft recipients and allograft rejection resistant to conventional immunosuppressive regimens; see also notes above
Cautions: see under Ciclosporin; also monitor ECG (**important:** also echocardiography, see CSM warning below), visual status, blood glucose, haematological and neurological parameters; **interactions:** Appendix 1 (tacrolimus)
DRIVING. May affect performance of skilled tasks (e.g. driving)
Contra-indications: hypersensitivity to macrolides; pregnancy (exclude before starting—if contraception needed non-hormonal methods should be used), breast-feeding; avoid concurrent administration with ciclosporin (care if patient has previously received ciclosporin)
Side-effects: include gastro-intestinal disturbances such as nausea, dyspepsia and ulceration; hypertension, angina, tachycardia, pleural and pericardial effusion, less frequently hypotension, arrhythmias, rarely ventricular or septal hypertrophy, cardiomyopathy (**important:** see CSM warning below) and pericarditis; tremor, headache, insomnia, anxiety, depression, encephalopathy and rarely agitation, somnolence, hallucinations, dizziness, decreased reflexes, migraine, convulsions, confusion, amblyopia, cataract, retinopathy, photophobia, deafness and tinnitus; haematological effects including leucocytosis, leucopenia, aplastic and haemolytic anaemia and rarely thrombocytopaenia; increased

serum creatinine and urea, less frequently kidney damage and renal failure; electrolyte disturbances including hypercalcaemia, hypokalaemia, hyperuricaemia, thyroid disorders, altered acid-base balance and glucose metabolism; pruritus, erythema, alopecia, sweating, hirsutism, photosensitivity; allergic reactions including anaphylaxis; gynaecomastia, oedema, hepatic dysfunction, cirrhosis, pancreatitis, weight and appetite changes, isolated cases of respiratory failure and pulmonary fibrosis

CSM Warning. Cardiomyopathy has been reported in children given tacrolimus after transplantation. Patients using the drug should be monitored carefully by echocardiography for hypertrophic changes; dose reduction or discontinuation should be considered if these occur

Dose: liver transplantation, starting 6 hours after transplantation, *by mouth*, 100–200 micrograms/kg daily in 2 divided doses *or by intravenous infusion* over 24 hours, 10–50 micrograms/kg; CHILD *by mouth*, 300 micrograms/kg daily in 2 divided doses *or by intravenous infusion* over 24 hours, 50 micrograms/kg

Renal transplantation, starting within 24 hours of transplantation, *by mouth*, 150–300 micrograms/kg daily in 2 divided doses *or by intravenous infusion* over 24 hours, 50–100 micrograms/kg; CHILD *by mouth*, 300 micrograms/kg daily in 2 divided doses *or by intravenous infusion* over 24 hours, 100 micrograms/kg

Maintenance treatment, dose adjusted according to response

Prograf® (Fujisawa) PoM
Capsules, tacrolimus 1 mg (white), net price 50-cap pack = £92.93, 100-cap pack = £185.86; 5 mg (greyish-red), 50-cap pack = £371.85. Label: 23, counselling, driving
Concentrate for intravenous infusion, tacrolimus 5 mg/mL. To be diluted before use. Net price 1-mL amp = £67.67
Note. Contains polyethoxylated castor oil which has been associated with anaphylaxis

8.2.3   Rituximab

Rituximab, a monoclonal antibody which causes lysis of B lymphocytes, has recently been introduced for the treatment of chemotherapy-resistant advanced follicular lymphoma. Full resuscitation facilities should be at hand and as with other cytotoxics, treatment should be undertaken under the close supervision of a specialist.

Rituximab should be used with caution in patients with a history of cardiovascular disease because exacerbation of angina, arrhythmia, and heart failure have been reported. Transient hypotension occurs frequently during infusion and antihypertensives may need to be withheld for 12 hours before infusion.

Infusion-related side-effects (including cytokine release syndrome) are reported commonly and occur predominantly during the first infusion; they include fever and chills, nausea and vomiting, allergic reactions (such as rash, pruritus, angioedema, bronchospasm and dyspnoea), flushing and tumour pain. Patients should be given an analgesic and an antihistamine before each dose of rituximab to reduce the incidence of these effects. Premedication with a corticosteroid should also be considered. The infusion may have to be stopped temporarily and the infusion-related effects treated—consult product literature for appropriate management. Evidence of pulmonary infiltration and features of tumour lysis syndrome should be sought if infusion-related effects occur.

Fatalities following **severe** cytokine release syndrome (characterised by severe dyspnoea) and associated with features of tumour lysis syndrome have occurred 1–2 hours after infusion of rituximab. Patients with a high tumour burden as well as those with pulmonary insufficiency or infiltration are at increased risk and should be monitored **very closely** (and a slower rate of infusion considered).

RITUXIMAB

Indications: see notes above

Cautions: see notes above—but for full details (including monitoring) consult product literature; pregnancy (Appendix 4)

Contra-indications: breast-feeding

Side-effects: see notes above—but for full details (including monitoring and management of side-effects) consult product literature

Mabthera® (Roche) ▼ PoM
Injection, rituximab 10 mg/mL, net price 10-mL vial = £174.63, 50-mL vial = £873.15. For intravenous infusion

8.2.4   Interferons

Interferons are naturally occurring proteins with complex effects on immunity and cell function.

Interferon alfa

Interferon alfa (formerly called leucocyte interferon or lymphoblastoid interferon) has shown some antitumour effect in certain lymphomas and solid tumours. Side-effects are dose-related, but commonly include nausea, influenza-like symptoms, lethargy, ocular side-effects and depression (suicidal behaviour reported). Myelosuppression may also occur, particularly affecting granulocyte counts. Cardiovascular problems (hypotension, hypertension, and arrhythmias), nephrotoxicity and hepatotoxicity have been reported. Other side-effects include hypersensitivity reactions, thyroid abnormalities, hyperglycaemia, psoriasiform rash, confusion, and coma and seizures (usually with high doses in the elderly).

INTERFERON ALFA

Indications: see under preparations

Cautions: consult product literature; **interactions:** Appendix 1 (interferons)

Contra-indications: consult product literature

Side-effects: see notes above and consult product literature

Dose: consult product literature

Intron A® (Schering-Plough) PoM

Injection, interferon alfa-2b (rbe) 10 million units/mL, net price 2.5-mL vial = £135.00. For subcutaneous or intravenous injection

Injection, powder for reconstitution, interferon alfa-2b (rbe), net price 1-million unit vial = £5.40; 3-million unit vial = £16.20; 5-million unit vial = £27.00; 10-million unit vial = £53.96 (all with injection equipment and water for injection). For subcutaneous or intravenous injection

Injection pen, interferon alfa-2b (rbe), net price 15 million units/mL, 1.5-mL cartridge = £97.20; 25 million units/mL, 1.5-mL cartridge = £162.00; 50 million units/mL, 1.5-mL cartridge = £324.00. For subcutaneous injection

Note. Each 1.5-mL multidose cartridge delivers 6 doses of 0.2 mL i.e. a total of 1.2 mL

For AIDS-related Kaposi's sarcoma, hairy cell leukaemia, follicular lymphoma, chronic myelogenous leukaemia, lymph or liver metastases of carcinoid tumour, chronic hepatitis B, chronic hepatitis C, adjunct in malignant melanoma and maintenance of remission in multiple myeloma

Roferon-A® (Roche) PoM

Injection, interferon alfa-2a (rbe). Net price 3 million units/mL, 1-mL vial = £16.20; 6 million units/mL, 0.5-mL (3 million-unit) prefilled syringe = £16.20, 3-mL (18 million-unit) vial = £97.19; 9 million units/mL, 0.5-mL (4.5 million-unit) prefilled syringe = £24.30; 12 million units/mL, 0.5-mL (6 million-unit) prefilled syringe = £32.39; 18 million units/mL, 0.5-mL (9 million-unit) prefilled syringe = £48.59, 1-mL (18 million-unit) vial = £97.19; 30 million units/mL, 0.6-mL (18 million-unit) cartridge = £101.77, for use with *Roferon* pen device. For subcutaneous injection (cartridges, vials, and prefilled syringes) and intramuscular injection (cartridges and vials)

For AIDS-related Kaposi's sarcoma, hairy cell leukaemia, chronic myelogenous leukaemia, recurrent or metastatic renal cell carcinoma, progressive cutaneous T-cell lymphoma, chronic hepatitis B and chronic hepatitis C, follicular non-Hodgkin's lymphoma, adjunct in malignant melanoma

Viraferon® (Schering-Plough) PoM

Injection, interferon alfa-2b (rbe) 6 million units/mL, net price 3-mL vial = £97.20. For subcutaneous injection

Injection pen, interferon alfa-2b (rbe), net price 15 million units/mL, 1.5-mL cartridge = £97.20; 25 million units/mL, 1.5-mL cartridge = £162.00. For subcutaneous injection

Note. 1.5-mL multidose cartridge delivers 6 doses of 0.2 mL each

For chronic hepatitis B and chronic hepatitis C

Interferon beta

Interferon beta (formerly called fibroblast interferon) is licensed for use in patients with *relapsing, remitting multiple sclerosis* (characterised by at least two attacks of neurological dysfunction over the previous two-year period, followed by complete or incomplete recovery) who are able to walk unaided. It is indicated for the reduction of frequency and degree of severity of clinical relapses. Not all patients respond and a deterioration in the bouts has been observed in some. Interferon beta-1b

is also licensed for use in patients with *secondary progressive multiple sclerosis*.

Interferon beta should not be used in those with a history of severe depressive illness (or of suicidal ideation), in those with inadequately controlled epilepsy, or in decompensated hepatic impairment; caution is advised in those with a history of these conditions or with cardiac disorders or myelosuppression. Most frequently reported side-effects include irritation at injection site (including inflammation, hypersensitivity, necrosis) and influenza-like symptoms (fever, chills, myalgia, or malaise) but these decrease over time; nausea and vomiting occur occasionally. Other side-effects include hypersensitivity reactions (including anaphylaxis and urticaria), raised liver enzymes (hepatitis reported rarely with interferon beta-1b), blood disorders, menstrual disorders, mood and personality changes, suicide attempts, confusion and convulsions; alopecia and thyroid dysfunction have been reported rarely with interferon beta-1b.

It is recommended that patients should be referred to a neurologist for a decision on whether treatment with interferon beta is indicated (see also Note below).

INTERFERON BETA

Indications: see notes above

Note. The Standing Medical Advisory Committee on the use of Interferon Beta-1b in Relapsing-Remitting Multiple Sclerosis in Adults has recommended that patients, in England and Wales, who apparently fulfil the indications for treatment should be referred to a neurologist for a decision on whether treatment in indicated. Similar advice has been provided in Scotland

Cautions; Contra-indications; Side-effects: see notes above—but for full details (including monitoring and dosage details) consult product literature; pregnancy (Appendix 4—advise contraceptive measures if appropriate), breast-feeding (Appendix 5)

■ Interferon beta-1a

Avonex® (Biogen) ▼ PoM

Injection, powder for reconstitution, interferon beta-1a. Net price 30-microgram (6 million unit) vial with diluent = £174.25. For intramuscular injection

Rebif® (Serono) ▼ PoM

Injection, interferon beta-1a, net price 22-microgram (6 million unit) prefilled syringe = £58.26; 44-microgram (12 million unit) prefilled syringe = £77.36. For subcutaneous injection

---

■ Interferon beta-1b

Betaferon® (Schering Health) ▼ PoM

Injection, powder for reconstitution, interferon beta-1b. Net price 300-microgram (9.6 million unit) vial with diluent = £51.06. For subcutaneous injection

---

8.2.5   Aldesleukin

Aldesleukin (recombinant interleukin-2) is licensed for use by subcutaneous injection in metastatic renal cell carcinoma; it is no longer given by intravenous infusion. Aldesleukin is a very toxic drug which, although responsible for tumour shrinkage in a small proportion of patients, has not been shown to increase survival. Toxicity is universal and often severe. A common acute problem is the development of a capillary leak syndrome causing pulmonary oedema and hypotension. Bone marrow, hepatic, renal, thyroid, and CNS toxicity is also common. It is for use in **specialist units only. Interactions:** Appendix 1 (aldesleukin)

Proleukin® (Chiron) PoM

Injection, powder for reconstitution, aldesleukin. Net price 18-million unit vial = £140.00

For metastatic renal cell carcinoma, **excluding** patients in whom all three of the following prognostic factors are present; performance status of Eastern Co-operative Oncology Group of 1 or greater, more than one organ with metastatic disease sites, and a period of less than 24 months between initial diagnosis of primary tumour and date of evaluation of treatment.

8.3	**Sex hormones and hormone antagonists in malignant disease**
8.3.1	Oestrogens
8.3.2	Progestogens
8.3.3	Androgens
8.3.4	Hormone antagonists

Hormonal manipulation has an important role in the treatment of metastatic breast, prostate, and endometrial cancer, and a more marginal role in the treatment of hypernephroma. These treatments are not curative, but may provide excellent palliation of symptoms in selected patients, sometimes for a period of years. Tumour response, and treatment toxicity should be carefully monitored and treatment changed if progression occurs or side-effects exceed benefit.

8.3.1   Oestrogens

Diethylstilbestrol (stilboestrol) is rarely used to treat prostate cancer because of its side-effects. It is occasionally used in postmenopausal women with breast cancer. Toxicity is common and dose-related side-effects include nausea, fluid retention, and venous and arterial thrombosis. Impotence and gynaecomastia always occur in men, and withdrawal bleeding may be a problem in women. Hypercalcaemia and bone pain may also occur in breast cancer.

Fosfestrol is also used for prostate cancer; it is activated by the enzyme acid phosphatase to produce diethylstilbestrol. Side-effects are as for diethylstilbestrol; in addition, perineal pain may complicate intravenous use.

Ethinylestradiol (ethinyloestradiol) is the most potent oestrogen available; unlike other oestrogens it is only slowly metabolised in the liver. It is used in breast cancer.

DIETHYLSTILBESTROL

(Stilboestrol)

Indications: see notes above

Cautions: cardiovascular disease; hepatic impairment

Side-effects: sodium retention with oedema, thromboembolism, jaundice, feminising effects in men; see also notes above

Dose: breast cancer, 10–20 mg daily
Prostate cancer, 1–3 mg daily

Diethylstilbestrol (Non-proprietary) PoM

Tablets, diethylstilbestrol 1 mg, net price 56 = £48.00; 5 mg, 28 = £36.00
Available from APS (*Apstil®*)

ETHINYLESTRADIOL

(Ethinyloestradiol)

Indications: see notes above; other indications (section 6.4.1.1)

Cautions: see under Diethylstilbestrol and notes above

Side-effects: see under Diethylstilbestrol and notes above

Dose: breast cancer, 1–3 mg daily

Preparations
Section 6.4.1.1

FOSFESTROL TETRASODIUM

Indications: prostate cancer

Cautions: see under Diethylstilbestrol and notes above

Side-effects: see under Diethylstilbestrol and notes above; nausea and vomiting; after intravenous injection, perineal irritation and pain in bony metastases

Dose: *by slow intravenous injection*, 600–1200 mg daily for at least 5 days; maintenance 300 mg 1–4 times weekly

By mouth, maintenance, initially up to 240 mg 3 times daily for 7 days then reducing over 14 days to 120–360 mg daily in divided doses

Honvan® (ASTA Medica) PoM

Tablets, f/c, fosfestrol tetrasodium 120 mg, net price 100-tab pack = £14.81
Note. Fosfestrol tetrasodium 100 mg tablets have now been replaced by 120 mg tablets
Injection, fosfestrol tetrasodium 60 mg/mL, net price 5-mL amp = £1.43

8.3.2   Progestogens

Progestogens are used largely as second- or third-line therapy in breast cancer. They are also used to treat endometrial cancer and renal cell carcinoma, but are little used for prostate cancer. **Medroxyprogesterone** or **megestrol** are usually chosen and can be given orally; high-dose or parenteral treatment cannot be recommended. Side-effects are mild but may include nausea, fluid retention, and weight gain.

GESTONORONE CAPROATE

(Gestronol Hexanoate)

Indications: see notes above; benign prostatic hypertrophy

Cautions: see under Medroxyprogesterone acetate (section 6.4.1.2) and notes above

Contra-indications: see under Medroxyprogesterone acetate (section 6.4.1.2) and notes above

Side-effects: see under Medroxyprogesterone acetate (section 6.4.1.2) and notes above

Dose: endometrial cancer, *by intramuscular injection*, 200–400 mg every 5–7 days

Benign prostatic hypertrophy, *by intramuscular injection*, 200 mg every week, increased to 300–400 mg every week if necessary

Gestonorone Caproate (Non-proprietary) PoM
Injection (oily), gestonorone caproate 100 mg/mL. Net price 2-mL amp = £12.50
Available from Cambridge

MEDROXYPROGESTERONE ACETATE

Indications: see notes above; other indications (section 6.4.1.2)

Cautions: see section 6.4.1.2 and notes above; **interactions:** Appendix 1 (progestogens)

Contra-indications: see section 6.4.1.2 and notes above

Side-effects: see section 6.4.1.2 and notes above; glucocorticoid effects at high dose may lead to a cushingoid syndrome

Dose: *by mouth*, endometrial, prostate, and renal cancer, 100–500 mg daily; breast cancer, various doses in range 0.4–1.5 g daily

By deep intramuscular injection into the gluteal muscle, various doses in range 1 g daily down to 250 mg weekly

Depo-Provera Oncology® (Pharmacia & Upjohn) PoM
Injection, medroxyprogesterone acetate 150 mg/mL. Net price 3.3-mL (500-mg) vial = £12.49

Farlutal® (Pharmacia & Upjohn) PoM
Tablets, both scored, medroxyprogesterone acetate 100 mg, net price 20 = £7.75; 250 mg, 50 = £48.45
Tablets, scored, medroxyprogesterone acetate 500 mg. Net price 56 = £108.52. Label: 27
Injection, medroxyprogesterone acetate 200 mg/mL. Net price 2.5-mL vial = £13.26

Provera® (Pharmacia & Upjohn) PoM
Tablets, medroxyprogesterone acetate 100 mg (scored), net price 60-tab pack = £23.86; 200 mg (scored), 30-tab pack = £23.60; 400 mg, 30-tab pack = £46.69
Tablets, medroxyprogesterone acetate 2.5 mg, 5 mg and 10 mg, see section 6.4.1.2

MEGESTROL ACETATE

Indications: see notes above

Cautions: see under Medroxyprogesterone acetate (section 6.4.1.2) and notes above

Contra-indications: see under Medroxyprogesterone acetate (section 6.4.1.2) and notes above

Side-effects: see under Medroxyprogesterone acetate (section 6.4.1.2) and notes above

Dose: breast cancer, 160 mg daily in single or divided doses; endometrial cancer, 40–320 mg daily in divided doses

Megace® (Bristol-Myers) PoM
Tablets, both scored, megestrol acetate 40 mg, net price 20 = £5.08; 160 mg (off-white), 30-tab pack = £29.30

NORETHISTERONE

Indications: see notes above; other indications, (section 6.4.1.2)

Cautions: see section 6.4.1.2 and notes above; **interactions:** Appendix 1 (progestogens)

Contra-indications: see section 6.4.1.2 and notes above

Side-effects: see section 6.4.1.2 and notes above

Dose: breast cancer, 40 mg daily, increased to 60 mg daily if required

Preparations
Section 6.4.1.2

8.3.3   Androgens

Testosterone esters (section 6.4.2) are occasionally still used as second- or third-line therapy for metastatic breast cancer.

8.3.4   Hormone antagonists

8.3.4.1   Breast cancer

The management of patients with breast cancer involves surgery, radiotherapy, drug therapy, or a combination of these. All women with invasive breast cancer should be considered for adjuvant therapy, which is determined by an assessment of the risk of recurrence, oestrogen-receptor status of the primary tumour, and menopausal status.

Tamoxifen is an oestrogen-receptor antagonist and at a dose of 20 mg daily is the adjuvant hormonal treatment of choice in women with oestrogen-receptor-positive breast cancer. This treatment delays the growth of metastases and increases survival; if tolerated it should be continued for at least 5 years.

Tamoxifen is also the hormonal treatment of choice in women with oestrogen-receptor-positive metastatic breast cancer. Approximately 60% of such patients respond to initial hormonal manipulation, whereas less than 10% of oestrogen-receptor-negative tumours respond.

Severe side-effects are unusual with tamoxifen but patients with bony metastases may experience an exacerbation of pain, sometimes associated with hypercalcaemia; this reaction commonly precedes tumour response. Amenorrhoea commonly develops in premenopausal women. For details of endometrial changes see under Cautions and for CSM advice see under Dose.

Patients with non-life-threatening metastases unresponsive to tamoxifen rarely respond to a secondary hormonal treatment. However, patients who initially respond to tamoxifen may respond to second-line hormone treatment. For premenopausal women ovarian ablation or a progestogen (section 8.3.2) can be used; for postmenopausal patients a progestogen or a newer aromatase inhibitor (see below) can be used. The newer aromatase inhibitors are well tolerated and are more effective than progestogens. Patients who respond can be given further hormone treatment on relapse; refractory disease is better treated with chemotherapy or managed with palliative therapy.

Toremifene, also an oestrogen-receptor antagonist, is licensed for hormone-dependent metastatic breast cancer in postmenopausal women.

Aminoglutethimide, an aromatase inhibitor, acts predominantly by blocking the conversion of androgens to oestrogens in the peripheral tissues; in breast cancer it has largely been replaced by the newer aromatase inhibitors which are better tolerated. Aminoglutethimide is also used as second-line treatment for prostate cancer (section 8.3.4.2). Aminoglutethimide may cause adrenal hypofunction and corticosteroid replacement therapy is necessary (section 6.3.1). Early toxicity is common and may include drowsiness, drug fever, and a morbilliform eruption; these side-effects generally settle spontaneously. Hepatic enzyme induction occurs, and may require modification of the doses of other drugs (e.g. oral anticoagulants).

Trilostane (section 6.7.3) is also indicated for postmenopausal breast cancer. It is quite well tolerated but diarrhoea and abdominal discomfort may be a problem. Like aminoglutethimide, trilostane may cause adrenal hypofunction and corticosteroid replacement therapy is needed.

Formestane, also an aromatase inhibitor, is indicated for breast cancer in women with natural or artificial postmenopausal status.

Anastrozole and **letrozole** are selective non-steroidal aromatase inhibitors used to treat advanced postmenopausal breast cancer. They are much better tolerated than aminoglutethimide and steroid replacement therapy is not necessary.

Goserelin (section 8.3.4.2), a gonadorelin analogue is now also indicated for management of advanced breast cancer in premenopausal women.

TAMOXIFEN

Indications: see under Dose and notes above

Cautions: occasional cystic ovarian swellings in premenopausal women, occasional hypercalcaemia if bony metastases; increased risk of thromboembolic events when used with cytotoxics; porphyria (section 9.8.2); **interactions:** Appendix 1 (tamoxifen)

ENDOMETRIAL CHANGES. An increased incidence of endometrial changes, including hyperplasia, polyps and cancer, has been reported in association with tamoxifen. Abnormal vaginal bleeding including menstrual irregularities, vaginal discharge and symptoms such as pelvic pain or pressure in those receiving (or who have previously received) tamoxifen should be promptly investigated.

Contra-indications: pregnancy (exclude before commencing and advise non-hormonal contra-

ception if appropriate—Appendix 4) and breast-feeding (Appendix 5)

Side-effects: hot flushes, vaginal bleeding (**important:** see also Cautions) or suppression of menstruation in some pre-menopausal women, vaginal discharge (**important:** see also Cautions), pruritus vulvae, gastro-intestinal disturbances, headache, light-headedness, tumour flare, falls in platelet counts; occasionally fluid retention, alopecia, rashes, uterine fibroids; also visual disturbances (including corneal changes, cataracts, retinopathy—usually with very high doses); leucopenia (sometimes with anaemia and thrombocytopenia), rarely neutropenia; hypertriglyceridaemia reported; thromboembolic events reported; liver enzyme changes (rarely fatty liver, cholestasis, hepatitis); rarely hypersensitivity reactions including angioedema, Stevens-Johnson syndrome, bullous pemphigoid; see also notes above

Dose: breast cancer, 20 mg daily

CSM ADVICE. The CSM has advised that tamoxifen in a dose of 20 mg daily substantially increases survival in early breast cancer, and that no further benefit has been demonstrated with higher doses. Patients should be told of the small risk of endometrial cancer (see under Cautions above) and encouraged to report relevant symptoms early. They can, however, be reassured that the benefits of treatment far outweigh the risks

Anovulatory infertility, 20 mg daily on second, third, fourth and fifth days of cycle; if necessary the daily dose may be increased to 40 mg then 80 mg for subsequent courses; if cycles irregular, start initial course on any day, with subsequent course starting 45 days later *or* on second day of cycle if menstruation occurs

Tamoxifen (Non-proprietary) PoM

Tablets, tamoxifen (as citrate) 10 mg, net price 30-tab pack = £3.88; 20 mg, 30-tab pack = £5.29; 40 mg, 30-tab pack = £12.86

Various strengths available from APS, Ashbourne (*Oestrifen®*), Berk (*Emblon®*), Cox, CP, Hillcross, Kent, Norton, Opus (*Fentamox®*), Pharmacia & Upjohn (*Tamofen®*)

Oral solution, tamoxifen (as citrate) 10 mg/5mL, net price 150 mL = £31.50

Available from Rosemont (*Soltamox®*)

Nolvadex® (Zeneca) PoM

Tablets, tamoxifen (as citrate) 10 mg, net price 30-tab pack = £5.78; 20 mg (*Nolvadex-D®*), 30-tab pack = £8.71; 40 mg (scored, *Nolvadex-Forte®*), 30-tab pack = £20.48

AMINOGLUTETHIMIDE

Indications: see notes above and under Dose

Cautions: see notes above; adrenal hypofunction (see below); monitor blood pressure, plasma electrolytes, blood counts, and thyroid function; **interactions:** Appendix 1 (aminoglutethimide)

ADRENAL HYPOFUNCTION. May cause adrenal hypofunction especially under conditions of stress (such as surgery, trauma, or acute illness), therefore corticosteroid replacement therapy is necessary (section 6.3.1). If a synthetic glucocorticoid such as dexamethasone is used instead of hydrocortisone a relatively high dose may be needed (metabolism of synthetic corticosteroids accelerated)

Contra-indications: pregnancy (advise non-hormonal contraceptive methods if appropriate) and breast-feeding; porphyria (section 9.8.2)

Side-effects: see notes above; drowsiness, lethargy, rash (sometimes with fever—usually in first 2 weeks and resolves despite continued administration); occasionally dizziness, nausea; other side-effects reported include ataxia, headache, depression, insomnia, pruritus, urticaria, diarrhoea, vomiting, constipation, anorexia, sweating, hypotension, adrenal insufficiency, hyponatraemia, hypoglycaemia, agranulocytosis, leucopenia, thrombocytopenia, hyperkalaemia, exfoliative dermatitis, Stevens-Johnson syndrome, hypothyroidism, inappropriate ADH-secretion, masculinisation and hirsutism in females, renal impairment, pancytopenia, anaemia, allergy, anaphylactic reactions, allergic alveolitis (withdraw immediately if suspected), cholestatic hepatitis, confusion

Dose: advanced breast and prostate cancer, 250 mg daily, increased once a week to max. 250 mg 4 times daily (in breast cancer 250 mg twice daily has proved sufficient in some patients; in prostate cancer up to 750 mg daily is usually satisfactory); given with a glucocorticoid (and sometimes with a mineralocorticoid as well)

Cushing's syndrome due to malignant disease, 250 mg daily, increased gradually to 1 g daily in divided doses (occasionally 1.5–2 g daily); glucocorticoid given only if necessary

Orimeten® (Novartis) PoM
Tablets, scored, aminoglutethimide 250 mg. Net price 56-tab pack = £20.22. Label: 2
Note. Tablets containing aminoglutethimide 250 mg are also available from Pharmacia & Upjohn

ANASTROZOLE

Indications: advanced breast cancer in postmenopausal women

Cautions: laboratory test for menopause if doubt

Contra-indications: pregnancy and breast-feeding; moderate or severe hepatic disease, moderate or severe renal impairment; not for premenopausal women

Side-effects: hot flushes, vaginal dryness, vaginal bleeding, hair thinning, anorexia, nausea, vomiting, diarrhoea, headache, rash; asthenia and somnolence—may initially affect ability to drive or operate machinery; slight increases in total cholesterol levels reported

Dose: 1 mg daily

Arimidex® (Zeneca) PoM
Tablets, f/c, anastrozole 1 mg. Net price 28-tab pack = £83.16

FORMESTANE

Indications: advanced breast cancer in women with natural or artificial postmenopausal status

Cautions: no studies performed in diabetes mellitus (monitor blood glucose)
DRIVING. Drowsiness may affect performance of skilled tasks (e.g. driving)

Contra-indications: not indicated for premenopausal women; pregnancy and breast-feeding

Side-effects: nausea, vomiting, rash, pruritus, exanthema, hot flushes; rarely, facial hypertrichosis, alopecia, lethargy, drowsiness, emotional lability, headache, dizziness, oedema of lower leg, thrombophlebitis, vaginal bleeding and inflammation, pelvic cramps, constipation, diarrhoea, arthralgia and exacerbation of bone pain, muscle cramps, sore throat, and anaphylactoid reaction; pain and irritation common at injection site (with occasional sterile abscess and rarely haematoma)

Dose: *by deep intramuscular injection* in the gluteal muscle, 250 mg every 2 weeks (alternate sites)

Lentaron® (Novartis) PoM
Injection, powder for reconstitution, formestane 250 mg. Net price 250-mg vial (with diluent) = £72.73. Counselling, driving

LETROZOLE

Indications: advanced breast cancer in postmenopausal women in whom other anti-oestrogen therapy has failed

Cautions: severe renal impairment

Contra-indications: severe hepatic impairment; not indicated for premenopausal women; pregnancy and breast-feeding

Side-effects: hot flushes, nausea, vomiting, dyspepsia, constipation, diarrhoea, abdominal pain, anorexia (and weight gain), dyspnoea, chest pain, coughing, dizziness, fatigue, headache, infection, musculoskeletal pain, peripheral oedema, rash, pruritus

Dose: 2.5 mg daily until tumour progression is evident

Femara® (Novartis) ▼ PoM
Tablets, f/c, letrozole 2.5 mg. Net price 14-tab pack = £41.58, 28-tab pack = £83.16

TOREMIFENE

Indications: hormone-dependent metastatic breast cancer in postmenopausal women

Cautions: hypercalcaemia may occur (especially if bone metastases and usually at beginning of treatment); **interactions:** Appendix 1 (toremifene)
ENDOMETRIAL CHANGES. There is a risk of increased endometrial changes including hyperplasia, polyps and cancer. Abnormal vaginal bleeding including menstrual irregularities, vaginal discharge and symptoms such as pelvic pain or pressure should be promptly investigated

Contra-indications: endometrial hyperplasia, severe hepatic impairment, history of severe thromboembolic disease; pregnancy and breast-feeding

Side-effects: hot flushes, vaginal bleeding or discharge (**important:** see also Cautions), dizziness, oedema, sweating, nausea, vomiting, chest or back pain, fatigue, headache, skin discoloration, weight increase, insomnia, constipation, dyspnoea, paresis, tremor, vertigo, pruritus, anorexia, corneal opacity (reversible), asthenia; thromboembolic events reported; rarely dermatitis, alopecia, emotional lability, depression, jaundice, stiffness

Dose: 60 mg daily

Fareston® (Orion) ▼ PoM
Tablets, toremifene (as citrate) 60 mg. Net price 30-tab pack = £30.37

8.3.4.2 Prostate cancer and gonadorelin analogues

Metastatic cancer of the prostate usually responds to hormonal treatment aimed at androgen depletion. The standard treatment is bilateral subcapsular orchidectomy, which commonly results in responses lasting 12–18 months. Alternatively, a gonadorelin analogue such as **buserelin**, **goserelin**, **leuprorelin**, or **triptorelin** may be given. Other therapies if disease progression occurs despite orchidectomy or treatment with a gonadorelin analogue, include the use of radiotherapy, strontium, antiandrogens, aminoglutethimide (section 8.3.4.1) or prednisolone (section 6.3.2). Such second-line treatment may palliate symptoms well, but rarely results in appreciable disease regression.

Gonadorelin analogues

Gonadorelin analogues are as effective as orchidectomy or **diethylstilbestrol** (section 8.3.1) but are expensive and require parenteral administration, at least initially. They cause initial stimulation then depression of luteinising hormone release by the pituitary. During the initial stage (1–2 weeks) increased production of testosterone by the testes may be associated with progression of prostate cancer. In susceptible patients this tumour 'flare' may cause spinal cord compression, ureteric obstruction or increased bone pain. When such problems are anticipated, alternative treatments (e.g. orchidectomy) or the additional use of an anti-androgen such as cyproterone acetate or flutamide (see below) are recommended; anti-androgen treatment should be started 3 days before the gonadorelin analogue and continued for 3 weeks. Gonadorelin analogues are also used in women for breast cancer (section 8.3.4.1) and other indications (section 6.7.2).

CAUTIONS. Men at risk of tumour 'flare' (see above) should be monitored closely during the first month of therapy. Caution is required in women with metabolic bone disease because decreases in bone mineral density may occur. The injection site should be rotated.

SIDE-EFFECTS. The gonadorelin analogues cause side-effects similar to the menopause in women and orchidectomy in men and include hot flushes and sweating, sexual dysfunction, vaginal dryness or bleeding, and gynaecomastia or changes in breast size. Signs and symptoms of prostate or breast cancer may worsen initially (managed in prostate cancer with anti-androgens, see above). Other side-effects include hypersensitivity reactions (rashes, pruritus, asthma, and rarely anaphylaxis), injection site reactions (see Cautions), headache (rarely migraine), visual disturbances, dizziness, arthralgia and possibly myalgia, hair loss, peripheral oedema, gastro-intestinal disturbances, weight changes, sleep disorders, and mood changes.

Anti-androgens

Cyproterone acetate, flutamide and **bicalutamide** are anti-androgens which can be used to cover the tumour 'flare' which may occur after commencing gonadorelin analogue administration. Cyproterone acetate and flutamide are also licensed for use alone in patients with metastatic prostate cancer refractory to gonadorelin analogue therapy. Bicalutamide is licensed for use alone in patients with locally advanced, non-metastatic prostate cancer.

BICALUTAMIDE

Indications: advanced prostate cancer, see also notes above

Cautions: hepatic impairment (Appendix 2), also consider periodic liver function tests; **interactions:** Appendix 1 (bicalutamide)

Side-effects: hot flushes, pruritus, breast tenderness, gynaecomastia, asthenia, somnolence; transient elevation of transaminase levels, cholestasis and jaundice (rarely hepatic failure); rarely thrombocytopenia, cardiovascular disorders (including angina, heart failure, conduction defects, arrhythmias and ECG changes); other effects (more common in elderly) include anorexia, dry mouth, dyspepsia, constipation, flatulence, dizziness, insomnia, decreased libido, impotence, dyspnoea, nocturia, alopecia, rashes, sweating, hyperglycaemia, peripheral oedema, weight changes, chest and abdominal pain

Dose: with orchidectomy or gonadorelin therapy, 50 mg daily (in gonadorelin therapy, started 3 days beforehand, see also notes above)

Locally advanced, non-metastatic prostate cancer, 150 mg once daily

Casodex® (Zeneca) PoM
Tablets, f/c, bicalutamide 50 mg, net price 28-tab pack = £128.00; 150 mg, 28-tab pack = £240.00

BUSERELIN

Indications: advanced prostate cancer; other indications (section 6.7.2)

Cautions: see notes above

Side-effects: see notes above; worsening hypertension, palpitations, glucose intolerance, altered blood lipids, elevated liver function tests, thrombocytopenia, leucopenia, nervousness, fatigue, memory and concentration disturbances, anxiety, increased thirst, hearing disorders; nasal irritation, nose bleeds and altered sense of taste and smell (spray formulation only)

Dose: *by subcutaneous injection*, 500 micrograms every 8 hours for 7 days, then *intranasally*, 1 spray into each nostril 6 times daily (see also notes above)

COUNSELLING. Avoid use of nasal decongestants before and for at least 30 minutes after treatment.

Suprefact® (Shire) PoM
Injection, buserelin 1 mg (as acetate)/mL. Net price 2 × 5.5-mL vial = £23.69
Nasal spray, buserelin 100 micrograms (as acetate)/metered spray. Net price treatment pack of 4 × 10-g bottle with spray pump = £87.68. Counselling, see above

CYPROTERONE ACETATE

Indications: prostate cancer, see under Dose and also notes above; other indications, see section 6.4.2

Cautions: in prostate cancer, blood counts initially and throughout treatment, hepatic impairment (Appendix 2); monitor hepatic function (liver function tests should be performed before treatment, see also under Side-effects below); monitor adrenocortical function regularly; risk of recurrence of thromboembolic disease; diabetes mellitus, sickle-cell anaemia, severe depression (in other indications some of these are contra-indicated, see section 6.4.2)

DRIVING. Fatigue and lassitude may impair performance of skilled tasks (e.g. driving)

Contra-indications: none in prostate cancer; for contra-indications relating to other indications see section 6.4.2

Side-effects: see section 6.4.2

HEPATOTOXICITY. Direct hepatic toxicity including jaundice, hepatitis and hepatic failure have been reported (usually after several months) in patients treated with cyproterone acetate 200–300 mg daily. Liver function tests should be performed before treatment and whenever symptoms suggestive of hepatotoxicity occur—if confirmed cyproterone should normally be withdrawn unless the hepatotoxicity can be explained by another cause such as metastatic disease (in which case cyproterone should be continued only if the perceived benefit exceeds the risk)

Dose: flare with initial gonadorelin therapy, 300 mg daily in 2–3 divided doses, reduced to 200 mg daily in 2–3 divided doses if necessary

Long-term palliative therapy where gonadorelin analogues or orchidectomy contra-indicated, not tolerated, or where oral therapy preferred, 200–300 mg daily in 2–3 divided doses

Hot flushes with gonadorelin therapy or after orchidectomy, initially 50 mg daily, adjusted according to response to 50–150 mg daily in 1–3 divided doses

Cyprostat® (Schering Health) PoM
Tablets, scored, cyproterone acetate 50 mg net price 168-tab pack = £96.70; 100 mg, 84-tab pack = £96.70. Label: 21

Note. Tablets containing cyproterone acetate 50 mg are also available from Cox, Generics, Hillcross

FLUTAMIDE

Indications: advanced prostate cancer, see also notes above

Cautions: cardiac disease (oedema reported); hepatic impairment (Appendix 2), also periodic liver function tests on long-term therapy and at the first sign or symptom indicating liver disorder (e.g. pruritus, dark urine, persistent anorexia, jaundice, abdominal pain, unexplained influenza-like symptoms); **interactions:** Appendix 1 (flutamide)

Side-effects: gynaecomastia (sometimes with galactorrhoea); nausea, vomiting, diarrhoea, increased appetite, insomnia, tiredness; other side-effects reported include decreased libido, inhibition of spermatogenesis, gastric and chest pain, headache, dizziness, oedema, blurred vision, thirst, rashes, pruritus, haemolytic anaemia, systemic lupus erythematosus-like syndrome, and lymphoedema; hepatic injury (with transaminase abnormalities, cholestatic jaundice, hepatic necrosis, encephalopathy and occasional fatality) reported

Dose: 250 mg 3 times daily (see also notes above)

Flutamide (Non-proprietary) PoM
Tablets, flutamide 250 mg. Net price 84-tab pack = £77.07

Available from Chiron (*Chimax®*), Cox, Generics, Hillcross, Orion

Drogenil® (Schering-Plough) PoM
Tablets, yellow, scored, flutamide 250 mg, net price 84-tab pack = £70.00

GOSERELIN

Indications: prostate cancer; advanced breast cancer; other indications (section 6.7.2)

Cautions: see notes above

Contra-indications: pregnancy and breast-feeding (Apendixes 4 and 5); undiagnosed vaginal bleeding

Side-effects: see notes above; also transient changes in blood pressure, rarely hypercalcaemia (in patients with metastatic breast cancer)

Dose: see under preparations below

Zoladex® (Zeneca) PoM
Implant, goserelin 3.6 mg (as acetate) in syringe applicator. Net price each = £122.27
Dose: advanced breast cancer and prostate cancer *by subcutaneous injection* into anterior abdominal wall, 3.6 mg every 28 days (see also notes above)

Zoladex® LA (Zeneca) PoM
Implant, goserelin 10.8 mg (as acetate) in syringe applicator. Net price each = £366.81
Dose: prostate cancer, *by subcutaneous injection* into anterior abdominal wall, 10.8 mg every 12 weeks (see also notes above)

LEUPRORELIN ACETATE

Indications: advanced prostate cancer; other indications (section 6.7.2)

Cautions: see notes above

Side-effects: see notes above; also fatigue, muscle weakness, paraesthesia, hypertension, palpitations; thrombocytopenia and leucopenia reported

Dose: see under preparations below

Prostap® SR (Wyeth) PoM
Injection (microsphere powder for reconstitution), leuprorelin acetate, net price 3.75-mg vial with 1-mL vehicle-filled syringe = £125.40
Dose: advanced prostate cancer and endometriosis, *by subcutaneous or by intramuscular injection*, 3.75 mg every 4 weeks (see also notes above)

Prostap® 3 (Wyeth) PoM
Injection (microsphere powder for reconstitution), leuprorelin acetate, net price 11.25-mg vial with 2-mL vehicle-filled syringe = £376.20
Dose: advanced prostate cancer, *by subcutaneous injection*, 11.25 mg every three months (see also notes above)

TRIPTORELIN

Indications: advanced prostate cancer; endometriosis (section 6.7.2)

Cautions: see notes above

Side-effects: see notes above; transient hypertension, dry mouth, excessive salivation, increased dysuria

Dose: *by intramuscular injection*, 3 mg every 4 weeks (see also notes above)

De-capeptyl® sr (Ipsen) PoM
Injection (copolymer microsphere powder for aqueous suspension), triptorelin. Net price 4.2-mg vial (with diluent) = £105.05

8.3.4.3 Somatostatin analogues

Octreotide and the recently introduced drug, **lanreotide** are analogues of the hypothalamic release-inhibiting hormone somatostatin. They are indicated for the relief of symptoms associated with neuroendocrine (particularly carcinoid) tumours and acromegaly. Octreotide is also licensed for the prevention of complications following pancreatic surgery; it may also be valuable in stopping variceal bleeding [unlicensed indication]—see also vasopressin and terlipressin (section 6.5.2).

CAUTIONS. Growth hormone-secreting pituitary tumours can expand causing serious complications; during treatment with somatostatin analogues patients should be monitored for signs of tumour expansion (e.g. visual field defects). Ultrasound examination of the gallbladder is recommended before treatment and at intervals of 6–12 months during treatment (avoid abrupt withdrawal of short-acting octreotide—see Side-effects below). In insulinoma an increase in the depth and duration of hypoglycaemia may occur (observe patients when initiating treatment and changing doses); in diabetes mellitus, insulin or oral antidiabetic requirements may be reduced. Thyroid function should be monitored on long-term therapy.

SIDE-EFFECTS. Gastro-intestinal disturbances including anorexia, nausea, vomiting, abdominal pain and bloating, flatulence, diarrhoea, and steatorrhoea may occur. Postprandial glucose tolerance may be impaired and rarely persistent hyperglycaemia occurs with chronic administration; hypoglycaemia has also been reported. Gallstones have been reported after long-term treatment (abrupt withdrawal of subcutaneous octreotide is associated with biliary colic and pancreatitis). Pain and irritation may occur at the injection site and sites should be rotated.

OCTREOTIDE

Indications: see under Dose

Cautions: see notes above; hepatic impairment (Appendix 2); pregnancy and breast-feeding (Appendixes 4 and 5); **interactions:** Appendix 1 (octreotide)

Side-effects: see notes above; rarely altered liver function tests, hepatitis, pancreatitis and transient alopecia

Dose: symptoms associated with carcinoid tumours with features of carcinoid syndrome, VIPomas, glucagonomas, *by subcutaneous injection*, initially 50 micrograms once or twice daily, gradually increased according to response to 200 micrograms 3 times daily (higher doses required exceptionally); maintenance doses variable; in carcinoid tumours discontinue after 1 week if no effect; if rapid response required, initial dose *by intravenous injection* (with ECG monitoring and after dilution to a concentration of 10–50% with sodium chloride 0.9% injection)

Acromegaly, short-term treatment before pituitary surgery *or* long-term treatment in those inadequately controlled by other treatment *or* until radiotherapy becomes fully effective *by subcutaneous injection*, 100–200 micrograms 3 times daily; discontinue if no improvement within 3 months

Prevention of complications following pancreatic surgery, consult product literature

Sandostatin® (Novartis) PoM
Injection, octreotide (as acetate)
50 micrograms/mL, 1-mL amp = £2.90;
100 micrograms/mL, 1-mL amp = £5.46;
200 micrograms/mL 5-mL vial = £54.39;
500 micrograms/mL, 1-mL amp = £26.45

■ Depot preparation
Sandostatin LAR® (Novartis) ▼ PoM
Injection (microsphere powder for aqueous suspension), octreotide (as acetate) 10-mg vial = £637.50; 20-mg vial = £850.00; 30-mg vial = £1062.50 (all supplied with diluent and syringe)
Dose: acromegaly and neuroendocrine tumours in patients adequately controlled on subcutaneous octreotide, *by deep intramuscular injection* (into the gluteal muscle), initially 20 mg every 4 weeks for 3 months, then adjusted according to symptoms and laboratory tests; max. 30 mg every 4 weeks
For acromegaly, start depot octreotide 1 day after the last dose of subcutaneous octreotide; for neuroendocrine tumours, continue subcutaneous octreotide for 2 weeks after first dose of depot octreotide

LANREOTIDE

Indications: see notes above

Cautions: see notes above; pregnancy and breast-feeding (Appendixes 4 and 5); **interactions:** Appendix 1 (lanreotide)

Side-effects: see notes above

Dose: acromegaly, *by intramuscular injection*, initially 30 mg every 14 days for 3 months; at 3 months increase dose if necessary to 30 mg every 7–10 days; if poor initial response before third fortnightly injection increase dose to 30 mg every 7–10 days

Neuroendocrine tumours, as for acromegaly; adjust dose interval according to symptoms

Somatuline® LA (Ipsen) ▼ PoM
Injection (copolymer microparticles for aqueous suspension), lanreotide (as acetate) 30-mg vial (with vehicle) = £334.25.

9: Nutrition and blood

9.1 Anaemias and some other blood disorders

9.1.1 Iron-deficiency anaemias
9.1.2 Drugs used in megaloblastic anaemias
9.1.3 Drugs used in hypoplastic, haemolytic, and renal anaemias
9.1.4 Drugs used in autoimmune thrombocytopenic purpura
9.1.5 G6PD deficiency
9.1.6 Drugs used in neutropenia

Before initiating treatment for anaemia it is essential to determine which type is present. Iron salts may be harmful and result in iron overload if given alone to patients with anaemias other than those due to iron deficiency.

9.1.1 Iron-deficiency anaemias

9.1.1.1 Oral iron
9.1.1.2 Parenteral iron

Treatment is only justified in the presence of a demonstrable iron-deficiency state. Before starting treatment, it is important to exclude any serious underlying cause of the anaemia (e.g. gastric erosion, colonic carcinoma).

Prophylaxis is justifiable in pregnancy only for women who have additional risk factors for iron deficiency (e.g. poor diet), menorrhagia, after subtotal or total gastrectomy, and in the management of low birth-weight infants such as premature babies, twins, and in infants delivered by caesarean section.

9.1.1.1 Oral iron

Iron salts should be given by mouth unless there are good reasons for using another route.

Ferrous salts show only marginal differences between one another in efficiency of absorption of iron, but ferric salts are much less well absorbed. Haemoglobin regeneration rate is little affected by the type of salt used provided sufficient iron is given, and in most patients the time factor is not critical. Choice of preparation is thus usually decided by incidence of side-effects and cost.

The oral dose of elemental iron for deficiency should be 100 to 200 mg daily. It is customary to give this as dried **ferrous sulphate**, 200 mg ($\equiv$ 65 mg elemental iron) three times daily; a dose of ferrous sulphate 200 mg once or twice daily may be effective for prophylaxis or for mild iron deficiency. If side-effects arise, dosage can be reduced or a change made to an alternative iron salt. It should be remembered, however, that an apparent improvement in tolerance on changing to another salt may be due to its lower content of elemental iron. The incidence of side-effects due to ferrous sulphate is no greater than with other iron salts when compared on the basis of equivalent amounts of elemental iron.

Iron content of different iron salts

Iron salt	Amount	Content of ferrous iron
Ferrous fumarate	200 mg	65 mg
Ferrous gluconate	300 mg	35 mg
Ferrous succinate	100 mg	35 mg
Ferrous sulphate	300 mg	60 mg
Ferrous sulphate, dried	200 mg	65 mg

THERAPEUTIC RESPONSE. The haemoglobin concentration should rise by about 100–200 mg per 100 mL (1–2 g per litre) per day *or* 2 g/100 mL (20 g/litre) over 3–4 weeks. After the haemoglobin has risen to normal, treatment should be continued for a further three months in an attempt to replenish the iron stores. Epithelial tissue changes such as atrophic glossitis and koilonychia are usually improved although the response is often slow.

COMPOUND PREPARATIONS. Some oral preparations contain ascorbic acid to aid absorption, or the iron is in the form of a chelate, which can be shown experimentally to produce a modest increase in absorption of iron. However, the therapeutic advantage is minimal and cost may be increased.

There is neither theoretical nor clinical justification for the inclusion of other therapeutically active ingredients, such as the B group of vitamins (except folic acid for pregnant women, see Iron and Folic Acid below and p. 412).

MODIFIED-RELEASE CAPSULES AND TABLETS. These are designed to release iron gradually as the capsule or tablet passes along the gut so that a smaller amount of iron is present in the lumen at any one time. It is claimed that each dose unit contains enough iron for 24 hours, thus permitting once daily dosage.

These preparations are likely to carry the iron past the first part of the duodenum into an area of the gut where conditions for iron absorption are poor. The low incidence of side-effects may well be because of the small amounts of iron available under these conditions and so the preparations have no therapeutic advantage and should not be used.

SIDE-EFFECTS. Because iron salts are astringent, gastro-intestinal irritation may occur. Nausea and epigastric pain are dose-related but the relationship between dose and altered bowel habit (constipation or diarrhoea) is less clear. Oral iron, particularly modified-release preparations, may exacerbate diarrhoea in patients with inflammatory bowel disease; care is also needed in patients with intestinal strictures and diverticulae.

Iron preparations taken orally may have a constipating effect particularly in older patients, occasionally leading to faecal impaction.

FERROUS SULPHATE

Indications: iron-deficiency anaemia
Cautions: pregnancy; **interactions:** Appendix 1 (iron)
Side-effects: see notes above
Dose: see under preparations below
COUNSELLING. Although iron preparations are best absorbed on an empty stomach they may be taken after food to reduce gastro-intestinal side-effects; they may discolour stools

Ferrous Sulphate (Non-proprietary)
Tablets, coated, dried ferrous sulphate 200 mg (65 mg iron), net price 20 = 53p
Dose: prophylactic, 1 tablet daily; therapeutic, 1 tablet 2–3 times daily

■ Modified-release preparations
Feospan® (Medeva) [NHS] [◀]
Spansule® (= capsules m/r), clear/red, enclosing green and brown pellets, dried ferrous sulphate 150 mg (47 mg iron). Net price 30-cap pack = £1.11. Label: 25
Dose: 1–2 capsules daily; CHILD over 1 year 1 capsule daily; can be opened and sprinkled on food

Ferrograd® (Abbott)
Filmtabs® (= tablets f/c), m/r, red, dried ferrous sulphate 325 mg (105 mg iron). Net price 30-tab pack = 54p. Label: 25
Dose: 1 tablet daily before food

Slow-Fe® (Novartis) [◀]
Tablets, m/r, dried ferrous sulphate 160 mg (50 mg iron). Net price 28-tab pack = 25p. Label: 25
Dose: prophylactic, 1 tablet daily; therapeutic, 2 tablets daily; CHILD over 6 years, 1 tablet daily

> [◀] denotes preparations that are considered to be less suitable for prescribing (see p. vi)

FERROUS FUMARATE

Indications: iron-deficiency anaemia
Cautions: pregnancy; **interactions:** Appendix 1 (iron)
Side-effects: see notes above
Dose: see under preparations below

Fersaday® (Goldshield)
Tablets, brown, f/c, ferrous fumarate 322 mg (100 mg iron). Net price 28-tab pack = 50p
Dose: prophylactic, 1 tablet daily; therapeutic, 1 tablet twice daily

Fersamal® (Goldshield)
Tablets, brown, ferrous fumarate 210 mg (68 mg iron). Net price 20 = 24p
Dose: 1–2 tablets 3 times daily
Syrup, brown, ferrous fumarate approx. 140 mg (45 mg iron)/5 mL. Net price 200 mL = £2.35
Dose: 10–20 mL twice daily; PREMATURE INFANT 0.6–2.4 mL/kg daily; CHILD up to 6 years 2.5–5 mL twice daily

Galfer® (Galen)
Capsules, red/green, ferrous fumarate 305 mg (100 mg iron). Net price 20 = 36p
Dose: 1 capsule 1–2 times daily before food
Syrup, brown, sugar-free ferrous fumarate 140 mg (45 mg iron)/5 mL. Net price 300 mL = £4.86
Dose: 10 mL 1–2 times daily before food; CHILD (full-term infant and young child) 2.5–5 mL 1–2 times daily

FERROUS GLUCONATE

Indications: iron-deficiency anaemia
Cautions: pregnancy; **interactions:** Appendix 1 (iron)
Side-effects: see notes above
Dose: see under preparation below

Ferrous Gluconate (Non-proprietary)
Tablets, red, coated, ferrous gluconate 300 mg
(35 mg iron). Net price 20 = 45p
Dose: prophylactic, 2 tablets daily before food; therapeutic, 4–6 tablets daily in divided doses before food;
CHILD 6–12 years, prophylactic and therapeutic, 1–3
tablets daily

FERROUS GLYCINE SULPHATE

Indications: iron-deficiency anaemia
Cautions: pregnancy; **interactions:** Appendix 1
(iron)
Side-effects: see notes above
Dose: see under preparation below

Plesmet® (Link)
Syrup, ferrous glycine sulphate equivalent to
25 mg iron/5 mL. Net price 100 mL = 62p
Dose: 5–10 mL 3 times daily; CHILD 2.5–5 mL 1–3
times daily, according to age

POLYSACCHARIDE-IRON COMPLEX

Indications: iron-deficiency anaemia
Cautions: pregnancy; **interactions:** Appendix 1
(iron)
Side-effects: see notes above
Dose: see under preparation below

Niferex® (Tillomed)
Elixir, brown, sugar-free, polysaccharide-iron
complex equivalent to 100 mg of iron/5 mL. Net
price 240-mL pack = £6.06; NHS * 30-mL dropper bottle for paediatric use = £2.16. Counselling,
use of dropper
Dose: prophylactic, 2.5 mL daily; therapeutic, 5 mL 1–2
times daily (once daily if required during second and
third trimester of pregnancy); PREMATURE INFANT and
INFANT, (from dropper bottle) 1 drop (approx.
500 micrograms iron) per 450 g body-weight 3 times
daily; CHILD 2–6 years 2.5 mL daily, 6–12 years 5 mL
daily
* except 30 mL paediatric dropper bottle for prophylaxis
and treatment of iron deficiency in infants born prematurely and endorsed 'SLS'

Niferex-150® (Tillomed) NHS
Capsules, brown/orange, polysaccharide-iron
complex equivalent to 150 mg of iron. Net price
20 = £2.74
Dose: therapeutic, 1 capsule daily

SODIUM FEREDETATE

(Sodium ironedetate)
Indications: iron-deficiency anaemia
Cautions: pregnancy; **interactions:** Appendix 1
(iron)
Side-effects: see notes above
Dose: see under preparation below

Sytron® (Link)
Elixir, sugar-free, sodium feredetate 190 mg equivalent to 27.5 mg of iron/5 mL. Net price 100 mL =
94p
Dose: 5 mL increasing gradually to 10 mL 3 times daily;
INFANT and PREMATURE INFANT 2.5 mL twice daily
(smaller doses should be used initially); CHILD 1–5 years
2.5 mL 3 times daily, 6–12 years 5 mL 3 times daily

Iron and folic acid

These preparations are used for the prevention of
iron and folic acid deficiences in pregnancy; they
should be distinguished from those used for the prevention of neural tube defects in women planning a
pregnancy (see p. 414).

It is important to note that the small doses of folic
acid contained in these preparations are inadequate
for the treatment of megaloblastic anaemias.

Fefol® (Medeva) NHS
Spansule® (= capsules m/r), clear/green, enclosing
brown, yellow, and white pellets, dried ferrous
sulphate 150 mg (47 mg iron), folic acid
500 micrograms. Net price 30-cap pack = £1.18.
Label: 25
Dose: 1 capsule daily

Ferrograd Folic® (Abbott)
Filmtabs® (= tablets f/c), red/yellow, dried ferrous
sulphate 325 mg (105 mg iron) for sustained
release, folic acid 350 micrograms. Net price 30-
tab pack = 54p. Label: 25
Dose: 1 tablet daily before food

Galfer FA® (Galen)
Capsules, red/yellow, ferrous fumarate 305 mg
(100 mg iron), folic acid 350 micrograms. Net
price 20 = 40p
Dose: 1 capsule daily before food

Lexpec with Iron-M® (Rosemont) PoM
Syrup, brown, sugar-free, ferric ammonium citrate
equivalent to 80 mg iron, folic acid
500 micrograms/5 mL. Net price 125 mL = £3.63
Dose: 5–10 mL daily before food
Note. *Lexpec with Iron-M®* contains five times less folic
acid than *Lexpec with Iron®*

Pregaday® (Medeva)
Tablets, brown, f/c, ferrous fumarate equivalent to
100 mg iron, folic acid 350 micrograms. Net price
28-tab pack = 51p
Dose: 1 tablet daily

Slow-Fe Folic® (Novartis) PoM
Tablets, m/r, ivory, f/c, dried ferrous sulphate
160 mg (50 mg iron), folic acid 400 micrograms.
Net price 28-tab pack = 28p. Label: 25
Dose: 1–2 tablets daily

■ Higher folic acid content

Appropriate in context of prevention of *recurrence of
neural tube defects*, see recommendations on p. 414. *Cautions:* theoretical possibility of masking anaemia due to
vitamin-B_{12} deficiency (which could allow vitamin-B_{12}
neuropathy to develop).

Ferfolic SV® (Sinclair) NHS PoM
Tablets, pink, ferrous gluconate 250 mg (30 mg
iron), folic acid 4 mg, ascorbic acid 10 mg. Net
price 20 = 40p
Dose: anaemia, 1–3 tablets daily after food
Prophylaxis of neural tube defects in women known to
be at risk, 1 tablet daily started before conception and
continued for at least first trimester; see also recommendations on p. 414

Lexpec with Iron® (Rosemont) PoM
Syrup, brown, sugar-free, ferric ammonium citrate
equivalent to 80 mg iron, folic acid 2.5 mg/5 mL.
Net price 150 mL = £4.35
Dose: 5–10 mL daily before food
Note. *Lexpec with Iron®* contains five times as much
folic acid as *Lexpec with Iron-M®*

Compound iron preparations

There is no justification for prescribing compound iron preparations, except for preparations of iron and folic acid for prophylactic use in pregnancy (see above).

Ferrous Sulphate Tablets, Compound, (Non-proprietary) NHS ▰
Tablets, green, s/c, dried ferrous sulphate equivalent to 170 mg of $FeSO_4$, copper sulphate 2.5 mg, manganese sulphate 2.5 mg. Net price 20 tabs = 48p
Dose: 1–2 tablets daily

Ferrograd C® (Abbott) NHS ▰
Filmtabs® (= tablets f/c), red, dried ferrous sulphate 325 mg (105 mg iron) for sustained release, ascorbic acid 500 mg (as sodium salt). Net price 30-tab pack = £1.68. Label: 25
Dose: 1 tablet daily before food

Givitol® (Galen) NHS ▰
Capsules, red/maroon, ferrous fumarate 305 mg (100 mg iron) with vitamins B group and C. Net price 20 = 82p
Dose: 1 capsule daily before food

▰ denotes preparations that are considered to be less suitable for prescribing (see p. vi)

9.1.1.2   Parenteral iron

The only valid reason for administering iron parenterally is failure of oral therapy due to lack of patient cooperation, severe gastro-intestinal side-effects, continuing severe blood loss or malabsorption. Provided that the oral iron preparation is taken reliably and is absorbed, then the haemoglobin response is not significantly faster with the parenteral route. The need for a more rapid cure of the anaemia is therefore not met by parenteral administration of iron.

A suitable parenteral preparation contains a complex of iron, sorbitol and citric acid as **iron sorbitol injection**. It is given by deep intramuscular injection and is **not** suitable for intravenous injection; the low mean molecular weight allows rapid absorption from the injection site but, excretion in the saliva and substantial urinary losses occur. To prevent leakage along the needle track with subsequent staining of the skin, intramuscular injections should be deep with suitable technique.

Iron sucrose a complex of ferric hydroxide and sucrose is given by either *slow intravenous injection* or by *intravenous infusion.* Patients should be given a small test dose initially.

IRON SUCROSE

A complex of ferric hydroxide with sucrose containing 2% (20 mg/mL) of iron
Indications: iron-deficiency anaemia
Cautions: oral iron therapy should not be given until 5 days after the last ferric hydroxide sucrose complex injection; facilities for cardio-pulmonary resuscitation must be at hand
Contra-indications: pregnancy; history of allergic disorders including asthma, eczema and anaphylaxis; liver disease; infection

Side-effects: nausea, vomiting, taste disturbances, headache, hypotension; less frequently paraesthesia, abdominal disorders, myalgia, fever, flushing, urticaria, peripheral oedema; rarely anaphylactoid reactions; injection site reactions including phlebitis reported
Dose: *by slow intravenous injection* or *by intravenous infusion,* calculated according to body-weight and iron deficit, consult product literature
CHILD not recommended

Venofer® (Syner-Med) ▼ PoM
Injection, iron (as iron sucrose) 20 mg/mL, net price 5-mL amp = £8.98

IRON SORBITOL

Colloidal solution of a complex of iron, sorbitol and citric acid, stabilised with dextrin and sorbitol; contains 5% (50 mg/mL) of iron
Indications: iron-deficiency anaemia
Cautions: oral iron should be stopped at least 24 hours before; history of allergic disorders including asthma; elderly, underweight or debilitated
Contra-indications: liver disease, kidney disease, untreated urinary-tract infections; early pregnancy; preferably avoid in patients with pre-existing cardiac abnormalities (e.g. angina or arrhythmias)
Side-effects: nausea, vomiting, diarrhoea, haematuria, taste disturbances, dizziness, flushing, myalgia; hypersensitivity reactions including urticaria and hypotension; occasionally severe arrhythmias; rarely anaphylactoid reactions; injection site reactions
Dose: *by deep intramuscular injection,* calculated according to body-weight and iron deficit, consult product literature

Jectofer® (Astra) PoM
Injection, iron sorbitol (iron 50 mg/mL). Net price 2-mL amp = 45p

9.1.2   Drugs used in megaloblastic anaemias

Most megaloblastic anaemias are due to lack of either vitamin B_{12} or folate and it is essential to establish in every case which deficiency is present and the underlying cause. In emergencies, where delay might be dangerous, it is sometimes necessary to administer both substances after the bone marrow test while plasma assay results are awaited. Normally, however, appropriate treatment should be instituted only when the results of tests are available.

The most common cause of megaloblastic anaemia in the UK is *pernicious anaemia* in which lack of gastric intrinsic factor due to an auto-immune gastritis causes malabsorption of vitamin B_{12}.

Vitamin B_{12} is also needed in the treatment of megaloblastosis due to *prolonged nitrous oxide anaesthesia,* which inactivates the vitamin, and in the rare syndrome of *congenital transcobalamin II deficiency.*

Vitamin B_{12} should be given prophylactically after *total gastrectomy* or *total ileal resection* (or after *partial gastrectomy* if a vitamin B$_{12}$ absorption test shows vitamin B$_{12}$ malabsorption).

Apart from dietary deficiency, all other causes of vitamin-B$_{12}$ deficiency are attributable to malabsorption. There is little place for the use of low-dose vitamin B$_{12}$ orally and none for vitamin B$_{12}$ intrinsic factor complexes given by mouth. Vitamin B$_{12}$ in larger oral doses of 1–2 mg daily [unlicensed] may be effective.

Hydroxocobalamin has completely replaced cyanocobalamin as the form of vitamin B$_{12}$ of choice for therapy; it is retained in the body longer than cyanocobalamin and thus for maintenance therapy can be given at intervals of up to 3 months. Treatment is generally initiated with frequent administration of intramuscular injections to replenish the depleted body stores. Thereafter, maintenance treatment, which is usually for life, can be instituted. There is no evidence that doses larger than those recommended provide any additional benefit in vitamin-B$_{12}$ neuropathy.

Folic acid has few indications for long-term therapy since most causes of folate deficiency are self-limiting or will yield to a short course of treatment. It should not be used in undiagnosed megaloblastic anaemia unless vitamin B$_{12}$ is administered concurrently otherwise neuropathy may be precipitated (see above).

In *folate-deficient megaloblastic anaemia* (e.g. due to poor nutrition, pregnancy, or antiepileptics), standard treatment to bring about a haematological remission and replenish body stores, is oral administration of folic acid 5 mg daily for 4 months; up to 15 mg daily may be necessary in malabsorption states.

For *prophylaxis in chronic haemolytic states or in renal dialysis*, it is sufficient to give folic acid 5 mg daily or even weekly, depending on the diet and the rate of haemolysis.

For *prophylaxis in pregnancy* the dose of folic acid is 200–500 micrograms daily (see Iron and Folic Acid, section 9.1.1.1). See also Prevention of Neural Tube Defects below.

Folinic acid is also effective in the treatment of folate-deficient megaloblastic anaemia but it is generally used in association with cytotoxic drugs (see section 8.1.3); it is given as calcium folinate.

PREVENTION OF NEURAL TUBE DEFECTS. Recommendations of an expert advisory group of the Department of Health include the advice that:

To prevent *recurrence of neural tube defect* (in a child of a man or woman with spina bifida or if there is a history of neural tube defect in a previous child) women who wish to become pregnant (or who are at risk of becoming pregnant) should be advised to take folic acid supplements at a dose of 5 mg daily (reduced to 4 mg daily if a suitable preparation becomes available); supplementation should continue until week 12 of pregnancy. Women receiving antiepileptic therapy need individual counselling by their doctor before starting folic acid.

To prevent *first occurrence of neural tube defect* women who are planning a pregnancy should be advised to take folic acid as a medicinal or food supplement at a dose of 400 micrograms daily before conception and during the first 12 weeks of pregnancy. Women who have not been taking supplements and who suspect they are pregnant should start at once and continue until week 12 of pregnancy.

There is **no** justification for prescribing multiple-ingredient vitamin preparations containing vitamin B$_{12}$ or folic acid.

HYDROXOCOBALAMIN

Indications: see under dose below

Cautions: should not be given before diagnosis fully established but see also notes above

Side-effects: itching, exanthema; fever, chills, hot flushes; nausea, dizziness; initial hypokalaemia; rarely acneiform and bullous eruptions; anaphylaxis

Dose: *by intramuscular injection*, pernicious anaemia and other macrocytic anaemias without neurological involvement, initially 0.25–1 mg on alternate days for 1–2 weeks, then 250 micrograms weekly until blood count within normal range, thereafter 1 mg every 2–3 months

Pernicious anaemia and other macrocytic anaemias with neurological involvement, initially 1 mg on alternate days until no further improvement, then 1 mg every 2 months

Prophylaxis of macrocytic anaemias associated with vitamin-B$_{12}$ deficiency, 1 mg every 2–3 months

Tobacco amblyopia and Leber's optic atrophy, initially 1 mg daily for 2 weeks, then 1 mg twice weekly until no further improvement, thereafter 1 mg every 1–3 months

CHILD, doses as for adult

Hydroxocobalamin (Non-proprietary) PoM
Injection, hydroxocobalamin 1 mg/mL. Net price 1-mL amp = £2.50
Note. The BP directs that when vitamin B$_{12}$ injection is prescribed or demanded hydroxocobalamin injection shall be dispensed or supplied
Available from Medeva (*Neo-Cytamen®* NHS), Gold-shield, Link (*Cobalin-H®* NHS)

CYANOCOBALAMIN

Indications: see notes above

Dose: *by mouth*, vitamin-B$_{12}$ deficiency of dietary origin, 50–150 micrograms or more daily taken between meals; CHILD 50–105 micrograms daily in 1–3 divided doses

By intramuscular injection, initially 1 mg repeated 10 times at intervals of 2–3 days, maintenance 1 mg every month, but see notes above

Cyanocobalamin (Non-proprietary)
Tablets NHS, cyanocobalamin 50 micrograms. Net price 50-tab pack = £2.77
* NHS except to treat or prevent vitamin-B$_{12}$ deficiency in a patient who is a vegan or who has a proven vitamin-B$_{12}$ deficiency of dietary origin and endorsed 'SLS'
Available from Goldshield (*Cytacon®* NHS)
Liquid NHS, cyanocobalamin 35 micrograms/5 mL. Net price 200 mL = £2.52
Available from Goldshield (*Cytacon®* NHS)
Injection PoM, cyanocobalamin 1 mg/mL. Net price 1-mL amp = £1.67
Note. The BP directs that when vitamin B$_{12}$ injection is prescribed or demanded hydroxocobalamin injection shall be dispensed or supplied
Available from Medeva (*Cytamen®* NHS)

FOLIC ACID

Indications: see notes above

Cautions: should never be given alone for pernicious anaemia and other vitamin B_{12}-deficiency states (may precipitate subacute combined degeneration of the spinal cord); **interactions:** Appendix 1 (folic acid and folinic acid)

Dose: initially, 5 mg daily for 4 months (see notes above); maintenance, 5 mg every 1–7 days depending on underlying disease; CHILD up to 1 year, 500 micrograms/kg daily; over 1 year, as adult dose

Prevention of neural tube defects, see notes above

¹ **Folic Acid** (Non-proprietary) PoM

Tablets, folic acid 400 micrograms, net price = 90-tab pack = £2.19; 5 mg, 20 = 12p

Note. 400-microgram tablets available from Lane (*Preconceive®*), 5-mg tablets available from various suppliers

1. Can be sold to the public provided daily doses do not exceed 500 micrograms

Syrup, folic acid 2.5 mg/5 mL, net price 150 mL = £9.74; 400 micrograms/5 mL, 150 mL = £1.56

Note. 2.5 mg/5 mL syrup available from Hillcross and Rosemont (*Lexpec®*, sugar-free); 400 micrograms/5 mL oral solution available from Rosemont (*Folicare®*)

9.1.3 Drugs used in hypoplastic, haemolytic, and renal anaemias

Anabolic steroids, pyridoxine, antilymphocyte immunoglobulin, and various corticosteroids are used in hypoplastic and haemolytic anaemias.

The appropriate use of **anabolic steroids** in the therapy of *aplastic anaemia* remains unclear. There is a wide variation in the reported successful responses. Occasional patients, however, do seem to derive benefit. Since nandrolone decanoate (section 6.4.3) requires intramuscular injection it is unsuitable in aplastic anaemia or cytotoxic aplasia because of the low platelet count. Oxymetholone tablets (available only on named-patient basis) may alternatively be used in aplastic anaemia. Controlled trials have shown that antilymphocyte globulin given by intravenous infusion produces a response in 50% of acquired cases; higher response rates have been reported when ciclosporin is given as well.

It is unlikely that dietary deprivation of **pyridoxine** (section 9.6.2) produces haematological effects in man. However, certain forms of *sideroblastic anaemia* respond to pharmacological doses, possibly reflecting its role as a co-enzyme during haemoglobin synthesis. Pyridoxine is indicated in both *idiopathic acquired* and *hereditary sideroblastic anaemias.* Although complete cures have not been reported, some increase in haemoglobin may occur; the dose required is usually high, up to 400 mg daily. *Reversible sideroblastic anaemias* respond to treatment of the underlying cause but in pregnancy, haemolytic anaemias, and alcohol dependence, or during isoniazid treatment, pyridoxine is also indicated.

Corticosteroids (see section 6.3) have an important place in the management of a wide variety of haematological disorders. They include conditions with an immune basis such as *auto-immune haemolytic anaemia, immune thrombocytopenias* and *neutropenias,* and *major transfusion reactions.* They are also used in chemotherapy schedules for many types of *lymphoma, lymphoid leukaemias,* and *paraproteinaemias,* including *myelomatosis.*

Erythropoietin

Epoetin (recombinant human erythropoietin) is used for the anaemia associated with erythropoietin deficiency in chronic renal failure, to increase the yield of autologous blood in normal individuals and to shorten the period of anaemia in patients receiving platinum-containing chemotherapy. The clinical efficacy of epoetin alfa and epoetin beta is similar. Epoetin beta is also used for the prevention of anaemia in premature infants of low birth-weight.

Other factors which contribute to the anaemia of chronic renal failure such as iron or folate deficiency should be corrected before treatment and monitored during therapy. Supplemental iron may improve the response in resistant patients. Aluminium toxicity, concurrent infection or other inflammatory disease may impair the response to epoetin.

EPOETIN ALFA and BETA

(Recombinant human erythropoietins)

Note. Although epoetin alfa and beta are clinically indistinguishable the prescriber must specify which is required

Indications: see under preparations, below

Cautions: inadequately treated or poorly controlled blood pressure (monitor closely blood pressure, haemoglobin, and electrolytes), interrupt treatment if blood pressure uncontrolled; sudden stabbing migraine-like pain is warning of hypertensive crisis; exclude other causes of anaemia (e.g. folic acid or vitamin B_{12} deficiency) and give iron supplements if necessary (see also notes above); ischaemic vascular disease; thrombocytosis (monitor platelet count for first 8 weeks); history of convulsions; malignant disease; chronic liver failure; increase in heparin dose may be needed; when used for anaemia before orthopaedic surgery avoid in cardiovascular disease including recent myocardial infarction or cerebrovascular accident; pregnancy and breast-feeding; **interactions:** Appendix 1 (epoetin)

Contra-indications: uncontrolled hypertension

Side-effects: dose-dependent increase in blood pressure or aggravation of hypertension; in isolated patients with normal or low blood pressure, hypertensive crisis with encephalopathy-like symptoms and generalised tonic-clonic seizures requiring immediate medical attention; dose-dependent increase in platelet count (but thrombocytosis rare) regressing during treatment; influenza-like symptoms (may be reduced if intravenous injection given over 5 minutes); shunt thrombosis especially if tendency to hypotension or arteriovenous shunt complications; isolated reports of hyperkalaemia, hyperphosphataemia, convulsions, skin reactions, palpebral oedema, anaphylaxis

Dose: aimed at increasing haemoglobin concentration at rate not exceeding 2 g/100 mL/month to stable level of 10–12 g/100 mL (9.5–11 g/100 mL in children); see under preparations, below

■ **Epoetin alfa**

Eprex® (Janssen-Cilag) PoM

Injection, epoetin alfa 2000 units/mL, net price
0.5-mL (1000-unit) vial = £8.38, 1-mL (2000-
unit) vial = £16.76; 4000 units/mL, 1-mL (4000-
unit) vial = £33.52; 10 000 units/mL, 1-mL
(10 000-unit) vial = £83.80

Injection, prefilled syringe, epoetin alfa, net price
1000 units = £8.38; 2000 units = £16.76; 3000 units
= £25.14; 4000 units = £33.52; 10 000 units =
£83.80. An auto-injector device is available for use
with 10 000-units prefilled syringes

Dose: anaemia associated with chronic renal failure in
patients on haemodialysis, *by subcutaneous injection*
(max. 1 mL per injection site) or *by intravenous injection* over 1–5 minutes, initially 50 units/kg 3 times
weekly adjusted according to response in steps of
25 units/kg 3 times weekly at intervals of 4 weeks; max.
600 units/kg weekly in 3 divided doses; maintenance
dose (when haemoglobin concentration of 10–12 g/
100 mL achieved), usually 33–100 units/kg 3 times
weekly *or* 50–150 units/kg twice weekly; CHILD (intravenous route only) initially as for adults; maintenance
dose (when haemoglobin concentration of 9.5–11 g/
100 mL achieved), under 10 kg usually 75–150 units/kg
3 times weekly, 10–30 kg usually 60–150 units/kg 3
times weekly, over 30 kg usually 30–100 units/kg 3
times weekly

Note. Subcutaneous dose generally about 20–30% lower
than intravenous; when changing route give same dose
then adjust according to weekly haemoglobin measurements

Anaemia associated with chronic renal failure in adults
on peritoneal dialysis, *by subcutaneous injection* (max.
1 mL per injection site), initially 50 units/kg twice
weekly adjusted according to response in steps of
25 units/kg twice weekly at intervals of 4 weeks; maintenance dose (when haemoglobin concentration of 10–
12 g/100 mL achieved), 25–50 units/kg twice weekly

Severe symptomatic anaemia of renal origin in adults
with renal insufficiency not yet on dialysis, preferably
by subcutaneous injection (max. 1 mL per injection site),
initially 50 units/kg 3 times weekly increased according
to response in steps of 25 units/kg 3 times weekly at
intervals of 4 weeks; maintenance dose (when haemoglobin concentration of 10–12 g/100 mL achieved), 17–
33 units/kg 3 times weekly; max. 600 units/kg weekly in
3 divided doses;

Anaemia in adults receiving platinum-containing chemotherapy, *by subcutaneous injection* (max. 1 mL per
injection site), initially 150 units/kg 3 times weekly,
increased if appropriate rise in haemoglobin (or reticulo-
cyte count) not achieved after 4 weeks to 300 units/kg 3
times weekly; discontinue if inadequate response after 4
weeks at higher dose; reduce dose by 25–50% if haemoglobin rise exceeds 2 g/100 mL per month; suspend if
haemoglobin exceeds 14 g/100 mL until it falls below
12 g/100 mL and reinstate with dose at 25% of previous dose; continue epoetin for 1 month after end of
chemotherapy

To increase yield of autologous blood (to avoid homologous blood) in predonation programme in moderate
anaemia *either* when large volume of blood required for
elective major surgery *or* if insufficient period to obtain
required volume of blood, *by intravenous injection* over
1–5 minutes, 600 units/kg twice weekly for 3 weeks
before surgery; consult product literature for details and
advice on ensuring high iron stores

Moderate anaemia (haemoglobin concentration 10–13 g/
100 mL) before elective orthopaedic surgery in adults
with expected moderate blood loss to reduce exposure to
homologous transfusion or if autologous transfusion
unavailable, *by subcutaneous injection* (max. 1 mL per

injection site), 600 units/kg every week for 3 weeks
before surgery and on day of surgery *or* 300 units/kg
daily for 15 days starting 10 days before surgery; consult
product literature for details

■ **Epoetin beta**

NeoRecormon® (Roche) ▼ PoM

Injection, powder for reconstitution, epoetin beta,
net price 500-unit vial = £4.19 (with water for
injection)

Note. Avoid contact of reconstituted injection with glass;
use only plastic materials

Injection, prefilled syringe, epoetin beta, net price
500 units = £4.19; 1000 units = £8.38; 2000 units
= £16.76; 3000 units = £25.14; 5000 units =
£41.90; 10 000 units = £83.80

Multidose injection, powder for reconstitution,
epoetin beta, net price 50 000-unit vial = £438.75;
100 000-unit vial = £838.01 (both with solvent)

Contra-indications: not for use in neonates owing to
presence of benzyl alcohol as additive

Note. Avoid contact of reconstituted injection with glass;
use only plastic materials

Reco-Pen, (for subcutaneous use), double-chamber cartridges (containing epoetin beta and solvent), net price 10 000-unit cartridge = £87.75;
20 000-unit cartridge = £175.50; for use with
Reco-Pen injection device, available free from
Roche; sterile needles for *Reco-pen*, net price 50-
needle pack = £5.10

Contra-indications: not for use in neonates owing to
presence of benzyl alcohol as additive

Dose: anaemia associated with chronic renal failure in
dialysis patients, symptomatic anaemia of renal origin in
patients not yet on dialysis, ADULT and CHILD

By subcutaneous injection, initially 60 units/kg weekly
(in 1–7 divided doses) for 4 weeks, increased according
to response at intervals of 4 weeks in steps of 60 units/
kg; maintenance dose (when haemoglobin concentration
of 10–12 g/100 mL achieved), initially reduce dose by
half then adjust according to response at intervals of 1–2
weeks; max. 720 units/kg weekly

By intravenous injection over 2 minutes, initially
40 units/kg 3 times weekly for 4 weeks, increased
according to response to 80 units/kg 3 times weekly with
further increases if needed at intervals of 4 weeks in
steps of 20 units/kg 3 times weekly; maintenance dose
(when haemoglobin concentration of 10–12 g/100 mL
achieved), initially reduce dose by half then adjust
according to response at intervals of 1–2 weeks; max.
720 units/kg weekly

Prevention of anaemias of prematurity in infants with
birth-weight of 0.75–1.5 kg and gestational age of less
than 34 weeks, *by subcutaneous injection* (of single-
dose, unpreserved injection), 250 units/kg 3 times
weekly preferably starting within 3 days of birth and
continued for 6 weeks

Anaemia in adults with solid tumours receiving platinum-containing chemotherapy, *by subcutaneous injection*, initially 450 units/kg weekly (in 3–7 divided
doses), increased if appropriate rise in haemoglobin not
achieved after 4 weeks to 900 units/kg weekly (in 3–7
divided doses); reduce dose by half if haemoglobin rise
exceeds 2 g/100 mL per month; suspend if haemoglobin
exceeds 14 g/100 mL until concentration falls below
12 g/100 mL and reinstate at 50% of the previous weekly
dose; continue for up to 3 weeks after end of chemotherapy

Note. If haemoglobin concentration falls by more than
1 g/100 mL in the first cycle of chemotherapy despite

treatment with epoetin beta, further treatment may not be effective

To increase yield of autologous blood (to avoid homologous blood) in predonation programme in moderate anaemia when blood conserving procedures are insufficient or unavailable, consult product literature

Iron overload

Severe tissue iron overload may occur in aplastic and other refractory anaemias, mainly as the result of repeated blood transfusions. It is a particular problem in refractory anaemias with hyperplastic bone marrow, especially *thalassaemia major*, where excessive iron absorption from the gut and inappropriate iron therapy may add to the tissue siderosis.

Iron overload associated with haemochromatosis may be treated with repeated venesection. Venesection may also be used for patients who have received multiple transfusions and whose bone marrow has recovered. Where venesection is contra-indicated, the long-term administration of the iron chelating compound **desferrioxamine mesilate** is useful. Subcutaneous infusions of desferrioxamine are given over 8–12 hours, 3–7 times a week. The dose should reflect the degree of iron overload. For children starting therapy (and who have low iron overload) the dose should not exceed 30 mg/kg. For established overload the dose is usually between 20 and 50 mg/kg daily. Desferrioxamine (up to 2 g per unit of blood) may also be given at the time of blood transfusion, provided that the desferrioxamine is **not** added to the blood and is **not** given through the same line as the blood (but the two may be given through the same cannula).

Iron excretion induced by desferrioxamine is enhanced by administration of ascorbic acid (vitamin C, section 9.6.3) in a dose of 200 mg daily (100 mg in infants); it should be given separately from food since it also enhances iron absorption. Ascorbic acid should not be given to patients with cardiac dysfunction; in patients with normal cardiac function ascorbic acid should be introduced 1 month after starting desferrioxamine.

Infusion of desferrioxamine may be used to treat *aluminium overload* in dialysis patients; theoretically 100 mg of desferrioxamine binds with 4.1 mg of aluminium.

Orally active iron chelators are under clinical study but are not available for general use.

DESFERRIOXAMINE MESILATE

(Deferoxamine Mesilate)

Indications: see notes above; iron poisoning, see Emergency Treatment of Poisoning

Cautions: renal impairment; eye and ear examinations before treatment and at 3-month intervals during treatment; aluminium-related encephalopathy (may exacerbate neurological dysfunction); pregnancy, breast-feeding; **interactions:** Appendix 1 (desferrioxamine)

Side-effects: gastro-intestinal disturbances; hepatic and renal impairment; arrhythmias, hypotension (especially when given too rapidly by intravenous injection); anaphylaxis; dizziness, convulsions; Yersinia infection more frequent; disturbances of hearing and vision (including lens opacity and retinopathy); skin reactions; pain on intramuscular injection; local irritation on subcutaneous infusion (usually if infusion concentration or dose too high)

Dose: see notes above; iron poisoning, see Emergency Treatment of Poisoning

Note. For full details and warnings relating to administration, consult product literature

Desferal® (Novartis) [PoM]

Injection, powder for reconstitution, desferrioxamine mesilate, net price 500-mg vial = £3.70

9.1.4 Drugs used in autoimmune thrombocytopenic purpura

It is usual to commence the treatment of autoimmune (idiopathic) thrombocytopenic purpura with corticosteroids, e.g. prednisolone 1 mg/kg daily, gradually reducing the dosage over the subsequent weeks. In patients who fail to achieve a satisfactory platelet count or relapse when corticosteroid dosage is reduced or withdrawn, splenectomy is considered.

Other therapy that has been tried in refractory cases includes azathioprine (section 8.2.1), cyclophosphamide (section 8.1.1), vincristine (section 8.1.4), ciclosporin (section 8.2.2), and danazol (section 6.7.2). Intravenous immunoglobulins (section 14.5), have also been used in refractory cases or where a temporary rapid rise in platelets is needed, as in pregnancy or pre-operatively. For patients with chronic severe thrombocytopenia refractory to other therapy, tranexamic acid (section 2.11) may be given to reduce the severity of haemorrhage.

9.1.5 G6PD deficiency

Glucose 6-phosphate dehydrogenase (G6PD) deficiency is highly prevalent in populations originating from most parts of Africa, from most parts of Asia, from Oceania, and from Southern Europe; it can also be encountered, rarely, in any other population.

Subjects with G6PD deficiency are susceptible to developing acute haemolytic anaemia on taking a number of common drugs. They are also susceptible to developing acute haemolytic anaemia upon ingestion of fava beans (broad beans, *Vicia faba*); this is termed *favism* and tends to be more severe in children or when the fresh fava beans are eaten raw.

When prescribing drugs for patients who are G6PD deficient, the following three points should be kept in mind:

1. G6PD deficiency is genetically heterogeneous; different genetic variants entail different susceptibility to the haemolytic risk from drugs; thus, a drug found to be safe in some G6PD-deficient subjects may not be equally safe in others;

2. no test specifically designed to identify potential risk in G6PD-deficient subjects is currently carried out by manufacturers;

3. the risk and severity of haemolysis is almost always dose-related.

The table below should be read with these points in mind. Whenever possible, a test for G6PD deficiency should be done before prescribing a drug in the list, especially if the patient belongs to a population group in which G6PD deficiency is common.

A very small group of G6PD-deficient individuals, with chronic non-spherocytic haemolytic anaemia, have haemolysis even in the absence of an exogenous trigger. These patients must be regarded as being at high risk of severe exacerbation of haemolysis following administration of any of the drugs listed below.

Drugs with definite risk of haemolysis in most G6PD-deficient subjects

Dapsone and other sulphones (higher doses for dermatitis herpetiformis more likely to cause problems)

Methylthioninium chloride (methylene blue)

Niridazole [not on UK market]

Nitrofurantoin

Pamaquin [not on UK market]

Primaquine (30 mg weekly for 8 weeks has been found to be without undue harmful effects in African and Asian people, see section 5.4.1)

Quinolones (including ciprofloxacin, nalidixic acid, norfloxacin, and ofloxacin)

Sulphonamides (including co-trimoxazole; some sulphonamides, e.g. sulfadiazine, have been tested and found not to be haemolytic in many G6PD-deficient subjects)

Drugs with possible risk of haemolysis in some G6PD-deficient subjects

Aspirin (acceptable in a dose of at least 1 g daily in most G6PD-deficient subjects)

Chloroquine (acceptable in acute malaria)

Menadione, water-soluble derivatives (e.g. menadiol sodium phosphate)

Probenecid

Quinidine (acceptable in acute malaria)

Quinine (acceptable in acute malaria)

Note. Mothballs may contain naphthalene which also causes haemolysis in subjects with G6PD-deficiency.

9.1.6   Drugs used in neutropenia

Recombinant human granulocyte-colony stimulating factor (rhG-CSF) stimulates the production of neutrophils and may reduce the duration of chemotherapy-induced neutropenia and thereby reduce the incidence of associated sepsis; there is as yet no evidence that it improves overall survival. **Filgrastim** (unglycosylated rhG-CSF) and **lenograstim** (glycosylated rhG-CSF) have similar effects; both have been used in a variety of clinical settings but they do not have any clear-cut routine indications. In congenital neutropenia filgrastim usually elevates the neutrophil count with appropriate clinical response. Prolonged use may be associated with an increased risk of myeloid malignancy.

Molgramostim (recombinant human granulocyte macrophage-colony stimulating factor) stimulates the production of all granulocytes and monocytes. It has more side-effects than granulocyte-colony stimulating factor and is ineffective in congenital neutropenia.

Treatment with recombinant human growth factors should only be prescribed by those experienced in their use.

For the use of **amifostine** in cytotoxic-induced neutropenic infection, see section 8.1.

FILGRASTIM

(Recombinant human granulocyte-colony stimulating factor, G-CSF)

Indications: (specialist use only) reduction in duration of neutropenia and incidence of febrile neutropenia in cytotoxic chemotherapy for malignancy (except chronic myeloid leukaemia and myelodysplastic syndromes); reduction in duration of neutropenia (and associated sequelae) in myeloablative therapy followed by bone-marrow transplantation; mobilisation of peripheral blood progenitor cells for harvesting and subsequent autologous infusion; severe congenital neutropenia, cyclic neutropenia, or idiopathic neutropenia and history of severe or recurrent infections (distinguish carefully from other haematological disorders, consult product literature)

Cautions: reduced myeloid precursors; monitor leucocyte count (discontinue treatment if leucocytosis, consult product literature); monitor platelet count and haemoglobin; regular morphological and cytogenetic bone-marrow examinations recommended in severe congenital neutropenia (possible risk of myelodysplastic syndromes or leukaemia); monitor spleen size; osteoporotic bone disease (monitor bone density if given for more than 6 months); does not prevent other toxic effects of high-dose chemotherapy; pregnancy, breast-feeding; **interactions:** Appendix 1 (filgrastim)

Contra-indications: severe congenital neutropenia (Kostman's syndrome) with abnormal cytogenetics

Side-effects: musculoskeletal pain, transient hypotension, disturbances in liver enzymes and serum uric acid; thrombocytopenia; urinary abnormalities including dysuria; allergic reactions (more common after intravenous infusion), proteinuria, haematuria, and transient decrease in blood glucose reported; cutaneous vasculitis also reported, also splenic enlargement, hepatomegaly, headache, diarrhoea, anaemia, epistaxis, alopecia, osteoporosis, and rash, reactions at injection site; rarely reported, exacerbation of rheumatoid arthritis, adult respiratory distress syndrome

Dose: cytotoxic-induced neutropenia, preferably *by subcutaneous injection or by intravenous infusion* (over 30 minutes), ADULT and CHILD, 500 000 units/kg daily started not less than 24 hours after cytotoxic chemotherapy, continued until neutrophil count in normal range, usually for up to 14 days (up to 38 days in acute myeloid leukaemia)

Myeloablative therapy followed by bone-marrow transplantation, *by intravenous infusion* over 30 minutes or over 24 hours *or by subcutaneous infusion* over 24 hours, 1 million units/kg daily, started not less than 24 hours following cytotoxic chemotherapy (and within 24 hours of bone-marrow infusion), then adjusted according to absolute neutrophil count (consult product literature)

Mobilisation of peripheral blood progenitor cells, used alone, *by subcutaneous injection or by subcutaneous infusion* over 24 hours, 1 million units/kg daily for 6 days; used following adjunctive myelosuppressive chemotherapy (to improve yield), *by subcutaneous injection*, 500 000 units/kg daily, started the day after completion of chemotherapy and continued until neutrophil count in normal range; for timing of leukapheresis consult product literature

Severe chronic neutropenia, *by subcutaneous injection*, ADULT and CHILD, in severe congenital neutropenia, initially 1.2 million units/kg daily in single or divided doses (initially 500 000 units/kg daily in idiopathic or cyclic neutropenia), adjusted according to response (consult product literature)

Neupogen® (Amgen) PoM

Injection, filgrastim 30 million units (300 micrograms)/mL; net price 1-mL vial or pre-filled syringe = £77.03, 1.6-mL (48 million-unit) vial or pre-filled syringe = £122.85

LENOGRASTIM

(Recombinant human granulocyte-colony stimulating factor, rHuG-CSF)

Indications: (specialist use only) reduction in the duration of neutropenia and associated complications following bone-marrow transplantation for non-myeloid malignancy or following treatment with cytotoxic chemotherapy associated with a significant incidence of febrile neutropenia; mobilisation of peripheral blood progenitor cells for harvesting and subsequent infusion

Cautions: see under Filgrastim; pre-malignant myeloid conditions; **interactions:** Appendix 1 (lenograstim)

Side-effects: see under Filgrastim; asthenia, abdominal pain and generalised pain reported in healthy donors

Dose: following bone-marrow transplantation, *by intravenous infusion*, ADULT and CHILD over 2 years 19.2 million units/m² daily started the day after transplantation, continued until neutrophil count stable in acceptable range (max. 28 days)

Cytotoxic-induced neutropenia, *by subcutaneous injection*, ADULT 19.2 million units/m² daily started the day after completion of chemotherapy, continued until neutrophil count stable in acceptable range (max. 28 days)

Mobilisation of peripheral blood progenitor cells, used alone, *by subcutaneous injection*, ADULT 1.28 million units/kg daily for 4–6 days (5–6 days in healthy donors); used following adjunctive myelosuppressive chemotherapy (to improve yield), *by subcutaneous injection*, 19.2 million units/m² daily, started the day after completion of chemotherapy and continued until neutrophil count in acceptable range; for timing of leukapheresis consult product literature

Granocyte® (Chugai) PoM

Injection, powder for reconstitution, lenograstim, net price 13.4 million-unit (105-microgram) vial = £42.00; 33.6 million-unit (263-microgram) vial = £77.03 (both with 1-mL amp or 1-mL prefilled syringe water for injections)

MOLGRAMOSTIM

(Recombinant human granulocyte macrophage-colony stimulating factor, GM-CSF)

Indications: (specialist use only) reduction of severity of neutropenia (and risk of infection) in cytotoxic chemotherapy; acceleration of myeloid recovery following bone-marrow transplantation; neutropenia in patients treated with ganciclovir in AIDS-related cytomegalovirus retinitis

Cautions: monitor serum albumin concentration and full blood count including differential white cell, platelet and haemoglobin; monitor closely patients with pulmonary disease; history of or predisposition to autoimmune disease; pregnancy and breast-feeding; not yet recommended for patients under 18 years

Contra-indications: myeloid malignancies

Side-effects: nausea, diarrhoea, vomiting, anorexia; dyspnoea; asthenia, fatigue; rash, fever, rigors, flushing, musculoskeletal pain; local reaction following subcutaneous injection; also reported, non-specific chest pain, stomatitis, headache, increased sweating, abdominal pain, pruritus, peripheral oedema, dizziness, paraesthesia, and myalgia; serious reactions reported include anaphylaxis, cardiac failure, capillary leak syndrome, cerebrovascular disorders, confusion, convulsions, hypotension, cardiac rhythm abnormalities, intracranial hypertension, pericardial effusion, pericarditis, pleural effusion, pulmonary oedema, syncope

Dose: (first dose under medical supervision)
Cytotoxic chemotherapy, *by subcutaneous injection*, 60 000–110 000 units/kg daily, starting 24 hours after last dose of chemotherapy, continued for 7–10 days

Bone-marrow transplantation, *by intravenous infusion*, 110 000 units/kg daily, starting day after transplantation, continued until absolute neutrophil count in desirable range (see product literature); max. duration of treatment 30 days

Adjunct in ganciclovir treatment, *by subcutaneous injection*, 60 000 units/kg daily for 5 days then adjusted to maintain desirable absolute neutrophil count and white blood cell count

Leucomax® (Novartis, Schering-Plough) ▼ PoM

Injection, powder for reconstitution, molgramostim, net price 1.67 million-unit (150-microgram) vial = £38.51; 3.33 million-unit (300-microgram) vial = £77.02; 4.44 million-unit (400 microgram) vial = £102.69

9.2   Fluids and electrolytes

9.2.1   Oral preparations for fluid and electrolyte imbalance

9.2.2   Parenteral preparations for fluid and electrolyte imbalance

The following tables give a selection of useful electrolyte values:

Electrolyte concentrations—intravenous fluids

Intravenous infusion	Millimoles per litre				
	Na$^+$	K$^+$	HCO$_3^-$	Cl$^-$	Ca^{2+}
Normal Plasma Values	142	4.5	26	103	2.5
Sodium Chloride 0.9%	150	—	—	150	—
Compound Sodium Lactate (Hartmann's)	131	5	29	111	2
Sodium Chloride 0.18% and Glucose 4%	30	—	—	30	—
Potassium Chloride 0.3% and Glucose 5%	—	40	—	40	—
Potassium Chloride 0.3% and Sodium Chloride 0.9%	150	40	—	190	—
To correct metabolic acidosis					
Sodium Bicarbonate 1.26%	150	—	150	—	—
Sodium Bicarbonate 8.4% for cardiac arrest	1000	—	1000	—	—
Sodium Lactate (m/6)	167	—	167	—	—

Electrolyte content—gastro-intestinal secretions

Type of fluid	Millimoles per litre				
	H$^+$	Na$^+$	K$^+$	HCO$_3^-$	Cl$^-$
Gastric	40–60	20–80	5–20	—	100–150
Biliary	—	120–140	5–15	30–50	80–120
Pancreatic	—	120–140	5–15	70–110	40–80
Small bowel	—	120–140	5–15	20–40	90–130

Faeces, vomit, or aspiration should be saved and analysed where possible if abnormal losses are suspected; where this is impracticable the approximations above may be helpful in planning replacement therapy

9.2.1   Oral preparations for fluid and electrolyte imbalance

9.2.1.1   Oral potassium

9.2.1.2   Oral sodium and water

9.2.1.3   Oral bicarbonate

Sodium and potassium salts, which may be given by mouth to prevent deficiencies or to treat established deficiencies of mild or moderate degree, are discussed in this section. Oral preparations for removing excess potassium and preparations for oral rehydration therapy are also included here. Oral bicarbonate, for metabolic acidosis, is also described in this section.

For reference to calcium, magnesium, and phosphate, see section 9.5.

9.2.1.1   Oral potassium

Compensation for potassium loss is especially necessary:

1. in those taking digoxin or anti-arrhythmic drugs, where potassium depletion may induce arrhythmias;
2. in patients in whom secondary hyperaldosteronism occurs, e.g. renal artery stenosis, cirrhosis of the liver, the nephrotic syndrome, and severe heart failure;
3. in patients with excessive losses of potassium in the faeces, e.g. chronic diarrhoea associated with intestinal malabsorption or laxative abuse.

Measures to compensate for potassium loss may also be required in the elderly since they frequently take inadequate amounts of potassium in the diet (but see below for **warning** on **renal insufficiency**). Measures may also be required during long-term administration of drugs known to induce potassium loss (e.g. corticosteroids). Potassium supplements are **seldom required** with the small doses of diuretics given to treat hypertension; **potassium-sparing diuretics** (rather than potassium supplements) are recommended for prevention of hypokalaemia due to diuretics such as furosemide (frusemide) or the thiazides when these are given to eliminate oedema.

DOSAGE. If potassium salts are used for the *prevention of hypokalaemia*, then doses of potassium chloride 2 to 4 g (approx. 25 to 50 mmol) daily by mouth are suitable in patients taking a normal diet. *Smaller doses* must be used if there is *renal insufficiency (common in the elderly)* otherwise there is **danger of hyperkalaemia**. Potassium salts cause nausea and vomiting therefore poor compliance is a major limitation to their effectiveness; where appropriate, potassium-sparing diuretics are preferable (see also above). When there is *established potassium depletion* larger doses may be necessary, the quantity depending on the severity of any continuing potassium loss (monitoring of plasma-potassium concentration and specialist advice would be required). Potassium depletion is frequently associated with chloride depletion and with metabolic alkalosis, and these disorders require correction.

ADMINISTRATION. Potassium salts are preferably given as a liquid (or effervescent) preparation, rather than modified-release tablets; they should be given as the chloride (the use of effervescent potassium tablets BPC 1968 should be restricted to *hyperchloraemic states*, section 9.2.1.3).

Salt substitutes. A number of salt substitutes which contain significant amounts of potassium chloride are readily available as health food products (e.g. *Losalt®* and *Ruthmol®*). These should not be used by patients with renal failure as potassium intoxication may result.

POTASSIUM CHLORIDE

Indications: potassium depletion (see notes above)

Cautions: elderly, mild to moderate renal impairment (close monitoring required), intestinal stricture, history of peptic ulcer, hiatus hernia (for sustained-release preparations); **important:** special hazard if given with drugs liable to raise plasma potassium concentration such as potassium-sparing diuretics, ACE inhibitors, or ciclosporin, for other **interactions:** Appendix 1 (potassium salts)

Contra-indications: severe renal impairment, plasma potassium concentrations above 5 mmol/litre

Side-effects: nausea and vomiting (severe symptoms may indicate obstruction), oesophageal or small bowel ulceration

Dose: see notes above

Note. Do not confuse Effervescent Potassium Tablets BPC 1968 (section 9.2.1.3) with effervescent potassium chloride tablets. Effervescent Potassium Tablets BPC 1968 do not contain chloride ions and their use should be restricted to hyperchloraemic states (section 9.2.1.3). Effervescent Potassium Chloride Tablets BP are usually available in two strengths, one containing 6.7 mmol each of K+ and Cl- (corresponding to *Kloref®*), the other containing 12 mmol K+ and 8 mmol Cl- (corresponding to *Sando-K®*). Generic prescriptions must specify the strength required.

Kay-Cee-L® (Geistlich)
Syrup, red, sugar-free, potassium chloride 7.5% (1 mmol/mL each of K+ and Cl-). Net price 500 mL = £2.86. Label: 21

Kloref® (Cox)
Tablets, effervescent, betaine hydrochloride, potassium benzoate, bicarbonate, and chloride, equivalent to potassium chloride 500 mg (6.7 mmol each of K+ and Cl-). Net price 50 = £1.90. Label: 13, 21

Kloref-S® (Cox)
Granules, effervescent, sugar-free, betaine hydrochloride, potassium bicarbonate and chloride equivalent to potassium chloride 1.5 g (20 mmol each of K+ and Cl-)/sachet. Net price 30 sachets = £3.95. Label: 13, 21

Sando-K® (HK Pharma)
Tablets, effervescent, potassium bicarbonate and chloride equivalent to potassium 470 mg (12 mmol of K+) and chloride 285 mg (8 mmol of Cl-). Net price 20 = £1.53. Label: 13, 21

■ Modified-release preparations
Avoid unless effervescent tablets or liquid preparations inappropriate

Slow-K® (Alliance) ▰▰
Tablets, m/r, orange, s/c, potassium chloride 600 mg (8 mmol each of K+ and Cl-). Net price 20 = 55p. Label: 25, 27, counselling, swallow whole with fluid during meals while sitting or standing

Potassium removal

Ion-exchange resins may be used to remove excess potassium in *mild hyperkalaemia* or in *moderate hyperkalaemia* when there are not ECG changes; intravenous therapy is required in emergencies (section 9.2.2).

POLYSTYRENE SULPHONATE RESINS

Indications: hyperkalaemia associated with anuria or severe oliguria, and in dialysis patients

Cautions: children (impaction of resin with excessive dosage or inadequate dilution); monitor for electrolyte disturbances (stop if plasma-potassium concentration below 5 mmol/litre); pregnancy and breast-feeding; sodium-containing resin in congestive heart failure, hypertension, renal impairment, and oedema

Contra-indications: obstructive bowel disease; oral administration or reduced gut motility in neonates; avoid calcium-containing resin in hyperparathyroidism, multiple myeloma, sarcoidosis, or metastatic carcinoma

Side-effects: rectal ulceration following rectal administration; colonic necrosis reported following enemas containing sorbitol; sodium retention, hypercalcaemia, gastric irritation, anorexia, nausea and vomiting, constipation (discontinue treatment—avoid magnesium-containing laxatives), diarrhoea; calcium-containing resin may cause hypercalcaemia (in dialysed patients and occasionally in those with renal impairment), hypomagnesaemia

Dose: *by mouth*, 15 g 3–4 times daily in water (not fruit squash which has a high potassium content) or as a paste; CHILD 0.5–1 g/kg daily in divided doses

By rectum, as an enema, 30 g in methylcellulose solution, retained for 9 hours followed by irrigation to remove resin from colon; NEONATE and CHILD, 0.5–1 g/kg daily

Calcium Resonium® (Sanofi-Synthelabo)
Powder, buff, calcium polystyrene sulphonate. Net price 300 g = £43.23. Label: 13

Resonium A® (Sanofi-Synthelabo)
Powder, buff, sodium polystyrene sulphonate. Net price 454 g = £58.53. Label: 13

9.2.1.2   Oral sodium and water

Sodium chloride is indicated in states of sodium depletion and usually needs to be given intravenously (section 9.2.2). In chronic conditions associated with mild or moderate degrees of sodium depletion, e.g. in salt-losing bowel or renal disease, oral supplements of sodium chloride or sodium bicarbonate (section 9.2.1.3), according to the acid-base status of the patient, may be sufficient.

SODIUM CHLORIDE

Indications: sodium depletion; see also section 9.2.2.

Slow Sodium® (HK Pharma)
Tablets, m/r, sodium chloride 600 mg (approx. 10 mmol each of Na+ and Cl-). Net price 100-tab pack = £6.05. Label: 25

Dose: prophylaxis of sodium chloride deficiency 4–8 tablets daily with water (in severe depletion up to max. 20 tablets daily)

Chronic renal salt wasting, up to 20 tablets daily with appropriate fluid intake

CHILD, according to requirements

Oral rehydration therapy (ORT)

As a worldwide problem *diarrhoea* is by far the most important indication for fluid and electrolyte replacement. Intestinal absorption of sodium and water is enhanced by glucose (and other carbohydrates). Replacement of fluid and electrolytes lost through diarrhoea can therefore be achieved by giving solutions containing sodium, potassium, and glucose or another carbohydrate such as rice starch.

Oral rehydration solutions should:

enhance the absorption of water and electrolytes;
replace the electrolyte deficit adequately and safely;
contain an alkalinising agent to counter acidosis;
be slightly hypo-osmolar (about 250 mmol/litre) to prevent the possible induction of osmotic diarrhoea;
be simple to use in hospital and at home;
be palatable and acceptable, especially to children;
be readily available.

It is the policy of the World Health Organization (WHO) to promote a single oral rehydration solution but to use it flexibly (e.g. by giving extra water between drinks of oral rehydration solution to moderately dehydrated infants).

Oral rehydration solutions used in the UK are lower in sodium (50–60 mmol/litre) than the WHO formulation since, in general, patients suffer less severe sodium loss.

Rehydration should be rapid over 3 to 4 hours (except in hypernatraemic dehydration in which case rehydration should occur more slowly over 12 hours). The patient should be reassessed after initial rehydration and if still dehydrated rapid fluid replacement should continue.

Once rehydration is complete further dehydration is prevented by encouraging the patient to drink normal volumes of an appropriate fluid and by replacing continuing losses with an oral rehydration solution; in infants, breast-feeding or formula feeds should be offered between oral rehydration drinks.

For intravenous rehydration see section 9.2.2.

ORAL REHYDRATION SALTS (ORS)

Indications: fluid and electrolyte loss in diarrhoea, see notes above

Dose: according to fluid loss, usually 200–400 mL solution after every loose motion; INFANT 1–1½ times usual feed volume; CHILD 200 mL after every loose motion

■ UK formulations

Note. After reconstitution any unused solution should be discarded no later than 1 hour after preparation unless stored in a refrigerator when it may be kept for up to 24 hours.

Proprietary brands of oral rehydration salts on sale to the public include *Boots Diareze Oral rehydration treatment.*

Diocalm Replenish® (SSL)

Oral powder, sodium chloride 350 mg, potassium chloride 300 mg, sodium citrate 590 mg, anhydrous glucose 4 g/sachet. Net price 5-sachet pack (orange-flavoured) = £1.72

Reconstitute one sachet with 200 mL of water (freshly boiled and cooled for infants)

Note. Five sachets reconstituted with 1 litre of water provide Na$^+$ 60 mmol, K$^+$ 20 mmol, Cl$^-$ 50 mmol, citrate 10 mmol, and glucose 111 mmol

Dioralyte® (Rhône-Poulenc Rorer)

Effervescent tablets, sodium chloride 117 mg, sodium bicarbonate 336 mg, potassium chloride 186 mg, citric acid anhydrous 384 mg, anhydrous glucose 1.62 g. Net price 10-tab pack (blackcurrant- or citrus-flavoured) = £1.42

Reconstitute 2 tablets with 200 mL of water (only for adults and for children over 1 year)

Note. Ten tablets when reconstituted with 1 litre of water provide Na$^+$ 60 mmol, K$^+$ 25 mmol, Cl$^-$ 45 mmol, citrate 20 mmol, and glucose 90 mmol

Oral powder, sodium chloride 470 mg, potassium chloride 300 mg, disodium hydrogen citrate 530 mg, glucose 3.56 g/sachet. Net price 20 sachet-pack (blackcurrant- or citrus-flavoured or natural) = £5.16

Reconstitute one sachet with 200 mL of water (freshly boiled and cooled for infants).

Note. Five sachets reconstituted with 1 litre of water provide Na$^+$ 60 mmol, K$^+$ 20 mmol, Cl$^-$ 60 mmol, citrate 10 mmol, and glucose 90 mmol

Dioralyte® Relief (Rhône-Poulenc Rorer)

Oral powder, sodium chloride 350 mg, potassium chloride 300 mg, sodium citrate 580 mg, cooked rice powder 6 g/sachet, net price 6-sachet pack (apricot-, blackcurrant- or raspberry-flavoured) = £1.92, 20-sachet pack (apricot-flavoured) = £6.19

Reconstitute one sachet with 200 mL of water (freshly boiled and cooled for infants)

Note. 5 sachets when reconstitued with 1 litre of water provide Na$^+$ 60 mmol, K$^+$ 20 mmol, Cl$^-$ 50 mmol and citrate 10 mmol; contains aspartame (section 9.4.1)

Electrolade® (Eastern)

Oral powder, sodium chloride 236 mg, potassium chloride 300 mg, sodium bicarbonate 500 mg, anhydrous glucose 4 g/sachet (banana-, blackcurrent-, melon-, or orange-flavoured). Net price 6-sachet (plain or multiflavoured) pack = £1.33, 20-sachet (single- or multiflavoured) pack = £4.99

Reconstitute one sachet with 200 mL of water (freshly boiled and cooled for infants)

Note. Five sachets when reconstituted with 1 litre of water provide Na$^+$ 50 mmol, K$^+$ 20 mmol, Cl$^-$ 40 mmol, HCO$_3^-$ 30 mmol, and glucose 111 mmol

Rehidrat® (Searle)

Oral powder, sodium chloride 440 mg, potassium chloride 380 mg, sodium bicarbonate 420 mg, citric acid 440 mg, glucose 4.09 g, sucrose 8.07 g, fructose 70 mg/sachet. Net price 24-sachet pack (orange, blackcurrant or lemon and lime flavour) = £6.44; 16-sachet pack (mixed flavours) = £4.29

Note. Lemon and lime version stains vomit green; blackcurrant version contains greater amounts of glucose (4.13 g) and sucrose (8.17 g), and less fructose (10 mg)

Reconstitute one sachet with 250 mL of water (freshly boiled and cooled for infants)

Note. Four sachets when reconstituted with 1 litre of water provide Na$^+$ 50 mmol, K$^+$ 20 mmol, Cl$^-$ 50 mmol, HCO$_3^-$ 20 mmol, citrate 9 mmol, glucose approx. 91 mmol, sucrose approx. 94 mmol, and fructose approx. 1–2 mmol

■ WHO formulation

Oral Rehydration Salts (Non-proprietary)

Oral powder, sodium chloride 3.5 g, potassium chloride 1.5 g, sodium citrate 2.9 g, anhydrous glucose 20 g. To be dissolved in sufficient water to produce 1 litre (providing Na$^+$ 90 mmol, K$^+$ 20 mmol, Cl$^-$ 80 mmol, citrate 10 mmol, glucose 111 mmol/litre)

Note. Recommended by the WHO and the United Nations Childrens Fund but not commonly used in the UK.

9.2.1.3   Oral bicarbonate

Sodium bicarbonate is given by mouth for *chronic acidotic states* such as uraemic acidosis or renal tubular acidosis. The dose for correction of metabolic acidosis is not predictable and the response must be assessed; 4.8 g daily (57 mmol each of Na$^+$ and HCO$_3^-$) or more may be required. For severe metabolic acidosis, sodium bicarbonate can be given intravenously (section 9.2.2).

Sodium bicarbonate may also be used to make the pH of the urine alkaline (see section 7.4.3); for use in dyspepsia see section 1.1.2.

Sodium supplements may increase blood pressure or cause fluid retention and pulmonary oedema in those at risk; hypokalaemia may be exacerbated.

Where *hyperchloraemic acidosis* is associated with potassium deficiency, as in some renal tubular and gastro-intestinal disorders it may be appropriate to give oral **potassium bicarbonate**, although acute or severe deficiency should be managed by intravenous therapy.

SODIUM BICARBONATE

Indications: see notes above
Cautions: see notes above; avoid in respiratory acidosis; **interactions:** Appendix 1 (antacids and adsorbents)
Dose: see notes above

Sodium Bicarbonate (Non-proprietary)
Capsules, sodium bicarbonate 500 mg (approx. 6 mmol each of Na$^+$ and HCO$_3^-$). Net price 20 = £6.11
Available from Generics, Norton
Tablets, sodium bicarbonate 600 mg, net price 20 tabs = 49p

POTASSIUM BICARBONATE

Indications: see notes above
Cautions: cardiac disease, renal impairment; **interactions:** Appendix 1 (potassium salts)
Contra-indications: hypochloraemia; plasma potassium concentration above 5 mmol/litre
Side-effects: nausea and vomiting
Dose: see notes above

Potassium Tablets, Effervescent (Non-proprietary)
Effervescent tablets, potassium bicarbonate 500 mg, potassium acid tartrate 300 mg, each tablet providing 6.5 mmol of K$^+$. To be dissolved in water before administration. Net price 100 = £4.53. Label: 13, 21
Available from Cox, Hillcross
Note. These tablets do not contain chloride; for effervescent tablets containing potassium and chloride, see under Potassium Chloride, section 9.2.1.1

Water

The term water used without qualification means either potable water freshly drawn direct from the public supply and suitable for drinking or freshly boiled and cooled purified water. The latter should be used if the public supply is from a local storage tank or if the potable water is unsuitable for a particular preparation. (Water for injections, section 9.2.2.)

<table>
<tr><td>9.2.2</td><td>**Parenteral preparations for fluid and electrolyte imbalance**</td></tr>
</table>

9.2.2.1 Electrolytes and water
9.2.2.2 Plasma and plasma substitutes

9.2.2.1   Electrolytes and water

Solutions of electrolytes are given intravenously, to meet normal fluid and electrolyte requirements or to replenish substantial deficits or continuing losses, when the patient is nauseated or vomiting and is unable to take adequate amounts by mouth. When intravenous administration is not possible large volumes of fluid can also be given subcutaneously by hypodermoclysis.

In an individual patient the nature and severity of the electrolyte imbalance must be assessed from the history and clinical and biochemical examination. Sodium, potassium, chloride, magnesium, phosphate, and water depletion can occur singly and in combination with or without disturbances of acid-base balance; for reference to the use of magnesium and phosphates, see section 9.5.

Isotonic solutions may be infused safely into a peripheral vein. Solutions more concentrated than plasma, for example 20% glucose are best given through an indwelling catheter positioned in a large vein.

Intravenous sodium

Sodium chloride in isotonic solution provides the most important extracellular ions in near physiological concentration and is indicated in *sodium depletion* which may arise from such conditions as gastro-enteritis, diabetic ketoacidosis, ileus, and ascites. In a severe deficit of from 4 to 8 litres, 2 to 3 litres of isotonic sodium chloride may be given over 2 to 3 hours; thereafter infusion can usually be at a slower rate. Excessive administration should be avoided; the jugular venous pressure should be assessed, the bases of the lungs should be examined for crepitations, and in elderly or seriously ill patients it is often helpful to monitor the right atrial (central) venous pressure.

To avoid the risk of osmotic demyelination syndrome, *chronic hyponatraemia* should be corrected slowly by limiting the rise in plasma-sodium concentration to no more than 10 mmol/litre in 24 hours.

Compound sodium lactate (Hartmann's solution) can be used instead of isotonic sodium chloride solution during surgery or in the initial management of the injured or wounded.

Sodium chloride and glucose solutions are indicated when there is combined *water and sodium depletion*. A 1:1 mixture of isotonic sodium chloride and 5% glucose allows some of the water (free of sodium) to enter body cells which suffer most from dehydration while the sodium salt with a volume of water determined by the normal plasma Na$^+$ remains extracellular. Combined sodium, potassium, chloride, and water depletion may occur, for example, with severe diarrhoea or persistent vomiting; replacement is carried out with sodium chloride intravenous infusion 0.9% and glucose intravenous infusion 5% with potassium as appropriate.

SODIUM CHLORIDE

Indications: electrolyte imbalance, also section 9.2.1.2
Cautions: restrict intake in impaired renal function, cardiac failure, hypertension, peripheral and pulmonary oedema, toxaemia of pregnancy
Side-effects: administration of large doses may give rise to sodium accumulation and oedema
Dose: see notes above

Sodium Chloride Intravenous Infusion (Non-proprietary) PoM
Intravenous infusion, usual strength sodium chloride 0.9% (9 g, 150 mmol each of Na$^+$ and Cl$^-$/litre), this strength being supplied when normal

saline for injection is requested. Net price 2-mL amp = 23p; 5-mL amp = 30p; 10-mL amp = 32p; 20-mL amp = 94p; 50-mL amp = £1.95

In hospitals, 500- and 1000-mL packs, and sometimes other sizes, are available

Note. The term 'normal saline' should **not** be used to describe sodium chloride intravenous infusion 0.9%; the term 'physiological saline' is acceptable but it is preferable to give the composition (i.e. sodium chloride intravenous infusion 0.9%).

■ With other ingredients

Sodium Chloride and Glucose Intravenous Infusion (Non-proprietary) [PoM]

Intravenous infusion, usual strength sodium chloride 0.18% (1.8 g, 30 mmol each of Na⁺ and Cl⁻/litre) and 4% of anhydrous glucose

In hospitals, 500- and 1000-mL packs, and sometimes other sizes are available

Ringer's Solution for Injection [PoM] calcium chloride (dihydrate) 322 micrograms, potassium chloride 300 micrograms, sodium chloride 8.6 mg/mL, providing the following ions (in mmol/litre), Ca²⁺ 2.2, K⁺ 4, Na⁺ 147, Cl⁻ 156

In hospitals, 500- and 1000-mL packs, and sometimes other sizes, are available

Sodium Lactate Intravenous Infusion, Compound (Non-proprietary) [PoM]

(Hartmann's Solution for Injection; Ringer-Lactate Solution for Injection),

Intravenous infusion, sodium chloride 0.6%, sodium lactate 0.25%, potassium chloride 0.04%, calcium chloride 0.027% (containing Na⁺ 131 mmol, K⁺ 5 mmol, Ca²⁺ 2 mmol, HCO₃⁻ (as lactate) 29 mmol, Cl⁻ 111 mmol/litre)

In hospitals, 500- and 1000-mL packs, and sometimes other sizes, are available

---

Intravenous glucose

Glucose solutions (5%) are mainly used to replace water deficits and should be given alone when there is no significant loss of electrolytes. Average water requirements in a healthy adult are 1.5 to 2.5 litres daily and this is needed to balance unavoidable losses of water through the skin and lungs and to provide sufficient for urinary excretion. Water depletion (dehydration) tends to occur when these losses are not matched by a comparable intake, as for example may occur in coma or dysphagia or in the aged or apathetic who may not drink water in sufficient amount on their own initiative.

Excessive loss of water without loss of electrolytes is uncommon, occurring in fevers, hyperthyroidism, and in uncommon water-losing renal states such as diabetes insipidus or hypercalcaemia. The volume of glucose solution needed to replace deficits varies with the severity of the disorder, but usually lies within the range of 2 to 6 litres.

Glucose solutions are also given in regimens with calcium, bicarbonate, and insulin for the emergency management of *hyperkalaemia.* They are also given, after correction of hyperglycaemia, during treatment of diabetic ketoacidosis, when they must be accompanied by continuing insulin infusion.

GLUCOSE

(Dextrose Monohydrate)

Note. Glucose BP is the monohydrate but Glucose Intravenous Infusion BP is a sterile solution of anhydrous

glucose or glucose monohydrate, potency being expressed in terms of anhydrous glucose

Indications: fluid replacement (see notes above), provision of energy (section 9.3)

Side-effects: glucose injections especially if hypertonic may have a low pH and may cause venous irritation and thrombophlebitis

Dose: water replacement, see notes above; energy source, 1–3 litres daily of 20–50% solution

Glucose Intravenous Infusion (Non-proprietary) [PoM]

Intravenous infusion, glucose or anhydrous glucose (potency expressed in terms of anhydrous glucose), usual strength 5% (50 mg/mL). 25% solution, net price 25-mL amp = £2.21; 50% solution, 25-mL amp = £3.11, 50-mL amp = £1.55

In hospitals, 500- and 1000-mL packs, and sometimes other sizes, are available; also available from Medeva (*Min-I-Jet® Glucose,* 50% in 10-mL and 50-mL disposable syringe).

Intravenous potassium

Potassium chloride and sodium chloride intravenous infusion and **potassium chloride and glucose** intravenous infusion are used to correct severe *hypokalaemia* and depletion and when sufficient potassium cannot be taken by mouth. Potassium chloride, as ampoules containing 1.5 g (20 mmol K⁺) in 10 mL,[1] should be added to 500 mL of sodium chloride 0.9% intravenous infusion and given slowly over 2 to 3 hours with specialist advice and ECG monitoring in difficult cases.[2] Repeated measurements of plasma potassium are necessary to determine whether further infusions are required and to avoid the development of hyperkalaemia; this is *especially liable to occur* in renal impairment.

POTASSIUM CHLORIDE

Indications: electrolyte imbalance; see also oral potassium supplements, section 9.2.1.1

Cautions: for intravenous infusion the concentration of solution should not usually exceed 3.2 g (43 mmol)/litre; specialist advice and ECG monitoring (see notes above)

Side-effects: rapid infusion toxic to heart

Dose: *by slow intravenous infusion,* depending on the deficit or the daily maintenance requirements, see also notes above

Potassium Chloride and Glucose Intravenous Infusion (Non-proprietary) [PoM]

Intravenous infusion, usual strength potassium chloride 0.3% (3 g, 40 mmol each of K⁺ and Cl⁻/litre) with 5% of anhydrous glucose

In hospitals, 500- and 1000-mL packs, and sometimes other sizes, are available

Potassium Chloride and Sodium Chloride Intravenous Infusion (Non-proprietary) [PoM]

Intravenous infusion, usual strength potassium chloride 0.3% (3 g/litre) and sodium chloride 0.9% (9 g/litre), containing 40 mmol of K⁺, 150 mmol of Na⁺, and 190 mmol of Cl⁻/litre

In hospitals, 500- and 1000-mL packs, and sometimes other sizes, are available

1. **Important**: mix infusion solution **thoroughly** after adding potassium chloride; use ready-prepared solutions when possible
2. Higher concentrations may be given in severe cases but require infusion pump control

Potassium Chloride, Sodium Chloride, and Glucose Intravenous Infusion (Non-proprietary) PoM

Intravenous infusion, sodium chloride 0.18% (1.8 g, 30 mmol of Na$^+$/litre) with 4% of anhydrous glucose and usually sufficient potassium chloride to provide 10–40 mmol of K$^+$/litre (to be specified by the prescriber)

In hospitals, 500- and 1000-mL packs, and sometimes other sizes, are available

Potassium Chloride Concentrate, Sterile (Non-proprietary) PoM

Sterile concentrate, potassium chloride 15% (150 mg, approximately 2 mmol each of K$^+$ and Cl$^-$/mL). Net price 10-mL amp = 45p

IMPORTANT. Must be diluted with **not less** than 50 times its volume of sodium chloride intravenous infusion 0.9% or other suitable diluent and **mixed well**

Solutions containing 10 and 20% of potassium chloride are also available in both 5- and 10-mL ampoules

---

Bicarbonate and lactate

Sodium bicarbonate is used to control severe *metabolic acidosis* (as in renal failure). Since this condition is usually attended by sodium depletion, it is reasonable to correct this first by the administration of isotonic sodium chloride intravenous infusion, provided the kidneys are not primarily affected and the degree of acidosis is not so severe as to impair renal function. In these circumstances, isotonic sodium chloride alone is usually effective as it restores the ability of the kidneys to generate bicarbonate. In renal acidosis or in severe metabolic acidosis of any origin (for example blood pH < 7.1) sodium bicarbonate (1.26%) may be infused with isotonic sodium chloride when the acidosis remains unresponsive to correction of anoxia or fluid depletion; a total volume of up to 6 litres (4 litres of sodium chloride and 2 litres of sodium bicarbonate) may be necessary in the adult. In severe shock due for example to cardiac arrest (see section 2.7), metabolic acidosis may develop without sodium depletion; in these circumstances sodium bicarbonate is best given in a small volume of hypertonic solution, such as 50 mL of 8.4% solution intravenously; plasma pH should be monitored.

Sodium bicarbonate infusion is also used in the emergency management of *hyperkalaemia* (see also under Glucose).

Sodium lactate intravenous infusion is obsolete in metabolic acidosis, and carries the risk of producing lactic acidosis, particularly in seriously ill patients with poor tissue perfusion or impaired hepatic function.

SODIUM BICARBONATE

Indications: metabolic acidosis

Dose: *by slow intravenous injection*, a strong solution (up to 8.4%), or *by continuous intravenous infusion*, a weaker solution (usually 1.26%), an amount appropriate to the body base deficit (see notes above)

Sodium Bicarbonate Intravenous Infusion PoM usual strength sodium bicarbonate 1.26% (12.6 g, 150 mmol each of Na$^+$ and HCO$_3^-$/litre); various other strengths available

In hospitals, 500- and 1000-mL packs, and sometimes other sizes, are available

Min-I-Jet® Sodium Bicarbonate (Medeva) PoM

Intravenous injection, sodium bicarbonate in disposable syringe, net price 4.2%, 10 mL = £4.81; 8.4%, 10 mL = £5.19, 50 mL = £7.75

SODIUM LACTATE ◢◤

Indications: see notes above

Sodium Lactate (Non-proprietary) PoM ◢◤

Intravenous infusion, sodium lactate M/6, contains the following ions (in mmol/litre), Na$^+$ 167, HCO$_3^-$ (as lactate) 167

> ◢◤ denotes preparations that are considered to be less suitable for prescribing (see p. vi)

Water

Water for Injections. PoM Net price 1-mL amp = 17p; 2-mL amp = 15p; 5-mL amp = 21p; 10-mL amp = 25p; 20-mL amp = 53p; 50-mL amp = £1.75

9.2.2.2   Plasma and plasma substitutes

Albumin solutions, prepared from whole blood, contain soluble proteins and electrolytes but no clotting factors, blood group antibodies, or plasma cholinesterases; they may be given without regard to the recipient's blood group.

Albumin solutions are used for the treatment of severe hypoproteinaemia, particularly when associated with a low plasma volume. Concentrated albumin solutions may also be used to obtain a diuresis in hypoalbuminaemic patients (e.g. in hepatic cirrhosis). The use of albumin solutions in acute plasma or blood loss may be wasteful; plasma substitutes are more appropriate. Albumin solutions have been linked with increased mortality in patients with hypovolaemia or hypoalbuminaemia such as those with acute blood loss or burns; it is uncertain whether albumin is responsible for the extra deaths.

> Plasma and plasma substitutes are often used in very ill patients whose condition is unstable. Therefore, close monitoring is required and fluid and electrolyte therapy should be adjusted according to the patient's condition at all times.

CSM advice. Following the publication of a meta-analysis in July 1998 concerning the safety of human albumin solution, the CSM has asked that product literature for albumin products should reflect the following:

- indications should focus on the use of albumin to replace lost fluids rather than the underlying cause of hypovolaemia; hypoalbuminaemia itself is not an appropriate indication;
- warnings should be added about the risks of hypervolaemia and cardiovascular overload, and the importance of monitoring patients receiving albumin to avoid these complications;
- special care is needed when administering albumin in conditions where capillary integrity is affected.

ALBUMIN SOLUTION

(Human Albumin Solution)

A solution containing protein derived from plasma, serum, or normal placentas; at least 95% of the protein is albumin. The solution may be isotonic (containing 4–5% protein) or concentrated (containing 15–25% protein).

Indications: see under preparations, below

Cautions: history of cardiac or circulatory disease (administer slowly to avoid rapid rise in blood pressure and cardiac failure, and monitor cardiovascular and respiratory function); correct dehydration when administering concentrated solution

Contra-indications: cardiac failure; severe anaemia

Side-effects: hypersensitivity reactions (including anaphylaxis) with nausea, vomiting, increased salivation, fever, tachycardia, hypotension and chills reported

■ Isotonic solutions

Indications: acute or sub-acute loss of plasma volume e.g. in burns, pancreatitis, trauma, and complications of surgery; plasma exchange

Available as: *Human Albumin Solution 4.5%* (50-, 100-, and 400-mL bottles—Hyland Immuno); *ALBA® 4.5%* (100- and 400-mL bottles— SNBTS); *Albutein® 5%* (250- and 500-mL vials—Grifols); *Zenalb® 4.5* (50-, 100-, 250-, and 500-mL bottles—BPL)

■ Concentrated solutions (20–25%)

Indications: severe hypoalbuminaemia associated with low plasma volume and generalised oedema where salt and water restriction with plasma volume expansion are required; adjunct in the treatment of hyperbilirubinaemia by exchange transfusion in the newborn

Available as: *Human Albumin Solution 20%* (10-, 50-, and 100-mL vials—Hyland Immuno); *ALBA® 20%* (100-mL vials—SNBTS); *Albutein® 20%* (50- and 100-mL vials—Grifols); *Albutein® 25%* (20-, 50-, and 100-mL vials—Grifols); *Zenalb® 20* (5-, 50-, and 100-mL bottles—BPL)

Plasma substitutes

Dextrans, **gelatin**, and the etherified starches, **hetastarch**, **hexastarch** and **pentastarch** are macromolecular substances which are metabolised slowly; they may be used at the outset to expand and maintain blood volume in shock arising from conditions such as burns or septicaemia. Plasma substitutes may be used as an immediate short-term measure to treat haemorrhage until blood is available. They are rarely needed when shock is due to sodium and water depletion because, in these circumstances, the shock responds to water and electrolyte repletion. See also section 2.7.1 for the management of shock.

Plasma substitutes should **not** be used to maintain plasma volume in conditions such as burns or peritonitis where there is loss of plasma protein, water and electrolytes over periods of several days or weeks. In these situations, plasma or plasma protein fractions containing large amounts of albumin should be given.

Large volumes of plasma substitutes can increase the risk of bleeding through depletion of coagulation factors.

Dextran 70 by intravenous infusion is used predominantly for volume expansion. Dextran 40 intravenous infusion is used in an attempt to improve peripheral blood flow in ischaemic disease of the limbs. Dextrans 40 and 70 have also been used in the prophylaxis of thromboembolism but are now rarely used for this purpose.

Dextrans may interfere with blood group crossmatching or biochemical measurements and these should be carried out before infusion is begun.

> Plasma and plasma substitutes are often used in very ill patients whose condition is unstable. Therefore, close monitoring is required and fluid and electrolyte therapy should be adjusted according to the patient's condition at all times.

CAUTIONS. Plasma substitutes should be used with caution in patients with cardiac disease or renal impairment; urine output should be monitored. Care should be taken to avoid haematocrit concentration from falling below 25–30% and the patient should be monitored for hypersensitivity reactions.

SIDE-EFFECTS. Hypersensitivity reactions may occur including, rarely, severe anaphylactoid reactions. Transient increase in bleeding time may occur.

DEXTRAN 40

Dextrans of weight average molecular weight about '40 000'

Indications: conditions associated with peripheral local slowing of the blood flow; prophylaxis of post-surgical thromboembolic disease (but see notes above)

Cautions: see notes above; can interfere with some laboratory tests (see also above); correct dehydration beforehand, give adequate fluids during therapy and, where possible, monitor central venous pressure

Side-effects: see notes above

Dose: *by intravenous infusion*, initially 500–1000 mL; further doses are given according to the patient's condition (see notes above)

Gentran 40® (Baxter) PoM

Intravenous infusion, dextran 40 intravenous infusion in glucose intravenous infusion 5% or in sodium chloride intravenous infusion 0.9%. Net price 500-mL bottle (both) = £4.56

Rheomacrodex® (Cambridge) PoM

Intravenous infusion, dextran 40 intravenous infusion in glucose intravenous infusion 5% or in sodium chloride intravenous infusion 0.9%. Net price 500-mL bottle (both) = £6.35

DEXTRAN 70

Dextrans of weight average molecular weight about '70 000'

Indications: short-term blood volume expansion; prophylaxis of post-surgical thromboembolic disease (but see notes above)

Cautions: see notes above; can interfere with some laboratory tests (see also above); where possible, monitor central venous pressure

Side-effects: see notes above

Dose: *by intravenous infusion*, after moderate to severe haemorrhage or in the shock phase of burn injury (initial 48 hours), 500–1000 mL rapidly initially followed by 500 mL later if necessary (see also notes above); total dosage should not exceed 20 mL/kg during initial 24 hours; CHILD total dosage should not exceed 20 mL/kg

Gentran 70® (Baxter) PoM

Intravenous infusion, dextran 70 intravenous infusion in glucose intravenous infusion 5% or in sodium chloride intravenous infusion 0.9%. Net price 500-mL bottle (both) = £4.78

GELATIN

Note. The gelatin is partially degraded

Indications: low blood volume

Cautions: see notes above

Side-effects: see notes above

Dose: *by intravenous infusion*, initially 500–1000 mL of a 3.5–4% solution (see notes above)

Gelofusine® (Braun) PoM

Intravenous infusion, succinylated gelatin (modified fluid gelatin, average molecular weight 30 000) 4%, sodium chloride 0.9%. Net price 500-mL bottle = £4.63

Haemaccel® (Hoechst Marion Roussel) PoM

Intravenous infusion, polygeline (degraded and modified gelatin, average molecular weight 30 000) 35 g, Na+ 145 mmol, K+ 5.1 mmol, Ca²⁺ 6.25 mmol, Cl⁻ 145 mmol/litre. Net price 500-mL bottle = £3.71

ETHERIFIED STARCH

A starch composed of more than 90% of amylopectin that has been etherified with hydroxyethyl groups; hetastarch has a higher degree of etherification than pentastarch

Indications: low blood volume

Cautions: see notes above; children

Side-effects: see notes above

Dose: see under preparations below

■ Hetastarch

Hespan® (Geistlich) PoM

Intravenous infusion, hetastarch (weight average molecular weight 450 000) 6% in sodium chloride intravenous infusion 0.9%. Net price 500-mL *Steriflex®* bag = £15.57

Dose: by intravenous infusion, 500–1000 mL; usual daily max. 1500 mL (see notes above)

■ Hexastarch

eloHAES® (Fresenius) PoM

Intravenous infusion, hexastarch (weight average molecular weight 200 000) 6% in sodium chloride intravenous infusion 0.9%. Net price 500-mL *Steriflex®* bag = £12.50

Dose: by intravenous infusion, 500–1000 mL; usual daily max. 1500 mL (see notes above)

■ Pentastarch

HAES-steril® (Fresenius) PoM

Intravenous infusion, pentastarch (weight average molecular weight 200 000), net price (both in sodium chloride intravenous infusion 0.9%) 6%, 500 mL = £10.50; 10%, 500 mL = £16.50

Dose: by intravenous infusion, pentastarch 6%, up to 2500 mL daily; pentastarch 10%, up to 1500 mL daily (see notes above)

Hemohes® (Braun) PoM

Intravenous infusion, pentastarch (weight average molecular weight 200 000), net price (both in sodium chloride intravenous infusion 0.9%) 6%, 500 mL = £12.50; 10%, 500 mL = £16.50

Dose: by intravenous infusion, pentastarch 6%, up to 2500 mL daily; pentastarch 10%, up to 1500 mL daily (see notes above)

Pentaspan® (Geistlich) PoM

Intravenous infusion, pentastarch (weight average molecular weight 250 000) 10% in sodium chloride intravenous infusion 0.9%. Net price 500-mL *Intraflex®* bag = £11.25

Dose: by intravenous infusion, 500–2000 mL; usual daily max. 2000 mL (see notes above)

9.3 Intravenous nutrition

When adequate feeding through the alimentary tract is not possible, nutrients may be given by intravenous infusion. This may be in addition to ordinary oral or tube feeding—**supplemental parenteral nutrition**, or may be the sole source of nutrition—**total parenteral nutrition** (TPN). Indications for this method include preparation of undernourished patients for surgery, chemotherapy, or radiation therapy; severe or prolonged disorders of the gastro-intestinal tract; major surgery, trauma, or burns; prolonged coma or refusal to eat; and some patients with renal or hepatic failure. The composition of proprietary preparations available is given in the table below.

Total parenteral nutrition requires the use of a solution containing amino acids, glucose, fat, electrolytes, trace elements, and vitamins. This is now commonly provided by the pharmacy in the form of the 3-litre bag. Loading doses of vitamin B₁₂ and folic acid are advised and other vitamins are given parenterally twice weekly.

The nutrition solution is infused through a central venous catheter inserted under full surgical precautions. Alternatively infusion through a peripheral vein is used for supplementary as well as total parenteral nutrition for periods of up to a month, depending on the availability of peripheral veins; factors prolonging cannula life and preventing thrombophlebitis include the use of soft polyurethane paediatric cannulae and use of feeds of low osmolality and neutral pH. Only nutritional fluids should be given by the dedicated intravenous line.

Before starting, the patient should be well oxygenated with a near normal circulating blood volume and attention should be given to renal function and acid-base status. Appropriate biochemical tests should have been carried out beforehand and serious deficits corrected. Nutritional and electrolyte status must be monitored throughout treatment.

Complications of long-term TPN include gall bladder sludging, gall stones, cholestasis and abnormal liver function tests. For details of the prevention and management of TPN complications, specialist literature should be consulted.

Protein is given as mixtures of essential and non-essential synthetic L-amino acids. Ideally, all essential amino acids should be included with a wide variety of non-essential ones to provide sufficient nitrogen together with electrolytes (see also section 9.2.2). Solutions vary in their composition of amino acids; they often contain an energy source (usually glucose) and electrolytes.

Energy is provided in a ratio of 0.6 to 1.1 megajoules (150–250 kcals) per gram of protein nitrogen. Energy requirements must be met if amino acids are to be utilised for tissue maintenance. A mixture of carbohydrate and fat energy sources (usually 30–50% as fat) gives better utilisation of amino acids than glucose alone.

Glucose is the preferred source of carbohydrate, but if more than 180 g is given per day frequent monitoring of blood glucose is required, and insulin may be necessary. Glucose in various strengths from 10 to 50% must be infused through a central venous catheter to avoid thrombosis.

In total parenteral nutrition regimens, it is necessary to provide adequate phosphate in order to allow phosphorylation of the glucose; between 20 and 30 mmol of phosphate is required daily.

Fructose and sorbitol have been used in an attempt to avoid the problem of hyperosmolar hyperglycaemic non-ketotic acidosis but other metabolic problems may occur, as with xylitol and ethanol which are now rarely used.

Fat emulsions have the advantages of a high energy to fluid volume ratio, neutral pH, and iso-osmolarity with plasma, and provide essential fatty acids. Several days of adaptation may be required to attain maximal utilisation. Reactions include occasional febrile episodes (usually only with 20% emulsions) and rare anaphylactic responses. Interference with biochemical measurements such as those for blood gases and calcium may occur if samples are taken before fat has been cleared. Daily checks are necessary to ensure complete clearance from the plasma in conditions where fat metabolism may be disturbed. **Additives may only be mixed with fat emulsions where compatibility is known**.

> **Administration.** Because of the complex requirements relating to parenteral nutrition full details relating to administration have been omitted. In all cases *product literature and other specialist literature should be consulted.*

Supplementary preparations

> Compatibility with the infusion solution must be acertained before adding supplementary preparations.

Addiphos® (Fresenius Kabi) [PoM]
Solution, sterile, phosphate 40 mmol, K⁺ 30 mmol, Na⁺ 30 mmol/20 mL. For addition to *Vamin®* solutions and glucose intravenous infusions. Net price 20-mL vial = £1.15

Additrace® (Fresenius Kabi) [PoM]
Solution, trace elements for addition to *Vamin®* solutions and glucose intravenous infusions, traces of Fe^{3+}, Zn^{2+}, Mn^{2+}, Cu^{2+}, Cr^{3+}, Se^{4+}, Mo^{6+}, F^-, I^-. For adults and children over 40 kg. Net price 10-mL amp = £1.75

Cernevit® (Baxter) [PoM]
Solution, *dl*-alpha tocopherol 11.2 units, ascorbic acid 125 mg, biotin 69 micrograms, colecalciferol 220 units, cyanocobalamin 6 micrograms, folic acid 414 micrograms, glycine 250 mg, nicotinamide 46 mg, pantothenic acid (as dexpanthenol) 17.25 mg, pyridoxine hydrochloride 5.5 mg, retinol (as palmitate) 3500 units, riboflavin (as dihydrated sodium phosphate) 4.14 mg, thiamine (as cocarboxylase tetrahydrate) 3.51 mg. Dissolve in 5 mL water for injections. Net price per vial = £2.90

Dipeptiven® (Fresenius Kabi) [PoM]
Solution, N(2)-L-alanyl-L-glutamine 200 mg/mL (providing L-alanine 82 mg, L-glutamine 134.6 mg). For addition to infusion solutions containing amino acids. Net price 50 mL = £25.00, 100 mL = £29.60
Dose: amino acid supplement for hypercatabolic or hypermetabolic states, 300–400 mg/kg daily; max. 400 mg/kg daily, dose not to exceed 20% of total amino acid intake

Multibionta® (Merck) [PoM]
Solution, ascorbic acid 500 mg, dexpanthenol 25 mg, nicotinamide 100 mg, pyridoxine hydrochloride 15 mg, riboflavin sodium phosphate 10 mg, thiamine hydrochloride 50 mg, tocopheryl acetate 5 mg, vitamin A 10 000 units. For addition to infusion solutions. Net price 10-mL amp = £1.61
Contra-indications: not for use in neonates owing to presence of benzyl alcohol as additive

Peditrace® (Fresenius Kabi) [PoM]
Solution, trace elements for addition to *Vaminolact®*, *Vamin® 14 Electrolyte-Free* solutions and glucose intravenous infusions, traces of Zn^{2+}, Cu^{2+}, Mn^{2+}, Se^{4+}, F^-, I^-. For use in infants (when kidney function established, usually second day of life) and children. Net price 10-mL vial = £3.10
Cautions: reduced biliary excretion especially in cholestatic liver disease or in markedly reduced urinary excretion (careful biochemical monitoring required); total parenteral nutrition exceeding 1 month (measure serum manganese concentration and check liver function before commencing treatment and regularly during treatment)—discontinue if manganese concentration raised or if cholestasis develops

Solivito N® (Fresenius Kabi) [PoM]
Solution, powder for reconstitution, biotin 60 micrograms, cyanocobalamin 5 micrograms, folic acid 400 micrograms, glycine 300 mg, nicotinamide 40 mg, pyridoxine hydrochloride 4.9 mg, riboflavin sodium phosphate 4.9 mg, sodium ascorbate 113 mg, sodium pantothenate 16.5 mg, thiamine mononitrate 3.1 mg. Dissolve in water for injections or glucose intravenous infusion for adding to glucose intravenous infusion or *Intralipid®*; dissolve in *Vitlipid N®* or *Intralipid®* for adding to *Intralipid®* only. Net price per vial = £1.75

Vitlipid N® (Fresenius Kabi) [PoM]
Emulsion, adult, vitamin A 330 units, ergocalciferol 20 units, *dl*-alpha tocopherol 1 unit, phytomenadione 15 micrograms/mL. For addition to *Intralipid®*. For adults and children over 11 years. Net price 10-mL amp = £1.71
Emulsion, infant, vitamin A 230 units, ergocalciferol 40 units, *dl*-alpha tocopherol 0.7 unit, phytomenadione 20 micrograms/mL. For addition to *Intralipid®*. Net price 10-mL amp = £1.71

Proprietary Infusion Fluids for Parenteral Feeding

Preparation	Nitrogen g/litre	[1]Energy kJ/litre	Electrolytes mmol/litre					Other components/litre
			K$^+$	Mg^{2+}	Na$^+$	Acet$^-$	Cl$^-$	
Aminoplasmal 5% E (Braun) Net price 500 mL = £9.02	8		25	2.6	43	59	29	dihydrogen phosphate 9 mmol, malic acid 1.01 g
Aminoplasmal 10% (Braun) Net price 500 mL = £17.06	16						57	
Aminoplex 12 (Geistlich) Net price 250 mL = £5.66; 500 mL = £10.80; 1000 mL = £19.07	12.44		30	2.5	35	5	67	malic acid 4.6 g
Aminoplex 24 (Geistlich) Net price 250 mL = £9.79; 500 mL = £17.28	24.9		30	2.5	35	5	67	malic acid 4.5 g
Aminoplex 24 Electrolyte-Free (Geistlich) Net price 250 mL = £9.79; 500 mL = £16.50	24.9							malic acid 9.5 g
Aminosteril 8 (Fresenius Kabi) Net price 500 mL = £7.95	7.95				55			
Aminosteril 14 (Fresenius Kabi) Net price 500 mL = £9.90; 1000 mL = £16.00	13.52				93			
Aminosteril 16 (Fresenius Kabi) Net price 500 mL = £10.90	15.9				109			
Clinimix N9G20E (Baxter) Net price (dual compartment bag of amino acids with electrolytes 1000 mL and glucose 20% with calcium 1000 mL) = £29.00	4.55	1680	30	2.5	35	50	40	Ca^{2+} 2.25 mmol, phosphate 15 mmol, anhydrous glucose 100 g
Clinimix N14G30E (Baxter) Net price (dual compartment bag of amino acids with electrolytes 1000 mL and glucose 30% with calcium 1000 mL) = £33.00	7	2520	30	2.5	35	70	40	Ca^{2+} 2.25 mmol, phosphate 15 mmol, anhydrous glucose 150 g
Clinomel N5-800 (Baxter) Net price (2000-mL triple compartment bag of amino acids with electrolytes 800 mL, glucose 25% with calcium 800 mL, lipid emulsion 20% 400 mL) = £66.00	4.8	3360	24	2	28	50	32	Ca^{2+} 1.8 mmol, phosphate 12 mmol, glycerol 5 g, soya oil 40 g, purified egg phospholipids 2.4 g, anhydrous glucose 200 g
Clinomel N6-900 (Baxter) Net price (2000-mL triple compartment bag of amino acids with electrolytes 800 mL, glucose 30% with calcium 800 mL, lipid emulsion 20% 400 mL) = £69.00	5.6	3696	24	2	28	56	32	Ca^{2+} 1.8 mmol, phosphate 12 mmol, glycerol 5 g, soya oil 40 g, purified egg phospholipids 2.4 g, anhydrous glucose 240 g
Clinomel N7-1000 (Baxter) Net price (2000-mL triple compartment bag of amino acids with electrolytes 800 mL, glucose 40% with calcium 800 mL, lipid emulsion 20% 400 mL) = £72.00	6.6	4368	24	2	28	60	32	Ca^{2+} 1.8 mmol, phosphate 12 mmol, glycerol 5 g, soya oil 40 g, purified egg phospholipids 2.4 g, anhydrous glucose 320 g
FreAmine III 8.5% (Fresenius Kabi) Net price 500 mL = £14.39; 1000 mL = £21.06	13.0				10	72	<3	phosphate 10 mmol
FreAmine III 10% (Fresenius Kabi) Net price 500 mL = £13.60; 1000 mL = £23.50	15.3				10	89	<3	phosphate 10 mmol
Glamin (Fresenius Kabi) Net price 250 mL = £14.16; 500 mL = £26.38; 1000 mL = £52.76	22.4				62			
GluCoplex 1000 (Geistlich) Net price 500 mL = £3.30; 1000 mL = £4.71		4200	30	2.5	50		67	dihydrogen phosphate 18 mmol, Zn^{2+} 0.046 mmol, anhydrous glucose 240 g
GluCoplex 1600 (Geistlich) Net price 500 mL = £3.64; 1000 mL = £4.88		6720	30	2.5	50		67	dihydrogen phosphate 18 mmol, Zn^{2+} 0.046 mmol, anhydrous glucose 400 g
Hepanutrin (Geistlich) Net price 500 mL = £15.74	15.6							
Hyperamine 30 (Braun) Net price 500 mL = £23.67	30				5			
Intrafusin 11 (Fresenius Kabi) Net price 1000 mL = £14.24	11.4		40	5	80		76	Ca^{2+} 3 mmol, phosphate 20 mmol, citrate 6 mmol
Intrafusin 22 (Fresenius Kabi) Net price 500 mL = £14.24	22.8							
Intralipid 10% (Fresenius Kabi) Net price 100 mL = £3.90; 500 mL = £8.58		4600						soya oil 100 g, glycerol 22 g, purified egg phospholipids 12 g, phosphate 15 mmol
Intralipid 20% (Fresenius Kabi) Net price 100 mL = £5.85; 250 mL = £9.65; 500 mL = £12.87		8400						soya oil 200 g, glycerol 22 g, purified egg phospholipids 12 g, phosphate 15 mmol

1. Excludes protein- or amino acid-derived energy

Note. 1000 kcal = 4200 kJ; 1000 kJ = 238.8 kcal. All entries are PoM

Proprietary Infusion Fluids for Parenteral Feeding

Preparation	Nitrogen g/litre	Energy[1] kJ/litre	K+	Mg2+	Na+	Acet-	Cl-	Other components/litre
Intralipid 30% (Fresenius Kabi) Net price 333 mL = £14.40		12600						soya oil 300 g, glycerol 16.7 g, purified egg phospholipids 12 g, phosphate 15 mmol
Ivelip 10% (Baxter) Net price 100 mL = £4.78; 500 mL = £9.51		4600						soya oil 100 g, glycerol 25 g
Ivelip 20% (Baxter) Net price 100 mL = £6.58; 500 mL = £14.53; 1000 mL = £25.84		8400						soya oil 200 g, glycerol 25 g
KabiMix 9 (Fresenius Kabi) Net price 2580 mL = £64.00	3.49	2600	23	1.9	31	21.3	31	Ca2+ 1.9 mmol, anhydrous glucose 58.14 g, phosphate 10.9 mmol, soya oil 38.76 g, glycerol 4.26 g, purified egg phospholipids 2.33 g
KabiMix 11 (Fresenius Kabi) Net price 2000 mL = £67.00	5.3	3500	23	2	31	34.9	31	Ca2+ 1.9 mmol, anhydrous glucose 116.28 g, phosphate 10.9 mmol, soya oil 38.76 g, glycerol 4.26 g, purified egg phospholipids 2.33 g
KabiMix 14 (Fresenius Kabi) Net price 2580 mL = £70.00	5.23	3570	23	1.9	31	34.9	31	Ca2+ 1.9 mmol, anhydrous glucose 116.28 g, phosphate 10.9 mmol, soya oil 38.76 g, glycerol 4.26 g, purified egg phospholipids 2.33 g
Lipofundin MCT/LCT 10% (Braun) Net price 100 mL = £7.70; 500 mL = £12.90		4430						soya oil 50 g, medium chain triglycerides 50 g
Lipofundin MCT/LCT 20% (Braun) Net price 100 mL = £8.79; 250 mL = £11.30; 500 mL = £19.18		8000						soya oil 100 g, medium chain triglycerides 100 g
Lipofundin N 10% (Braun) Net price 100 mL = £7.10; 250 mL = £9.50; 500 mL = £11.76		4470						soya oil 100 g, glycerol 25 g, egg lecithin 8 g
Lipofundin N 20% (Braun) Net price 100 mL = £8.10; 250 mL = £9.99; 500 mL = £15.38		8520						soya oil 200 g, glycerol 25 g, egg lecithin 12 g
Lipovenos 10% (Fresenius Kabi) Net price 500 mL = £9.50		4600						fractionated soya oil 100 g, egg lecithin 12 g, glycerol 25 g
Lipovenos 20% (Fresenius Kabi) Net price 100 mL = £4.90; 250 mL = £5.60; 500 mL = £14.50		8400						fractionated soya oil 200 g, egg lecithin 12 g, glycerol 25 g
Nutracel 400 (Baxter) Net price 500 mL = £2.54		3400		18		0.16	66	Ca2+ 15 mmol, Mn2+ 0.01 mmol, Zn2+ 0.08 mmol, anhydrous glucose 200 g
Nutracel 800 (Baxter) Net price 1000 mL = £4.39		3400		9		0.08	33	Ca2+ 7.5 mmol, Mn2+ 0.005 mmol, Zn2+ 0.04 mmol, anhydrous glucose 200 g
NuTRIflex Lipid peri (Braun) Net price (triple compartment bag of amino acids 500 mL or 1000 mL; glucose 500 mL or 1000 mL; lipid emulsion 20% 250 mL or 500 mL) 1250 mL = £43.38, 2500 mL = £65.05	4.56	2664	24	2.4	40	32	38.4	Ca2+ 2.4 mmol, Zn2+ 0.024 mmol, phosphate 6 mmol, anhydrous glucose 64 g, soya oil 20 g, medium chain triglycerides 20 g
NuTRIflex Lipid plus (Braun) Net price (triple compartment bag of amino acids 500 mL, 750 mL or 1000 mL; glucose 500 mL, 750 mL or 1000 mL; lipid emulsion 20% 250 mL, 375 mL or 500 mL) 1250 mL = £47.17, 1875 mL = £60.23, 2500 mL = £69.27	5.44	3600	28	3.2	40	36	36	Ca2+ 3.2 mmol, Zn2+ 0.024 mmol, phosphate 12 mmol, anhydrous glucose 120 g, soya oil 20 g, medium chain triglycerides 20 g
NuTRIflex Lipid plus without Electrolytes (Braun) Net price (triple compartment bag of amino acids 500 mL, 750 mL or 1000 mL; glucose 500 mL, 750 mL or 1000 mL; lipid emulsion 20% 250 mL, 375 mL or 500 mL) 1250 mL = £47.17, 1875 mL = £60.23, 2500 mL = £69.27	5.44	3600						anhydrous glucose 120 g, soya oil 20 g, medium chain triglycerides 20 g

1. Excludes protein- or amino acid-derived energy

Note. 1000 kcal = 4200 kJ; 1000 kJ = 238.8 kcal. All entries are PoM

Proprietary Infusion Fluids for Parenteral Feeding

Preparation	Nitrogen g/litre	[1]Energy kJ/litre	Electrolytes mmol/litre					Other components/litre
			K$^+$	Mg^{2+}	Na$^+$	Acet$^-$	Cl$^-$	
NuTRIflex Lipid special (Braun) Net price (triple compartment bag of amino acids 500 mL, 750 mL or 1000 mL; glucose 500 mL, 750 mL or 1000 mL; lipid emulsion 20% 250 mL, 375 mL or 500 mL) 1250 mL = £57.69, 1875 mL = £75.58, 2500 mL = £89.21	8	4004	37.6	4.24	53.6	48	48	Ca^{2+} 4.24 mmol, Zn^{2+} 0.032 mmol, phosphate 16 mmol, anhydrous glucose 144 g, soya 144 g, medium chain triglycerides 20 g
NuTRIflex Lipid special without Electrolytes (Braun) Net price (triple compartment bag of amino acids 500 mL, 750 mL or 1000 mL; glucose 500 mL, 750 mL or 1000 mL; lipid emulsion 20% 250 mL, 375 mL or 500 mL) 1250 mL = £57.69, 1875 mL = £75.58, 2500 mL = £89.21	8	4004						anhydrous glucose 144 g, soya oil 20 g, medium chain triglycerides 20 g
Nutriflex Basal (Braun) Net price (dual compartment bag of 800 mL and 1200 mL) = £28.35	4.6	2095	30	5.7	49.9	35	50	Ca^{2+} 3.6 mmol, phosphate 12.8 mmol, anhydrous glucose 125 g
Nutriflex Peri (Braun) Net price (dual compartment bag of 800 mL and 1200 mL) = £33.00	5.7	1340	15	4	27	19.5	31.6	Ca^{2+} 2.5 mmol, phosphate 5.7 mmol, anhydrous glucose 80 g
Nutriflex Plus (Braun) Net price (dual compartment bag of 800 mL and 1200 mL) = £39.18	6.8	2510	25	5.7	37.2	22.9	35.5	Ca^{2+} 3.6 mmol, phosphate 20 mmol, anhydrous glucose 150 g
Nutriflex Special (Braun) Net price (dual compartment bag of 750 mL and 750 mL) = £43.30	10	4020	25.7	5	40.5	22	49.5	Ca^{2+} 4.1 mmol, phosphate 15 mmol, anhydrous glucose 240 g
Plasma-Lyte 148 (water) (Baxter) Net price 1000 mL = £1.59			5	1.5	140	27	98	gluconate 23 mmol
Plasma-Lyte 148 (dextrose 5%) (Baxter) Net price 1000 mL = £1.59		840	5	1.5	140	27	98	gluconate 23 mmol, anhydrous glucose 50 g
Plasma-Lyte M (dextrose 5%) (Baxter) Net price 1000 mL = £1.33		840	16	1.5	40	12	40	Ca^{2+} 2.5 mmol, lactate 12 mmol, anhydrous glucose 50 g
[2]Primene 10% (Baxter) Net price 100 mL = £6.05; 250 mL = £8.29	15						15.6	
Synthamin 9 (Baxter) Net price 500 mL = £6.97; 1000 mL = £12.92	9.1		60	5	70	100	70	acid phosphate 30 mmol
Synthamin 14 (Baxter) Net price 500 mL = £10.09; 1000 mL = £17.94; 3000 mL = £51.29	14.0		60	5	70	140	70	acid phosphate 30 mmol
Synthamin 14 without electrolytes (Baxter) Net price 500 mL = £10.34; 1000 mL = £18.33	14.0				68	34		
Synthamin 17 (Baxter) Net price 500 mL = £13.26; 1000 mL = £24.08	16.5		60	5	70	150	70	acid phosphate 30 mmol
Synthamin 17 without electrolytes (Baxter) Net price 500 mL = £13.26	16.5				82	40		
Vamin 9 (Fresenius Kabi) Net price 500 mL = £5.85; 1000 mL = £10.04	9.4		20	1.5	50		50	Ca^{2+} 2.5 mmol
Vamin 9 Glucose (Fresenius Kabi) Net price 100 mL = £3.02; 500 mL = £6.14; 1000 mL = £11.02	9.4	1700	20	1.5	50		50	Ca^{2+} 2.5 mmol, anhydrous glucose 100 g
Vamin 14 (Fresenius Kabi) Net price 500 mL = £8.63; 1000 mL = £14.67	13.5		50	8	100	135	100	Ca^{2+} 5 mmol, SO$_4^{2-}$ 8 mmol
Vamin 14 (Electrolyte-Free) (Fresenius Kabi) Net price 500 mL = £8.29; 1000 mL = £14.67	13.5				90			
Vamin 18 (Electrolyte-Free) (Fresenius Kabi) Net price 500 mL = £10.97; 1000 mL = £19.74	18				110			
Vaminolact (Fresenius Kabi) Net price 100 mL = £3.36; 500 mL = £7.75	9.3							
Vitrimix KV (Fresenius Kabi) Net price (combined pack of Intralipid 20% 250 mL and Vamin 9 glucose 750 mL) = £19.40	7.0	3340	15	1.1	38		38	Ca^{2+} 1.9 mmol, anhydrous glucose 75 g, soya oil 50 g, purified egg phospholipids 3 g, glycerol 5.5 g, phosphate 3.75 mmol

1. Excludes protein- or amino acid-derived energy

2. For use in neonates and children only

Note. 1000 kcal = 4200 kJ; 1000 kJ = 238.8 kcal. All entries are PoM

9.4   Oral nutrition
9.4.1   Foods for special diets
9.4.2   Enteral nutrition

9.4.1   Foods for special diets

These are preparations that have been modified to eliminate a particular constituent from a food or are nutrient mixtures formulated as substitutes for the food. They are for patients who either cannot tolerate or cannot metabolise certain common constituents of food.

PHENYLKETONURIA. Phenylketonuria (phenyla-laninaemia), which results from the inability to metabolise phenylalanine, is managed by restricting its dietary intake to a small amount sufficient for tissue building and repair. Aspartame (as a sweetener in some foods and medicines) contributes to the phenylalanine intake and may affect control of phenylketonuria. Where the presence of aspartame is specified in the product literature this is indicated in the BNF against the preparation.

COELIAC DISEASE. Coeliac disease, which results from an intolerance to gluten, is managed by completely eliminating gluten from the diet.

> **ACBS.** In certain clinical conditions some foods may have the characteristics of drugs and the Advisory Committee on Borderline Substances advises as to the circumstances in which such foods may be regarded as drugs and so can be prescribed in the NHS. Prescriptions for these foods issued in accordance with the advice of this committee and endorsed 'ACBS' will normally not be investigated. See Appendix 7 for details of these foods and a listing by clinical condition (consult Drug Tariff for late amendments).

■ Preparations
For preparations on the ACBS list see Appendix 7
Forceval Protein Powder® (Unigreg)
Powder, strawberry, vanilla and natural flavours, protein (calcium caseinate, providing all essential amino acids) 55%, carbohydrate 30%, with vitamins, minerals, trace elements, fat and low electrolytes (lactose- and gluten-free), net price 14 × 30-g sachets = £17.92; chocolate flavour (as above but protein content is 45%), 14 × 36-g sachets = £17.92. For hypoproteinaemia, malabsorption states and as an adjunct to nutritional support. Not to be prescribed for any CHILD under 2 years or for those with renal or hepatic failure; unsuitable as a sole source of nutrition

9.4.2   Enteral nutrition

The body's reserves of protein rapidly become exhausted in severely ill patients, especially during chronic illness or in those with severe burns, extensive trauma, pancreatitis, or intestinal fistula. Much can be achieved by frequent meals and by persuading the patient to take supplementary snacks of ordinary food between the meals.

However, extra calories, protein, other nutrients, and vitamins are often best given by supplementing

ordinary meals with sip or tube feeds of one of the nutritionally complete foods.

When patients cannot feed normally at all, for example patients with severe facial injury, oesophageal obstruction, or coma, a diet composed solely of nutritionally complete foods must be given. This is planned by a dietitian who will take into account the protein and total energy requirement of the patient and decide on the form and relative contribution of carbohydrate and fat to the energy requirements.

There are a number of nutritionally complete foods available and their use reduces an otherwise heavy workload in hospital or in the home. Most contain protein derived from milk or soya. Some contain protein hydrolysates or free amino acids and are only appropriate for patients who have diminished ability to break down protein, as may be the case in inflammatory bowel disease or pancreatic insufficiency.

Even when nutritionally complete feeds are being given it may be important to monitor water and electrolyte balance. Extra minerals (e.g. magnesium and zinc) may be needed in patients where gastrointestinal secretions are being lost. Additional vitamins may also be needed. Regular haematological and biochemical tests may be needed particularly in the unstable patient.

Some feeds are supplemented with vitamin K; for drug interactions of vitamin K see Appendix 1 (vitamins).

CHILDREN. Infants and young children have special requirements and in most situations liquid feeds prepared for adults are totally unsuitable and should not be given. Expert advice should be sought.

■ Preparations
See Appendix 7

9.5   Minerals
9.5.1   Calcium and magnesium
9.5.2   Phosphorus
9.5.3   Fluoride
9.5.4   Zinc

See section 9.1.1 for iron salts.

9.5.1   Calcium and magnesium
9.5.1.1   Calcium supplements
9.5.1.2   Hypercalcaemia
9.5.1.3   Magnesium

9.5.1.1   Calcium supplements

Calcium supplements are usually only required where dietary calcium intake is deficient. This dietary requirement varies with age and is relatively greater in childhood, pregnancy, and lactation, due to an increased demand, and in old age, due to impaired absorption. In osteoporosis, a calcium intake which is double the recommended daily amount (RDA) reduces the rate of bone loss. If the actual dietary intake is less than the RDA, a supplement of as much as 40 mmol is appropriate.

In hypocalcaemic tetany an initial intravenous injection of 10 mL (2.25 mmol) of calcium gluconate injection 10% should be followed by the continuous infusion of about 40 mL (9 mmol) daily, but plasma calcium should be monitored. This regimen can also be used, immediately but temporarily, to reduce the toxic effects of hyperkalaemia.

Calcium may also be used in cardiac resuscitation (section 2.7.3).

CALCIUM SALTS

Indications: see notes above; calcium deficiency

Cautions: renal impairment; sarcoidosis; **interactions:** Appendix 1 (calcium salts)

Contra-indications: conditions associated with hypercalcaemia and hypercalciuria (eg. some forms of malignant disease)

Side-effects: mild gastro-intestinal disturbances; bradycardia, arrhythmias, and irritation after intravenous injection

Dose: *by mouth*, daily in divided doses, see notes above

By slow intravenous injection, acute hypocalcaemia, calcium gluconate 1–2 g (2.25–4.5 mmol of Ca^{2+})

CHILD obtain paediatric advice

■ Oral preparations

Calcium Gluconate (Non-proprietary)
Tablets, calcium gluconate 600 mg (53.4 mg calcium or 1.35 mmol Ca^{2+}), net price 20 = 78p. Label: 24

Effervescent tablets, calcium gluconate 1 g (89 mg calcium or 2.25 mmol Ca^{2+}), net price 100 = £11.49. Label: 13

Note. Each tablet usually contains 4.46 mmol Na^+

Calcium Lactate (Non-proprietary)
Tablets, calcium lactate 300 mg (39 mg calcium or 1 mmol Ca^{2+}), net price 20 = 25p

Cacit® (Procter & Gamble Pharm.)
Tablets, effervescent, pink, calcium carbonate 1.25 g, providing calcium citrate when dispersed in water (500 mg calcium or 12.6 mmol Ca^{2+}), net price 76-tab pack = £10.88. Label: 13

Calcette® (Ashbourne)
Tablets (chewable), calcium carbonate 1.25 g (500 mg calcium or 12.6 mmol Ca^{2+}), net price 100-tab pack = £8.98. Label: 24
Excipients: include aspartame

Calcichew® (Shire)
Tablets (chewable), calcium carbonate 1.25 g (500 mg calcium or 12.6 mmol Ca^{2+}), net price 100-tab pack = £9.82
Forte tablets (chewable), calcium carbonate 2.5 g (1 g calcium or 25 mmol Ca^{2+}), net price 100-tab pack = £21.94. Label: 24
Excipients: include aspartame

Calcidrink® (Shire)
Granules, effervescent, calcium carbonate 2.52 g (1 g calcium or 25 mmol Ca^{2+}). Net price 30-sachet pack = £8.48. Label: 13

Calcium-500 (Martindale)
Tablets, pink, f/c, calcium carbonate 1.25 g (500 mg calcium or 12.5 mmol Ca^{2+}). Net price 100-tab pack = £10.17. Label: 25

Calcium-Sandoz® (Alliance)
Syrup, calcium glubionate 1.09 g, calcium lactobionate 723 mg (108.3 mg calcium or 2.7 mmol Ca^{2+})/5 mL. Net price 300 mL = £3.48

Ossopan® (Sanofi-Synthelabo)
Tablets, buff, f/c, hydroxyapatite 830 mg (178 mg calcium or 4.4 mmol Ca^{2+}). Net price 50 = £10.09
Granules, brown, hydroxyapatite 3.32 g (712 mg calcium or 17.8 mmol Ca^{2+})/sachet. Net price 28-sachet pack = £18.04

Ostram® (Merck)
Powder, calcium phosphate 3.3 g (1.2 g calcium or 29.9 mmol Ca^{2+})/sachet. Net price 30-sachet pack = £5.95. Label: 13

Sandocal® (Novartis)
Sandocal-400 tablets, effervescent, calcium lactate gluconate 930 mg, calcium carbonate 700 mg, anhydrous citric acid 1.189 g, providing calcium 400 mg (10 mmol Ca^{2+}). Net price 5 × 20-tab pack = £7.20. Label: 13
Sandocal-1000 tablets, effervescent, calcium lactate gluconate 2.327 g, calcium carbonate 1.75 g, anhydrous citric acid 2.973 g providing 1 g calcium (25 mmol Ca^{2+}). Net price 3 × 10-tab pack = £6.45. Label: 13

Titralac®, section 9.5.2.2

■ Parenteral preparations

Calcium Gluconate (Non-proprietary) PoM
Injection, calcium gluconate 10% (8.9 mg calcium or 220 micromol Ca^{2+}/mL). Net price 10-mL amp = 57p
Available from Antigen, Phoenix

Calcium Chloride (Non-proprietary) PoM
Injection, calcium chloride 100 mg/mL (27.3 mg calcium or 680 micromol Ca^{2+}/mL). Net price 10-mL disposable syringe = £4.02
Available from Aurum, Medeva (Min-I-Jet® Calcium Chloride 10%)

■ With vitamin D
Section 9.6.4

9.5.1.2   Hypercalcaemia

Severe hypercalcaemia calls for urgent treatment before detailed investigation of the cause. Dehydration should be corrected first with intravenous infusion of **sodium chloride 0.9%**. Drugs (such as thiazides and vitamin D compounds) which promote hypercalcaemia, should be discontinued and dietary calcium should be restricted.

If *severe hypercalcaemia persists* drugs which inhibit mobilisation of calcium from the skeleton may be required. The **bisphosphonates** are useful and disodium pamidronate (section 6.6.2) is probably the most effective.

Corticosteroids (section 6.3) are widely given, but may only be useful where hypercalcaemia is due to sarcoidosis or vitamin D intoxication; they often take several days to achieve the desired effect.

Calcitonin (section 6.6.1) is relatively non-toxic but is expensive and its effect can wear off after a few days despite continued use; it is rarely effective where bisphosphonates have failed to reduce serum calcium adequately.

Intravenous chelating drugs such as **trisodium edetate** are rarely used; they usually cause pain in the limb receiving the infusion and may cause renal damage.

After treatment of severe hypercalcaemia the underlying cause must be established. *Further treatment* is governed by the same principles as for initial therapy. Salt and water depletion and drugs promoting hypercalcaemia should be avoided; oral administration of a bisphosphonate may be useful. **Sodium cellulose phosphate**, which binds calcium in the gut, is rarely helpful, and any associated increase in serum phosphate may be harmful. Similarly, oral and intravenous phosphate may only achieve a reduction in serum calcium by precipitating calcium phosphate in the tissues, resulting in nephrocalcinosis and impairment of renal function. Parathyroidectomy may be indicated for hyperparathyroidism.

SODIUM CELLULOSE PHOSPHATE

Indications: reduction of calcium absorption from food in conditions such as hypercalciuria and hypercalcaemia (but see also notes above)
Cautions: renal impairment (avoid if severe); pregnancy and breast-feeding; growing children
Contra-indications: congestive heart failure and other conditions in which low sodium intake essential, severe renal impairment
Side-effects: occasional diarrhoea; magnesium deficiency reported
Dose: 5 g 3 times daily with meals; CHILD 10 g daily in 3 divided doses with meals

Calcisorb® (3M)
Sachets, sodium cellulose phosphate 5 g. Net price 90-sachet pack = £17.88. Label: 13, 21, counselling, may be sprinkled on food

> denotes preparations that are considered to be less suitable for prescribing (see p. vi)

TRISODIUM EDETATE

Indications: hypercalcaemia (but see notes above); lime burns in the eye (see under Preparations)
Cautions: repeated plasma-calcium determinations important; caution in tuberculosis; avoid rapid infusion, see under Dose
Contra-indications: impaired renal function
Side-effects: nausea, diarrhoea, cramp; in overdosage renal damage
Dose: hypercalcaemia, *by intravenous infusion* over 2–3 hours, up to 70 mg/kg daily; CHILD up to 60 mg/kg daily
IMPORTANT. Ensure rate of infusion and concentration correct (see Appendix 6); too rapid a rate or too high a concentration is extremely hazardous and repeated measurements of plasma calcium concentrations are important for control and maintenance of near normal ionised calcium concentrations. Decrease infusion rate on signs of increased muscle reactivity; discontinue if tetany occurs and restart cautiously only after plasma ionised and total calcium concentrations indicate need for further treatment (and tetany has stopped)

Limclair® (Sinclair) PoM
Injection, trisodium edetate 200 mg/mL. For dilution and use as an intravenous infusion. Net price 5-mL amp = £4.76
Note. For topical use in the eye, dilute 1 mL to 50 mL with sterile purified water

Magnesium is an essential constituent of many enzyme systems, particularly those involved in energy generation; the largest stores are in the skeleton.

Magnesium salts are not well absorbed from the gastro-intestinal tract which explains the use of magnesium sulphate (section 1.6.4) as an osmotic laxative.

Magnesium is mainly excreted by the kidneys and is therefore retained in renal failure although significant *hypermagnesaemia* (causing muscle weakness and arrhythmias) is rare.

HYPOMAGNESAEMIA. Since magnesium is secreted in large amounts in the gastro-intestinal fluid, excessive losses in diarrhoea, stoma or fistula are the most common of the causes of *hypomagnesaemia*; deficiency may also occur in alcoholism or diuretic therapy and it has been reported after prolonged treatment with aminoglycosides. Hypomagnesaemia often causes secondary hypocalcaemia (with which it may be confused) and also hypokalaemia and hyponatraemia.

Symptomatic *hypomagnesaemia* is associated with a deficit of 0.5–1 mmol/kg; up to 160 mmol Mg^{2+} over up to 5 days may be required to replace the deficit (allowing for urinary losses). Magnesium is given initially by intravenous infusion or by intramuscular injection of **magnesium sulphate**; the intramuscular injection is painful. Plasma magnesium concentrations should be measured to determine the rate and duration of infusion and the dose should be reduced in renal impairment. To prevent *recurrence of the deficit*, magnesium may be given by mouth in a dose of 24 mmol Mg^{2+} daily in divided doses; a suitable preparation is magnesium glycerophosphate tablets [not licensed, available from IDIS]. For maintenance (e.g. in intravenous nutrition), parenteral doses of magnesium are of the order of 10–20 mmol Mg^{2+} daily (often about 12 mmol Mg^{2+} daily).

ARRHYTHMIAS. Magnesium sulphate has also been recommended for the emergency treatment of *serious arrhythmias*, especially in the presence of hypokalaemia (when hypomagnesaemia may also be present) and when salvos of rapid ventricular tachycardia show the characteristic twisting wave front known as *torsades de pointes*. The usual dose of magnesium sulphate is intravenous injection of 8 mmol Mg^{2+} over 10–15 minutes (repeated once if necessary).

MYOCARDIAL INFARCTION. Evidence suggesting a sustained reduction in mortality in patients with *suspected myocardial infarction* given an initial intravenous injection of magnesium sulphate 8 mmol Mg^{2+} over 20 minutes followed by an intravenous infusion of 65–72 mmol Mg^{2+} over the following 24 hours, has not been borne out by a larger study. Some workers, however, continue to hold the view that magnesium is beneficial if given immediately (and for as long as there is a likelihood of reperfusion taking place).

ECLAMPSIA. Magnesium sulphate has been shown to have a major role in *eclampsia* for the prevention of recurrent seizures. Regimens in the UK may vary between hospitals but typically involve initial intravenous administration of magnesium sulphate 4 g (approx. 16 mmol Mg^{2+}) over 5–10 minutes followed by intravenous infusion at a rate of 1 g (approx. 4 mmol Mg^{2+}) every hour for at least 24 hours after the last seizure; recurrence of seizures may require an additional intravenous bolus of 2 g (approx. 8 mmol Mg^{2+}). Monitoring of blood pressure, respiratory rate and urinary output is carried out, as is monitoring for clinical signs of overdosage (loss of patellar reflexes, weakness, nausea, sensation of warmth, flushing, drowsiness, double vision, and slurred speech—calcium gluconate injection is used for the management of magnesium toxicity).

MAGNESIUM SULPHATE

Indications: see notes above; constipation (section 1.6.4); paste for boils (section 13.10.5)

Cautions: see notes above; hepatic impairment (Appendix 2); renal impairment (risk of accumulation); in severe hypomagnesaemia administer initially via controlled infusion device (preferably syringe pump); **interactions:** Appendix 1 (magnesium salts)

Side-effects: generally associated with hypermagnesaemia, nausea, vomiting, thirst, flushing of skin, hypotension, arrhythmias, coma, respiratory depression, drowsiness, confusion, loss of tendon reflexes, muscle weakness; colic and diarrhoea following oral administration

Dose: see notes above

Magnesium Sulphate (Non-proprietary) PoM
Injection, magnesium sulphate 50% (approx. 2 mmol Mg^{2+}/mL), net price 2-mL (1-g) amp = £3.43; 10 mL (5-g) amp = £3.05
Available from Aurum, Medeva

9.5.2   Phosphorus

9.5.1   Phosphate supplements
9.5.2.2   Phosphate-binding agents

9.5.2.1   Phosphate supplements

Oral phosphate supplements may be required in addition to vitamin D in a small minority of patients with hypophosphataemic vitamin D-resistant rickets. Diarrhoea is a common side-effect and should prompt a reduction in dosage.

Phosphate infusion is occasionally needed in alcohol dependence or in phosphate deficiency arising from use of parenteral nutrition deficient in phosphate supplements; phosphate depletion also occurs in severe diabetic ketoacidosis. For *established hypophosphataemia*, monobasic potassium phosphate may be infused at a maximum rate of 9 mmol every 12 hours. Excessive doses of phosphates may cause hypocalcaemia and metastatic calcification; it is **essential** to monitor closely plasma concentrations of calcium, phosphate, potassium, and other electrolytes.

For phosphate requirements in *total parenteral nutrition* regimens, see section 9.3.

Phosphate-Sandoz® (HK Pharma)
Tablets, effervescent, anhydrous sodium acid phosphate 1.936 g, sodium bicarbonate 350 mg, potassium bicarbonate 315 mg, equivalent to phosphorus 500 mg (16.1 mmol phosphate), sodium 468.8 mg (20.4 mmol Na^+), potassium 123 mg (3.1 mmol K^+). Net price 20 = £3.29. Label: 13
Dose: hypercalcaemia, up to 6 tablets daily adjusted according to response; CHILD under 5 years up to 3 tablets daily
Vitamin D-resistant hypophosphataemic osteomalacia, 4–6 tablets daily; CHILD under 5 years 2–3 tablets daily

9.5.2.2   Phosphate-binding agents

Aluminium-containing and calcium-containing antacids are used as phosphate-binding agents in the management of hyperphosphataemia complicating renal failure. Calcium-containing phosphate-binding agents are contra-indicated in hypercalcaemia or hypercalciuria. Phosphate-binding agents which contain aluminium may increase plasma aluminium in dialysis patients.

ALUMINIUM HYDROXIDE

Indications: hyperphosphataemia; dyspepsia (section 1.1.1)

Cautions: hyperaluminaemia; porphyria (section 9.8.2); see also notes above; **interactions:** Appendix 1 (antacids)

Side-effects: see section 1.1.1

Aluminium Hydroxide (Non-proprietary)
Mixture (gel), about 4% w/w Al_2O_3 in water. Net price 200 mL = 41p
Dose: hyperphosphataemia, 20–100 mL according to requirements of patient
Note. The brand name *Aludrox®* NHS (Pfizer Consumer) is used for aluminium hydroxide mixture, net price 200 mL = £1.28. For *Aludrox®* NHS tablets see preparations with magnesium, section 1.1.1

Alu-Cap® (3M)
Capsules, green/red, dried aluminium hydroxide 475 mg (low Na^+). Net price 120-cap pack = £4.03
Dose: phosphate-binding agent in renal failure, 4–20 capsules daily in divided doses with meals

CALCIUM SALTS

Indications: hyperphosphataemia

Cautions: see notes above; **interactions:** Appendix 1 (calcium salts)

Side-effects: hypercalcaemia

Calcette®, section 9.5.1.1
Calcichew®, section 9.5.1.1
Calcium-500, section 9.5.1.1

Phosex® (Vitaline)
Tablets, yellow, calcium acetate 1 g (250 mg calcium or 6.2 mmol Ca^{2+}), net price 180-tab pack = £19.79. Label: 25
Dose: phosphate-binding agent (with meals) in renal failure, according to the requirements of the patient

Titralac® (3M)
Tablets, calcium carbonate 420 mg (168 mg calcium or 4.2 mmol Ca^{2+}), glycine 180 mg. Net price 180-tab pack = £2.81
COUNSELLING. May be chewed, crushed or swallowed whole
Dose: calcium supplement, or phosphate-binding agent (with meals) in renal failure, according to the requirements of the patient

9.5.3   Fluoride

Availability of adequate fluoride confers significant resistance to dental caries. It is now considered that the topical action of fluoride on enamel and plaque is more important than the systemic effect.

Where the natural fluoride content of the drinking water is significantly less than 1 mg per litre (one part per million) artificial fluoridation is the most economical method of supplementing fluoride intake.

Daily administration of tablets or drops is a suitable alternative, but systemic fluoride supplements should not be prescribed without reference to the fluoride content of the local water supply; they are not advisable when the water contains more than 700 micrograms per litre (0.7 parts per million). In addition, infants need not receive fluoride supplements until the age of 6 months.

Use of dentifrices which incorporate sodium fluoride or monofluorophosphate is also a convenient source of fluoride.

Individuals who are either particularly caries prone or medically compromised may be given additional protection by use of fluoride rinses or by application of fluoride gels. Rinses may be used daily or weekly; daily use of a less concentrated rinse is more effective than weekly use of a more concentrated one. High-strength gels must be applied on a regular basis under professional supervision; extreme caution is necessary to prevent the child from swallowing any excess. Less concentrated gels have recently become available for home use. Varnishes are also available and are particularly valuable for young or handicapped children since they adhere to the teeth and set in the presence of moisture.

FLUORIDES

Note. Sodium fluoride 2.2 mg provides approx. 1 mg fluoride ion
Indications: prophylaxis of dental caries—see notes above
Contra-indications: not for areas where drinking water is fluoridated
Side-effects: occasional white flecks on teeth with recommended doses; rarely yellowish-brown discoloration if recommended doses are exceeded
Dose: expressed as fluoride ion (F$^-$):
Water content less than 300 micrograms F$^-$/litre (0.3 parts per million), CHILD up to 6 months none; 6 months–3 years 250 micrograms F$^-$ daily, 3–6 years 500 micrograms F$^-$ daily, over 6 years 1 mg F$^-$ daily
Water content between 300 and 700 micrograms F$^-$/litre (0.3–0.7 parts per million), CHILD up to 3 years none, 3–6 years 250 micrograms F$^-$ daily, over 6 years 500 micrograms F$^-$ daily

Water content above 700 micrograms F$^-$/litre (0.7 parts per million), supplements not advised
Note. These doses reflect the recommendations of the British Dental Association, the British Society of Paediatric Dentistry and the British Association for the Study of Community Dentistry (*Br Dent J* 1997; **182:** 6–7)

■ Tablets
COUNSELLING. Tablets should be sucked or dissolved in the mouth and taken preferably in the evening
There are arrangements for health authorities to supply fluoride tablets in the course of pre-school dental schemes, and they may also be supplied in school dental schemes.

En-De-Kay® (Manx)
Fluotabs 2–4 years, natural orange-flavoured, scored, sodium fluoride 1.1 mg (500 micrograms F$^-$). Net price 200-tab pack = £1.83
Fluotabs 4+ years, natural orange-flavoured, scored, sodium fluoride 2.2 mg (1 mg F$^-$). Net price 200-tab pack = £1.83

Fluor-a-day® (Dental Health)
Tablets, buff, sodium fluoride 1.1 mg (500 micrograms F$^-$), net price 200-tab pack = £1.77; 2.2 mg (1 mg F$^-$), 200-tab pack = £1.77

FluoriGard® (Colgate-Palmolive)
Tablets 0.5, purple, grape-flavoured, scored, sodium fluoride 1.1 mg (500 micrograms F$^-$). Net price 200-tab pack = £1.91
Tablets 1.0, orange, orange-flavoured, scored, sodium fluoride 2.2 mg (1 mg F$^-$). Net price 200-tab pack = £1.91

■ Oral drops
Note. Fluoride supplements not considered necessary below 6 months of age (see notes above)
En-De-Kay® (Manx)
Fluodrops® (= paediatric drops), sugar-free, sodium fluoride 550 micrograms (250 micrograms F$^-$)/0.15 mL. Net price 60 mL = £1.62
Note. Corresponds to Sodium Fluoride Oral Drops DPF 0.37% equivalent to sodium fluoride 80 micrograms (F$^-$ 36 micrograms)/drop

■ Mouthwashes
Rinse mouth for 1 minute and spit out
COUNSELLING. Avoid eating, drinking, or rinsing mouth for 15 minutes after use
Duraphat® (Colgate-Palmolive)
Weekly dental rinse (= mouthwash), blue, sodium fluoride 0.2%. Net price 150 mL = £2.42. Counselling, see above
CHILD 6 years and over, for *weekly* use, rinse with 10 mL

En-De-Kay® (Manx)
Daily fluoride mouthrinse (= mouthwash), blue, sodium fluoride 0.05%. Net price 250 mL = £1.81
CHILD 6 years and over, for *daily* use, rinse with 10 mL
[PoM] *Fluorinse* (= mouthwash), red, sodium fluoride 2%. Net price 100 mL = £3.97. Counselling, see above
CHILD 8 years and over, for *daily* use, dilute 5 drops to 10 mL of water; for *weekly* use, dilute 20 drops to 10 mL

FluoriGard® (Colgate-Palmolive)
Daily dental rinse (= mouthwash), blue, sodium fluoride 0.05%. Net price 500 mL = £3.11. Counselling, see above
CHILD 6 years and over, for *daily* use, rinse with 10 mL

■ Gels

FluoriGard® (Colgate-Palmolive)
Gel-Kam (= gel), stannous fluoride 0.4% in glycerol basis. Net price 100 mL = £3.05. Counselling, see below

ADULT and CHILD 3 years and over, for *daily* use, using a toothbrush, apply onto all tooth surfaces

COUNSELLING. Swish between teeth for 1 minute before spitting out. Avoid eating, drinking, or rinsing mouth for at least 30 minutes after use

9.5.4　Zinc

Oral zinc therapy should only be given when there is good evidence of deficiency (hypoproteinaemia spuriously lowers plasma-zinc concentrations). Zinc deficiency can occur in individuals on inadequate diets, in malabsorption, with increased body loss due to trauma, burns and protein-losing conditions, and during intravenous feeding. Therapy should continue until clinical improvement occurs and be replaced by dietary measures unless there is severe malabsorption, metabolic disease, or continuing zinc loss. Side-effects of zinc salts are abdominal pain and dyspepsia.

ZINC SALTS

Indications: see notes above
Cautions: see notes above; **interactions:** Appendix 1 (zinc)
Side-effects: see notes above

Solvazinc® (Thames)
Effervescent tablets, yellow-white, zinc sulphate monohydrate 125 mg (45 mg zinc). Net price 30 = £4.32. Label: 13, 21
Dose: ADULT and CHILD over 30 kg, 1 tablet in water 1–3 times daily after food; CHILD under 10 kg, ½ tablet daily; 10–30 kg, ½ tablet 1–3 times daily

9.6　Vitamins

9.6.1	Vitamin A
9.6.2	Vitamin B group
9.6.3	Vitamin C
9.6.4	Vitamin D
9.6.5	Vitamin E
9.6.6	Vitamin K
9.6.7	Multivitamin preparations

Vitamins are used for the prevention and treatment of specific deficiency states or where the diet is known to be inadequate; they may be prescribed in the NHS to prevent or treat deficiency but not as dietary supplements.

Their use as general 'pick-me-ups' is of unproven value and, in the case of preparations containing vitamin A or D, may actually be harmful if patients take more than the prescribed dose. The 'fad' for mega-vitamin therapy with water-soluble vitamins, such as ascorbic acid and pyridoxine, is unscientific and can be harmful.

Dietary reference values for vitamins are available in the Department of Health publication:

Dietary Reference Values for Food Energy and Nutrients for the United Kingdom: Report of the Panel on Dietary Reference Values of the Committee on Medical Aspects of Food Policy. *Report on Health and Social Subjects 41*. London: HMSO, 1991

9.6.1　Vitamin A

Deficiency of vitamin A (retinol) is associated with ocular defects (particularly xerophthalmia) and an increased susceptibility to infections, but deficiency is rare in Britain (even in disorders of fat absorption). Despite initial epidemiological evidence suggesting that vitamin A or carotene may have a protective effect against some epithelial cancers, the claims have not been substantiated.

Massive overdose can cause rough skin, dry hair, an enlarged liver, and a raised erythrocyte sedimentation rate and raised serum calcium and serum alkaline phosphatase concentrations.

In view of evidence suggesting that high levels of vitamin A may cause birth defects, women who are (or may become) pregnant are advised not to take vitamin A supplements (including tablets and fish-liver oil drops), except on the advice of a doctor or an antenatal clinic; nor should they eat liver or products such as liver paté or liver sausage.

VITAMIN A

(Retinol)
Indications: see notes above
Cautions: see notes above
Side-effects: see notes above
Dose: see notes above and under preparations

■ Vitamins A and D

Halibut-liver Oil (Non-proprietary)
Capsules, vitamin A 4000 units [also contains vitamin D]. Net price 20 = 22p
Available from Thornton & Ross

Vitamins A and D (Non-proprietary)
Capsules, vitamin A 4000 units, vitamin D 400 units. Net price 20 = 50p
Available from CP

Halycitrol® (LAB) [NHS]
Emulsion, vitamin A 4600 units, vitamin D 380 units/5 mL. Net price 114 mL = £1.50
Dose: 5 mL daily but see notes above

■ Vitamins A, C and D

Mothers' and Children's Vitamin Drops
(Cupal)
Oral drops, vitamin A 5000 units, vitamin D 2000 units, ascorbic acid 150 mg/mL
Available free of charge to pregnant women and children aged under 5 years in families receiving Income Support or an income-based Jobseeker's Allowance under the Welfare Food Scheme. If prescribed, prescription needs to be endorsed 'ACBS'. Otherwise available direct to the public from maternity and child health clinics
Dose: pregnant and nursing mothers and CHILD 1 month–5 years, 5 drops daily (5 drops contain vitamin A approx. 700 units, ascorbic acid approx. 20 mg, vitamin D approx. 300 units)
Note. Recommended by the Department of Health for routine supplementation in all pregnant women and children from 1 year to 5 years. For breast-fed baby whose mother was in good vitamin status during pregnancy, supplementation may begin at 6 months of age; where there is doubt about the mother's vitamin status during pregnancy, supplementation should begin at 1 month of age; a baby consuming 500 mL infant formula feed or follow-on formula feed daily does not need vitamin supplementation because the formula feeds are fortified with vitamin D

Vitamin Tablets (with Calcium and Iodine) for Nursing Mothers (Sussex)

Tablets, orange, s/c, vitamin A (as retinyl acetate) 8 mg, ascorbic acid 60 mg, ergocalciferol 400 units, calcium hydrogen phosphate 190 mg (40 mg calcium or 1 mmol Ca^{2+}), potassium iodide 130 micrograms

Recommended by the Department of Health for routine supplementation in nursing mothers. Free of charge to nursing mothers with children aged under 1 year in families receiving Income Support or an income-based Jobseeker's Allowance under the Welfare Food Scheme. If prescribed, prescription needs to be endorsed 'ACBS'. Otherwise available direct to the public from maternity and child health clinics

Dose: one tablet daily

Note. Women who are (or may become) pregnant are advised not to take this supplement except on the advice of a doctor or antenatal clinic

■ Vitamin A injection

Vitamin A Palmitate (Cambridge) PoM

Injection, vitamin A (retinol) 50 000 units (as palmitate)/mL. Net price 2-mL amp = £3.45

Dose: by deep intramuscular injection, deficiency, 100 000 units monthly, increased to weekly in acute deficiency states; courses no longer than 6 weeks with 2-week interval

Liver disease, 100 000 units every 2–4 months

INFANT under 1 year and CHILD 50 000 units monthly

Note. Contains polyethoxylated castor oil which has been associated with anaphylaxis; do **not** mix or dilute

Cautions: children, liver disease (specialist use), see also notes above

---

9.6.2   Vitamin B group

Deficiency of the B vitamins, other than deficiency of vitamin B_{12} (section 9.1.2) is rare in Britain and is usually treated by preparations containing thiamine (B_1), riboflavin (B_2), and nicotinamide, which is used in preference to nicotinic acid, as it does not cause vasodilatation. Other members (or substances traditionally classified as members) of the vitamin B complex such as aminobenzoic acid, biotin, choline, inositol, and pantothenic acid or panthenol may be included in vitamin B preparations but there is no evidence of their value.

The severe deficiency states Wernicke's encephalopathy and Korsakoff's psychosis, especially as seen in chronic alcoholism, are best treated by the parenteral administration of B vitamins (*Pabrinex®*); anaphylaxis has been reported with these preparations (see CSM advice, below).

As with other vitamins of the B group, pyridoxine (B_6) deficiency is rare, but it may occur during isoniazid therapy and is characterised by peripheral neuritis. High doses of pyridoxine are given in some metabolic disorders, such as hyperoxaluria, and it is also used in sideroblastic anaemia (section 9.1.3). Pyridoxine has been tried in a wide variety of other disorders, including the premenstrual syndrome, but there is little sound evidence to support the claims, and overdosage induces toxic effects.

Nicotinic acid inhibits the synthesis of cholesterol and triglyceride (see section 2.12). Folic acid and vitamin B_{12} are used in the treatment of megaloblastic anaemia (section 9.1.2). Folinic acid (available as calcium folinate) is used in association with cytotoxic therapy (section 8.1.3).

RIBOFLAVIN

(Riboflavine, vitamin B_2)

Indications: see notes above

Preparations

Injections of vitamins B and C, see under Thiamine

■ Oral vitamin B complex preparations, see below

THIAMINE

(Vitamin B_1)

Indications: see notes above

Cautions: anaphylactic shock may occasionally follow injection (see CSM advice below)

Dose: mild chronic deficiency, 10–25 mg daily; severe deficiency, 200–300 mg daily

---

> **CSM advice**
>
> Since potentially serious allergic adverse reactions may occur during, or shortly after, administration, the CSM has recommended that:
>
> 1. Use be restricted to patients in whom parenteral treatment is essential;
>
> 2. Intravenous injections should be administered slowly (over 10 minutes);
>
> 3. Facilities for treating anaphylaxis should be available when administered.

Thiamine (Non-proprietary)

Tablets, thiamine hydrochloride 50 mg, net price 20 = 34p; 100 mg, 20 = 54p

Available from Roche Consumer Health (*Benerva®* NHS)

Pabrinex® (Link) PoM

Parenteral vitamins B and C for rapid correction of severe depletion or malabsorption (e.g in alcoholism, after acute infections, postoperatively, or in psychiatric states), maintenance of vitamins B and C in chronic intermittent haemodialysis

Dose: see CSM advice above

Coma or delirium from alcohol, from opioids, or from barbiturates, collapse following narcosis, by intravenous injection or infusion of *I/V High potency*, 2-3 pairs every 8 hours

Psychosis following narcosis or electroconvulsive therapy, toxicity from acute infections, by intravenous injection or infusion of *I/V High potency* or by deep intramuscular injection into the gluteal muscle of *I/M High potency*, 1 pair twice daily for up to 7 days

Haemodialysis, by intravenous infusion of *I/V High potency* (in sodium chloride intravenous infusion 0.9%) 1 pair every 2 weeks

I/M High potency injection, for intramuscular use only, ascorbic acid 500 mg, nicotinamide 160 mg, pyridoxine hydrochloride 50 mg, riboflavin 4 mg, thiamine hydrochloride 250 mg/7 mL. Net price 7 mL (in 2 amps) = £1.86

I/V High potency injection, for intravenous use only, ascorbic acid 500 mg, anhydrous glucose 1 g, nicotinamide 160 mg, pyridoxine hydrochloride 50 mg, riboflavin 4 mg, thiamine hydrochloride 250 mg/10 mL. Net price 10 mL (in 2 amps) = £1.66

■ Oral vitamin B complex preparations, see below

PYRIDOXINE HYDROCHLORIDE
(Vitamin B$_6$)
Indications: see under Dose
Cautions: interactions: Appendix 1 (vitamins)
Dose: deficiency states, 20–50 mg up to 3 times daily
Isoniazid neuropathy, prophylaxis 10 mg daily (but preparation of suitable strength not available); therapeutic, 50 mg three times daily
Idiopathic sideroblastic anaemia, 100–400 mg daily in divided doses
Premenstrual syndrome, 50–100 mg daily (but see notes above)

> **Important.** Concerns about possible toxicity resulting from prolonged use of pyridoxine (vitamin B$_6$) at high dosage have not yet been resolved. The Royal Pharmaceutical Society of Great Britain has advised that pharmacists should consider how to advise customers requesting preparations containing higher doses and that they should decide their own policy on the display of products containing more than 10 mg per daily dose of pyridoxine.

Pyridoxine (Non-proprietary)
Tablets, pyridoxine hydrochloride 20 mg, net price 20 = 34p; 50 mg, 20 = 29p
Available from Cox, CP, Hillcross
Orovite Complement B6® (SSL) ▣
Tablets, m/r, yellow, pyridoxine hydrochloride 100 mg. Net price 28-tab pack = £2.33. Label: 25

■ Injections of vitamins B and C, see under Thiamine

NICOTINAMIDE
Indications: see notes above; acne vulgaris, see section 13.6.1

Nicotinamide (Non-proprietary)
Tablets, nicotinamide 50 mg. Net price 20 = £1.32

■ Injections of vitamins B and C, see under Thiamine

Oral vitamin B complex preparations

Note. Other multivitamin preparations are in section 9.6.7.
Vitamin B Tablets, Compound ◤ nicotinamide 15 mg, riboflavin 1 mg, thiamine hydrochloride 1 mg. Net price 20 = 7p
Dose: prophylactic, 1–2 tablets daily
Vitamin B Tablets, Compound, Strong ◤
brown, f/c or s/c, nicotinamide 20 mg, pyridoxine hydrochloride 2 mg, riboflavin 2 mg, thiamine hydrochloride 5 mg. Net price 20 = 15p
Dose: treatment of vitamin-B deficiency, 1–2 tablets 3 times daily
Vigranon B® (Wallace Mfg) ▣ ◤
Syrup, thiamine hydrochloride 5 mg, riboflavin 2 mg, nicotinamide 20 mg, pyridoxine hydrochloride 2 mg, panthenol 3 mg/5 mL. Net price 150 mL = £2.02

> ◤ denotes preparations that are considered to be less suitable for prescribing (see p. vi)

Other compounds

Potassium aminobenzoate has been used in the treatment of various disorders associated with excessive fibrosis such as scleroderma but its therapeutic value is **doubtful**.

Potaba® (Glenwood) ▣
Capsules, potassium aminobenzoate 500 mg. Net price 20 = £1.42. Label: 21
Tablets, potassium aminobenzoate 500 mg. Net price 20 = £1.00. Label: 21
Envules® (= powder in sachets), potassium aminobenzoate 3 g. Net price 40 sachets = £15.37. Label: 13, 21
Dose: Peyronie's disease, scleroderma, 12 g daily in divided doses after food

> ◤ denotes preparations that are considered to be less suitable for prescribing (see p. vi)

9.6.3   Vitamin C
(Ascorbic acid)

Vitamin C therapy is essential in scurvy, but less florid manifestations of vitamin C deficiency are commonly found, especially in the elderly. It is rarely necessary to prescribe more than 100 mg daily except early in the treatment of scurvy.

Claims that vitamin C ameliorates colds or promotes wound healing have not been proved.

ASCORBIC ACID
Indications: prevention and treatment of scurvy
Dose: prophylactic, 25–75 mg daily; therapeutic, not less than 250 mg daily in divided doses

Ascorbic Acid (Non-proprietary)
Tablets, ascorbic acid 50 mg, net price 20 = 7p; 100 mg, 20 = 20p; 200 mg, 20 = 38p; 500 mg (label: 24), 20 = 90p
Available from Cox, Roche Consumer Health (*Redoxon®* ▣)
Tablets ▣, effervescent, ascorbic acid 1 g. Net price 10-tab pack = £1.23. Label: 13
Available from Roche Consumer Health (*Redoxon®* ▣)
Injection, ascorbic acid 100 mg/mL. Net price 5-mL amp = £2.28

■ For children's welfare vitamin drops containing vitamin C with A and D, see vitamin A

9.6.4   Vitamin D

Note. The term Vitamin D is used for a range of compounds which possess the property of preventing or curing rickets. They include ergocalciferol (calciferol, vitamin D$_2$), colecalciferol (vitamin D$_3$), dihydrotachysterol, alfacalcidol (1α-hydroxycolecalciferol), and calcitriol (1,25-dihydroxycolecalciferol).

Simple vitamin D deficiency can be prevented by taking an oral supplement of only 10 micrograms (400 units) of ergocalciferol (calciferol, vitamin D$_2$) daily. Vitamin D deficiency is not uncommon in Asians consuming unleavened bread and in the elderly living alone and can be prevented by taking an oral supplement of 20 micrograms (800 units) of ergocalciferol daily. Since there is no plain tablet of this strength available **calcium and ergocalciferol tablets** can be given (although the calcium is unnecessary).

Vitamin D deficiency caused by *intestinal malabsorption* or *chronic liver disease* usually requires vitamin D in pharmacological doses, such as **calciferol tablets** up to 1 mg (40 000 units) daily; the hypocalcaemia of *hypoparathyroidism* often requires doses of up to 2.5 mg (100 000 units) daily in order to achieve normocalcaemia. The newer vitamin D derivatives, **alfacalcidol** and **calcitriol**, have a shorter duration of action, and therefore have the advantage that problems associated with hypercalcaemia due to excessive dosage are shorter lasting and easier to treat.

Vitamin D requires hydroxylation by the kidney to its active form therefore the hydroxylated derivatives **alfacalcidol** or **calcitriol** should be prescribed if patients with *severe renal impairment* require vitamin D therapy. Calcitriol is also licensed for the management of postmenopausal osteoporosis.

Important. All patients receiving pharmacological doses of vitamin D should have the plasma-calcium concentration checked at intervals (initially weekly) and whenever nausea or vomiting are present. Breast milk from women taking pharmacological doses of vitamin D may cause hypercalcaemia if given to an infant.

ERGOCALCIFEROL
(Calciferol, Vitamin D_2)

Indications: see notes above

Cautions: take care to ensure correct dose in infants; monitor plasma calcium in patients receiving high doses and in renal impairment

Contra-indications: hypercalcaemia; metastatic calcification

Side-effects: symptoms of overdosage include anorexia, lassitude, nausea and vomiting, diarrhoea, weight loss, polyuria, sweating, headache, thirst, vertigo, and raised concentrations of calcium and phosphate in plasma and urine

Dose: see notes above

■ Daily supplements

Note. There is no plain vitamin D tablet available for treating simple deficiency (see notes above). Alternatives include vitamins capsules (see 9.6.7), preparations of vitamins A and D (see 9.6.1), and calcium and ergocalciferol tablets (see below).

Calcium and Ergocalciferol (Non-proprietary)
(Calcium and Vitamin D)
Tablets, calcium lactate 300 mg, calcium phosphate 150 mg (97 mg calcium or 2.4 mmol Ca^{2+}), ergocalciferol 10 micrograms (400 units). Net price 20 = 25p. Counselling, crush before administration or may be chewed

Adcal-D₃® (Strakan)
Tablets (chewable), calcium carbonate 1.5 g (600 mg calcium or 15.1 mmol Ca^{2+}), colecalciferol 10 micrograms (400 units), net price 100-tab pack = £7.50. Label: 24

Cacit® D3 (Procter & Gamble Pharm.)
Granules, effervescent, calcium carbonate 1.25 g (500 mg calcium or 12.6 mmol Ca^{2+}), colecalciferol 11 micrograms (440 units)/sachet. Net price 30-sachet pack = £3.91. Label: 13

Calceos® (Thames)
Tablets (chewable), calcium carbonate 1.25 g (500 mg calcium or 12.6 mmol Ca $^{2+}$), colecalciferol 10 micrograms (400 units). Net price 60-tab pack = £8.00. Label: 24

Calcichew® D3 (Shire)
Tablets (chewable), calcium carbonate 1.25 g (500 mg calcium or 12.6 mmol Ca^{2+}), colecalciferol 5 micrograms (200 units). Net price 100-tab pack = £15.02. Label: 24
Excipients: include aspartame

Calcichew® D3 Forte (Shire)
Tablets (chewable), calcium carbonate 1.25 g (500 mg calcium or 12.6 mmol Ca^{2+}), colecalciferol 10 micrograms (400 units). Net price 100-tab pack = £9.50. Label: 24.
Excipients: include aspartame

■ Pharmacological strengths (see notes above)

Calciferol (Non-proprietary)
Tablets, colecalciferol or ergocalciferol 250 micrograms (10 000 units), net price 20 = £4.83; 1.25 mg (50 000 units) may also be available
Available from Norton

Note. The BP directs that when calciferol tablets qualified by a descriptor relating to strength (such as 'high strength') are prescribed or demanded, the intention of the prescriber or purchaser with respect to the strength expressed in micrograms or milligrams per tablet should be ascertained. To avoid **errors** arising from the use of such titles prescribers are required to **abandon** them and **specify strength required**

Injection ▣PoM▣, colecalciferol or ergocalciferol, 7.5 mg (300 000 units)/mL in oil. Net price 1-mL amp = £5.92, 2-mL amp = £7.07

ALFACALCIDOL
(1α-Hydroxycholecalciferol)

Indications: see notes above

Cautions: see under Ergocalciferol

Contra-indications: see under Ergocalciferol

Side-effects: see under Ergocalciferol

Dose: *by mouth or by intravenous injection* over 30 seconds, ADULT and CHILD over 20 kg, initially 1 microgram daily (elderly 500 nanograms), adjusted to avoid hypercalcaemia; maintenance, usually 0.25–1 microgram daily; NEONATE and PREMATURE INFANT initially 50–100 nanograms/kg daily, CHILD under 20 kg initially 50 nanograms/kg daily

AlfaD® (Berk) ▣PoM▣
Capsules, alfacalcidol 250 nanograms (pink), net price 30-cap pack = £3.37; 1 microgram (orange), 30-cap pack = £10.06
Excipients: include arachis (peanut) oil

One-Alpha® (Leo) ▣PoM▣
Capsules, alfacalcidol 250 nanograms, net price 30-cap pack = £3.37; 1 microgram (brown), 30-cap pack = £10.06
Excipients: include sesame oil
Solution, sugar-free, alfacalcidol 200 nanograms/mL. Net price 60 mL = £14.51 (with oral syringe)
Injection, alfacalcidol 2 micrograms/mL, net price 0.5-mL amp = £2.32, 1-mL amp = £4.42
Note. Contains propylene glycol and should be used with caution in small premature infants

CALCITRIOL

(1,25-Dihydroxycholecalciferol)

Indications: see notes above

Cautions: see under Ergocalciferol; monitor plasma calcium and creatinine during dosage titration

Contra-indications: see under Ergocalciferol

Side-effects: see under Ergocalciferol

Dose: see under preparations below

Calcijex® (Abbott) ‖PoM‖
Injection, calcitriol 1 microgram/mL, net price 1-mL amp = £5.71; 2 micrograms/mL, 1-mL amp = £11.42
Dose: hypocalcaemia in dialysis patients with chronic renal failure, by intravenous injection (or injection through catheter) after haemodialysis, initially 500 nanograms (approx. 10 nanograms/kg) 3 times a week, increased if necessary in steps of 250–500 nanograms at intervals of 2–4 weeks; usual dose 0.5–3 micrograms 3 times a week; CHILD not established

Rocaltrol® (Roche) ‖PoM‖
Capsules, calcitriol 250 nanograms (red/white), net price 20 = £4.12; 500 nanograms (red), 20 = £7.36
Dose: renal osteodystrophy, ADULT, initially 250 nanograms daily, or on alternate days (in patients with normal or only slightly reduced plasma calcium), increased if necessary within 2–4 weeks in steps of 250 nanograms at intervals of 2–4 weeks; usual dose 0.5–1 microgram daily; CHILD not established
Established postmenopausal osteoporosis, 250 nanograms twice daily (monitor plasma calcium and creatinine, consult product literature)

COLECALCIFEROL

(Cholecalciferol, vitamin D₃)

Indications: see under Ergocalciferol—alternative to ergocalciferol in calciferol tablets and injection

Cautions: see under Ergocalciferol

Contra-indications: see under Ergocalciferol

Side-effects: see under Ergocalciferol

DIHYDROTACHYSTEROL

Indications: see under Ergocalciferol

Cautions: see under Ergocalciferol

Contra-indications: see under Ergocalciferol

Side-effects: see under Ergocalciferol

AT 10® (Intrapharm)
Oral solution, dihydrotachysterol 250 micrograms/mL. Net price 15-mL dropper bottle = £22.87
Note. Contains arachis (peanut) oil
Dose: acute, chronic, and latent forms of hypocalcaemic tetany due to hypoparathyroidism, consult product literature

9.6.5   Vitamin E

(Tocopherols)

The daily requirement of vitamin E has not been well defined but is probably about 3 to 15 mg daily. There is little evidence that oral supplements of vitamin E are essential in adults, even where there is fat malabsorption secondary to cholestasis. In young children with congenital cholestasis, abnormally low vitamin E concentrations may be found in association with neuromuscular abnormalities, which usually respond only to the parenteral administration of vitamin E.

Vitamin E has been tried for various other conditions but there is little scientific evidence of its value.

ALPHA TOCOPHERYL ACETATE

Indications: see notes above

Cautions: predisposition to thrombosis; increased risk of necrotising enterocolitis in premature infants weighing less than 1.5 kg

Side-effects: diarrhoea and abdominal pain with doses more than 1 g daily

Vitamin E Suspension (Cambridge)
Suspension, alpha tocopheryl acetate 500 mg/5 mL. Net price 100 mL = £14.79
Dose: malabsorption in cystic fibrosis, 100–200 mg daily; CHILD under 1 year 50 mg daily; 1 year and over, 100 mg daily
Malabsorption in abetalipoproteinaemia, ADULT and CHILD 50–100 mg/kg daily
Malabsorption in chronic cholestasis, INFANT 150–200 mg/kg daily
Note. Tablets containing tocopheryl acetate 50 mg and 200 mg available from Roche Consumer Health (*Ephynal®*)

9.6.6   Vitamin K

Vitamin K is necessary for the production of blood clotting factors and proteins necessary for the normal calcification of bone.

Because vitamin K is fat soluble, patients with fat malabsorption, especially in biliary obstruction or hepatic disease, may become deficient. For oral administration to prevent vitamin-K deficiency in malabsorption syndromes, a water-soluble preparation, **menadiol sodium phosphate** must be used; the usual dose is about 10 mg daily.

Oral coumarin anticoagulants act by interfering with vitamin K metabolism in the hepatic cells and their effects can be antagonised by giving vitamin K; for British Society for Haematology Guidelines, see section 2.8.2.

VITAMIN K DEFICIENCY BLEEDING. Infants are relatively deficient in vitamin K and those who do not receive supplements of vitamin K are at risk of serious bleeds including intracranial bleeding. The Chief Medical Officer and the Chief Nursing Officer have recommended that all newborn babies should receive vitamin K to prevent vitamin K deficiency bleeding (haemorrhagic disease of the newborn). An appropriate regimen should be selected after discussion with parents in the antenatal period.

Vitamin K (as **phytomenadione**) 1 mg may be given by a single intramuscular injection at birth; this prevents vitamin K deficiency bleeding in virtually all babies. Fears about the safety of parenteral vitamin K appear to be unfounded.

Alternatively, vitamin K may be given by mouth, and arrangements must be in place to ensure the appropriate regimen is followed. Two doses of a colloidal (mixed micelle) preparation of phytomenadione 2 mg should be given in the first week. For breast-fed babies, a third dose of phytomenadione 2 mg is given at 1 month of age; the third dose is omitted in formula-fed babies because formula feeds contain vitamin K.

MENADIOL SODIUM PHOSPHATE

Indications: see notes above
Cautions: G6PD deficiency (section 9.1.5) and vitamin E deficiency (risk of haemolysis); **interactions:** Appendix 1 (vitamins)
Contra-indications: neonates and infants, late pregnancy
Dose: see notes above

Menadiol Phosphate (Non-proprietary)
Tablets, menadiol sodium phosphate equivalent to 10 mg of menadiol phosphate. Net price 100-tab pack = £32.33
Available from Cambridge

PHYTOMENADIONE

(Vitamin K$_1$)
Indications: see notes above
Cautions: intravenous injections should be given very slowly (see also below); **interactions:** Appendix 1 (vitamins)
Dose: see notes above

Konakion® (Roche)
Tablets, s/c, phytomenadione 10 mg, net price 10-tab pack = £1.77. To be chewed or allowed to dissolve slowly in the mouth (Label: 24)
Injection PoM, phytomenadione 2 mg/mL, net price 0.5-mL amp = 23p
Note. Contains polyethoxylated castor oil which has been associated with anaphylaxis; should not be diluted therefore **not** for intravenous infusion—for intramuscular or slow intravenous injection

■ Colloidal formulation
Konakion® MM (Roche) PoM
Injection, phytomenadione 10 mg/mL in a mixed micelles vehicle. Net price 1-mL amp = 43p
Excipients: include glycocholic acid 54.6 mg/amp, lecithin
Cautions: reduce dose in elderly; liver impairment (glycocholic acid may displace bilirubin); reports of anaphylactoid reactions
Note. Konakion® MM may be administered by slow intravenous injection or by intravenous infusion in glucose 5% (see Appendix 6); **not** for intramuscular injection

Konakion® MM Paediatric (Roche) PoM
Injection, phytomenadione 10 mg/mL. Net price 0.2-mL amp = £1.55
Excipients: include glycocholic acid 10.9 mg/amp, lecithin
Cautions: parenteral administration in premature infants of less than 2.5 kg (increased risk of kernicterus)
Note. Konakion® MM Paediatric may be administered *by mouth* or *by intramuscular injection* or *by intravenous injection*

Multivitamin preparations

Vitamins Capsules, ascorbic acid 15 mg, nicotinamide 7.5 mg, riboflavin 500 micrograms, thiamine hydrochloride 1 mg, vitamin A 2500 units, vitamin D 300 units. Net price 20 = 21p

Abidec® (W-L)
Drops, vitamins A, B group, C, and D. Net price 25 mL (with dropper) = £1.84

Dalivit® (Eastern)
Oral drops, vitamins A, B group, C, and D, net price 25 mL = £1.60, 50 mL = £2.86

Vitamin and mineral supplements and adjuncts to synthetic diets

Forceval® (Unigreg)
Capsules, brown/red, vitamins (ascorbic acid 60 mg, biotin 100 micrograms, cyanocobalamin 3 micrograms, folic acid 400 micrograms, nicotinamide 18 mg, pantothenic acid 4 mg, pyridoxine 2 mg, riboflavin 1.6 mg, thiamine 1.2 mg, vitamin A 2500 units, vitamin D$_2$ 400 units, vitamin E 10 mg, minerals and trace elements (calcium 100 mg, chromium 200 micrograms, copper 2 mg, iodine 140 micrograms, iron 12 mg, magnesium 30 mg, manganese 3 mg, molybdenum 250 micrograms, phosphorus 77 mg, potassium 4 mg, selenium 50 micrograms, zinc 15 mg). Net price 30-cap pack = £5.39, 45-cap pack = £7.70; 90-cap pack = £14.70
Dose: vitamin and mineral deficiency and as adjunct in synthetic diets, 1 capsule daily
Junior capsules, brown, vitamins (ascorbic acid 25 mg, biotin 50 micrograms, cyanocobalamin 2 micrograms, folic acid 100 micrograms, nicotinamide 7.5 mg, pantothenic acid 2 mg, pyridoxine 1 mg, riboflavin 1 mg, thiamine 1.5 mg, vitamin A 1250 units, vitamin D$_2$ 200 units, vitamin E 5 mg, vitamin K$_1$ 25 micrograms), minerals and trace elements (chromium 50 micrograms, copper 1 mg, iodine 75 micrograms, iron 5 mg, magnesium 1 mg, manganese 1.25 mg, molybdenum 50 micrograms, selenium 25 micrograms, zinc 5 mg). Net price 30-cap pack = £4.05, 60-cap pack = £7.70
Dose: vitamin and mineral deficiency and as adjunct in synthetic diets, CHILD over 5 years, 2 capsules daily

Ketovite® (Paines & Byrne)
Tablets PoM, yellow, ascorbic acid 16.6 mg, riboflavin 1 mg, thiamine hydrochloride 1 mg, pyridoxine hydrochloride 330 micrograms, nicotinamide 3.3 mg, calcium pantothenate 1.16 mg, alpha tocopheryl acetate 5 mg, inositol 50 mg, biotin 170 micrograms, folic acid 250 micrograms, acetomenaphthone 500 micrograms. Net price 100-tab pack = £4.17
Dose: prevention of deficiency in disorders of carbohydrate or amino acid metabolism, 1 tablet 3 times daily; with *Ketovite® Liquid* as vitamin supplement with synthetic diets

Liquid, pink, sugar-free, vitamin A 2500 units, ergocalciferol 400 units, choline chloride 150 mg, cyanocobalamin 12.5 micrograms/5 mL. Net price 150-mL pack = £2.70
Dose: prevention of deficiency in disorders of carbohydrate or amino acid metabolism, 5 mL daily; with *Ketovite® Tablets* as vitamin supplement with synthetic diets

---

Bitters and tonics

Mixtures containing simple and aromatic bitters, such as alkaline gentian mixture, are traditional remedies for loss of appetite. All depend on suggestion.

Gentian Mixture, Acid, BP
Mixture, concentrated compound gentian infusion 10%, dilute hydrochloric acid 5% in a suitable vehicle. Extemporaneous preparations should be recently prepared according to the following formula: concentrated compound gentian infusion 1 mL, dilute hydrochloric acid 0.5 mL, double-strength chloroform water 5 mL, water to 10 mL
Dose: 10 mL 3 times daily in water before meals

Gentian Mixture, Alkaline, BP
(Alkaline Gentian Oral Solution)
Mixture, concentrated compound gentian infusion 10%, sodium bicarbonate 5% in a suitable vehicle. Extemporaneous preparations should be recently prepared according to the following formula: concentrated compound gentian infusion 1 mL, sodium bicarbonate 500 mg, double-strength chloroform water 5 mL, water to 10 mL
Dose: 10 mL 3 times daily in water before meals

Effico® (Pharmax) NHS ▭
Tonic, green, thiamine hydrochloride 180 micrograms, nicotinamide 2.1 mg, caffeine 20.2 mg, compound gentian infusion 0.31 mL/ 5 mL. Net price 300-mL pack = £2.10, 500-mL pack = £2.79

Labiton® (LAB) NHS ▭
Tonic, brown, thiamine hydrochloride 375 micrograms, caffeine 3.5 mg, kola nut dried extract 3.025 mg, alcohol 1.4 mL/5 mL. Net price 200 mL = £2.22

Metatone® (W-L) NHS ▭
Tonic, thiamine hydrochloride 500 micrograms, calcium glycerophosphate 45.6 mg, manganese glycerophosphate 5.7 mg, potassium glycerophosphate 45.6 mg, sodium glycerophosphate 22.8 mg/5 mL. Net price 300 mL = £2.68

▭ denotes preparations that are considered to be less suitable for prescribing (see p. vi)

9.8   Metabolic disorders

9.8.1   Wilson's disease, carnitine deficiency, Gaucher's disease and nephropathic cystinosis
9.8.2   Acute porphyrias

This section covers drugs used in metabolic disorders and not readily classified elsewhere.

9.8.1   Wilson's disease, carnitine deficiency, Gaucher's disease, and nephropathic cystinosis

Wilson's disease

Penicillamine (see also section 10.1.3) is used in Wilson's disease (hepatolenticular degeneration) to aid the elimination of copper ions. See below for other indications.

Trientine is used for the treatment of Wilson's disease only, in patients intolerant of penicillamine; it is **not** an alternative to penicillamine for rheumatoid arthritis or cystinuria.

PENICILLAMINE

Indications: see under Dose below
Cautions: see section 10.1.3
Contra-indications: see section 10.1.3
Side-effects: see section 10.1.3
Dose: Wilson's disease, 1.5–2 g daily in divided doses before food; max. 2 g daily for 1 year; maintenance 0.75–1 g daily; ELDERLY 20 mg/kg daily in divided doses, adjusted according to response; CHILD up to 20 mg/kg daily in divided doses, minimum 500 mg daily
Autoimmune hepatitis (used rarely; after disease controlled with corticosteroids), initially 500 mg daily in divided doses increased slowly over 3 months; usual maintenance dose 1.25 g daily; ELDERLY not recommended
Cystinuria, therapeutic, 1–3 g daily in divided doses before food, adjusted to maintain urinary cystine below 200 mg/litre; prophylactic (maintain urinary cystine below 300 mg/litre) 0.5–1 g at bedtime; maintain adequate fluid intake (at least 3 litres daily); CHILD and ELDERLY minimum dose to maintain urinary cystine below 200 mg/litre
Severe active rheumatoid arthritis, section 10.1.3
Copper and lead poisoning, see Emergency Treatment of Poisoning

Preparations
Section 10.1.3

TRIENTINE DIHYDROCHLORIDE

Indications: Wilson's disease in patients intolerant of penicillamine
Cautions: see notes above; pregnancy; **interactions:** Appendix 1 (trientine)
Side-effects: nausea; penicillamine-induced systemic lupus erythematosus may not resolve on transfer to trientine
Dose: 1.2–2.4 g daily in 2–4 divided doses before food

Trientine Dihydrochloride Capsules,▼ PoM
trientine dihydrochloride 300 mg. Label: 6, 22
Available from K & K-Greeff
Note. The CSM has requested that in addition to the usual CSM reporting request special records should also be kept by the pharmacist

Carnitine deficiency

Carnitine is available for the management of primary carnitine deficiency due to inborn errors of metabolism or of secondary deficiency in haemodialysis patients.

CARNITINE

Indications: primary and secondary carnitine deficiency
Cautions: renal impairment; monitoring of free and acyl carnitine in blood and urine recommended; pregnancy (but appropriate to use) and breast-feeding
Side-effects: nausea, vomiting, abdominal pain, diarrhoea, body odour; side-effects may be dose-related—monitor tolerance during first week and after any dose increase

Dose: primary deficiency, *by mouth*, up to 200 mg/kg daily in 2–4 divided doses; higher doses of up to 400 mg/kg daily occasionally required; *by intravenous injection*, up to 100 mg/kg daily in 3–4 divided doses

Secondary deficiency, *by intravenous injection*, 20 mg/kg after each dialysis session (dosage adjusted according to carnitine concentration); maintenance, *by mouth*, 1 g daily

Carnitor® (Shire) PoM
Oral liquid, L-carnitine 1 g/10-mL single-dose bottle. Net price 10 × 10-mL single-dose bottle = £35.00
Paediatric solution, L-carnitine 30%. Net price 20 mL = £21.00
Injection, L-carnitine 200 mg/mL. Net price 5-mL amp = £11.90

Gaucher's disease

Imiglucerase, an enzyme produced by recombinant DNA technology, is administered as enzyme replacement therapy in Gaucher's disease, a familial disorder affecting principally the liver, spleen, bone marrow, and lymph nodes.

IMIGLUCERASE

Indications: (specialist use only) type I Gaucher's disease
Cautions: pregnancy and breast-feeding; monitor for imiglucerase antibodies; when stabilised monitor all parameters and response to treatment at intervals of 6–12 months
Side-effects: pruritus, pain, swelling or sterile abscess at injection site; hypersensitivity reactions; also reported nausea, vomiting, diarrhoea, abdominal pain, fatigue, headache, dizziness, fever, rash
Dose: *by intravenous infusion*, initially 60 units/kg once every 2 weeks (2.5 units/kg 3 times a week or 15 units/kg once every 2 weeks may improve haematological parameters and organomegaly, but not bone parameters); maintenance, adjust dose according to response

Cerezyme® (Genzyme) PoM
Intravenous infusion, powder for reconstitution, imiglucerase, net price 200-unit vial = £595.00

Nephropathic cystinosis

Mercapatamine (Cysteamine) is available for the treatment of nephropathic cystinosis.

MERCAPTAMINE
(Cysteamine)
Indications: (specialist use only) nephropathic cystinosis
Cautions: leucocyte-cystine concentration and haematological monitoring required—consult product literature; dose of phosphate supplement may need to be adjusted
Contra-indications: pregnancy and breast-feeding; hypersensitivity to mercaptamine or penicillamine

Side-effects: breath and body odour, nausea, vomiting, diarrhoea, anorexia, lethargy, fever, rash; also reported dehydration, hypertension, abdominal discomfort, gastroenteritis, drowsiness, encephalopathy, headache, nervousness, depression; anaemia, leucopenia, increases in liver enzymes; rarely gastro-intestinal ulceration and bleeding, seizures, hallucinations, urticaria, interstitial nephritis
Dose: initial doses should be one-sixth to one-quarter of the expected maintenance dose, increased gradually over 4–6 weeks
Maintenance, ADULT and CHILD over 50 kg bodyweight, 2 g daily in 4 divided doses
CHILD up to 12 years, 1.3 g/m² (approx. 50 mg/kg) daily in 4 divided doses

Cystagon® (Orphan Europe) ▼ PoM
Capsules, mercaptamine 50 mg, net price 100-cap pack = £44.00; 150 mg, 100-cap pack = £125.00
Note. CHILD under 6 years at risk of aspiration, capsules can be opened and contents sprinkled on food (at a temperature suitable for eating); avoid adding to acidic drinks (e.g. orange juice)

9.8.2   Acute porphyrias

The acute porphyrias (acute intermittent porphyria, variegate porphyria, hereditary coproporphyria and 5-aminolaevulinic dehydratase deficiency porphyria) are hereditary disorders of haem biosynthesis; they have a prevalence of about 1 in 10 000 of the population.

Great care must be taken when prescribing for patients with acute porphyria since many drugs can induce acute porphyric crises. Since acute porphyrias are hereditary, relatives of affected individuals should be screened and advised about the potential danger of certain drugs.

Haem arginate (*Normosang®*, Orphan Europe) is administered by short intravenous infusion as haem replacement in moderate, severe or unremitting acute porphyria crises. Supplies may be obtained outside office hours from the on-call pharmacist at:

University Hospital of Wales,
Cardiff   (029) 2074 7747
St. James's University Hospital,
Leeds   (0113) 243 3144
                              or   (0113) 283 7010
St Thomas's Hospital,
London   (020) 7928 9292

Further information may be obtained from:
Welsh Drug Information Centre
University Hospital of Wales
Cardiff CF4 4XW
Telephone (029) 2074 2979

HAEM ARGINATE

(Human hemin)

Indications: acute porphyrias (acute intermittent porphyria, porphyria variegata, hereditary copro-porphyria)

Cautions: pregnancy and breast feeding

Side-effects: rarely hypersensitivity reactions and fever; pain and thrombophlebitis at injection site

Dose: *by intravenous infusion*, ADULT and CHILD 3 mg/kg once daily (max. 250 mg daily) for 4 days; if response inadequate, repeat 4-day course with close biochemical monitoring

Normosang® (Orphan Europe) ▼ [PoM]
Concentrate for intravenous infusion, haem arginate 25 mg/mL, net price 10-mL amp = £281.25

Drugs unsafe for use in acute porphyrias

The following list contains drugs on the UK market that have been classified as 'unsafe' in porphyria because they have been shown to be porphyrinogenic in animals or *in vitro*, or have been associated with acute attacks in patients.

Note. Quite modest changes in chemical structure can lead to changes in porphyrinogenicity but where possible general statements have been made about groups of drugs; these should be checked first

Drug groups (please check first)

Amphetamines	Ergot Derivatives[7]
Anabolic Steroids	Gold Salts
Antidepressants[1]	Hormone Replacement
Antihistamines[2]	Therapy
Barbiturates[3]	Menopausal Steroids
Benzodiazepines[4]	Progestogens[5]
Cephalosporins	Sulphonamides[8]
Contraceptives, steroid[5]	Sulphonylureas[9]
Diuretics[6]	

Individual Drugs (please check groups above first)

Alcohol	Ketoconazole
Alcuronium	Lidocaine (lignocaine)[14]
Aluminium-containing	Loxapine
Antacids[10]	Mebeverine
Aminoglutethimide	Mefenamic Acid
Amiodarone	Meprobamate
Azapropazone	Methotrexate
Baclofen	Methyldopa
Bromocriptine	Metoclopramide[15]
Busulfan	Metyrapone
Captopril	Miconazole
Carbamazepine	Mifepristone
Carisoprodol	Minoxidil[15]
Chloral Hydrate[11]	Nalidixic Acid
Chlorambucil	Nifedipine
Chloramphenicol	Nitrofurantoin
Chloroform[12]	Orphenadrine
Clonidine	Oxybutynin
Cocaine	Oxycodone
Colistin	Oxymetazoline
Cyclophosphamide	Oxytetracycline
Cycloserine	Pentazocine[13]
Ciclosporin	Phenoxybenzamine
Danazol	Phenylbutazone
Dapsone	Phenytoin
Dexfenfluramine	Piroxicam
Dextropropoxyphene[13]	Prilocaine
Diclofenac	Probenecid
Doxycycline	Pyrazinamide
Econazole	Ranitidine
Enflurane	Rifabutin[16]
Erythromycin	Rifampicin[16]
Etamsylate	Simvastatin
Ethionamide	Sulfinpyrazone
Ethosuximide	Sulpiride
Etomidate	Tamoxifen
Fenfluramine	Theophylline[17]
Flucloxacillin	Thioridazine
Flupentixol	Tinidazole
Griseofulvin	Trimethoprim
Halothane	Triclofos[11]
Hydralazine	Valproate[4]
Hyoscine	Verapamil
Isometheptene Mucate	Zuclopenthixol
Isoniazid	

1. Includes tricyclic (and related) and MAOIs.
2. Most antihistamines should be avoided but cetirizine, chlorphenamine, cyclizine, diphenhydramine, doxylamine, ketotifen, loratadine, and alimemazine (trimeprazine) thought to be safe.
3. Includes methohexital, primidone, and thiopental.
4. Status epilepticus has been treated successfully with intravenous diazepam; temazepam is thought to be safe; where essential, seizure prophylaxis has been undertaken with clonazepam or valproate.
5. Progestogens are more porphyrinogenic than oestrogens; oestrogens may be safe at least in replacement doses. Progestogens should be avoided whenever possible by all women susceptible to acute porphyria; however, where non-hormonal contraception is inappropriate, progestogens may be used with extreme caution if the potential benefit outweighs risk. The risk of an acute attack is greatest in women who have had a previous attack or are aged under 30 years. Long-acting progestogen preparations should never be used in those at risk of acute porphyria.
6. Acetazolamide, amiloride, bumetanide, cyclopenthiazide and triamterene have been used.
7. Includes ergometrine (oxytocin probably safe), lisuride and pergolide.
8. Includes co-trimoxazole and sulfasalazine.
9. Glipizide is thought to be safe
10. Absorption limited but magnesium-containing antacids preferable.
11. Although evidence of hazard is uncertain, manufacturer advises avoid
12. Small amounts in medicines probably safe.
13. Morphine, diamorphine, codeine, dihydrocodeine, and pethidine are thought to be safe.
14. Bupivacaine is thought to be safe and lidocaine (lignocaine) may be used with caution.
15. May be used with caution if safer alternative not available.
16. Rifamycins have been used in a few patients without evidence of harm—use with caution if safer alternative not available.
17. Includes aminophylline.

10: Musculoskeletal and joint diseases

For treatment of septic arthritis see section 5.1, table 1.

10.1   Drugs used in rheumatic diseases and gout

10.1.1   Non-steroidal anti-inflammatory drugs

10.1.2   Corticosteroids

10.1.3   Drugs which suppress the rheumatic disease process

10.1.4   Drugs for treatment of gout

Rheumatoid arthritis and other inflammatory disorders

Most rheumatic diseases require symptomatic treatment to relieve pain. A non-steroidal anti-inflammatory drug (NSAID) is indicated when pain and stiffness are due to inflammatory rheumatic disease. Drugs are also available which may affect the disease process itself and favourably influence the outcome (section 10.1.3). For rheumatoid arthritis these include penicillamine, gold salts, antimalarials (chloroquine and hydroxychloroquine), immunosuppressants (azathioprine, ciclosporin, cyclophosphamide, and methotrexate), and sulfasalazine—they are sometimes known as second-line or disease-modifying antirheumatic drugs; recent evidence has suggested that corticosteroids may also be able to reduce the rate of joint destruction (section 10.1.2.1). Drugs which may affect the disease process in psoriatic arthritis include gold salts, azathioprine, and methotrexate (section 10.1.3) and for gout they include uricosuric drugs and allopurinol (section 10.1.4).

Osteoarthritis

In osteoarthritis (sometimes called degenerative joint disease or osteoarthrosis) non-drug measures such as weight reduction and exercise should be encouraged. For pain relief in osteoarthritis and soft-tissue lesions, paracetamol (section 4.7.1) is often adequate and should be used first. Alternatively a low-dose NSAID (e.g. ibuprofen up to 1.2 g daily) may be used. If pain relief with either drug is inadequate, both paracetamol (in a full dose of 4 g daily) and a low-dose NSAID may be required; if necessary the dose of the NSAID may need to be increased or a low dose of an opioid analgesic given with paracetamol (as co-codamol 8/500 or co-dydramol 10/500).

Topical treatment including application of an NSAID or capsaicin 0.025% (section 10.3.2) may provide some pain relief in osteoarthritis.

Intra-articular corticosteroid injections (section 10.1.2.2) may produce temporary benefit in osteoarthritis, especially if associated with soft-tissue inflammation. Hyaluronic acid and its derivatives have recently become available for osteoarthritis of the knee. Sodium hyaluronate (*Hyalgan®*, Shire) and hylan G-F 20 (*Synvisc®*, Biomatrix) are injected intra-articularly to supplement natural hyaluronic acid in the synovial fluid.

10.1.1 Non-steroidal anti-inflammatory drugs

In *single doses* non-steroidal anti-inflammatory drugs (NSAIDs) have analgesic activity comparable to that of paracetamol (section 4.7.1), but paracetamol is preferred, particularly in the elderly (see also Prescribing for the elderly, p. 16).

In regular *full dosage* NSAIDs have both a lasting analgesic and an anti-inflammatory effect which makes them particularly useful for the treatment of continuous or regular pain associated with inflammation. Therefore, although paracetamol often gives adequate pain control in osteoarthritis, NSAIDs are more appropriate than paracetamol or the opioid analgesics in the *inflammatory arthritides* (e.g. rheumatoid arthritis) and in some cases of *advanced osteoarthritis*. They may also be of benefit in the less well defined conditions of *back pain* and *soft-tissue disorders*.

CHOICE. Differences in anti-inflammatory activity between different NSAIDs are small, but there is considerable variation in individual patient tolerance and response. About 60% of patients will respond to any NSAID; of the others, those who do not respond to one may well respond to another. A full analgesic effect should normally be obtained within a week, whereas an anti-inflammatory effect may not be achieved (or may not be clinically assessable) for up to 3 weeks. If appropriate responses are not obtained within these times, another NSAID should be tried.

The main differences between NSAIDs are in the incidence and type of side-effects. Before treatment is started the prescriber should weigh efficacy against possible side-effects.

NSAIDs vary in their selectivity for inhibiting different types of cyclo-oxygenase; selective inhibition of cyclo-oxygenase 2 is claimed to improve gastro-intestinal tolerance but this remains unproven. A number of other factors also determine susceptibility to gastro-intestinal effects and an NSAID should be chosen on the basis of the incidence of gastro-intestinal and other side-effects.

Ibuprofen is a propionic acid derivative with anti-inflammatory, analgesic, and antipyretic properties. It has fewer side-effects than other NSAIDs but its anti-inflammatory properties are weaker. Doses of 1.6 to 2.4 g daily are needed for rheumatoid arthritis and it is unsuitable for conditions where inflammation is prominent such as acute gout.

Other propionic acid derivatives:

Naproxen has emerged as one of the first choices as it combines good efficacy with a low incidence of side-effects (but more than ibuprofen, see CSM comment below) and administration is only twice daily.

Fenbufen is claimed to be associated with less gastro-intestinal bleeding, but there is a high risk of rashes (see p. 451).

Fenoprofen is as effective as naproxen, and **flurbiprofen** may be slightly more effective. Both are associated with slightly greater gastro-intestinal side-effects than ibuprofen.

Ketoprofen has anti-inflammatory properties similar to ibuprofen and has more side-effects (see also CSM comment below). **Dexketoprofen**, an isomer of ketoprofen, has been introduced for the short-term relief of mild to moderate pain.

Tiaprofenic acid is as effective as naproxen; it has more side-effects than ibuprofen (**important:** reports of severe cystitis, see CSM advice on p. 455).

Drugs with properties similar to those of propionic acid derivatives:

Azapropazone is similar in effect to naproxen; it has a tendency to cause rashes and is associated with an increased risk of severe gastro-intestinal toxicity (**important:** see CSM restrictions on p. 449).

Diclofenac and **aceclofenac** have actions similar to that of naproxen; their side-effects are also similar to naproxen.

Diflunisal is an aspirin derivative but its clinical effect more closely resembles that of the propionic acid derivatives than that of its parent compound. Its long duration of action allows twice-daily administration.

Etodolac is comparable in effect to naproxen; side-effects appear to be comparable to those of ibuprofen but long-term data are awaited.

Indometacin (indomethacin) has an action equal to or superior to that of naproxen, but with a high incidence of side-effects including headaches, dizziness, and gastro-intestinal disturbances (see also CSM comment below).

Ketorolac is used in the short-term management of moderate to severe postoperative pain (section 15.1.4.2)

Mefenamic acid is a related analgesic but its anti-inflammatory properties are minor and side-effects differ in that diarrhoea and occasionally haemolytic anaemia may occur which necessitate discontinuation of treatment.

Meloxicam has recently been introduced for the short-term treatment of osteoarthritis and long-term treatment of rheumatoid arthritis.

Nabumetone is comparable in effect to naproxen.

Phenylbutazone is a potent anti-inflammatory drug but because of occasional serious side-effects its use is limited to the hospital treatment of ankylosing spondylitis; prolonged administration may be necessary but it should not be used unless other drugs have failed.

Piroxicam is as effective as naproxen and has a prolonged duration of action which permits once-daily administration. It has more gastro-intestinal side-effects than ibuprofen, especially in the elderly (see also CSM comment below).

Rofecoxib has been introduced recently for symptomatic relief in osteoarthritis

Sulindac is similar in tolerance to naproxen.

Tenoxicam is similar in activity and tolerance to naproxen. Its long half-life allows once-daily administration.

Tolfenamic acid is indicated for the treatment of migraine (section 4.7.4.1)

CAUTIONS AND CONTRA-INDICATIONS. NSAIDs should be used with caution in the elderly (risk of serious side-effects and fatalities, see also Prescribing for the elderly p. 16), in allergic disorders (they are **contra-indicated** in patients with a history of hypersensitivity to aspirin or any other NSAID—which includes those in whom attacks of asthma, angioedema, urticaria or rhinitis have been precipitated by aspirin or any other NSAID), during pregnancy and breast-feeding (see Appendixes 4 and 5), and in coagulation defects.

In patients with renal, cardiac, or hepatic impairment caution is required since the use of NSAIDs may result in deterioration of renal function (see also under Side-effects, below and Appendixes 2 and 3); the dose should be kept as **low as possible** and renal function should be **monitored**.

NSAIDs should not be given to patients with active peptic ulceration (see also **CSM advice** below). While it is preferable to avoid them in patients with current or previous gastro-intestinal ulceration or bleeding, and to withdraw them if gastro-intestinal lesions develop, nevertheless patients with serious rheumatic diseases (e.g. rheumatoid arthritis) are usually dependent on NSAIDs for effective relief of pain and stiffness. For advice on the prophylaxis and treatment of NSAID-associated peptic ulcers, see section 1.3.

For **interactions** of NSAIDs, see Appendix 1 (NSAIDs)

SIDE-EFFECTS. The side-effects of NSAIDs vary in severity and frequency. Gastro-intestinal discomfort, nausea, diarrhoea, and occasionally bleeding and ulceration occur (see also CSM advice below); dyspepsia may be minimised by taking these drugs with food or milk. Other side-effects include hypersensitivity reactions (particularly rashes, angioedema, and bronchospasm—see CSM advice below), headache, dizziness, vertigo, hearing disturbances such as tinnitus, photosensitivity, and haematuria. Blood disorders have also occurred. Fluid retention may occur (rarely precipitating congestive heart failure in elderly patients). Renal failure may be provoked by NSAIDs especially in patients with pre-existing renal impairment (**important**, see also under Cautions above). Rarely, papillary necrosis or interstitial fibrosis associated with NSAIDs may lead to renal failure. Hepatic damage, alveolitis, pulmonary eosinophilia, pancreatitis, eye changes, Stevens-Johnson syndrome and toxic epidermal necrolysis are other rare side-effects. Induction of or exacerbation of colitis has been reported. Aseptic meningitis has been reported rarely with NSAIDs; patients with connective tissue disorders such as systemic lupus erythematosus may be especially susceptible.

Overdosage: see Emergency Treatment of Poisoning, p. 21.

CSM advice (g.i. side-effects)

Recent evidence on the relative safety of 7 oral NSAIDs has indicated differences in the risks of serious upper gastro-intestinal side-effects. **Azapropazone** is associated with the *highest risk* (**important:** see also restrictions on p. 449) and **ibuprofen** with the *lowest*; **piroxicam, ketoprofen, indometacin, naproxen** and **diclofenac** are associated with *intermediate risks* (possibly higher in the case of piroxicam). There are insufficient data to reach clear conclusions on other available oral NSAIDs.

Recommendations are that NSAIDs associated with low risk should *generally be preferred*, to start at the *lowest recommended dose, not to use more than one* oral NSAID at a time, and to remember that all NSAIDs are *contra-indicated* in patients with peptic ulceration.

Previous recommendations of the CSM have included the advice that in patients with a history of peptic ulcer disease and in the elderly, NSAIDs should be given only after other forms of treatment have been carefully considered.

CSM warning (asthma)

Any degree of worsening of asthma may be related to the ingestion of NSAIDs, either prescribed or (in the case of ibuprofen and others) purchased over the counter.

IBUPROFEN

Indications: pain and inflammation in rheumatic disease (including juvenile arthritis) and other musculoskeletal disorders; mild to moderate pain including dysmenorrhoea; postoperative analgesia; migraine; fever and pain in children

Cautions: see notes above; **interactions:** Appendix 1 (NSAIDs)

Contra-indications: see notes above;

Side-effects: see notes above; **overdosage:** see Emergency Treatment of Poisoning, p. 21

Dose: initially 1.2–1.8 g daily in 3–4 divided doses preferably after food; increased if necessary to max. of 2.4 g daily; maintenance dose of 0.6–1.2 g daily may be adequate

Juvenile rheumatoid arthritis, CHILD over 7 kg bodyweight 30–40 mg/kg daily in 3–4 divided doses

Fever and pain in children, CHILD over 7 kg bodyweight 20–30 mg/kg daily in divided doses *or* 1–2 years 50 mg 3–4 times daily, 3–7 years 100 mg 3–4 times daily, 8–12 years 200 mg 3–4 times daily

Ibuprofen (Non-proprietary) PoM
Tablets, coated, ibuprofen 200 mg, net price 84-tab pack = £4.00; 400 mg, 84-tab pack = £5.05; 600 mg, 20 = £1.90. Label: 21

Various strengths available from APS, Ashbourne (*Arthrofen®*), Berk (*Lidifen®*), Cox, CP, DDSA (*Ebufac®*), Kent, Norton, Ranbaxy (*Rimafen®*), Pharmacia & Upjohn (*Motrin®*, including an 800-mg strength)

Oral suspension, ibuprofen 100 mg/5 mL, net price 100 mL = £1.88, 150 mL = £2.81. Label: 21

Note. Sugar-free versions are available and can be ordered by specifying 'sugar-free' on the prescription Available from Crookes (*Nurofen® for Children Sugar Free*), Galpharm (*Galprofen®*)

Note. Proprietary brands of ibuprofen preparations are on sale to the public; brand names include, Advil®, Anadin Ibuprofen®, Anadin Ultra®, Boots Children's 6 years Plus Fever & Pain Relief®, Cuprofen®, Galprofen®, Hedex® Ibuprofen, Ibrufhalal®, Ibufem®, Inoven®, Junifen®, Librofem®, Migrafen®, Novaprin®, Nurofen®, Obifen®, Pacifene®, PhorPain®, Proflex®, Relcofen®; compound proprietary preparations containing ibuprofen include Advil® Cold and Sinus (ibuprofen, pseudoephedrine), Lemsip® Power + (ibuprofen, pseudoephedrine), Nurofen® Cold & Flu (ibuprofen, pseudoephedrine), Nurofen® Plus (ibuprofen, codeine), Solpaflex® (ibuprofen, codeine)

Brufen® (Knoll) PoM
Tablets, all magenta, ibuprofen 200 mg (s/c), net price 20 = 68p; 400 mg (s/c), 20 = £1.28; 600 mg (f/c), 20 = £2.04. Label: 21
Syrup, orange, ibuprofen 100 mg/5 mL. Net price 500 mL = £8.07. Label: 21
Granules, effervescent, ibuprofen 600 mg/sachet. Net price 20-sachet pack = £5.67. Label: 13, 21
Note. Contains sodium approx. 9 mmol/sachet
Topical preparations: section 10.3.2

■ Modified release
Brufen Retard® (Knoll) PoM
Tablets, m/r, f/c, ibuprofen 800 mg, net price 56-tab pack = £9.65. Label: 25, 27
Dose: 2 tablets daily as a single dose, preferably in the early evening, increased in severe cases to 3 tablets daily in 2 divided doses; CHILD not recommended

Fenbid® (Goldshield) PoM
Spansule® (= capsule m/r), maroon/pink, enclosing off-white pellets, ibuprofen 300 mg. Net price 120-cap pack = £9.64. Label: 25
Dose: 1–3 capsules every 12 hours; CHILD not recommended

■ With codeine
For an adverse comment on compound analgesic preparations, see p. 204. For details of the **side-effects, cautions**, and **contra-indications** of opioid analgesics, see p. 210 (**important:** the elderly are particularly susceptible to opioid side-effects).
Codafen Continus® (Napp) PoM ▭
Tablets, white/pink, ibuprofen 300 mg (m/r), codeine phosphate 20 mg. Net price 56-tab pack = £6.01; 112-tab pack = £12.00. Label: 2, 21, 25
Dose: 1–2 tablets every 12 hours; max. 3 tablets every 12 hours; CHILD not recommended

▭ denotes preparations that are considered to be less suitable for prescribing (see p. vi)

ACECLOFENAC
Indications: pain and inflammation in rheumatoid arthritis, osteoarthritis and ankylosing spondylitis
Cautions: see notes above; avoid in porphyria (section 9.8.2); **interactions:** Appendix 1 (NSAIDs)
Contra-indications: see notes above
Side-effects: see notes above
Dose: 100 mg twice daily (reduce to 100 mg daily initially in hepatic impairment); CHILD not recommended

Preservex® (UCB Pharma) ▼ PoM
Tablets, f/c, aceclofenac 100 mg, net price 60-tab pack = £14.95. Label: 21

ACEMETACIN
(Glycolic acid ester of indometacin)
Indications: pain and inflammation in rheumatic disease and other musculoskeletal disorders; post-operative analgesia
Cautions: see under Indometacin and notes above
DRIVING. Dizziness may affect performance of skilled tasks (e.g. driving)
Contra-indications: see under Indometacin and notes above
Side-effects: see under Indometacin and notes above

Dose: 120 mg daily in divided doses with food, increased if necessary to 180 mg daily; CHILD not recommended

Emflex® (Merck) PoM
Capsules, yellow/orange, acemetacin 60 mg, net price 90-cap pack = £20.93. Label: 21, counselling, driving

AZAPROPAZONE
Indications: see under CSM restrictions, below
CSM RESTRICTIONS. CSM *has restricted* azapropazone to use in rheumatoid arthritis, ankylosing spondylitis and acute gout only when other NSAIDs have been tried and failed, *has* **contra-indicated** it in patients with a history of peptic ulceration, and *has reduced* the maximum daily dose to 600 mg for rheumatoid arthritis and ankylosing spondylitis in patients over 60 years
Cautions: see notes above; avoid in porphyria (section 9.8.2); **interactions:** Appendix 1 (NSAIDs)
Contra-indications: see notes above; history of peptic ulceration, inflammatory bowel disease or blood disorder; for specific restrictions and contra-indications relating to renal impairment see under Dose
Side-effects: see notes above; photosensitivity, see CSM advice below
PHOTOSENSITIVITY. CSM has reminded of need to advise patients taking azapropazone to avoid direct exposure to sunlight (or to use sunblock preparations)
Dose:
Rheumatoid arthritis and ankylosing spondylitis, 1.2 g daily in 2 or 4 divided doses; in renal impairment or in elderly 300 mg twice daily, avoid altogether in severe renal impairment; CHILD not recommended
Acute gout (always ensure increased fluid intake), 1.8 g daily in divided doses until acute symptoms subside (usually by day 4) *then* 1.2 g daily in divided doses until symptoms resolve—consider appropriate alternative therapy if they persist; in mild renal impairment or in elderly, 1.8 g daily for first 24 hours then 1.2 g daily in divided doses reducing to max. 600 mg daily in divided doses as soon as possible (preferably by day 4) *then* continuing only until acute symptoms resolve—consider appropriate alternative therapy if they persist, and *avoid altogether for gout* in moderate to severe renal impairment and *avoid for gout in elderly* even in mild renal impairment; CHILD not recommended

Rheumox® (Goldshield) PoM
Capsules, orange, azapropazone 300 mg. Net price 112-cap pack = £17.16. Label: 11 (also photosensitivity counselling, see above), 21
Tablets, orange, f/c, scored, azapropazone 600 mg. Net price 112-tab pack = £29.03. Label: 11 (also photosensitivity counselling, see above), 21

DEXKETOPROFEN
Indications: short-term treatment of mild to moderate pain including dysmenorrhoea
Cautions: see notes above; **interactions:** Appendix 1 (NSAIDs)
Contra-indications: see notes above
Side-effects: see notes above

Dose: 12.5 mg every 4–6 hours *or* 25 mg every 8 hours; max. 75 mg daily; ELDERLY initially max. 50 mg daily; CHILD not recommended

Keral® (Menarini) ▼ PoM
Tablets, f/c, scored, dexketoprofen (as trometamol) 25 mg, net price 20-tab pack = £3.90; 50-tab pack = £9.75. Label: 22

DICLOFENAC SODIUM

Indications: pain and inflammation in rheumatic disease (including juvenile arthritis) and other musculoskeletal disorders; acute gout; postoperative pain
Cautions: see notes above; **interactions:** Appendix 1 (NSAIDs)
Contra-indications: see notes above; porphyria (section 9.8.2)
INTRAVENOUS USE. Additional contra-indications include concomitant NSAID or anticoagulant use (including low-dose heparin), history of haemorrhagic diathesis, history of confirmed or suspected cerebrovascular bleeding, operations with high risk of haemorrhage, history of asthma, moderate or severe renal impairment, hypovolaemia, dehydration
Side-effects: see notes above; suppositories may cause rectal irritation
Dose: *by mouth*, 75–150 mg daily in 2–3 divided doses, preferably after food
By deep intramuscular injection into the gluteal muscle, acute exacerbations and post-operative, 75 mg once daily (twice daily in severe cases) for max. of 2 days
Ureteric colic, 75 mg then a further 75 mg after 30 minutes if necessary
By intravenous infusion (in hospital setting), 75 mg repeated if necessary after 4–6 hours for max. 2 days
Prevention of postoperative pain, initially after surgery 25–50 mg over 15–60 minutes then 5 mg/ hour for max. 2 days
By rectum in suppositories, 75–150 mg daily in divided doses
Max. total daily dose by any route 150 mg
CHILD 1–12 years, juvenile arthritis, *by mouth or by rectum*, 1–3 mg/kg daily in divided doses (25 mg e/c tablets, 12.5 mg and 25 mg suppositories only)

Diclofenac Sodium (Non-proprietary) PoM
Tablets, both e/c, diclofenac sodium 25 mg, net price 20 = 67p; 50 mg, 20 = £1.22. Label: 5, 25
Available from APS, Arun (*Diclovol®*), Ashbourne (*Diclozip®*), Berk (*Flamrase®*), Cox, Dexcel Pharma (*Dicloflex®*), Eastern (*Volraman®*), Goldshield (*Acoflam®*), Kent (*Enzed®*), Lagap, Norton, Sterwin, Trinity (*Lofensaid®*)
Injection, diclofenac sodium 25 mg/mL. Net price 3-mL amp = 83p
Available from Antigen
Note. Licensed for intramuscular use
Voltarol® (Novartis) PoM
Tablets, both e/c, diclofenac sodium 25 mg (yellow), net price 84-tab pack = £3.94; 50 mg (brown), 84-tab pack = £6.13. Label: 5, 25
Dispersible tablets, sugar-free, pink, diclofenac, equivalent to diclofenac sodium 50 mg, net price 21-tab pack = £5.15. Label: 13, 21
Note. Voltarol Dispersible tablets are more suitable for **short-term** use in acute conditions for which treatment required for no more than 3 months (no information on use beyond 3 months)

Injection, diclofenac sodium 25 mg/mL. Net price 3-mL amp = 83p
Suppositories, diclofenac sodium 12.5 mg, net price 10 = 65p; 25 mg, 10 = £1.15; 50 mg, 10 = £1.89; 100 mg, 10 = £3.38
Emulgel® gel, section 10.3.2

■ Diclofenac potassium

Voltarol Rapid® (Novartis) PoM
Tablets, s/c, diclofenac potassium 25 mg (red), net price 28-tab pack = £3.05; 50 mg (brown), 28-tab pack = £5.85
Dose: rheumatic disease, musculoskeletal disorders, acute gout, post-operative pain, 75–150 mg daily in 2–3 divided doses; CHILD over 14 years, 75–100 mg daily in 2–3 divided doses
Migraine, 50 mg at onset, repeated after 2 hours if necessary then after 4–6 hours; max. 200 mg in 24 hours; CHILD not recommended

■ Modified release

Diclomax SR® (Parke-Davis) PoM
Capsules, m/r, yellow, diclofenac sodium 75 mg. Net price 56-cap pack = £13.01. Label: 21, 25
Dose: 1 capsule 1–2 times daily *or* 2 capsules once daily, preferably with food; CHILD not recommended

Diclomax Retard® (Parke-Davis) PoM
Capsules, m/r, diclofenac sodium 100 mg. Net price 28-tab pack = £9.36. Label: 21, 25
Dose: 1 capsule daily preferably with food; CHILD not recommended

Motifene® 75 mg (Sankyo) PoM
Capsules, e/c, m/r, diclofenac sodium 75 mg (enclosing e/c pellets containing diclofenac sodium 25 mg and m/r pellets containing diclofenac sodium 50 mg). Net price 56-cap pack = £14.99. Label: 25
Dose: 1 capsule 1-2 times daily; CHILD not recommended

Voltarol® 75 mg SR (Novartis) PoM
Tablets, m/r, pink, diclofenac sodium 75 mg. Net price 28-tab pack = £8.68; 56-tab pack = £17.35. Label: 21, 25
Dose: 75 mg 1–2 times daily preferably with food; CHILD not recommended
Note. Modified-release tablets containing diclofenac sodium 75 mg available from Arun (*Diclovol®SR*), Bartholomew Rhodes (*Diclotard® 75 MR*), Cox (*Flamatak® 75 MR*), Dexcel Pharma (*Dicloflex® 75 SR*), Goldshield (*Acoflam® 75 SR*), Hillcross (*Dexomon® 75 SR*), Lagap (*Rhumalgan® CR*), Norton, Pharmacia & Upjohn (*Flexotard® MR 75*), Sovereign (*Rheumatac® Retard 75*), Sterwin (*Slofenac® SR*), Trinity (*Lofensaid® Retard 75, Volsaid® Retard 75*)

Voltarol® Retard (Novartis) PoM
Tablets, m/r, red, diclofenac sodium 100 mg. Net price 28-tab pack = £12.72. Label: 21, 25
Dose: 1 tablet daily preferably with food; CHILD not recommended
Note. Modified-release tablets containing diclofenac sodium 100 mg available from APS, Arun (*Diclovol®Retard*), Berk (*Flamrase® SR¹*), Cox (*Flamatak® 100 MR*), Dexcel Pharma (*Dicloflex® Retard*), Genus (*Digenac® XL¹*), Goldshield (*Acoflam® Retard*), Hillcross (*Dexomon® Retard 100*), Lagap (*Rhumalgan® CR*), Norton, Pharmacia & Upjohn (*Flexotard® MR 100*), Sterwin (*Slofenac® SR*), Trinity (*Lofensaid® Retard 100, Volsaid® Retard 100*)
1. Also licensed for dysmenorrhoea and associated menorrhagia

■ With misoprostol

For **cautions**, **contra-indications**, and **side-effects** of misoprostol, see section 1.3.4

Arthrotec® (Searle) PoM

Arthrotec® 50 tablets, diclofenac sodium (in e/c core) 50 mg, misoprostol 200 micrograms. Net price 60-tab pack = £13.31; 140-tab pack = £31.06 (hosp. only). Label: 21, 25

Dose: prophylaxis against NSAID-induced gastroduodenal ulceration in patients requiring diclofenac for rheumatoid arthritis or osteoarthritis, 1 tablet 2–3 times daily with food; CHILD not recommended

Arthrotec® 75 tablets, diclofenac sodium (in e/c core) 75 mg, misoprostol 200 micrograms. Net price 60-tab pack = £17.59. Label: 21, 25

Dose: prophylaxis against NSAID-induced gastroduodenal ulceration in patients requiring diclofenac for rheumatoid arthritis or osteoarthritis, 1 tablet twice daily with food; CHILD not recommended

DIFLUNISAL

Indications: pain and inflammation in rheumatic disease and other musculoskeletal disorders; mild to moderate pain including dysmenorrhoea

Cautions: see notes above; **interactions:** Appendix 1 (NSAIDs)

Contra-indications: see notes above

Side-effects: see notes above

Dose: mild to moderate pain, initially 1 g, then 500 mg every 12 hours (increased to max. 500 mg every 8 hours if necessary)

Osteoarthritis, rheumatoid arthritis, 0.5–1 g daily as a single daily dose *or* in 2 divided doses

Dysmenorrhoea, initially 1 g, then 500 mg every 12 hours

CHILD not recommended

Dolobid® (MSD) PoM

Tablets, both f/c, diflunisal 250 mg (peach), net price 20 = £1.80; 500 mg (orange), 20 = £3.61. Label: 21, 25, counselling, avoid aluminium hydroxide

ETODOLAC

Indications: pain and inflammation in rheumatoid arthritis and osteoarthritis

Cautions: see notes above; **interactions:** Appendix 1 (NSAIDs)

Contra-indications: see notes above

Side-effects: see notes above

Dose: 600 mg daily; CHILD not recommended

Lodine SR® (Monmouth) PoM

Tablets, m/r, light-grey, etodolac 600 mg. Net price 30-tab pack = £15.50. Label: 25

FENBUFEN

Indications: pain and inflammation in rheumatic disease and other musculoskeletal disorders

Cautions: see notes above; **interactions:** Appendix 1 (NSAIDs)

Contra-indications: see notes above

Side-effects: see notes above, but also high risk of rashes (discontinue immediately); erythema multiforme and Stevens-Johnson syndrome reported; also allergic interstitial lung disorders (may follow rashes)

Dose: 300 mg in the morning and 600 mg at bedtime *or* 450 mg twice daily; CHILD under 14 years not recommended

Fenbufen (Non-proprietary) PoM

Capsules, fenbufen 300 mg, net price 84-cap pack = £17.27. Label: 21

Available from Ashbourne (*Fenbuzip®*), Genus, Hillcross, Kent, Norton

Tablets, fenbufen 300 mg, net price 84-tab pack = £13.19; 450 mg, 56-tab pack = £13.17. Label: 21

Available from Ashbourne (*Fenbuzip®*), Cox, Generics, Genus, Hillcross, Kent, Norton, Sterwin

Lederfen® (Lederle) PoM

Capsules, dark blue, fenbufen 300 mg. Net price 84-cap pack = £18.83. Label: 21

Tablets, both light blue, f/c, fenbufen 300 mg, net price 84-tab pack = £18.83; 450 mg, 56-tab pack = £18.83. Label: 21

FENOPROFEN

Indications: pain and inflammation in rheumatic disease and other musculoskeletal disorders; mild to moderate pain

Cautions: see notes above; **interactions:** Appendix 1 (NSAIDs)

Contra-indications: see notes above

Side-effects: see notes above; upper respiratory-tract infection, nasopharyngitis, and cystitis also reported

Dose: 300–600 mg 3–4 times daily with food; max. 3 g daily; CHILD not recommended

Fenopron® (Typharm) PoM

Tablets, both orange, fenoprofen (as calcium salt) 300 mg (*Fenopron® 300*), net price 100-tab pack = £9.45; 600 mg (*Fenopron® 600*, scored), 100-tab pack = £18.29. Label: 21

FLURBIPROFEN

Indications: pain and inflammation in rheumatic disease and other musculoskeletal disorders; mild to moderate pain including dysmenorrhoea; migraine; postoperative analgesia; relief of sore throat (section 12.3.1)

Cautions: see notes above; **interactions:** Appendix 1 (NSAIDs)

Contra-indications: see notes above

Side-effects: see notes above; suppositories may cause rectal irritation

Dose: *by mouth or by rectum* in suppositories, 150–200 mg, daily in divided doses, increased in acute conditions to 300 mg daily

Dysmenorrhoea, initially 100 mg, then 50–100 mg every 4–6 hours; max. 300 mg daily

CHILD not recommended

Froben® (Knoll) PoM

Tablets, both yellow, s/c, flurbiprofen 50 mg, net price 20 = £1.82; 100 mg, 20 = £3.44. Label: 21

Note. Flurbiprofen tablets also available from Cox, Kent, Norton

Suppositories, flurbiprofen 100 mg. Net price 12 = £2.90

■ Modified release

Froben SR® (Knoll) PoM

Capsules, m/r, yellow, enclosing off-white beads, flurbiprofen 200 mg. Net price 30-cap pack = £10.88. Label: 21, 25

Dose: rheumatic disease, 1 capsule daily, preferably in the evening; CHILD not recommended

INDOMETACIN
(Indomethacin)

Indications: pain and moderate to severe inflammation in rheumatic disease and other acute musculoskeletal disorders; acute gout; dysmenorrhoea; closure of ductus arteriosus (section 7.1.1.1)

Cautions: see notes above; epilepsy, parkinsonism, psychiatric disturbances; during prolonged therapy ophthalmic and blood examinations particularly advisable; avoid rectal administration in proctitis and haemorrhoids; **interactions:** Appendix 1 (NSAIDs)

DRIVING. Dizziness may affect performance of skilled tasks (e.g. driving)

Contra-indications: see notes above

Side-effects: see notes above; frequently gastrointestinal disturbances (including diarrhoea), headache, dizziness, and light-headedness; gastro-intestinal ulceration and bleeding; rarely, drowsiness, confusion, insomnia, convulsions, psychiatric disturbances, depression, syncope, blood disorders (particularly thrombocytopenia), hypertension, hyperglycaemia, blurred vision, corneal deposits, peripheral neuropathy, and intestinal strictures; suppositories may cause rectal irritation and occasional bleeding

Dose: *by mouth*, rheumatic disease, 50–200 mg daily in divided doses, with food; CHILD not recommended

Acute gout, 150–200 mg daily in divided doses

Dysmenorrhoea, up to 75 mg daily

By rectum in suppositories, 100 mg at night and in the morning if required; CHILD not recommended

Combined oral and rectal treatment, max. total daily dose 150–200 mg

Indometacin (Non-proprietary) PoM

Capsules, indometacin 25 mg, net price 20 = 20p; 50 mg, 20 = 39p. Label: 21, counselling, driving, see above

Available from APS, Ashbourne (*Indomax®*), Cox, Kent, MSD (*Indocid®*), Ranbaxy (*Rimacid®*)

Suspension, sugar-free, indometacin 25 mg/5 mL. Net price 200 mL = £3.12. Label: 21, counselling, driving, see above

Available from MSD (*Indocid®*)

Suppositories, indometacin 100 mg. Net price 10 = £1.39. Counselling, driving, see above

Available from Cox, MSD (*Indocid®*), Norton

■ Modified release

Indometacin m/r preparations PoM

Capsules, m/r, indometacin 75 mg. Net price 20 = £3.94. Label: 21, 25, counselling, driving, see above

Dose: 1 capsule 1–2 times daily; CHILD not recommended

Available from Ashbourne (*Indomax 75 SR®*), Bartholomew Rhodes (*Indotard MR®*), Cox (*Pardelprin®*), Generics (*Slo-Indo®*), Hillcross (*Rheumacin LA®*), Lagap (*Indolar SR®*), MSD (*Indocid-R®*), Pharmacia & Upjohn (*Indomod®*; also 25-mg strength)

Tablets, m/r, indometacin 25 mg (*Flexin-25 Continus®*, green), net price 56-tab pack = £6.83; 50 mg (*Flexin-50 Continus®*, red), 28-tab pack = £6.83; 75 mg (*Flexin-75 Continus®*, yellow), 28-tab pack = £9.75. Label: 21, 25, counselling, driving, see above

Dose: initially 75 mg daily, adjusted in steps of 25–50 mg; range 25–200 mg daily in 1–2 divided doses; dysmenorrhoea, up to 75 mg daily; CHILD not recommended

Available from Napp

KETOPROFEN

Indications: pain and mild inflammation in rheumatic disease and other musculoskeletal disorders, and after orthopaedic surgery; acute gout; dysmenorrhoea

Cautions: see notes above; **interactions:** Appendix 1 (NSAIDs)

Contra-indications: see notes above

Side-effects: see notes above; pain may occur at injection site (occasionally tissue damage); suppositories may cause rectal irritation

Dose: *by mouth*, rheumatic disease, 100–200 mg daily in 2–4 divided doses with food; CHILD not recommended

Pain and dysmenorrhoea, 50 mg up to 3 times daily; CHILD not recommended

By rectum in suppositories, rheumatic disease, 100 mg at bedtime; CHILD not recommended

Combined oral and rectal treatment, max. total daily dose 200 mg

By deep intramuscular injection into the gluteal muscle, 50–100 mg every 4 hours (max. 200 mg in 24 hours) for up to 3 days; CHILD not recommended

Ketoprofen (Non-proprietary) PoM

Capsules, ketoprofen 50 mg, net price 100-cap pack = £15.62; 100 mg, 100-cap pack = £27.34. Label: 21

Available from Lagap

Orudis® (Hawgreen) PoM

Capsules, ketoprofen 50 mg (green/purple), net price 112-cap pack = £17.28; 100 mg (pink), 56-cap pack = £17.33. Label: 21

Suppositories, ketoprofen 100 mg. Net price 10 = £7.44

Oruvail® (Hawgreen) PoM

Injection, ketoprofen 50 mg /mL. Net price 2-mL amp = £1.20

Gel, section 10.3.2

■ Modified release

Oruvail® (Hawgreen) PoM

Capsules, all m/r, enclosing white pellets, ketoprofen 100 mg (pink/purple), net price 56-cap pack = £26.77; 150 mg (pink), 28-cap pack = £15.28; 200 mg (pink/white), 28-cap pack = £26.69. Label: 21, 25

Dose: 100–200 mg once daily with food; CHILD not recommended

Note. Modified-release capsules containing ketoprofen 100 mg and 200 mg also available from APS (*Ketovail®*), Ashbourne (*Ketozip XL®*-200 mg), Cox (*Jomethid XL®*-200 mg), Galen (*Ketotard® 200XL*), Lagap (*Larafen CR®*-200 mg), Tillomed (*Ketil CR*), Trinity (*Fenoket®*-200 mg, *Ketocid®*-200 mg)

MEFENAMIC ACID

Indications: mild to moderate pain in rheumatoid arthritis (including juvenile arthritis), osteoarthritis, and related conditions; dysmenorrhoea and menorrhagia

Cautions: see notes above; porphyria (section 9.8.2); **interactions:** Appendix 1 (NSAIDs)

Contra-indications: see notes above; inflammatory bowel disease

Side-effects: see notes above; drowsiness; diarrhoea or rashes (withdraw treatment); thrombocytopenia, positive Coombs' test, haemolytic anaemia and aplastic anaemia reported; convulsions in overdosage

Dose: 500 mg 3 times daily preferably after food; CHILD over 6 months, 25 mg/kg daily in divided doses for not longer than 7 days, except in juvenile arthritis

Mefenamic Acid (Non-proprietary) PoM
Capsules, mefenamic acid 250 mg. Net price 20 = £1.41. Label: 21
Available from APS, Ashbourne (*Dysman 250®*), Cox, Elan (*Ponstan®*), Kent, Norton, Sterwin
Tablets, mefenamic acid 500 mg, net price 20 = £1.63. Label: 21
Available from APS, Ashbourne (*Dysman 500®*), Cox, Elan (*Ponstan Forte®*), Norton
Paediatric oral suspension, mefenamic acid 50 mg/5 mL. Net price 125 mL = £3.37. Label: 21
Available from Elan (*Ponstan®*)

MELOXICAM

Indications: pain and inflammation in rheumatic disease; exacerbation of osteoarthritis (short-term); ankylosing spondylitis

Cautions: see notes above; avoid rectal administration in proctitis or haemorrhoids; **interactions:** Appendix 1 (NSAIDs)

Contra-indications: see notes above; renal failure (unless receiving dialysis)

Side-effects: see notes above

Dose: *by mouth*, osteoarthritis, 7.5 mg daily with food, increased if necessary to max. 15 mg once daily
Rheumatoid arthritis and ankylosing spondylitis, 15 mg once daily with food (7.5 mg daily in elderly)
By rectum, in suppositories, osteoarthritis, 7.5 mg daily; rheumatoid arthritis, 15 mg once daily (7.5 mg daily in elderly); ankylosing spondylitis, 15 mg once daily
CHILD under 15 years not recommended

Mobic® (Boehringer Ingelheim) ▼ PoM
Tablets, both yellow, scored, meloxicam 7.5 mg, net price 30-tab pack = £10.00; 15 mg, 30-tab pack = £13.90. Label: 21
Suppositories, meloxicam 7.5 mg, net price 12 = £4.00; 15 mg, 12 = £6.00

NABUMETONE

Indications: pain and inflammation in osteoarthritis and rheumatoid arthritis

Cautions: see notes above; **interactions:** Appendix 1 (NSAIDs)

Contra-indications: see notes above

Side-effects: see notes above

Dose: 1 g at night, in severe conditions 0.5–1 g in morning as well; elderly 0.5–1 g daily; CHILD not recommended

Nabumetone (Non-proprietary) PoM
Tablets, 500 mg, net price 56-tab pack = £18.11
Available from Cox

Relifex® (SmithKline Beecham) PoM
Tablets, red, f/c, nabumetone 500 mg. Net price 56-tab pack = £18.11. Label: 21, 25
Suspension, sugar-free, nabumetone 500 mg/5 mL. Net price 300-mL pack = £25.22. Label: 21

NAPROXEN

Indications: pain and inflammation in rheumatic disease (including juvenile arthritis) and other musculoskeletal disorders; dysmenorrhoea; acute gout

Cautions: see notes above; **interactions:** Appendix 1 (NSAIDs)

Contra-indications: see notes above

Side-effects: see notes above; suppositories may cause rectal irritation and occasional bleeding

Dose: *by mouth*, 0.5–1 g daily in 2 divided doses *or* 1 g once daily; CHILD (over 5 years), juvenile arthritis, 10 mg/kg daily in 2 divided doses
Acute musculoskeletal disorders and dysmenorrhoea, 500 mg initially, then 250 mg every 6–8 hours as required; max. dose after first day 1.25 g daily; CHILD under 16 years not recommended
Acute gout, 750 mg initially, then 250 mg every 8 hours until attack has passed; CHILD under 16 years not recommended
By rectum in suppositories, 500 mg at bedtime; if necessary 500 mg in morning as well; CHILD under 16 years not recommended

Naproxen (Non-proprietary) PoM
Tablets, naproxen 250 mg, net price 20 = £1.25; 500 mg, 28-tab pack = £3.47. Label: 21
Available from APS, Ashbourne (*Arthrosin®*), Berk (*Timpron®*), Cox, CP (*Arthroxen®*), Hillcross, Norton, Sterwin
Tablets, e/c, naproxen 250 mg, net price 56-tab pack = £5.00; 500 mg, 56-tab pack = £9.16. Label: 5, 25
Available from APS, Berk (*Timpron® EC*), Generics, Norton

Naprosyn® (Roche) PoM
Tablets, all scored, naproxen 250 mg (buff), net price 56-tab pack = £4.89; 500 mg (buff), 56-tab pack = £9.77. Label: 21
Tablets, e/c, (*Naprosyn EC®*), naproxen 250 mg, net price 56-tab pack = £4.89; 375 mg, 56-tab pack = £7.33; 500 mg, 56-tab pack = £9.77. Label: 5, 25
Suspension, orange, naproxen 125 mg/5 mL. Contains about 1.7 mmol Na⁺/5 mL. Net price 240 mL = £3.65. Label: 21
Suppositories, naproxen 500 mg. Net price 10 = £2.28

Nycopren® (Ardern) PoM
Tablets, both e/c, naproxen 250 mg, net price 56-tab pack = £5.79; 500 mg, 56-tab pack = £11.58. Label: 5, 25

Synflex® (Roche) PoM

Tablets, blue, naproxen sodium 275 mg. Net price 60-tab pack = £8.11. Label: 21

Note. 275 mg naproxen sodium ≡ 250 mg naproxen
Dose: musculoskeletal disorders, postoperative analgesia, 550 mg twice daily when necessary, preferably after food; max. 1.1 g daily; CHILD under 16 years not recommended
Dysmenorrhoea and acute gout, initially 550 mg then 275 mg every 6–8 hours as required; max. of 1.375 g on first day and 1.1 g daily thereafter; CHILD under 16 years not recommended
Migraine, 825 mg at onset, then 275–550 mg at least 30 minutes after initial dose; max 1.375 g in 24 hours; CHILD under 16 years not recommended

■ Modified release
Naprosyn® S/R (Roche) PoM

Tablets, m/r, f/c, scored, naproxen 500 mg (as sodium salt), net price 56-tab pack = £14.60. Label: 25
Dose: rheumatic and musculoskeletal disorders, 1–2 tablets once daily; CHILD under 16 years not recommended

■ With misoprostol
For **cautions**, **contra-indications**, and **side-effects** of misoprostol, see section 1.3.4

Condrotec® (Searle) PoM

Tablets, f/c, off-white/yellow, naproxen 500 mg, misoprostol 200 micrograms, net price 60-tab pack = £17.59. Label: 21
Dose: patients requiring naproxen for rheumatoid arthritis, osteoarthritis, or ankylosing spondylitis, with prophylaxis against NSAID-induced gastroduodenal ulceration, 1 tablet twice daily with food; CHILD not recommended

Napratec® (Searle) PoM

Combination pack, 56 yellow scored tablets, naproxen 500 mg; 56 white scored tablets, misoprostol 200 micrograms. Net price = £19.80. Label: 21
Dose: patients requiring naproxen for rheumatoid arthritis, osteoarthritis, or ankylosing spondylitis, with prophylaxis against NSAID-induced gastroduodenal ulceration, 1 naproxen 500-mg tablet and 1 misoprostol 200-microgram tablet taken together twice daily with food; CHILD not recommended

PHENYLBUTAZONE ▭

Indications: ankylosing spondylitis when other therapy unsuitable
Cautions: blood counts before and during treatment if for more than 7 days; elderly (reduce dose); breast-feeding; allergic disorders (see also under Contra-indications), withdraw if acute pulmonary syndrome including fever and dyspnoea; see also notes above; **interactions:** Appendix 1 (NSAIDs)
COUNSELLING. Warn patient to tell doctor immediately if sore throat, mouth ulcers, bruising, fever, malaise, rash, or non-specific illness develops
Contra-indications: cardiovascular disease, pulmonary, renal and hepatic impairment; pregnancy; history of peptic ulceration, of gastro-intestinal haemorrhage, inflammatory bowel disease, or of blood disorders (including coagulation defects); history of hypersensitivity precipitated by aspirin or other NSAIDs (see also below); porphyria (section 9.8.2); Sjögren's syndrome; thyroid disease; children under 14
HYPERSENSITIVITY. NSAIDs are **contra-indicated** in history of hypersensitivity to aspirin or to any other NSAID—*which includes those* in whom attacks of *asthma, angioedema, urticaria or rhinitis* have been precipitated by aspirin or any other NSAID

Side-effects: see notes above; parotitis, stomatitis, goitre, pancreatitis, hepatitis, nephritis, visual disturbances; rarely leucopenia, thrombocytopenia, agranulocytosis, aplastic anaemia, Stevens-Johnson syndrome, toxic epidermal necrolysis, pulmonary toxicity
Dose: initially 200 mg 2–3 times daily for 2 days, with or after food, then reduced to minimum effective, usually 100 mg 2–3 times daily; CHILD under 14 years not recommended

Butacote® (Novartis) PoM ▭

Tablets, light blue, e/c, s/c, phenylbutazone 100 mg, net price 20 = 40p (hosp. only). Label: 5, 21, 25, counselling, blood disorder symptoms (see above)

▭ denotes preparations that are considered to be less suitable for prescribing (see p. vi)

PIROXICAM

Indications: pain and inflammation in rheumatic disease (including juvenile arthritis) and other musculoskeletal disorders; acute gout
Cautions: see notes above; avoid in porphyria (section 9.8.2); **interactions:** Appendix 1 (NSAIDs)
Contra-indications: see notes above
Side-effects: see notes above; pain at injection site (occasionally tissue damage); suppositories may cause rectal irritation and occasional bleeding
Dose: *by mouth or by rectum*, rheumatic disease, initially 20 mg daily, maintenance 10–30 mg daily, in single or divided doses
CHILD (over 6 years) *by mouth*, juvenile arthritis, less than 15 kg, 5 mg daily; 16–25 kg, 10 mg; 26–45 kg, 15 mg; over 46 kg, 20 mg
Acute musculoskeletal disorders, 40 mg daily in single or divided doses for 2 days, then 20 mg daily for 7–14 days; CHILD not recommended
Acute gout, 40 mg initially, then 40 mg daily in single or divided doses for 4–6 days; CHILD not recommended
By deep intramuscular injection into gluteal muscle, for initial treatment of acute conditions, as dose by mouth (on short-term basis); CHILD not recommended

Piroxicam (Non-proprietary) PoM

Capsules, piroxicam 10 mg, net price 20 = £1.19; 20 mg, 20 = £2.67. Label: 21
Available from APS, Ashbourne (*Pirozip®*), Berk (*Flamatrol®*), Cox, Hillcross, Kent (*Kentene®*), Norton

Feldene® (Pfizer) PoM

Capsules, piroxicam 10 mg (maroon/blue), net price 56-cap pack = £6.00; 20 mg (maroon), 28-cap pack = £6.00. Label: 21
Tablets, (*Feldene Melt®*), piroxicam 20 mg, net price 28-tab pack = £9.83. Label: 10 patient information leaflet, 21
Excipients: include aspartame equivalent to phenylalanine 140 micrograms/tablet (section 9.4.1)
Note. Feldene Melt® tablets can be taken by placing on tongue or by swallowing
Dispersible tablets, piroxicam 10 mg (scored), net price 56-tab pack = £9.75; 20 mg, 28-tab pack = £9.75. Label: 13, 21
Note. Piroxicam dispersible tablets also available from Hillcross
Injection, piroxicam 20 mg/mL. Net price 1-mL amp = 70p

Suppositories, piroxicam 20 mg. Net price 10 = £5.20

Gel, section 10.3.2

Brexidol® (Trinity) PoM
Tablets, yellow, scored, piroxicam (as betadex) 20 mg, net price 30-tab pack = £12.22. Label: 21
Dose: osteoarthritis, rheumatic disease and acute musculoskeletal disorders, 1 tablet daily (may be halved in elderly); CHILD not recommended

ROFECOXIB

Indications: pain and inflammation in osteoarthritis

Cautions: see notes above; **interactions**: Appendix 1 (NSAIDs)

Contra-indications: see notes above; renal impairment (creatinine clearance less than 30 mL/minute); inflammatory bowel disease; severe congestive heart failure

Side-effects: see notes above; mouth ulcers, chest pain, weight gain, sleep disturbance, depression, atopic eczema, and muscle cramps reported; raised liver enzymes (discontinue if persistently high)

Dose: 12.5 mg daily, increased if necessary to max. 25 mg once daily; CHILD not recommended

Vioxx® (MSD) ▼ PoM
Tablets, rofecoxib 12.5 mg (ivory), net price 28-tab pack = £21.58; 25 mg (yellow), 28-tab pack = £21.58
Suspension, sugar-free, yellow, strawberry-flavoured, rofecoxib 12.5 mg/5 mL, net price 150 mL = £23.12; 25 mg/5 mL, 150 mL = £23.12

SULINDAC

Indications: pain and inflammation in rheumatic disease and other musculoskeletal disorders; acute gout

Cautions: see notes above; history of renal stones and ensure adequate hydration; **interactions:** Appendix 1 (NSAIDs)

Contra-indications: see notes above

Side-effects: see notes above; urine discoloration occasionally reported

Dose: 200 mg twice daily with food (may be reduced according to response); max. 400 mg daily; acute gout should respond within 7 days; limit treatment of peri-articular disorders to 7–10 days; CHILD not recommended

Clinoril® (MSD) PoM
Tablets, both yellow, scored, sulindac 100 mg, net price 20 = £2.24; 200 mg, 20 = £4.32. Label: 21
Note. Sulindac tablets also available from Generics

TENOXICAM

Indications: pain and inflammation in rheumatic disease and other musculoskeletal disorders

Cautions: see notes above; **interactions:** Appendix 1 (NSAIDs)

Contra-indications: see notes above

Side-effects: see notes above

Dose: *by mouth*, rheumatic disease, 20 mg daily; CHILD not recommended
Acute musculoskeletal disorders, 20 mg daily for 7 days; max. 14 days; CHILD not recommended
By intravenous or intramuscular injection, for initial treatment for 1–2 days, as dose by mouth; CHILD not recommended

Mobiflex® (Roche) PoM
Tablets, red-brown, f/c, tenoxicam 20 mg. Net price 28-tab pack = £13.47. Label: 21
Injection, powder for reconstitution, tenoxicam 20 mg. Net price per amp (with solvent) = 87p

TIAPROFENIC ACID

Indications: pain and inflammation in rheumatic disease and other musculoskeletal disorders

Cautions: see notes above; **interactions:** Appendix 1 (NSAIDs)

Contra-indications: see notes above; active bladder or prostate disease (or symptoms) and history of recurrent urinary-tract disorders—if urinary symptoms develop discontinue immediately and perform urine tests and culture; see also CSM advice below

CSM ADVICE. Following reports of **severe cystitis** CSM has recommended that tiaprofenic acid should not be given to patients with urinary-tract disorders and should be stopped if urinary symptoms develop. Patients should be advised to stop taking tiaprofenic acid and to report to their doctor promptly if they develop urinary-tract symptoms (such as increased frequency, nocturia, urgency, pain on urinating, or blood in urine)

Side-effects: see notes above

Dose: 600 mg daily in 2–3 divided doses; CHILD not recommended

Tiaprofenic Acid (Non-proprietary) PoM
Tablets, tiaprofenic acid 200 mg, net price 84-tab pack = £21.45; 300 mg, 56-tab pack = £21.45. Label: 21
Available from Cox

Surgam® (Florizel) PoM
Tablets, tiaprofenic acid 200 mg, net price 84-tab pack = £20.48; 300 mg, 56-tab pack = £20.48. Label: 21

■ Modified release

Surgam SA® (Florizel) PoM
Capsules, m/r, maroon/pink enclosing white pellets, tiaprofenic acid 300 mg. Net price 56-cap pack = £20.48. Label: 25
Dose: 2 capsules once daily; CHILD not recommended

Aspirin and the salicylates

Aspirin was the traditional first choice anti-inflammatory analgesic but most physicians now prefer to start treatment with another NSAID which may be better tolerated and more convenient for the patient.

In regular high dosage aspirin has about the same anti-inflammatory effect as other NSAIDs. The required dose for active inflammatory joint disease is at least 3.6 g daily. There is little anti-inflammatory effect with less than 3 g daily. Gastro-intestinal side-effects such as nausea, dyspepsia, and gastro-intestinal bleeding may occur with any dosage of aspirin but anti-inflammatory doses are associated with a much higher incidence of side-effects. Anti-inflammatory doses of aspirin may also cause mild chronic salicylate intoxication (salicylism) characterised by dizziness, tinnitus, and deafness; these symptoms may be controlled by reducing the dosage.

ASPIRIN

(Acetylsalicylic Acid)

Indications: pain and inflammation in rheumatic disease and other musculoskeletal disorders (including juvenile arthritis); see also section 4.7.1; antiplatelet (section 2.9)

Cautions: asthma, allergic disease, uncontrolled hypertension, hepatic or renal impairment (avoid if severe), dehydration, pregnancy (particularly at term; see also Appendix 4), elderly; G6PD-deficiency (section 9.1.5); **interactions:** Appendix 1 (aspirin)

REYE'S SYNDROME. Owing to an association with Reye's syndrome aspirin-containing preparations should not be given to children under 12 years, unless specifically indicated, e.g. for juvenile arthritis (Still's disease). It is **important** to advise families that aspirin is not a suitable medicine for children with minor illnesses.

Contra-indications: gastro-intestinal ulceration; children under 12 years (except for juvenile arthritis) and breast-feeding (association with Reye's syndrome, see above); haemophilia and other bleeding disorders; not for treatment of gout

HYPERSENSITIVITY. Aspirin and other NSAIDs **contra-indicated** in history of hypersensitivity to aspirin or any other NSAID—which includes those in whom attacks of asthma, angioedema, urticaria or rhinitis have been precipitated by aspirin or any other NSAID

Side-effects: common with anti-inflammatory doses; gastro-intestinal discomfort or nausea, ulceration with occult bleeding (but occasionally major haemorrhage); also other haemorrhage (e.g. subconjunctival); hearing disturbances such as tinnitus (leading rarely to deafness), vertigo, confusion, hypersensitivity reactions (angioedema, bronchospasm and rashes); increased bleeding time; rarely oedema, myocarditis, blood disorders, particularly thrombocytopenia; **overdosage:** see Emergency Treatment of Poisoning, p. 21

Dose: 0.3–1 g every 4 hours after food; max. in acute conditions 8 g daily; CHILD, juvenile arthritis, up to 80 mg/kg daily in 5–6 divided doses after food, increased in acute exacerbations to 130 mg/kg

Note. High doses of aspirin are very rarely required and are now given under specialist supervision only, and with plasma monitoring (especially in children)

Preparations

Section 4.7.1

BENORILATE

(Benorylate)

(Aspirin-paracetamol ester; 2 g benorilate is equivalent to approximately 1.15 g aspirin and 970 mg paracetamol)

Indications: pain and inflammation in rheumatic disease and other musculoskeletal disorders; mild to moderate pain; pyrexia

Cautions: see under Aspirin (above) and Paracetamol (section 4.7.1)

Contra-indications: see under Aspirin (above) and Paracetamol (section 4.7.1)

Side-effects: see under Aspirin (above) and Paracetamol (section 4.7.1)

Dose: rheumatic disease, 4–8 g daily divided into 2–3 doses; max. 6 g daily for elderly; CHILD not recommended

Mild to moderate pain, 2 g twice daily preferably after food; CHILD not recommended

Benoral® (Sanofi-Synthelabo)

Tablets, benorilate 750 mg. Net price 100-tab pack = £8.67. Label: 21, 31

Granules, benorilate 2 g/sachet. Net price 60 sachet-pack = £13.77. Label: 13, 21, 31

Suspension, sugar-free, benorilate 2 g/5 mL. Net price 300 mL = £11.86. Label: 21, 31

10.1.2   Corticosteroids

10.1.2.1   Systemic corticosteroids

The general actions and uses of the corticosteroids are described in section 6.3. Treatment with corticosteroids in rheumatic diseases should be reserved for specific indications, e.g. when other anti-inflammatory drugs are unsuccessful.

In severe, possibly life-threatening, situations a high initial dose of corticosteroid is given to induce remission and the dose then gradually reduced to the lowest maintenance dose that will control the disease or, if possible, discontinued altogether. A major problem is that relapse may occur as dosage reduction is made, particularly if this is carried out too rapidly. The tendency is therefore to increase and maintain dosage and consequently the patient becomes dependent on corticosteroids. For this reason pulse doses of corticosteroids (e.g. methylprednisolone (as sodium succinate) up to 1 g intravenously on three consecutive days) is in current use to suppress highly active inflammatory disease while longer term and slower acting medication is being commenced.

Prednisolone is used for most purposes; it has the advantage over the more potent corticosteroids (see section 6.3.2) of permitting finer dosage adjustments. To minimise side-effects the maintenance dose of prednisolone should be kept as low as possible, usually 7.5 mg daily. Recent evidence has suggested that prednisolone 7.5 mg daily may substantially reduce the rate of joint destruction in moderate to severe *rheumatoid arthritis* of less than 2 years duration. The reduction in joint destruction must be distinguished from mere symptomatic improvement (which lasts only 6 to 12 months at this dose) and care should be taken to avoid increasing the dosage beyond 7.5 mg daily. Current evidence supports maintenance of this anti-erosive dose for 2–4 years only, after which, treatment should be tapered off to avoid possible long-term adverse effects.

Polymyalgia rheumatica and *giant cell (temporal) arteritis* are always treated with corticosteroids. The usual initial dose of prednisolone in polymyalgia rheumatica is 10 to 15 mg daily and in giant cell arteritis 40 to 60 mg daily (the higher dose being used if visual symptoms occur). Treatment should be continued until remission of disease activity and doses then gradually reduced to a maintenance level of about 7.5–10 mg daily. Relapse is common if therapy is stopped within 3 years but most patients can discontinue treatment after approximately 3 to 6 years after which recurrences become rare.

Polyarteritis nodosa and *polymyositis* are usually treated with corticosteroids. An initial dose of 60 mg of prednisolone daily is often used and reduced to a maintenance dose of 10 to 15 mg daily.

Systemic lupus erythematosus is treated with corticosteroids when necessary using a similar dosage regimen to that for polyarteritis nodosa and polymyositis (above). Patients with pleurisy, pericarditis, or other systemic manifestations will respond to corticosteroids. It may then be possible to reduce the dosage; alternate-day treatment is sometimes adequate, and the drug may be gradually withdrawn. In some mild cases corticosteroid treatment may be stopped after a few months. Many mild cases of systemic lupus erythematosus do not require corticosteroid treatment. Alternative treatment with anti-inflammatory analgesics, and possibly chloroquine, should be considered.

Ankylosing spondylitis should not be treated with long-term corticosteroids; rarely, pulse doses may be needed and may be useful in extremely active disease that does not respond to conventional treatment.

10.1.2.2 Local corticosteroid injections

Corticosteroids are injected locally for an anti-inflammatory effect. In inflammatory conditions of the joints, particularly in rheumatoid arthritis, they are given by *intra-articular injection* to relieve pain, increase mobility, and reduce deformity in one or a few joints. Full aseptic precautions are essential; infected areas should be avoided. Occasionally an acute inflammatory reaction develops after an intra-articular or soft-tissue injection of a corticosteroid. This may be a reaction to the microcrystalline suspension of the corticosteroid used, but must be distinguished from sepsis introduced into the injection site. An almost insoluble compound such as triamcinolone hexacetonide has a long-acting (depot) effect and is preferred for intra-articular injection.

Smaller amounts of corticosteroids may also be injected directly into soft tissues for the relief of inflammation in conditions such as *tennis* or *golfer's elbow* or *compression neuropathies*. In *tendinitis*, injections should be made into the tendon sheath and not directly into the tendon (due to the absence of a true tendon sheath, the Achilles tendon should not be injected). A soluble preparation (e.g. containing betamethasone or dexamethasone sodium phosphate) is preferred for injection into the carpal tunnel.

Hydrocortisone acetate or one of the synthetic analogues such as triamcinolone hexacetonide is generally used for local injection. The risk of necrosis and muscle wasting in small areas may be slightly increased with triamcinolone; flushing has been reported with intra-articular corticosteroid injections. Charcot-like arthropathies have also been reported (particularly following repeated intra-articular injections).

Corticosteroid injections are also injected into soft tissues for the treatment of skin lesions (see section 13.4).

LOCAL CORTICOSTEROID INJECTIONS

Indications: local inflammation of joints and soft tissues (for details, consult product literature)

Cautions: see notes above and consult product literature; see also section 6.3.2

Contra-indications: see notes above and consult product literature

Side-effects: see notes above and consult product literature

Dose: see under preparations

■ Dose calculated as dexamethasone sodium phosphate

Dexamethasone (Organon) PoM

Injection, dexamethasone sodium phosphate 5 mg/mL (≡ dexamethasone 4 mg/mL ≡ dexamethasone phosphate 4.8 mg/mL). Net price 1-mL amp = 83p; 2-mL vial = £1.27

Dose: by intra-articular or intrasynovial injection (for details consult product literature), 0.4–4 mg (calculated as dexamethasone sodium phosphate) according to size; where appropriate may be repeated at intervals of 3–21 days according to response

■ Dose calculated as dexamethasone phosphate

Decadron® (MSD) PoM

Injection, dexamethasone phosphate 4 mg /mL (≡ dexamethasone 3.33 mg/mL ≡ dexamethasone sodium phosphate 4.17 mg/mL). Net price 2-mL vial = £1.76

Dose: by intra-articular or intrasynovial injection (for details consult product literature), 0.4–4 mg (calculated as dexamethasone phosphate) according to size (*soft-tissue infiltration* 2–6 mg); where appropriate may be repeated at intervals of 3–21 days; also for *intralesional injection*

Note. Injection containing Dexamethasone phosphate 4 mg/mL (as sodium phosphate) is also available from Faulding DBL

■ Hydrocortisone acetate

Hydrocortistab® (Sovereign) PoM

Injection, (aqueous suspension), hydrocortisone acetate 25 mg/mL. Net price 1-mL amp = £4.77

Dose: by intra-articular or intrasynovial injection (for details consult product literature), 5–50 mg according to size; where appropriate may be repeated at intervals of 21 days; not more than 3 joints should be treated on any one day; CHILD 5–30 mg (divided)

■ Methylprednisolone acetate

Depo-Medrone® (Pharmacia & Upjohn) PoM

Injection (aqueous suspension), methylprednisolone acetate 40 mg/mL. Net price 1-mL vial = £2.70; 2-mL vial = £4.87; 3-mL vial = £7.05

Dose: by intra-articular or intrasynovial injection (for details consult product literature), 4–80 mg, according to size; where appropriate may be repeated at intervals of 7–35 days; also for *intralesional injection*

Depo-Medrone® with Lidocaine (Pharmacia & Upjohn) PoM

Injection (aqueous suspension), methylprednisolone acetate 40 mg, lidocaine hydrochloride 10 mg/mL. Net price 1-mL vial = £2.61; 2-mL vial = £4.68

Dose: by intra-articular or intrasynovial injection (for details consult product literature), 4–80 mg, according to size; where appropriate may be repeated at intervals of 7–35 days

■ Prednisolone acetate

Deltastab® (Sovereign) PoM

Injection (aqueous suspension), prednisolone acetate 25 mg/mL. Net price 1-mL amp = £4.77

Dose: by intra-articular or intrasynovial injection (for details consult product literature), 5–25 mg according to size; not more than 3 joints should be treated on any one day; where appropriate may be repeated when relapse occurs

For *intramuscular injection*, see section 6.3.2

■ Triamcinolone acetonide

Adcortyl® Intra-articular/Intradermal (Squibb) PoM

Injection (aqueous suspension), triamcinolone acetonide 10 mg/mL. Net price 1-mL amp = £1.02; 5-mL vial = £4.14

Dose: by intra-articular injection or intrasynovial injection (for details consult product literature), 2.5–15 mg according to size (for larger doses use *Kenalog®*); where appropriate may be repeated when relapse occurs

By intradermal injection, (for details consult product literature): 2–3 mg; max. 5 mg at any one site (total max. 30 mg); where appropriate may be repeated at intervals of 1–2 weeks

CHILD under 6 years not recommended

Kenalog® Intra-articular/Intramuscular (Squibb) PoM

Injection (aqueous suspension), triamcinolone acetonide 40 mg/mL. Net price 1-mL vial = £1.70

Dose: by intra-articular or intrasynovial injection (for details consult product literature), 5–40 mg according to size; total max. 80 mg (for doses below 5 mg use *Adcortyl® Intra-articular/Intradermal*); where appropriate may be repeated when relapse occurs; CHILD under 6 years not recommended

For *intramuscular injection,* see section 6.3.2

■ Triamcinolone hexacetonide

Lederspan® (Lederle) PoM

Injection (aqueous suspension), triamcinolone hexacetonide 5 mg/mL. Net price 5-mL vial = £3.14

Dose: by intralesional injection (for details consult product literature), up to 500 micrograms/square inch of affected skin

Injection (aqueous suspension), triamcinolone hexacetonide 20 mg/mL. Net price 1-mL vial = £2.73; 5 mL vial = £10.62

Dose: by intra-articular or intrasynovial injection (for details consult product literature), 2–30 mg according to size; where appropriate may be repeated at intervals of 21–28 days; for *intralesional injection,* see above

10.1.3   Drugs which suppress the rheumatic disease process

Certain drugs such as gold, penicillamine, hydroxychloroquine, chloroquine, immunosuppressants, and sulfasalazine may suppress the disease process in *rheumatoid arthritis,* as may gold and immunosuppressants in *psoriatic arthritis.* They are sometimes known as second-line or disease-modifying antirheumatic drugs (DMARDs). Unlike NSAIDs they do not produce an immediate therapeutic effect but require 4 to 6 months of treatment for a full response. If one of these drugs does not lead to objective benefit within 6 months, it should be discontinued.

These drugs may improve not only the symptoms and signs of inflammatory joint disease but also extra-articular manifestations such as vasculitis. They reduce the erythrocyte sedimentation rate and sometimes the titre of rheumatoid factor. Some (e.g. ciclosporin) may retard erosive damage as judged radiologically.

These drugs are used in rheumatoid arthritis where treatment with NSAIDs alone provides inad-

equate control. Since, in the first few months, the course of rheumatoid arthritis is unpredictable, it is usual to delay treatment for about 6 months depending on the progress of the disease, but treatment should be initiated if severe symptoms persist.

Penicillamine and immunosuppressants are also sometimes used in rheumatoid arthritis where there are troublesome extra-articular features such as vasculitis, and in patients who are taking excessive doses of corticosteroids. Where the response is satisfactory there is often a striking reduction in requirements of both corticosteroids and other drugs. Gold and penicillamine are effective in *palindromic rheumatism* and chloroquine is sometimes used to treat *systemic* and *discoid lupus erythematosus.*

JUVENILE IDIOPATHIC ARTHRITIS. Gold, penicillamine, and related drugs may also be used to treat *juvenile idiopathic arthritis* (juvenile chronic arthritis) when indications are similar.

Gold

Gold may be given by intramuscular injection as sodium aurothiomalate or by mouth as auranofin.

Sodium aurothiomalate must be given by deep intramuscular injection and the area gently massaged. A test dose of 10 mg must be given followed by doses of 50 mg at weekly intervals until there is definite evidence of remission. Benefit is not to be expected until about 300 to 500 mg has been given; if there is no remission after 1 g has been given it should be discontinued. In patients who do respond, the interval between injections is then gradually increased to 4 weeks and treatment is continued for up to 5 years after complete remission. If relapse occurs the dosage frequency may be immediately increased to 50 mg weekly and only once control has been obtained again should the dosage frequency be decreased; if no response is seen within 2 months, alternative treatment should be sought. It is important to avoid complete relapse since second courses of gold are not usually effective. Children may be given 1 mg/kg weekly to a maximum of 50 mg weekly, the intervals being gradually increased to 4 weeks according to response; an initial test dose is given corresponding to one-tenth to one-fifth of the calculated dose.

Auranofin is given by mouth. If there is no response after 9 months treatment should be discontinued.

Gold therapy should be discontinued in the presence of blood disorders or proteinuria (associated with immune complex nephritis) which is repeatedly above 300 mg/litre without other cause (such as urinary-tract infection). Urine tests and full blood counts (including total and differential white cell and platelet counts) must therefore be performed before starting treatment with gold and before each intramuscular injection; in the case of oral treatment the urine and blood tests should be carried out monthly. Rashes with pruritus often occur after 2 to 6 months of intramuscular treatment and may necessitate discontinuation of treatment; the most common side-effect of oral therapy, diarrhoea with or without nausea or abdominal pain, may respond to bulking agents (such as bran) or temporary reduction in dosage.

SODIUM AUROTHIOMALATE

Indications: active progressive rheumatoid arthritis, juvenile arthritis

Cautions: see notes above; renal and hepatic impairment, elderly, history of urticaria, eczema, colitis, drugs which cause blood disorders; annual chest X-ray; **interactions:** Appendix 1 (gold)

Contra-indications: severe renal and hepatic disease (see notes above); history of blood disorders or bone marrow aplasia, exfoliative dermatitis, systemic lupus erythematosus, necrotising enterocolitis, pulmonary fibrosis; pregnancy and breast-feeding (Appendixes 4 and 5); porphyria (section 9.8.2)

Side-effects: severe reactions (occasionally fatal) in up to 5% of patients; mouth ulcers, skin reactions (including, on prolonged parenteral treatment, irreversible pigmentation in sun-exposed areas), proteinuria, blood disorders (sometimes sudden and fatal); rarely colitis, peripheral neuritis, pulmonary fibrosis, hepatotoxicity with cholestatic jaundice, nephrotic syndrome, alopecia

Dose: *by deep intramuscular injection,* administered on expert advice, see notes above

COUNSELLING. Warn patient to tell doctor immediately if sore throat, fever, infection, non-specific illness, unexplained bleeding and bruising, purpura, mouth ulcers, metallic taste, or rashes develop; also ask patients to report immediately any breathlessness or cough

Myocrisin® (JHC) [PoM]

Injection, sodium aurothiomalate 20 mg/mL, net price 0.5-mL (10-mg) amp = £3.16; 40 mg/mL, 0.5-mL (20-mg) amp = £4.60; 100 mg/mL, 0.5-mL (50-mg) amp = £9.36. Counselling, blood disorder symptoms

AURANOFIN

Indications: active progressive rheumatoid arthritis

Cautions: see under Sodium Aurothiomalate; also caution in inflammatory bowel disease

BLOOD COUNTS. Withdraw if platelet count falls below 100 000/mm³ or if signs and symptoms suggestive of thrombocytopenia occur, see also notes above

Contra-indications: see under Sodium Aurothiomalate

Side-effects: diarrhoea most common (reduced by bulking agents such as bran); see also under Sodium Aurothiomalate

Dose: administered on expert advice, 6 mg daily (initially in 2 divided doses then if tolerated as single dose), if response inadequate after 6 months, increase to 9 mg daily (in 3 divided doses), discontinue if no response after a further 3 months; CHILD not recommended

COUNSELLING. Warn patient to tell doctor immediately if sore throat, fever, infection, non-specific illness, unexplained bleeding and bruising, purpura, mouth ulcers, metallic taste, or rashes develop; also ask patients to report immediately any breathlessness or cough

Note. The package insert for *Ridaura®* also advises that patients must also report immediately if conjunctivitis or hair loss develops

Ridaura® (Yamanouchi) [PoM]

Tablets, pale yellow, f/c, auranofin 3 mg. Net price 60-tab pack = £22.40. Label: 21, counselling, blood disorder symptoms (see above)

Penicillamine

Penicillamine has a similar action to gold, and more patients are able to continue treatment than with gold but side-effects occur frequently. Penicillamine should be discontinued if there is no improvement within 1 year.

Patients should be warned not to expect improvement for at least 6 to 12 weeks after treatment is initiated. If remission has been sustained for 6 months, reduction of dosage by 125 to 250 mg every 12 weeks may be attempted.

Blood counts, including platelets, and urine examinations should be carried out before starting treatment and then every 1 or 2 weeks for the first 2 months then every 4 weeks to detect blood disorders and proteinuria (they should also be carried out in the week after any dose increase). A reduction in platelet count calls for discontinuation with subsequent re-introduction at a lower dosage and then, if possible, gradual increase. Proteinuria, associated with immune complex nephritis, occurs in up to 30% of patients, but may resolve despite continuation of treatment; treatment may be continued provided that renal function tests remain normal, oedema is absent, and the 24-hour urinary excretion of protein does not exceed 2 g.

Nausea may occur but is not usually a problem provided that penicillamine is taken before food or on retiring and that low initial doses are used and only gradually increased. Loss of taste may occur about 6 weeks after treatment is started but usually returns 6 weeks later irrespective of whether or not treatment is discontinued; mineral supplements are not recommended. Rashes are a common side-effect. Those which occur in the first few months of treatment disappear when the drug is stopped and treatment may then be re-introduced at a lower dose level and gradually increased. Late rashes are more resistant and often necessitate discontinuation of treatment.

Patients who are hypersensitive to penicillin may react rarely to penicillamine.

PENICILLAMINE

Indications: see notes above and under Dose

Cautions: see notes above; renal impairment (Appendix 3), pregnancy (Appendix 4); avoid concurrent gold, chloroquine, hydroxychloroquine, or immunosuppressive treatment; avoid oral iron within 2 hours of a dose; **interactions:** Appendix 1 (penicillamine)

BLOOD COUNTS and URINE TESTS. See notes above. Longer intervals may be adequate in cystinuria and Wilson's disease. Consider withdrawal if platelet count falls below 120 000/mm³ or white blood cells below 2500/mm³ or if 3 successive falls within reference range (can restart at reduced dose when counts return to within reference range but permanent withdrawal necessary if recurrence of neutropenia or thrombocytopenia)

COUNSELLING. Warn patient to tell doctor immediately if sore throat, fever, infection, non-specific illness, unexplained bleeding and bruising, purpura, mouth ulcers, or rashes develop

Contra-indications: hypersensitivity (except in life-threatening situation when desensitisation may be attempted—consult product literature); lupus erythematosus

Side-effects: (see also notes above) initially nausea, anorexia, fever, and skin reactions; taste loss (mineral supplements not recommended); blood disorders including thrombocytopenia, neutropenia, agranulocytosis and aplastic anaemia; proteinuria, rarely haematuria (withdraw immediately); haemolytic anaemia, nephrotic syndrome, lupus erythematosus-like syndrome, myasthenia gravis-like syndrome, polymyositis (rarely with cardiac involvement), dermatomyositis, mouth ulcers, stomatitis, alopecia, bronchiolitis and pneumonitis, pemphigus, Goodpasture's syndrome, and Stevens-Johnson syndrome also reported; male and female breast enlargement reported; in non-rheumatoid conditions rheumatoid arthritis-like syndrome also reported; late rashes (reduce dose or withdraw treatment)

Dose: severe active rheumatoid arthritis, administered on expert advice, ADULT initially 125–250 mg daily before food for 1 month increased by similar amounts at intervals of not less than 4 weeks to usual maintenance of 500–750 mg daily in divided doses; max. 1.5 g daily; ELDERLY initially up to 125 mg daily before food for 1 month increased by similar amounts at intervals of not less than 4 weeks; max. 1 g daily; CHILD maintenance of 15–20 mg/kg daily (initial dose lower and increased at intervals of 4 weeks over a period of 3-6 months)

Wilson's disease, chronic active hepatitis, and cystinuria, section 9.8.1

Copper and lead poisoning, see Emergency Treatment of Poisoning, p. 26

Penicillamine (Non-proprietary) [PoM]
Tablets, penicillamine 125 mg, net price 20 = £1.85; 250 mg, 20 = £3.32. Label: 6, 22, counselling, blood disorder symptoms (see above)
Available from APS, Cox, Hillcross, Norton

Distamine® (Dista) [PoM]
Tablets, all f/c, penicillamine 125 mg, net price 20 = £2.17; 250 mg, 20 = £3.74. Label: 6, 22, counselling, blood disorder symptoms (see above)

Antimalarials

The antimalarials **chloroquine** and **hydroxychloroquine** have a similar action to gold or penicillamine. The antimalarials should not be used for psoriatic arthritis.

Chloroquine and hydroxychloroquine are better tolerated than gold or penicillamine. Retinopathy (see below) occurs rarely provided that the recommended doses are not exceeded; in the elderly it is difficult to distinguish drug-induced retinopathy from ageing changes.

Mepacrine (section 5.4.4) is sometimes used in discoid lupus erythematosus [unlicensed].

CAUTIONS. Chloroquine and hydroxychloroquine should be used with caution in hepatic impairment and in renal impairment (Appendix 3). Manufacturers recommend regular ophthalmological examination but the evidence of practical value is unsatisfactory (see advice of Royal College of Ophthalmologists, below). Hydroxychloroquine should be avoided in pregnancy and breast-feeding; chloroquine can, however, be used for malaria during pregnancy and breast-feeding. Both should be used with caution in neurological disorders (especially in those with a history of epilepsy), in severe gastro-intestinal disorders, in G6PD deficiency (section 9.1.5), in porphyria, and in the elderly (see also above). Chloroquine and hydroxychloroquine may exacerbate psoriasis and aggravate myasthenia gravis. Concurrent use of hepatotoxic drugs should be avoided; other **interactions**: Appendix 1 (chloroquine and hydroxychloroquine).

Advice of Royal College of Ophthalmologists
The Royal College of Ophthalmologists has advised that a screening protocol for chloroquine should be negotiated with local ophthalmologists; no screening is recommended for mepacrine because it is not thought to be associated with ophthalmological effects. The following recommendations relate to hydroxychloroquine.
Before treatment:
• Assess renal and liver function (adjust dose if impaired)
• Ask patient about visual impairment (not corrected by glasses). If impairment or eye disease present, assessment by an optometrist is advised and any abnormality should be referred to an ophthalmologist
• Record near visual acuity of each eye (with glasses where appropriate) using a standard reading chart
• Initiate hydroxychloroquine treatment if no abnormality detected (at a dose not exceeding hydroxychloroquine sulphate 6.5 mg/kg daily)
During treatment:
• Ask patient about visual symptoms and monitor visual acuity annually using the standard reading chart
• Refer to ophthalmologist if visual acuity changes or if vision blurred and warn patient to stop treatment and seek prescribing doctor's advice
• A child treated for juvenile arthritis should receive slit-lamp examination routinely to check for uveitis
• If long-term treatment is required (more than 5 years), individual arrangement should be agreed with the local ophthalmologist
Note. To avoid excessive dosage in obese patients, the dose of hydroxychloroquine and chloroquine should be calculated on the basis of lean body weight. Ocular toxicity is unlikely with chloroquine phosphate not exceeding 4 mg/kg daily (equivalent to chloroquine base approx. 2.5 mg/kg daily)

SIDE-EFFECTS. The side-effects of chloroquine and hydroxychloroquine include gastro-intestinal disturbances, headache and skin reactions (rashes, pruritus); those occurring less frequently include ECG changes, convulsions, visual changes, retinal damage (see above), keratopathy, ototoxicity, hair depigmentation, hair loss, and discoloration of skin and mucous membranes. Side-effects that occur rarely include blood disorders (including thrombocytopenia, agranulocytosis, and aplastic anaemia), mental changes (including emotional disturbances and psychosis), myopathy (including cardiomyopathy), acute generalised exanthematous pustulosis, exfoliative dermatitis, Stevens-Johnson syndrome, and hepatic damage. **Important**: very toxic in overdosage—immediate advice from poisons centres essential (see also p. 23).

CHLOROQUINE

Indications: active rheumatoid arthritis (including juvenile arthritis), systemic and discoid lupus erythematosus; malaria (section 5.4.1)
Cautions: see notes above
Side-effects: see notes above

Dose: administered on expert advice, chloroquine (base) 150 mg daily; max. 2.5 mg/kg daily, see recommendations above; CHILD, up to 3 mg/kg daily

Note. Chloroquine base 150 mg ≡ chloroquine sulphate 200 mg ≡ chloroquine phosphate 250 mg (approx.).

Preparations
See section 5.4.1

HYDROXYCHLOROQUINE SULPHATE

Indications: active rheumatoid arthritis (including juvenile arthritis), systemic and discoid lupus erythematosus

Cautions: see notes above

Side-effects: see notes above

Dose: administered on expert advice, initially 400 mg daily in divided doses; maintenance 200–400 mg daily; max. 6.5 mg/kg daily (but not exceeding 400 mg daily), see recommendations above; CHILD, up to 6.5 mg/kg daily (max. 400 mg daily)

Plaquenil® (Sanofi-Synthelabo) [PoM]
Tablets, orange, f/c, hydroxychloroquine sulphate 200 mg. Net price 60-tab pack = £20.23. Label: 5, 21

Immunosuppressants

When used in *rheumatoid arthritis* **immunosuppressants** have a similar action to gold and are useful alternatives in cases that have failed to respond to gold, penicillamine, chloroquine, or hydroxychloroquine.

Azathioprine is usually given in a dose of 1.5 to 2.5 mg/kg daily in divided doses. Blood counts are needed to detect possible neutropenia or thrombocytopenia (usually resolved by reducing the dose). Nausea, vomiting, and diarrhoea may occur, usually starting early during the course of treatment, and may necessitate withdrawal of the drug; herpes zoster infection may also occur.

Methotrexate is usually given in an initial dose of 2.5 mg by mouth once a week, increased slowly to a maximum of 15 mg once a week (occasionally 20 mg), subject to regular full blood counts (including differential white cell count and platelet count), renal and liver-function tests. In patients who experience gastro-intestinal side-effects with methotrexate, folic acid 5 mg every week may help to reduce the frequency of such side-effects.

Leflunomide, which acts on the immune system, has been introduced recently as a disease-modifying antirheumatic drug; it should be prescribed by specialists. Its therapeutic effect starts after 4–6 weeks and improvement may continue for a further 4–6 months. The active metabolite of leflunomide persists for a long period; active procedures to wash the drug out are required in case of serious adverse effects, before starting treatment with another disease-modifying antirheumatic drug, or, in men or women, before conception. Side-effects of leflunomide include bone marrow toxicity; its immunosuppressive effects increase the risk of infection and malignancy.

Ciclosporin (cyclosporin) is licensed for severe active rheumatoid arthritis when conventional second-line therapy is inappropriate or ineffective. There is some evidence that ciclosporin may retard the rate of erosive progression and improve symptom control in patients only partially responsive to methotrexate.

Cyclophosphamide (section 8.1.1) may be used at a dose of 1 to 1.5 mg/kg daily by mouth for rheumatoid arthritis with severe systemic manifestations [unlicensed indication]; it is toxic and regular blood counts (including platelet count) should be carried out. Cyclophosphamide may also be given intravenously in a dose of 0.5 to 1 g (with prophylactic mesna) for *severe systemic rheumatoid arthritis* and for other connective tissue diseases (especially with active vasculitis), repeated initially at fortnightly then at monthly intervals (according to clinical response and haematological monitoring).

Immunosuppressants are also used in the management of severe cases of *systemic lupus erythematosus* and other connective tissue disorders. They are often given in conjunction with corticosteroids for patients with severe or progressive renal disease though the evidence for their benefit is doubtful. They may be used in cases of *polymyositis* which are resistant to corticosteroids. They are used for their corticosteroid-sparing effect in patients whose corticosteroid requirements are excessive. **Azathioprine** is usually used.

Azathioprine and methotrexate are used in the treatment of *psoriatic arthropathy* [unlicensed indication] for severe or progressive cases which are not controlled with anti-inflammatory drugs.

AZATHIOPRINE

Indications: see notes above; transplantation rejection, see section 8.2.1

Cautions: see section 8.2.1

Contra-indications: see section 8.2.1

Side-effects: see section 8.2.1

Dose: *by mouth,* initially, rarely more than 3 mg/kg daily, reduced according to response; maintenance 1–3 mg/kg daily; consider withdrawal if no improvement within 3 months

Preparations
Section 8.2.1

CICLOSPORIN
(Cyclosporin)

Indications: severe active rheumatoid arthritis when conventional second-line therapy inappropriate or ineffective; graft-versus-host disease (section 8.2.2); atopic dermatitis and psoriasis (section 13.5.2).

Cautions: see section 8.2.2

ADDITIONAL CAUTIONS IN RHEUMATOID ARTHRITIS. *Contra-indicated* in abnormal renal function, uncontrolled hypertension (see also below), uncontrolled infections, and malignancy. Measure serum creatinine at least twice before treatment and monitor every 2 weeks for first 3 months, then every 4 weeks (or more frequently if dose increased or concomitant NSAIDs introduced or increased (see also *interactions:* Appendix 1 (ciclosporin)), reduce dose if serum creatinine increases more than 30% above baseline in more than 1 measurement; if above 50%, reduce dose by 50% (even if within normal range) and discontinue if reduction not successful within 1 month; monitor blood pressure (discontinue if hypertension develops that cannot be controlled by antihypertensive therapy); monitor hepatic function if concomitant NSAIDs given.

Side-effects: see section 8.2.2

Dose: *by mouth*, administered in accordance with expert advice, initially 2.5 mg/kg daily in 2 divided doses, if necessary increased gradually after 6 weeks; max. 4 mg/kg daily (discontinue if response insufficient after 3 months); dose adjusted according to response for maintenance and treatment reviewed after 6 months (continue only if benefits outweigh risks); CHILD and under 18 years, not recommended

IMPORTANT. For preparations and counselling and for advice on conversion between the preparations, see section 8.2.2

Preparations
Section 8.2.2

LEFLUNOMIDE

Indications: active rheumatoid arthritis

Cautions: renal impairment (Appendix 3); impaired bone-marrow function including anaemia, leucopenia or thrombocytopenia (avoid if significant and due to causes other than rheumatoid arthritis); history of tuberculosis; exclude pregnancy before treatment; effective contraception essential during treatment and for at least 2 years after treatment in women and at least 3 months after treatment in men (plasma concentration monitoring required; waiting time before conception may be reduced with washout procedures—consult product literature and see below); monitor full blood count (including differential white cell count and platelet count) before treatment and every 2 weeks for 6 months then every 8 weeks; monitor liver function—discontinue if significantly raised liver enzymes; monitor blood pressure; washout procedures recommended for serious adverse effects and before transferring to other disease modifying antirheumatic drugs (consult product literature and see below); **interactions:** Appendix 1 (leflunomide)

WASHOUT PROCEDURE. To aid drug elimination in case of serious adverse-effect, before starting another disease-modifying antirheumatic drug, or before conception (see also Appendix 4), stop treatment and give *either* colestyramine 8 g 3 times daily for 11 days *or* activated charcoal 50 g 4 times daily for 11 days; the concentration of the active metabolite after washout should be less than 20 micrograms/litre (measured on 2 occasions 14 days apart) in men or women before conception—consult product literature

Contra-indications: severe immunodeficiency; serious infection; hepatic impairment; severe hypoproteinaemia; pregnancy (**important teratogenic risk:** see Cautions and Appendix 4); breast-feeding (Appendix 5)

Side-effects: diarrhoea, nausea, vomiting, anorexia, oral mucosal disorders, abdominal pain, weight loss; increase in blood pressure; headache, dizziness, asthenia, paraesthesia; tenosynovitis; alopecia, eczema, dry skin, rash, pruritus; leucopenia; rarely taste disturbances, anxiety, tendon rupture, urticaria, anaemia, thrombocytopenia, eosinophilia, hyperlipidaemia, hypokalaemia, hypophosphataemia, hepatic dysfunction; also reported, anaphylaxis, pancytopenia, Stevens-Johnson syndrome, toxic epidermal necrolysis (discontinue and initiate washout procedure—consult product literature)

Dose: initially 100 mg once daily for 3 days then maintenance, 10–20 mg once daily

Arava® (Hoechst Marion Roussel) ▼ PoM
Tablets, f/c, leflunomide 10 mg, net price 30-tab pack = £46.50; 20 mg (ochre), 30-tab pack = £46.50; 100 mg, 3-tab pack = £23.25. Label: 4

METHOTREXATE

Indications: severe active rheumatoid arthritis unresponsive to conventional therapy; malignant disease (section 8.1.3); psoriasis (section 13.5.2)

Cautions: see section 13.5.2

PULMONARY TOXICITY. Pulmonary toxicity may be a special problem in rheumatoid arthritis (patient to contact doctor immediately if dyspnoea or cough). For other special warnings, including CSM advice and counselling advice relating to interaction with aspirin and NSAIDs, see Methotrexate, section 13.5.2.

Contra-indications: see section 13.5.2

Side-effects: see section 13.5.2

Dose: *by mouth*, 7.5 mg once weekly (as a single dose *or* divided into 3 doses of 2.5 mg given at intervals of 12 hours), adjusted according to response; max. total weekly dose 20 mg

IMPORTANT. Note that the above dose is a **weekly** dose

Preparations
Section 8.1.3

Sulfasalazine

Sulfasalazine (sulphasalazine) has a beneficial effect in suppressing the inflammatory activity of rheumatoid arthritis. Side-effects include rashes, gastro-intestinal intolerance and, especially in patients with rheumatoid arthritis, occasional leucopenia, neutropenia, and thrombocytopenia. These haematological abnormalities occur usually in the first 3 to 6 months of treatment and are reversible on cessation of treatment. Close monitoring of full blood counts (including differential white cell count and platelet count) is necessary initially, and at monthly intervals during the first 3 months (liver function tests also being performed at monthly intervals for the first 3 months). Although the manufacturer recommends renal function tests, evidence of practical value is unsatisfactory.

SULFASALAZINE
(Sulphasalazine)

Indications: active rheumatoid arthritis; ulcerative colitis, see section 1.5 and notes above

Cautions: see section 1.5 and notes above

The CSM has recommended that patients should be advised to report any unexplained bleeding, bruising, purpura, sore throat, fever or malaise. A blood count should be performed and the drug stopped immediately if there is suspicion of a blood dyscrasia.

Contra-indications: see section 1.5 and notes above

Side-effects: see section 1.5 and notes above

Dose: *by mouth*, administered on expert advice, as enteric-coated tablets, initially 500 mg daily, increased by 500 mg at intervals of 1 week to a max. of 2–3 g daily in divided doses

Sulfasalazine (Non-proprietary) PoM
Tablets, e/c, sulfasalazine 500 mg. Net price 112-tab pack = £12.11. Label: 5, 14, 25, counselling, blood disorder symptoms (see CSM recommendation above), contact lenses may be stained
Available from Cox (*Sulazine EC®*)

Salazopyrin EN-Tabs® (Pharmacia & Upjohn) PoM
Tablets, e/c, yellow, f/c, sulfasalazine 500 mg. Net price 112-tab pack = £12.11. Label: 5, 14, 21, 25, counselling, blood disorder symptoms (see CSM recommendation above), contact lenses may be stained

10.1.4 Drugs for treatment of gout

It is important to distinguish drugs used for the treatment of acute attacks of gout from those used in the long-term control of the disease. The latter exacerbate and prolong the acute manifestations if started during an attack.

Acute attacks of gout

Acute attacks of gout are usually treated with high doses of **NSAIDs** such as diclofenac, indometacin, ketoprofen, naproxen, piroxicam, or sulindac (section 10.1.1). The use of azapropazone should be restricted to patients in whom less toxic drugs have been ineffective (**important**: see CSM restrictions on p. 449). Colchicine is an alternative. Aspirin is *not* indicated in gout. Allopurinol and uricosurics are not effective in treating an acute attack and may prolong it indefinitely if started during the acute episode.

Colchicine is probably as effective as NSAIDs. Its use is limited by the development of toxicity at higher doses, but it is of value in patients with heart failure since, unlike NSAIDs, it does not induce fluid retention; moreover it can be given to patients receiving anticoagulants.

COLCHICINE

Indications: acute gout, short-term prophylaxis during initial therapy with allopurinol and uricosuric drugs; prophylaxis of familial Mediterranean fever (recurrent polyserositis) [unlicensed]

Cautions: elderly, gastro-intestinal disease, cardiac, hepatic and renal impairment; **interactions:** Appendix 1 (colchicine)

Contra-indications: pregnancy and breast-feeding

Side-effects: most common are nausea, vomiting, and abdominal pain; excessive doses may also cause profuse diarrhoea, gastro-intestinal haemorrhage, rashes, renal and hepatic damage. Rarely peripheral neuritis, myopathy, alopecia, and with prolonged treatment blood disorders

Dose: treatment of gout, 1 mg initially, followed by 500 micrograms every 2–3 hours until relief of pain is obtained or vomiting or diarrhoea occurs, or until a total dose of 6 mg has been reached; the course should not be repeated within 3 days
Prevention of gout attacks during initial treatment with allopurinol or uricosuric drugs, 500 micrograms 2–3 times daily

Prophylaxis of familial Mediterranean fever [unlicensed], 0.5–2 mg daily

Colchicine (Non-proprietary) PoM
Tablets, colchicine 500 micrograms, net price 20 = £4.04
Available from CP

Long-term control of gout

Frequent recurrence of acute attacks of gout may call for the initiation of long-term ('interval') treatment. For long-term control of gout the formation of uric acid from purines may be reduced with the **xanthine-oxidase inhibitor** allopurinol, or the **uricosuric drugs** probenecid or sulfinpyrazone may be used to increase the excretion of uric acid in the urine. Treatment should be continued indefinitely to prevent further attacks of gout by correcting the hyperuricaemia. These drugs should never be started during an acute attack. The initiation of treatment may precipitate an acute attack therefore colchicine or an anti-inflammatory analgesic should be used as a prophylactic and continued for at least one month after the hyperuricaemia has been corrected (usually about 3 months of prophylaxis). However, if an acute attack develops during treatment, then the treatment should continue at the same dosage and the acute attack treated in its own right.

Allopurinol is a well tolerated drug which is widely used. It is especially useful in patients with renal impairment or urate stones where uricosuric drugs cannot be used; it is *not* indicated for the treatment of asymptomatic hyperuricaemia. It is usually given once daily, since the active metabolite of allopurinol has a long half-life, but doses over 300 mg daily should be divided. It may occasionally cause rashes.

Probenecid and **sulfinpyrazone** (sulphinpyrazone) can be used instead of allopurinol, or in conjunction with it in cases that are resistant to treatment.

Aspirin and salicylates antagonise the uricosuric drugs; they do not antagonise allopurinol but are nevertheless *not* indicated in gout.

Crystallisation of urate in the urine may occur with the uricosuric drugs and it is important to ensure an adequate urine output especially in the first few weeks of treatment. As an additional precaution the urine may be rendered alkaline.

ALLOPURINOL

Indications: prophylaxis of gout and of uric acid and calcium oxalate renal stones

Cautions: administer prophylactic colchicine or NSAID (*not* aspirin or salicylates) until at least 1 month after hyperuricaemia corrected; ensure adequate fluid intake (2 litres/day); hepatic and renal impairment (see Appendix 3); in neoplastic conditions treatment with allopurinol (if required) should be commenced before cytotoxic drugs are given; pregnancy and breast-feeding; **interactions:** Appendix 1 (allopurinol)

Contra-indications: not a treatment for acute gout but continue if attack develops when already receiving allopurinol, and treat attack separately (see notes above)

Side-effects: rashes (**withdraw** therapy; if rash mild re-introduce cautiously but **discontinue** immediately if recurrence—hypersensitivity reactions occur rarely and include exfoliation, fever, lymphadenopathy, arthralgia, and eosinophilia resembling Stevens-Johnson or Lyell's syndrome, vasculitis, hepatitis, interstitial nephritis and very rarely epilepsy); gastro-intestinal disorders; rarely malaise, headache, vertigo, drowsiness, visual and taste disturbances, hypertension, symptomless xanthine deposits in muscle, alopecia, hepatotoxicity, paraesthesia and neuropathy, blood disorders (including leucopenia, thrombocytopenia, haemoytic anaemia and aplastic anaemia)

Dose: initially 100–300 mg daily as a single dose, preferably after food, then adjusted according to plasma or urinary uric acid concentration; usual maintenance dose in mild conditions 100–200 mg daily, in moderately severe conditions 300–600 mg daily, in severe conditions 700–900 mg daily; doses over 300 mg daily given in divided doses; CHILD (in neoplastic conditions, enzyme disorders) 10–20 mg/kg daily *or* 100–400 mg daily

Allopurinol (Non-proprietary) PoM

Tablets, allopurinol 100 mg, net price 28-tab pack = £2.06; 300 mg, 28-tab pack = £6.40. Label: 8, 21, 27

Available from APS, Ashbourne (*Xanthomax®*), Berk (*Caplenal®*), Cox, CP, DDSA (*Cosuric®*), Hillcross, Kent, Norton, Ranbaxy (*Rimapurinol®*)

Zyloric® (GlaxoWellcome) PoM

Tablets, allopurinol 100 mg, net price 100-tab pack = £10.96; 300 mg, 28-tab pack = £7.86. Label: 8, 21, 27

PROBENECID

Indications: gout prophylaxis (to correct hyperuricaemia); reduction of tubular excretion of penicillins and certain cephalosporins (section 5.1)

Cautions: see notes above; during initial therapy give prophylactic colchicine or NSAID (*not* aspirin or salicylates), ensure adequate fluid intake (about 2 litres daily) and render urine alkaline if uric acid overload is high; peptic ulceration, renal impairment (avoid if severe); transient false-positive Benedict's test; G6PD-deficiency (section 9.1.5); **interactions:** Appendix 1 (probenecid)

Contra-indications: history of blood disorders, nephrolithiasis, porphyria (section 9.8.2), acute gout attack; avoid aspirin and salicylates

Side-effects: gastro-intestinal disturbances, urinary frequency, headache, flushing, dizziness, alopecia, anaemia, haemolytic anaemia, sore gums; hypersensitivity reactions including anaphylaxis, dermatitis, pruritus, urticaria, fever and Stevens-Johnson syndrome; rarely nephrotic syndrome, hepatic necrosis, leucopenia, aplastic anaemia; toxic epidermal necrolysis reported with concurrent colchicine

Dose: uricosuric therapy, initially 250 mg twice daily after food, increased after a week to 500 mg twice daily then up to 2 g daily in 2–4 divided doses according to plasma-uric acid concentration and reduced for maintenance

Benemid® (MSD) PoM

Tablets, scored, probenecid 500 mg. Net price 20 = 66p. Label: 12, 21, 27

SULFINPYRAZONE

(Sulphinpyrazone)

Indications: gout prophylaxis, hyperuricaemia

Cautions: see under Probenecid; regular blood counts advisable; cardiac disease (may cause salt and water retention); **interactions:** Appendix 1 (sulfinpyrazone)

Contra-indications: see under Probenecid; avoid in hypersensitivity to NSAIDs

Side-effects: gastro-intestinal disturbances, occasionally allergic skin reactions, salt and water retention; rarely blood disorders, gastro-intestinal ulceration and bleeding, acute renal failure, raised liver enzymes, jaundice and hepatitis

Dose: initially 100–200 mg daily with food (or milk) increasing over 2–3 weeks to 600 mg daily (rarely 800 mg daily), continued until serum uric acid concentration normal then reduced for maintenance (maintenance dose may be as low as 200 mg daily)

Anturan® (Novartis) PoM

Tablets, both yellow, s/c, sulfinpyrazone 100 mg, net price 84-tab pack = £3.93; 200 mg, 84-tab pack = £7.82. Label: 12, 21

10.2 Drugs used in neuromuscular disorders

10.2.1 Drugs which enhance neuromuscular transmission

Anticholinesterases are used as first-line treatment in *myasthenia gravis*.

Corticosteroids are only given concomitantly if anticholinesterase treatment is failing.

Plasmapheresis may produce temporary remission in otherwise unresponsive patients.

Anticholinesterases

Anticholinesterase drugs enhance neuromuscular transmission in voluntary and involuntary muscle in myasthenia gravis. They prolong the action of acetylcholine by inhibiting the action of the enzyme acetylcholinesterase. Excessive dosage of these drugs may impair neuromuscular transmission and precipitate 'cholinergic crises' by causing a depolarising block. This may be difficult to distinguish from a worsening myasthenic state.

Muscarinic side-effects of anticholinesterases include increased sweating, salivary, and gastric secretion, also increased gastro-intestinal and uterine motility, and bradycardia. These parasympathomimetic effects are antagonised by atropine.

Edrophonium has a very brief action and is therefore used mainly for the diagnosis of myasthenia gravis. A single test-dose usually causes substantial improvement in muscle power (lasting about 5 minutes) in patients with the disease (if respiration already impaired, *only* in conjunction with someone skilled at intubation).

Edrophonium can also be used to determine whether a patient with myasthenia is receiving inadequate or excessive treatment with cholinergic drugs. If treatment is excessive an injection of edrophonium will either have no effect or will intensify symptoms (if respiration already impaired, *only* in conjunction with someone skilled at intubation). Conversely, transient improvement may be seen if the patient is being inadequately treated. The test is best performed just before the next dose of anticholinesterase.

Neostigmine produces a therapeutic effect for up to 4 hours. Its pronounced muscarinic action is a disadvantage, and simultaneous administration of an antimuscarinic drug such as atropine or propantheline may be required to prevent colic, excessive salivation, or diarrhoea. In severe disease neostigmine may be given every 2 hours. The maximum that most patients can tolerate is 180 mg daily.

Pyridostigmine is less powerful and slower in action than neostigmine but it has a longer duration of action. It is preferable to neostigmine because of its smoother action and the need for less frequent dosage. It is particularly preferred in patients whose muscles are weak on wakening. It has a comparatively mild gastro-intestinal effect but an antimuscarinic drug may still be required. It is inadvisable to exceed a daily dose of 720 mg.

Distigmine has the longest action but the danger of a 'cholinergic crisis' caused by accumulation of the drug is greater than with shorter-acting drugs.

Neostigmine and edrophonium are also used to reverse the actions of the non-depolarising muscle relaxants (see section 15.1.6).

NEOSTIGMINE

Indications: myasthenia gravis; other indications (section 15.1.6)

Cautions: asthma (*extreme* caution), bradycardia, recent myocardial infarction, epilepsy, hypotension, parkinsonism, vagotonia, peptic ulceration, renal impairment, pregnancy and breastfeeding. Atropine or other antidote to muscarinic effects may be necessary (particularly when neostigmine is given by injection), but it should not be given routinely as it may mask signs of overdosage; **interactions:** Appendix 1 (parasympathomimetics)

Contra-indications: intestinal or urinary obstruction

Side-effects: nausea, vomiting, increased salivation, diarrhoea, abdominal cramps (more marked with higher doses). Signs of overdosage are increased gastro-intestinal discomfort, bronchial secretions, and sweating, involuntary defaecation and micturition, miosis, nystagmus, bradycardia, hypotension, agitation, excessive dreaming, and weakness eventually leading to fasciculation and paralysis

Dose: *by mouth*, neostigmine bromide 15–30 mg at suitable intervals throughout day, total daily dose 75–300 mg (but see also notes above); NEONATE 1–5 mg every 4 hours, half an hour before feeds; CHILD up to 6 years initially 7.5 mg, 6–12 years initially 15 mg, usual total daily dose 15–90 mg

By subcutaneous or intramuscular injection, neostigmine metilsulfate 1–2.5 mg at suitable inter-

vals throughout day (usual total daily dose 5–20 mg); NEONATE 50–250 micrograms every 4 hours half an hour before feeds; CHILD 200–500 micrograms as required

Neostigmine (Non-proprietary) ☐PoM☐
Tablets, scored, neostigmine bromide 15 mg. Net price 20 = £2.86
Available from Cambridge
Injection, neostigmine metilsulfate 2.5 mg/mL. Net price 1-mL amp = 50p
Available from Antigen, Phoenix

DISTIGMINE BROMIDE

Indications: myasthenia gravis; urinary retention and other indications, see section 7.4.1

Cautions; Contra-indications; Side-effects: see under Neostigmine

Dose: initially 5 mg daily half an hour before breakfast, increased at intervals of 3–4 days if necessary to a max. of 20 mg daily; CHILD up to 10 mg daily according to age

Preparations
Section 7.4.1

EDROPHONIUM CHLORIDE

Indications: see under Dose and notes above; reversal of non-depolarising neuromuscular blockade and diagnosis of dual block (section 15.1.6)

Cautions; Contra-indications; Side-effects: see under Neostigmine; have resuscitation facilities; *extreme* caution in respiratory distress (see notes above) and in asthma

Note. Severe cholinergic reactions can be counteracted by injection of atropine sulphate (which should always be available)

Dose: diagnosis of myasthenia gravis, *by intravenous injection*, 2 mg followed after 30 seconds (if no adverse reaction has occurred) by 8 mg; in adults without suitable veins, *by intramuscular injection*, 10 mg

Detection of overdosage or underdosage of cholinergic drugs, *by intravenous injection*, 2 mg (best before next dose of anticholinesterase, see notes above)

CHILD *by intravenous injection*, 20 micrograms/kg followed after 30 seconds (if no adverse reaction has occurred) by 80 micrograms/kg

Edrophonium (Non-proprietary) ☐PoM☐
Injection, edrophonium chloride 10 mg/mL. Net price 1-mL amp = £4.58
Available from Cambridge

PYRIDOSTIGMINE BROMIDE

Indications: myasthenia gravis

Cautions; Contra-indications; Side-effects: see under Neostigmine; weaker muscarinic action

Dose: *by mouth*, 30–120 mg at suitable intervals throughout day, total daily dose 0.3–1.2 g (but see also notes above); NEONATE 5–10 mg every 4 hours, 30–60 minutes before feeds; CHILD up to 6 years initially 30 mg, 6–12 years initially 60 mg, usual total daily dose 30–360 mg

Mestinon® (ICN) ☐PoM☐
Tablets, scored, pyridostigmine bromide 60 mg. Net price 20 = £5.02

Immunosuppressant therapy

Corticosteroids (section 6.3) are established as treatment for myasthenia gravis where *thymectomy* is inadvisable or to reduce the risk of surgery beforehand. The initial dose may be high (up to 100 mg **prednisolone** daily) but most advise starting with a smaller dose (20 mg prednisolone daily) and gradually increasing it. There is grave risk of exacerbation of the myasthenia during the initial stages of therapy, particularly in the first 2-3 weeks, therefore inpatient supervision is essential. Improvement usually begins after about 2 weeks on the high-dose regimen. In some patients a prolonged remission may be induced, but often patients need a maintenance dose of 10–40 mg prednisolone daily; alternate-day therapy is popular. Patients who need a corticosteroid may benefit from the addition of **azathioprine** (section 8.2.1) in a dose of 2 mg/kg daily which may allow a reduction in corticosteroid dosage.

10.2.2 Skeletal muscle relaxants

Drugs described below are used for the relief of chronic muscle spasm or spasticity; they are not indicated for spasm associated with minor injuries. They act principally on the central nervous system with the exception of dantrolene which has a peripheral site of action. They differ in action from the muscle relaxants used in anaesthesia (section 15.1.5) which block transmission at the neuromuscular junction.

The underlying cause of spasticity should be treated and any aggravating factors (e.g. pressure sores, infection) remedied. Skeletal muscle relaxants are effective in most forms of spasticity except the rare alpha variety. The major disadvantage of treatment with these drugs is that reduction in muscle tone can cause a loss of splinting action of the spastic leg and trunk muscles and sometimes lead to an increase in disability.

Dantrolene acts directly on skeletal muscle and produces fewer central adverse effects making it a drug of choice. The dose should be increased slowly.

Baclofen inhibits transmission at spinal level and also depresses the central nervous system. The dose should be increased slowly to avoid the major side-effects of sedation and hypotonia (other adverse events are uncommon).

Diazepam may also be used. Sedation and, occasionally, extensor hypotonus are disadvantages. Other benzodiazepines also have muscle-relaxant properties. Muscle-relaxant doses of benzodiazepines are similar to anxiolytic doses (section 4.1.2).

Tizanidine is a newly introduced alpha$_2$-adrenoceptor agonist indicated for spasticity associated with multiple sclerosis or spinal cord injury.

BACLOFEN

Indications: chronic severe spasticity resulting from disorders such as multiple sclerosis or traumatic partial section of spinal cord

Cautions: psychiatric illness, cerebrovascular disease, elderly; respiratory, hepatic or renal impairment, epilepsy; history of peptic ulcer; hypertonic

bladder sphincter; pregnancy (see Appendix 4); avoid abrupt withdrawal (may precipitate autonomic dysreflexia, see also CSM advice below); porphyria (section 9.8.2); **interactions:** Appendix 1 (muscle relaxants)

WITHDRAWAL. The CSM has advised that serious side-effects can occur with abrupt withdrawal; to minimise risk, therapy should be discontinued by gradual dose reduction over at least 1–2 weeks (longer if symptoms occur)

DRIVING. Drowsiness may affect performance of skilled tasks (e.g. driving); effects of alcohol enhanced

Contra-indications: peptic ulceration

Side-effects: frequently sedation, drowsiness, nausea; occasionally lightheadedness, lassitude, confusion, dizziness, ataxia, hallucinations, headache, euphoria, insomnia, depression, tremor, nystagmus, paraesthesia, convulsions, muscular pain and weakness, respiratory or cardiovascular depression, hypotension, dry mouth, gastro-intestinal and urinary disturbances; rarely visual disorders, taste alterations, increased sweating, rash, blood sugar changes, altered liver function tests, and paradoxical increase in spasticity

Dose: *by mouth*, 5 mg 3 times daily, preferably after food, gradually increased; max. 100 mg daily; CHILD 0.75–2 mg/kg daily (over 10 years, max. 2.5 mg/kg daily) *or* 2.5 mg 4 times daily increased gradually according to age to maintenance: 1–2 years 10–20 mg daily, 2–6 years 20–30 mg daily, 6–10 years 30–60 mg daily

By intrathecal injection, see preparation below

Baclofen (Non-proprietary) PoM

Tablets, baclofen 10 mg. Net price 20 = £1.15. Label: 2, 8

Available from APS, Ashbourne (*Baclospas®*), Berk (*Balgifen®*), Cox, Hillcross, Lagap, Norton

Lioresal® (Novartis) PoM

Tablets, scored, baclofen 10 mg. Net price 84-tab pack = £9.03. Label: 2, 8
    Excipients: include gluten

Liquid, sugar-free, baclofen 5 mg/5 mL. Net price 300 mL = £7.46. Label: 2, 8

■ By intrathecal injection

Lioresal® (Novartis) PoM

Intrathecal injection, baclofen, 50 micrograms/mL, net price 1-mL amp (for test dose) = £2.50; 500 micrograms/mL, 20-mL amp (for use with implantable pump) = £55.55; 2 mg/mL, 5-mL amp (for use with implantable pump) = £55.55

Important: consult product literature for full instructions on dose testing and titration—it is important that patients are monitored closely in an appropriately equipped and staffed environment during screening and immediately following pump implantation, and that resuscitation equipment is available for immediate use

Dose: by intrathecal injection, specialist use only, severe chronic spasticity unresponsive to oral antispastic drugs (or where side-effects of oral therapy unacceptable), initial *test dose* (with resuscitation equipment to hand, see also above) 25–50 micrograms over at least 1 minute via catheter or lumbar puncture, increased in steps to max. 100 micrograms to determine appropriate dose *then dose-titration phase*, most often using infusion pump (implanted into chest wall or abdominal wall tissues in experienced centres only) to establish *appropriate maintenance dose* (ranging from 10 micrograms to 1.2 mg daily; usual range 300–800 micrograms daily) retaining some spasticity to avoid sensation of paralysis; CHILD under 18 years, not recommended

DANTROLENE SODIUM

Indications: chronic severe spasticity of voluntary muscle; malignant hyperthermia (section 15.1.8)

Cautions: impaired cardiac and pulmonary function; test liver function before and at intervals during therapy; therapeutic effect may take a few weeks to develop but if treatment is ineffective it should be discontinued after 4–6 weeks. Avoid when spasticity is useful, for example, locomotion; **interactions:** Appendix 1 (muscle relaxants)

DRIVING. Drowsiness may affect performance of skilled tasks (e.g. driving); effects of alcohol enhanced

Contra-indications: hepatic impairment (may cause severe liver damage); acute muscle spasm

Side-effects: transient drowsiness, dizziness, weakness, malaise, fatigue, diarrhoea (withdraw if severe, discontinue treatment if recurs on re-introduction), anorexia, nausea, headache, rash; less frequently constipation, dysphagia, speech and visual disturbances, confusion, nervousness, insomnia, depression, seizures, chills, fever, increased urinary frequency; rarely, tachycardia, erratic blood pressure, dyspnoea, haematuria, possible crystalluria, urinary incontinence or retention, pleural effusion, pericarditis, dose-related hepatotoxicity (occasionally fatal) may be more common in women over 30 especially those taking oestrogens

Dose: initially 25 mg daily, may be increased at weekly intervals to max. of 100 mg 4 times daily; usual dose 75 mg 3 times daily; CHILD not recommended

Dantrium® (Procter & Gamble Pharm.) [PoM]
Capsules, both orange/brown, dantrolene sodium 25 mg, net price 20 = £2.53; 100 mg, 20 = £8.85. Label: 2

DIAZEPAM

Indications: muscle spasm of varied aetiology, including tetanus; other indications (section 4.1.2, section 4.8, section 15.1.4.1)

Cautions; Contra-indications; Side-effects: see section 4.1.2; also hypotonia; special precautions for intravenous injection (section 4.8.2)

Dose: *by mouth*, 2–15 mg daily in divided doses, increased if necessary in spastic conditions to 60 mg daily according to response

Cerebral spasticity in selected cases, CHILD 2–40 mg daily in divided doses

By intramuscular or by slow intravenous injection (into a large vein at a rate of not more than 5 mg/minute), in acute muscle spasm, 10 mg repeated if necessary after 4 hours

Note. Only use intramuscular route when oral and intravenous routes not possible; special precautions for intravenous injection see section 4.8.2

Tetanus, ADULT and CHILD, *by intravenous injection*, 100–300 micrograms/kg repeated every 1–4 hours; *by intravenous infusion (or by nasoduodenal tube)*, 3–10 mg/kg over 24 hours, adjusted according to response

Preparations
Section 4.1.2

TIZANIDINE

Indications: spasticity associated with multiple sclerosis or spinal cord injury or disease

Cautions: elderly, renal impairment (Appendix 3), pregnancy and breast-feeding, monitor liver function monthly for first 4 months and in those who develop unexplained nausea, anorexia or fatigue; **interactions:** Appendix 1 (muscle relaxants)

DRIVING Drowsiness may affect performance of skilled tasks (e.g. driving); effects of alcohol enhanced

Contra-indications: severe hepatic impairment

Side-effects: drowsiness, fatigue, dizziness, dry mouth, nausea, gastro-intestinal disturbances, hypotension; also reported, bradycardia, insomnia, hallucinations and altered liver enzymes (discontinue if persistently raised—consult product literature); rarely acute hepatitis

Dose: initially 2 mg daily as a single dose increased according to response at intervals of at least 3–4 days in steps of 2 mg daily (and given in divided doses) usually up to 24 mg daily in 3–4 divided doses; max. 36 mg daily; CHILD not recommended

Zanaflex® (Elan) ▼ [PoM]
Tablets, scored, tizanidine (as hydrochloride) 2 mg, net price 120-tab pack = £71.76; 4 mg, 120-tab pack = £89.70. Label: 2

Other muscle relaxants

The clinical efficacy of carisoprodol, meprobamate (section 4.1.2), and methocarbamol as muscle relaxants is **not** well established although they have been included in compound analgesic preparations.

CARISOPRODOL [less suitable]

Indications: short-term symptomatic relief of muscle spasm (but see notes above)

Cautions; Contra-indications; Side-effects: see under Meprobamate, section 4.1.2; drowsiness is common; avoid in porphyria (section 9.8.2)

Dose: 350 mg 3 times daily; ELDERLY half adult dose or less

Carisoma® (Pharmax) [PoM] [less suitable]
Tablets, carisoprodol 125 mg, net price 100 = £7.10; 350 mg, 100 = £7.95. Label: 2

> [less suitable icon] denotes preparations that are considered to be less suitable for prescribing (see p. vi)

METHOCARBAMOL [less suitable]

Indications: short-term symptomatic relief of muscle spasm (but see notes above)

Cautions: hepatic and renal impairment (avoid injection in renal impairment); **interactions:** Appendix 1 (Muscle Relaxants)

DRIVING. Drowsiness may affect performance of skilled tasks (e.g. driving); effects of alcohol enhanced

Contra-indications: coma or pre-coma, brain damage, epilepsy, myasthenia gravis

Side-effects: lassitude, light-headedness, dizziness, restlessness, anxiety, confusion, drowsiness, nausea, allergic rash or angioedema, convulsions
Dose: *by mouth*, 1.5 g 4 times daily (elderly 750 mg or less); may be reduced to 750 mg 3 times daily

Robaxin® (Shire) PoM ▭
750 Tablets, scored, methocarbamol 750 mg. Net price 20 = £2.53. Label: 2

▭ denotes preparations that are considered to be less suitable for prescribing (see p. vi)

Nocturnal leg cramps

Quinine salts (section 5.4.1) 200–300 mg at bedtime are effective in reducing the frequency of nocturnal leg cramps by about 25% in ambulatory patients. It may take up to 4 weeks for improvement to become apparent and it is then given on a continuous basis if there is benefit. Patients should be monitored closely during the early stages for adverse effects as well as for benefit. Treatment should be interrupted at intervals of approximately 3 months to assess the need for further quinine treatment. Quinine is very toxic in overdosage and accidental fatalities have occurred in children (see also below).

QUININE
Indications; Dose: see notes above; malaria (section 5.4.1)
Cautions; Contra-indications; Side-effects: see section 5.4.1; **important:** very toxic in **overdosage**—immediate advice from poison centres essential (see also p. 19)

Preparations
Section 5.4.1

10.3 Drugs for the relief of soft-tissue inflammation

10.3.1   Enzymes
10.3.2   Rubefacients and other topical antirheumatics

Extravasation

Local guidelines for the management of extravasation should be followed where they exist or specialist advice sought.

Extravasation injury follows leakage of drugs or intravenous fluids from the veins or inadvertent administration into the subcutaneous or subdermal tissue. It must be dealt with **promptly** to prevent tissue necrosis.

Acidic or alkaline preparations and those with an osmolarity greater than that of plasma can cause extravasation injury and excipients including alcohol and polyethylene glycol have also been implicated. Cytotoxic drugs commonly cause extravasation injury. In addition, certain patients

such as the very young and the elderly are at increased risk. Those receiving anticoagulants are more likely to lose blood into surrounding tissues if extravasation occurs whilst those receiving sedatives or analgesics may not notice the early signs or symptoms of extravasation.

PREVENTION OF EXTRAVASATION. Precautions should be taken to avoid extravasation; ideally, drugs liable to cause extravasation injury should be given through a central line and patients receiving repeated doses of hazardous drugs peripherally should have the cannula resited at regular intervals. Attention should be paid to the manufacturers' recommendations for administration. Placing a glyceryl trinitrate patch (section 2.6.1) distal to the cannula may improve the patency of the vessel in patients with small veins or in those whose veins are prone to collapse.

Patients should be asked to report any pain or burning at the site of injection immediately.

MANAGEMENT OF EXTRAVASATION. If extravasation is suspected the infusion should be stopped immediately but the cannula should not be removed until after an attempt has been made to aspirate the area (through the cannula) in order to remove as much of the drug as possible. Aspiration is sometimes possible if the extravasation presents with a raised bleb or blister at the injection site and is surrounded by hardened tissue, but it is often unsuccessful if the tissue is soft or soggy. Corticosteroids are usually given to treat inflammation, although there is little evidence to support their use in extravasation. Hydrocortisone or dexamethasone (section 6.3.2) may be given either locally by subcutaneous injection or intravenously at a site distant from the injury. Antihistamines (section 3.4.1) and analgesics (section 4.7) may be required for symptom relief.

The management of extravasation beyond these measures is not well standardised and calls for specialist advice. Treatment depends on the nature of the offending substance; one approach is to localise and neutralise the substance whereas another is to spread and dilute it. The first method may be appropriate following extravasation of vesicant drugs and involves administration of an antidote (if available) and the application of cold compresses 3–4 times a day (consult specialist literature for details of specific antidotes). Spreading and diluting the offending substance involves infiltrating the area with physiological saline, applying warm compresses, elevating the affected limb, and administering hyaluronidase (section 10.3.1). A saline flush-out technique (involving flushing the subcutaneous tissue with physiological saline) may be effective but requires specialist advice. Hyaluronidase should **not** be administered following extravasation of vesicant drugs (unless it is either a specific antidote or used in the saline flush-out technique).

10.3.1   Enzymes

Hyaluronidase is used to render the tissues more easily permeable to injected fluids, e.g. for introduction of fluids by subcutaneous infusion (termed hypodermoclysis).

HYALURONIDASE

Indications: enhance permeation of subcutaneous or intramuscular injections, local anaesthetics and subcutaneous infusions; promote resorption of excess fluids and blood

Cautions: infants or elderly (control speed and total volume and avoid overhydration especially in renal impairment)

Contra-indications: do not apply direct to cornea; avoid sites where infection or malignancy; not for anaesthesia in unexplained premature labour; not to be used to reduce swelling of bites or stings; not for intravenous administration

Side-effects: occasional severe allergy

Dose: With subcutaneous or intramuscular injection, 1500 units dissolved directly in solution to be injected (ensure compatibility)

With local anaesthetics, 1500 units mixed with local anaesthetic solution (ophthalmology, 15 units/mL)

Hypodermoclysis, 1500 units dissolved in 1 mL water for injections or 0.9% sodium chloride injection, administered before start of 500–1000 mL infusion fluid

Extravasation or haematoma, 1500 units dissolved in 1 mL water for injections or 0.9% sodium chloride injection, infiltrated into affected area (as soon as possible after extravasation)

Hyalase® (CP) [PoM]

Injection, powder for reconstitution, hyaluronidase (ovine). Net price 1500-unit amp = £7.60

10.3.2   Rubefacients and other topical antirheumatics

Rubefacients act by counter-irritation. Pain, whether superficial or deep-seated, is relieved by any method which itself produces irritation of the skin. Counter-irritation is comforting in painful lesions of the muscles, tendons, and joints, and in non-articular rheumatism. Rubefacients probably all act through the same essential mechanism and differ mainly in intensity and duration of action.

Topical **NSAIDs** (e.g. felbinac, ibuprofen, ketoprofen and piroxicam) may provide some slight relief of pain in musculoskeletal conditions.

Topical NSAIDs and counter-irritants

CAUTIONS. Apply with gentle massage only. Avoid contact with eyes, mucous membranes, and inflamed or broken skin; discontinue if rash develops. Hands should be washed immediately after use. Not for use with occlusive dressings. Topical application of large amounts may result in systemic effects including hypersensitivity and asthma (renal disease has also been reported). Not generally suitable for children. Patient packs carry a **warning** to avoid during **pregnancy** or **breast-feeding**.

HYPERSENSITIVITY. For NSAID hypersensitivity and asthma warning, see pp. 447-8

PHOTOSENSITIVITY. Patients should be advised against excessive exposure to sunlight of area treated in order to avoid possibility of photosensitivity

Algesal® (Solvay)
Cream, diethylamine salicylate 10%. Net price 50 g = 75p
Apply three times daily
Excipients: include fragrance

Balmosa® (Pharmax)
Cream, camphor 4%, capsicum oleoresin 0.035%, menthol 2%, methyl salicylate 4%. Net price 40 g = 68p
Excipients: include wool fat

Difflam® (3M)
Cream, benzydamine hydrochloride 3%. Net price 100 g = £6.69
Apply 3–6 times daily for up to 10 days
Excipients: include propylene glycol, hydroxybenzoates (parabens), fragrance

Feldene® (Pfizer) [PoM]
Gel, piroxicam 0.5%. Net price 60 g = £5.00; 112 g = £7.84 (also 7.5 g starter pack, hosp. only)
Apply 3–4 times daily; therapy should be reviewed after 4 weeks
Excipients: include benzyl alcohol, propylene glycol

Fenbid® Forte Gel (Goldshield) [PoM]
Gel, ibuprofen 10%, net price 100 g = £6.50
Apply up to 4 times daily; therapy should be reviewed after 14 days
Excipients: include benzyl alcohol

Ibugel® (Dermal)
Gel, ibuprofen 5%. Net price 100 g = £5.95
Apply up to 3 times daily
Excipients: include propylene glycol

Ibumousse® (Dermal)
Foam, ibuprofen 5%, net price 125 g = £6.58. Label: 15
Apply 3–4 times daily
Excipients: include propylene glycol

Ibuspray® (Dermal)
Spray application, ibuprofen 5%. Net price 100-mL = £6.95. Label: 15
Apply 3-4 times daily
Excipients: none as listed in section 13.1.3

Intralgin® (3M)
Gel, benzocaine 2%, salicylamide 5% in an alcoholic vehicle. Net price 50 g = 47p
Excipients: none as listed in section 13.1.3

Movelat® (Sankyo)
Cream, mucopolysaccharide polysulphate (heparinoid) 0.2%, salicylic acid 2%, thymol 0.1%. Net price 100 g = £4.14
Apply up to 4 times daily
Excipients: none as listed in section 13.1.3
Gel, mucopolysaccharide polysulphate (heparinoid) 0.2%, salicylic acid 2%. Net price 100 g = £4.14
Apply up to 4 times daily
Excipients: include disodium edetate, fragrance

Oruvail® (Rhône-Poulenc Rorer) [PoM]
Gel, ketoprofen 2.5%. Net price 100 g = £6.78
Apply 2–4 times daily for up to 7 days (usual recommended dose 15 g daily)
Excipients: include fragrance

Powergel® (Searle) [PoM]
Gel, ketoprofen 2.5%. Net price 50 g = £3.25; 100 g = £6.25; Twinpack (2 × 50-g pack) = £6.50
Apply 2–3 times daily for up to max. 10 days
Excipients: include hydroxybenzoates (parabens), fragrance

Proflex® (Novartis Consumer Health)
Cream, ibuprofen 5%. Net price 100 g = £6.50
Apply 3–4 times daily
Excipients: include hydroxybenzoates (parabens), propylene glycol

Transvasin® (SSL)

Cream, ethyl nicotinate 2%, hexyl nicotinate 2%, thurfyl salicylate 14%. Net price 40 g = 89p; 80 g = £1.51
Apply at least twice daily

Excipients: include hydroxybenzoates (parabens), polysorbate, fragrance

Spray application, hydroxyethyl salicylate 5%, diethylamine salicylate 5%, methyl nicotinate 1%. Net price 125 mL = £1.64

Traxam® (Whitehall) [PoM]

Foam, felbinac 3.17%. Net price 100 g = £7.00. Label:15

Excipients: none as listed in section 13.1.3

Gel, felbinac 3%. Net price 100 g = £7.00
Apply 2–4 times daily; max. 25 g daily; therapy should be reviewed after 14 days

Excipients: none as listed in section 13.1.3

Note. Felbinac is an active metabolite of the NSAID fenbufen

Voltarol Emulgel® (Novartis) [PoM]

Gel, diclofenac diethylammonium salt 1.16% (equivalent to diclofenac sodium 1%). Net price 20 g (hosp. only) = £1.55; 100 g = £7.00
Apply 3–4 times daily; therapy should be reviewed after 14 days (or after 28 days for osteoarthritis)

Excipients: include propylene glycol, fragrance

Topical NSAIDs and counter-irritants on sale to the public together with their significant ingredients include:

Algesal® (diethylamine salicylate), **Algipan Rub®** (capsicin, glycol salicylate, methyl nicotinate),
Balmosa® (camphor, capsicum oleoresin, menthol, methyl salicylate), **Bengués Balsam®** (menthol, methyl salicylate), **BN Liniment®** (turpentine oil, strong ammonia solution, ammonium chloride), **Boots Muscular Pain Relief Gel®** (ketoprofen), **Boots Pain Relief Balm®** (ethyl nicotinate, glycol monosalicylate, nonylic acid vanillylamide), **Boots Pain Relief Embrocation®** (camphor, turpentine oil), **Boots Pain Relief Warming Spray®** (camphor, ethyl nicotinate, methyl salicylate),
Cremalgin® (capsicin, glycol salicylate, methyl nicotinate), **Cuprofen® Ibutop® Gel** (ibuprofen)
Deep Freeze Cold Gel® (menthol), **Deep Freeze Spray®** (levomenthol), **Deep Heat Extra Strength®**, **Deep Heat Massage Liniment®**, **Deep Heat Maximum®**, **Deep Heat Pre–Sport Rub®** (menthol, methyl salicylate), **Deep Heat Rub®** (eucalyptus oil, menthol, menthyl salicylate, turpentine oil), **Deep Heat Spray ®** (glycol salicylate, ethyl salicylate, methyl salicylate, methyl nicotinate), **Deep Relief®** (ibuprofen, menthol), **Difflam® Cream** (benzydamine), **Dubam Cream®** (methyl salicylate, menthol, cineole), **Dubam Spray®** (ethyl salicylate, methyl salicylate, glycol salicylate, methyl nicotinate)
Elliman's Universal Embrocation® (acetic acid, turpentine oil)
Feldene P® Gel (piroxicam), **Fenbid®** Gel (ibuprofen), **Fiery Jack Cream®** (capsicum oleoresin, diethylamine salicylate, glycol salicylate, methyl nicotinate), **Fiery Jack Ointment®** (capsicum oleoresin)
Goddard's White Oil Embrocation® (dilute acetic acid, dilute ammonia solution, turpentine oil)
Hansaplast® Thermo Plaster (capsaicinoids, colophony)
Ibuleve®, **Ibuleve Mousse®**, **Ibuleve Sports Gel®** (ibuprofen), **Intralgin®** (benzocaine, salicylamide)
Lloyds Cream® (diethyl salicylate)
Mentholatum® Ibuprofen Gel (ibuprofen), **Movelat® Relief Cream** (mucopolysaccharide polysulphate, salicylic acid, thymol), **Movelat® Relief Gel** (mucopolysaccharide polysulphate, salicylic acid)
Nasciodine® (camphor, iodine, menthol, methyl salicylate, turpentine oil), **Nella Red Oil®** (clove oil, mustard oil, methyl nicotinate), **Nurofen Muscular Pain Relief Gel®** (ibuprofen)
Oruvail® Gel (ketoprofen 30-g tube; 100-g tube prescribable on NHS [PoM]
PR Freeze Spray® (dimethylether, dimethoxymethane), **PR Heat Spray®** (ethyl nicotinate, methyl salicylate, camphor); **Proflex Cream®** (ibuprofen), **Proflex Pain Relief Gel®** (ibuprofen)

Radian®-B Ibuprofen Gel (ibuprofen), **Radian®-B Muscle Lotion**, **Radian®-B Heat Spray** (ammonium salicylate, camphor, menthol, salicylic acid), **Radian®-B Muscle Rub** (camphor, capsicin, menthol, methyl salicylate), **Ralgex Cream®** (capsicin, glycol monosalicylate, methyl nicotinate), **Ralgex Freeze Spray®** (dimethyl ether, glycol monosalicylate, isopentane), **Ralgex® Ibutop® Gel** (ibuprofen), **Ralgex Low Odour Spray®** (glycol monosalicylate, methyl nicotinate), **Ralgex Spray®** (ethyl salicylate, methyl salicylate, glycol monosalicylate, methyl nicotinate), **Ralgex Stick®** (capsicin, ethyl salicylate, methyl salicylate, glycol salicylate, menthol)
Salonair® (benzyl nicotinate, camphor, glycol salicylate, menthol, methyl salicylate, squalane), **Salonpas Plasters®** (glycol salicylate, methyl salicylate), **Solpaflex® Gel** (ketoprofen)
Tiger Balm Red Extra Strength® (camphor, clove oil, cajuput oil, cinnamon oil, menthol, peppermint oil), **Tiger Balm®** (cajuput oil, camphor, clove oil, menthol, peppermint oil), **Transvasin Cream®** (ethyl nicotinate, hexyl nicotinate, thurfyl salicylate), **Transvasin Spray®** (diethylamine salicylate, hydroxyethyl salicylate, methyl salicylate), **Traxam Pain Relief®** (felbinac)
Zam–Buk® (camphor, eucalyptus oil, thyme oil, colophony)

Capsaicin

See also Cautions above, Topical NSAIDs and Counter-irritants

Axsain® (Elan) [PoM]
Cream, capsaicin 0.075%. Net price 45 g = £15.04. For post-herpetic neuralgia (**important: after** lesions have healed), apply up to 3–4 times daily; for painful diabetic neuropathy, under supervision of hospital consultant, apply 3–4 times daily for 8 weeks then review

Zacin® (Elan) [PoM]
Cream, capsaicin 0.025%. Net price 45 g = £15.04.
Symptomatic relief in osteoarthritis, apply 4 times daily

Poultices

Kaolin Poultice ▬◢ , heavy kaolin 52.7%, thymol 0.05%, boric acid 4.5%, peppermint oil 0.05%, methyl salicylate 0.2%, glycerol 42.5%. Net price 200 g = £1.91
Warm and apply directly or between layers of muslin; avoid application of overheated poultice

Kaolin Poultice K/L Pack® (K/L) ▬◢
Kaolin poultice. Net price 4 × 100-g pouches = £5.50

▬◢ denotes preparations that are considered to be less suitable for prescribing (see p. vi)

11: Eye

11.1 Administration of drugs to the eye

EYE DROPS AND EYE OINTMENTS. When administered in the form of eye drops, drugs penetrate the globe, probably through the cornea. However, systemic effects, which are usually undesirable, may well arise from absorption of drugs into the general circulation via conjunctival vessels or from the nasal mucosa after the excess of the preparation has drained down through the tear ducts; nasal drainage of drugs is much more often associated with eye drops than with eye ointments. For example, a beta-blocker administered as eye drops may induce bronchospasm or bradycardia in susceptible individuals. The extent of systemic absorption following ocular administration is highly variable.

Eye drops are generally instilled into the pocket formed by gently pulling down the lower eyelid and keeping the eye closed for as long as possible after application, preferably 1–2 minutes; one drop is all that is needed. A small amount of eye ointment is applied similarly; the ointment melts rapidly and blinking helps to spread it.

When two different preparations in the form of eye drops are required at the same time of day, for example pilocarpine and timolol in glaucoma, dilution and overflow may occur when one immediately follows the other. The patient should therefore leave an interval of 5 minutes.

Generally it is inadvisable for patients to continue to wear contact lenses, particularly hydrophilic (soft) contact lenses when receiving eye drops. For warnings relating to eye drops and contact lenses, see section 11.9.

EYE LOTIONS. These are solutions for the irrigation of the conjunctival sac. They act mechanically to flush out irritants or foreign bodies as a first-aid treatment. Sterile sodium chloride 0.9% solution (section 11.8.1) is usually used. Clean water will suffice in an emergency.

OTHER PREPARATIONS. Subconjunctival injection may be used to administer anti-infective drugs, mydriatics, or corticosteroids for conditions not responding to topical therapy. The drug diffuses through the cornea and sclera to the anterior and posterior chambers and vitreous humour. However, because the dose-volume is limited (usually not more than 1 mL), this route is suitable only for drugs which are readily soluble.

Drugs such as antibiotics and corticosteroids may be administered systemically to treat an eye condition.

Suitable plastic devices which gradually release a specified amount of drug over a period of, say, 1 week are also used (e.g. *Ocusert®*).

PRESERVATIVES AND SENSITISERS. Information on preservatives and on substances identified as skin sensitisers (see section 13.1.3) is provided under preparation entries.

11.2 Control of microbial contamination

Preparations for the eye should be sterile when issued. Eye drops in multiple-application containers include preservative but care should be taken to avoid contamination of the contents during use.

Eye drops in multiple-application containers for *domiciliary use* should not be used for more than 4 weeks after first opening (unless otherwise stated).

Eye drops for use in *hospital wards* are normally discarded 1 week after first opening. Individual containers should be provided for each patient. Containers used before an operation should be discarded at the time of the operation and fresh containers supplied. A fresh supply should also be provided upon discharge from hospital; it may be acceptable in specialist ophthalmology units to issue on discharge eye drop bottles that have been in use for the patient for less than 36 hours.

Eye drops used in *out-patient departments* should be discarded at the end of each day. In clinics for eye diseases and in accident and emergency departments, where the dangers of infection are high, single-application packs should be used; if a multiple-application pack is used, it should be discarded after single use.

Diagnostic dyes (e.g. fluorescein) should be used only from single-application packs.

In *eye surgery* it is wise to use single-application containers. Preparations used during intra-ocular procedures and others that may penetrate into the anterior chamber must be isotonic and without preservatives and buffered if necessary to a neutral pH. Large volume intravenous infusion preparations are not suitable for this purpose. For all surgical procedures, a previously unopened container is used for each patient.

11.3 Anti-infective eye preparations

11.3.1	Antibacterials
11.3.2	Antifungals
11.3.3	Antivirals

EYE INFECTIONS. Most acute superficial eye infections can be treated topically. Blepharitis and conjunctivitis are often caused by staphylococci; keratitis and endophthalmitis may be bacterial, viral, or fungal.

Bacterial *blepharitis* is treated by application of an antibacterial eye ointment to the conjunctival sac or to the lid margins. Systemic treatment may occasionally be required and is usually undertaken after culturing organisms from the lid margin and determining their antibiotic sensitivity; antibiotics such as the tetracyclines given for 3 months or longer may be appropriate.

Acute *infective conjunctivitis* is treated with antibacterial eye drops and eye ointment. A poor response might indicate viral or allergic conjunctivitis. *Gonococcal conjunctivitis* is treated with systemic and topical antibiotics.

Corneal ulcer and *keratitis* require specialist treatment and may call for subconjunctival or systemic administration of antibiotics.

Endophthalmitis is a medical emergency which also calls for specialist management and often requires parenteral, subconjunctival, or intra-ocular administration of antibiotics.

For reference to the treatment of *crab lice of the eyelashes*, see section 13.10.4

11.3.1 Antibacterials

Bacterial infections are generally treated topically with eye drops and eye ointments. Systemic administration is sometimes appropriate in blepharitis. In intra-ocular infection, a variety of routes (intracorneal, intravitreal and systemic) may be used.

Chloramphenicol has a broad spectrum of activity and is the drug of choice for *superficial eye infections*. Chloramphenicol eye drops are well tolerated and the recommendation that chloramphenicol eye drops should be avoided because of an increased risk of aplastic anaemia is not well founded.

Other antibiotics with a broad spectrum of activity include **framycetin**, **gentamicin**, and **neomycin**, and also **ciprofloxacin**, **ofloxacin** and the recently introduced **lomefloxacin**. Gentamicin, ciprofloxacin and ofloxacin are effective for infections caused by *Pseudomonas aeruginosa*.

Ciprofloxacin eye drops are licensed for *corneal ulcers*; intensive application (especially in the first 2 days) is required throughout the day and night.

Chlortetracycline is used in the treatment of *chlamydial infections* including *trachoma* (consult World Health Organization guidelines).

Fusidic acid is useful for staphylococcal infections.

Propamidine isetionate is of little value in bacterial infections but is specific for the rare but potentially devastating condition of *acanthamoeba keratitis* (see also section 11.9).

WITH CORTICOSTEROIDS. Many antibiotic preparations also incorporate a corticosteroid but such mixtures should **not** be used unless a patient is under close specialist supervision. In particular they should not be prescribed for undiagnosed 'red eye' which is sometimes caused by the herpes simplex virus and may be difficult to diagnose (section 11.4).

ADMINISTRATION
Eye drops. Apply 1 drop at least every 2 hours then reduce frequency as infection is controlled and continue for 48 hours after healing.
Eye ointment. Apply *either* at night (if eye drops used during the day) *or* 3–4 times daily (if eye ointment used alone).

CHLORAMPHENICOL

Indications: see notes above
Side-effects: transient stinging; see also notes above
Administration: see notes above

Chloramphenicol (Non-proprietary) PoM
Eye drops, chloramphenicol 0.5%. Net price 10 mL = 81p
Eye ointment, chloramphenicol 1%. Net price 4 g = £1.10

Chloromycetin® (Goldshield) [PoM]
Redidrops (= eye drops), chloramphenicol 0.5%.
Net price 5 mL = £1.65; 10 mL = £2.01
Excipients: include phenylmercuric acetate
Ophthalmic ointment (= eye ointment), chloramphenicol 1%. Net price 4 g = £2.01

Sno Phenicol® (Chauvin) [PoM]
Eye drops, chloramphenicol 0.5%, in a viscous
vehicle. Net price 10 mL = £1.08
Excipients: include chlorhexidine acetate

■ Single use
Minims® Chloramphenicol (Chauvin) [PoM]
Eye drops, chloramphenicol 0.5%. Net price 20 ×
0.5 mL = £4.92

CHLORTETRACYCLINE

Indications: local treatment of infections, including trachoma (see notes above)
Administration: see notes above

Aureomycin® (Lederle) [PoM]
Ophthalmic ointment (= eye ointment), chlortetracycline hydrochloride 1%. Net price 3.5 g = 92p

CIPROFLOXACIN

Indications: superficial bacterial infections, see
notes above; corneal ulcers
Cautions: not recommended for children under 1
year; pregnancy and breast-feeding
Side-effects: local burning and itching; lid margin
crusting; hyperaemia; bad taste; corneal staining,
keratitis, lid oedema, tearing, photophobia, corneal
infiltrates; nausea and visual disturbances reported
Administration: superficial bacterial infection,
see notes above
  Corneal ulcer, apply throughout day and night,
first day 2 drops every 15 minutes for 6 hours
then every 30 minutes for the rest of the day, second day apply 2 drops every hour, third to fourteenth days apply 2 drops every 4 hours; if longer
treatment required physician to decide frequency
(max. duration of treatment 21 days)

Ciloxan® (Alcon) [PoM]
Ophthalmic solution (= eye drops), ciprofloxacin
(as hydrochloride) 0.3%. Net price 5 mL = £4.94
Excipients: include benzalkonium chloride

FRAMYCETIN SULPHATE

Indications: see notes above
Administration: see notes above

Soframycin® (Florizel) [PoM]
Eye drops, framycetin sulphate 0.5%. Net price
10 mL = £4.62 .
Excipients: include benzalkonium chloride
Eye ointment, framycetin sulphate 0.5%. Net price
5 g = £2.52

FUSIDIC ACID

Indications: see notes above
Administration: see under preparation below

Fucithalmic® (Leo) [PoM]
Eye drops, m/r, fusidic acid 1% in gel basis (liquifies on contact with eye). Net price 5 g = £2.09
Excipients: include benzalkonium chloride, disodium edetate
Apply twice daily

GENTAMICIN

Indications: see notes above
Administration: see notes above

Cidomycin® (Hoechst Marion Roussel) [PoM]
Drops (for ear or eye), gentamicin 0.3% (as sulphate). Net price 8 mL = £1.31
Excipients: include benzalkonium chloride, disodium edetate

Garamycin® (Schering-Plough) [PoM]
Drops (for ear or eye), gentamicin 0.3% (as sulphate). Net price 10 mL = £1.79
Excipients: include benzalkonium chloride

Genticin® (Roche) [PoM]
Drops (for ear or eye), gentamicin 0.3% (as sulphate). Net price 10 mL = £1.91
Excipients: include benzalkonium chloride

■ Single use
Minims® Gentamicin (Chauvin) [PoM]
Eye drops, gentamicin 0.3% (as sulphate). Net
price 20 × 0.5 mL = £5.75

LOMEFLOXACIN

Indications: see notes above
Cautions: pregnancy and breast-feeding
Side-effects: local irritation; rarely hypersensitivity reactions
Administration: initially apply every 5 minutes
for 20 minutes (5 doses), then twice daily for 7–9
days

Okacyn® (CIBA Vision) ▼ [PoM]
Eye drops, lomefloxacin (as hydrochloride) 0.3%,
net price 5 mL = £4.90
Excipients: include benzalkonium chloride, disodium edetate

NEOMYCIN SULPHATE

Indications: see notes above
Administration: see notes above

Neomycin (Non-proprietary) [PoM]
Eye drops, neomycin sulphate 0.5% (3500 units/
mL). Net price 10 mL = £2.81
Available from Martindale
Eye ointment, neomycin sulphate 0.5%
(3500 units/g). Net price 3 g = £2.24
Available from Martindale

Neosporin® (Dominion) [PoM]
Eye drops, gramicidin 25 units, neomycin sulphate
1700 units, polymyxin B sulphate 5000 units/mL.
Net price 5 mL = £5.12
Excipients: include thiomersal
Apply 2–4 times daily or more frequently if required

■ Single use
Minims® Neomycin Sulphate (Chauvin) [PoM]
Eye drops, neomycin sulphate 0.5%. Net price 20
× 0.5 mL = £5.75
Excipients: include disodium edetate

OFLOXACIN

Indications: see notes above
Cautions: pregnancy and breast-feeding; not to be
used for more than 10 days
Side-effects: local irritation including photophobia; dizziness, numbness, nausea and headache
reported
Administration: see notes above

Exocin® (Allergan) PoM
Ophthalmic solution (= eye drops), ofloxacin 0.3%. Net price 5 mL = £2.17
Excipients: include benzalkonium chloride

POLYMYXIN B SULPHATE

Indications: see notes above
Administration: see notes above

Polyfax® (Dominion) PoM
Eye ointment, polymyxin B sulphate 10 000 units, bacitracin zinc 500 units/g. Net price 4 g = £3.26
Polytrim® (Dominion) PoM
Eye drops, trimethoprim 0.1%, polymyxin B sulphate 10 000 units/mL. Net price 5 mL = £3.05
Excipients: include thiomersal
Eye ointment, trimethoprim 0.5%, polymyxin B sulphate 10 000 units/g. Net price 4 g = £3.05

PROPAMIDINE ISETIONATE

Indications: local treatment of infections (but see notes above)

Brolene® (Rhône-Poulenc Rorer)
Eye drops, propamidine isetionate 0.1%. Net price 10 mL = £2.35
Apply 4 times daily
Excipients: include benzalkonium chloride
Note. Eye drops containing propamidine isetionate 0.1% also available from Typharm (*Golden Eye Drops*)
Eye ointment, dibromopropamidine isetionate 0.15%. Net price 5 g = £2.47
Apply 1–2 times daily
Note. Eye ointment containing dibromopropamidine isetionate 0.15% also available from Typharm (*Golden Eye Ointment*)

11.3.2 Antifungals

Fungal infections of the cornea are rare but can occur after agricultural injuries, especially in hot and humid climates. Orbital mycosis is rare, and when it occurs is usually due to direct spread of infection from the paranasal sinuses. Increasing age, debility, or immunosuppression may encourage fungal proliferation. The spread of infection via the bloodstream occasionally produces a metastatic endophthalmitis.

Many different fungi are capable of producing ocular infection; they may be identified by appropriate laboratory procedures.

Antifungal preparations for the eye are not generally available. Treatment will normally be carried out at specialist centres, but requests for information about supplies of preparations not available commercially should be addressed to the local Health Authority (or equivalent in Scotland or Northern Ireland), or to the nearest hospital ophthalmology unit, or to Moorfields Eye Hospital, City Road, London EC1V 2PD (tel. (020) 7253 3411).

11.3.3 Antivirals

Herpes simplex infections producing, for example, dendritic corneal ulcer can be treated with **aciclovir**. For systemic treatment of cytomegalovirus retinitis, see section 5.3.

ACICLOVIR
(Acyclovir)
Indications: local treatment of herpes simplex infections
Side-effects: mild stinging and local inflammation reported
Administration: apply 5 times daily (continue for at least 3 days after complete healing)

Zovirax® (GlaxoWellcome) PoM
Eye ointment, aciclovir 3%. Net price 4.5 g = £10.67
Tablets and *injection*, see section 5.3
Cream, see section 13.10.3

11.4 Corticosteroids and other anti-inflammatory preparations

11.4.1   Corticosteroids
11.4.2   Other anti-inflammatory preparations

11.4.1 Corticosteroids

Corticosteroids administered locally (as eye drops, eye ointments or subconjunctival injection) or by mouth have an important place in treating anterior segment inflammation, including that which results from surgery.

Topical corticosteroids should normally only be used under expert supervision; three main dangers are associated with their use:

- a 'red eye', where the diagnosis is unconfirmed, may be due to herpes simplex virus, and a corticosteroid may aggravate the condition, leading to corneal ulceration, with possible damage to vision and even loss of the eye. Bacterial, fungal and amoebic infections pose a similar hazard;
- 'steroid glaucoma' may follow the use of corticosteroid eye preparations in susceptible individuals;
- a 'steroid cataract' may follow prolonged use.

Other side-effects include thinning of the cornea and sclera.

Use of a combination product containing a corticosteroid with an anti-infective is rarely justified.

Systemic corticosteroids (section 6.3.2) may be useful for ocular conditions. The risk of producing a 'steroid cataract' is very high (75%) if the equivalent of more than 15 mg prednisolone is given daily for several years.

BETAMETHASONE

Indications: local treatment of inflammation (short-term)
Cautions: see notes above
Side-effects: see notes above
Administration: apply eye drops every 1–2 hours until controlled then reduce frequency, eye ointment 2–4 times daily or at night when used with eye drops

Betnesol® (Medeva) PoM
Drops (for ear, eye, or nose), betamethasone sodium phosphate 0.1%. Net price 10 mL = £1.31
Excipients: include benzalkonium chloride, disodium edetate
Eye ointment, betamethasone sodium phosphate 0.1%. Net price 3 g = 56p

Betnesol-N® (Medeva) PoM ▰
Drops (for ear, eye, or nose), see section 12.1.1
Eye ointment, betamethasone sodium phosphate 0.1%, neomycin sulphate 0.5%. Net price 3 g = 64p

Vista-Methasone® (Martindale) PoM
Drops (for ear, eye, or nose), betamethasone sodium phosphate 0.1%. Net price 5 mL = £1.10; 10 mL = £1.25
Excipients: include benzalkonium chloride

Vista-Methasone N® (Martindale) PoM ▰
Drops (for ear, eye, or nose), see section 12.1.1

CLOBETASONE BUTYRATE

Indications: local treatment of inflammation (short-term)
Cautions: see notes above
Side-effects: see notes above
Administration: apply eye drops 4 times daily; severe conditions every 1–2 hours until controlled then reduce frequency

Cloburate® (Dominion) PoM
Eye drops, clobetasone butyrate 0.1%. Net price 10 mL = £2.72
Excipients: include benzalkonium chloride

DEXAMETHASONE

Indications: local treatment of inflammation (short-term)
Cautions: see notes above
Side-effects: see notes above
Administration: apply eye drops 4–6 times daily; severe conditions every 30–60 minutes until controlled then reduce frequency

Maxidex® (Alcon) PoM
Eye drops, dexamethasone 0.1%, hypromellose 0.5%. Net price 5 mL = £1.49; 10 mL = £2.95
Excipients: include benzalkonium chloride, disodium edetate, polysorbate 80

Maxitrol® (Alcon) PoM ▰
Eye drops, dexamethasone 0.1%, hypromellose 0.5%, neomycin 0.35% (as sulphate), polymyxin B sulphate 6000 units/mL. Net price 5 mL = £1.77
Excipients: include benzalkonium chloride, polysorbate 20
Eye ointment, dexamethasone 0.1%, neomycin 0.35% (as sulphate), polymyxin B sulphate 6000 units/g. Net price 3.5 g = £1.52
Excipients: include hydroxybenzoates (parabens), wool fat

Sofradex® (Florizel) PoM ▰
Drops and ointment (for ear or eye), see section 12.1.1

■ Single use
Minims® Dexamethasone (Chauvin) PoM
Eye drops, dexamethasone sodium phosphate 0.1%. Net price 20 × 0.5 mL = £6.95
Excipients: include disodium edetate

▰ denotes preparations that are considered to be less suitable for prescribing (see p. vi)

FLUOROMETHOLONE

Indications: local treatment of inflammation (short-term)
Cautions: see notes above
Side-effects: see notes above
Administration: apply eye drops 2–4 times daily (initially every hour for 24–48 hours then reduce frequency)

FML® (Allergan) PoM
Ophthalmic suspension (= eye drops), fluorometholone 0.1%, polyvinyl alcohol (*Liquifilm®*) 1.4%. Net price 5 mL = £1.71; 10 mL = £2.95
Excipients: include benzalkonium chloride, disodium edetate, polysorbate 80

FML-Neo® (Allergan) PoM ▰
Eye drops, fluorometholone 0.1%, neomycin sulphate 0.5%, polyvinyl alcohol (*Liquifilm®*) 1.4%. Net price 5 mL = £2.08
Excipients: include benzalkonium chloride, disodium edetate, polysorbate 80

HYDROCORTISONE ACETATE

Indications: local treatment of inflammation (short-term)
Cautions: see notes above
Side-effects: see notes above

Hydrocortisone (Non-proprietary) PoM
Eye drops, hydrocortisone acetate 1%. Net price 10 mL = £3.21
Available from Martindale
Eye ointment, hydrocortisone acetate 0.5%, net price 3 g = £2.10; 1%, 3 g = £2.12; 2.5%, 3 g = £2.16
Available from Martindale

Neo-Cortef® (Dominion) PoM ▰
Drops and *ointment* (for ear or eye), see section 12.1.1
Note. Eye drops containing hydrocortisone acetate 1.5% and neomycin sulphate 0.5% also available from Martindale

PREDNISOLONE

Indications: local treatment of inflammation (short-term)
Cautions: see notes above
Side-effects: see notes above
Administration: apply eye drops every 1–2 hours until controlled then reduce frequency

Pred Forte® (Allergan) PoM
Eye drops, prednisolone acetate 1%. Net price 5 mL = £1.52; 10 mL = £3.05
Excipients: include benzalkonium chloride, disodium edetate, polysorbate 80
Apply 2–4 times daily

Predsol® (Medeva) PoM
Drops (for ear or eye), prednisolone sodium phosphate 0.5%. Net price 10 mL = £1.31
Excipients: include benzalkonium chloride, disodium edetate

Predsol-N® (Medeva) PoM ▰
Drops (for ear or eye), see section 12.1.1

■ Single use
Minims® Prednisolone (Chauvin) PoM
Eye drops, prednisolone sodium phosphate 0.5%. Net price 20 × 0.5 mL = £5.75
Excipients: include disodium edetate

RIMEXOLONE

Indications: local treatment of inflammation (short-term)
Cautions: see notes above
Side-effects: see notes above
Administration: postoperative inflammation, apply 4 times daily for 2 weeks, beginning 24 hours after surgery
Steroid-responsive inflammation, apply at least 4 times daily for up to 4 weeks
Uveitis, apply every hour during daytime in week 1, then every 2 hours in week 2, then 4 times daily in week 3, then twice daily for first 4 days of week 4, then once daily for remaining 3 days of week 4

Vexol® (Alcon) ▼ PoM
Eye drops, rimexolone 1%, net price 5 mL = £5.95
Excipients: include benzalkonium chloride, disodium edetate, polysorbate 80

11.4.2 Other anti-inflammatory preparations

Other preparations used for the topical treatment of inflammation and allergic conjunctivitis include antihistamines, lodoxamide, and sodium cromoglicate.

Topical preparations of **antihistamines** such as eye drops containing **antazoline** (with xylometazoline as *Otrivine-Antistin®*), **azelastine** and **levocabastine** may be used for allergic conjunctivitis.

Sodium cromoglicate (sodium cromoglycate) and **nedocromil sodium** eye drops may be useful for vernal keratoconjunctivitis and other allergic forms of conjunctivitis.

Lodoxamide eye drops are used for allergic conjunctival conditions including seasonal allergic conjunctivitis.

Emedastine eye drops have been introduced recently for seasonal allergic conjunctivitis.

ANTAZOLINE SULPHATE

Indications: allergic conjunctivitis

Otrivine-Antistin® (CIBA Vision)
Eye drops, antazoline sulphate 0.5%, xylometazoline hydrochloride 0.05%. Net price 10 mL = £2.30
Excipients: include benzalkonium chloride, disodium edetate
Apply 2–3 times daily
Note. Xylometazoline is a sympathomimetic; it should be avoided in angle-closure glaucoma and absorption may result in systemic side-effects and the possibility of interaction with other drugs

AZELASTINE HYDROCHLORIDE

Indications: seasonal allergic conjunctivitis
Side-effects: mild transient irritation; bitter taste reported
Administration: ADULT and CHILD over 12 years, apply twice daily, increased if necessary to 4 times daily

Optilast® (ASTA Medica) ▼ PoM
Eye drops, azelastine hydrochloride 0.05%. Net price 6 mL = £6.88
Excipients: include benzalkonium chloride, disodium edetate

EMEDASTINE

Indications: seasonal allergic conjunctivitis
Side-effects: transient burning or stinging; blurred vision, local oedema, keratitis, irritation, dry eye, lacrimation, corneal infiltrates (discontinue) and staining; photophobia; headache, and rhinitis occasionally reported
Administration: ADULT and CHILD over 3 years, apply twice daily

Emadine® (Alcon) ▼ PoM
Eye drops, emedastine 0.05% (as difumarate), net price 5 mL = £7.69
Excipients: include benzalkonium chloride

LEVOCABASTINE

Indications: seasonal allergic conjunctivitis
Side-effects: local irritation, blurred vision, local oedema, urticaria; dyspnoea, headache, drowsiness
Administration: ADULT and CHILD over 9 years, apply twice daily, increased if necessary to 3–4 times daily, discontinue if no improvement within 3 days; max. 4 weeks treatment per year

[1]**Livostin®** (CIBA Vision) PoM
Eye drops, levocabastine 0.05% (as hydrochloride). Net price 4 mL = £8.49
Excipients: include benzalkonium chloride, disodium edetate, polysorbate 80, propylene glycol
1. Levocabastine 0.05% eye drops can be sold to the public (in max. pack size of 4 mL) for treatment of seasonal allergic conjunctivitis in adults and children over 12 years; proprietary brands on sale to the public include *Livostin®Direct* eye drops

LODOXAMIDE

Indications: allergic conjunctivitis
Side-effects: mild transient burning, stinging, itching, and lacrimation; flushing and dizziness reported
Administration: ADULT and CHILD over 4 years, apply eye drops 4 times daily

Alomide® (Alcon) PoM
Ophthalmic solution (= eye drops), lodoxamide 0.1% (as trometamol). Net price 10 mL = £5.48
Excipients: include benzalkonium chloride, disodium edetate

NEDOCROMIL SODIUM

Indications: allergic conjunctivitis; vernal keratoconjunctivitis
Side-effects: transient burning and stinging; distinctive taste reported
Administration: seasonal and perennial conjunctivitis, ADULT and CHILD over 6 years, apply twice daily increased if necessary to 4 times daily; max. 12 weeks treatment for seasonal allergic conjunctivitis
Vernal keratoconjunctivitis, ADULT and CHILD over 6 years, apply 4 times daily

Rapitil® (Rhône-Poulenc Rorer) PoM
Eye drops, nedocromil sodium 2%. Net price 5 mL = £9.75
Excipients: include benzalkonium chloride, disodium edetate

SODIUM CROMOGLICATE

(Sodium cromoglycate)

Indications: allergic conjunctivitis; vernal kerato-conjunctivitis

Side-effects: transient burning and stinging

Administration: apply eye drops 4 times daily, eye ointment 2–3 times daily

¹**Sodium Cromoglicate** (Non-proprietary) PoM
Eye drops, sodium cromoglicate 2%. Net price 13.5 mL = £2.32

Available from Baker Norton (*Hay-Crom® Aqueous*), Cox, Dominion, Rhône-Poulenc Rorer (*Opticrom® Aqueous*), Opus (*Viz-on®*), Pharma-Global (*Vividrin®*)

1. Sodium cromoglicate 2% eye drops can be sold to the public (in max. pack size of 10 mL) for treatment of acute seasonal and perennial allergic conjunctivitis; proprietary brands on sale to the public include *Boots Hayfever Relief*, *Clariteyes®*, *Opticrom® Allergy*, and *Optrex® Hayfever Allergy*

11.5 Mydriatics and cycloplegics

Antimuscarinics dilate the pupil and paralyse the ciliary muscle; they vary in potency and duration of action.

Short-acting, relatively weak mydriatics, such as **tropicamide** 0.5%, facilitate the examination of the fundus of the eye. **Cyclopentolate** 1% or **atropine** are preferable for producing cycloplegia for refraction in young children. Atropine 1% (in ointment form) is sometimes preferred for children under 5 years of age. Atropine, which has a longer duration of action, is also used for the treatment of anterior uveitis mainly to prevent posterior synechiae, often with phenylephrine 10% eye drops (2.5% in children, the elderly, and those with cardiac disease). **Homatropine** 1% is also used in the treatment of anterior segment inflammation, and may be preferred for its shorter duration of action.

CAUTIONS. Darkly pigmented iris is more resistant to pupillary dilatation and caution should be exercised to avoid overdosage. Mydriasis may precipitate acute angle-closure glaucoma in a very few patients, usually aged over 60 years and hypermetropic (long-sighted), who are predisposed to the condition because of a shallow anterior chamber. Phenylephrine may interact with systemically administered monoamine-oxidase inhibitors; other **interactions**: Appendix 1 (sympathomimetics).

DRIVING. Patients should be warned not to drive for 1–2 hours after mydriasis.

SIDE-EFFECTS. Ocular side-effects of mydriatics and cycloplegics include transient stinging and raised intra-ocular pressure; on prolonged administration, local irritation, hyperaemia, oedema and conjunctivitis may occur. Contact dermatitis (conjunctivitis) is not uncommon with the antimuscarinic mydriatic drugs, especially atropine.

Toxic systemic reactions to atropine and cyclopentolate may occur in the very young and the very old; see under Atropine Sulphate (section 1.2) for systemic side-effects of antimuscarinic drugs.

Antimuscarinics

ATROPINE SULPHATE

Indications: refraction procedures in young children; anterior uveitis—see also notes above

Cautions: risk of systemic effects with eye drops in infants under 3 months—eye ointment preferred; see also notes above

Side-effects: see notes above

Atropine (Non-proprietary) PoM
Eye drops, atropine sulphate 0.5%, net price 10 mL = £2.15; 1%, 10 mL = 82p
Available from Martindale
Eye ointment, atropine sulphate 1%. Net price 3 g = £2.51
Available from Martindale

Isopto Atropine® (Alcon) PoM
Eye drops, atropine sulphate 1%, hypromellose 0.5%. Net price 5 mL = 99p
Excipients: include benzalkonium chloride

■ Single use

Minims® Atropine Sulphate (Chauvin) PoM
Eye drops, atropine sulphate 1%. Net price 20 × 0.5 mL = £4.92

CYCLOPENTOLATE HYDROCHLORIDE

Indications: see notes above
Cautions: see notes above
Side-effects: see notes above

Mydrilate® (Boehringer Ingelheim) PoM
Eye drops, cyclopentolate hydrochloride 0.5%, net price 5 mL = 73p; 1%, 5 mL = 98p
Excipients: include benzalkonium chloride

■ Single use

Minims® Cyclopentolate (Chauvin) PoM
Eye drops, cyclopentolate hydrochloride 0.5 and 1%. Net price 20 × 0.5 mL (both) = £4.92

HOMATROPINE HYDROBROMIDE

Indications: see notes above
Cautions: see notes above
Side-effects: see notes above

Homatropine (Non-proprietary) PoM
Eye drops, homatropine hydrobromide 1%, net price 10 mL = £1.86; 2%, 10 mL = £2.04
Available from Martindale

■ Single use

Minims® Homatropine Hydrobromide (Chauvin) PoM
Eye drops, homatropine hydrobromide 2%. Net price 20 × 0.5 mL = £5.75

TROPICAMIDE

Indications: see notes above
Cautions: see notes above
Side-effects: see notes above

Mydriacyl® (Alcon) <u>PoM</u>
Eye drops, tropicamide 0.5%, net price 5 mL =
£1.36; 1%, 5 mL = £1.68
Excipients: include benzalkonium chloride, disodium edetate

■ Single use
Minims® Tropicamide (Chauvin) <u>PoM</u>
Eye drops, tropicamide 0.5 and 1%. Net price 20 ×
0.5 mL (both) = £5.75

Sympathomimetics

PHENYLEPHRINE HYDROCHLORIDE

Indications: mydriasis; see also notes above
Cautions: children and elderly (avoid 10%
strength); cardiovascular disease (avoid or use
2.5% strength only); tachycardia; hyperthyroidism; diabetes; see also notes above
Contra-indications: angle-closure glaucoma
Side-effects: eye pain and stinging; blurred vision,
photophobia; systemic effects include arrhythmias, hypertension, coronary artery spasm

Phenylephrine (Non-proprietary)
Eye drops, phenylephrine hydrochloride 10%. Net
price 10 mL = £2.93
Available from Martindale
See also under Hypromellose (section 11.8.1)

■ Single use
Minims® Phenylephrine Hydrochloride
(Chauvin)
Eye drops, phenylephrine hydrochloride 2.5%, net
price 20 × 0.5 mL = £5.75; 10%, 20 × 0.5 mL =
£5.75
Excipients: include disodium edetate

11.6 Treatment of glaucoma

Glaucoma is usually (but not always) associated
with an abnormally high intra-ocular pressure; it
may result in blindness. The rise in pressure is
almost always due to reduced outflow of aqueous
humour, the inflow remaining constant. Treatment
is aimed at reducing intra-ocular pressure.

Probably the commonest condition is *chronic
simple glaucoma* where the obstruction is in the
trabecular meshwork. It is commonly first treated
with a topical beta-blocker and other drugs added as
necessary to control the intra-ocular pressure e.g.
adrenaline or pilocarpine.

Dorzolamide, a topical carbonic anhydrase inhibitor, can be used as an alternative to topical beta-
blockers or as an adjunct to them. Acetazolamide is
a carbonic anhydrase inhibitor which is given by
mouth.

Brimonidine, a selective alpha$_2$-adrenoceptor
stimulant, is licensed for open-angle glaucoma and
ocular hypertension when other drugs are inappropriate.

Apraclonidine (section 11.8.2) is an alpha$_2$-
adrenoceptor stimulant which reduces the rate of
production of aqueous humour.

Latanoprost is a prostaglandin analogue which
increases the uveoscleral outflow of aqueous

humour. It is indicated for open-angle glaucoma
and ocular hypertension in patients for whom other
drugs are inappropriate.

In emergency or before surgery, mannitol 20%
(up to max. of 500 mL) should be given by slow
intravenous infusion until the intra-ocular pressure
has been satisfactorily reduced. Acetazolamide by
intravenous injection may also be used for the
emergency management of raised intra-ocular pressure.

If supplementary topical treatment is required
after *iridectomy* or a drainage operation in either
open-angle or angle-closure glaucoma, a beta-
blocker is preferred to pilocarpine. This is because
of the risk that posterior synechiae will be formed
as a result of the miotic effect of pilocarpine, especially in angle-closure glaucoma.

Miotics

The small pupil is an unfortunate side-effect of
these drugs (except when pilocarpine is used temporarily before an operation for *angle-closure
glaucoma*). They act by opening up the inefficient
drainage channels in the trabecular meshwork
resulting from contraction or spasm of the ciliary
muscle.

Miotics used in the management of raised intra-
ocular pressure include carbachol and pilocarpine;
ecothiopate iodide (as *Phospholine Iodide®*,
Dominion) is no longer on the UK market but is
still available on a named-patient basis for use
under expert supervision.

CAUTIONS. A darkly pigmented iris may require
higher concentration of the miotic or more frequent
administration and care should be taken to avoid
overdosage. Retinal detachment has occurred in
susceptible individuals and those with retinal disease; therefore fundus examination is advised
before starting treatment with a miotic. Care is also
required in conjunctival or corneal damage. Intra-
ocular pressure and visual fields should be monitored in those with chronic simple glaucoma and
those receiving long-term treatment with a miotic.
Miotics should be used with caution in cardiac disease, hypertension, asthma, peptic ulceration,
urinary-tract obstruction, and Parkinson's disease.
COUNSELLING. Blurred vision may affect performance of
skilled tasks (e.g. driving) particularly at night or in
reduced lighting

CONTRA-INDICATIONS. Miotics are contra-indicated in conditions where pupillary constriction is
undesirable such as anterior iritis, anterior uveitis and
some forms of secondary glaucoma. They should be
avoided in acute inflammatory disease of the anterior segment.

SIDE-EFFECTS. Ciliary spasm leads to headache
and browache which may be more severe in the initial 2–4 weeks of treatment (a particular disadvantage in patients under 40 years of age). Ocular side-
effects include burning, itching, smarting, blurred
vision, conjunctival vascular congestion, myopia,
lens changes with chronic use, vitreous haemorrhage, and pupillary block. Systemic side-effects
(see under Parasympathomimetics, section 7.4.1)
are rare following application to the eye.

CARBACHOL

Indications: see notes above
Cautions: see notes above
Contra-indications: see notes above
Side-effects: see notes above
Administration: apply eye drops up to 4 times daily

Isopto Carbachol® (Alcon) PoM
Eye drops, carbachol 3%, hypromellose 1%. Net price 10 mL = £1.76
Excipients: include benzalkonium chloride

PILOCARPINE

Indications: see notes above; dry mouth (section 12.3.5)
Cautions: see notes above
Contra-indications: see notes above
Side-effects: see notes above
Administration: apply eye drops up to 4 times daily

Pilocarpine Hydrochloride (Non-proprietary) PoM
Eye drops, pilocarpine hydrochloride 0.5%, net price 10 mL = £1.34; 1%, 10 mL = 98p; 2%, 10 mL = £1.11; 3%, 10 mL = £1.36; 4%, 10 mL = £1.53
Available from Cox, Hillcross, Martindale

Isopto Carpine® (Alcon) PoM
Eye drops, all with hypromellose 0.5%; pilocarpine hydrochloride 0.5%, net price 10 mL = 73p; 1%, 10 mL = 81p; 2%, 10 mL = 90p; 3%, 10 mL = 97p; 4%, 10 mL = £1.04
Excipients: include benzalkonium chloride

■ Single use
Minims® Pilocarpine Nitrate (Chauvin) PoM
Eye drops, pilocarpine nitrate 1, 2, and 4%, net price 20 × 0.5 mL (all) = £4.92

■ Long acting
Ocusert® (Dominion) PoM
Pilo-20 ocular insert, pilocarpine 20 micrograms released per hour for 1 week, net price pack of 8 inserts = £33.50. Counselling, method of use
Pilo-40 ocular insert, pilocarpine 40 micrograms released per hour for 1 week, net price pack of 8 inserts = £39.06. Counselling, method of use

Pilogel® (Alcon) PoM
Ophthalmic gel, pilocarpine hydrochloride 4%, carbomer 940 (polyacrylic acid) 3.5%, net price 5 g = £6.86
Excipients: include benzalkonium chloride, disodium edetate
Apply 1–1.5 cm gel once daily at bedtime

Sympathomimetics

Adrenaline (**epinephrine**) probably acts both by reducing the rate of production of aqueous humour and by increasing the outflow through the trabecular meshwork. It is contra-indicated in angle-closure glaucoma because it is a mydriatic, unless an iridectomy has been carried out. Side-effects include severe smarting and redness of the eye; adrenaline should be used with caution in patients with hypertension and heart disease.

Dipivefrine is a pro-drug of adrenaline. It is claimed to pass more rapidly through the cornea and is then converted to the active form.

Guanethidine enhances and prolongs the effects of adrenaline. Prolonged use, particularly of the higher strength, may result in conjunctival fibrosis with secondary corneal changes; the conjunctiva and cornea should be examined at least every six months.

Brimonidine, a selective alpha$_2$-adrenoceptor stimulant, is licensed for the reduction of intra-ocular pressure in open-angle glaucoma or ocular hypertension in patients for whom beta-blockers are inappropriate; it may also be used as adjunctive therapy when intra-ocular pressure is inadequately controlled by a beta-blocker alone.

Apraclonidine (section 11.8.2) is another alpha$_2$-adrenoceptor stimulant. Eye drops containing apraclonidine 0.5% are used for a short term to delay laser treatment or surgery for glaucoma in patients not adequately controlled by another drug; eye drops containing 1% are used for control of intra-ocular pressure after anterior segment laser surgery.

ADRENALINE/EPINEPHRINE

Indications: see notes above
Contra-indications: see notes above
Side-effects: see notes above
Administration: apply eye drops 1–2 times daily

Eppy® (Chauvin) PoM
Eye drops, adrenaline 1%, net price 7.5 mL = £4.06
Excipients: include benzalkonium chloride, also acetylcysteine as antioxidant

Simplene® (Chauvin) PoM
Eye drops, adrenaline, in a viscous vehicle, 0.5%, net price 7.5 mL = £3.45; 1%, 7.5 mL = £3.79
Excipients: include benzalkonium chloride, also acetylcysteine as antioxidant

BRIMONIDINE TARTRATE

Indications: adjunct to beta-blockers or used alone in raised intra-ocular pressure in ocular hypertension or open-angle glaucoma in patients unresponsive to beta-blockers or if beta-blockers contra-indicated
Cautions: severe cardiovascular disease; cerebral or coronary insufficiency, Raynaud's syndrome, postural hypotension, depression, hepatic or renal impairment; pregnancy, breast-feeding; **interactions:** Appendix 1 (alpha$_2$-adrenoceptor stimulants)
DRIVING. Drowsiness may affect performance of skilled tasks (e.g. driving)
Side-effects: ocular reactions include hyperaemia, burning, stinging, blurring, pruritus, allergy, and conjunctival follicles; occasionally corneal erosion and staining, photophobia, eyelid inflammation, conjunctivitis; headache, dry mouth, taste alteration, fatigue, dizziness, drowsiness reported; rarely depression, nasal dryness, palpitations, and hypersensitivity reactions
Administration: apply one drop twice daily

Alphagan® (Allergan) ▼ PoM
Eye drops, brimonidine tartrate 0.2%, net price 5 mL = £10.31
Excipients: include benzalkonium chloride

DIPIVEFRINE HYDROCHLORIDE

Indications: as for Adrenaline/Epinephrine, see notes above
Contra-indications: see notes above
Side-effects: see notes above
Administration: apply 1 drop twice daily

Propine® (Allergan) [PoM]
Eye drops, dipivefrine hydrochloride 0.1%, net price 5 mL = £3.81, 10 mL = £4.77
Excipients: include benzalkonium chloride, disodium edetate

GUANETHIDINE MONOSULPHATE

Indications: see notes above
Cautions: see notes above
Administration: apply eye drops 1–2 times daily

Ganda® (Chauvin) [PoM]
Eye drops '1 + 0.2', guanethidine monosulphate 1%, adrenaline 0.2% in a viscous vehicle, net price 7.5 mL = £4.49
Excipients: include benzalkonium chloride
Eye drops '3 + 0.5', guanethidine monosulphate 3%, adrenaline 0.5% in a viscous vehicle, net price 7.5 mL = £5.86
Excipients: include benzalkonium chloride

Beta-blockers

Topical application of a beta-blocker to the eye reduces intra-ocular pressure effectively in *chronic simple glaucoma*, probably by reducing the rate of production of aqueous humour. Administration by mouth also reduces intra-ocular pressure but this route is not used since side-effects may be troublesome.

Beta-blockers used as eye drops include **betaxolol**, **carteolol**, **levobunolol**, **metipranolol**, and **timolol**.

CAUTIONS, CONTRA-INDICATIONS AND SIDE-EFFECTS. Systemic absorption may follow topical application therefore eye drops containing a beta-blocker are contra-indicated in patients with bradycardia, heart block, or uncontrolled heart failure. **Important:** for a warning to avoid in asthma see CSM advice below. Consider also other cautions, contra-indications and side-effects of beta-blockers (p. 76). Local side-effects of eye drops include ocular stinging, burning, pain, itching, erythema, dry eyes and allergic blepharoconjunctivitis; occasionally corneal disorders have been reported.

CSM advice. The CSM has advised that beta-blockers, even those with apparent cardioselectivity, should not be used in patients with asthma or a history of obstructive airways disease, unless no alternative treatment is available. In such cases the risk of inducing bronchospasm should be appreciated and appropriate precautions taken.

INTERACTIONS. Since systemic absorption may follow topical application the possibility of interactions, in particular, with drugs such as verapamil should be borne in mind. See also Appendix 1 (beta-blockers).

BETAXOLOL HYDROCHLORIDE

Indications: see notes above
Cautions: see notes above
Contra-indications: see notes above
Side-effects: see notes above
Administration: apply eye drops twice daily

Betoptic® (Alcon) [PoM]
Ophthalmic solution (= eye drops), betaxolol (as hydrochloride) 0.5%, net price 5 mL = £4.23
Excipients: include benzalkonium chloride, disodium edetate
Ophthalmic suspension (= eye drops), m/r, betaxolol (as hydrochloride) 0.25%, net price 5 mL = £4.77
Excipients: include benzalkonium chloride, disodium edetate
Unit dose eye drop suspension, m/r, betaxolol (as hydrochloride) 0.25%, net price 50 × 0.25 mL = £14.49

CARTEOLOL HYDROCHLORIDE

Indications: see notes above
Cautions: see notes above
Contra-indications: see notes above
Side-effects: see notes above
Administration: apply eye drops twice daily

Teoptic® (CIBA Vision) [PoM]
Eye drops, carteolol hydrochloride 1%, net price 5 mL = £4.60; 2%, 5 mL = £5.40
Excipients: include benzalkonium chloride

LEVOBUNOLOL HYDROCHLORIDE

Indications: see notes above
Cautions: see notes above
Contra-indications: see notes above
Side-effects: see notes above; anterior uveitis occasionally reported
Administration: apply eye drops once or twice daily

Betagan® (Allergan) [PoM]
Eye drops, levobunolol hydrochloride 0.5%, polyvinyl alcohol (*Liquifilm®*) 1.4%. Net price 5-mL= £4.66, triple pack (3 × 5 mL) = £11.89
Excipients: include benzalkonium chloride, disodium edetate
Unit dose eye drops, levobunolol hydrochloride 0.5%, polyvinyl alcohol (*Liquifilm®*) 1.4%. Net price 30 × 0.4 mL = £9.98
Excipients: include disodium edetate

METIPRANOLOL

Indications: see notes above but in chronic open-angle glaucoma **restricted** to patients allergic to preservatives or to those wearing soft contact lenses (in whom benzalkonium chloride should be avoided)
Cautions: see notes above
Contra-indications: see notes above
Side-effects: see notes above; granulomatous anterior uveitis reported (discontinue treatment)
Administration: apply eye drops twice daily

Minims® Metipranolol (Chauvin) [PoM]
Eye drops, metipranolol 0.1%, net price 20 × 0.5 mL = £10.19; 0.3%, 20 × 0.5 mL = £11.09

TIMOLOL MALEATE

Indications: see notes above
Cautions: see notes above
Contra-indications: see notes above
Side-effects: see notes above
Administration: apply eye drops twice daily; long acting preparations, see under preparations below

Timolol (Non-proprietary) [PoM]
Eye drops, timolol (as maleate) 0.25%, net price 5 mL = £4.23; 0.5%, 5 mL = £4.57
Available from APS, Bioglan, Cox, Hillcross, Lagap, Martindale, Norton, Opus (*Glau-opt®*)

Timoptol® (MSD) [PoM]
Eye drops, in Ocumeter® metered-dose unit, timolol (as maleate) 0.25%, net price 5 mL = £3.55; 0.5%, 5 mL = £3.55
Excipients: include benzalkonium chloride
Unit dose eye drops, timolol (as maleate) 0.25%, net price 30 × 0.2 mL = £9.60; 0.5%, 30 × 0.2 mL = £10.97

■ Long acting

Timoptol®-LA (MSD) [PoM]
Ophthalmic gel-forming solution (= eye drops), timolol (as maleate) 0.25%, net price 2.5 mL = £3.55; 0.5%, 2.5 mL = £3.55
Excipients: include benzododecinium bromide
Apply eye drops once daily

■ With dorzolamide
See under Dorzolamide

Carbonic anhydrase inhibitors and systemic drugs

The **carbonic anhydrase inhibitors**, acetazolamide and dorzolamide, reduce intra-ocular pressure by reducing aqueous humour production. Systemic use also produces weak diuresis.

Acetazolamide is given by mouth or by intravenous injection (intramuscular injections are painful because of the alkaline pH of the solution). Acetazolamide is a sulphonamide; blood disorders, rashes and other sulphonamide-related side-effects occur occasionally. It is not generally recommended for long-term use but electrolyte disturbances and metabolic acidosis that occur may be corrected by administering potassium bicarbonate (as effervescent potassium tablets, section 9.2.1.3).

Dorzolamide, a topical carbonic anhydrase inhibitor, is licensed for use in patients resistant to beta-blockers or those in whom beta-blockers are contra-indicated. It is used alone or as an adjunct to a topical beta-blocker. Systemic absorption may rarely give rise to sulphonamide-like side-effects and may require discontinuation if severe.

The **osmotic diuretics**, intravenous hypertonic **mannitol**, or **glycerol** by mouth, are useful short-term ocular hypotensive drugs.

ACETAZOLAMIDE

Indications: reduction of intra-ocular pressure in open-angle glaucoma, secondary glaucoma, and peri-operatively in angle-closure glaucoma; diuresis (section 2.2.7); epilepsy

Cautions: not generally recommended for prolonged use but if given monitor blood count and plasma electrolyte concentration; pulmonary obstruction (risk of acidosis); elderly; pregnancy and breast-feeding; avoid extravasation at injection site (risk of necrosis); **interactions:** Appendix 1 (diuretics)

Contra-indications: hypokalaemia, hyponatraemia, hyperchloraemic acidosis; severe hepatic impairment; renal impairment; sulphonamide hypersensitivity

Side-effects: nausea, vomiting, diarrhoea, taste disturbance; loss of appetite, paraesthesia, flushing, headache, dizziness, fatigue, irritability, depression; thirst, polyuria; reduced libido; metabolic acidosis and electrolyte disturbances on long-term therapy; occasionally, drowsiness, confusion, hearing disturbances, urticaria, malaena, glycosuria, haematuria, abnormal liver function, renal calculi, blood disorders including agranulocytosis and thrombocytopenia, rashes including Stevens-Johnson syndrome and toxic epidermal necrolysis; rarely, photosensitivity, liver damage, flaccid paralysis, convulsions; transient myopia reported

Dose: glaucoma, *by mouth or by intravenous injection*, 0.25–1 g daily in divided doses
Epilepsy, 0.25–1 g daily in divided doses; CHILD 8–30 mg/kg daily, max. 750 mg daily
By intramuscular injection, as for intravenous injection but preferably avoided because of alkalinity

Diamox® (Wyeth) [PoM]
Tablets, acetazolamide 250 mg. Net price 112-tab pack = £11.53. Label: 3
Sodium Parenteral (= injection), powder for reconstitution, acetazolamide (as sodium salt). Net price 500-mg vial = £14.76

Diamox® SR (Wyeth) [PoM]
Capsules, m/r, two-tone orange, enclosing orange f/c pellets, acetazolamide 250 mg. Net price 28-cap pack = £10.50. Label: 3, 25
Dose: glaucoma, 1–2 capsules daily

DORZOLAMIDE

Indications: adjunct to beta-blockers or used alone in raised intra-ocular pressure in ocular hypertension, open-angle glaucoma, or pseudoexfoliative glaucoma in patients unresponsive to beta-blockers or if beta-blockers contra-indicated

Cautions: hepatic impairment; systemic absorption follows topical application; **interactions:** Appendix 1 (dorzolamide)

Contra-indications: severe renal impairment or hyperchloraemic acidosis; pregnancy and breast-feeding

Side-effects: burning, stinging and itching of the eye, bitter taste, blurred vision, tearing, conjunctivitis, superficial punctate keratitis, eyelid inflammation, anterior uveitis, transient myopia; headache, dizziness, paraesthesia, asthenia, nausea; rash and allergic reactions (including urticaria, angioedema, bronchosopasm); urolithiasis

Administration: used alone, apply 3 times daily; with topical beta-blocker, apply twice daily

Trusopt® (MSD) [PoM]
Ophthalmic solution (= eye drops), dorzolamide (as hydrochloride) 2%, net price 5 mL = £9.31
Excipients: include benzalkonium chloride

■ With timolol

For cautions, contra-indications, and side-effects of timolol, see section 11.6, Beta-blockers

Cosopt® (MSD) ▼ PoM

Ophthalmic solution (= eye drops), dorzolamide (as hydrochloride) 2%, timolol (as maleate) 0.5%, net price 5 mL = £13.50

Excipients: include benzalkonium chloride

For raised intra-ocular pressure in open-angle glaucoma, or pseudoexfoliative glaucoma when beta-blockers alone not adequate, apply twice daily

Prostaglandin analogue

Latanoprost, a recently introduced prostaglandin analogue, increases uveoscleral outflow. It is indicated for open-angle glaucoma and ocular hypertension when other drugs are inappropriate; there is little experience of its use in other variants of glaucoma. Patients should be monitored for any changes to eye coloration since latanoprost may increase the brown pigment in the iris; particular care is required in those with mixed coloured irides and those receiving treatment to one eye only.

LATANOPROST

Indications: raised intra-ocular pressure in open-angle glaucoma and ocular hypertension in patients intolerant or unresponsive to other drugs

Cautions: before initiating treatment, advise patients of possible change in eye colour; monitor for eye colour change; brittle or severe asthma; not to be used within 5 minutes of use of thiomersal-containing preparations; manufacturer advises avoid in pregnancy and in breast-feeding

Side-effects: brown pigmentation particularly in those with mixed coloured irides (withdraw treatment if possible); ocular irritation; darkening, thickening and lengthening of eye lashes; conjunctival hyperaemia; transient punctate epithelial erosions; macular oedema, iritis and uveitis reported rarely; darkening of palpebral skin reported very rarely

Administration: apply 1 drop once daily, preferably in the evening

Xalatan® (Pharmacia & Upjohn) ▼ PoM

Eye-drops, latanoprost 50 micrograms/mL, net price 2.5 mL = £15.28

Excipients: include benzalkonium chloride

11.7   Local anaesthetics

Oxybuprocaine and tetracaine (amethocaine) are probably the most widely used topical local anaesthetics. Proxymetacaine causes less initial stinging and is useful for children. Oxybuprocaine or a combined preparation of lidocaine (lignocaine) and fluorescein is used for tonometry. Tetracaine produces a more profound anaesthesia and is suitable for use before minor surgical procedures, such as the removal of corneal sutures. It has a temporary disruptive effect on the corneal epithelium. Lidocaine, with or without adrenaline (epinephrine), is injected into the eyelids for minor surgery, while retrobulbar or peribulbar injections are used for surgery of the globe itself. Local anaesthetics should never be used for the management of ocular symptoms.

LIDOCAINE HYDROCHLORIDE/ LIGNOCAINE HYDROCHLORIDE

Indications: local anaesthetic

Minims® Lignocaine and Fluorescein (Chauvin) PoM

Eye drops, lidocaine hydrochloride 4%, fluorescein sodium 0.25%. Net price 20 × 0.5 mL = £6.93

OXYBUPROCAINE HYDROCHLORIDE

Indications: local anaesthetic

Minims® Benoxinate (Oxybuprocaine) Hydrochloride (Chauvin) PoM

Eye drops, oxybuprocaine hydrochloride 0.4%. Net price 20 × 0.5 mL = £4.92

PROXYMETACAINE HYDROCHLORIDE

Indications: local anaesthetic

Minims® Proxymetacaine Hydrochloride (Chauvin) PoM

Eye drops, proxymetacaine hydrochloride 0.5%. Net price 20 × 0.5 mL = £6.95

■ With fluorescein

Minims® Proxymetacaine and Fluorescein (Chauvin) PoM

Eye drops, proxymetacaine hydrochloride 0.5%, fluorescein sodium 0.25%. Net price 20 × 0.5 mL = £7.95

TETRACAINE HYDROCHLORIDE/ AMETHOCAINE HYDROCHLORIDE

Indications: local anaesthetic

Minims® Amethocaine Hydrochloride (Chauvin) PoM

Eye drops, tetracaine hydrochloride 0.5 and 1%. Net price 20 × 0.5 mL (both) = £5.75

11.8   Miscellaneous ophthalmic preparations

11.8.1   Tear deficiency, ocular lubricants and astringents

11.8.2   Ocular diagnostic and peri-operative preparations

Certain eye drops, e.g. amphotericin, ceftazidime, cefuroxime, colistin, desferrioxamine, dexamethasone, gentamicin and vancomycin may be prepared aseptically from material supplied for injection; for details on preparation of trisodium edetate eye drops see section 9.5.1.2.

11.8.1 Tear deficiency, ocular lubricants, and astringents

Chronic soreness of the eyes associated with reduced or abnormal tear secretion (e.g. in Sjögren's syndrome) often responds to tear replacement therapy. The severity of the condition and patient preference will often guide the choice of preparation.

Hypromellose is the traditional choice of treatment for tear deficiency. It may need to be instilled frequently (e.g. hourly) for adequate relief. Ocular surface mucin is often abnormal in tear deficiency and the combination of hypromellose with a mucolytic such as **acetylcysteine** can be helpful.

The ability of **carbomers** to cling to the eye surface may help reduce frequency of application to 4 times daily.

Polyvinyl alcohol increases the persistence of the tear film and is useful when the ocular surface mucin is reduced.

Povidone eye drops are also used in the management of tear deficiency.

Sodium chloride 0.9% drops are sometimes useful in tear deficiency, and can be used as 'comfort drops' by contact lens wearers, and to facilitate lens removal.

Eye ointments containing **paraffin** may be used to lubricate the eye surface, especially in cases of recurrent corneal epithelial erosion. They may cause temporary visual disturbance and are best suited for application before sleep. Ointments should not be used during contact lens wear.

Zinc sulphate is a traditional astringent that is now little used.

ACETYLCYSTEINE

Indications: tear deficiency, impaired or abnormal mucus production
Administration: apply eye drops 3–4 times daily

Ilube® (Alcon) [PoM]
Eye drops, acetylcysteine 5%, hypromellose 0.35%. Net price 10 mL = £4.63
Excipients: include benzalkonium chloride, disodium edetate

CARBOMERS
(Polyacrylic acid)
Synthetic high molecular weight polymers of acrylic acid cross-linked with either allyl ethers of sucrose or allyl ethers of pentaerithrityl
Indications: dry eyes including keratoconjunctivitis sicca, unstable tear film
Administration: apply 3–4 times daily or as required

GelTears® (Chauvin)
Gel (= eye drops), carbomer 940 (polyacrylic acid) 0.2%. Net price 10 g = £2.90
Excipients: include benzalkonium chloride

Viscotears® (CIBA Vision)
Liquid gel (= eye drops), carbomer 940 (polyacrylic acid) 0.2%. Net price 10 g = £2.85
Excipients: include cetrimide, disodium edetate

HYDROXYETHYLCELLULOSE
Indications: tear deficiency

Minims® Artificial Tears (Chauvin)
Eye drops, hydroxyethylcellulose 0.44%. Net price 20 × 0.5 mL = £5.75

HYPROMELLOSE
Indications: tear deficiency

Hypromellose (Non-proprietary)
Eye drops, hypromellose 0.3%, net price 10 mL = 95p
Available from Cox, Martindale, Norton

Isopto Alkaline® (Alcon)
Eye drops, hypromellose 1%, net price 10 mL = 99p
Excipients: include benzalkonium chloride

Isopto Plain® (Alcon)
Eye drops, hypromellose 0.5%, net price 10 mL = 85p
Excipients: include benzalkonium chloride

Moisture-eyes® (Co-Pharma)
Eye drops, hypromellose 0.3% (buffered), net price 10 mL = £1.13
Excipients: include benzalkonium chloride

Tears Naturale® (Alcon)
Eye drops, dextran '70' 0.1%, hypromellose 0.3%, net price 15 mL = £1.68
Excipients: include benzalkonium chloride, disodium edetate

■ Single use
Artelac® SDU (Pharma-Global)
Eye drops, hypromellose 0.32%, net price 30 × 0.5 mL = £9.95

■ With phenylephrine
Note. Phenylephrine (section 11.5) acts to constrict conjunctival vessels, thus producing a whiter eye; it is not recommended for prolonged use

Isopto Frin® (Alcon) [image]
Eye drops, phenylephrine hydrochloride 0.12%, hypromellose 0.5%, net price 10 mL = £1.14
Excipients: include benzethonium chloride
Temporary relief of redness due to minor irritation, apply up to 4 times daily

▰ denotes preparations that are considered to be less suitable for prescribing (see p. vi)

LIQUID PARAFFIN
Indications: dry eye conditions

Lacri-Lube® (Allergan)
Eye ointment, white soft paraffin 57.3%, liquid paraffin 42.5%, wool alcohols 0.2%. Net price 3.5 g = £1.90, 5 g = £2.47

Lubri-Tears® (Alcon)
Eye ointment, white soft paraffin 60%, liquid paraffin 30%, wool fat 10%. Net price 5 g = £2.29

PARAFFIN, YELLOW, SOFT
Indications: see notes above

Simple Eye Ointment, liquid paraffin 10%, wool fat 10%, in yellow soft paraffin. Net price 4 g = £2.45
Available from Martindale

POLYVINYL ALCOHOL

Indications: tear deficiency

Hypotears® (CIBA Vision)
Eye drops, macrogol '8000' 2%, polyvinyl alcohol 1%. Net price 15 mL = £1.09
Excipients: include benzalkonium chloride, disodium edetate

Liquifilm Tears® (Allergan)
Ophthalmic solution (= eye drops), polyvinyl alcohol 1.4%. Net price 15 mL = £1.61
Excipients: include benzalkonium chloride, disodium edetate
Ophthalmic solution (= eye drops), polyvinyl alcohol 1.4%, povidone 0.6%. Net price 30 × 0.4 mL = £5.35

Sno Tears® (Chauvin)
Eye drops, polyvinyl alcohol 1.4%. Net price 10 mL = £1.10
Excipients: include benzalkonium chloride, disodium edetate

POVIDONE

Indications: dry eye conditions
Administration: apply 4 times daily or as required

Oculotect® (CIBA Vision)
Eye drops, povidone 5%. Net price 20 × 0.4 mL = £3.40

SODIUM CHLORIDE

Indications: irrigation, including first-aid removal of harmful substances

Sodium Chloride 0.9% Solutions
See section 13.11.1
Balanced Salt Solution
Solution (sterile), sodium chloride 0.64%, sodium acetate 0.39%, sodium citrate 0.17%, calcium chloride 0.048%, magnesium chloride 0.03%, potassium chloride 0.075%
For intra-ocular or topical irrigation during surgical procedures
Available from Alcon (15 mL, 250 mL and 500 mL) and from CIBA Vision (*Iocare®*, 15 mL and 500 mL)

■ Single use
Minims® Sodium Chloride (Chauvin)
Eye drops, sodium chloride 0.9%. Net price 20 × 0.5 mL = £4.92

ZINC SULPHATE

Indications: see notes above
Cautions: see notes above

Zinc Sulphate (Non-proprietary)
Eye drops, zinc sulphate 0.25%. Net price 10 mL = £2.76
Available from Martindale

| 11.8.2 | Ocular diagnostic and peri-operative preparations |

Ocular diagnostic preparations

Fluorescein sodium and **rose bengal** are used in diagnostic procedures and for locating damaged areas of the cornea due to injury or disease. Rose bengal is more efficient for the diagnosis of conjunctival epithelial damage but it stings excessively unless a local anaesthetic is instilled beforehand.

FLUORESCEIN SODIUM

Indications: detection of lesions and foreign bodies

Minims® Fluorescein Sodium (Chauvin)
Eye drops, fluorescein sodium 1 or 2%. Net price 20 × 0.5 mL (both) = £4.92

■ With local anaesthetic
Section 11.7

ROSE BENGAL

Indications: detection of lesions and foreign bodies

Minims® Rose Bengal (Chauvin)
Eye drops, rose bengal 1%. Net price 20 × 0.5 mL = £5.75

Ocular peri-operative drugs

Drugs used to prepare the eye for surgery and drugs that are injected into the anterior chamber at the time of surgery are included here. Sodium hyaluronate preparations (*Healonid®*, Pharmacia & Upjohn; *Ophthalin®*, CIBA Vision) are used during surgical procedures on the eye.

Special presentations of **sodium chloride 0.9%** solution are used routinely in intra-ocular surgery (section 11.8.1).

ACETYLCHOLINE CHLORIDE

Indications: cataract surgery, penetrating keratoplasty, iridectomy, and other anterior segment surgery requiring rapid complete miosis

Miochol® (CIBA Vision) [PoM]
Solution for intra-ocular irrigation, acetylcholine chloride 1%, mannitol 3% when reconstituted. Net price 2 mL-vial = £8.32

APRACLONIDINE

Note. Apraclonidine is a derivative of clonidine
Indications: control of intra-ocular pressure
Cautions: history of angina, severe coronary insufficiency, recent myocardial infarction, cardiac failure, cerebrovascular disease, vasovagal attack, chronic renal failure; depression; pregnancy and breast-feeding; monitor intra-ocular pressure and visual fields; loss of effect may occur over time; suspend treatment if reduction in vision occurs in end-stage glaucoma; exaggerated reduction in intra-ocular pressure following peri-operative use should be closely monitored; **interactions:** Appendix 1 (alpha$_2$-adrenoceptor stimulants)
DRIVING. Drowsiness may affect performance of skilled tasks (e.g. driving)
Contra-indications: history of severe or unstable and uncontrolled cardiovascular disease
Side-effects: dry mouth, taste disturbance; hyperaemia, ocular pruritus, discomfort and tearing (withdraw if ocular intolerance including oedema of lids and conjunctiva); headache, asthenia, dry nose; lid retraction, conjunctival blanching and mydriasis reported after peri-operative use; since absorption may follow topical application systemic effects (see Clonidine Hydrochloride, section 2.5.2) may occur
Administration: see under preparations below

Iopidine® (Alcon) [PoM]

Ophthalmic solution (= eye drops), apraclonidine 1% (as hydrochloride). Net price 12 × 2 single use 0.25-mL units = £81.90

Administration: control or prevention of postoperative elevation of intra-ocular pressure after anterior segment laser surgery, apply 1 drop 1 hour before laser procedure then 1 drop immediately after completion of procedure; CHILD not recommended

Iopidine 0.5% ophthalmic solution (= eye drops), apraclonidine 0.5% (as hydrochloride). Net price 5 mL = £11.45

Excipients: include benzalkonium chloride

Administration: short-term adjunctive treatment of chronic glaucoma in patients not adequately controlled by another drug (see note below), apply 1 drop 3 times daily usually for max. 1 month; CHILD not recommended

Note. May not provide additional benefit if patient already using two drugs that suppress the production of aqueous humour

---

DICLOFENAC SODIUM

Indications: inhibition of intraoperative miosis during cataract surgery (but does not possess intrinsic mydriatic properties); postoperative inflammation in cataract surgery; pain in corneal epithelial defects after photorefractive keratectomy or accidental trauma

Voltarol® Ophtha (CIBA Vision) [PoM]

Eye drops, diclofenac sodium 0.1%. Net price pack of 5 single-dose units = £4.00, 40 single-dose units = £32.00

FLURBIPROFEN SODIUM

Indications: inhibition of intraoperative miosis (but does not possess intrinsic mydriatic properties); anterior segment inflammation following postoperative and post-laser trabeculoplasty when corticosteroids contra-indicated

Ocufen® (Allergan) [PoM]

Ophthalmic solution (= eye drops), flurbiprofen sodium 0.03%, polyvinyl alcohol (Liquifilm®) 1.4%. Net price 40 × 0.4 mL = £37.15

KETOROLAC TROMETAMOL

Indications: prophylaxis and reduction of inflammation and associated symptoms following ocular surgery

Acular® (Allergan) [PoM]

Eye drops, ketorolac trometamol 0.5%. Net price 5 mL = £6.68

Excipients: include benzalkonium chloride, disodium edetate

11.9   Contact lenses

Note. Some recommendations in this section involve non-licensed indications.

For cosmetic reasons many people prefer to wear contact lenses rather than spectacles; contact lenses are also sometimes required for medical indications. Visual defects are corrected by either rigid ('hard' or gas permeable) lenses or soft (hydrogel) lenses; soft lenses are the most popular type, because they are the most comfortable, though they may not give the best vision. Lenses should usually be worn for a specified number of hours each day. Continuous (extended) wear involves much greater risks to eye health and is not recommended except where medically indicated.

Contact lenses require meticulous care. Poor compliance with directions for use, and with daily cleaning and disinfection, may result in complications which include ulcerative keratitis, conjunctival problems (such as purulent or papillary conjunctivitis). One-day disposable lenses, which are worn only once and therefore require no maintenance or storage, are becoming increasingly popular.

Acanthamoeba keratitis, a sight-threatening condition, is associated with ineffective lens cleaning and disinfection or the use of contaminated lens cases. The condition is especially associated with the use of soft lenses (including frequently replaced lenses). Acanthamoeba keratitis is treated by specialists with intensive use of polihexanide (polyhexamethylene biguanide), propamidine isetionate, chlorhexidine and neomycin drops, sometimes in combination.

CONTACT LENSES AND DRUG TREATMENT. Special care is required in prescribing eye preparations for contact lens users. Some drugs and preservatives in eye preparations can accumulate in hydrogel lenses and may induce toxic reactions. Therefore, unless medically indicated, the lenses should be removed before instillation and not worn during the period of treatment. Alternatively, unpreserved drops can be used. Eye drops may, however, be instilled over rigid corneal contact lenses. Ointment preparations should never be used in conjunction with contact lens wear.

Many drugs given systemically can also have adverse effects on contact lens wear. These include oral contraceptives (particularly those with a higher oestrogen content), drugs which reduce blink rate (e.g. anxiolytics, hypnotics, antihistamines, and muscle relaxants), drugs which reduce tear production (e.g. antihistamines, antimuscarinics, phenothiazines and related drugs, some beta-blockers, diuretics, and tricyclic antidepressants), and drugs which increase lacrimation (including ephedrine and hydralazine). Other drugs that may affect contact lens wear are isotretinoin (may cause conjunctival inflammation), primidone (may cause ocular or eyelid oedema), aspirin (salicylic acid appears in tears and may be absorbed by contact lenses—leading to irritation), and rifampicin and sulfasalazine (may discolour lenses).

12: Ear, nose, and oropharynx

12.1 Drugs acting on the ear

12.1.1   Otitis externa

12.1.2   Otitis media

12.1.3   Removal of ear wax

12.1.1 Otitis externa

Otitis externa is an inflammatory reaction of the meatal skin. It is important to exclude an underlying chronic otitis media before treatment is commenced. Many cases recover after thorough cleansing of the external ear canal by suction, dry mopping, or gentle syringing. A frequent problem in resistant cases is the difficulty in applying lotions and ointments satisfactorily to the relatively inaccessible affected skin. The most effective method is to introduce a ribbon gauze dressing soaked with **corticosteroid** ear drops or with an astringent such as **aluminium acetate** solution. When this is not practical, the ear should be gently cleansed with a probe covered in cotton wool and the patient encouraged to lie with the affected ear uppermost for ten minutes after the canal has been filled with a liberal quantity of the appropriate solution.

If infection is present, a topical anti-infective which is not used systemically (such as **neomycin** or **clioquinol**) may be used, but for only about a week as excessive use may result in fungal infections; these may be difficult to treat and require expert advice. Sensitivity to the anti-infective or solvent may occur and resistance to antibacterials is a possibility with prolonged use. **Chloramphenicol** may also be used but the ear drops contain propylene glycol and cause sensitivity in about 10% of patients (the eye ointment can be used instead [unlicensed indication]). Solutions containing an anti-infective and a corticosteroid (such as *Locorten-Vioform®*) are used for treating cases where infection is present with inflammation and eczema. In view of reports of ototoxicity in patients with a perforated tympanic membrane (eardrum), the CSM has issued a reminder that treatment with a topical aminoglycoside antibiotic is contra-indicated in those with a tympanic perforation.

An acute infection may cause severe pain and a systemic antibiotic is required with a simple analgesic such as paracetamol. When a resistant staphylococcal infection (a boil) is present in the external auditory meatus, **flucloxacillin** is the drug of choice (section 5.1, table 1); **ciprofloxacin** (or an aminoglycoside) may be needed in pseudomonal infections which may occur if the patient has diabetes or is immunocompromised.

The skin of the pinna adjacent to the ear canal is often affected by eczema. Topical corticosteroid creams and ointments (see section 13.4) are then required, but prolonged use should be avoided.

Astringent preparations

ALUMINIUM ACETATE

Indications: inflammation in otitis externa (see notes above)

Administration: insert into meatus or apply on a gauze wick which should be kept saturated with the ear drops

Aluminium Acetate (Non-proprietary)
Ear drops 13%, aluminium sulphate 2.25 g, calcium carbonate 1 g, tartaric acid 450 mg, acetic acid (33%) 2.5 mL, purified water 7.5 mL
Available from manufacturers of 'special order' products
Ear drops 8%, dilute 8 parts aluminium acetate ear drops (13%) with 5 parts purified water. Must be freshly prepared

Anti-inflammatory preparations

BETAMETHASONE SODIUM PHOSPHATE

Indications: eczematous inflammation in otitis externa (see notes above)
Cautions: avoid prolonged use
Contra-indications: untreated infection
Side-effects: local sensitivity reactions

Betnesol® (Medeva) [PoM]
Drops (for ear, eye, or nose), betamethasone sodium phosphate 0.1%. Net price 10 mL = £1.31
Excipients: include benzalkonium chloride
Ear, apply 2–3 drops every 2–3 hours; reduce frequency when relief obtained; *eye*, see section 11.4.1; *nose*, see section 12.2.1

Vista-Methasone® (Martindale) [PoM]
Drops (for ear, eye, or nose), betamethasone sodium phosphate 0.1%. Net price 5 mL = £1.15; 10 mL = £1.31
Excipients: include benzalkonium chloride
Ear, apply 2–3 drops every 3–4 hours; reduce frequency when relief obtained; *eye*, see section 11.4.1; *nose*, see section 12.2.1

■ With antibacterial

Betnesol-N® (Medeva) [PoM]
Drops (for ear, eye, or nose), betamethasone sodium phosphate 0.1%, neomycin sulphate 0.5%. Net price 10 mL = £1.35
Excipients: include benzalkonium chloride
Ear, apply 2–3 drops 3–4 times daily; *eye*, see section 11.4.1; *nose*, section 12.2.3

Vista-Methasone N® (Martindale) [PoM]
Drops (for ear, eye, or nose), betamethasone sodium phosphate 0.1%, neomycin sulphate 0.5%. Net price 5 mL = £1.17; 10 mL = £1.29
Excipients: include thiomersal
Ear, apply 2–3 drops every 3–4 hours; reduce frequency when relief obtained; *eye*, see section 11.4.1; *nose*, section 12.2.3

DEXAMETHASONE

Indications: eczematous inflammation in otitis externa (see notes above)
Cautions: avoid prolonged use
Contra-indications: untreated infection
Side-effects: local sensitivity reactions

■ With antibacterial

Otomize® (Stafford-Miller) [PoM]
Ear spray, dexamethasone 0.1%, neomycin sulphate 3250 units/mL, glacial acetic acid 2%. Net price 5-mL pump-action aerosol unit = £3.85
Apply 1 metered spray into the ear 3 times daily

Sofradex® (Florizel) [PoM] [▬▬]
Drops (for ear or eye), dexamethasone (as sodium metasulphobenzoate) 0.05%, framycetin sulphate 0.5%, gramicidin 0.005%. Net price 10 mL = £5.21
Ear, apply 2–3 drops 3–4 times daily; *eye*, see section 11.4.1
Ointment (for ear or eye), dexamethasone 0.05%, framycetin sulphate 0.5%, gramicidin 0.005%. Net price 5 g = £3.72
Ear, apply 1–2 times daily; *eye*, see section 11.4.1

FLUMETASONE PIVALATE
(Flumethasone Pivalate)

Indications: eczematous inflammation in otitis externa (see notes above)
Cautions: avoid prolonged use
Contra-indications: untreated infection
Side-effects: local sensitivity reactions

■ With antibacterial

Locorten-Vioform® (Novartis Consumer Health) [PoM]
Ear drops, flumetasone pivalate 0.02%, clioquinol 1%. Net price 7.5 mL = £1.02
Apply 2–3 drops into the ear twice daily for up to 7–10 days; not recommended for child under 2 years

HYDROCORTISONE

Indications: eczematous inflammation in otitis externa (see notes above)
Cautions: avoid prolonged use
Contra-indications: untreated infection
Side-effects: local sensitivity reactions

■ With antibacterial

Gentisone HC® (Roche) [PoM]
Ear drops, hydrocortisone acetate 1%, gentamicin 0.3% (as sulphate). Net price 10 mL = £3.97
Excipients: include benzalkonium chloride
Apply 2–4 drops into the ear 3–4 times daily and at night

Neo-Cortef® (Dominion) [PoM]
Drops (for ear or eye), hydrocortisone acetate 1.5%, neomycin sulphate 0.5%. Net price 10 mL = £4.11
Excipients: include miripirium chloride (myristyl-gamma-picolinium chloride)
Note. Ear drops containing hydrocortisone acetate 1.5% and neomycin sulphate 0.5% are also available from Martindale
Ear, apply 2–3 drops 3–4 times daily; *eye*, see section 11.4.1
Ointment (for ear or eye), hydrocortisone acetate 1.5%, neomycin sulphate 0.5%. Net price 3.9 g = £1.53
Ear, apply 1–2 times daily; *eye*, see section 11.4.1

Otosporin® (GlaxoWellcome) [PoM] [▬▬]
Ear drops, hydrocortisone 1%, neomycin sulphate 3400 units, polymyxin B sulphate 10 000 units/mL. Net price 5 mL = £2.15; 10 mL = £4.30
Apply 3 drops into the ear 3–4 times daily

[▬▬] denotes preparations that are considered to be less suitable for prescribing (see p. vi)

PREDNISOLONE SODIUM PHOSPHATE

Indications: eczematous inflammation in otitis externa (see notes above)
Cautions: avoid prolonged use
Contra-indications: untreated infection
Side-effects: local sensitivity reactions

Predsol® (Medeva) PoM
Drops (for ear or eye), prednisolone sodium phosphate 0.5%. Net price 10 mL = £1.31
Excipients: include benzalkonium chloride
Ear, apply 2–3 drops every 2–3 hours; reduce frequency when relief obtained; _eye_, see section 11.4.1

■ With antibacterial

Predsol-N® (Medeva) PoM
Drops (for ear or eye), prednisolone sodium phosphate 0.5%, neomycin sulphate 0.5%. Net price 10 mL = £1.20
Excipients: include benzalkonium chloride
Ear, apply 2–3 drops 3–4 times daily; _eye_, see section 11.4.1

TRIAMCINOLONE ACETONIDE

Indications: eczematous inflammation in otitis externa (see notes above)
Cautions: avoid prolonged use
Contra-indications: untreated infection
Side-effects: local sensitivity reactions

■ With antibacterial

Audicort® (Wyeth) PoM
Ear drops, triamcinolone acetonide 0.1%, neomycin (as neomycin undecenoate) 0.35%. Net price 10 mL = £4.73
Apply 2–5 drops into the ear 3–4 times daily; CHILD not recommended

Tri-Adcortyl Otic® (Squibb) PoM [≡]
Ear ointment, triamcinolone acetonide 0.1%, gramicidin 0.025%, neomycin 0.25% (as sulphate), nystatin 100 000 units/g in _Plastibase®_. Net price 10 g = £1.58
Apply into the ear 2–4 times daily

Anti-infective preparations

CHLORAMPHENICOL [≡]

Indications: bacterial infection in otitis externa (but see notes above)
Cautions: avoid prolonged use (see notes above)
Side-effects: high incidence of sensitivity reactions to vehicle

Chloramphenicol (Non-proprietary) PoM [≡]
Ear drops, chloramphenicol in propylene glycol, net price 5%, 10 mL = £1.40; 10%, 10 mL = £1.43
Available from Martindale
Apply 2–3 drops into the ear 2–3 times daily

[≡] denotes preparations that are considered to be less suitable for prescribing (see p. vi)

CLIOQUINOL

Indications: mild bacterial or fungal infections in otitis externa (see notes above)
Cautions: avoid prolonged use (see notes above)
Contra-indications: perforated tympanic membrane
Side-effects: local sensitivity; stains skin and clothing

■ With corticosteroid
Locorten-Vioform®, PoM see Flumetasone

CLOTRIMAZOLE

Indications: fungal infection in otitis externa (see notes above)
Side-effects: occasional local irritation or sensitivity

Canesten® (Bayer Consumer Care)
Solution, clotrimazole 1% in polyethylene glycol (macrogol 400). Net price 20 mL = £2.43
Ear, apply 2–3 times daily continuing for at least 14 days after disappearance of infection; _skin_, see section 13.10.2

FRAMYCETIN SULPHATE

Indications: see under Gentamicin
Cautions: see under Gentamicin
Contra-indications: perforated tympanic membrane (see notes above)
Side-effects: local sensitivity

■ With corticosteroid
Sofradex®, PoM see Dexamethasone

GENTAMICIN

Indications: bacterial infection in otitis externa (see notes above)
Cautions: avoid prolonged use (see notes above)
Contra-indications: perforated tympanic membrane (see notes above)
Side-effects: local sensitivity

Cidomycin® (Hoechst Marion Roussel) PoM
Drops (for ear or eye), gentamicin 0.3% (as sulphate). Net price 8 mL = £1.31
Excipients: include benzalkonium chloride, disodium edetate
Ear, apply 2–4 drops 3–4 times daily and at night; _eye_, see section 11.3.1

Garamycin® (Schering-Plough) PoM
Drops (for ear or eye), gentamicin 0.3% (as sulphate). Net price 10 mL = £1.79
Excipients: include benzalkonium chloride
Ear, apply 3–4 drops 3–4 times daily; reduce frequency when relief obtained; _eye_, see section 11.3.1

Genticin® (Roche) PoM
Drops (for ear or eye), gentamicin 0.3% (as sulphate). Net price 10 mL = £1.91
Excipients: include benzalkonium chloride
Ear, apply 2–3 drops 3–4 times daily and at night; _eye_, see section 11.3.1

■ With corticosteroid
Gentisone HC®, PoM see Hydrocortisone

NEOMYCIN SULPHATE

Indications: bacterial infection in otitis externa (see notes above)
Cautions: avoid prolonged use (see notes above)
Contra-indications: perforated tympanic membrane (see notes above)
Side-effects: local sensitivity

■ With corticosteroid
Audicort®, PoM see Triamcinolone
Betnesol-N®, PoM see Betamethasone
Neo-Cortef®, PoM see Hydrocortisone
Otomize®, PoM see Dexamethasone
Otosporin®, PoM see Hydrocortisone
Predsol-N®, PoM see Prednisolone
Tri-Adcortyl Otic®, PoM see Triamcinolone
Vista-Methasone N®, PoM see Betamethasone

Other aural preparations

Choline salicylate is a mild analgesic but it is of doubtful value when applied topically.

Audax® (SSL) NHS ▭
Ear drops, choline salicylate 20%, glycerol 12.6%. Net price 10 mL = £2.27

▭ denotes preparations that are considered to be less suitable for prescribing (see p. vi)

Otitis media

Acute otitis media is the commonest cause of severe pain in small children and recurrent attacks, especially in infants, are particularly distressing. *Otitis media with effusion* ('glue ear') is present in about 10% of the child population and in 90% of children with cleft palates; this condition should be referred to hospital because of the risk of permanent damage to middle ear function and impaired language development. Chronic otitis media is thought to be a result of untreated or resistant cases of otitis media with effusion.

Local treatment of *acute otitis media* is ineffective and there is no place for drops containing a local anaesthetic. Many attacks are viral in origin and need only treatment with a **simple analgesic** such as paracetamol for pain. Severe bacterial infection should be treated with **systemic antibiotics**; bacterial examination of any discharge is helpful in selecting the appropriate treatment (section 5.1, table 1). Again, simple analgesics such as paracetamol are used to relieve pain. In *recurrent acute otitis media* a daily dose of a prophylactic antibiotic (trimethoprim or erythromycin) during the winter months can be tried.

The organisms recovered from patients with *chronic otitis media* are often opportunists living in the debris, keratin, and necrotic bone present in the middle ear and mastoid. Thorough cleansing with an aural suction tube may completely resolve infection of many years duration. Acute exacerbations of chronic infection may require systemic antibiotics (section 5.1, table 1). A swab should be taken to determine the organism present and its antibiotic

sensitivity. Presence of *Pseudomonas aeruginosa* and *Proteus* spp. requires treatment with parenteral antibiotics. Local debridement of the meatal and middle ear contents may then be followed by topical treatment with ribbon gauze dressings as for otitis externa (section 12.1.1). This is particularly true with infections in mastoid cavities when dusting powders can also be tried.

The CSM has issued a reminder (section 12.1.1) that topical treatment with ototoxic antibiotics is contra-indicated in the presence of a perforation.

Removal of ear wax

Wax is a normal bodily secretion which provides a protective film on the meatal skin and need only be removed if it causes deafness or interferes with a proper view of the ear drum. As a general rule syringing is best avoided in patients with a history of recurring otitis externa, a perforated ear drum, or previous ear surgery. A person who has hearing in one ear only should not have that ear syringed because even a very slight risk of damage is unacceptable in this situation.

Wax may be removed by syringing with water (warmed to body temperature). If necessary, wax can be softened before syringing with simple remedies such as **sodium bicarbonate** ear drops, **olive oil** ear drops or **almond oil** ear drops, which are safe, effective and inexpensive. If the wax is hard and impacted the drops may be used twice daily for a few days before syringing; otherwise the wax may be softened on the day of syringing. The patient should lie with the affected ear uppermost for 5 to 10 minutes after a generous amount of the softening remedy has been introduced into the ear. Some proprietary preparations containing organic solvents can cause irritation of the meatal skin, and in most cases the simple remedies indicated above are just as effective and less likely to cause irritation. Docusate sodium or urea–hydrogen peroxide are ingredients in a number of proprietary preparations.

Almond Oil (Non-proprietary)
Ear drops, almond oil in a suitable container
Allow to warm to room temperature before use

Olive Oil (Non-proprietary)
Ear drops, olive oil in a suitable container
Allow to warm to room temperature before use

Sodium Bicarbonate (Non-proprietary)
Ear drops, sodium bicarbonate 5%, net price 10 mL = £1.21
Available from Thornton & Ross

Cerumol® (LAB) ▭
Ear drops, chlorobutanol 5%, paradichlorobenzene 2%, arachis (peanut) oil 57.3%. Net price 11 mL = £1.45

Exterol® (Dermal) ▭
Ear drops, urea–hydrogen peroxide complex 5% in glycerol. Net price 8 mL = £1.97

Molcer® (Wallace Mfg) ▭
Ear drops, docusate sodium 5%. Net price 15 mL = £1.32

Otex® (DDD) ◼◼◼◼
Ear drops, urea–hydrogen peroxide 5%. Net price
8 mL = £2.45

Waxsol® (Norgine) ◼◼◼◼
Ear drops, docusate sodium 0.5%. Net price
10 mL = 95p

◼◼◼◼ denotes preparations that are considered to
be less suitable for prescribing (see p. vi)

12.2 Drugs acting on the nose

12.2.1 Drugs used in nasal allergy
12.2.2 Topical nasal decongestants
12.2.3 Nasal preparations for infection and
        epistaxis

Rhinitis is often self-limiting and sinusitis is best
treated with systemic antibiotics (section 5.1, table
1). There are few indications for nasal sprays and
drops except in allergic rhinitis (section 12.2.1).
Many nasal preparations contain sympathomimetic
drugs which may damage the nasal cilia (section
12.2.2). Douching the nose with salt and water is
not recommended for the treatment of chronic rhinitis. However some ENT departments use saline
sniffs for a short period after endonasal surgery.

NASAL POLYPS. Short-term use of corticosteroid
nasal drops helps to produce significant shrinkage
of nasal polyps; to be effective, the drops must be
administered with the patient in the 'head down'
position. The reduction in swelling can be maintained by continuing treatment with a corticosteroid
nasal spray.

12.2.1 Drugs used in nasal allergy

Mild cases of allergic rhinitis are controlled by topical **nasal corticosteroids** or **oral antihistamines**
(section 3.4.1); **systemic nasal decongestants** are
of doubtful value (section 3.10).

More persistent symptoms and nasal congestion
can be relieved by topical nasal **corticosteroids** and
cromoglicate (cromoglycate); topical antihistamines (azelastine and levocabastine) are also used
in allergic rhinitis. In seasonal allergic rhinitis (e.g.
hay fever), treatment should begin 2 to 3 weeks
before the season commences and may have to be
continued for several months; treatment may be
required for years in perennial rhinitis.

In allergic rhinitis, topical preparations of corticosteroids and cromoglicate have a well-established
role; although it may be less effective, cromoglicate
is often the first choice in children. Topical antihistamines are considered less effective than topical
corticosteroids but probably more effective than
cromoglicate.

Very disabling symptoms occasionally justify the
use of **systemic corticosteroids** for short periods
(section 6.3), for example in students taking important examinations. They may also be used at the
beginning of a course of treatment with a corticosteroid spray to relieve severe mucosal oedema and
allow the spray to penetrate the nasal cavity.

Antihistamines

AZELASTINE HYDROCHLORIDE
Indications: allergic rhinitis
Side-effects: irritation of nasal mucosa; taste dis-
turbance

▎**Rhinolast®** (ASTA Medica) PoM
Aqueous nasal spray, azelastine hydrochloride
140 micrograms (0.14 mL)/metered spray. Net
price 20 mL (with metered pump) = £11.92
Excipients: include benzalkonium chloride, sodium edetate
ADULT and CHILD over 5 years, apply 140 micrograms
(1 spray) into each nostril twice daily
1. Can be sold to the public for nasal administration in
aqueous form (other than by aerosol) if supplied for the
treatment of seasonal allergic rhinitis in adults and children over 12 years, subject to max. single dose of
140 micrograms per nostril, max. daily dose of
280 micrograms per nostril, and a pack size limit of 36
doses; a proprietary brand (*Rhinolast® Hayfever*) is on
sale to the public

LEVOCABASTINE
Indications: treatment of allergic rhinitis
Cautions: renal impairment (see Appendix 3)
Side-effects: nasal irritation; hypersensitivity
reactions, headache, fatigue, drowsiness reported

▎**Livostin®** (CIBA Vision) PoM
Aqueous nasal spray, levocabastine (as hydrochloride) 0.05%. Net price 10-mL spray pump =
£8.90
Excipients: include propylene glycol, polysorbate 80 and benzalkonium chloride
ADULT and CHILD 9 years and over, apply 2 sprays into
each nostril twice daily, increased if necessary to 3–4
times daily; max. period of treatment 4 weeks
1. Can be sold to the public for nasal administration if
supplied for the symptomatic treatment of seasonal
allergic rhinitis in adults and children over 12 years subject to max. strength of levocabastine 0.05% and a pack
size of 10 mL; proprietary brands on sale to the public
include *Livostin® Direct Nasal Spray*

Corticosteroids

Nasal preparations containing corticosteroids
(beclometasone, betamethasone, budesonide, flunisolide, fluticasone, mometasone, and triamcinolone) have a useful role in the prophylaxis and
treatment of allergic rhinitis (see notes above).

CAUTIONS. Corticosteroid nasal preparations
should be avoided in the presence of untreated nasal
infections, and also after nasal surgery (until healing has occurred); they should also be avoided in
pulmonary tuberculosis. Patients transferred from
systemic corticosteroids may experience exacerbation of some symptoms. Systemic absorption may
follow nasal administration particularly if high
doses are used or if treatment is prolonged; for cautions and side-effects of systemic corticosteroids,
see section 6.3.2. The CSM recommends that the
height of children receiving prolonged treatment
with nasal corticosteroids is monitored; if growth is
slowed, referral to a paediatrician should be considered.

SIDE-EFFECTS. Local side-effects include dryness, irritation of nose and throat, epistaxis and rarely ulceration; nasal septal perforation (usually following nasal surgery) and raised intra-ocular pressure or glaucoma may also occur rarely. Smell and taste disturbances may also occur. Hypersensitivity reactions, including bronchospasm, have been reported.

BECLOMETASONE DIPROPIONATE

(Beclomethasone Dipropionate)

Indications: prophylaxis and treatment of allergic and vasomotor rhinitis

Cautions: see notes above

Side-effects: see notes above

Dose: ADULT and CHILD over 6 years, apply 100 micrograms (2 sprays) into each nostril twice daily *or* 50 micrograms (1 spray) into each nostril 3–4 times daily; max. total 400 micrograms (8 sprays) daily; when symptoms controlled, dose reduced to 50 micrograms (1 spray) into each nostril twice daily

¹**Beclometasone** (Non-proprietary) PoM

Nasal spray, beclometasone dipropionate 50 micrograms/metered spray. Net price 200-spray unit = £3.15

Available from Ashbourne (*Zonivent®*), Baker Norton (*Nasobec Aqueous®*), Cox, Galen (*Beclo-aqua® 50*), Generics

1. Can be sold to the public for nasal administration (other than by aerosol) if supplied for the prevention and treatment of allergic rhinitis in adults over 18 years subject to max. single dose of 100 micrograms per nostril, max. daily dose of 200 micrograms per nostril for max. period of 3 months, and a pack size of 5.6 mg; proprietary brands on sale to the public include *Beconase® Allergy, Boots Hayfever Relief®, Nasobec® Hayfever*

Beconase® (A&H) PoM

Nasal spray (aqueous suspension), beclometasone dipropionate 50 micrograms/metered spray. Net price 200-spray unit with applicator = £4.01
Excipients: include benzalkonium chloride, polysorbate 80

BETAMETHASONE SODIUM PHOSPHATE

Indications: non-infected inflammatory conditions of nose

Cautions: see notes above

Side-effects: see notes above

Betnesol® (Medeva) PoM

Drops (for ear, eye, or nose), betamethasone sodium phosphate 0.1%. Net price 10 mL = £1.31
Excipients: include benzalkonium chloride
Nose, apply 2–3 drops into each nostril 2–3 times daily; *ear*, section 12.1.1; *eye*, see section 11.4.1

Vista-Methasone® (Martindale) PoM

Drops (for ear, eye, or nose), betamethasone sodium phosphate 0.1%. Net price 5 mL = £1.15, 10 mL = £1.31
Excipients: include benzalkonium chloride
Nose, apply 2–3 drops into each nostril twice daily; *ear*, section 12.1.1; *eye*, see section 11.4.1

BUDESONIDE

Indications: prophylaxis and treatment of allergic and vasomotor rhinitis; nasal polyps

Cautions: see notes above

Side-effects: see notes above

¹**Rhinocort Aqua®** (Astra) PoM

Nasal spray, budesonide 100 micrograms/metered spray. Net price 100-spray unit = £5.85
Excipients: include disodium edetate, polysorbate 80, potassium sorbate

Rhinitis, ADULT and CHILD over 12 years, apply 200 micrograms (2 sprays) into each nostril once daily in the morning *or* 100 micrograms (1 spray) into each nostril twice daily; when control achieved reduce to 100 micrograms (1 spray) into each nostril once daily

Nasal polyps, ADULT and CHILD over 12 years, 100 micrograms (1 spray) into each nostril twice daily for up to 3 months

1. Can be sold to the public for nasal administration (other than by aerosol) if supplied for the prevention and treatment of seasonal allergic rhinitis in adults over 18 years subject to max. single dose of 200 micrograms per nostril, max. daily dose of 200 micrograms per nostril for max. period of 3 months, and a pack size of 10 mg

DEXAMETHASONE ISONICOTINATE

Indications: treatment of allergic rhinitis

Cautions: see notes above; avoid contact with eyes

Side-effects: see notes above

■ With sympathomimetic

For cautions and side-effects of sympathomimetics see Ephedrine Hydrochloride, section 12.2.2

Dexa-Rhinaspray Duo® (Boehringer Ingelheim) PoM

Nasal spray, dexamethasone isonicotinate 20 micrograms, tramazoline hydrochloride 120 micrograms/metered spray. Net price 110-dose unit = £2.15
Excipients: include polysorbate 80

Allergic rhinitis, ADULT and CHILD over 12 years, apply 1 spray into each nostril 2–3 times daily, max. 6 times daily; max. duration 14 days; CHILD 5–12 years 1 spray into each nostril up to twice daily; under 5 years not recommended

FLUNISOLIDE

Indications: prophylaxis and treatment of allergic rhinitis

Cautions: see notes above

Side-effects: see notes above

¹**Syntaris®** (Roche) PoM

Aqueous nasal spray, flunisolide 25 micrograms/metered spray. Net price 240-spray unit with pump and applicator = £5.25
Excipients: include benzalkonium chloride, butylated hydroxytoluene, disodium edetate, polysorbates, propylene glycol

ADULT, apply 50 micrograms (2 sprays) into each nostril twice daily, increased if necessary to max. 3 times daily then reduced for maintenance; CHILD 5–14 years initially 25 micrograms (1 spray) into each nostril up to 3 times daily

1. Flunisolide non-pressurised nasal spray can be sold to the public (in max. pack size of 6 mg) for the prevention and treatment (in adults over 18 years) of seasonal allergic rhinitis, including hayfever; max. dose 50 micrograms per nostril and max. daily dose 100 micrograms per nostril for max. period of 3 months

FLUTICASONE PROPIONATE

Indications: see under preparations below

Cautions: see notes above

Side-effects: see notes above

Flixonase® (A&H) [PoM]

Aqueous nasal spray, fluticasone propionate
50 micrograms/metered spray. Net price 120-
spray unit with applicator = £11.43
Excipients: include benzalkonium chloride, polysorbate 80
Prophylaxis and treatment of allergic rhinitis, ADULT
and CHILD over 12 years, apply 100 micrograms (2
sprays) into each nostril once daily, preferably in the
morning, increased to twice daily if required; max. total
400 micrograms (8 sprays) daily; CHILD 4–11 years,
50 micrograms (1 spray) into each nostril once daily,
increased to twice daily if required; max. total
200 micrograms (4 sprays) daily

Flixonase Nasule® (A&H) ▼ [PoM]

Nasal drops, fluticasone propionate
400 micrograms/unit dose, net price 28 × 0.4 mL-
units = £13.48
Excipients: include polysorbate 20
Nasal polyps, apply approx. 6 drops into each nostril
once or twice daily, consider alternative treatment if no
improvement after 4–6 weeks; CHILD not recommended

MOMETASONE FUROATE

Indications: prophylaxis and treatment of allergic
rhinitis
Cautions: see notes above
Side-effects: see notes above

Nasonex® (Schering-Plough) ▼ [PoM]

Aqueous nasal spray, mometasone furoate
50 micrograms/metered spray. Net price 140-
spray unit = £10.92
Excipients: include benzalkonium chloride, polysorbate 80
ADULT and CHILD 12 years and over, apply
100 micrograms (2 sprays) into each nostril once daily,
increased if necessary to max. 200 micrograms (4
sprays) into each nostril once daily; when control
achieved reduce to 50 micrograms (1 spray) into each
nostril once daily; CHILD 6–11 years, 50 micrograms (1
spray) into each nostril once daily

TRIAMCINOLONE ACETONIDE

Indications: prophylaxis and treatment of allergic
rhinitis
Cautions: see notes above
Side-effects: see notes above

Nasacort® (Rhône-Poulenc Rorer) [PoM]

Aqueous nasal spray, triamcinolone acetonide
55 micrograms/metered spray. Net price 120-
spray unit = £9.60
Excipients: include benzalkonium chloride, disodium edetate,
polysorbate 80
ADULT and CHILD over 12 years apply 110 micrograms
(2 sprays) into each nostril once daily; when control
achieved, reduce to 55 micrograms (1 spray) into each
nostril once daily; CHILD 6–12 years, 55 micrograms (1
spray) into each nostril once daily

Cromoglicate

SODIUM CROMOGLICATE

(Sodium Cromoglycate)
Indications: prophylaxis of allergic rhinitis
Side-effects: local irritation; rarely transient
bronchospasm

Rynacrom® (Pantheon)

4% aqueous nasal spray, sodium cromoglicate 4%
(5.2 mg/squeeze). Net price 22 mL with pump =
£19.10
Excipients: include benzalkonium chloride
ADULT and CHILD, apply 1 squeeze into each nostril 2–4
times daily

Vividrin® (Pharma-Global)

Nasal spray, sodium cromoglicate 2%. Net price
15 mL = £5.45
Excipients: include benzalkonium chloride
ADULT and CHILD, apply 1 spray into each nostril 4–6
times daily

■ With sympathomimetic

Rynacrom Compound® (Pantheon)

Nasal spray, sodium cromoglicate 2% (2.6 mg/
metered spray) and xylometazoline hydrochloride
0.025% (32.5 micrograms/metered spray). Net
price 26 mL with pump = £14.33
Excipients: include benzalkonium chloride
Apply 1 spray into each nostril 4 times daily
Note. A proprietary brand of sodium cromoglicate 2%
and xylometazoline hydrochloride 0.025% (*Rynacrom
Allergy®*) is on sale to the public

12.2.2   Topical nasal decongestants

The nasal mucosa is sensitive to changes in atmos-
pheric temperature and humidity and these alone
may cause slight nasal congestion. The nose and
nasal sinuses produce a litre of mucus in 24 hours
and much of this finds its way silently into the
stomach via the nasopharynx. Slight changes in the
nasal airway, accompanied by an awareness of
mucus passing along the nasopharynx causes some
patients to be inaccurately diagnosed as suffering
from chronic sinusitis. These symptoms are particularly noticeable in the later stages of the common
cold. **Sodium chloride** 0.9% given as nasal drops
may relieve nasal congestion by helping to liquefy
mucous secretions. Corticosteroid nasal drops produce shrinkage of nasal polyps (section 12.2).

Symptoms of nasal congestion associated with
vasomotor rhinitis and the common cold can be
relieved by the short-term use (usually not longer
than 7 days) of decongestant nasal drops and
sprays. These all contain sympathomimetic drugs
which exert their effect by vasoconstriction of the
mucosal blood vessels which in turn reduces
oedema of the nasal mucosa. They are of limited
value because they can give rise to a rebound congestion (rhinitis medicamentosa) on withdrawal,
due to a secondary vasodilation with a subsequent
temporary increase in nasal congestion. This in turn
tempts the further use of the decongestant, leading
to a vicious cycle of events. **Ephedrine nasal
drops** is the safest sympathomimetic preparation
and can give relief for several hours. The more
potent sympathomimetic drugs oxymetazoline, and
xylometazoline are more likely to cause a rebound
effect. **All** of these preparations may cause a hypertensive crisis if used during treatment with a
monoamine-oxidase inhibitor.

Non-allergic watery rhinorrhoea often responds
well to treatment with **ipratropium bromide**.

Inhalations of **warm moist air** are useful in the
treatment of symptoms of acute infective conditions, and the use of compounds containing volatile

substances such as menthol and eucalyptus may encourage their use (section 3.8). There is no evidence that nasal preparations containing antihistamines and anti-infective agents have any therapeutic effect.

Systemic nasal decongestants—see section 3.10.

Sympathomimetics

EPHEDRINE HYDROCHLORIDE

Indications: nasal congestion
Cautions: avoid excessive or prolonged use; caution in infants under 3 months (no good evidence of value—if irritation occurs might narrow nasal passage); **interactions:** Appendix 1 (sympathomimetics)
Side-effects: local irritation; after excessive use tolerance with diminished effect, rebound congestion
Administration: see below

Ephedrine (Non-proprietary)
Nasal drops, ephedrine hydrochloride 0.5%, net price 10 mL = £1.08; 1%, 10 mL = £1.15
Note. The BP directs that if no strength is specified 0.5% drops should be supplied
Instil 1–2 drops into each nostril up to 3 or 4 times daily when required

XYLOMETAZOLINE HYDROCHLORIDE

Indications: nasal congestion
Cautions: see under Ephedrine Hydrochloride
Side-effects: see under Ephedrine Hydrochloride

Xylometazoline Nasal Drops, xylometazoline hydrochloride 0.1%, net price 10 mL = £1.63
Instil 2–3 drops into each nostril 2–3 times daily when required; max. duration 7 days; not recommended for children under 12 years
Xylometazoline Nasal Drops, Paediatric, xylometazoline hydrochloride 0.05%, net price 10 mL = £1.53
CHILD over 3 months instil 1–2 drops into each nostril 1–2 times daily when required (not recommended for infants under 3 months of age, doctor's advice only under 2 years); max. duration 7 days
Note. The brand name *Otrivine®* [NHS] is used for xylometazoline adult nasal drops 0.1%, children's nasal drops 0.05%, and adult nasal spray 0.1%
Sympathomimetic nasal preparations on sale to the public (not prescribable on the NHS) include:

Afrazine® (oxymetazoline), **Dristan®** (oxymetazoline), **Fenox®** (phenylephrine), **Nazo-Mist®** (xylometazoline), **Otrivine®** (xylometazoline—prescribable in non-proprietary form as nasal drops, see above), **Sudafed®** nasal spray (oxymetazoline), **Vicks Sinex®** (oxymetazoline)

Antimuscarinic

IPRATROPIUM BROMIDE

Indications: rhinorrhoea associated with allergic and non-allergic rhinitis
Cautions: see section 3.1.2; avoid spraying near eyes
Side-effects: nasal dryness and epistaxis
Administration: apply 42 micrograms (2 sprays) into each nostril 2–3 times daily; CHILD under 12 years not recommended

Rinatec® (Boehringer Ingelheim) [PoM]
Nasal spray 0.03%, ipratropium bromide 21 micrograms/metered spray. Net price 180-dose unit = £4.55
Excipients: include benzalkonium chloride

12.2.3   Nasal preparations for infection and epistaxis

There is **no** evidence that topical anti-infective nasal preparations have any therapeutic value in rhinitis or sinusitis; for elimination of nasal staphylococci, see below.

Systemic treatment of sinusitis—see section 5.1, table 1.

Betnesol-N® (Medeva) [PoM] ▰
Drops (for ear, eye, or nose), betamethasone sodium phosphate 0.1%, neomycin sulphate 0.5%. Net price 10 mL = £1.35
Excipients: include benzalkonium chloride
Nose, apply 2–3 drops into nostril 2–3 times daily; *eye,* see section 11.4.1; *ear,* see section 12.1.1

¹ **Locabiotal®** (Servier) [NHS] [PoM] ▰
Spray, fusafungine 500 micrograms/metered spray. Net price 50-spray unit with nasal (yellow) and oral (white) adapters = £1.55
Excipients: include alcohol
1. [NHS] Except for treatment of infections and inflammation of the oropharynx and endorsed 'SLS'
Infection and inflammation of upper respiratory tract (but not recommended, see notes above), 1 spray into each nostril or into mouth every 4 hours; CHILD 1 spray into each nostril or into mouth every 6 hours; withdraw if no improvement after 7 days

Vista-Methasone N® (Martindale) [PoM] ▰
Drops (for ear, eye, or nose), betamethasone sodium phosphate 0.1%, neomycin sulphate 0.5%. Net price 5 mL = £1.17, 10 mL = £1.29
Excipients: include thiomersal
Nose, apply 2–3 drops into each nostril twice daily; *eye,* see section 11.4.1; *ear,* see section 12.1.1

> ▰ denotes preparations that are considered to be less suitable for prescribing (see p. vi)

Nasal staphylococci

Elimination of organisms such as staphylococci from the nasal vestibule can be achieved by the use of a cream containing **chlorhexidine and neomycin** (*Naseptin®*), but re-colonisation frequently occurs. Coagulase-positive staphylococci are present in the noses of 40% of the population.

A nasal ointment containing **mupirocin** is also available; it should probably be held in reserve for resistant cases. In hospital, mupirocin nasal ointment should be reserved for the eradication (in both patients and staff) of nasal carriage of methicillin-resistant *Staphylococcus aureus* (MRSA). The ointment should be applied 3 times daily for 5 days and a sample taken 2 days after treatment to confirm eradication. The course may be repeated if the sample is positive (and the throat is not colonised). To avoid the development of resistance, the treatment course should not exceed 7 days and the course should not be repeated on more than one occasion. If the MRSA strain is mupirocin-resistant or does not respond after 2 courses, consider alternative products such as chlorhexidine and neomycin cream.

Bactroban Nasal® (Beecham) PoM
Nasal ointment, mupirocin 2% (as calcium salt) in
white soft paraffin basis. Net price 3 g = £6.24
For eradication of nasal carriage of staphylococci,
including methicillin-resistant *Staphylococcus aureus*
(MRSA), apply 2–3 times daily to the inner surface of
each nostril

Naseptin® (Alliance) PoM
Cream, chlorhexidine hydrochloride 0.1%, neomycin sulphate 3250 units/g. Net price 15 g =
£1.48
Excipients: include arachis (peanut) oil
For eradication of nasal carriage of staphylococci, apply
to nostrils 4 times daily for 10 days; for preventing nasal
carriage of staphylococci apply to nostrils twice daily

Epistaxis

Bismuth iodoform paraffin paste (BIPP) is used
for packing cavities after ear, nose and oropharyngeal surgery as a mild disinfectant and astringent; it
is also used to pack nasal cavities in acute epistaxis.
It is available either as a paste, to be applied to ribbon gauze packing, or as BIPP-impregnated ribbon
gauze.

BISMUTH SUBNITRATE AND IODOFORM

Indications: packing cavities after ear, nose or
oropharyngeal surgery; epistaxis
Cautions: hyperthyroidism
Side-effects: erythematous rash (discontinue use);
encephalopathy reported only with large packs or
when placed directly on neural tissue

Bismuth Subnitrate and Iodoform (Non-
proprietary)
Paste, 30-g sachet, net price = £9.50; 30-g tube =
£14.95
Available from Aurum, Oxford Pharmaceuticals
(*OxBipp®*)
Impregnated gauze, sterile, net price 1.25 cm ×
100 cm, 10 = £89.70; 1.25 cm × 125 cm, 5 =
£44.85; 1.25 cm × 200 cm, 5 = £62.05; 1.25 cm ×
300 cm, 5 = £81.15; 2.5 cm × 100 cm, 10 =
£97.20; 2.5 cm × 125 cm, 5 = £48.60; 2.5 cm ×
200 cm, 5 = £70.35; 2.5 cm × 300 cm, 5 = £92.55
Available from Aurum, Oxford Pharmaceuticals
(*OxBipp-G®*)

12.3   Drugs acting on the oropharynx

12.3.1	Drugs for oral ulceration and inflammation
12.3.2	Oropharyngeal anti-infective drugs
12.3.3	Lozenges and sprays
12.3.4	Mouthwashes, gargles, and dentifrices
12.3.5	Treatment of dry mouth

12.3.1   Drugs for oral ulceration and inflammation

Ulceration of the oral mucosa may be caused by
trauma (physical or chemical), recurrent aphthae,
infections, carcinoma, dermatological disorders,
nutritional deficiencies, gastro-intestinal disease,
haematopoietic disorders, and drug therapy. It is
important to establish the diagnosis in each case as
the majority of these lesions require specific management in addition to local treatment. Patients with
an unexplained mouth ulcer of more than 3 weeks'
duration require urgent referral to hospital to
exclude oral cancer. Local treatment aims at protecting the ulcerated area, or at relieving pain or
reducing inflammation.

SIMPLE MOUTHWASHES. A **saline** or **compound
thymol glycerin** mouthwash (section 12.3.4) may
relieve the pain of traumatic ulceration. The
mouthwash is made up with warm water and used
at frequent intervals until the discomfort and swelling subsides.

ANTISEPTIC MOUTHWASHES. Secondary bacterial infection may be a feature of any mucosal ulceration; it can increase discomfort and delay healing.
Use of a **chlorhexidine** or **povidone–iodine**
mouthwash (section 12.3.4) is often beneficial and
may accelerate healing of recurrent aphthae.

MECHANICAL PROTECTION. **Carmellose gelatin paste** may relieve some discomfort arising
from ulceration by protecting the ulcer site. The
paste adheres to the mucosa, but is difficult to apply
effectively to some parts of the mouth.

CORTICOSTEROIDS. Topical corticosteroid therapy may be used for some forms of oral ulceration.
In the case of aphthous ulcers it is most effective if
applied in the 'prodromal' phase.
    Thrush or other types of candidiasis are recog-
nised complications of corticosteroid treatment.
    Hydrocortisone lozenges are allowed to dissolve
next to an ulcer and are useful in recurrent aphthae,
erosive lichen planus, discoid lupus erythematosus,
and benign mucous membrane pemphigoid.
    Triamcinolone dental paste is designed to keep
the corticosteroid in contact with the mucosa for
long enough to permit penetration of the lesion, but
is difficult for patients to apply properly.
    Systemic corticosteroid therapy is reserved for
severe conditions such as pemphigus vulgaris (section 6.3.4).

LOCAL ANALGESICS. Local analgesics have a
limited role in the management of oral ulceration.
When applied topically their action is of a relatively
short duration so that analgesia cannot be maintained continuously throughout the day. The main
indication for a topical local analgesic is to relieve
the pain of otherwise intractable oral ulceration particularly when it is due to major aphthae. For this
purpose lidocaine (lignocaine) 5% ointment or lozenges containing a local anaesthetic are applied to
the ulcer. When local anaesthetics are used in the
mouth care must be taken not to produce anaesthesia of the pharynx before meals as this might
lead to choking.
    Benzydamine mouthwash or spray may be useful
in palliating the discomfort associated with a variety
of ulcerative conditions. It has also been found to be
effective in reducing the discomfort of post-irradia-
tion mucositis. Some patients find the full-strength
mouthwash causes some stinging and, for them, it
should be diluted with an equal volume of water.
Flurbiprofen lozenges have been introduced
recently; they are licensed for the relief of sore throat.

Choline salicylate dental gel has some analgesic action and may provide relief for recurrent aphthae, but excessive application or confinement under a denture irritates the mucosa and can itself cause ulceration. Benefit in teething may merely be due to pressure of application (comparable with biting a teething ring); excessive use can lead to salicylate poisoning.

OTHER PREPARATIONS. **Carbenoxolone** gel or mouthwash may be of some value. **Tetracycline** rinsed in the mouth may also be of value.

BENZYDAMINE HYDROCHLORIDE

Indications: painful inflammatory conditions of oropharynx
Side-effects: occasional numbness or stinging

Difflam® (3M)
Oral rinse, green, benzydamine hydrochloride 0.15%. Net price 300 mL = £3.92
Rinse or gargle, using 15 mL (diluted with water if stinging occurs) every 1½–3 hours as required, usually for not more than 7 days; not suitable for children aged 12 years or under
Spray, benzydamine hydrochloride 0.15%. Net price 30-mL unit = £3.41
ADULT, 4–8 puffs onto affected area every 1½–3 hours; CHILD under 6 years 1 puff per 4 kg to max. 4 puffs every 1½–3 hours; 6–12 years 4 puffs every 1½–3 hours

CARBENOXOLONE SODIUM

Indications: mild oral and perioral lesions

Bioral Gel® (Merck Consumer Health)
Gel, carbenoxolone sodium 2% in adhesive basis. Net price 5 g = £2.30
Apply after meals and at bedtime

Bioplex® (Cortecs) [PoM]
Mouthwash granules, carbenoxolone sodium 1% (20 mg/sachet). Net price 24 × 2-g sachets = £7.23
For mouth ulcers, rinse with 1 sachet in 30–50 mL of warm water 3 times daily and at bedtime

CARMELLOSE SODIUM

Indications: mechanical protection of oral and perioral lesions

Orabase® (ConvaTec)
Oral paste, carmellose sodium 16.7%, pectin 16.7%, gelatin 16.7%, in *Plastibase*®. Net price 30 g = £1.78; 100 g = £3.96
Apply a thin layer when necessary after meals

Orahesive® (ConvaTec)
Powder, carmellose sodium, pectin, gelatin, equal parts. Net price 25 g = £2.06
Sprinkle on the affected area

CORTICOSTEROIDS

Indications: oral and perioral lesions
Contra-indications: untreated oral infection
Side-effects: occasional exacerbation of local infection

¹**Adcortyl in Orabase**® (Squibb) [PoM]
Oral paste, triamcinolone acetonide 0.1% in adhesive basis. Net price 10 g = £1.27
ADULT and CHILD, apply a thin layer 2–4 times daily; do not rub in; use limited to 5 days for children and short-term use also advised for elderly
1. A 5-g tube (*Adcortyl in Orabase® for Mouth Ulcers*) is on sale to the public for the treatment of common mouth ulcers for max. 5 days

Corlan® (Medeva)
Pellets (= lozenges), hydrocortisone 2.5 mg (as sodium succinate). Net price 20 = £1.40
Note. Supplies may be difficult to obtain
ADULT and CHILD, 1 lozenge 4 times daily, allowed to dissolve slowly in the mouth in contact with the ulcer; if ulcers recur rapidly treatment may be continued for a period at reduced dosage

FLURBIPROFEN

Indications: relief of sore throat
Cautions: see section 10.1.1
Contra-indications: see section 10.1.1
Side-effects: taste disturbance, mouth ulcers (move lozenge around mouth); see also section 10.1.1

Strefen® (Crookes) [PoM]
Lozenges, flurbiprofen 8.75 mg, net price 16 = £2.00
Allow 1 lozenge to dissolve slowly in the mouth every 3–6 hours, max. 5 lozenges in 24 hours; CHILD under 12 years not recommended

LOCAL ANAESTHETICS

Indications: relief of pain in oral lesions
Cautions: avoid prolonged use; hypersensitivity

Preparations
Local anaesthetics are included in some mouth ulcer preparations, for details see below
Local anaesthetics are also included in some throat lozenges and sprays, see section 12.3.3

Preparations (including teething gels) containing local anaesthetics include: *Anbesol*®, *Calgel*®, *Dentinox*®, *Rinstead*®, *Rinstead*® *Contact Pastilles*, *Woodward's*®, *Ulc-Aid*®

SALICYLATES

Indications: mild oral and perioral lesions
Cautions: frequent application, especially in children, may give rise to salicylate poisoning
Note. CSM warning on aspirin and Reye's syndrome does not apply to non-aspirin salicylates or to topical preparations such as teething gels

■ Choline salicylate
Choline Salicylate Dental Gel, BP
Oral gel, choline salicylate 8.7% in a flavoured gel basis
Available as *Bonjela*® (R&C), net price 15 g (sugar-free) = £1.59; *Dinnefords Teejel*® (SSL), 10 g = £1.17
Apply ½-inch of gel with gentle massage not more often than every 3 hours; CHILD over 4 months ¼-inch of gel not more often than every 3 hours; max. 6 applications daily

■ Salicylic acid

Pyralvex® (Norgine)

Oral paint, brown, rhubarb extract (anthraquinone glycosides 0.5%), salicylic acid 1%. Net price 10 mL with brush = £1.41

Apply 3–4 times daily; CHILD under 12 years not recommended

TETRACYCLINE

Indications: severe recurrent aphthous ulceration; oral herpes (section 12.3.2)

Side-effects: fungal superinfection
For side-effects, cautions and contra-indications relating to systemic administration of tetracyclines see section 5.1.3

Local application
For preparation of a mouthwash, the contents of a 250–mg tetracycline capsule (see section 5.1.3) can be stirred into a small amount of water, then held in the mouth for 2–3 minutes 3-4 times daily usually for 3 days; longer courses are sometimes used (but precautions may be required to avoid oral thrush, section 12.3.2); it should preferably not be swallowed [unlicensed indication]
Note. Tetracycline stains teeth; avoid in children under 12 years of age

The following list includes topical treatments for mouth ulcers on sale to the public, together with their significant ingredients:

Adcortyl in Orabase® for Mouth Ulcers (triamcinolone acetonide), **Anbesol®** (cetylpyridinium, chlorocresol, lidocaine (lignocaine)), **Bansor®** (cetrimide), **Bioral Gel®** (carbenoxolone), **Bonjela gel®** (choline salicylate), **Bonjela pastilles®** (aminoacridine (aminacrine), lidocaine (lignocaine)), **Dinnefords Teejel®** (choline salicylate), **Frador®** (chlorobutanol, menthol), **Medijel®** (aminoacridine (aminacrine), lidocaine (lignocaine)), **Oragard®** (cetylpyridinium, lidocaine (lignocaine)), **Pyralvex®** (anthraquinone glycoside, salicylic acid), **Rinstead gel®** (benzocaine, chloroxylenol), **Rinstead pastilles®** (chloroxylenol, menthol)

12.3.2 Oropharyngeal anti-infective drugs

The most common cause of a sore throat is a viral infection which does not benefit from anti-infective treatment. Streptococcal sore throats require systemic **penicillin** therapy (section 5.1, table 1). Acute ulcerative gingivitis (Vincent's infection) responds to systemic **metronidazole** 200 mg 3 times daily for 3 days (section 5.1.11).

Preparations administered in the dental surgery for the local treatment of periodontal disease include gels of metronidazole (*Elyzol®*, Dumex) and of minocycline (*Dentomycin®*, Blackwell).

Fungal infections

Candida albicans may cause thrush and other forms of stomatitis which are sometimes associated with the use of broad-spectrum antibiotics or of cytotoxics; withdrawing the causative drug may lead to rapid resolution. Otherwise, an antifungal drug may be effective.

Of the antifungal drugs used for mouth infections, **amphotericin** and **nystatin** are not absorbed from the gastro-intestinal tract and are used by local application in the mouth. **Miconazole** occupies an intermediate position since it is used by local application in the mouth but is also absorbed to the extent that potential interactions need to be considered. **Fluconazole** and **itraconazole** are absorbed when taken by mouth and are available for administration by mouth for oropharyngeal candidiasis (section 5.2).

AMPHOTERICIN

Indications: oral and perioral fungal infections

Side-effects: mild gastro-intestinal disturbances reported

Fungilin® (Squibb) PoM
Lozenges, yellow, amphotericin 10 mg. Net price 60-lozenge pack = £3.95. Label: 9, 24, counselling, after food

Allow 1 lozenge to dissolve slowly in the mouth 4 times daily for 10–15 days (continued for 48 hours after lesions have resolved); increase to 8 daily if infection severe

Oral suspension, yellow, sugar-free, amphotericin 100 mg/mL. Net price 12 mL with pipette = £2.31. Label: 9, counselling, use of pipette, hold in mouth, after food

Place 1 mL in the mouth after food and retain near lesions 4 times daily for 14 days (continued for 48 hours after lesions have resolved)

MICONAZOLE

Indications: see under Preparations; intestinal fungal infections (section 5.2)

Cautions: pregnancy and breast-feeding; avoid in porphyria (section 9.8.2); **interactions:** Appendix 1 (antifungals, imidazole and triazole)

Contra-indications: hepatic impairment

Side-effects: nausea and vomiting, diarrhoea (with long-term treatment); rarely allergic reactions; isolated reports of hepatitis

¹**Daktarin®** (Janssen-Cilag) PoM
Oral gel, sugar-free, orange-flavoured, miconazole 24 mg/mL. Net price 15-g tube = £2.27, 80-g tube = £5.00. Label: 9, counselling, hold in mouth, after food

Prevention and treatment of oral fungal infections, place 5–10 mL in the mouth after food and retain near lesions 4 times daily; CHILD under 2 years 2.5 mL twice daily, 2–6 years 5 mL twice daily, over 6 years 5 mL 4 times daily; treatment continued for 48 hours after lesions have resolved
Localised lesions, smear small amount of gel on affected area with clean finger (dental prostheses should be removed at night and brushed with gel)
1. 15-g tube can be sold to the public

Dumicoat® (Dumex) PoM
Denture lacquer, miconazole 50 mg/g. Net price pack of 3 × 1-g bottles (with brushes and cleansing tissues) = £13.50. Label: 10 patient information leaflet

Candida-associated denture stomatitis, apply contents of 1 bottle to upper surface of upper denture after thorough cleansing, allow to dry, and replace; repeat twice at intervals of 1 week

NYSTATIN

Indications: oral and perioral fungal infections

Side-effects: oral irritation and sensitisation, nausea reported; see also section 5.2

Dose: (as pastilles or as suspension) 100 000 units 4 times daily after food, usually for 7 days (continued for 48 hours after lesions have resolved)

Note. Immunosuppressed patients may require higher doses (e.g. 500 000 units 4 times daily)

Nystatin (Non-proprietary) PoM

Oral suspension, nystatin 100 000 units/mL. Net price 30 mL = £2.20. Label: 9, counselling, hold in mouth, after food

Available from Hillcross, Rosemont (*Nystamont®*, sugar-free)

Nystan® (Squibb) PoM

Pastilles, yellow/brown, nystatin 100 000 units. Net price 28-pastille pack = £3.24. Label: 9, 24, counselling, after food

Oral suspension, yellow, nystatin 100 000 units/mL. Net price 30 mL with pipette = £2.05. Label: 9, counselling, use of pipette, hold in mouth, after food

---

Viral infections

The management of herpes infections of the mouth is a soft diet, adequate fluid intake, analgesics as required, and the use of **chlorhexidine** mouthwash (section 12.3.4) to control plaque accumulation if toothbrushing is painful. In the case of severe herpetic stomatitis, systemic **aciclovir** is required (section 5.3).

Herpes infections of the mouth may also respond to **tetracycline** (section 12.3.1) rinsed in the mouth.

Idoxuridine 0.1% paint has been superseded by more effective preparations.

12.3.3 Lozenges and sprays

There is no convincing evidence that antiseptic lozenges and sprays have a beneficial action and they sometimes irritate and cause sore tongue and sore lips. Some of these preparations also contain local anaesthetics which relieve pain but may cause sensitisation.

The following list includes throat lozenges and sprays on sale to the public, together with their significant ingredients.

AAA® (benzocaine), **Beechams Throat Plus®** (benzalkonium, hexylresorcinol), **Bradosol®** (benzalkonium), **Bradosol Plus®** (domiphen, lidocaine (lignocaine)), **Dequacaine®** (benzocaine, dequalinium), **Dequadin®** (dequalinium), **Eludril®** spray (tetracaine (amethocaine), chlorhexidine), **Labosept®** (dequalinium), **Meggezones®** (menthol), **Mentholatum®** lozenges (amylmetacresol, menthol), **Merocaine®** (benzocaine, cetylpyridinium), **Merocets®** lozenges (cetylpyridinium), **Merothol®** lozenges (cetylpyridinium, menthol), **Strepsils®** lozenges (amylmetacresol, dichlorobenzyl alcohol), **Strepsils Extra®** lozenges (hexylresorcinol, menthol), **Strepsils Pain Relief Plus®** lozenges (amylmetacresol, dichlorobenzyl alcohol, lidocaine (lignocaine)), **Strepsils Pain Relief Spray®** (lidocaine (lignocaine)), **TCP®** pastilles (phenols), **Tyrozets®** (benzocaine, tyrothricin), **Valda®** (menthol, thymol), **Vicks Ultra Chloraseptic®** (benzocaine)

12.3.4 Mouthwashes, gargles, and dentifrices

Mouthwashes have a mechanical cleansing action and freshen the mouth. Warm **compound sodium chloride mouthwash** or **compound thymol glycerin** is as useful as any.

Mouthwashes containing an oxidising agent, such as **hydrogen peroxide**, may be useful in the treatment of acute ulcerative gingivitis (Vincent's infection) since the organisms involved are anaerobes. It also has a mechanical cleansing effect due to frothing when in contact with oral debris. **Sodium perborate** is similar in effect to hydrogen peroxide.

There is evidence that **chlorhexidine** has a specific effect in inhibiting the formation of plaque on teeth. A chlorhexidine mouthwash may be useful as an adjunct to other oral hygiene measures for oral infection or when toothbrushing is not possible.

Povidone–iodine mouthwash is useful for mucosal infections but does not inhibit plaque accumulation. It should not be used for periods longer than 14 days because a significant amount of iodine is absorbed.

There is no convincing evidence that gargles are effective.

CETYLPYRIDINIUM CHLORIDE

Indications: oral hygiene

Merocet® (SSL)

Solution (= mouthwash or gargle), yellow, cetylpyridinium chloride 0.05%. Net price 200 mL = £1.90

To be used undiluted or diluted with an equal volume of warm water

---

CHLORHEXIDINE GLUCONATE

Indications: see under preparations below

Side-effects: mucosal irritation (discontinue if desquamation); reversible brown staining of teeth, parotid gland swelling reported

Note. Chlorhexidine gluconate may be incompatible with some ingredients in toothpaste; leave an interval of at least 30 minutes between using mouthwash and toothpaste

Chlorhexidine (Non-proprietary)

Mouthwash, chlorhexidine gluconate 0.2%, net price 300 mL = £1.93

Oral hygiene and plaque inhibition, rinse mouth with 10 mL for about 1 minute twice daily

Denture stomatitis, cleanse and soak dentures in mouthwash solution for 15 minutes twice daily

Available from Blackwell (original, aniseed-, or mint-flavoured)

Chlorohex® (Colgate-Palmolive)

Chlorohex 1200® mouthwash, chlorhexidine gluconate 0.12% (mint-flavoured). Net price 300 mL = £2.20

Oral hygiene and plaque inhibition, rinse mouth with 15 mL for about 30 seconds twice daily

Chlorohex 2000® mouthwash, chlorhexidine gluconate 0.2% (mint-flavoured). Net price 300 mL = £2.20
Oral hygiene and plaque inhibition, rinse mouth with 10 mL for about 1 minute twice daily
Denture stomatitis, cleanse and soak dentures in mouthwash solution for 15 minutes twice daily

Corsodyl® (SmithKline Beecham Healthcare)
Dental gel, chlorhexidine gluconate 1%. Net price 50 g = £1.21
Oral hygiene and plaque inhibition, brush on the teeth once or twice daily
Mouthwash, chlorhexidine gluconate 0.2%. Net price 300 mL (original or mint) = £1.93, 600 mL (mint) = £3.85
Oral hygiene and plaque inhibition, rinse mouth with 10 mL for about 1 minute twice daily
Oral spray, chlorhexidine gluconate 0.2% (mint-flavoured). Net price 60 mL = £4.10
Oral hygiene and plaque inhibition, apply as required to tooth and gingival surfaces using up to max. 12 actuations (approx. 0.14 mL/actutation) twice daily

HEXETIDINE
Indications: oral hygiene

Oraldene® (Warner Lambert)
Mouthwash or *gargle*, red, hexetidine 0.1%. Net price 100 mL = £1.13; 200 mL = £2.02
Use 15 mL undiluted 2–3 times daily

OXIDISING AGENTS
Indications: oral hygiene, see notes above

Hydrogen Peroxide Mouthwash, DPF [1], consists of Hydrogen Peroxide Solution 6% (≡approx. 20 volume) BP
Rinse the mouth for 2–3 minutes with 15 mL in half a tumblerful of warm water 2–3 times daily
1. Included in the BP

Peroxyl ® (Colgate-Palmolive)
Mouthwash, hydrogen peroxide 1.5%, net price 250 mL = £2.04
Rinse the mouth with 10 mL for about 1 minute up to 4 times daily (after meals and at bedtime)

Bocasan® (Oral B Labs)
Mouthwash, sodium perborate 68.6% (buffered). Net price 20 × 1.7-g sachet pack = £1.77
Use 1 sachet in 30 mL of water 3 times daily after meals
Cautions: do not use for longer than 7 days because of possible absorption of borate; not recommended in renal impairment or for children under 5 years

POVIDONE–IODINE
Indications: oral hygiene
Cautions: pregnancy; breast-feeding; see also notes above
Contra-indications: avoid regular use in patients with thyroid disorders or those receiving lithium therapy
Side-effects: idiosyncratic mucosal irritation and hypersensitivity reactions; may interfere with thyroid-function tests and with tests for occult blood

Betadine® (SSL)
Mouthwash or *gargle*, amber, povidone-iodine 1%. Net price 250 mL = £1.12
Adults and children over 6 years, up to 10 mL undiluted or diluted with an equal quantity of warm water for up to 30 seconds up to 4 times daily for up to 14 days

SODIUM CHLORIDE
Indications: oral hygiene, see notes above

Sodium Chloride Mouthwash, Compound, BP
Mouthwash, sodium bicarbonate 1%, sodium chloride 1.5% in a suitable vehicle with a peppermint flavour.
Extemporaneous preparations should be prepared according to the following formula: sodium chloride 1.5 g, sodium bicarbonate 1 g, concentrated peppermint emulsion 2.5 mL, double-strength chloroform water 50 mL, water to 100 mL
To be diluted with an equal volume of warm water

THYMOL
Indications: oral hygiene, see notes above

Compound Thymol Glycerin, BP 1988,
glycerol 10%, thymol 0.05% with colouring and flavouring
To be used undiluted or diluted with 3 volumes of warm water
Mouthwash Solution-tablets, consist of tablets which may contain antimicrobial, colouring, and flavouring agents in a suitable soluble effervescent basis to make a mouthwash suitable for dental purposes.
Dissolve 1 tablet in a tumblerful of warm water

12.3.5 Treatment of dry mouth

Xerostomia (dry mouth) may be caused by drugs with antimuscarinic (anticholinergic) side-effects (e.g. antispasmodics, tricyclic antidepressants, and some antipsychotics), by irradiation of the head and neck region or by damage to or disease of the salivary glands. Patients with a persistently dry mouth may develop a burning or scalded sensation and have poor oral hygiene; they may develop *increased dental caries, periodontol disease, intolerance of dentures,* and *oral infections* (particularly candidiasis). Dry mouth may be relieved in many patients by simple measures such as frequent sips of cool drinks or sucking pieces of ice or sugar-free fruit pastilles.

An **artificial saliva** can provide useful relief of dry mouth. A properly balanced artificial saliva should be of a neutral pH and contain electrolytes (including fluoride) to correspond approximately to the composition of saliva. Of the proprietary preparations available, *Luborant®* is licensed for any condition giving rise to a dry mouth; *Saliva Orthana®, Salivace®, Saliveze®, Glandosane®* and *Oralbalance®* have ACBS approval for dry mouth associated only with radiotherapy or sicca syndrome. *Salivix®* pastilles, which act locally as salivary stimulants, are also available and have similar ACBS approval.

Pilocarpine tablets are restricted to use in xerostomia following irradiation for head and neck cancer. They are effective only in patients who have some residual salivary gland function, and therefore should be withdrawn if there is no response.

Local treatment

Glandosane® (Fresenius)

Aerosol spray, carmellose sodium 500 mg, sorbitol 1.5 g, potassium chloride 60 mg, sodium chloride 42.2 mg, magnesium chloride 2.6 mg, calcium chloride 7.3 mg, and dipotassium hydrogen phosphate 17.1 mg/50 g. Net price 50-mL unit (neutral, lemon or peppermint flavoured) = £4.15

ACBS: patients suffering from dry mouth as a result of having (or having undergone) radiotherapy, or sicca syndrome, spray onto oral and pharyngeal mucosa as required

Luborant® (Antigen)

Oral spray, pink, sorbitol 1.8 g, carmellose sodium (sodium carboxymethylcellulose) 390 mg, dibasic potassium phosphate 48.23 mg, potassium chloride 37.5 mg, monobasic potassium phosphate 21.97 mg, calcium chloride 9.972 mg, magnesium chloride 3.528 mg, sodium fluoride 258 micrograms/60 mL, with preservatives and colouring agents. Net price 60-mL unit = £3.96

Saliva deficiency, 2–3 sprays onto oral mucosa up to 4 times daily, or as directed

Oralbalance® (Laclede)

Saliva replacement gel, lactoperoxidase, glucose oxidase, xylitol in a gel basis. Net price 50-g tube = £3.60

ACBS: patients suffering from dry mouth as a result of having (or having undergone) radiotherapy, or sicca syndrome, apply to gums and tongue as required

Saliva Orthana® (Nycomed)

Oral spray, gastric mucin 3.5%, xylitol 2%, sodium fluoride 4.2 mg/litre, with preservatives and flavouring agents. Net price 50-mL bottle = £3.80; 450-mL refill = £25.10

Lozenges, mucin 65 mg, xylitol 59 mg, in a sorbitol basis. Net price 45-lozenge pack = £3.03

ACBS: patients suffering from dry mouth as a result of having (or having undergone) radiotherapy, or sicca syndrome, spray 2–3 times onto oral and pharyngeal mucosa, when required

Note. Saliva Orthana® lozenges do not contain fluoride

Salivace® (Penn)

Oral spray, carmellose sodium (sodium carboxymethylcellulose), xylitol, calcium chloride, dibasic potassium phosphate, sodium chloride, potassium chloride, and methyl hydroxybenzoate. Net price 100 mL = £4.95

ACBS: patients suffering from dry mouth as a result of having (or having undergone) radiotherapy, or sicca syndrome, 1–2 sprays onto oral mucosa as required

Saliveze® (Wyvern)

Oral spray, carmellose sodium (sodium carboxymethylcellulose), calcium chloride, magnesium chloride, potassium chloride, sodium chloride, and dibasic sodium phosphate. Net price 50-mL bottle (mint-flavoured) = £3.50

ACBS: patients suffering from dry mouth as a result of having (or having undergone) radiotherapy, or sicca syndrome, 1 spray onto oral mucosa as required

Salivix® (Cortecs)

Pastilles, sugar-free, reddish-amber, acacia, malic acid and other ingredients. Net price 50-pastille pack = £2.86

ACBS: patients suffering from dry mouth as a result of having (or having undergone) radiotherapy, or sicca syndrome, suck 1 pastille when required

Systemic treatment

PILOCARPINE HYDROCHLORIDE

Indications: symptoms of salivary gland hypofunction in xerostomia following irradiation for head and neck cancer (see also notes above)

Cautions: close medical supervision in asthma (avoid if uncontrolled, see Contra-indications) and in cardiovascular disease; cholelithiasis or biliary-tract disease, peptic ulcer, hepatic impairment (reduce initial dose), renal impairment; risk of increased urethral smooth muscle tone and renal colic; eye examinations before treatment (decreased visual acuity more likely at night and in patients with central lens changes); maintain adequate fluid intake to avoid dehydration associated with excessive sweating; cognitive or psychiatric disturbances; **interactions:** Appendix 1 (parasympathomimetics)

COUNSELLING. Blurred vision may affect ability to drive, particularly at night, and to perform hazardous activities in reduced lighting

Contra-indications: uncontrolled asthma and chronic obstructive pulmonary disease (increased bronchial secretions and increased airways resistance); acute iritis, angle-closure glaucoma; pregnancy and breast-feeding

Side-effects: sweating; also chills, diarrhoea, nausea, vomiting, lacrimation, abdominal pain, amblyopia, hypertension, constipation, abnormal vision (see Counselling), dizziness, rhinitis, asthenia, increased urinary frequency, headache, dyspepsia, vasodilatation, flushing; other possible side-effects include: respiratory distress, gastro-intestinal spasm, AV block, tachycardia, bradycardia, other arrhythmias, hypotension, shock, confusion, tremors

Dose: 5 mg 3 times daily with or immediately after meals (last dose always with evening meal); if dose tolerated but response not sufficient after 4–8 weeks, may be increased to max. 30 mg daily in divided doses (but associated with increased side-effects); discontinue if no improvement after 3 months; CHILD not recommended

Salagen® (Chiron) PoM

Tablets, f/c, pilocarpine hydrochloride 5 mg. Net price 84-tab pack = £51.43. Label: 21, 27, counselling, driving

13: Skin

13.1   Management of skin conditions

13.1.1   Vehicles

Both vehicle and active ingredients are important in the treatment of skin conditions; the vehicle alone may have more than a mere placebo effect. The vehicle affects the degree of hydration of the skin, has a mild anti-inflammatory effect, and aids the penetration of active drug in the preparation.

Applications are usually viscous solutions, emulsions, or suspensions for application to the skin.

Collodions are painted on the skin and allowed to dry to leave a flexible film over the site of application.

Creams are emulsions of oil and water and are generally well absorbed into the skin. They may contain an antimicrobial preservative unless the active ingredient or basis has sufficient intrinsic bactericidal or fungicidal activity. Generally, creams are cosmetically more acceptable than ointments because they are less greasy and easier to apply.

Dusting powders are used only rarely. They reduce friction between opposing skin surfaces. Dusting powders should not be applied to moist areas because they tend to cake and abrade the skin. Talc is a lubricant but it does not absorb moisture whereas starch is less lubricant but absorbs water.

Gels consist of active ingredients in suitable hydrophilic or hydrophobic bases; they generally have a high water content. Gels are suitable for application to the face and scalp.

Lotions have a cooling effect and may be preferred to ointments or creams for application over a hairy area. Lotions in alcoholic basis can cause stinging if used on broken skin. *Shake lotions* (such as calamine lotion) contain insoluble powders which leave a deposit on the skin surface.

Ointments are greasy preparations which are normally anhydrous and insoluble in water, and are more occlusive than creams. They are particularly suitable for chronic, dry lesions. The most commonly used ointment bases consist of soft paraffin or a combination of soft, liquid and hard paraffin. Some ointment bases have both *hydrophilic and lipophilic* properties; they may have occlusive properties on the skin surface, encourage hydration, and also be miscible with water; they often have a mild anti-inflammatory effect. *Water-soluble ointments* contain macrogols which are freely soluble in water and are therefore readily washed off; they have a limited but useful application in circumstances where ready removal is desirable.

Pastes are stiff preparations containing a high proportion of finely powdered solids such as zinc oxide and starch suspended in an ointment. They are used for circumscribed lesions such as those which occur in lichen simplex, chronic eczema, or psoriasis. They are less occlusive than ointments and can be used to protect inflamed, lichenified, or excoriated skin.

DILUTION. The BP directs that creams and ointments should **not** normally be diluted but that should dilution be necessary care should be taken, in particular, to prevent microbial contamination. The appropriate diluent should be used and heating should be avoided during mixing; excessive dilution may affect the stability of some creams. Diluted creams should normally be used within 2 weeks of their preparation.

13.1.2 Suitable quantities for prescribing

Suitable quantities of dermatological preparations to be prescribed for specific areas of the body are:

	Creams and Ointments	Lotions
Face	15 to 30 g	100 mL
Both hands	25 to 50 g	200 mL
Scalp	50 to 100 g	200 mL
Both arms or both legs	100 to 200 g	200 mL
Trunk	400 g	500 mL
Groins and genitalia	15 to 25 g	100 mL

These amounts are usually suitable for an adult for twice daily application for 1 week. The recommendations do not apply to corticosteroid preparations—for suitable quantities of corticosteroid preparations see section 13.4

13.1.3 Excipients and sensitisation

The following excipients in topical preparations may be associated with sensitisation, particularly of eczematous skin. Details of whether they are contained in preparations listed in the BNF are given after the preparation entry.

Beeswax	Fragrances
Benzyl alcohol	Hydroxybenzoates (parabens)
Butylated hydroxyanisole	Isopropyl palmitate
Butylated hydroxytoluene	Polysorbates
Chlorocresol	Propylene glycol
Edetic acid (EDTA)	Sorbic acid
Ethylenediamine	Wool fat and related substances including lanolin[1]

13.2 Emollient and barrier preparations

13.2.1   Emollients
13.2.2   Barrier preparations

BORDERLINE SUBSTANCES. The preparations marked 'ACBS' are regarded as drugs when prescribed in accordance with the advice of the Advisory Committee on Borderline Substances for the clinical conditions listed. Prescriptions issued in accordance with this advice and endorsed 'ACBS' will normally not be investigated. See Appendix 7 for listing by clinical condition.

1. Purified versions of wool fat have reduced the problem

13.2.1 Emollients

Emollients soothe, smooth and hydrate the skin and are indicated for all dry or scaling disorders. Their effects are short-lived and they should be applied frequently even after improvement occurs. They are useful in dry and eczematous disorders, and to a lesser extent in psoriasis (section 13.5.2). Light emollients such as **aqueous cream** are suitable for many patients with dry skin but a wide range of more greasy preparations including **white soft paraffin**, **emulsifying ointment**, and a mixture of **white soft paraffin** and **liquid paraffin** are available; the severity of the condition, patient preference and site of application will often guide the choice of emollient; emollients should be applied in the direction of hair growth. Some ingredients may rarely cause sensitisation (section 13.1.3) and this should be suspected if an eczematous reaction occurs.

Preparations containing an antibacterial should be avoided unless infection is present (section 13.10) or is a frequent complication.

Urea is employed as a hydrating agent. It is used in scaling conditions and may be useful in elderly patients. It is occasionally used with other topical agents such as corticosteroids to enhance penetration.

Aqueous Cream, BP, emulsifying ointment 30%, [1]phenoxyethanol 1% in freshly boiled and cooled purified water. Net price 100 g = 22p
1. The BP permits use of alternative antimicrobials provided their identity and concentration are stated on the label

Emulsifying Ointment, BP, emulsifying wax 30%, white soft paraffin 50%, liquid paraffin 20%. Net price 100 g = 30p

Hydrous Ointment, BP (oily cream), dried magnesium sulphate 0.5%, phenoxyethanol 1%, wool alcohols ointment 50%, in freshly boiled and cooled purified water. Net price 100 g = 44p

Paraffin, White Soft, BP (white petroleum jelly). Net price 100 g = 32p

Paraffin, Yellow Soft, BP (yellow petroleum jelly). Net price 100 g = 33p

Alcoderm® (Galderma)
Cream, containing liquid paraffin, cetyl alcohol, stearyl alcohol, sodium lauryl sulphate, carbomer, triethanolamine, sorbitan stearate, sorbitol, spermaceti, silicone fluid. Net price 60 g = £2.40
For dry skin conditions
Excipients: include hydroxybenzoates (parabens), isopropyl palmitate
Lotion, water-miscible, ingredients as above. Net price 200 mL = £4.77
For dry skin conditions

Aveeno® (Bioglan)
Cream, colloidal oatmeal in emollient basis. Net price 100 mL = £3.78
ACBS: For endogenous and exogenous eczema, xeroderma, ichthyosis, and senile pruritus (pruritus of the elderly) associated with dry skin
Excipients: include benzyl alcohol, isopropyl palmitate

Dermamist® (Yamanouchi)
Spray application, white soft paraffin 10% in a basis containing liquid paraffin, fractionated coconut oil. Net price 250-mL pressurised aerosol unit = £9.17
For dry skin conditions including eczema, ichthyosis, pruritus of the elderly
Caution: flammable
Excipients: none as listed in section 13.1.3

Diprobase® (Schering-Plough)

Cream, cetomacrogol 2.25%, cetostearyl alcohol 7.2%, liquid paraffin 6%, white soft paraffin 15%, water-miscible basis used for *Diprosone®* cream. Net price 50 g = £1.54; 500-g dispenser = £6.61
For dry skin conditions
Excipients: include chlorocresol

Ointment, liquid paraffin 5%, white soft paraffin 95%, basis used for *Diprosone®* ointment. Net price 50 g = £1.54
For dry skin conditions
Excipients: none as listed in section 13.1.3

Drapolene® —section 13.2.2

E45® (Crookes)

Cream, light liquid paraffin 12.6%, white soft paraffin 14.5%, hypoallergenic hydrous wool fat (hypoallergenic lanolin) 1% in self-emulsifying monostearin, net price 50 g = £1.18, 125 g = £2.39, 500 g = £5.61
For dry skin conditions
Excipients: include hydroxybenzoates (parabens)

Emollient Wash Cream, soap substitute, zinc oxide 5% in an emollient basis, net price 250-mL pump pack = £2.75
ACBS: for endogenous and exogenous eczema, xeroderma, ichthyosis and senile pruritus (pruritus of the elderly) associated with dry skin
Excipients: none as listed in section 13.1.3

Lotion, light liquid paraffin 4%, cetomacrogol, white soft paraffin 10%, hypoallergenic anhydrous wool fat (hypoallergenic lanolin) 1% in glyceryl monostearate, net price 200 mL = £2.17, 500-mL pump pack = £4.08
ACBS: for symptomatic relief of dry skin conditions, such as those associated with atopic eczema and contact dermatitis
Excipients: include isopropyl palmitate, hydroxybenzoates (parabens), benzyl alcohol

Epaderm® (SSL)

Ointment, emulsifying wax 30%, yellow soft paraffin 30%, liquid paraffin 40%, net price 125 g = £3.67; 500 g = £6.21
For use as an emollient or soap substitute
Excipients: none as listed in section 13.1.3

Hewletts Cream® (Kestrel)

Cream, hydrous wool fat 4%, zinc oxide 8%, arachis (peanut) oil, oleic acid, white soft paraffin. Net price 35 g = £1.19; 400 g = £4.85
For nursing hygiene and care of skin, and chapped hands
Excipients: include fragrance

Hydromol® (Quinoderm Ltd)

Cream, arachis (peanut) oil 10%, isopropyl myristate 5%, liquid paraffin 10%, sodium pyrrolidone carboxylate 2.5%, sodium lactate 1%. Net price 50 g = £2.04; 100 g = £3.80; 500 g = £12.60
For dry skin conditions
Excipients: include hydroxybenzoates (parabens)

Kamillosan® (Goldshield)

Ointment, chamomile extracts 10.5% in a basis containing wool fat. Net price 30 g = £1.50; 50 g = £2.50
For nappy rash, sore nipples and chapped hands
Excipients: include beeswax, hydroxybenzoates (parabens)

Keri® (Bristol-Myers)

Lotion, mineral oil 16%, with lanolin oil. Net price 190-mL pump pack = £3.56; 380-mL pump pack = £5.81
For dry skin conditions and nappy rash
Excipients: include hydroxybenzoates (parabens), propylene glycol, fragrance

LactiCare® (Stiefel)

Lotion, lactic acid 5%, sodium pyrrolidone carboxylate 2.5%. Net price 150 mL = £3.19
For dry skin conditions
Excipients: include isopropyl palmitate, fragrance

Lipobase® (Yamanouchi)

Cream, fatty cream basis used for *Locoid Lipocream®*. Net price 50 g = £1.85
Excipients: include hydroxybenzoates (parabens)

Morhulin® (SSL)

Ointment, cod-liver oil 11.4%, zinc oxide 38%, in a basis containing liquid paraffin and yellow soft paraffin. Net price 50 g = £1.19; 350 g = £5.65
For minor wounds, varicose ulcers, pressure sores, eczema and nappy rash
Excipients: include wool fat derivative

Neutrogena® Dermatological Cream (J&J)

Cream, glycerol 40% in an emollient basis. Net price 100 g = £3.67
For dry skin conditions
Excipients: include hydroxybenzoates (parabens)

Oilatum® (Stiefel)

Cream, arachis (peanut) oil 21%. Net price 40 g = £1.79; 80 g = £2.78
For dry skin conditions
Excipients: include fragrance

Shower emollient (gel), light liquid paraffin 70%. Net price 125 g = £4.84
For dry skin conditions including dermatitis
Excipients: include fragrance

Ultrabase® (Schering Health)

Cream, water-miscible, containing liquid paraffin and white soft paraffin. Net price 50 g = £1.05; 500-g dispenser = £6.89
For dry skin conditions
Excipients: include hydroxybenzoates (parabens), disodium edetate, fragrance

Unguentum M® (Crookes)

Cream, cetostearyl alcohol, glyceryl monostearate, saturated neutral oil, liquid paraffin, white soft paraffin, colloidal anhydrous silica, net price 50 g = £1.59, 100 g = £3.13, 200-mL dispenser = £6.19, 500 g = £9.55
For dry skin conditions and nappy rash
Excipients: include polysorbate 40, propylene glycol, sorbic acid

Vaseline Dermacare® (Elida Faberge)

Cream, dimeticone 1%, white soft paraffin 15%. Net price 150 mL = £2.11
ACBS: for endogenous and exogenous eczema, xeroderma, ichthyosis and senile pruritus (pruritus of the elderly) associated with dry skin
Excipients: include hydroxybenzoates (parabens)

Lotion, dimeticone 1%, liquid paraffin 4%, white soft paraffin 5% in an emollient basis. Net price 75 mL = £1.18; 200 mL = £2.29
ACBS: as for *Vaseline Dermacare® Cream*
Excipients: include disodium edetate, hydroxybenzoates (parabens), wool fat

■ Preparations containing urea

Aquadrate® (Procter & Gamble Pharm.)

Cream, urea 10%. Net price 30 g = £1.18; 100 g = £3.54
For dry, scaling and itching skin, apply thinly and rub into area when required
Excipients: none as listed in section 13.1.3

Balneum® Plus (Crookes)

Cream, urea 5%, lauromacrogols 3%. Net price 100 g = £5.58
For dry, scaling and itching skin, apply twice daily
Excipients: include benzyl alcohol, polysorbates

Calmurid® (Galderma)

Cream, urea 10%, lactic acid 5%. Diluent aqueous cream, life of diluted cream 14 days. Net price 100 g = £4.75; 500-g dispenser = £21.48

For dry, scaling and itching skin, apply a thick layer for 3–5 minutes, massage into area, and remove excess, usually twice daily. Use half-strength cream for 1 week if stinging occurs

Excipients: none as listed in section 13.1.3

E45® Itch Relief Cream (Crookes)

Cream, urea 5%, lauromacrogols 3%, net price 50 g = £2.10

For dry, scaling, and itching skin, apply twice a day

Excipients: include benzyl alcohol, polysorbates

Eucerin® (Beiersdorf)

Cream, urea 10%, net price 50 mL = £3.52, 150 mL = £8.57

For dry skin conditions including eczema, ichthyosis, xeroderma, hyperkeratosis, apply thinly and rub into area twice daily

Excipients: include benzyl alcohol, isopropyl palmitate, wool fat

Lotion, urea 10%, net price 150 mL = £3.36, 250 mL = £4.28

For dry skin conditions including eczema, ichthyosis, xeroderma, hyperkeratosis, apply sparingly and rub into area twice daily

Excipients: include benzyl alcohol, isopropyl palmitate

Nutraplus® (Galderma)

Cream, urea 10%. Net price 100 g = £4.37

For dry, scaling and itching skin, apply 2–3 times daily

Excipients: include hydroxybenzoates (parabens), propylene glycol

■ With antimicrobials

Dermol® (Dermal)

Dermol® 500 Lotion, benzalkonium chloride 0.1%, chlorhexidine hydrochloride 0.1%, liquid paraffin 2.5%, isopropyl myristate 2.5%, net price 500-mL dispenser = £6.79

For dry and pruritic skin conditions including eczema and dermatitis, use directly on the skin or as soap substitute

Excipients: none as listed in section 13.1.3

Dermol® 600 Bath Emollient, benzalkonium chloride 0.5%, liquid paraffin 25%, isopropyl myristate 25%, net price 600 mL = £8.49

For dry and pruritic skin conditions including eczema and dermatitis, add up to 30 mL/bath (infant up to 15 mL)

Excipients: include polysorbate 60

Dermol® 200 Shower Emollient, benzalkonium chloride 0.1%, chlorhexidine hydrochloride 0.1%, liquid paraffin 2.5%, isopropyl myristate 2.5%, net price 200 mL = £3.99

For dry and pruritic skin conditions including eczema and dermatitis, use directly on the skin or as soap substitute

Excipients: none as listed in section 13.1.3

13.2.1.1 Emollient bath additives

Alpha Keri Bath® (Bristol-Myers)

Bath oil, liquid paraffin 91.7%, oil-soluble fraction of wool fat 3%. Net price 240 mL = £3.45; 480 mL = £6.43

For dry skin conditions including ichthyosis and pruritus of the elderly, add 10–20 mL/bath (infants 5 mL)

Excipients: include fragrance

Aveeno® (Bioglan)

Aveeno® Bath oil, colloidal oatmeal, white oat fraction in emollient basis. Net price 250 mL = £4.28

ACBS: for endogenous and exogenous eczema, xeroderma, ichthyosis, and senile pruritus (pruritus of the elderly) associated with dry skin, add 30 mL/bath

Excipients: include beeswax, fragrance

Aveeno Oilated® Bath additive, oatmeal, white oat fraction in emollient basis. Net price 10 × 50-g sachets = £7.30

ACBS: as for Aveeno® Bath oil; add 1 sachet/bath (infants half sachet)

Excipients: none as listed in section 13.1.3

Balneum® (Crookes)

Balneum® bath oil, soya oil 84.75%, net price 200 mL = £2.79, 500 mL = £6.06, 1 litre = £11.70

For dry skin conditions including those associated with dermatitis and eczema; add 20 mL/bath (infant 5 mL)

Excipients: include butylated hydroxytoluene, propylene glycol, fragrance

Balneum Plus® bath oil, soya oil 82.95%, mixed lauromacrogols 15%, net price 500 mL = £7.50

For dry skin conditions including those associated with dermatitis and eczema where pruritus also experienced; add 20 mL/bath (infant 5 mL)

Excipients: include butylated hydroxytoluene, propylene glycol, fragrance

Diprobath® (Schering-Plough)

Bath additive, isopropyl myristate 39%, light liquid paraffin 46%. Net price 500 mL = £7.50

For dry skin conditions including dermatitis and eczema; add 25 mL/bath (infant 10 mL)

Excipients: none as listed in section 13.1.3

E45® (Crookes)

Emollient bath oil, cetyl dimeticone 5%, liquid paraffin, net price 250 mL = £2.75, 500 mL = £4.57

ACBS: for endogenous and exogenous eczema, xeroderma, ichthyosis, and senile pruritus (pruritus of the elderly) associated with dry skin; add 15 mL/bath (child 5–10 mL)

Excipients: none as listed in section 13.1.3

Emmolate® (Bio-Medical)

Bath oil, acetylated wool alcohols 5%, liquid paraffin 65%. Net price 200 mL = £2.25

For contact dermatitis, dry skin conditions including ichthyosis and pruritus of the elderly; add 15–20 mL/bath (infant and child 5–10 mL)

Excipients: none as listed in section 13.1.3

Emulsiderm® (Dermal)

Liquid emulsion, liquid paraffin 25%, isopropyl myristate 25%, benzalkonium chloride 0.5%. Net price 300 mL (with 15-mL measure) = £4.33; 1 litre (with 30-mL measure) = £13.49

For dry skin conditions including eczema and ichthyosis; add 7–30 mL/bath

Excipients: include polysorbate 60

Eurax® (Novartis Consumer Health)

Dermatological bath oil, acetylated wool alcohols 5%, light liquid paraffin 65%. Net price 200 mL = £3.19

For dry skin conditions including dermatitis, pruritus of the elderly and ichthyosis; add 15–20 mL/bath (infant and child 5–10 mL)

Hydromol Emollient® (Quinoderm Ltd)

Bath additive, isopropyl myristate 13%, light liquid paraffin 37.8%. Net price 150 mL = £1.87; 350 mL = £3.80; 1 litre = £9.00

For dry skin conditions including eczema, ichthyosis and pruritus of the elderly; add 1–3 capfuls/bath (infant ½–2 capfuls)

Excipients: none as listed in section 13.1.3

Oilatum® (Stiefel)

Oilatum® Emollient bath additive (emulsion), acetylated wool alcohols 5%, liquid paraffin 63.4%. Net price 250 mL = £2.75; 500 mL = £4.57

For dry skin conditions including dermatitis, pruritus of the elderly and ichthyosis; add 5–15 mL/bath (infant 2.5–10 mL)

Excipients: include isopropyl palmitate, fragrance

Oilatum® Fragrance Free bath additive, light liquid paraffin 63.4%, net price 500 mL = £5.75

For dry skin conditions including dermatitis, pruritus of the elderly and ichthyosis; add 1–3 capfuls/bath (infant ½–2 capfuls)

Excipients: include wool fat, isopropyl palmitate

Oilatum® Plus bath additive, benzalkonium chloride 6%, triclosan 2%, light liquid paraffin 52.5%. Net price 500 mL = £7.86, 1 litre = £15.30

For topical treatment of eczema including eczema at risk from infection; add 1–2 capfuls/bath (infant over 6 months 1 mL)

Excipients: include wool fat, isopropyl palmitate

13.2.2   Barrier preparations

Barrier preparations often contain water-repellent substances such as **dimeticone** (dimethicone) or other silicones. They are used for areas around stomas, pressure areas in the elderly, bedsores, etc. They are no substitute for adequate nursing care, and it is doubtful if they are any more effective than the traditional compound **zinc ointments**.

NAPPY RASH. Barrier creams and ointments are used for protection against nappy rash which is usually a local dermatitis. The first line of treatment is to ensure that nappies are changed frequently, and that tightly fitting water-proof pants are avoided. The rash may clear when left exposed to the air and a barrier preparation may be helpful. If the rash is associated with a fungal infection, an antifungal cream such as clotrimazole cream (section 13.10.2) is useful. A mild corticosteroid such as hydrocortisone 1% may be useful but treatment should be limited to a week or less; the occlusive effect of nappies and water-proof pants may increase absorption (for cautions, see Hydrocortisone p. 507).

Zinc Cream, BP, zinc oxide 32%, arachis (peanut) oil 32%, calcium hydroxide 0.045%, oleic acid 0.5%, wool fat 8%, in freshly boiled and cooled purified water. Net price 50 g = 47p

For nappy and urinary rash and eczematous conditions

Zinc Ointment, BP, zinc oxide 15%, in Simple Ointment BP 1988 (which contains wool fat 5%, hard paraffin 5%, cetostearyl alcohol 5%, white soft paraffin 85%). Net price 25 g = 14p

For nappy and urinary rash and eczematous conditions

Zinc and Castor Oil Ointment, BP, zinc oxide 7.5%, castor oil 50%, arachis (peanut) oil 30.5%, white beeswax 10%, cetostearyl alcohol 2%. Net price 25 g = 14p

For nappy and urinary rash

Conotrane® (Yamanouchi)

Cream, benzalkonium chloride 0.1%, dimeticone '350' 22%. Net price 100 g = 66p; 500 g = £3.12

For nappy and urinary rash and pressure sores

Excipients: include fragrance

Drapolene® (Warner Lambert)

Cream, benzalkonium chloride 0.01%, cetrimide 0.2% in a basis containing white soft paraffin, cetyl alcohol and wool fat. Net price 100 g = £1.37; 200 g = £2.23; 350 g = £3.66

For nappy and urinary rash; minor wounds

Excipients: include chlorocresol

Medicaid® (Eastern)

Cream, cetrimide 0.5% in a basis containing light liquid paraffin, white soft paraffin, cetostearyl alcohol, glyceryl monostearate, net price 50 g = £1.49

For nappy rash, minor burns and abrasions

Excipients: include wool fat, hydroxybenzoates (parabens), perfume

Metanium® (Roche Consumer Health)

Ointment, titanium dioxide 20%, titanium peroxide 5%, titanium salicylate 3% in a basis containing dimeticone, light liquid paraffin, white soft paraffin, and benzoin tincture. Net price 30 g = £1.65

For nappy rash and related disorders

Excipients: none as listed in section 13.1.3

Siopel® (Bioglan)

Barrier cream, dimeticone '1000' 10%, cetrimide 0.3%, arachis (peanut) oil. Net price 50 g = 86p

For protection against water-soluble irritants

Excipients: include butylated hydroxytoluene, hydroxybenzoates (parabens)

Sprilon® (S&N Hlth.)

Spray application, dimeticone 1.04%, zinc oxide 12.5%, in a basis containing wool alcohols, cetostearyl alcohol, dextran, white soft paraffin, liquid paraffin, propellants. Net price 115-g pressurised aerosol unit = £3.54

For urinary rash, pressure sores, leg ulcers, moist eczema, fissures, fistulae and ileostomy care

Caution: flammable

Excipients: include hydroxybenzoates (parabens), wool fat

Sudocrem® (Pharmax)

Cream, benzyl alcohol 0.39%, benzyl benzoate 1.01%, benzyl cinnamate 0.15%, hydrous wool fat (hypoallergenic lanolin) 4%, zinc oxide 15.25%. Net price 30 g = 83p, 60 g = 89p, 125 g = £1.46, 250 g = £2.50, 400 g = £3.70

For nappy rash and pressure sores

Excipients: include beeswax (synthetic), polysorbates, propylene glycol, fragrance

Vasogen® (Pharmax)

Barrier cream, dimeticone 20%, calamine 1.5%, zinc oxide 7.5%. Net price 50 g = 70p; 100 g = £1.20

For nappy rash, pressure sores, ileostomy and colostomy care

Excipients: include hydroxybenzoates (parabens), wool fat

13.3   Topical local anaesthetics and antipruritics

Pruritus may be caused by systemic disease (such as drug hypersensitivity, obstructive jaundice, endocrine disease, and certain malignant diseases) as well as by skin disease (e.g. psoriasis, eczema, urticaria, and scabies). Where possible the underlying causes should be treated. An **emollient** (section 13.2.1) may be of value where the pruritus is associated with dry skin. Pruritus that occurs in otherwise healthy elderly people can also be treated with an emollient. For advice on the treatment of pruritus in palliative care, see Prescribing in Palliative Care, p. 14.

Preparations containing **crotamiton** are sometimes used but are of uncertain value. Preparations containing **calamine** are often ineffective.

A topical preparation containing **doxepin** 5% has been introduced recently for the relief of pruritus in eczema; it can cause drowsiness and there may be a risk of sensitisation.

Pruritus is common in biliary obstruction, especially in primary biliary cirrhosis and drug-induced cholestasis. Oral administration of **colestyramine** (cholestyramine) is the treatment of choice (section 2.12).

Topical antihistamines and local anaesthetics are only marginally effective and may occasionally cause sensitisation. A short course of a topical corticosteroid is appropriate in treating *insect stings*. Insect stings should not be treated with calamine preparations.

A short treatment with a **sedating antihistamine** (section 3.4.1) may help in insect stings and in intractable pruritus where sedation is desirable.

For preparations used in *pruritus ani*, see section 1.7.1.

CALAMINE

Indications: pruritus

Calamine (Non-proprietary)
Aqueous cream, calamine 4%, zinc oxide 3%, liquid paraffin 20%, self-emulsifying glyceryl monostearate 5%, cetomacrogol emulsifying wax 5%, phenoxyethanol 0.5%, freshly boiled and cooled purified water 62.5%. Net price 100 mL = 60p
Lotion (= cutaneous suspension), calamine 15%, zinc oxide 5%, glycerol 5%, bentonite 3%, sodium citrate 0.5%, liquefied phenol 0.5%, in freshly boiled and cooled purified water. Net price 200 mL = 62p
Oily lotion (BP 1980), calamine 5%, arachis (peanut) oil 50%, oleic acid 0.5%, wool fat 1%, in calcium hydroxide solution. Net price 200 mL = £1.06

CROTAMITON

Indications: pruritus (including pruritus after scabies—section 13.10.4); see notes above
Cautions: avoid use near eyes and broken skin; use on doctor's advice for children under 3 years
Contra-indications: acute exudative dermatoses
Administration: pruritus, apply 2–3 times daily; CHILD below 3 years, apply once daily

Eurax® (Novartis Consumer Health)
Cream, crotamiton 10%. Net price 30 g = £2.16; 100 g = £3.73
Excipients: include beeswax, hydroxybenzoates (parabens), fragrance
Lotion, crotamiton 10%. Net price 100 mL = £2.80
Excipients: include propylene glycol, sorbic acid, fragrance

DOXEPIN HYDROCHLORIDE

Indications: pruritus in eczema; depressive illness (section 4.3.1)
Cautions: glaucoma, urinary retention, severe liver impairment, mania; avoid application to large areas; pregnancy and breast-feeding; **interactions:** Appendix 1 (antidepressants, tricyclic)
DRIVING. Drowsiness may affect performance of skilled tasks (e.g. driving); effects of alcohol enhanced

Side-effects: drowsiness; local burning, stinging, irritation, tingling and rash; dry mouth and other systemic side-effects reported (section 4.3.1)
Administration: apply thinly 3–4 times daily; usual max. 3 g per application; usual total max. 12 g daily; coverage should be less than 10% of body surface area; CHILD under 12 years not recommended

Xepin® (Bioglan) [PoM]
Cream, doxepin hydrochloride 5%, net price 30 g = £12.61. Label: 2, 10 patient information leaflet
Excipients:include benzyl alcohol

TOPICAL LOCAL ANAESTHETICS

Indications: relief of local pain, see notes above. See section 15.2 for use in surface anaesthesia
Cautions: occasionally cause hypersensitivity
Note. Topical local anaesthetic preparations may be absorbed, especially through mucosal surfaces, therefore excessive application should be avoided and they should preferably not be used for more than about 3 days; not generally suitable for young children

The following is a list of topical local anaesthetic preparations on sale to the public, together with their significant ingredients:
Anethaine® (tetracaine (amethocaine)), **Anthisan® Plus** (benzocaine, mepyramine), **BurnEze®** (benzocaine), **Dermidex®** (lidocaine (lignocaine), alcloxa, cetrimide, chlorbutanol), **Dettol® Antiseptic Pain Relief spray** (lidocaine (lignocaine)), **Lanacane® cream** (benzocaine, chlorothymol), **Solarcaine®** (benzocaine, triclosan), **Solarcaine® gel** (lidocaine (lignocaine)), **Vagisil® cream** (lidocaine (lignocaine)), **Wasp–Eze® spray** (benzocaine, mepyramine)

TOPICAL ANTIHISTAMINES

Indications: see notes above
Cautions: may cause hypersensitivity; avoid in eczema; photosensitivity (diphenhydramine); not recommended for longer than 3 days

The following is a list of topical antihistamine preparations on sale to the public, together with their significant ingredients:
Anthisan® (mepyramine), **Anthisan® Plus** (mepyramine, benzocaine), **Boots Bite & Sting Relief Antihistamine cream** (mepyramine), **Caladryl®** (diphenhydramine, calamine, camphor), **R.B.C.®** (antazoline, calamine, camphor, cetrimide, menthol), **Wasp–Eze® ointment** (antazoline), **Wasp–Eze® spray** (mepyramine, benzocaine)

> denotes preparations that are considered to be less suitable for prescribing (see p. vi)

13.4 Topical corticosteroids

Topical corticosteroids are used for the treatment of inflammatory conditions of the skin other than those due to an infection, in particular the *eczematous disorders* (for further details see section 13.5.1). Corticosteroids suppress various components of the inflammatory reaction while in use; they are in no sense curative, and when treatment is discontinued a rebound exacerbation of the condition may occur. They are indicated for the relief of symptoms and for the suppression of signs of the disorder when potentially less harmful measures are ineffective.

Topical corticosteroids are of no value in the treatment of *urticaria* and they are **contra-indicated** in *rosacea*; they may worsen ulcerated or secondarily infected lesions. They should not be used indiscriminately in *pruritus* (where they will only benefit if inflammation is causing the itch) and are **not** recommended for *acne vulgaris*.

Systemic or potent topical corticosteroids should be avoided or given only under specialist supervision *in psoriasis* because, although they may suppress the psoriasis in the short term, relapse or vigorous rebound occurs on withdrawal (sometimes precipitating severe pustular psoriasis). Topical use of potent corticosteroids on widespread psoriasis also leads to systemic as well as to local side-effects. It is reasonable, however, to prescribe a weaker corticosteroid (such as hydrocortisone) for short periods (perhaps up to 4 weeks) for *flexural* and *facial psoriasis* (**important:** not more potent than hydrocortisone 1% on the face). In the case of *scalp psoriasis* it is reasonable to use a more potent corticosteroid such as betamethasone or fluocinonide.

In general, the most potent topical corticosteroids should be reserved for recalcitrant dermatoses such as *chronic discoid lupus erythematosus, lichen simplex chronicus, hypertrophic lichen planus*, and *palmoplantar pustulosis*. With rare exceptions, potent corticosteroids should not be used on the face as they may precipitate a rosacea-like disorder, perioral dermatitis, and cause skin atrophy.

Intralesional corticosteroid injections (section 10.1.2.2) are more effective than the very potent topical corticosteroid preparations and they should be reserved for severe cases where there are localised lesions (such as *keloid scars, hypertrophic lichen planus*, or *localised alopecia areata*) and topical treatment has failed. Their effects may last for several weeks or even months. Particular care is needed to inject accurately into the lesion in order to avoid severe skin atrophy and loss of pigmentation.

SIDE-EFFECTS. Unlike the *potent* and *very potent* groups, the *moderate* and *mild* groups are rarely associated with side-effects. The more potent the preparation the more care is required, as absorption through the skin can cause severe pituitary-adrenal-axis suppression and Cushing's syndrome (section 6.3.2), both of which depend on the area of the body treated and the duration of the treatment. Absorption is greatest from areas of thin skin, raw surfaces, and intertriginous areas, and is increased by occlusion.

Local side-effects include:

(a)   spread and worsening of untreated infection;

(b)   thinning of the skin which may be restored over a period of time after stopping although the original structure may never return;

(c)   irreversible striae atrophicae and telangiectasia;

(d)   contact dermatitis;

(e)   perioral dermatitis, an inflammatory papular disorder on the face of young women;

(f)   acne at the site of application in some patients;

(g)   mild depigmentation which may be reversible

CHOICE OF FORMULATION. *Water-miscible* creams are suitable for moist or weeping lesions whereas *ointments* are generally chosen for dry, lichenified or scaly lesions or where a more occlusive effect is required. *Lotions* may be useful when minimal application to a large or hair-bearing area is required or for the treatment of exudative lesions. *Occlusive polythene or hydrocolloid dressings* increase absorption, but also increase the risk of side-effects; they are therefore used only under supervision on a short-term basis for very thick areas of skin (such as the palms and soles). The *inclusion of urea* or *salicylic acid* increases the penetration of the corticosteroid.

TOPICAL CORTICOSTEROID POTENCIES

Potency	Examples
Mild	Hydrocortisone 1%
Moderately potent	Clobetasone butyrate 0.05%
Potent	Betamethasone 0.1% (as valerate)
	Hydrocortisone butyrate
Very potent	Clobetasol propionate 0.05%

The preparation containing the **least potent** drug at the lowest strength which is effective is the one of choice; dilution should be avoided whenever possible.

APPLICATION. Corticosteroid preparations should normally be applied once or twice daily. It is not necessary to apply them more frequently.

The length of a corticosteroid cream or ointment expelled from a tube may be used to specify the quantity to be applied to a given area of skin. This length may be measured in terms of a *fingertip unit* (the distance from the tip of the adult index finger to the first crease). One fingertip unit (approximately 500 mg) is sufficient to cover an area that is twice that of the flat adult hand.

Suitable quantities of corticosteroid preparations to be prescribed for specific areas of the body are:

	Creams and Ointments
Face and neck	15 to 30 g
Both hands	15 to 30 g
Scalp	15 to 30 g
Both arms	30 to 60 g
Both legs	100 g
Trunk	100 g
Groins and genitalia	15 to 30 g

These amounts are usually suitable for an adult for twice daily application for 1 week

CHILDREN. Children, especially babies, are particularly susceptible to side-effects. The more potent corticosteroids are **contra-indicated** in infants under 1 year, and in general should be **avoided** in paediatric treatment or if necessary used with great care for short periods. A mild corticosteroid such as hydrocortisone 1% ointment or cream is useful for treating nappy rash (section 13.2.2) and for atopic eczema in childhood (but see caution below).

COMPOUND PREPARATIONS. The advantages of including other substances (such as antibacterials or antifungals) with corticosteroids in topical preparations are debatable, but they may have a place where there is associated bacterial or fungal infection.

HYDROCORTISONE

Indications: mild inflammatory skin disorders such as eczemas (but for over-the-counter preparations, see below); nappy rash, see notes above and section 13.2.2

Cautions: see notes above; also avoid prolonged use in infants and children (extreme caution in dermatoses of infancy including nappy rash—where possible treatment should be limited to 5–7 days), avoid prolonged use on the face (and keep away from eyes); more potent corticosteroids **contra-indicated** in infants under 1 year (see also notes above)

PSORIASIS. Risks of more potent corticosteroids in psoriasis include possibility of rebound relapse, development of generalised pustular psoriasis, and local and systemic toxicity, see also section 13.5.2; they are specifically **contra-indicated** in widespread plaque psoriasis

Contra-indications: untreated bacterial, fungal, or viral skin lesions; rosacea (acne rosacea), perioral dermatitis; not recommended for acne vulgaris (more potent corticosteroids specifically **contra-indicated**)

Side-effects: see notes above

Administration: apply thinly 1–2 times daily

Hydrocortisone (Non-proprietary) PoM
Cream, hydrocortisone 0.5%, net price, 15 g = 38p; 30 g = 60p; 1%, 15 g = 42p. Label: 28. Potency: mild

Ointment, hydrocortisone 0.5%, net price 15 g = 38p; 30 g = 60p; 1%, 15 g = 38p. Label: 28. Potency: mild

When hydrocortisone cream or ointment is prescribed and no strength is stated, the 1% strength should be supplied

Over–the–counter products. The following is a list of skin creams and ointments that contain hydrocortisone (alone or with other ingredients) that can be sold to the public: **Dermacort®** (hydrocortisone 0.1%, cream), **Eurax Hc®** (hydrocortisone 0.25%; crotamiton 10%, cream), **Hc45®** (hydrocortisone acetate 1%, cream), **Lanacort®** (hydrocortisone acetate 1%, cream and ointment), **Zenoxone®** (hydrocortisone 1%, cream). They can be sold to the public for treatment of allergic contact dermatitis, irritant dermatitis, insect bite reactions and mild to moderate eczema

Cautions: not for children under 10 years or in pregnancy, without medical advice

Contra-indications: eyes/face, anogenital region, broken or infected skin (including cold sores, acne, and athlete's foot)

Administration: apply sparingly over small area 1–2 times daily for max. of 1 week

■ Proprietary hydrocortisone preparations
Note. The following preparations are PoM; those on sale to the public (with restrictions) are specified above.

Dioderm® (Dermal) PoM
Cream, hydrocortisone 0.1%. Net price 30 g = £2.69. Label: 28. Potency: mild
Excipients: include propylene glycol
Note. Although this contains only 0.1% hydrocortisone, the formulation is designed to provide a clinical activity comparable to that of Hydrocortisone Cream 1% BP

Efcortelan® (GlaxoWellcome) PoM
Cream, hydrocortisone 0.5%, net price, 30 g = 60p; 1%, 30 g = 74p; 2.5%, 30 g = £1.66. Label: 28. Potency: mild
Excipients: include chlorocresol

Ointment, hydrocortisone 0.5%, net price, 30 g = 60p; 1%, 30 g = 74p; 2.5%, 30 g = £1.66. Label: 28. Potency: mild
Excipients: none as listed in section 13.1.3

Mildison® (Yamanouchi) PoM
Lipocream, hydrocortisone 1%. Net price 30 g = £2.19. Label: 28. Potency: mild
Excipients: include hydroxybenzoates (parabens)

■ Compound preparations
Note. Compound preparations with coal tar, section 13.5.2

Alphaderm® (Procter & Gamble Pharm.) PoM
Cream, hydrocortisone 1%, urea 10%. Net price 30 g = £1.75; 100 g = £5.42. Label: 28. Potency: moderate
Excipients: none as listed in section 13.1.3

Calmurid HC® (Galderma) PoM
Cream, hydrocortisone 1%, urea 10%, lactic acid 5%. Net price 30 g = £2.33; 100 g = £7.30. Label: 28. Potency: moderate
Excipients: none as listed in section 13.1.3
Note. Manufacturer advises dilute to half-strength with aqueous cream for 1 week if stinging occurs then transfer to undiluted preparation (but see section 13.1.1 for advice to avoid dilution where possible)

Eurax-Hydrocortisone® (Novartis Consumer Health) PoM
Cream, hydrocortisone 0.25%, crotamiton 10%. Net price 30 g = 91p. Label: 28. Potency: mild
Excipients: include hydroxybenzoates (parabens), propylene glycol, fragrance
Note. A 15-g tube is on sale to the public for treatment of contact dermatitis and insect bites (*Eurax Hc®*)

■ With antimicrobials
See notes above for comment on compound preparations

Canesten HC® (Bayer Consumer Care) PoM
Cream, hydrocortisone 1%, clotrimazole 1%, net price 30 g = £2.17. Label: 28. Potency: mild
Excipients: include benzyl alcohol
Note. A 15-g tube is on sale to the public for the treatment of athlete's foot and fungal infection of skin folds with associated inflammation (*Canesten® Hydrocortisone*)

Daktacort® (Janssen-Cilag) PoM
Cream, hydrocortisone 1%, miconazole nitrate 2%. Net price 30 g = £2.24. Label: 28. Potency: mild
Excipients: include butylated hydroxyanisole, disodium edetate
Ointment, hydrocortisone 1%, miconazole nitrate 2%. Net price 30 g = £2.25. Label: 28. Potency: mild
Excipients: none as listed in section 13.1.3

Econacort® (Squibb) PoM
Cream, hydrocortisone 1%, econazole nitrate 1%. Net price 30 g = £2.25. Label: 28. Potency: mild
Excipients: include hydroxyanisole

Fucidin H® (Leo) PoM
Cream, hydrocortisone acetate 1%, fusidic acid 2%. Net price 15 g = £3.08; 30 g = £5.30. Label: 28. Potency: mild
Excipients: include butylated hydroxyanisole, potassium sorbate
Gel, hydrocortisone acetate 1%, fusidic acid 2%. Net price 15 g = £2.71; 30 g = £4.71. Label: 28. Potency: mild
Excipients: include hydroxybenzoates (parabens), polysorbate 80
Ointment, hydrocortisone acetate 1%, sodium fusidate 2%. Net price 15 g = £2.51; 30 g = £4.35. Label: 28. Potency: mild
Excipients: include wool fat

Gregoderm® (Unigreg) PoM
Ointment, hydrocortisone 1%, neomycin sulphate
0.4%, nystatin 100 000 units/g, polymyxin B sulphate 7250 units/g. Net price 15 g = £2.51. Label:
28. Potency: mild
Excipients: none as listed in section 13.1.3

Nystaform-HC® (Bayer) PoM
Cream, hydrocortisone 0.5%, nystatin
100 000 units/g, chlorhexidine hydrochloride 1%.
Net price 30 g = £2.66. Label: 28. Potency: mild
Excipients: include benzyl alcohol, polysorbate '60'
Ointment, hydrocortisone 1%, nystatin
100 000 units/g, chlorhexidine acetate 1%. Net
price 30 g = £2.66. Label: 28. Potency: mild
Excipients: none as listed in section 13.1.3

Quinocort® (Quinoderm Ltd) PoM
Cream, hydrocortisone 1%, potassium hydroxy-
quinoline sulphate 0.5%. Net price 30 g = £1.56.
Label: 28. Potency: mild
Excipients: include edetic acid (EDTA), chlorocresol

Terra-Cortril® (Pfizer) PoM
Topical ointment, hydrocortisone 1%, oxytetracycline 3% (as hydrochloride). Net price 15 g =
£1.01; 30 g = £1.82. Label: 28. Potency: mild
Excipients: none as listed in section 13.1.3

Terra-Cortril Nystatin® (Pfizer) PoM
Cream, hydrocortisone 1%, nystatin 100 000 units/
g, oxytetracycline 3% (as calcium salt). Net price
30 g = £2.01. Label: 28. Potency: mild
Excipients: include hydroxybenzoates (parabens), polysorbate,
propylene glycol, fragrance

Timodine® (R&C) PoM
Cream, hydrocortisone 0.5%, nystatin
100 000 units/g, benzalkonium chloride solution
0.2%, dimeticone '350' 10%. Net price 30 g =
£2.38. Label: 28. Potency: mild
Excipients: include butylated hydroxyanisole, hydroxybenzoates
(parabens), sorbic acid

Vioform-Hydrocortisone® (Novartis Consumer
Health) PoM
Cream, hydrocortisone 1%, clioquinol 3%. Net
price 30 g = £1.53. Label: 28. Potency: mild
Excipients: none as listed in section 13.1.3
Ointment, hydrocortisone 1%, clioquinol 3%. Net
price 30 g = £1.53. Label:28. Potency: mild
Excipients: none as listed in section 13.1.3
Caution: stains clothing

HYDROCORTISONE BUTYRATE

Indications: severe inflammatory skin disorders
such as eczemas unresponsive to less potent corticosteroids; psoriasis, see notes above
Cautions: see under Hydrocortisone and notes
above
Contra-indications: see under Hydrocortisone
and notes above
Side-effects: see under Hydrocortisone and notes
above
Administration: apply thinly 1–2 times daily

Locoid® (Yamanouchi) PoM
Cream, hydrocortisone butyrate 0.1%. Net price
30 g = £2.04; 100 g = £6.26. Label: 28. Potency:
potent
Excipients: include hydroxybenzoates (parabens)
Lipocream, hydrocortisone butyrate 0.1%. Net
price 30 g = £2.14; 100 g = £6.56. Label: 28.
Potency: potent
Excipients: include hydroxybenzoates (parabens)
Note. For bland cream basis see *Lipobase®*, section
13.2.1

Ointment, hydrocortisone butyrate 0.1%. Net price
30 g = £2.04; 100 g = £6.26. Label: 28. Potency:
potent
Excipients: none as listed in section 13.1.3
Scalp lotion, hydrocortisone butyrate 0.1%, in an
aqueous isopropyl alcohol basis. Net price
100 mL = £8.83. Label: 15, 28. Potency: potent
Excipients: none as listed in section 13.1.3

Locoid Crelo® (Yamanouchi) PoM
Lotion (topical emulsion), hydrocortisone butyrate
0.1% in a water-miscible basis. Net price 100 g
(with applicator nozzle) = £7.50. Label: 28.
Potency: potent
Excipients: include hydroxybenzoates (parabens), propylene glycol

■ With antimicrobials
See notes above for comment on compound preparations

Locoid C® (Yamanouchi) PoM
Cream, hydrocortisone butyrate 0.1%, chlorquinal-
dol 3%. Net price 30 g = £2.67. Label: 28.
Potency: potent
Excipients: none as listed in section 13.1.3
Caution: causes staining
Ointment, ingredients as for cream, in a greasy
basis. Net price 30 g = £2.67. Label: 28. Potency:
potent
Excipients: none as listed in section 13.1.3
Caution: causes staining

ALCLOMETASONE DIPROPIONATE

Indications: inflammatory skin disorders such as
eczemas
Cautions: see under Hydrocortisone and notes
above
Contra-indications: see under Hydrocortisone
and notes above
Side-effects: see under Hydrocortisone and notes
above
Administration: apply thinly 1–2 times daily

Modrasone® (Dominion) PoM
Cream, alclometasone dipropionate 0.05%. Net
price 50 g = £2.82. Label: 28. Potency: moderate
Excipients: include chlorocresol, propylene glycol
Ointment, alclometasone dipropionate 0.05%. Net
price 50 g = £2.82. Label: 28. Potency: moderate
Excipients: include beeswax, propylene glycol

BECLOMETASONE DIPROPIONATE

(Beclomethasone dipropionate)
Indications: severe inflammatory skin disorders
such as eczemas unresponsive to less potent corticosteroids; psoriasis, see notes above
Cautions: see under Hydrocortisone and notes
above
Contra-indications: see under Hydrocortisone
and notes above
Side-effects: see under Hydrocortisone and notes
above
Administration: apply thinly 1–2 times daily

Propaderm® (GlaxoWellcome) PoM
Cream, beclometasone dipropionate 0.025%. Net
price 30 g = £1.58. Label: 28. Potency: potent
Excipients: include chlorocresol
Ointment, beclometasone dipropionate 0.025%.
Net price 30 g = £1.58. Label: 28. Potency: potent
Excipients: include propylene glycol

BETAMETHASONE ESTERS

Indications: severe inflammatory skin disorders such as eczemas unresponsive to less potent corticosteroids; psoriasis, see notes above

Cautions: see under Hydrocortisone and notes above; use of more than 100 g per week of 0.1% preparation likely to cause adrenal suppression

Contra-indications: see under Hydrocortisone and notes above

Side-effects: see under Hydrocortisone and notes above

Administration: apply thinly 1–2 times daily

Betamethasone Valerate (Non-proprietary) PoM
Cream, betamethasone 0.1% (as valerate). Net price 30 g = £1.40. Label: 28. Potency: potent
Ointment, betamethasone 0.1% (as valerate). Net price 30 g = £1.40. Label: 28. Potency: potent

Betacap® (Dermal) PoM
Scalp application, betamethasone 0.1% (as valerate) in a water-miscible basis containing coconut oil derivative. Net price 100 mL = £4.22. Label: 15, 28. Potency: potent
Excipients: none as listed in section 13.1.3

Betnovate® (GlaxoWellcome) PoM
Cream, betamethasone 0.1% (as valerate), in a water-miscible basis. Net price 30 g = £1.40; 100 g = £3.95. Label: 28. Potency: potent
Excipients: include chlorocresol
Ointment, betamethasone 0.1% (as valerate), in an anhydrous paraffin basis. Net price 30 g = £1.40; 100 g = £3.95. Label: 28. Potency: potent
Excipients: none as listed in section 13.1.3
Lotion, betamethasone 0.1% (as valerate). Net price 100 mL = £4.75. Label: 28. Potency: potent
Excipients: include hydroxybenzoates (parabens)
Scalp application, betamethasone 0.1% (as valerate) in a water-miscible basis. Net price 100 mL = £4.42. Label: 15, 28. Potency: potent
Excipients: none as listed in section 13.1.3

Betnovate-RD® (GlaxoWellcome) PoM
Cream, betamethasone 0.025% (as valerate) in a water-miscible basis (1 in 4 dilution of Betnovate® cream). Net price 100 g = £3.26. Label: 28. Potency: moderate
Excipients: include chlorocresol
Ointment, betamethasone 0.025% (as valerate) in an anhydrous paraffin basis (1 in 4 dilution of Betnovate® ointment). Net price 100 g = £3.26. Label: 28. Potency: moderate
Excipients: none as listed in section 13.1.3

Bettamousse® (Medeva) PoM
Foam (= scalp application), betamethasone valerate 0.12% (≡ betamethasone 0.1%). Net price 100 g = £7.50. Label: 28. Potency: potent
Excipients: include polysorbate 60, propylene glycol
Caution: flammable

Diprosone® (Schering-Plough) PoM
Cream, betamethasone 0.05% (as dipropionate). Net price 30 g = £2.41; 100 g = £6.84. Label: 28. Potency: potent
Excipients: include chlorocresol
Ointment, betamethasone 0.05% (as dipropionate). Net price 30 g = £2.41; 100 g = £6.84. Label: 28. Potency: potent
Excipients: none as listed in section 13.1.3

Lotion, betamethasone 0.05% (as dipropionate). Net price 30 mL = £3.04; 100 mL = £8.71. Label: 28. Potency: potent
Excipients: none as listed in section 13.1.3

■ **With salicylic acid**
See notes above for comment on compound preparations

Diprosalic® (Schering-Plough) PoM
Ointment, betamethasone 0.05% (as dipropionate), salicylic acid 3%. Net price 30 g = £3.30; 100 g = £9.50. Label: 28. Potency: potent
Excipients: none as listed in section 13.1.3
Apply thinly 1–2 times daily; max. 60 g per week
Scalp application, betamethasone 0.05% (as dipropionate), salicylic acid 2%, in an alcoholic basis. Net price 100 mL = £10.50. Label: 28. Potency: potent
Excipients: include disodium edetate
Apply a few drops 1–2 times daily

■ **With antimicrobials**
See notes above for comment on compound preparations

Betnovate-C® (GlaxoWellcome) PoM
Cream, betamethasone 0.1% (as valerate), clioquinol 3%. Net price 30 g = £1.72. Label: 28. Potency: potent
Excipients: include chlorocresol
Caution: stains clothing
Ointment, betamethasone 0.1% (as valerate), clioquinol 3%. Net price 30 g = £1.72. Label: 28. Potency: potent
Excipients: none as listed in section 13.1.3
Caution: stains clothing

Betnovate-N® (GlaxoWellcome) PoM
Cream, betamethasone 0.1% (as valerate), neomycin sulphate 0.5%. Net price 30 g = £1.72; 100 g = £4.77. Label: 28. Potency: potent
Excipients: include chlorocresol
Ointment, betamethasone 0.1% (as valerate), neomycin sulphate 0.5%. Net price 30 g = £1.72; 100 g = £4.77. Label: 28. Potency: potent
Excipients: none as listed in section 13.1.3

Fucibet® (Leo) PoM
Cream, betamethasone 0.1% (as valerate), fusidic acid 2%. Net price 15 g = £3.57; 30 g = £6.04; 60 g = £12.07. Label: 28. Potency: potent
Excipients: include chlorocresol

Lotriderm® (Dominion) PoM
Cream, betamethasone 0.05% (as dipropionate), clotrimazole 1%. Net price 15 g = £3.25. Label: 28. Potency: potent
Excipients: include benzyl alcohol, propylene glycol

CLOBETASOL PROPIONATE

Indications: short-term treatment only of severe resistant inflammatory skin disorders such as recalcitrant eczemas unresponsive to less potent corticosteroids; psoriasis, see notes above

Cautions: see under Hydrocortisone and notes above; max. 50 g of 0.05% preparation per week

Contra-indications: see under Hydrocortisone and notes above

Side-effects: see under Hydrocortisone and notes above

Administration: apply thinly 1–2 times daily for up to 4 weeks

Dermovate® (GlaxoWellcome) PoM
Cream, clobetasol propionate 0.05%. Net price
30 g = £2.56; 100 g = £7.52. Label: 28. Potency:
very potent
Excipients: include beeswax (or beeswax substitute), chlorocresol, propylene glycol
Ointment, clobetasol propionate 0.05%. Net price
30 g = £2.56; 100 g = £7.52. Label: 28. Potency:
very potent
Excipients: include propylene glycol
Scalp application, clobetasol propionate 0.05%, in
a thickened alcoholic basis. Net price 30 mL =
£2.93; 100 mL = £9.91. Label: 15, 28. Potency:
very potent
Excipients: none as listed in section 13.1.3

■ With antimicrobials
See notes above for comment on compound preparations
Dermovate-NN® (GlaxoWellcome) PoM
Cream, clobetasol propionate 0.05%, neomycin
sulphate 0.5%, nystatin 100 000 units/g. Net price
30 g = £3.50. Label: 28. Potency: very potent
Excipients: include beeswax substitute
Ointment, ingredients as for cream, in a paraffin
basis. Net price 30 g = £3.50. Label: 28. Potency:
very potent
Excipients: none as listed in section 13.1.3

CLOBETASONE BUTYRATE

Indications: eczemas and dermatitis of all types;
maintenance between courses of more potent corticosteroids
Cautions: see under Hydrocortisone and notes
above
Contra-indications: see under Hydrocortisone
and notes above
Side-effects: see under Hydrocortisone and notes
above
Administration: apply thinly 1–2 times daily

Eumovate® (GlaxoWellcome) PoM
Cream, clobetasone butyrate 0.05%. Net price 30 g =
£1.76; 100 g = £5.16. Label: 28. Potency: moderate
Excipients: include beeswax substitute, chlorocresol
Ointment, clobetasone butyrate 0.05%. Net price
30 g = £1.76; 100 g = £5.16. Label: 28. Potency:
moderate
Excipients: none as listed in section 13.1.3

■ With antimicrobials
See notes above for comment on compound preparations
Trimovate® (GlaxoWellcome) PoM
Cream, clobetasone butyrate 0.05%, oxytetra-
cycline 3% (as calcium salt), nystatin
100 000 units/g. Net price 30 g = £3.13. Label: 28.
Potency: moderate
Excipients: include chlorocresol
Caution: stains clothing

DESOXIMETASONE
(Desoxymethasone)
Indications: severe acute inflammatory, allergic,
and chronic skin disorders; psoriasis, see notes
above
Cautions: see under Hydrocortisone and notes
above
Contra-indications: see under Hydrocortisone
and notes above
Side-effects: see under Hydrocortisone and notes
above
Administration: apply thinly 1–2 times daily

Stiedex® (Stiefel) PoM
LP Oily cream, desoximetasone 0.05%. Net price
30 g = £2.73; 100 g = £8.19. Label:28. Potency:
moderate
Excipients: include edetic acid (EDTA), wool fat
Lotion, desoximetasone 0.25%, salicylic acid 1%.
Net price 50 mL = £7.69. Label: 28. Potency:
potent
Excipients: include disodium edetate, propylene glycol

DIFLUCORTOLONE VALERATE

Indications: severe inflammatory skin disorders
such as eczemas unresponsive to less potent corticosteroids; high strength (0.3%), short-term treatment of severe exacerbations; psoriasis, see notes
above
Cautions: see under Hydrocortisone and notes
above; max. 60 g of 0.3% per week
Contra-indications: see under Hydrocortisone
and notes above
Side-effects: see under Hydrocortisone and notes
above
Administration: apply thinly 1–2 times daily for
up to 4 weeks (0.1% preparations) or 2 weeks
(0.3% preparations), reducing strength as condition responds

Nerisone® (Schering Health) PoM
Cream, diflucortolone valerate 0.1%. Net price
30 g = £1.59. Label: 28. Potency: potent
Excipients: include disodium edetate, hydroxybenzoates
(parabens)
Oily cream, diflucortolone valerate 0.1%. Net
price 30 g = £2.56. Label: 28. Potency: potent
Excipients: include beeswax
Ointment, diflucortolone valerate 0.1%. Net price
30 g = £1.59. Label: 28. Potency: potent
Excipients: none as listed in section 13.1.3
Nerisone Forte® (Schering Health) PoM
Oily cream, diflucortolone valerate 0.3%. Net
price 15 g = £2.09. Label: 28. Potency: very
potent
Excipients: include beeswax
Ointment, diflucortolone valerate 0.3%. Net price
15 g = £2.09. Label: 28. Potency: very potent
Excipients: none as listed in section 13.1.3

FLUDROXYCORTIDE/
FLURANDRENOLONE

Indications: inflammatory skin disorders such as
eczemas
Cautions: see under Hydrocortisone and notes
above
Contra-indications: see under Hydrocortisone
and notes above
Side-effects: see under Hydrocortisone and notes
above
Administration: apply thinly 1–2 times daily,
reducing strength as condition responds

Haelan® (Typharm) PoM
Cream, fludroxycortide 0.0125%. Net price 60 g =
£3.26. Label: 28. Potency: moderate
Excipients: include propylene glycol
Ointment, fludroxycortide 0.0125%. Net price 60 g
= £3.26. Label: 28. Potency: moderate
Excipients: include beeswax, polysorbate
Tape, polythene adhesive film impregnated with
fludroxycortide 4 micrograms /cm². Net price

7.5 cm × 50 cm = £5.67; 7.5 cm × 200 cm = £19.07

For chronic localised recalcitrant dermatoses (but not acute or weeping), cut tape to fit lesion, apply to clean, dry skin shorn of hair, usually for 12 of each 24 hours

Note. Haelan® Tape cannot be prescribed on form FP10 (GP10 in Scotland) since it is not reimbursable

FLUOCINOLONE ACETONIDE

Indications: inflammatory skin disorders such as eczemas; psoriasis, see notes above

Cautions: see under Hydrocortisone and notes above

Contra-indications: see under Hydrocortisone and notes above

Side-effects: see under Hydrocortisone and notes above

Administration: apply thinly 1–2 times daily, reducing strength as condition responds

Synalar® (Bioglan) PoM
Cream, fluocinolone acetonide 0.025%. Net price 30 g = £1.34. Label: 28. Potency: potent
Excipients: include benzyl alcohol, polysorbates, propylene glycol
Gel, fluocinolone acetonide 0.025%. Net price 30 g = £1.98. For use on scalp and other hairy areas. Label: 28. Potency: potent
Excipients: include hydroxybenzoates (parabens), propylene glycol
Ointment, fluocinolone acetonide 0.025%. Net price 30 g = £1.37. Label: 28. Potency: potent
Excipients: include propylene glycol, wool fat

Synalar 1 in 4 Dilution® (Bioglan) PoM
Cream, fluocinolone acetonide 0.00625%. Net price 50 g = £1.56. Label: 28. Potency: moderate
Excipients: include benzyl alcohol, polysorbates, propylene glycol
Ointment, fluocinolone acetonide 0.00625%. Net price 50 g = £1.56. Label: 28. Potency: moderate
Excipients: include propylene glycol, wool fat

Synalar 1 in 10 Dilution® (Bioglan) PoM
Cream, fluocinolone acetonide 0.0025%. Net price 50 g = £1.48. Label: 28. Potency: mild
Excipients: include benzyl alcohol, polysorbates, propylene glycol

■ With antibacterials
See notes above for comment on compound preparations

Synalar C® (Bioglan) PoM
Cream, fluocinolone acetonide 0.025%, clioquinol 3%. Net price 15 g = 86p. Label: 28. Potency: potent
Excipients: include disodium edetate, hydroxybenzoates (parabens), polysorbates, propylene glycol
Ointment, ingredients as for cream. Net price 15 g = 86p. Label: 28. Potency: potent.
Caution: stains clothing
Excipients: include propylene glycol, wool fat

Synalar N® (Bioglan) PoM
Cream, fluocinolone acetonide 0.025%, neomycin sulphate 0.5%. Net price 30 g = £1.41. Label: 28. Potency: potent
Excipients: include hydroxybenzoates (parabens), polysorbates, propylene glycol
Ointment, ingredients as for cream, in a greasy basis. Net price 30 g = £1.41. Label: 28. Potency: potent
Excipients: include propylene glycol, wool fat

FLUOCINONIDE

Indications: severe inflammatory skin disorders such as eczemas unresponsive to less potent corticosteroids; psoriasis, see notes above

Cautions: see under Hydrocortisone and notes above

Contra-indications: see under Hydrocortisone and notes above

Side-effects: see under Hydrocortisone and notes above

Administration: apply thinly 1–2 times daily

Metosyn® (Bioglan) PoM
FAPG cream, fluocinonide 0.05%. Net price 25 g = £1.17; 100 g = £3.95. Label: 28. Potency: potent
Excipients: include propylene glycol
Ointment, fluocinonide 0.05%. Net price 25 g = £1.04; 100 g = £3.90. Label: 28. Potency: potent
Excipients: include propylene glycol, wool fat

FLUOCORTOLONE

Indications: severe inflammatory skin disorders such as eczemas unresponsive to less potent corticosteroids; psoriasis, see notes above

Cautions: see under Hydrocortisone and notes above

Contra-indications: see under Hydrocortisone and notes above

Side-effects: see under Hydrocortisone and notes above

Administration: apply thinly 1–2 times daily, reducing strength as condition responds

Ultralanum Plain® (Schering Health) PoM
Cream, fluocortolone hexanoate 0.25%, fluocortolone pivalate 0.25%. Net price 50 g = £2.95. Label: 28. Potency: moderate
Excipients: include disodium edetate, hydroxybenzoates (parabens), fragrance
Ointment, fluocortolone 0.25%, fluocortolone hexanoate 0.25%. Net price 50 g = £2.95. Label: 28. Potency: moderate
Excipients: include wool fat, fragrance

FLUTICASONE PROPIONATE

Indications: inflammatory skin disorders such as dermatitis and eczemas unresponsive to less potent corticosteroids

Cautions: see under Hydrocortisone and notes above

Contra-indications: see under Hydrocortisone and notes above

Side-effects: see under Hydrocortisone and notes above

Administration: apply cream thinly once daily *or* ointment twice daily

Cutivate® (GlaxoWellcome) PoM
Cream, fluticasone propionate 0.05%. Net price 15 g = £2.35; 50 g = £6.95. Label: 28. Potency: potent
Excipients: include propylene glycol
Ointment, fluticasone propionate 0.005%. Net price 15 g = £2.35, 50 g = £6.95. Label: 28. Potency: potent
Excipients: include propylene glycol

HALCINONIDE

Indications: short-term treatment only of severe resistant inflammatory skin disorders such as recalcitrant eczemas unresponsive to less potent corticosteroids; psoriasis, see notes above

Cautions: see under Hydrocortisone and notes above

Contra-indications: see under Hydrocortisone and notes above

Side-effects: see under Hydrocortisone and notes above

Administration: apply thinly 1–2 times daily

Halciderm Topical® (Squibb) PoM
Cream, halcinonide 0.1%. Net price 30 g = £3.40. Label: 28. Potency: very potent
Excipients: include propylene glycol

MOMETASONE FUROATE

Indications: severe inflammatory skin disorders such as eczemas unresponsive to less potent corticosteroids; psoriasis, see notes above

Cautions: see under Hydrocortisone and notes above

Contra-indications: see under Hydrocortisone and notes above

Side-effects: see under Hydrocortisone and notes above

Administration: apply thinly once daily (to scalp in case of lotion)

Elocon® (Schering-Plough) PoM
Cream, mometasone furoate 0.1%. Net price 30 g = £4.88; 100 g = £14.05. Label: 28. Potency: potent
Excipients: none as listed in section 13.1.3
Ointment, mometasone furoate 0.1%. Net price 30 g = £4.88; 100 g = £14.05. Label: 28. Potency: potent
Excipients: none as listed in section 13.1.3
Scalp lotion, mometasone furoate 0.1% in an aqueous isopropyl alcohol basis. Net price 30 mL = £4.88. Label: 28. Potency: potent
Excipients: include propylene glycol

TRIAMCINOLONE ACETONIDE

Indications: severe inflammatory skin disorders such as eczemas unresponsive to less potent corticosteroids; psoriasis, see notes above

Cautions: see under Hydrocortisone and notes above

Contra-indications: see under Hydrocortisone and notes above

Side-effects: see under Hydrocortisone and notes above

Administration: apply thinly 1–2 times daily

Adcortyl® (Squibb) PoM
Cream, triamcinolone acetonide 0.1%. Net price 30 g = £1.59. Label: 28. Potency: potent
Excipients: include benzyl alcohol, propylene glycol
Ointment, triamcinolone acetonide 0.1%. Net price 30 g = £1.59. Label: 28. Potency: potent
Excipients: none as listed in section 13.1.3

■ **With antimicrobials**
See notes above for comment on compound preparations

Adcortyl with Graneodin® (Squibb) PoM
Cream, triamcinolone acetonide 0.1%, gramicidin 0.025%, neomycin (as sulphate) 0.25% . Net price 25 g = £3.00. Label: 28. Potency: potent
Excipients: include benzyl alcohol, propylene glycol

Aureocort® (Lederle) PoM
Ointment, triamcinolone acetonide 0.1%, chlortetracycline hydrochloride 3%, in an anhydrous greasy basis containing wool fat and white soft paraffin. Net price 15 g = £2.70. Label: 28. Potency: potent
Excipients: include hydroxybenzoates (parabens), wool fat
Caution: stains clothing

Nystadermal® (Squibb) PoM
Cream, triamcinolone acetonide 0.1%, nystatin 100 000 units/g. Net price 15 g = £2.27. Label: 28. Potency: potent
Excipients: include benzyl alcohol, propylene glycol, fragrance

Pevaryl TC® (Janssen-Cilag) PoM
Cream, triamcinolone 0.1%, econazole nitrate 1%. Net price 15 g = £4.00. Label: 28. Potency: potent
Excipients: include butylated hydroxyanisole, disodium edetate, benzoic acid

Tri-Adcortyl® (Squibb) PoM
Cream, triamcinolone acetonide 0.1%, gramicidin 0.025%, neomycin (as sulphate) 0.25%, nystatin 100 000 units/g. Net price 30 g = £3.15. Label: 28. Potency: potent
Excipients: include benzyl alcohol, ethylenediamine, propylene glycol, fragrance
Ointment, triamcinolone acetonide 0.1%, gramicidin 0.025%, neomycin (as sulphate) 0.25%, nystatin 100 000 units/g. Net price 30 g = £3.15. Label: 28. Potency: potent
Excipients: none as listed in section 13.1.3
Note. Not recommended owing to presence of ethylenediamine in the cream and also because combination of antibiotic with antifungal not considered useful in either the cream or ointment

▅▅ denotes preparations that are considered to be less suitable for prescribing (see p. vi)

13.5   Preparations for eczema and psoriasis

13.5.1   Preparations for eczema
13.5.2   Preparations for psoriasis

13.5.1   Preparations for eczema

An eczematous disorder (dermatitis) is a cutaneous reaction characterised by inflammation and itching. Where possible, the cause (e.g. household detergent) should be established and removed; a patient with suspected contact dermatitis should be patch tested to establish the diagnosis. *Atopic eczema* is the most common form of eczema and usually requires regular application of an **emollient** (section 13.2.1) with short courses of a **mild to moderate topical corticosteroid** (section 13.4); the topical corticosteroid chosen should always be the least potent that is effective. In *mild to moderate atopic eczema* use of the topical corticosteroid should be restricted to periods of one to two weeks, in conjunction with regular use of an **emollient** (section 13.2.1). *Severe atopic eczema* on the limbs or body (or a flare-up of mild to moderate eczema) may require application of a **potent or moderately potent corticosteroid** for the first one to two weeks, followed by a **weaker preparation** as the condition improves; an **emollient** should also be used.

If itching in eczema is a major problem, consideration should be given to administration of a sedating **antihistamine** by mouth; at recommended doses, non-sedating antihistamines are of less value than the sedating antihistamines.

Dry, fissured, scaly lesions are treated with bland **emollients** (section 13.2.1) which are often all that is necessary to allay irritation and permit healing. Preparations such as **aqueous cream** or **emulsifying ointment** should be used as soap substitutes for hand washing and in the bath; patients should be advised to rub the preparation onto the skin before rinsing off completely. The addition of a bath oil may also be helpful (section 13.2.1.1).

Weeping eczemas may be treated with topical corticosteroid creams (section 13.4) ; they are, however, commonly secondarily infected and swabs should be taken for culture and sensitivity testing. Topical or oral antibiotics, or antiseptic soaks (such as potassium permanganate 0.01% applied for no longer than 48 hours) can be used.

Coal tar (section 13.5.2) is used occasionally in chronic atopic eczema.

Ichthammol is usually used in chronic lichenified forms of eczema or to control pruritus. It can be applied to flexures of the limbs as **zinc paste and ichthammol bandage** (Appendix 8).

Ciclosporin (cyclosporin) (section 13.5.2) is now available for *severe resistant atopic dermatitis*; its use calls for specialist care in a hospital context.

Gamolenic acid has been claimed to improve atopic eczema. However, the evidence in favour of a useful therapeutic effect is scant.

For comment on the role of **corticosteroids** in eczema see section 13.4.

ICHTHAMMOL

Indications: chronic lichenified eczema
Side-effects: skin irritation
Administration: apply 1–3 times daily

Ichthammol Ointment, BP 1980, ichthammol 10%, yellow soft paraffin 45%, wool fat 45%. Net price 25 g = 22p
Zinc and Ichthammol Cream, BP, ichthammol 5%, cetostearyl alcohol 3%, wool fat 10%, in zinc cream. Net price 100 g = 75p
Zinc Paste and Ichthammol Bandage, BP (*Ichthopaste®*, *Ichthaband®*), see Appendix 8 (section A8.2.9)

GAMOLENIC ACID

Indications: symptomatic relief of atopic eczema (but see notes above); mastalgia (section 6.7.2)
Cautions: history of epilepsy, concomitant treatment with epileptogenic drugs e.g. phenothiazines; pregnancy
Side-effects: occasional nausea, indigestion, headache; rarely hypersensitivity reactions including rash, urticaria, pruritus and abdominal pain

Dose: 160–240 mg twice daily; CHILD 1–12 years, 80–160 mg twice daily
COUNSELLING. Capsules may be swallowed whole (except *Epogam®* paediatric capsules, see below), or cut open and contents swallowed directly or mixed with milk or taken on bread

Gamolenic Acid (Non-proprietary) PoM
Capsules, gamolenic acid 40 mg in evening primrose oil, net price 240-cap pack = £23.31. Counselling, see above.
Excipients: include vitamin E
Available from Norton
Epogam® (Searle) PoM
Epogam® 40 capsules, gamolenic acid 40 mg in evening primrose oil. Net price 240-cap pack = £23.31. Counselling, see above
Excipients: include vitamin E
Epogam® 80 capsules, gamolenic acid 80 mg in evening primrose oil. Net price 120-cap pack = £23.31. Counselling, see above
Excipients: include vitamin E
Epogam® paediatric capsules, gamolenic acid 80 mg in evening primrose oil. Net price 60-cap pack = £14.72. Counselling, see below
Excipients: include vitamin E
COUNSELLING. *Epogam®* paediatric capsules must *not* be swallowed whole, but cut open at the 'snip-off' neck and contents swallowed directly or mixed with milk or taken on bread

Seborrhoeic dermatitis

Seborrhoeic dermatitis (seborrhoeic eczema) is often associated with malassezia (pityrosporum) infection. Seborrhoeic dermatitis may respond *either* to a **mild topical corticosteroid** (section 13.4), *or* to a **topical antifungal** such as ketoconazole cream (section 13.10.2) *or* to a combination of both. Topical application of **lithium succinate and zinc sulphate** ointment has also been shown to be effective. **Coal tar**, **salicylic acid**, and **sulphur** preparations (section 13.5.2) are also used for seborrhoeic dermatitis of the scalp.

Seborrhoeic dermatitis of the scalp (including dandruff) is managed with topical scalp preparations, see section 13.9

LITHIUM SUCCINATE

Indications: seborrhoeic dermatitis
Cautions: may exacerbate psoriasis; avoid eyes, mucous membranes
Side-effects: occasional skin irritation
Administration: initially apply thinly twice daily, then reduce; CHILD under 12 years not recommended

Efalith® (Scotia) PoM
Ointment, lithium succinate 8%, zinc sulphate 0.05%. Net price 20 g = £3.00
Excipients: include wool fat derivative

13.5.2 Preparations for psoriasis

Psoriasis is characterised by epidermal thickening and scaling. It commonly affects extensor surfaces and the scalp. For mild conditions, treatment, other than reassurance and an **emollient**, may be unnecessary.

In more troublesome cases of psoriasis, local application of salicylic acid, coal tar, calcipotriol, or dithranol may have a beneficial effect.

Salicylic acid may be used in all hyperkeratotic and scaling conditions to enhance the rate of loss of surface scale. Preparations containing salicylic acid 2% are used initially and then gradually increased to concentrations of 3 to 6%. Side-effects are few but include irritation, or, when large areas are treated, salicylate toxicity.

Coal tar is more active than salicylic acid and has anti-inflammatory and antiscaling properties. It is used in psoriasis and occasionally in *chronic atopic eczema*. The formulation and strength chosen depends on patient acceptability, severity and site of the condition; the 'thicker' the patch of eczema or psoriasis the stronger the concentration of coal tar required. **Coal tar paste** or **zinc and coal tar paste** are generally suitable for most cases but are limited by their unpleasant appearance and smell and they may not be used on the face. Some of the newer preparations are more acceptable. Mild coal tar preparations may be suitable for treating the face. **Zinc paste and coal tar bandage** (Appendix 8 section A8.2.9) is useful for treating the limbs. **Tar shampoos** are described in section 13.9. When lesions are extensive coal tar baths are useful. Combinations of coal tar with zinc or salicylic acid have little advantage over the simpler preparations. Preparations containing hydrocortisone and coal tar may be useful in eczemas.

Dithranol is very effective in psoriasis. The preparation is applied carefully to the lesion. Usual concentrations are 0.1–3% and should normally only be applied for short contact periods of 30–60 minutes (**important:** if using above 0.1% the sensitivity of the skin must first be tested—further increases must be gradual). Dithranol must be used with caution as it can cause quite severe skin irritation (especially to perilesional skin). For this reason it must be applied only to the lesions and it is customary to start with low concentrations (e.g. 0.1%) and gradually build up (e.g. every 7 days) to the maximum concentration which produces a therapeutic effect without irritation. It should not be applied to flexural areas since burning may occur. Hands should be washed thoroughly after use. Some patients are intolerant to dithranol even in low concentrations; it is important to recognise them early in treatment because continued use can result in their psoriasis becoming unstable. Fair skin is more sensitive than dark skin. Proprietary preparations may be more convenient as they may cause less staining than dithranol paste. *Ingram's method* of applying dithranol is sometimes used in hospital. The patient soaks in a warm bath containing coal tar solution 1 in 800 and after drying is exposed to ultraviolet radiation B (UVB) to produce minimal erythema. **Dithranol paste** is applied to the lesions and the normal skin protected by applying talc and stockinette dressings. The procedure is repeated daily.

UVB phototherapy is also effective by itself in mild to moderate, guttate or chronic plaque psoriasis.

Calcipotriol is a vitamin D derivative that is now widely used for topical application for plaque psoriasis; a scalp solution is also used for scalp psoriasis. Advantages are that it does not have an unpleasant smell and does not stain clothing. **Tacalcitol**, another vitamin D analogue, has been introduced recently for once-daily application in the treatment of plaque psoriasis.

Tazarotene is a retinoid introduced recently for topical use in mild to moderate plaque psoriasis affecting up to 10% of skin area.

PUVA, photochemotherapy combining a psoralen with long-wave ultraviolet irradiation (UVA), is effective in some patients with psoriasis; special lamps are required. The psoralen, generally methoxsalen [unlicensed] is used to enhance the therapeutic effect of the irradiation; it may be administered either by mouth or topically. Treatment is available in hospital dermatology centres; it has to be carefully regulated, owing to the short-term hazard of severe burning and the long-term hazards of accelerated ageing of the skin, the development of skin cancer and, unless protected, cataract formation.

Acitretin is a retinoid given by mouth for the treatment of *severe resistant or complicated psoriasis* and some of the *congenital disorders of keratinisation* including Darier's disease (keratosis follicularis). It is a metabolite of **etretinate** (which it has replaced). It should be prescribed **only** by, or under the supervision of, a consultant dermatologist and is available to hospitals (or specified retail pharmacies) **only**. It is a retinoid (a vitamin A derivative) with marked effects on keratinising epithelia. A therapeutic effect occurs after 2 to 4 weeks with maximum benefit after 4 to 6 weeks. Acitretin treats only manifestations not the ultimate causes of these diseases, but treatment should be limited to a period of 6 to 9 months with a 3- to 4-month rest period before repeating treatment. Most patients suffer from dryness and cracking of the lips. Other side-effects include a mild transient increase in the rate of hair fall (reversible on withdrawal), occasional generalised pruritus, paronychia, and nose bleeds. There is a tendency for the plasma lipids to rise in some patients. Acitretin is **teratogenic** and must be **avoided** in pregnancy. Contraceptive measures must be taken at least **1 month before** and during treatment by women who may become pregnant and for at least **two years after** a course of the drug.

An antimetabolite, usually **methotrexate**, may also be used for *severe resistant psoriasis*, but this must again always be done under hospital supervision, the dose being adjusted according to severity of the condition and in accordance with haematological and biochemical measurements; the usual dose is 10 to 25 mg of methotrexate once weekly, by mouth.

Ciclosporin (cyclosporin) is now also available for *severe resistant psoriasis* and once again its use calls for specialist care in a hospital context.

For comment on the limited role of **corticosteroids** in psoriasis, see section 13.4.

Topical preparations for psoriasis

CALCIPOTRIOL

Indications: plaque psoriasis

Cautions: pregnancy; avoid use on face and inadvertent transfer to other body areas; wash hands thoroughly after application; risk of hypercalcaemia if max. recommended weekly dose exceeded (reported with less in generalised pustular or erythrodermic exfoliative psoriasis)

Contra-indications: disorders of calcium metabolism

Side-effects: local irritation; also dermatitis, pruritus, erythema, aggravation of psoriasis, photosensitivity; rarely facial or perioral dermatitis; hypercalcaemia (see Cautions)

Administration: *cream* or *ointment* apply once or twice daily; max. 100 g weekly (less with *scalp solution*, see below); CHILD over 6 years, apply twice daily; 6–12 years max. 50 g weekly; over 12 years max. 75 g weekly

Note. Patient information leaflets for *Dovonex*® cream and ointment advise liberal application (but note max. recommended weekly dose, above)

Dovonex® (Leo) [PoM]

Cream, calcipotriol 50 micrograms/g, net price 30 g = £7.78, 60 g = £15.57, 120 g = £28.08
Excipients: include disodium edetate

Ointment, calcipotriol 50 micrograms/g, net price 30 g = £7.78, 60 g = £15.57, 120 g = £28.08
Excipients: include disodium edetate, propylene glycol

Scalp solution, calcipotriol 50 micrograms/mL, net price 60 mL = £21.28, 120 mL = £42.45
Excipients: include propylene glycol
Scalp psoriasis, apply to scalp twice daily; max. 60 mL weekly (less with cream or ointment, see below); CHILD not recommended

MAX. WHEN PREPARATIONS USED TOGETHER. Max. total calcipotriol 5 mg in any one week (e.g. scalp solution 60 mL with cream or ointment 30 g *or* cream or ointment 60 g with scalp solution 30 mL)

TACALCITOL

Indications: plaque psoriasis

Cautions: pregnancy; avoid use on scalp, contact with eyes and inadvertent transfer to other body areas; wash hands thoroughly after application; risk of hypercalcaemia in generalised pustular or erythrodermic exfoliative psoriasis; monitor plasma calcium if risk of hypercalcaemia or in renal impairment; may be degraded by UV light (including sunlight)

Contra-indications: disorders of calcium metabolism including hypercalcaemia (see Cautions)

Side-effects: local irritation including itching, erythema, burning, paraesthesia; rarely contact dermatitis, worsening of psoriasis

Administration: apply daily preferably at bedtime; max. 5 g daily; usual max. 2 courses of 12 weeks per year; CHILD not recommended

Curatoderm® (Crookes) [PoM]

Ointment, tacalcitol (as monohydrate) 4 micrograms/g, net price 30 g = £15.09, 60 g = £26.06
Excipients: none as listed in section 13.1.3

TAZAROTENE

Indications: mild to moderate plaque psoriasis affecting up to 10% of skin area

Cautions: advise patients to wash hands immediately after use, avoid contact with eyes, face, intertriginous areas, hair-covered scalp, eczematous or inflamed skin; avoid excessive exposure to UV light (including sunlight, solariums, PUVA or UVB treatment); do not apply emollients or cosmetics within 1 hour of application

Contra-indications: pregnancy—advise women of child-bearing age to ensure adequate contraceptive protection; breast-feeding

Side-effects: local irritation (more common with higher concentration and may require discontinuation), burning, erythema, desquamation, non-specific rash, contact dermatitis, and worsening of psoriasis; rarely stinging and inflamed, dry or painful skin

Administration: apply once daily in the evening usually for up to 12 weeks; CHILD under 18 years not recommended

Zorac® (Bioglan) ▼ [PoM]

Gel, tazarotene 0.05%, net price 30 g = £14.09, 60 g = £26.26; 0.1%, 30 g = £14.80, 60 g = £27.70
Excipients: include benzyl alcohol, butylated hydroxyanisole, butylated hydroxytoluene, disodium edetate, polysorbate 40

COAL TAR

Indications: psoriasis and occasionally chronic atopic eczema

Cautions: avoid eyes, mucosa, genital or rectal areas, and broken or inflamed skin; use suitable chemical protection gloves for extemporaneous preparation

Contra-indications: not for use in sore, acute, or pustular psoriasis or in presence of infection

Side-effects: skin irritation and acne-like eruptions, photosensitivity; stains skin, hair, and fabric

Administration: apply 1–3 times daily starting with low-strength preparations

Note. For shampoo preparations see section 13.9; impregnated dressings see Appendix 8 (section A8.2.9)

■ Non-proprietary preparations
May be difficult to obtain—moreover some patients may find newer proprietary preparations more acceptable

Calamine and Coal Tar Ointment, BP, calamine 12.5 g, strong coal tar solution 2.5 g, zinc oxide 12.5 g, hydrous wool fat 25 g, white soft paraffin 47.5 g
Apply 1–2 times daily

Coal Tar and Salicylic Acid Ointment, BP, coal tar 2 g, salicylic acid 2 g, emulsifying wax 11.4 g, white soft paraffin 19 g, coconut oil 54 g, polysorbate '80' 4 g, liquid paraffin 7.6 g
Apply 1–2 times daily

Coal Tar Paste, BP, strong coal tar solution 7.5%, in compound zinc paste
Apply 1–2 times daily

Zinc and Coal Tar Paste, BP, zinc oxide 6%, coal tar 6%, emulsifying wax 5%, starch 38%, yellow soft paraffin 45%
Apply 1–2 times daily

■ Proprietary preparations
Alphosyl® (Stafford-Miller)

Cream, coal tar extract 5%, allantoin 2%, in a vanishing-cream basis. Net price 100 g = £1.66
Excipients: include beeswax, hydroxybenzoates (parabens), isopropyl palmitate, propylene glycol
Psoriasis, apply to skin 2–4 times daily

Lotion, coal tar extract 5%, allantoin 2%. Net price 250 mL = £1.50
Excipients: include isopropyl palmitate, propylene glycol
Psoriasis, apply to skin or scalp 2–4 times daily

Carbo-Dome® (Lagap)

Cream, coal tar solution 10%, in a water-miscible basis. Net price 30 g = £4.77; 100 g = £10.50

Excipients: include beeswax, hydroxybenzoates (parabens)

Psoriasis, apply to skin 2–3 times daily

Clinitar® (CHS)

Cream, coal tar extract 1%. Net price 100 g = £10.99

Excipients: include isopropyl palmitate, propylene glycol

Psoriasis and eczema, apply to skin 1–2 times daily

Exorex® (Pharmax)

Lotion, prepared coal tar 1% in an emollient basis, net price 100 mL = £8.65; 250 mL = £17.33

Excipients: include hydroxybenzoates (parabens), polysorbate 80

Psoriasis, apply to skin or scalp 2–3 times daily. Dilute with a few drops of water before application to children and elderly

Gelcosal® (Quinoderm Ltd)

Gel, strong coal tar solution 5%, pine tar 5%, salicylic acid 2%. Net price 50 g = £3.40

Excipients: none as listed in section 13.1.3

Psoriasis and chronic scaling dermatitis, apply to skin twice daily

Gelcotar® (Quinoderm Ltd)

Gel, strong coal tar solution 5%, pine tar 5%. Net price 50 g = £3.06; 500 g = £15.87

Excipients: none as listed in section 13.1.3

Psoriasis and chronic dermatitis, apply to skin twice daily

Liquid, see section 13.9

Pragmatar® (Alliance)

Cream, cetyl alcohol-coal tar distillate 4%, salicylic acid 3%, sulphur (precipitated) 3%. Net price 25 g = £3.12; 100 g = £10.07

Excipients: include fragrance

Scaly skin disorders, apply thinly once daily; dandruff and other seborrhoeic conditions, apply to scalp once weekly or in severe cases daily. Dilute with a few drops of water before application to infants

Psoriderm® (Dermal)

Cream, coal tar 6%, lecithin 0.4%. Net price 225 mL = £3.55

Excipients: include hydroxybenzoates (parabens), isopropyl palmitate, propylene glycol

Psoriasis, apply to skin or scalp twice daily

Scalp lotion—section 13.9

■ Bath preparations

Coal Tar Solution, BP, coal tar 20%, polysorbate '80' 5%, in alcohol (96%). Net price 100 mL = 79p

Use 100 mL in a bath

Note. Strong Coal Tar Solution BP contains coal tar 40%

Polytar Emollient® (Stiefel)

Bath additive, coal tar solution 2.5%, arachis (peanut) oil extract of coal tar 7.5%, tar 7.5%, cade oil 7.5%, liquid paraffin 35%. Net price 350 mL = £4.87, 500 mL = £6.50

Excipients: include isopropyl palmitate

Psoriasis, eczema, atopic and pruritic dermatoses, use 2–4 capfuls (15–30 mL) in bath and soak for 20 minutes

Psoriderm® (Dermal)

Bath emulsion, coal tar 40%. Net price 200 mL = £3.09

Excipients: include polysorbate 20

Psoriasis, use 30 mL in a bath and soak for 5 minutes

■ With corticosteroids

Alphosyl HC® (Stafford-Miller) [PoM]

Cream, coal tar extract 5%, hydrocortisone 0.5%, allantoin 2%, net price 100 g = £3.22. Label: 28. Potency: mild

Excipients: include beeswax, hydroxybenzoates (parabens), isopropyl palmitate, wool fat

Psoriasis, apply thinly 1–2 times daily; CHILD under 5 years not recommended

DITHRANOL

Indications: subacute and chronic psoriasis, see notes above

Cautions: avoid use near eyes and sensitive areas of skin; see also notes above

Contra-indications: hypersensitivity; acute and pustular psoriasis

Side-effects: local burning sensation and irritation; stains skin, hair, and fabrics

Administration: see notes above and under preparations

Note. Some of these dithranol preparations also contain coal tar or salicylic acid—for cautions and side-effects see under Coal Tar (above) or under Salicylic Acid

*****Dithranol Ointment, BP** [PoM] dithranol, in yellow soft paraffin; usual strengths 0.1–2%. Part of basis may be replaced by hard paraffin if a stiffer preparation is required. Label: 28

* [PoM] if dithranol content more than 1%, otherwise may be sold to the public

Dithranol Paste, BP, dithranol in zinc and salicylic acid (Lassar's) paste. Usual strengths 0.1–1% of dithranol. Label: 28

Dithrocream® (Dermal)

Cream, dithranol 0.1%, net price 50 g = £4.24; 0.25%, 50 g = £4.55; 0.5%, 50 g = £5.24; 1%, 50 g = £6.10; [PoM] 2%, 50 g = £7.64. Label: 28. For application to skin or scalp; 0.1–0.5% suitable for overnight treatment, 1–2% for max. 1 hour

Excipients: include chlorocresol, salicylic acid

Micanol® (Medeva)

Cream, dithranol 1% in a lipid-stabilised basis, net price 50 g = £7.98; [PoM] 3%, 50 g = £9.94. Label: 28

For application to skin, for up to 30 minutes, if necessary 3% cream may be used under medical supervision; apply to scalp for up to 30 minutes

Note. At the end of contact time use plenty of lukewarm (not hot) water to rinse off cream; soap should not be used

Excipients: none as listed in section 13.1.3

Psorin® (Cortecs)

Ointment, dithranol 0.11%, crude coal tar 1%, salicylic acid 1.6%. Net price 50 g = £5.30, 100 g = £10.50. Label: 28. For application to skin up to twice daily

Excipients: include beeswax, wool fat

Scalp gel, dithranol 0.25%, salicylic acid 1.6% in gel basis contaning methyl salicylate. Net price 50 g = £3.98. Label: 28. For application to scalp, initially apply on alternate days for 10–20 minutes; may be increased to daily application for max. 1 hour and then wash off

Excipients: none as listed in section 13.1.3

SALICYLIC ACID

For coal tar preparations containing salicylic acid, see under Coal Tar p. 515; for dithranol preparations containing salicylic acid see under Dithranol, above

Indications: hyperkeratotic skin disorders

Cautions: see notes above; avoid broken or inflamed skin

SALICYLATE TOXICITY. If large areas of skin are treated, salicylate toxicity may be a hazard

Side-effects: sensitivity, excessive drying, irritation, systemic effects after widespread use (see under Cautions)

Salicylic Acid Collodion, BP —section 13.7

Salicylic Acid Ointment, BP, salicylic acid 2%, in wool alcohols ointment. Net price 25 g = 18p
Apply twice daily

Zinc and Salicylic Acid Paste, BP (Lassar's Paste), zinc oxide 24%, salicylic acid 2%, starch 24%, white soft paraffin 50%. Net price 25 g = 14p
Apply twice daily

Oral retinoids for psoriasis

ACITRETIN

Note. Acitretin is a metabolite of etretinate

Indications: severe extensive psoriasis resistant to other forms of therapy; palmoplantar pustular psoriasis; severe congenital ichthyosis; severe Darier's disease (keratosis follicularis)

Cautions: exclude pregnancy before starting— patients should avoid pregnancy at least 1 month before, during, and for at least 2 years after treatment, should avoid tetracycline, high doses of vitamin A (more than 4000–5000 units daily) and use of keratolytics, and should not donate blood during or for at least 1 year after stopping therapy (teratogenic risk); monitor hepatic function and plasma lipids at start, 1 month after initiating treatment, and then at intervals of 3 months; diabetes (can alter glucose tolerance—initial frequent blood glucose checks); radiographic assessment on long-term treatment; investigate atypical musculoskeletal symptoms; not recommended for children except under exceptional circumstances (premature epiphyseal closure reported); patients should avoid excessive exposure to sunlight and unsupervised use of sunlamps; **interactions:** Appendix 1 (retinoids)

Contra-indications: hepatic and renal impairment; pregnancy (**important teratogenic risk:** see Cautions and Appendix 4); breast-feeding

Side-effects: (mainly dose-related) dryness of mucous membranes (sometimes erosion), of skin (sometimes scaling, thinning, erythema especially of face, and pruritus), and of conjunctiva (sometimes conjunctivitis and decreased tolerance of contact lenses); other side-effects reported include palmoplantar exfoliation, epistaxis, epidermal fragility, paronychia, granulomatous lesions, reversible hair thinning and alopecia, myalgia and arthralgia, occasional nausea, headache, malaise, drowsiness and sweating; benign intracranial hypertension (**avoid** concomitant tetracyclines); photosensitivity, mood changes and blood disorders (including thrombocytopenia and anaemia) reported for etretinate, raised liver enzymes, rarely jaundice and hepatitis (**avoid** concomitant methotrexate); raised triglycerides; decreased night vision reported; skeletal hyperostosis and extraosseous calcification reported following long-term administration of etretinate (and premature epiphyseal closure in children, see Cautions)

Dose: administered in accordance with expert advice, initially 25–30 mg daily (Darier's disease 10 mg daily) for 2–4 weeks, then adjusted according to response, usually within range 25–50 mg daily (in some cases up to max. 75 mg daily) for further 6–8 weeks (in Darier's disease and ichthyosis not more than 50 mg daily for up to 6 months); CHILD (**important:** exceptional circumstances only, see Cautions), 500 micrograms/kg daily (occasionally up to 1 mg/kg daily to max. 35 mg daily for limited periods) with careful monitoring of musculoskeletal development

Neotigason® (Roche) [PoM]
Capsules, acitretin 10 mg (brown/white), net price 56-cap pack = £25.34; 25 mg (brown/yellow), 56-cap pack = £58.80 (**hosp. or specified retail pharmacy only**—consult product literature for details, specialist dermatological supervision). Label: 10 patient information leaflet, 21

Oral immunosuppressants for psoriasis

CICLOSPORIN

(Cyclosporin)

Indications: see under Dose; transplantation and graft-versus-host disease (section 8.2.2)

Cautions: see section 8.2.2

ADDITIONAL CAUTIONS IN ATOPIC DERMATITIS AND PSORIASIS. ***Contra-indicated*** in abnormal renal function, hypertension not under control (see also below), infections not under control, and malignancy (see also below). Dermatological and physical examination, including blood pressure and renal function measurements required at least twice before starting; discontinue if hypertension develops that cannot be controlled by dose reduction or antihypertensive therapy; avoid excessive exposure to sunlight and use of UVB or PUVA; *in atopic dermatitis,* also allow herpes simplex infections to clear before starting (if they occur during treatment withdraw if severe); *Staphylococcus aureus* skin infections not absolute contra-indication providing controlled (but avoid erythromycin unless no other alternative—see also **interactions:** Appendix 1 (ciclosporin)); monitor serum creatinine every 2 weeks throughout; *in psoriasis,* also exclude malignancies (including those of skin and cervix) before starting (biopsy any lesions not typical of psoriasis) and treat patients with malignant or pre-malignant conditions of skin only after appropriate treatment (and if no other option); monitor serum creatinine every 2 weeks for first 3 months then every 2 months (monthly if dose more than 2.5 mg/kg daily), reducing dose by 25–50% if increases more than 30% above baseline (even if within normal range) and discontinuing if reduction not successful within 1 month; also discontinue if lymphoproliferative disorder develops

Side-effects: see section 8.2.2

Dose: ADULT over 16 years *by mouth*, administered in accordance with expert advice

Short-term treatment (max. 8 weeks) of severe atopic dermatitis where conventional therapy ineffective or inappropriate, initially 2.5 mg/kg daily in 2 divided doses, if good initial response not achieved within 2 weeks, increase rapidly to max. 5 mg/kg daily; initial dose of 5 mg/kg daily in 2 divided doses if very severe; CHILD under 16 years not recommended

Severe psoriasis where conventional therapy ineffective or inappropriate, initially 2.5 mg/kg daily in 2 divided doses, increased gradually to max. 5 mg/kg daily if no improvement within 1 month (discontinue if response still insufficient after 6 weeks); initial dose of 5 mg/kg daily justified if condition requires rapid improvement; CHILD under 16 years not recommended

IMPORTANT. For preparations and counselling and for advice on conversion between the preparations, see section 8.2.2

Preparations

Section 8.2.2

METHOTREXATE

Indications: severe uncontrolled psoriasis unresponsive to conventional therapy (specialist use only); malignant disease (section 8.1.3); rheumatoid arthritis (section 10.1.3)

Cautions; Contra-indications; Side-effects: see also notes above, section 8.1.3, and product literature; investigations required before starting include full blood count, renal function tests (**contra-indicated** if significant impairment, see section 8.1.3 and Appendix 3), liver function tests (**contra-indicated** if abnormalities, see below and Appendix 2), followed by close monitoring during treatment (see also CSM advice, below); **contra-indicated** in pregnancy (following administration to woman or man, avoid conception for **at least 6 months** after stopping) and breast-feeding (see Cytotoxic drugs, Appendixes 4 and 5) and immunodeficiency syndromes; may decrease male or female fertility (effect may be reversible); extreme caution in peptic ulceration, ulcerative colitis, diarrhoea and ulcerative stomatitis (withdraw if stomatitis develops—may be first sign of gastro-intestinal toxicity); photosensitivity—lesions of psoriasis aggravated by UV radiation (skin ulceration reported); **interactions:** see below and Appendix 1 (methotrexate)

CSM ADVICE. In view of reports of blood dyscrasias (including fatalities) and liver cirrhosis with low-dose methotrexate, the CSM has advised:

- full blood count and renal and liver function tests before starting treatment and repeated weekly until therapy stabilised, thereafter patients should be monitored every 2–3 months

- patients should report all symptoms and signs suggestive of infection, especially sore throat

Treatment with folinic acid (as calcium folinate, section 8.1.3) may be required in acute toxicity

BLOOD COUNT. Haematopoietic suppression may occur abruptly; factors likely to increase toxicity include advanced age, renal impairment and concomitant administration of another anti-folate drug. Any profound drop in white cell or platelet count calls for immediate withdrawal of methotrexate and introduction of supportive therapy

LIVER TOXICITY. Liver cirrhosis reported. Treatment should not be started or should be discontinued if any abnormality of liver function tests or liver biopsy is present or develops during therapy. Abnormalities may return to normal within 2 weeks after which treatment may be recommenced if judged appropriate

PULMONARY TOXICITY. May be special problem in rheumatoid arthritis (patient to contact doctor immediately if dyspnoea or cough)

ASPIRIN and other NSAIDs. If aspirin or other NSAIDs are given concurrently the dose of methotrexate should be carefully monitored. Patients should be advised to avoid self-medication with over-the-counter aspirin or ibuprofen

Dose: *by mouth*, 10–25 mg once weekly, adjusted according to response; ELDERLY consider dose reduction (extreme caution); CHILD not recommended

IMPORTANT. Note that the above dose is a **weekly** dose

Preparations

Section 8.1.3

13.6   Acne and rosacea

| 13.6.1 | Topical preparations for acne |
| 13.6.2 | Oral preparations for acne |

ACNE. Treatment of acne should be commenced early to prevent scarring. Patients should be counselled that an improvement may not be seen for at least a couple of months. The choice of treatment depends on whether the acne is predominantly inflammatory or comedonal and its severity.

Mild to moderate acne is generally treated with topical preparations (section 13.6.1). Systemic treatment (section 13.6.2) with oral antibiotics is generally used for *moderate to severe acne* or where topical preparations are not tolerated or are ineffective or where application to the site is difficult. Other oral preparations used for acne include the hormone treatment co-cyprindiol (cyproterone acetate with ethinylestradiol).

Severe acne, acne unresponsive to prolonged courses of oral antibiotics, scarring, or acne associated with psychological problems calls for early referral to a consultant dermatologist who may prescribe isotretinoin for administration by mouth.

ROSACEA. Rosacea is not comedonal (but may exist with acne which may be comedonal). The pustules and papules of rosacea respond to topical metronidazole (section 13.10.1.2) or to oral administration of oxytetracycline or tetracycline 500 mg twice daily (section 5.1.3) or of erythromycin 500 mg twice daily (section 5.1.5); courses usually last 6–12 weeks and are repeated intermittently. Alternatively, doxycycline (section 5.1.3) in a dose of 50 mg twice daily for 2–4 weeks followed by 50 mg once daily for a further 8 weeks may be used if oxytetracycline or tetracycline is inappropriate. Isotretinoin is occasionally given in refractory cases [unlicensed indication]. Camouflagers (section 13.8.2) may be required for the redness.

13.6.1 Topical preparations for acne

Significant comedonal acne responds well to topical retinoids (see p. 520), whereas both comedones and inflamed lesions respond well to benzoyl peroxide or azelaic acid (see below). Alternatively, topical application of an antibiotic such as erythromycin or clindamycin may be effective for inflammatory or comedonal acne. If topical preparations prove inadequate oral preparations may be needed (section 13.6.2).

Benzoyl peroxide and azelaic acid

Benzoyl peroxide is effective in mild to moderate acne. Both comedones and inflamed lesions respond well to benzoyl peroxide. The lower concentrations seem to be as effective as higher concentrations in reducing inflammation. It is usual to start with a lower strength and to increase the concentration of benzoyl peroxide gradually. Adverse effects include local skin irritation, particularly when therapy is initiated, but the scaling and redness often subside with treatment continued at a reduced frequency of application. If the acne does not respond after 2 months then use of a topical antibiotic should be considered.

Azelaic acid has antimicrobial and anticomedonal properties. It may be an alternative to benzoyl peroxide or to a topical retinoid for treating mild to moderate comedonal acne, particularly of the face. Some patients prefer it because it is less likely to cause local irritation than benzoyl peroxide.

BENZOYL PEROXIDE

Indications: acne vulgaris

Cautions: avoid contact with eyes, mouth, and mucous membranes; may bleach fabrics and hair; avoid excessive exposure to sunlight

Side-effects: skin irritation (reduce frequency or suspend use)

Administration: apply 1–2 times daily, starting treatment with lower-strength preparations

Acnecide® (Galderma)
Gel, benzoyl peroxide, in an aqueous gel basis, 5%, net price 60 g = £3.00; 10%, 60 g = £3.30
Excipients: include propylene glycol

Brevoxyl® (Stiefel)
Cream, benzoyl peroxide, in an aqueous basis, 4%, net price 40 g = £3.30
Excipients: include fragrance

Nericur® (Schering Health)
Gel, benzoyl peroxide, in an aqueous gel basis, 5%, net price 30 g = £1.45; 10%, 30 g = £1.60
Excipients: include propylene glycol

PanOxyl® (Stiefel)
Aquagel (= aqueous gel), benzoyl peroxide 2.5%, net price 40 g = £1.76; 5%, 40 g = £1.92; 10%, 40 g = £2.07
Excipients: include propylene glycol
Cream, benzoyl peroxide, in a non-greasy basis, 5%, net price 40 g = £1.51
Excipients: include isopropyl palmitate, propylene glycol

Gel, benzoyl peroxide, in an aqueous alcoholic basis, 5%, net price 40 g = £1.51; 10%, 40 g = £1.69
Excipients: include fragrance
Lotion, benzoyl peroxide, in a non-greasy basis, 5% , net price 30 mL = £1.45; 10%, 30 mL = £1.45
Excipients: include isopropyl palmitate, propylene glycol
Wash, benzoyl peroxide, in a detergent basis, 10%, net price 150 mL = £4.00
Excipients: none as listed in section 13.1.3

■ With antimicrobials

Acnidazil® (J&J MSD)
Cream, benzoyl peroxide 5%, miconazole nitrate 2%. Net price 15 g = £2.33; 30 g = £3.55
Excipients: include polysorbate 20, propylene glycol

Benzamycin® (Bioglan) [PoM]
Gel, pack for reconstitution, providing erythromycin 3% and benzoyl peroxide 5% in an alcoholic basis. Net price per pack to provide 23.3 g = £7.94, 46.6 g = £15.27
Excipients: none as listed in section 13.1.3
Apply twice daily (very fair skin, initially once daily at night)

Quinoderm® (Quinoderm Ltd)
Cream, benzoyl peroxide 5%, potassium hydroxyquinoline sulphate 0.5%, in an astringent vanishing-cream basis. Net price 50 g = £2.21
Excipients: include edetic acid (EDTA)
Cream, benzoyl peroxide 10%, potassium hydroxyquinoline sulphate 0.5%, in an astringent vanishing-cream basis. Net price 25 g = £1.30; 50 g = £2.49
Excipients: include edetic acid (EDTA)
Lotio-gel, benzoyl peroxide 5%, potassium hydroxyquinoline sulphate 0.5%, in an astringent creamy basis. Net price 30 mL = £1.47
Excipients: include edetic acid (EDTA)

AZELAIC ACID

Indications: acne vulgaris

Cautions: pregnancy, breast-feeding; avoid contact with eyes

Side-effects: local irritation (reduce frequency or discontinue use temporarily); rarely photosensitisation

Skinoren® (Schering Health) [PoM]
Cream, azelaic acid 20%, net price 30 g = £5.00
Excipients: include propylene glycol
Apply twice daily (sensitive skin, once daily for first week). Extended treatment may be required but manufacturer advises period of treatment should not exceed 6 months

Topical antibiotics for acne

For many patients with mild to moderate inflammatory acne, topical antibiotics may be no more effective than topical benzoyl peroxide or tretinoin. Topical antibiotics are probably best reserved for patients who wish to avoid oral antibiotics or who cannot tolerate oral antibiotics. Topical preparations of **erythromycin** and **clindamycin** are effective for inflammatory acne; topical preparations of tetracycline may be effective. Topical antibiotics can produce mild irritation of the skin, and on rare occasions cause sensitisation.

Antibiotic resistance of *Propionibacterium acnes* is increasing; there is cross-resistance between erythromycin and clindamycin. To avoid development of resistance:

- when possible use non-antibiotic antimicrobials (such as benzoyl peroxide or azelaic acid);
- avoid concomitant treatment with different oral and topical antibiotics;
- if a particular antibiotic is effective, use it for repeat courses if needed;
- do not continue treatment for longer than necessary (however, treatment with a topical preparation should be continued for at least 6 months);
- short intervening courses of topical antibacterial drugs (such as benzoyl peroxide or azelaic acid) may help to eliminate any resistant propionibacteria

ANTIBIOTICS

Indications: acne vulgaris

Cautions: some manufacturers advise preparations containing alcohol are not suitable for use with benzoyl peroxide

PoM **Benzamycin®** see under Benzoyl Peroxide above

Dalacin T® (Pharmacia & Upjohn) PoM
Topical solution, clindamycin (as phosphate) 1%, in an aqueous alcoholic basis. Net price (both with applicator) 30 mL = £4.34; 50 mL = £7.23
Excipients: include propylene glycol
Apply twice daily

Lotion, clindamycin (as phosphate) 1% in an aqueous basis. Net price 30 mL = £5.08; 50 mL = £8.47
Excipients: include hydroxybenzoates (parabens)
Apply twice daily

Eryacne® (Galderma) PoM
Gel, erythromycin in an alcoholic basis, 2% (*Eryacne® 2*), net price 30 g = £4.97; 4% (*Eryacne® 4*), 30 g = £4.97
Excipients: include butylated hydroxytoluene
Apply twice daily starting with 4% for 4 weeks then reducing to 2% if condition improves

Stiemycin® (Stiefel) PoM
Solution, erythromycin 2% in an alcoholic basis. Net price 50 mL = £8.60
Excipients: include propylene glycol
Apply twice daily

Topicycline® (Monmouth) PoM
Solution, powder for reconstitution, tetracycline hydrochloride, 4-epitetracycline hydrochloride, providing tetracycline hydrochloride 2.2 mg/mL when reconstituted with solvent containing *n*-decyl methyl sulphoxide and citric acid in 40% alcohol. Net price per pack of powder and solvent to provide 70 mL = £6.15
Excipients: none as listed in section 13.1.3
Apply twice daily

Zineryt® (Yamanouchi) PoM
Topical solution, powder for reconstitution, erythromycin 40 mg/mL, zinc acetate 12 mg/mL when reconstituted with solvent containing ethanol. Net price per pack of powder and solvent to provide 30 mL = £7.09; 90 mL = £20.62
Excipients: none as listed in section 13.1.3
Apply twice daily

Topical retinoids and related preparations for acne

Tretinoin and its isomer **isotretinoin** are useful in treating comedonal acne but patients should be warned that some redness and skin peeling might occur initially but settles with time. Several months of treatment may be needed to achieve an optimal response and the treatment should be continued until no new lesions develop.

Topical **isotretinoin** is licensed to treat non-inflammatory and inflammatory lesions in patients with mild to moderate acne. Isotretinoin is also given by mouth; see section 13.6.2 for **warnings** relating to use by mouth.

Adapalene is a recently introduced retinoid-like drug indicated for mild to moderate acne. It may be less irritant than other topical retinoids.

CAUTIONS. Topical retinoids should be avoided in severe acne involving large areas. Contact with eyes, nostrils, mouth and mucous membranes, eczematous, broken or sunburned skin should be avoided. These drugs should be used with caution in sensitive areas such as the neck, and accumulation in angles of the nose should be avoided. Exposure to UV light (including sunlight, solariums) should be avoided; if sun exposure is unavoidable, an appropriate sunscreen or protective clothing should be used. Use of retinoids with abrasive cleaners, comedogenic or astringent cosmetics should be avoided. Allow peeling (e.g resulting from use of benzoyl peroxide) to subside before using a topical retinoid; alternating a preparation that causes peeling with a topical retinoid may give rise to contact dermatitis (reduce frequency of retinoid application).

CONTRA-INDICATIONS. Topical retinoids are contra-indicated in pregnancy (Appendix 4); women of child-bearing age should take adequate contraceptive precautions; topical retinoids should be avoided in breast-feeding (Appendix 5). Tretinoin is contra-indicated in personal or familial history of cutaneous epithelioma.

SIDE-EFFECTS. Local reactions include burning, erythema, stinging, pruritus, dry or peeling skin (discontinue if severe). Increased sensitivity to UVB light or sunlight occurs. Temporary changes of skin pigmentation have been reported. Eye irritation and oedema, and blistering or crusting of skin have been reported rarely.

ADAPALENE

Indications: mild to moderate acne
Cautions: see notes above
Contra-indications: see notes above
Side-effects: see notes above
Administration: apply thinly once daily before retiring

Differin® (Galderma) PoM
Cream, adapalene 0.1%, net price 30 g = £8.00
Excipients: include disodium edetate, hydroxybenzoates (parabens)
Gel, adapalene 0.1%, net price 30 g = £8.00
Excipients: include disodium edetate, hydroxybenzoates (parabens), propylene glycol

TRETINOIN

Note. Tretinoin is the acid form of vitamin A

Indications: see under preparations below; photo-damage (section 13.8.1); malignant disease (section 8.1.5)

Cautions: see notes above

Contra-indications: see notes above

Side-effects: see notes above

Administration: see under preparations below

Retin-A® (Janssen-Cilag) PoM
Cream, tretinoin 0.025%, net price 60 g = £6.03
Acne vulgaris, for dry or fair skin, apply thinly 1–2 times daily
Excipients: include butylated hydroxytoluene, sorbic acid

Gel, tretinoin 0.01%, net price 60 g = £6.03; 0.025%, 60 g = £6.03
Acne vulgaris and other keratotic conditions, apply thinly 1–2 times daily
Excipients: include butylated hydroxytoluene

Lotion, tretinoin 0.025%. Net price 100 mL = £6.94
Acne vulgaris, for application to large areas such as the back, apply thinly 1–2 times daily
Excipients: include butylated hydroxytoluene

Acticin® (Strakan) PoM
Cream, tretinoin 0.025%, net price 45 g = £7.50
Acne vulgaris, for dry or fair skin, apply thinly once daily before retiring to bed
Excipients: include butylated hydroxytoluene, propylene glycol, sorbic acid

Gel, tretinoin 0.025% in an alcoholic basis, net price 45 g = £7.50
Acne vulgaris, for oily or dark skin, apply thinly once daily before retiring to bed
Excipients: include butylated hydroxytoluene

ISOTRETINOIN

Note. Isotretinoin is an isomer of tretinoin

Indications; Cautions; Contra-indications; Side-effects: (*after topical application* **only**): see notes above

IMPORTANT. For **indications, cautions, contra-indications** and **side-effects** of isotretinoin **when given by mouth**, see pp. 522-3

Administration: apply thinly 1–2 times daily

Isotrex® (Stiefel) PoM
Gel, isotretinoin 0.05%, net price 30 g = £6.65. Label: 10 patient information leaflet
Excipients: include butylated hydroxytoluene

■ With antibacterial

Isotrexin® (Stiefel) PoM
Gel, isotretinoin 0.05%, erythromycin 2% in ethanolic basis, net price 30 g = £8.36. Label: 10 patient information leaflet
Excipients: include butylated hydroxytoluene

Other topical preparations for acne

Salicylic acid is available in various preparations for sale direct to the public for the treatment of mild acne.

Preparations containing **sulphur** and **abrasive agents** are not considered beneficial in acne.

Topical **corticosteroids** should **not** be used in acne.

A topical preparation of **nicotinamide** is available for inflammatory acne.

ABRASIVE AGENTS ▱

Indications: acne vulgaris (but see notes above)

Cautions: avoid contact with eyes; discontinue use temporarily if skin becomes irritated

Contra-indications: superficial venules, telangiectasia

Brasivol® (Stiefel) ▱
Paste No. 1, aluminium oxide 38.09% in fine particles, in a soap-detergent basis; *Paste No. 2*, aluminium oxide 52.2% in medium particles, net price 75 g (both) = £2.49
Excipients: include fragrance
Use instead of soap 1–3 times daily, starting with *No.1*

Ionax Scrub® (Galderma) NHS ▱
Gel, polyethylene granules 21.9%, benzalkonium chloride 0.25% in a foaming aqueous alcoholic basis. Net price 60 g = £3.13
Excipients: include propylene glycol
Use instead of soap 1–2 times daily

CORTICOSTEROIDS

Indications: use in acne not recommended (see notes above)

Cautions: see section 13.4 and notes above

Contra-indications: see section 13.4 and notes above

Side-effects: see section 13.4 and notes above

Actinac® (Peckforton) PoM ▱
Lotion (powder for reconstitution with solvent), chloramphenicol 40 mg, hydrocortisone acetate 40 mg, allantoin 24 mg, butoxyethyl nicotinate 24 mg, precipitated sulphur 320 mg/g. Discard after 21 days. Net price 2 × 6.25-g bottles powder with 2 × 20-mL bottles solvent = £9.30. Label: 28. Potency: mild
Excipients: none as listed in section 13.1.3

NICOTINAMIDE

Indications: see under preparation

Cautions: avoid contact with eyes and mucous membranes (including nose and mouth); reduce frequency of application if excessive dryness, irritation or peeling

Side-effects: dryness of skin; also pruritus, erythema, burning and irritation

Papulex® (Pharmagenix)
Gel, nicotinamide 4%. Net price 60 g = £7.98
Excipients: none as listed in section 13.1.3
Inflammatory acne vulgaris, apply twice daily; reduce to once daily or on alternate days if irritation occurs

SALICYLIC ACID ▱

Indications: acne vulgaris; psoriasis (section 13.5.2); warts and calluses (section 13.7)

Cautions: avoid contact with mouth, eyes, mucous membranes; systemic effects after excessive use (see section 10.1.1)

Side-effects: local irritation

Acnisal® (DermaPharm) ▱
Topical solution, salicylic acid 2% in a detergent and emollient basis. Net price 177 mL = £4.13.
Use up to 3 times daily
Excipients: include benzyl alcohol

SULPHUR ◼

Cautions: avoid contact with eyes, mouth, and mucous membranes; causes skin irritation

■ With resorcinol

Prolonged application of resorcinol may interfere with thyroid function therefore not recommended

Eskamel® (Goldshield) NHS ◼

Cream, resorcinol 2%, sulphur 8%, in a non-greasy flesh-coloured basis. Net price 25 g = £2.52

Excipients: include propylene glycol, fragrance

■ With salicylic acid

See above for cautions relating to salicylic acid

Salicylic Acid and Sulphur Cream, BP 1980, ◼ salicylic acid 2%, precipitated sulphur 2%, in aqueous cream

Salicylic Acid and Sulphur Ointment, BPC, ◼ salicylic acid 3%, precipitated sulphur 3%, in hydrous ointment (oily cream)

◼ denotes preparations that are considered to be less suitable for prescribing (see p. vi)

13.6.2 Oral preparations for acne

Oral antibiotics for acne

Systemic antibacterial treatment is useful for inflammatory acne if topical treatment is not adequately effective or if it is inappropriate. Anticomedonal treatment (e.g. with topical benzoyl peroxide) may also be required.

Either **oxytetracycline** or **tetracycline** (section 5.1.3) is usually given for acne in a dose of 500 mg twice daily. If there is no improvement after the first 3 months another oral antibiotic should be used. Maximum improvement usually occurs after 4 to 6 months but in more severe cases treatment may need to be continued for 2 years or longer.

Doxycycline and **minocycline** (section 5.1.3) are alternatives to tetracycline. Doxycycline may be used in a dosage of 100 mg daily. Minocycline offers less likelihood of bacterial resistance but may sometimes cause irreversible pigmentation; it is given in a dosage of 100 mg daily (in one or two divided doses).

Erythromycin in a dose of 500 mg twice daily is an alternative for the management of acne but propionibacteria strains resistant to erythromycin are becoming widespread and this may explain poor response.

Concomitant use of different topical and systemic antibiotics is undesirable owing to the increased likelihood of the development of bacterial resistance.

Hormone treatment for acne

Co-cyprindiol (cyproterone acetate with ethinylestradiol) contains an anti-androgen. It is no more effective than an oral broad spectrum antibiotic but is useful in women who also wish to receive oral contraception.

Improvement of acne probably occurs because of decreased sebum secretion which is under androgen control. Some women with moderately severe hirsutism may also benefit as hair growth is also androgen-dependent. Its contra-indications include pregnancy and a predisposition to thrombosis.

CO-CYPRINDIOL

A mixture of cyproterone acetate and ethinylestradiol in the mass proportions 2000 parts to 35 parts, respectively

Indications: severe acne in women refractory to prolonged oral antibiotic therapy (but see notes above)

Cautions: see under Combined Oral Contraceptives (section 7.3.1)

Contra-indications: see under Combined Oral Contraceptives (section 7.3.1)

Side-effects: see under Combined Oral Contraceptives (section 7.3.1)

Dianette® (Schering Health) PoM

Tablets, beige, s/c, co-cyprindiol 2000/35 (cyproterone acetate 2 mg, ethinylestradiol 35 micrograms), net price 21-tab pack = £4.32

Dose: 1 tablet daily for 21 days starting on day 1 of menstrual cycle and repeated after a 7-day interval, usually for several months; withdraw when acne or hirsutism completely resolved (repeat courses may be given if recurrence)

Oral retinoid for acne

The retinoid **isotretinoin** (*Roaccutane®*) reduces sebum secretion. It is used for the systemic treatment of nodulo-cystic and conglobate acne, severe acne, scarring, acne which has not responded to an adequate course of a systemic antibiotic, or acne which is associated with psychological problems. It is also useful in women who develop acne in the third or fourth decades of life, since late onset acne is frequently unresponsive to antibiotics.

Isotretinoin is a toxic drug that should be prescribed **only** by, or under the supervision of, a consultant dermatologist. It is given for at least 16 weeks; repeat courses are not normally required.

Side-effects of isotretinoin include severe dryness of the skin and mucous membranes, nose bleeds, and joint pains. The drug is **teratogenic** and must **not** be given to women of child-bearing age unless they practise effective contraception and then only after detailed assessment and explanation by the physician (see under Cautions below).

ISOTRETINOIN

Note. Isotretinoin is an isomer of tretinoin

Indications: see notes above

Cautions: exclude pregnancy before starting (perform pregnancy test 2–3 days before expected menstruation, start treatment on day 2 or 3 of menstrual cycle)—effective contraception must be practised at least 1 month before, during, and for at least 1 month after treatment; avoid blood donation during treatment and for at least 1 month after treatment; history of depression; measure hepatic function and plasma lipids before treatment, 1 month after starting and then every 3 months; diabetes; dry eye syndrome (associated with risk of keratitis); avoid keratolytics; **interactions:** Appendix 1 (retinoids)

WAX EPILATION AND DERMABRASION. Warn patient to avoid wax epilation during treatment and for 5–6 months after stopping (risk of epidermal stripping); avoid dermabrasion during treatment and for 5–6 months after stopping (risk of scarring)

Contra-indications: pregnancy (**important teratogenic risk:** see Cautions and Appendix 4); breast-feeding; renal or hepatic impairment; hypervitaminosis A, hyperlipidaemia

Side-effects: dryness of skin (with scaling, thinning, erythema, pruritus), epidermal fragility (trauma may cause blistering); rarely acne fulminans, facial hyperpigmentation; dryness of nasal mucosa (with mild epistaxis), of pharyngeal mucosa (with hoarseness), of conjunctiva (sometimes conjunctivitis), decreased tolerance to contact lenses and rarely keratitis; visual disturbances (papilloedema, optic neuritis, corneal opacities, cataracts, decreased night vision, photophobia, blurred vision)—expert referral and consider withdrawal; hair thinning (reversible on withdrawal) or (rarely) hirsutism; nausea, headache, malaise, drowsiness, sweating; benign intracranial hypertension (avoid concomitant tetracyclines); myalgia and arthralgia; raised serum creatinine concentrations reported; rarely jaundice and hepatitis; raised plasma triglycerides and cholesterol (risk of pancreatitis if triglycerides above 8 g/litre); allergic vasculitis and granulomatous lesions reported, other side-effects reported include hearing deficiency, mood changes (severe depression), convulsions, menstrual irregularities, hyperuricaemia, inflammatory bowel disease, paronychia and Gram-positive infections, tendinitis, bone changes (including early epiphyseal closure and skeletal hyperostosis following long-term administration), thrombocytopenia, thrombocytosis, neutropenia and anaemia, lymphadenopathy, and haematuria and proteinuria

Dose: initially 500 micrograms/kg daily (in 1–2 divided doses) with food for 4 weeks; if good response continue for further 8–12 weeks; if little response, increase to 1 mg/kg daily for 8–12 weeks; if intolerant, reduce dose to 100–200 micrograms/kg daily

Roaccutane® (Roche) PoM
Capsules, isotretinoin 5 mg (red-violet/white), net price 56-cap pack = £18.22; 20 mg (red-violet/white), 56-cap pack = £50.21(**hosp. or specified retail pharmacy only**). Label: 10, patient information card, 21

13.7 Preparations for warts and calluses

Warts (verrucas) are caused by a human papillomavirus, which most frequently affects the hands, feet (plantar warts), and the anogenital region (see below); treatment usually relies on local tissue destruction. Warts may regress on their own and treatment is required only if the warts are painful, unsightly, persistent, or cause distress.

Preparations of **salicylic acid, formaldehyde, gluteraldehyde** or **silver nitrate** are available for purchase by the public; they are suitable for the removal of warts on hands and feet. **Salicylic acid** is a useful keratolytic which may be considered first; it is also suitable for the removal of *corns and calluses*. Colloidal preparations of salicylic acid are available but some patients may develop an allergy to colophony in the formulation. An ointment combining **salicylic acid** with **podophyllum resin** (*Posalfilin®*) is available for treating plantar warts.

SALICYLIC ACID

Indications: see under preparations
Cautions: protect surrounding skin and avoid broken skin; not suitable for application to face, anogenital region, or large areas
Contra-indications: diabetes or if peripheral blood circulation impaired
Side-effects: skin irritation, see notes above
ADMINISTRATION. Advise patient to apply carefully to wart and to protect surrounding skin (e.g. with soft paraffin or specially designed plaster); rub wart surface gently with file or pumice stone once weekly; treatment may need to be continued for up to 3 months

Salicylic Acid Collodion, BP, salicylic acid 12%, in flexible collodion. Label: 15. For warts and calluses, apply daily or on alternate days

Cuplex® (S&N Hlth.)
Gel, salicylic acid 11%, lactic acid 4%, copper acetate (= Cu^{2+} 0.0011%), in a collodion basis. Net price 5 g = £2.33. Label: 15. For plantar and mosaic warts, corns, and calluses, apply twice daily

Duofilm® (Stiefel)
Paint, salicylic acid 16.7%, lactic acid 16.7%, in flexible collodion. Net price 15 mL (with applicator) = £1.95. Label: 15. For plantar and mosaic warts, apply daily

Occlusal® (DermaPharm)
Application, salicylic acid 26% in polyacrylic solution. Net price 10 mL (with applicator) = £2.98. Label : 15. For common and plantar warts, apply daily

Salactol® (Dermal)
Paint, salicylic acid 16.7%, lactic acid 16.7%, in flexible collodion. Net price 10 mL (with applicator) = £1.93. Label: 15. For warts, particularly plantar warts, verrucas, corns, and calluses, apply daily

Salatac® (Dermal)
Gel, salicylic acid 12%, lactic acid 4% in a collodion basis. Net price 8 g (with applicator) = £3.36. Label: 15. For warts, verrucas, corns, and calluses, apply daily

Verrugon® (Pickles)
Ointment, salicylic acid 50% in a paraffin basis. Net price 6 g = £2.33. For plantar warts, apply daily

■ With podophyllum
Posalfilin® (Norgine)
Ointment, podophyllum resin 20%, salicylic acid 25%. Net price 10 g = £3.12. For plantar warts apply daily
Note. Owing to the salicylic acid content, not suitable for anogenital warts; owing to the podophyllum content also contra-indicated in pregnancy and breast-feeding

FORMALDEHYDE

Indications: see under preparations
Cautions: see under Salicylic Acid
Contra-indications: see under Salicylic Acid
Side-effects: see under Salicylic Acid

Formaldehyde Lotion, formaldehyde solution, BP, 3 mL, water to 100 mL. For plantar warts, applied to wart-bearing region for 15–20 minutes at night as a soak

Veracur® (Typharm)
Gel, formaldehyde 0.75% in a water-miscible gel basis. Net price 15 g = £2.41. For warts, particularly plantar warts, apply twice daily

GLUTARALDEHYDE

Indications: warts, particularly plantar warts
Cautions: protect surrounding skin; not for application to face, mucosa, or anogenital areas
Side-effects: rashes, skin irritation (discontinue if severe); stains skin brown
Administration: apply twice daily (see also under Salicylic acid)

Glutarol® (Dermal)
Solution (= application), glutaraldehyde 10%. Net price 10 mL (with applicator) = £2.33

SILVER NITRATE

Indications: see under preparation
Cautions: protect surrounding skin and avoid broken skin; not suitable for application to face, anogenital region, or large areas
Side-effects: stains skin and fabric
Administration: see under preparation; instructions in proprietary packs generally incorporate advice to remove dead skin before use by gentle filing and to cover with adhesive dressing after application

AVOCA® (Bray)
Caustic pencil, tip containing silver nitrate 95%, potassium nitrate 5%, net price, treatment pack (including emery file, 6 adhesive dressings and protector pads) = £1.66. For common warts and verrucas, apply moistened caustic pencil tip for 1–2 minutes; repeat after 24 hours up to max. 3 applications for warts *or* max. 6 applications for verrucas

Anogenital warts

The treatment of anogenital warts (condylomata acuminata) should accompany screening for other sexually transmitted diseases. **Podophyllum** and **podophyllotoxin** (the major active ingredient of podophyllum) may be used for *soft, non-keratinised* external anogenital warts; these preparations can cause considerable irritation of the treated area and severe toxicity on excessive application. Patients with a limited number of external warts or *keratinised* lesions may be better treated with cryotherapy or other forms of physical ablation.

Imiquimod cream has been introduced for the treatment of external anogenital warts; it may be used for both keratinised and non-keratinised lesions.

Inosine pranobex (section 5.3) is licensed for adjunctive treatment of genital warts but its effectiveness has not been established.

IMIQUIMOD

Indications: external genital and perianal warts
Cautions: avoid normal skin, inflamed skin and open wounds; not suitable for internal genital

warts; uncircumcised males (risk of phimosis or stricture of foreskin); pregnancy (Appendix 4); breast-feeding (Appendix 5)
Side-effects: local reactions including itching, pain, erythema, erosion, oedema, and excoriation; rarely local ulceration and scabbing
Dose: apply thinly 3 times a week at night until lesions resolve (max. 16 weeks); CHILD not recommended
  IMPORTANT. Should be rubbed in and allowed to stay on the treated area for 6–10 hours then washed off with mild soap and water (uncircumcised males treating warts under foreskin should wash the area daily). The cream should be washed off before sexual contact

Aldara® (3M) ▼ PoM
Cream, imiquimod 5%, net price 12-sachet pack = £55.18. Label: 10 patient information leaflet
  Excipients: include benzyl alcohol, hydroxybenzoates (parabens), polysorbate 60
  Condoms: effect on latex condoms and diaphragms not yet known

PODOPHYLLUM

Indications: see under preparations
Cautions: avoid normal skin and open wounds; keep away from face; very irritant to eyes; **important:** see also warnings below
Contra-indications: pregnancy and breast-feeding; children
Side-effects: see notes above

Podophyllin Paint, Compound, BP, PoM
(podophyllum resin 15% in compound benzoin tincture), podophyllum resin 1.5 g, compound benzoin tincture to 10 mL; 5 mL to be dispensed unless otherwise directed. Label: 15
  External genital warts, applied weekly in genitourinary clinic (or at a general practitioner's surgery by trained nurses after screening for other sexually transmitted diseases)
  IMPORTANT. Should be allowed to stay on the treated area for not longer than 6 hours and then washed off. Care should be taken to avoid splashing the surrounding skin during application (which must be covered with soft paraffin as a protection). Where there are a large number of warts only a few should be treated at any one time as **severe toxicity** caused by absorption of podophyllin has been reported

■ Podophyllotoxin
Condyline® (Ardern) PoM
Solution, podophyllotoxin 0.5% in alcoholic basis. Net price 3.5 mL (with applicators) = £14.49. Label: 15
  Condylomata acuminata affecting the penis or the female external genitalia, apply twice daily for 3 consecutive days; treatment may be repeated at weekly intervals if necessary for a total of five 3-day treatment courses; direct medical supervision for lesions in the female and for lesions greater than 4 cm² in the male; max. 50 single applications ('loops') per session (consult product literature)

Warticon® (Perstorp) PoM
Cream, podophyllotoxin 0.15%. Net price 5 g (with mirror) = £16.62
  Condylomata acuminata affecting the penis or the female external genitalia, apply twice daily for 3 consecutive days; treatment may be repeated at weekly intervals if necessary for a total of four 3-day treatment courses; direct medical supervision for lesions greater than 4 cm²

Solution, blue, podophyllotoxin 0.5% in alcoholic basis. Net price 3 mL (with applicators— *Warticon*® [for men]; with applicators and mirror— *Warticon Fem*® [for women]) = £13.85. Label: 15

Condylomata acuminata affecting the penis or the female external genitalia, apply twice daily for 3 consecutive days; treatment may be repeated at weekly intervals if necessary for a total of four 3-day treatment courses; direct medical supervision for lesions greater than 4 cm²; max. 50 single applications ('loops') per session (consult product literature)

13.8 Sunscreens and camouflagers

13.8.1   Sunscreening preparations
13.8.2   Camouflagers

13.8.1 Sunscreening preparations

Solar ultraviolet irradiation can be harmful to the skin. It is responsible for disorders such as *polymorphic light eruption, solar urticaria*, and the various *cutaneous porphyrias*. It also provokes (or at least aggravates) disorders such as *rosacea* and *lupus erythematosus*. It may also cause photosensitivity in patients taking some drugs such as demeclocycline, phenothiazines, or amiodarone. All these conditions (as well as *sunburn*) may occur after relatively short periods of exposure to the sun. Exposure over longer periods may cause more serious problems. Both *melanoma* and *non-melanoma skin cancer* are now thought to be caused in many instances by solar ultraviolet irradiation. Exposure to the sun may also cause the skin to wrinkle and develop other signs *associated with ageing*. Solar ultraviolet irradiation also provokes attacks of *recurrent herpes labialis* (although it is not known whether the effect of sunlight exposure is local or systemic).

Solar ultraviolet radiation is approximately 200–400 nm in wavelength. The medium wavelengths (280–310 nm, known as UVB) cause sunburn and contribute to the long-term changes responsible for skin cancer and ageing. The long wavelengths (310–400 nm, known as UVA) do not cause sunburn but are responsible for many *photosensitivity reactions* and *photodermatoses*; they also seem to contribute to long-term damage and to be involved in the pathogenesis of *skin cancer* and *photodamage*.

Sunscreen preparations contain substances that protect the skin against UVB and hence guard against sunburn. The sun protection factor (SPF, usually indicated in the preparation title) provides guidance on the degree of protection offered against UVB; it indicates the multiples of protection provided against burning, compared with unprotected skin; for example, an SPF of 8 should enable a person to remain 8 times longer in the sun without burning. Such preparations, however, do not prevent long-term damage associated with UVA, which might not become apparent for 10 to 20 years. Preparations that also contain reflective substances, such as titanium dioxide, provide the most effective protection against UVA. Some products now indicate the degree of protection offered against UVA with a

star rating system. This system does not refer to an absolute measure but indicates the protection against UVA relative to protection against UVB for the same product. Four stars indicate that the product offers a balanced amount of UVA and UVB protection; products with three, two, or one star rating indicate that the protection offered is greater against UVB than UVA. However the usefulness of the star rating system remains controversial.

Some sunscreens, particularly aminobenzoates, may rarely cause photosensitivity reactions. Bergamot oil (which contains 5-methoxypsoralen) occasionally causes photosensitisation with subsequent pigmentation; it is suspected of increasing the incidence of skin cancers, but this has not been established.

BORDERLINE SUBSTANCES. The preparations marked 'ACBS' are regarded as drugs when prescribed for skin protection against ultraviolet radiation in abnormal cutaneous photosensitivity resulting from genetic disorders or photodermatoses, including vitiligo and those resulting from radiotherapy; chronic or recurrent herpes simplex labialis. Preparations with SPF less than 15 are no longer prescribable. See also Appendix 7.

Ambre Solaire® (Garnier)
Total sunblock cream (UVA and UVB protection; UVB-SPF60), avobenzone 3.5%, 4-methylbenzylidene camphor 5%, terephthalylidene dicamphor sulphonic acid 3.25%, titanium dioxide 4.1%. Net price 50 mL = £5.52. ACBS
Excipients: include disodium edetate, hydroxybenzoates (parabens)

Coppertone® (SSL)
Ultrashade 23 lotion (UVA and UVB protection; UVB-SPF23), ethylhexyl *p*-methoxycinnamate 7.5%, oxybenzone 3%, padimate-O 2.5%. Net price 150 mL = £4.46. ACBS
Excipients: include hydroxybenzoates (parabens), wool fat, fragrance

E45 Sun® (Crookes)
Lotion (UVA and UVB protection; UVB-SPF 15), water-resistant, titanium dioxide 2%, zinc oxide 13.5%. Net price 150 mL = £5.74. ACBS
Excipients: include hydroxybenzoates (parabens), isopropyl palmitate
Lotion (UVA and UVB protection; UVB-SPF 25), water-resistant, titanium dioxide 3.6%, zinc oxide 14%. Net price 150 mL = £6.12. ACBS
Excipients: include hydroxybenzoates (parabens), isopropyl palmitate
Sunblock lotion (UVA and UVB protection; UVB-SPF 50), water-resistant, titanium dioxide 6.4%, zinc oxide 16%. Net price 150 mL = £6.63. ACBS
Excipients: include hydroxybenzoates (parabens), isopropyl palmitate

Piz Buin® (Novartis Consumer Health)
Sunblock lotion (UVA and UVB protection; UVB-SPF 20), ethylhexyl *p*-methoxycinnamate 7.5%, avobenzone 1.5%, titanium dioxide 3%. Net price 200 mL = £7.35. ACBS
Excipients: include hydroxybenzoates (parabens), propylene glycol, fragrance

RoC Total Sunblock® (J&J)
Cream (UVA and UVB protection; UVB-SPF 25), containing avobenzone 2%, ethylhexyl *p*-methoxycinnamate 7.5%, titanium dioxide 5.5%. Net price 50 mL = £4.06. ACBS
Excipients: include beeswax, hydroxybenzoates (parabens)

Spectraban® (Stiefel)
Lotion (UVB protection; UVB-SPF 25), amino-benzoic acid 5%, padimate-O 3.2%, in an alcoholic basis. Net price 150 mL = £3.45. ACBS
Excipients: include fragrance
Caution: flammable; stains clothing
Ultra lotion (UVA and UVB protection; UVB-SPF 28), water resistant, avobenzone 2%, oxybenzone 3%, padimate-O 8%, titanium dioxide 2%. Net price 150 mL = £5.45. ACBS
Excipients: include benzyl alcohol, disodium edetate, sorbic acid, fragrance

Uvistat® (Windsor)
Lipscreen (UVA and UVB protection; UVB-SPF 15), ethylhexyl *p*-methoxycinnamate 3%, avobenzone 4%. Net price 5-g stick = £1.65. ACBS
Excipients: include butylated hydroxyanisole, fragrance
Babysun cream (UVA and UVB protection; UVB-SPF 22), water-resistant, ethylhexyl *p*-methoxycinnamate 7%, avobenzone 4%, titanium dioxide 4.5%. Net price 50 g = £3.63, 100 g = £5.10. ACBS
Excipients: include disodium edetate, hydroxybenzoates (parabens), fragrance
Cream (UVA and UVB protection; UVB-SPF 22 but marketed as 'factor 20'), water-resistant, ethylhexyl *p*-methoxycinnamate 7%, avobenzone 4%, titanium dioxide 4.5%. Net price 100 g = £5.10. ACBS
Excipients: include disodium edetate, hydroxybenzoates (parabens), fragrance
Lotion (UVA and UVB protection; UVB-SPF 25), tinted, water-resistant, methylbenzylidene camphor 6%, avobenzone 4%, titanium dioxide 4%. Net price 200 mL = £5.08. ACBS
Excipients: include edetic acid (EDTA), hydroxybenzoates (parabens), fragrance
Ultrablock cream (UVA and UVB protection; UVB-SPF 30), ethylhexyl *p*-methoxycinnamate 7.5%, avobenzone 4%, titanium dioxide 6.5%. Net price 50 g = £4.08. ACBS
Excipients: include disodium edetate, hydroxybenzoates (parabens), fragrance

Photodamage

Application of tretinoin 0.05% cream is reported to be associated with gradual improvement in photodamaged skin (usually within 3–4 months of starting).

TRETINOIN

Note. Tretinoin is the acid form of vitamin A
Indications: mottled hyperpigmentation, roughness and fine wrinkling of photodamaged skin due to chronic sun exposure; acne vulgaris (section 13.6); malignant disease (section 8.1.5)
Cautions: see section 13.6.1
Contra-indications: see section 13.6.1
Side-effects: see section 13.6.1
Administration: apply thinly at night, then reduce to 1–3 nights weekly

Retinova® (Janssen-Cilag) [NHS] [PoM]
Cream, tretinoin 0.05%, net price 20 g = £13.75.
Excipients: include fragrance

13.8.2   Camouflagers

Disfigurement of the skin can be very distressing to patients and have a marked psychological effect. In skilled hands, or with experience, these preparations can be very effective in concealing scars and

birthmarks. The depigmented patches in vitiligo are also very disfiguring and camouflage creams are of great cosmetic value.

BORDERLINE SUBSTANCES. The preparations marked 'ACBS' are regarded as drugs when prescribed for postoperative scars and other deformities and as an adjunctive therapy in the relief of emotional disturbances due to disfiguring skin disease, such as vitiligo. See also Appendix 7.

Boots Covering Cream® (Boots)
Cream (2 shades). Net price 50 g = £3.15. ACBS
Excipients: include hydroxybenzoates (parabens)

Covermark® (Epiderm)
Classic foundation (masking cream, 10 shades). Net price 12 g = £11.23. ACBS
Excipients: include beeswax, hydroxybenzoates (parabens), fragrance
Finishing powder. Net price 75 g = £9.50. ACBS
Excipients: include beeswax, hydroxybenzoates (parabens), fragrance

Dermablend® (Brodie & Stone)
Cover creme. Net price 10.7 g (15 shades) = £7.02; 28.4 g (11 shades)= £11.11. ACBS
Excipients: include beeswax, hydroxybenzoates (parabens)
Leg and body cover, (9 shades). Net price 64 g = £10.23. ACBS
Excipients: include beeswax, hydroxybenzoates (parabens)
Setting powder. Net price 28 g = £9.65. ACBS
Excipients: include hydroxybenzoates (parabens)

Dermacolor® (Fox)
Camouflage creme, (30 shades). Net price 30 g = £7.25. ACBS
Excipients: include beeswax, wool fat, fragrance
Fixing powder, (5 shades). Net price 60 g = £5.88. ACBS
Excipients: include fragrance

Keromask® (Network)
Masking cream, (2 shades). Net price 15 mL = £5.42. ACBS
Excipients: include butylated hydroxyanisole, hydroxybenzoates (parabens), wool fat
Finishing powder. Net price 25 g = £5.42. ACBS
Excipients: none as listed in section 13.1.3

Veil® (Blake)
Cover cream, (20 shades), net price 19 g = £5.96, 44 g = £9.65, 70 g = £13.90. ACBS
Excipients: include hydroxybenzoates (parabens), wool fat derivative
Finishing powder, translucent, net price 35 g = £5.96. ACBS
Excipients: include butylated hydroxyanisole, hydroxybenzoates (parabens)

13.9   Shampoos and some other scalp preparations

Dandruff is considered to be a mild form of seborrhoeic dermatitis (see also section 13.5.1). The treatment of choice is the frequent use of a mild detergent shampoo generally once or twice weekly; this rids the scalp of scale but does not have a therapeutic effect in itself. Shampoos containing antimicrobial agents such as **pyrithione zinc** (which are widely available) and **selenium sulphide** may have beneficial effects. Shampoos containing **tar** extracts may be useful and they are also used in *psoriasis.* **Ketoconazole** shampoo is probably the most effective.

For more severe conditions, **ketoconazole** shampoo may be used on the scalp. **Corticosteroid** gels and lotions (section 13.4) can also be used.

Shampoos containing **coal tar** and **salicylic acid** may also be useful. Patients who do not respond to these treatments may need to be referred to exclude the possibility of other skin conditions.

Cradle cap in infants may be treated with **olive oil** or **arachis oil** (ground-nut oil, peanut oil) applications followed by shampooing.

See also section 13.5 (psoriasis and eczema), section 13.10.4 (lice), and section 13.10.2 (ringworm).

Alphosyl 2 in 1® (Stafford-Miller)
Shampoo, alcoholic coal tar extract 5%. Net price 125 mL = £1.81; 250 mL = £3.43
Excipients: include hydroxybenzoates (parabens), fragrance
Dandruff, use once or twice weekly as necessary; psoriasis, seborrhoeic dermatitis, scaling and itching, use every 2–3 days

Betadine® (SSL)
Scalp and skin cleanser—section 13.11.4
Shampoo solution, povidone–iodine 4%, in a surfactant solution. Net price 250 mL = £2.32
Excipients: include fragrance
Seborrhoeic scalp conditions associated with excessive dandruff, pruritus, scaling, exudation and erythema, infected scalp lesions (recurrent furunculosis, infective folliculitis, impetigo), apply 1–2 times weekly; CHILD under 2 years not recommended

Capasal® (Dermal)
Shampoo, coal tar 1%, coconut oil 1%, salicylic acid 0.5%. Net price 250 mL = £5.28
Excipients: none as listed in section 13.1.3
Scaly scalp disorders including psoriasis, seborrhoeic dermatitis, dandruff, and cradle cap, apply daily as necessary

Ceanel Concentrate® (Quinoderm Ltd)
Shampoo, cetrimide 10%, undecenoic acid 1%, phenylethyl alcohol 7.5%. Net price 50 mL = £1.30; 150 mL = £3.40; 500 mL = £9.80
Excipients: none as listed in section 13.1.3
Scalp psoriasis, seborrhoeic dermatitis, dandruff, apply 3 times in first week then twice weekly

Clinitar® (CHS)
Shampoo solution, coal tar extract 2%. Net price 100 g = £2.50
Excipients: include polysorbates, fragrance
Scalp psoriasis, seborrhoeic dermatitis, and dandruff, apply up to 3 times weekly

Cocois® (Medeva)
Scalp ointment, coal tar solution 12%, salicylic acid 2%, precipitated sulphur 4%, in a coconut oil emollient basis. Net price 40 g (with applicator nozzle) = £5.04; 100 g = £9.46
Excipients: none as listed in section 13.1.3
Scaly scalp disorders including psoriasis, eczema, seborrhoeic dermatitis and dandruff, apply to scalp once weekly as necessary (if severe use daily for first 3–7 days), shampoo off after 1 hour; CHILD 6–12 years, medical supervision required (not recommended under 6 years)

Gelcotar® (Quinoderm Ltd)
Liquid, strong coal tar solution 1.25%, cade oil 0.5%, in a shampoo basis. Net price 150 mL = £1.67; 350 mL = £3.32
Excipients: include chlorocresol
Scalp psoriasis, seborrhoeic dermatitis, and dandruff, apply twice weekly
Gel, see section 13.5.2

Ionil T® (Galderma)
Shampoo application, benzalkonium chloride 0.2%, coal tar solution 4.25%, salicylic acid 2% in an alcoholic basis. Net price 200 mL = £2.56
Excipients: include disodium edetate
Scalp psoriasis, seborrhoeic dermatitis, apply 1–2 times weekly; CHILD under 12 years not recommended

Lenium® (Janssen-Cilag)
Cream, selenium sulphide 2.5%. Net price 42 g = £1.28; 100 g = £1.97
Excipients: include fragrance
Seborrhoeic dermatitis and dandruff, apply twice weekly for 2 weeks then once weekly for 2 weeks and then as necessary
Caution: avoid using 48 hours before or after applying hair colouring or waving preparations

Meted® (DermaPharm)
Shampoo, salicylic acid 3%, sulphur 5%. Net price 120 mL = £3.90
Excipients: include fragrance
Scaly scalp disorders including psoriasis, seborrhoeic dermatitis, and dandruff, apply at least twice weekly

Nizoral® (Janssen-Cilag) [PoM]
Shampoo, ketoconazole 2%. Net price 120 mL = £5.84
Excipients: none as listed in section 13.1.3
For seborrhoeic dermatitis and dandruff apply twice weekly for 2–4 weeks, for pityriasis versicolor once daily for max. 5 days
Note. Can be sold to the public for the prevention and treatment of dandruff and seborrhoeic dermatitis of the scalp as a shampoo formulation containing ketoconazole max. 2%, in a pack containing max.120 mL and labelled to show a max. frequency of application of once every 3 days; a brand on sale to the public is *Nizoral® Dandruff Shampoo*; *Neutrogena® Long Lasting Dandruff Control Shampoo* containing ketoconazole 1% is available as a cosmetic.

Pentrax® (DermaPharm)
Shampoo, coal tar 4.3%. Net price 120 mL = £3.90
Excipients: none as listed in section 13.1.3
Scaly scalp disorders including psoriasis, seborrhoeic dermatitis, and dandruff, apply at least twice weekly

Polytar® (Stiefel)
Liquid, arachis (peanut) oil extract of crude coal tar 0.3%, cade oil 0.3%, coal tar solution 0.1%, oleyl alcohol 1%, tar 0.3%. Net price 250 mL = £2.23
Excipients: include polysorbate 80, fragrance
Scalp disorders including psoriasis, seborrhoea, eczema, pruritus and dandruff, apply 1–2 times weekly

Polytar AF® (Stiefel)
Shampoo, arachis (peanut) oil extract of coal tar 0.3%, cade oil 0.3%, coal tar solution 0.1%, pine tar 0.3%, pyrithione zinc 1%. Net price 150 mL = £4.40
Excipients: include fragrance
Scaly scalp disorders including psoriasis, seborrhoeic dermatitis, and dandruff, apply 2–3 times weekly for at least 3 weeks

Polytar Plus® (Stiefel)
Liquid, ingredients as *Polytar®* liquid with hydrolysed animal protein 3%. Net price 500 mL = £4.40
Excipients: include polysorbate 80, fragrance
Scalp disorders including psoriasis, seborrhoea, eczema, pruritus and dandruff, apply 1–2 times weekly

Pragmatar® —section 13.5.2

Psoriderm® (Dermal)
Scalp lotion (= shampoo), coal tar 2.5%, lecithin 0.3%. Net price 250 mL = £5.33
Excipients: include disodium edetate
Scalp psoriasis, use as necessary

Selsun® (Abbott)

Shampoo application, selenium sulphide 2.5%. Net price 50 mL = £1.44; 100 mL = £1.96; 150 mL = £2.75

Excipients: include fragrance

Seborrhoeic dermatitis and dandruff, apply twice weekly for 2 weeks then once weekly for 2 weeks and then as necessary; CHILD under 5 years not recommended; pityriasis versicolor, section 13.10.2 [unlicensed indication]

Caution: avoid using 48 hours before or after applying hair colouring or waving preparations

T/Gel® (Neutrogena)

Shampoo, coal tar extract 2%. Net price 125 mL = £2.80; 250 mL = £4.46

Excipients: include hydroxybenzoates (parabens), tetrasodium edetate, fragrance

Scalp psoriasis, seborrhoeic dermatitis, dandruff, apply as necessary

Male-pattern baldness

Topical application of **minoxidil** may stimulate limited hair growth in a small proportion of adults but only for as long as it is used.

MINOXIDIL

Indications: male-pattern baldness (men and women)

Cautions: see section 2.5.1 (only about 1.4–1.7% absorbed); monitor hypertensive patients closely; avoid contact with eyes, mouth and mucous membranes, broken, infected, or inflamed skin; avoid inhalation of spray mist; avoid topical drugs which enhance absorption

Contra-indications: see section 2.5.1

Side-effects: see section 2.5.1; irritant dermatitis, allergic contact dermatitis

Administration: apply 1 mL twice daily to dry hair and scalp (discontinue if no improvement after 1 year); 5% strength for use in men only

Regaine® (Pharmacia & Upjohn) NHS

Regaine® Regular Strength topical solution, minoxidil 2% in an aqueous alcoholic basis. Net price 60-mL bottle with applicators = £14.16

Excipients: include propylene glycol

Regaine® Extra Strength topical solution, minoxidil 5% in an aqueous alcoholic basis. Net price 60-mL bottle with applicators = £17.00; 3 × 60-mL bottles = £34.03

Excipients: include propylene glycol

Cautions: flammable; wash hands after application

13.10   Anti-infective skin preparations

13.10.1   Antibacterial preparations

For many skin infections such as *erysipelas* and *cellulitis* systemic antibacterial treatment is the method of choice because the infection is too deeply sited for adequate penetration of topical preparations. For details of suitable treatment see section 5.1, table 1.

Impetigo may be treated by topical application of **fusidic acid** or **mupirocin** or, if widespread, with oral administration of **flucloxacillin** or **erythromycin** (section 5.1, table 1). Mild antiseptics such as **povidone–iodine** (section 13.11.4) are used to soften crusts and exudate.

Although there are a great many antibacterial drugs presented in topical preparations some are potentially hazardous and frequently their use is not necessary if adequate hygienic measures can be taken. Moreover not all skin conditions that are oozing, crusted, or characterised by pustules are actually infected. Topical antibiotics should be **avoided** on *leg ulcers* unless used in short courses for defined infections; treatment of bacterial colonisation is generally inappropriate.

To minimise the development of resistant organisms it is advisable to limit the choice of antibiotics applied topically to those not used systemically. Unfortunately some of these, for example neomycin, may cause sensitisation, and there is cross-sensitivity with other aminoglycoside antibiotics, such as gentamicin. If *large areas of skin* are being treated, ototoxicity may also be a hazard with aminoglycoside antibiotics (and also with polymyxins), particularly in children, in the elderly, and in those with renal impairment. *Resistant organisms* are more common in hospitals, and whenever possible swabs for bacteriological examination should be taken before beginning treatment.

Mupirocin is not related to any other antibiotic in use; it is effective for skin infections, particularly those due to Gram positive organisms but it is not indicated for pseudomonal infection. Although *Staphylococcus aureus* strains with low level resistance to mupirocin are emerging, it is generally useful when there is resistant infection. To avoid the development of resistance it should not be used for longer than 10 days and its use in hospital should if possible be avoided.

Silver sulfadiazine (silver sulphadiazine) is used in the treatment of infected burns.

13.10.1.1   Antibacterial preparations only used topically

FRAMYCETIN SULPHATE

Indications: bacterial skin infections

Cautions: treatment of large areas (risk of ototoxicity particularly in children, elderly, and in renal impairment)

Side-effects: sensitisation (see also notes above)

Sofra-Tulle® *see* Framycetin Gauze Dressing, Appendix 8 (section A8.1.10)

MUPIROCIN

Indications: bacterial skin infections (see also notes above)

Administration: apply up to 3 times daily for up to 10 days

Bactroban® (Beecham) [PoM]
Ointment, mupirocin 2%. Net price 15 g = £4.71
Excipients: none as listed in section 13.1.3
Note. Manufacturer advises: contains macrogol therefore caution in renal impairment; may sting
Nasal ointment, see section 12.2.3

NEOMYCIN SULPHATE

Indications: bacterial skin infections
Cautions: large areas, see below
LARGE AREAS. If large areas of skin are being treated ototoxicity may be a hazard, particularly in children, in the elderly, and in those with renal impairment
Side-effects: sensitisation (see also notes above)

Neomycin Cream BPC [PoM] ▄▄▄
Cream, neomycin sulphate 0.5%, cetomacrogol emulsifying ointment 30%, chlorocresol 0.1%, disodium edetate 0.01%, in freshly boiled and cooled purified water. Net price 15 g = £1.07
Apply up to 3 times daily (short-term use)

Cicatrin® (GlaxoWellcome) [PoM]
Cream, neomycin sulphate 3300 units, bacitracin zinc 250 units, cysteine 2 mg, glycine 10 mg, threonine 1 mg/g. Net price 15 g = 90p; 30 g = £1.80
Excipients: include wool fat derivative
Superficial bacterial infection of skin, apply up to 3 times daily; ADULT max. 60 g daily for 3 weeks; do not repeat for at least 3 months; CHILD reduced dose
Dusting powder, neomycin sulphate 3300 units, bacitracin zinc 250 units, cysteine 2 mg, glycine 10 mg, threonine 1 mg/g. Net price 15 g = 90p; 50 g = £3.00
Excipients: none as listed in section 13.1.3
Superficial bacterial infection of skin, apply up to 3 times daily, ADULT max. 50 g daily for 4 weeks; do not repeat for at least 3 months; CHILD reduced dose

Graneodin® (Squibb) [PoM]
Ointment, neomycin sulphate 0.25%, gramicidin 0.025%. Net price 25 g = £1.47
Excipients: none as listed in section 13.1.3
Superficial bacterial infection of skin, apply 2–4 times daily (for max. 7 days—possibly longer for sycosis barbae)

▄▄▄ denotes preparations that are considered to be less suitable for prescribing (see p. vi)

POLYMYXINS

(Includes colistin sulphate and polymyxin B sulphate)
Indications: bacterial skin infections
Cautions: treatment of large areas (risk of ototoxicity particularly in children, elderly, and in renal impairment)
Side-effects: sensitisation (see also notes above)

Polyfax® (Dominion) [PoM]
Ointment, polymyxin B sulphate 10 000 units, bacitracin zinc 500 units/g. Net price 20 g = £4.62
Excipients: none as listed in section 13.1.3
Apply 3 times daily

Colomycin® (Pharmax) [PoM]
Powder, sterile, for making topical preparations (usually 1%), colistin sulphate. Net price 1-g vial = £19.24

SILVER SULFADIAZINE

(Silver sulphadiazine)
Indications: prophylaxis and treatment of infection in burn wounds; as an adjunct to short-term treatment of infection in leg ulcers and pressure sores; as an adjunct to prophylaxis of infection in

skin graft donor sites and extensive abrasions; for conservative management of finger-tip injuries
Cautions: hepatic and renal impairment; G6PD deficiency; pregnancy and breast-feeding (avoid in late pregnancy and in neonate—see also Appendix 4); may inactivate enzymatic debriding agents therefore concomitant use may be inappropriate; for large amounts see also **interactions:** Appendix 1 (co-trimoxazole and sulphonamides)
LARGE AREAS. Plasma-sulfadiazine concentrations may approach therapeutic levels with *side-effects* and *interactions* as for sulphonamides (see section 5.1.8) if large areas of skin are treated. Owing to the association of sulphonamides with severe blood and skin disorders treatment should be stopped immediately if blood disorders or rashes develop—but leucopenia developing 2–3 days after starting treatment of burns patients is reported usually to be self-limiting and silver sulfadiazine need not usually be discontinued provided blood counts are monitored carefully to ensure return to normality within a few days. Argyria may also occur if large areas of skin are treated (or if application is prolonged).
Contra-indications: pregnancy and breast-feeding; sensitivity to sulphonamides; not recommended for neonates (see also Appendix 4)
Side-effects: allergic reactions including burning, itching and rashes; argyria reported following prolonged use; leucopenia reported (monitor blood levels)

Flamazine® (S&N Hlth.) [PoM]
Cream, silver sulfadiazine 1%. Net price 50 g = £4.11; 250 g = £11.00; 500 g = £19.48
Excipients: include polysorbates, propylene glycol
In burns apply daily with sterile applicator or more frequently if volume of exudate large; in leg ulcers daily (or every 48 hours—not recommended for leg or pressure ulcers that are very exudative); in finger-tip injuries apply every 2–3 days—for details see product literature

13.10.1.2 Antibacterial preparations also used systemically

CHLORTETRACYCLINE HYDROCHLORIDE

Indications: bacterial skin infections (see notes above)
Cautions: see notes above; overgrowth with non-susceptible organisms; stains clothing
Side-effects: rarely hypersensitivity reactions
Administration: apply 1–3 times daily

Aureomycin® (Lederle) [PoM]
Ointment, chlortetracycline hydrochloride 3%. Net price 30 g = £1.77
Excipients: include wool fat

FUSIDIC ACID

Indications: staphylococcal skin infections
Cautions: see notes above; avoid contact with eyes
Side-effects: rarely hypersensitivity reactions
Administration: apply 3–4 times daily

Fucidin® (Leo) [PoM]
Cream, fusidic acid 2%. Net price 15 g = £2.74; 30 g = £4.62
Excipients: include butylated hydroxyanisole
Gel, fusidic acid 2%. Net price 15 g = £2.37; 30 g = £4.10
Excipients: include hydroxybenzoates (parabens), polysorbate 80

Ointment, sodium fusidate 2%. Net price 15 g =
£2.23; 30 g = £3.79
Excipients: include wool fat
Fucidin Intertulle® PoM *see* Appendix 8 (section A8.1.10)

METRONIDAZOLE

Indications: see under preparations
Cautions: avoid exposure to strong sunlight or UV light
Side-effects: local skin irritation
Administration: see under preparations

■ Rosacea (see also section 13.6)

Metrogel® (Novartis) PoM
Gel, metronidazole 0.75%. Net price 40 g =
£17.36. Label: 10 patient information leaflet
Excipients: include hydroxybenzoates (parabens), propylene glycol
Administration: acute inflammatory exacerbations of
acne rosacea, apply thinly twice daily for 8–9 weeks;
avoid contact with eyes

Noritate® (Kestrel) PoM
Cream, metronidazole 1%, net price 30 g = £19.08.
Label: 10 patient information leaflet
Excipients: include hydroxybenzoates (parabens)
Administration: acne rosacea, apply once daily for 8
weeks; avoid contact with eyes

Rozex® (Stafford-Miller) PoM
Cream, metronidazole 0.75%, net price 30 g =
£11.46. Label: 10 patient information leaflet
Excipients: include benzyl alcohol, isopropyl palmitate
Gel, metronidazole 0.75%. Net price 30 g =
£11.46. Label: 10 patient information leaflet
Excipients: include disodium edetate, hydroxybenzoates
(parabens), propylene glycol
Administration: inflammatory papules, pustules and erythema of acne rosacea, apply twice daily for 3–4
months; avoid contact with eyes

■ Malodorous tumours and skin ulcers

Anabact® (Bioglan) PoM
Gel, metronidazole 0.75%, net price 15 g = £4.47,
30 g = £7.89
Excipients: include hydroxybenzoates (parabens), propylene glycol
Administration: malodorous fungating tumours and malodorous gravitational and decubitus ulcers, apply to
clean wound 1–2 times daily and cover with non-adherent dressing

Metrotop® (SSL) PoM
Gel, metronidazole 0.8%, net price 15 g = £4.73,
30 g = £8.36
Excipients: none as listed in section 13.1.3
Administration: malodorous fungating tumours and malodorous gravitational and decubitus ulcers, apply to clean
wound 1–2 times daily and cover (flat wounds, apply liberally; cavities, smear on paraffin gauze and pack loosely)

TETRACYCLINE HYDROCHLORIDE

Indications: see under Chlortetracycline Hydrochloride
Cautions: see under Chlortetracycline Hydrochloride
Side-effects: see under Chlortetracycline Hydrochloride
Administration: apply 1–3 times daily

Achromycin® (Lederle) PoM
Ointment, tetracycline hydrochloride 3%. Net
price 30 g = £1.44
Excipients: include wool fat

13.10.2 Antifungal preparations

Ideally skin scrapings should be examined to confirm diagnosis before treatment is begun. Widespread or intractable fungal infections are treated
systemically (see section 5.2). Most localised infections are treated with the topical preparations
described below.

Most ringworm infections, including tinea pedis,
can be treated adequately with topical preparations.
The imidazoles **clotrimazole**, **econazole**, **miconazole** and **sulconazole** are all effective and commonly used. Nail ringworm (tinea unguium) and
scalp ringworm (*T. capitis*) are treated systemically
(section 5.2). **Amorolfine** is a newly introduced
antifungal that differs chemically from other antifungals and has some activity against moulds. It is
available as a cream for fungal skin infections and a
lacquer for fungal nail infections. **Terbinafine** has
also been recently introduced in the form of a
cream; it is also available for systemic administration (section 5.2). Combinations of imidazoles and
weak corticosteroids may be of use in the treatment
of eczematous intertrigo and, in the first few days
only, of a severely inflamed patch of ringworm.
Compound benzoic acid ointment (Whitfield's
ointment) was also quite effective but was cosmetically less acceptable than the proprietary preparations and is rarely used. The **undecenoates** are less
effective in treating ringworm infections. Proprietary preparations containing **tolnaftate** are on sale
to the public.

Pityriasis versicolor (tinea versicolor) may be
treated topically with a 3-day course of **selenium
sulphide** shampoo repeated after a month; it is
applied to the scalp and affected areas and left on
overnight. Topical **imidazoles** (clotrimazole, ketoconazole, and miconazole) and topical **terbinafine**
are alternatives but large quantities may be
required. Pityriasis versicolor may be treated systemically with **itraconazole**; **fluconazole** is an
alternative. Relapse is common, especially in
immunocompromised individuals (section 5.2)

Candidal skin infections may also be treated by
topical application with the broad-spectrum antifungals, clotrimazole, econazole, and miconazole.
Oral preparations of some antifungals are now also
available (section 5.2), but should preferably be
reserved for those who are resistant to (or intolerant
of) topical preparations. **Nystatin** preparations are
also equally as effective in candidiasis although
they are ineffective against infections due to
dermatophyte fungi (tinea).

Lotions or sprays are generally chosen for application to large and hairy areas. Ointments are best
avoided on moist surfaces because of their occlusive properties. Nail lacquers and paints may be
effective for early fungal dystrophy of the nails and
should be considered when up to 2 nails are affected
(or where systemic therapy is contra-indicated).
Dusting-powders have no place in the treatment of
fungal infections, except for toiletry or cosmetic
purposes, as they are therapeutically ineffective and
may cause skin irritation.

AMOROLFINE

Indications: see under preparations
Cautions: pregnancy, breast-feeding; avoid eyes, ears, and mucous membranes
Side-effects: occasional transient burning sensation, erythema, pruritus

Loceryl® (Galderma) PoM
Cream, amorolfine (as hydrochloride) 0.25%. Net price 20 g = £4.83. Label: 10 patient information leaflet
Excipients: include disodium edetate
Administration: fungal skin infections, apply once daily after cleansing in the evening for at least 2–3 weeks (up to 6 weeks for foot mycosis) continuing for 3–5 days after lesions have healed

Nail lacquer, amorolfine (as hydrochloride) 5%. Net price 5-mL pack (with nail files, spatulas and cleansing swabs) = £29.94. Label: 10 patient information leaflet
Administration: fungal nail infections, apply to infected nails 1–2 times weekly after filing and cleansing; allow to dry (approx. 3 minutes); treat finger nails for 6 months, toe nails for 9–12 months (review at intervals of 3 months); avoid nail varnish or artificial nails during treatment

BENZOIC ACID

Indications: ringworm (tinea), but see notes above

Benzoic Acid Ointment, Compound, BP
(Whitfield's ointment), benzoic acid 6%, salicylic acid 3%, in emulsifying ointment
Apply twice daily

BENZOYL PEROXIDE

Indications: fungal skin infections, particularly tinea pedis

Quinoped® (Quinoderm Ltd)
Cream, benzoyl peroxide 5%, potassium hydroxyquinoline sulphate 0.5%, in an astringent basis. Net price 25 g = £1.23
Excipients: include edetic acid (EDTA)
Apply twice daily

CLOTRIMAZOLE

Indications: fungal skin infections
Side-effects: occasional skin irritation or sensitivity
Administration: apply 2–3 times daily continuing for 14 days after lesions have healed

Clotrimazole (Non-proprietary)
Cream, clotrimazole 1%, net price 20 g = £2.14
Available from CP, Cox, Generics; proprietary brands on sale to the public include *Canesten® AF* and *Mycil Gold®*

Canesten® (Bayer Consumer Care)
Cream, clotrimazole 1%, net price 20 g = £2.14, 50 g = £4.44
Excipients: include benzyl alcohol, polysorbate 60
Solution, clotrimazole 1% in macrogol 400 (polyethylene glycol 400), net price 20 mL = £2.43. For hairy areas
Excipients: none as listed in section 13.1.3
Spray, clotrimazole 1%, in 30% isopropyl alcohol, net price 40-mL atomiser = £4.99. Label: 15. For large or hairy areas
Excipients: include propylene glycol
Dusting powder, clotrimazole 1%, net price 30 g = £1.52
Excipients: none as listed in section 13.1.3

Masnoderm® (Dominion)
Cream, clotrimazole 1%. Net price 20 g = £1.47
Excipients: include benzyl alcohol, polysorbates

ECONAZOLE NITRATE

Indications; Side-effects: see under Clotrimazole
Administration: apply 2–3 times daily continuing for 14 days after lesions have healed

Ecostatin® (Squibb)
Cream, econazole nitrate 1%. Net price 15 g = £1.49; 30 g = £2.75
Excipients: include butylated hydroxyanisole, fragrance

Pevaryl® (Janssen-Cilag)
Cream, econazole nitrate 1%. Net price 30 g = £2.65
Excipients: include butylated hydroxyanisole, fragrance
Lotion, econazole nitrate 1%. Net price 30 mL = £3.33
Excipients: include butylated hydroxyanisole, fragrance

KETOCONAZOLE

Indications; Side-effects: see under Clotrimazole

Nizoral® (Janssen-Cilag) PoM
*Cream NHS, ketoconazole 2%. Net price 30 g = £3.81
Excipients: include polysorbates, propylene glycol
Apply 1–2 times daily, continuing for a few days after lesions have healed
* NHS except for seborrhoeic dermatitis and pityriasis versicolor and endorsed 'SLS'

MICONAZOLE NITRATE

Indications; Side-effects: see under Clotrimazole
Administration: apply twice daily continuing for 10 days after lesions have healed; nail infections, apply daily under occlusive dressing

Daktarin® (Janssen-Cilag)
Cream, miconazole nitrate 2%. Net price 30 g = £2.07
Excipients: include butylated hydroxyanisole
Dusting powder, NHS miconazole nitrate 2%. Net price 20 g = £1.81
Excipients: none as listed in section 13.1.3
Spray powder, miconazole nitrate 0.16%, in an aerosol basis. Net price 100 g = £2.27
Excipients: none as listed in section 13.1.3

NYSTATIN

Indications: skin infections due to *Candida* spp.
Administration: apply 2–4 times daily, continuing for 7 days after lesions have healed

Nystaform® (Bayer) PoM
Cream, nystatin 100 000 units/g, chlorhexidine hydrochloride 1%. Net price 30 g = £2.62
Excipients: include benzyl alcohol, polysorbate 60

Nystan® (Squibb) PoM
Cream, nystatin 100 000 units/g. Net price 30 g = £2.18
Excipients: include benzyl alcohol, propylene glycol, fragrance
Ointment, nystatin 100 000 units/g, in *Plastibase®*. Net price 30 g = £1.75
Excipients: none as listed in section 13.1.3

Tinaderm-M® (Schering-Plough) [PoM]
Cream, nystatin 100 000 units/g, tolnaftate 1%. Net price 20 g = £1.83. For *Candida* infections and tinea
Excipients: include butylated hydroxytoluene, hydroxybenzoates (parabens), fragrance

SALICYLIC ACID

Indications: fungal nail infections, particularly tinea
Side-effects: hypersensitivity reactions

Phytex® (Pharmax) [▨]
Paint, salicylic acid 1.46% (total combined), tannic acid 4.89% and boric acid 3.12% (as borotannic complex), in a vehicle containing alcohol and ethyl acetate. Net price 25 mL (with brush) = £1.29. For fungal nail infections (onychomycosis)
Excipients: none as listed in section 13.1.3
Apply twice daily
Caution: flammable; avoid in pregnancy and children under 5 years

▨ denotes preparations that are considered to be less suitable for prescribing (see p. vi)

SULCONAZOLE NITRATE

Indications; Side-effects: see under Clotrimazole
Cautions: avoid contact with eyes (lens changes in *animals* after high oral doses)

Exelderm® (Bioglan) [PoM]
Cream, sulconazole nitrate 1%. Net price 30 g = £2.10
Apply 1–2 times daily continuing for 2–3 weeks after lesions have healed
Excipients: include polysorbates, propylene glycol

TERBINAFINE

Indications: fungal skin infections
Cautions: pregnancy, breast-feeding; avoid contact with eyes
Side-effects: redness, itching, or stinging; rarely allergic reactions (discontinue)

Lamisil® (Novartis) [PoM]
Cream, terbinafine hydrochloride 1%. Net price 15 g = £4.86; 30 g = £8.76
Apply thinly 1–2 times daily for up to 1 week in tinea pedis, 1–2 weeks in tinea corporis and tinea cruris, 2 weeks in cutaneous candidiasis and pityriasis versicolor; review after 2 weeks; CHILD not recommended
Excipients: include benzyl alcohol, polysorbate 60
Tablets, see section 5.2

TIOCONAZOLE

Indications: see under preparation
Side-effects: local irritation, usually during first week of treatment; discontinue if sensitivity reaction develops

Trosyl® (Pfizer) [PoM]
Nail solution, tioconazole 28%. Net price 12 mL (with applicator brush) = £27.38
Excipients: none as listed in section 13.1.3
Administration: fungal nail infections, apply to nails and surrounding skin twice daily for up to 6 months (may be extended to 12 months)

UNDECENOATES

Indications: skin infections, particularly tinea pedis

Monphytol® (LAB) [▨]
Paint, methyl undecenoate 5%, propyl undecenoate 0.7%, salicylic acid 3%, methyl salicylate 25%, propyl salicylate 5%, chlorbutanol 3%. Net price 18 mL (with brush) = £1.61. For fungal (particularly nail) infections
Excipients: none as listed in section 13.1.3
Apply twice daily

Mycota® (SSL)
Cream, zinc undecenoate 20%, undecenoic acid 5%. Net price 25 g = £1.10
Excipients: include fragrance
Dusting powder, zinc undecenoate 20%, undecenoic acid 2%. Net price 70 g = £1.61
Excipients: include fragrance
Spray application, undecenoic acid 2.5%, dichlorophen 0.25% (pressurised aerosol pack). Net price 100 mL = £1.73
Excipients: include fragrance
Apply 1–2 times daily

13.10.3 Antiviral preparations

Aciclovir cream is indicated for the treatment of initial and recurrent labial and genital *herpes simplex infections*; treatment should begin as early as possible. Systemic treatment is necessary for buccal or vaginal infections; *herpes zoster (shingles)* also requires systemic treatment (for details of systemic use see section 5.3). **Penciclovir** cream has been introduced recently; it is indicated for the treatment of labial *herpes simplex infection*.

Idoxuridine solution (5% in dimethyl sulfoxide) is of little value.

ACICLOVIR

(Acyclovir)
Indications: see notes above
Cautions: avoid contact with eyes and mucous membranes
Side-effects: transient stinging or burning; occasionally erythema or drying of the skin
Administration: apply to lesions every 4 hours (5 times daily) for 5 days, started at first sign of attack

Aciclovir (Non-proprietary) [PoM]
Cream, aciclovir 5%, net price 2 g = £4.02, 10 g = £11.85
Excipients: include propylene glycol
Available from Cox (*excipients* also include sorbic acid), Genus, Pharmacia & Upjohn

Zovirax® (GlaxoWellcome) [PoM]
Cream, aciclovir 5%. Net price 2 g = £5.29; 10 g = £15.94
Excipients: include propylene glycol
Note. A 2-g tube and a pump pack are on sale to the public for the treatment of cold sores (*Zovirax*® *Cold Sore Cream*); other brands on sale to the public include *Boots Avert*®, *Herpetad*®, *Soothelip*® and *Virasorb*®
Eye ointment, section 11.3.3
Tablets, section 5.3

PENCICLOVIR

Indications: see notes above
Cautions: avoid contact with eyes and mucous membranes
Side-effects: transient stinging, burning, numbness

Vectavir® (SmithKline Beecham) ▼ PoM
Cream, penciclovir 1%. Net price 2 g = £4.20
Administration: Herpes labialis, apply to lesions every 2 hours during waking hours for 4 days, starting at first sign of attack; CHILD under 16 years, not recommended
Excipients: include propylene glycol

IDOXURIDINE IN DIMETHYL SULFOXIDE ▬◢

Indications: of little value, see notes above
Cautions: avoid contact with the eyes, mucous membranes, and textiles; breast-feeding (may taste unpleasant)
Contra-indications: pregnancy (toxicity in *animal* studies); **not** to be used in mouth
Side-effects: stinging on application, changes in taste; overuse may cause maceration

Herpid® (Yamanouchi) PoM ▬◢
Application, idoxuridine 5% in dimethyl sulfoxide. Net price 5 mL (with applicator) = £5.63
Administration: herpes simplex or herpes zoster, apply to lesions 4 times daily for 4 days, starting at first sign of attack; CHILD under 12 years, not recommended

▬◢ denotes preparations that are considered to be less suitable for prescribing (see p. vi)

13.10.4 Parasiticidal preparations

Suitable quantities of parasiticidal preparations to be prescribed for specific areas of the body in adults are:

	Skin creams	Lotions	Cream rinses
Scalp (headlice)	—	50 mL	50–100 mL
Body (scabies)	30–60 g	100 mL	—
Body (crab lice)	30–60 g	100 mL	—

These amounts are usually suitable for an adult for single application.

Scabies

Malathion and **permethrin** are used for *scabies (Sarcoptes scabiei).*

Aqueous preparations are preferable to alcoholic lotions, which are not recommended owing to irritation of excoriated skin and the genitalia.

Older preparations include benzyl benzoate, which is an irritant and should be avoided in children. Lindane and sulfiram (monosulfiram) have been discontinued.

Ivermectin (*Mectizan®*, MSD, not on UK market) in a single dose of 200 micrograms/kg by mouth has been used, in combination with topical drugs, for treatment of hyperkeratotic scabies that does not respond to topical treatment alone.

APPLICATION. Although acaricides have traditionally been applied after a hot bath, this is **not** necessary and there is even evidence that a hot bath may increase absorption into the bloodstream, removing them from their site of action on the skin.

All members of the affected household should be treated. Treatment should be applied to the whole body paying particular attention to the webs of the fingers and toes and brushing lotion under the ends of the nails. In the case of infants and young children (up to the age of about 2 years), the elderly, the immunocompromised, and those who have experienced treatment failure, application should be extended to the scalp, neck, face, and ears. Providing they are applied properly, malathion and permethrin need only be applied once; in the case of benzyl benzoate up to 3 applications on consecutive days may be needed. It is important to warn users **not** to wash their hands since this would require re-application. Patients with hyperkeratotic (crusted or 'Norwegian') scabies may require 2 or 3 applications of acaricide on consecutive days to ensure that enough penetrates the skin crusts to kill all the mites.

ITCHING. The *itch of scabies* persists for some weeks after the infestation has been eliminated and antipruritic treatment may be required. Application of **crotamiton** can be used to control itching after treatment with more effective acaricides, but caution is necessary if the skin is excoriated. Oral administration of a **sedating antihistamine** (section 3.4.1) at night may also be useful.

Head lice

Carbaryl, **malathion**, and the **pyrethroids** (permethrin and phenothrin) are effective against *head lice* (*Pediculus humanus capitis*) but lice in some districts have developed resistance; resistance to two or more parasiticidal preparations has also been reported. Head lice infestation (pediculosis) should be treated using lotion, liquid or cream rinse formulations. Shampoos are diluted too much in use to be effective. Alcoholic formulations are effective but aqueous formulations are preferred in severe eczema and for asthmatic patients and small children. A contact time of 12 hours or overnight treatment is recommended for lotions and liquids; a 2-hour treatment is no longer regarded as sufficient to ensure death of eggs. Shorter application times are recommended for permethrin rinse and phenothrin foam application.

In general, a course of treatment for head lice should be 2 applications of product 7 days apart to prevent lice emerging from any eggs that survive the first application.

The policy of rotating insecticides on a district-wide basis is now considered outmoded. To overcome the development of resistance, a mosaic strategy is required whereby, if a course of treatment fails to cure, a different insecticide is used for the next course.

A **head lice repellant** containing piperonal 2% (*Rappell®*) is on sale to the public.

WET COMBING METHODS. Several products are available which require the use of a plastic detection comb and hair conditioner. The methods typically involve meticulous combing with the detection comb (probably for at least 30 minutes each time) over the whole scalp at 4-day intervals for a minimum of 2 weeks. There is no published evidence of the efficacy of these methods.

Crab lice

Carbaryl [unlicensed for crab lice], **phenothrin**, and **malathion** are effective for *crab lice (Pthirus pubis)*. An aqueous preparation should be applied to **all** parts of the body (not merely the groins and axillae) for 12 hours or overnight; a second treatment is preferable after 7 days to kill lice emerging from surviving eggs. Alcoholic lotions are not recommended (owing to irritation of excoriated skin and the genitalia).

Aqueous **malathion** lotion is effective for *crab lice of the eye lashes* (but does not have a product licence for this indication).

Benzyl benzoate

Benzyl benzoate is effective for *scabies* but is not a first-choice for *scabies* (see notes above).

BENZYL BENZOATE

Indications: scabies (but see notes above)
Cautions: children (not recommended, see also under Administration, below), avoid contact with eyes and mucous membranes; do not use on broken or secondarily infected skin; pregnancy and breast-feeding
Side-effects: skin irritation, burning sensation especially on genitalia and excoriations, occasionally rashes
Administration: apply over the whole body; repeat without bathing on the following day and wash off 24 hours later; a third application may be required in some cases
Note. Not recommended for children—dilution to reduce irritant effect also reduces efficacy. Some manufacturers recommend application to the body but to exclude the head and neck, but in the elderly, the immunocompromised and those who have experienced treatment failure, application may need to be extended to the scalp, neck, face, and ears

Benzyl Benzoate Application, BP (Non-proprietary)
Application, benzyl benzoate 25% in an emulsion basis. Net price 500 mL = £2.44
Available from CP, Norton, Rhône-Poulenc Rorer (*Ascabiol®*, *excipients: include* triethanolamine)

Carbaryl

Carbaryl is recommended for *head lice*; an aqueous solution is recommended for *crab lice* (see notes above) but a suitable product is not currently licensed for this indication. In the light of experimental data in *animals* it would be prudent to consider carbaryl as a potential human carcinogen and it has been restricted to prescription only use. The Department of Health has emphasised that the risk is a theoretical one and that any risk from the intermittent use of head lice preparations is likely to be exceedingly small.

CARBARYL

(Carbaril)
Indications: see notes above and under preparations
Cautions: avoid contact with eyes; do not use on broken or secondarily infected skin; do not use more than once a week for 3 weeks at a time; children under 6 months, medical supervision required; alcoholic lotions **not** recommended for pediculosis in asthma, in severe eczema or in small children

Side-effects: skin irritation
Administration: rub into dry hair and scalp, allow to dry naturally, shampoo after 12 hours, and comb wet hair (see also notes above)

Carylderm® (SSL) [PoM]
Liquid, carbaryl 1% in an aqueous basis. Net price 50 mL = £2.28; 200 mL = £5.85. For head lice
Excipients: include hydroxybenzoates (parabens)
Lotion, carbaryl 0.5%, in an alcoholic basis. Net price 55 mL = £2.28; 160 mL = £5.85. Label: 15. For head lice (alcoholic, see notes above)
Excipients: include fragrance

Malathion

Malathion is recommended for *scabies, head lice* and *crab lice* (for details see notes above).

The risk of systemic effects associated with 1–2 applications of malathion is considered to be very low; however applications repeated at intervals of less than 1 week *or* application for more than 3 consecutive weeks should be **avoided** since the likelihood of eradication of lice is not increased.

MALATHION

Indications: see notes above and under preparations
Cautions: avoid contact with eyes; do not use on broken or secondarily infected skin; do not use more than once a week for 3 weeks at a time; children under 6 months, medical supervision required; alcoholic lotions **not** recommended for head lice in severe eczema, asthma or in small children, or for scabies or crab lice (see notes above)
Side-effects: skin irritation
Administration: head lice, rub 0.5% preparation into dry hair and scalp, allow to dry naturally, remove by washing after 12 hours (see also notes above) *or* apply 1% shampoo to wet hair and rinse after 5 minutes, repeat, comb wet hair; repeat twice at intervals of 3 days
Crab lice, apply 0.5% aqueous preparation over whole body, allow to dry naturally, wash off after 12 hours or overnight
Scabies, apply 0.5% preparation over whole body, and wash off after 24 hours; if hands are washed with soap within 24 hours, they should be retreated; see also notes above
Note. For scabies manufacturer recommends application to the body but not necessarily to the head and neck. In the case of young children, however, application may need to be extended to the scalp, neck, face, and ears; this extended application may also be necessary for the elderly, for the immunocompromised and for those who have experienced treatment failure

Derbac-M® (SSL)
Liquid, malathion 0.5% in an aqueous basis, net price 50 mL = £2.05, 200 mL = £5.28. For crab lice, head lice and scabies
Excipients: include hydroxybenzoates (parabens), fragrance
Prioderm® (SSL)
Lotion, malathion 0.5%, in an alcoholic basis, net price 50 mL = £2.05, 200 mL = £4.62. Label: 15. For crab lice, head lice and scabies (alcoholic, see notes above)
Excipients: include fragrance

Cream shampoo ⟨NHS⟩, malathion 1%. Net price
40 g = £2.50. For crab lice and head lice
  Excipients: include hydroxybenzoates (parabens), sodium edetate, wool fat, fragrance

Quellada M® (Stafford-Miller)
Liquid, malathion 0.5% in an aqueous basis, net
price 50 mL = £1.85, 200 mL = £4.62. For crab
lice, head lice and scabies
  Excipients: include hydroxybenzoates (parabens), fragrance
Cream shampoo, malathion 1%, net price 40 g =
£2.18. For crab lice and head lice
  Excipients: include hydroxybenzoates (parabens), sodium edetate, wool fat, fragrance

Suleo-M® (SSL)
Lotion, malathion 0.5%, in an alcoholic basis, net
price 50 mL = £2.05, 200 mL = £5.28. Label: 15.
For head lice (alcoholic, see notes above)
  Excipients: include fragrance

Permethrin

Permethrin is effective for *scabies* and *head lice*
(for details see notes above).

PERMETHRIN

Indications: see notes above and under preparations

Cautions: avoid contact with eyes; do not use on
broken or secondarily infected skin; pregnancy
and breast-feeding; children under 6 months,
medical supervision required for cream rinse
(head lice); children aged 2 months–2 years, medical supervision required for dermal cream
(scabies)

Side-effects: pruritus, erythema, and stinging;
rarely rashes and oedema

Administration: see under preparations

Lyclear® Creme Rinse (Warner Lambert)
Cream rinse, permethrin 1% in basis containing
isopropyl alcohol 20%, net price 59 mL = £2.26, 2
× 59-mL pack = £4.17
  Administration: head lice, apply to clean damp hair and
  rinse after 10 minutes
  Note. Not affected by chlorine in swimming pools

Lyclear® Dermal Cream (Kestrel)
Dermal cream, permethrin 5%. Net price 30 g =
£5.52. Label: 10 patient information leaflet
  Excipients: include butylated hydroxytoluene, wool fat derivative
  Administration: scabies, apply over whole body and
  wash off after 8–12 hours; CHILD (see also Cautions,
  above) apply over whole body including face, neck,
  scalp and ears. If hands are washed with soap within 8
  hours of application, they should be treated again with
  cream (see notes above)
  Note. Manufacturer recommends application to the body
  but to exclude head and neck. In the case of young children, however, application may need to be extended to
  the scalp, neck, face, and ears; this extended application
  may also be necessary for the elderly, for the immunocompromised and for those who have experienced treatment failure.
  Larger patients may require up to two 30-g packs for
  adequate treatment.

Phenothrin

Phenothrin is recommended for *head lice* and *crab
lice* (for details see notes above).

PHENOTHRIN

Indications: see notes above and under preparations

Cautions: avoid contact with eyes; do not use on
broken or secondarily infected skin; do not use
more than once a week for 3 weeks at a time; children under 6 months, medical supervision
required; alcoholic preparations **not** recommended for head lice in severe eczema, in asthma,
in small children, or for scabies or crab lice (see
notes above)

Side-effects: skin irritation

Administration: see under preparations

Full Marks® (SSL)
Liquid, phenothrin 0.5% in an aqueous basis, net
price 50 mL = £2.05, 200 mL = £5.28
  Excipients: include hydroxybenzoates (parabens), fragrance
  Administration: head lice, apply to dry hair, allow to dry
  naturally; shampoo after 12 hours or next day, comb wet
  hair
Lotion, phenothrin 0.2% in basis containing isopropyl alcohol 69.3%, net price 55 mL = £2.05,
160 mL = £4.62. Label: 15
  Excipients: include fragrance
  Administration: crab lice and head lice (alcoholic, see
  above), apply to dry hair, allow to dry naturally; shampoo after 2 hours, comb wet hair
Mousse (= foam application), phenothrin 0.5% in
an alcoholic basis, net price 50 g = £2.28, 150 g =
£5.28. Label: 15
  Excipients: none as listed in section 13.1.3
  Administration: head lice (alcoholic, see above), apply
  to dry hair; shampoo after 30 minutes, comb wet hair

13.10.5 Preparations for minor cuts and abrasions

Some of the preparations listed are used in minor
burns, and abrasions. They are applied as necessary.
Preparations containing camphor and sulphonamides should be **avoided**. Preparations such as
magnesium sulphate paste are also listed but are now
rarely used to treat carbuncles and boils as these are
best treated with antibiotics (section 5.1.1.2).

Cetrimide Cream, BP, cetrimide 0.5% in a suitable water-miscible basis such as cetostearyl
alcohol 5%, liquid paraffin 50% in freshly boiled
and cooled purified water. Net price 50 g = 66p

Chlorhexidine Cream, BP 1988, chlorhexidine gluconate solution usually 5% (≡ chlorhexidine gluconate 1%), cetomacrogol emulsifying
wax 25%, liquid paraffin 10%, in purified water,
freshly boiled and cooled

Proflavine Cream, BPC, proflavine hemisul-
phate 0.1%, yellow beeswax 2.5%, chlorocresol
0.1%, liquid paraffin 67.3%, freshly boiled and
cooled purified water 25%, wool fat 5%. Net
price 100 mL = 50p
  Caution: stains clothing

■ Preparations for boils

Magnesium Sulphate Paste, BP, dried magnesium sulphate 45 g, glycerol 55 g, phenol 500 mg.
Net price 25 g = 51p; 50 g = 59p. Should be
stirred before use
Apply under dressing

Collodion

Flexible collodion may be used to seal minor cuts and wounds that have partially healed.

Collodion, Flexible, BP, castor oil 2.5%, colophony 2.5% in a collodion basis, prepared by dissolving pyroxylin (10%) in a mixture of 3 volumes of ether and 1 volume of alcohol (90%). Net price 10 mL = 20p. Label: 15 (**important**: very highly inflammable)

Surgical tissue adhesive

Enbucrilate is used as a tissue adhesive for closure of minor skin wounds. It is for use in hospitals only.

Indermil® (Sherwood Davis & Geck)
Tissue adhesive, sterile, enbucrilate, net price 5 × 500-mg units = £39.38, 20 × 500-mg units = £152.25, 5-g vial = £17.33

Histoacryl® (Braun)
Tissue adhesive, sterile, enbucrilate, net price 5 × 200-mg unit (blue) = £31.75, 10 × 200-mg unit (blue) = £59.00, 5 × 500-mg unit (clear or blue) = £33.00, 10 × 500-mg unit (blue) = £61.00

13.11 Disinfectants and cleansers

13.11.1	Alcohols and saline
13.11.2	Chlorhexidine salts
13.11.3	Cationic surfactants and soaps
13.11.4	Chlorine and iodine
13.11.5	Phenolics
13.11.6	Astringents, oxidisers, and dyes
13.11.7	Preparations for promotion of wound healing

The choice of *cleanser* is an important factor in treating skin conditions. For example, scaling disorders are best treated with **emulsifying ointment** (section 13.2.1) or other cleansers that do not irritate the skin.

Sodium chloride solution 0.9% is suitable for general cleansing of skin and wounds.

Useful *disinfectants* for skin cleansing include **cetrimide** (which has useful detergent properties), **chlorhexidine** and **potassium permanganate solution** 1 in 10 000. **Povidone–iodine** is preferred to chlorinated solutions (such as dilute sodium hypochlorite solution) which are too irritant and are no longer recommended. Topical preparations of **hexachlorophene** (hexachlorophane) should be used with caution in neonates and should **not** be used on large raw surfaces.

Astringent preparations, such as **potassium permanganate** solution are useful for oozing eczematous reactions (section 13.5.1). Silver nitrate lotion is now rarely used as it stains the skin black and may cause toxic effects if used for prolonged periods.

13.11.1 Alcohols and saline

ALCOHOL

Indications: skin preparation before injection
Cautions: flammable; avoid broken skin; patients have suffered severe burns when diathermy has been preceded by application of alcoholic skin disinfectants

Industrial Methylated Spirit, BP
Mixture of 19 volumes of ethanol (absolute alcohol) of an appropriate strength with 1 volume of approved wood naphtha and is Industrial Methylated Spirit of the quality known either as '66 OP' or as '74 OP'
Net price 100 mL = 26p. Label: 15

Surgical Spirit, BP, methyl salicylate 0.5 mL, diethyl phthalate 2%, castor oil 2.5%, in industrial methylated spirit. Net price 100 mL = 19p. Label: 15

SODIUM CHLORIDE

Indications: see notes above

Sodium Chloride (Non-proprietary)
Solution (sterile), sodium chloride 0.9%, net price 10 × 10-mL unit = £3.18; 10 × 20-mL unit = £9.39; 10 × 30-mL unit = £3.00
Available from GBM, Generics (20-mL vial only)

Askina® (Braun)
Askina® Spray, solution in aerosol can (sterile), sodium chloride 0.9% (buffered), net price 120-mL can = £2.45, 250-mL can = £2.75, 350-mL can = £3.20
Askina® Jet, solution (sterile), sodium chloride 0.9%, net price 24 × 10-mL unit = £5.52, 24 × 20-mL unit = £6.24, 24 × 30-mL unit = £7.20

Irriclens® (ConvaTec)
Solution in aerosol can, (sterile), sodium chloride 0.9%. Net price 240-mL can = £2.75

Normasol® (SSL)
Solution (sterile), sodium chloride 0.9%. Net price 25 × 25-mL sachet = £5.85; 10 × 100-mL sachet = £7.16
See also section 11.8.2

Sterac® Sodium Chloride (Galen)
Solution (sterile), sodium chloride 0.9%. Net price 150 mL = 83p

Steripod® Sodium Chloride (SSL)
Steripod® sodium chloride 0.9% solution (sterile), sodium chloride 0.9%. Net price 25 × 20-mL sachet = £6.83

Saline Steripoules® (Bartholomew Rhodes)
Solution (sterile), sodium chloride 0.9%. Net price 25 × 20-mL unit = £6.83

13.11.2 Chlorhexidine salts

CHLORHEXIDINE

Indications: see under preparations; bladder irrigation and catheter patency solutions (see section 7.4.4)
Cautions: avoid contact with eyes, brain, meninges and middle ear; not for use in body cavities; alcoholic solutions not suitable before diathermy
Side-effects: occasional sensitivity

Chlorhexidine 0.05% (Baxter)
2000 Solution (sterile), pink, chlorhexidine acetate 0.05%. Net price 500 mL = 72p, 1000 mL = 77p
For cleansing and disinfecting wounds and burns

Cepton® (Eastern)
Skin wash (= solution), red, chlorhexidine gluconate 1%, net price 150 mL = £3.25
For use as skin wash in acne
Lotion, blue, chlorhexidine gluconate 0.1%, net price 150 mL = £3.25
For skin disinfection in acne

CX Antiseptic Dusting Powder® (Adams)
Dusting powder, sterile, chlorhexidine acetate 1%. Net price 15 g = £2.25
For skin disinfection and antisepsis

Hibiscrub® (Zeneca)
Cleansing solution, red, chlorhexidine gluconate solution 20% (≡ 4% chlorhexidine gluconate), perfumed, in a surfactant solution, net price 250 mL = £1.05; 500 mL = £1.54, 5 litres = £12.11
Use instead of soap for pre-operative hand and skin preparation and for general hand and skin antisepsis

Hibisol® (Zeneca)
Solution, chlorhexidine gluconate solution 2.5% (≡ 0.5% chlorhexidine gluconate), in isopropyl alcohol 70% with emollients. Net price 500 mL = £1.60
To be used undiluted for hand and skin disinfection

Hibitane Obstetric® (Bioglan)
Cream, chlorhexidine gluconate solution 5% (≡ 1% chlorhexidine gluconate), in a pourable water-miscible basis. Net price 250 mL = 98p.
For use in obstetrics and gynaecology as an antiseptic and lubricant (for application to skin around vulva and perineum and to hands of midwife or doctor)

Hydrex® (Adams)
Solution, chlorhexidine gluconate solution 2.5% (≡ chlorhexidine gluconate 0.5%), in an alcoholic solution, net price 600 mL (clear) = £1.40, 2 litre = £4.60; 600 mL (pink) = £1.40, 2 litre = £4.60; 600 mL (blue) = £1.50
For pre-operative skin disinfection
Note. Flammable
Surgical scrub, chlorhexidine gluconate 4% in an alcoholic solution, net price 250 mL = 95p, 500 mL = £1.45, 5 litre = £11.60
For pre-operative hand and skin preparation and for general hand disinfection

pHiso-Med® (Sanofi-Synthelabo) NHS
Solution, chlorhexidine gluconate 4% in an emulsion basis. Net price 150 mL = £4.64.
For use as a soap substitute in acne and seborrhoeic conditions; for bathing babies in maternity units (as 1 in 10 dilution) to prevent cross-infection and for pre-operative hand and skin preparation

Sterexidine® (Galen)
Solution (sterile), chlorhexidine gluconate 0.02%. Net price 150 mL = 83p
For disinfection and wound cleansing

Steripod® Chlorhexidine (SSL)
Steripod® Chlorhexidine solution, chlorhexidine gluconate solution 0.25% (≡ chlorhexidine gluconate 0.05%). Net price 25 × 20-mL vials = £6.52
For swabbing wounds and burns

Unisept® (SSL)
Solution (sterile), pink, chlorhexidine gluconate 0.05%. Net price 25 × 25-mL sachet = £5.59; 6 × 100-mL sachet = £4.30
For cleansing and disinfecting wounds and burns and swabbing in obstetrics

∎ With cetrimide

Steripod® Chlorhexidine/Cetrimide (SSL)
Steripod® Chlorhexidine/Cetrimide solution, chlorhexidine gluconate solution 0.075% (≡ chlorhexidine gluconate 0.015%), cetrimide 0.15%. Net price 25 × 20-mL vials = £6.83
For cleansing and disinfecting wounds and burns

Tisept® (SSL)
Solution (sterile), yellow, chlorhexidine gluconate 0.015%, cetrimide 0.15%. Net price 25 × 25-mL sachet = £5.59; 6 × 100-mL sachet = £4.30
To be used undiluted for general skin disinfection and wound cleansing

Travasept 100® (Baxter)
Solution (sterile), yellow, chlorhexidine acetate 0.015%, cetrimide 0.15%. Net price 500 mL = 72p; 1000 mL = 77p
To be used undiluted in skin disinfection such as wound cleansing and obstetrics

Concentrates

Hibitane 5% Concentrate® (Bioglan)
Solution, red, chlorhexidine gluconate solution 25% (≡ 5% chlorhexidine gluconate), in a perfumed aqueous solution. Net price 5 litres = £11.46
To be used diluted 1 in 10 (0.5%) with alcohol 70% for pre-operative skin preparation, or 1 in 100 (0.05%) with water for general skin disinfection
Note. Alcoholic solutions not suitable before diathermy (see Alcohol, above)

∎ With cetrimide

Hibicet Hospital Concentrate® (Zeneca)
Solution, orange, chlorhexidine gluconate solution 7.5% (≡ chlorhexidine gluconate 1.5%), cetrimide 15%. Net price 5 litres = £8.16
To be used diluted 1 in 100 (1%) to 1 in 30 with water for skin disinfection and wound cleansing, and diluted 1 in 30 in alcohol 70% for pre-operative skin preparation
Note. Alcoholic solutions not suitable before diathermy (see Alcohol, above)

13.11.3 Cationic surfactants and soaps

CETRIMIDE

Indications: skin disinfection
Cautions: avoid contact with eyes; avoid use in body cavities
Side-effects: skin irritation and occasionally sensitisation

Preparations
Ingredient of *Hibicet Hospital Concentrate®*, *Steripod®*, *Tisept®*, and *Travasept® 100*, see above

SOFT SOAP

Indications: removal of adherent crusts

Soap Spirit, BP, soft soap 65% in alcohol (90%). Net price 100 mL = 40p

Chlorine and iodine

CHLORINATED SOLUTIONS ◣

Cautions: bleaches fabric; irritant (protect surrounding tissues with soft paraffin)

Chlorinated Soda Solution, Surgical, BPC ◣ (Dakin's Solution), boric acid, chlorinated lime, sodium carbonate, sufficient of each to provide a solution containing 0.5% of available chlorine in purified water, freshly boiled and cooled. Net price 500 mL = 75p. Has been used undiluted for cleansing wounds and ulcers but no longer recommended (too irritant)

Chlorasol® (SSL) [NHS] ◣
Solution (sterile), sodium hypochlorite, containing 0.3% available chlorine. Net price 25 × 25-mL sachets = £8.49
Irritant therefore no longer recommended

◣ denotes preparations that are considered to be less suitable for prescribing (see p. vi)

IODINE COMPOUNDS

Indications: skin disinfection

Cautions: pregnancy, breast-feeding; broken skin (see below); renal impairment (see Appendix 3)
LARGE OPEN WOUNDS. The application of povidone-iodine to large wounds or severe burns may produce systemic adverse effects such as metabolic acidosis, hypernatraemia and impairment of renal function.

Contra-indications: avoid regular use in patients with thyroid disorders or those receiving lithium therapy

Side-effects: rarely sensitivity; may interfere with thyroid function tests

Betadine® (SSL)
Antiseptic paint, povidone-iodine 10% in an alcoholic solution. Net price 8 mL (with applicator brush) = £1.01
Apply undiluted to minor wounds and infections, twice daily
Alcoholic solution, povidone-iodine 10%. Net price 500 mL = £1.91
To be applied undiluted in pre- and post-operative skin disinfection; CHILD not recommended for regular use in neonates (and contra-indicated in very low birthweight infants)
Note. Flammable—caution in procedures involving hot wire cautery and diathermy
Antiseptic solution, povidone-iodine 10% in aqueous solution. Net price 500 mL = £1.75
To be applied undiluted in pre- and post-operative skin disinfection; CHILD not recommended for regular use in neonates (and contra-indicated in very low birthweight infants)
Note. Not for body cavity irrigation
Dry powder spray, povidone-iodine 2.5% in a pressurised aerosol unit. Net price 150-g unit = £2.79
For skin disinfection, particularly minor wounds and infections; CHILD under 2 years not recommended
Note. Not for use in serous cavities

Ointment, povidone-iodine 10%, in a water-miscible basis, net price 20 g = £1.45; 80 g = £2.92
For skin disinfection, particularly minor wounds and infections; CHILD under 2 years not recommended
Excipients: none as listed in section 13.1.3
Scalp and skin cleanser solution, povidone-iodine 7.5%, in a surfactant basis. Net price 250 mL = £2.43
Use for seborrhoeic conditions of scalp and acne vulgaris of face and neck 1–2 times daily; CHILD under 2 years not recommended
Skin cleanser solution, povidone-iodine 4%, in a surfactant basis. Net price 250 mL = £2.14
For infective conditions of the skin. Retain on skin for 3–5 minutes before rinsing; repeat twice daily; CHILD under 2 years not recommended
Surgical scrub, povidone-iodine 7.5%, in a non-ionic surfactant basis. Net price 500 mL = £1.58
To be used as a pre-operative scrub for hands and skin; CHILD not recommended for regular use in neonates (and contra-indicated in very low birthweight infants)

Savlon® Dry Powder (Novartis Consumer Health)
Savlon® Dry powder spray, povidone-iodine 1.14% in a pressurised aerosol unit. Net price 50-mL unit = £2.14
For minor wounds

Videne® (Adams)
Alcoholic tincture, povidone-iodine 10%, net price 500 mL = £1.68
To be applied undiluted in pre-operative skin disinfection
Antiseptic solution, povidone-iodine 10% in aqueous solution, net price 500 mL = £1.54
To be applied undiluted in pre-operative skin disinfection and general antisepsis
Surgical scrub, povidone-iodine 7.5% in aqueous solution, net price 500 mL = £1.45
To be used as a pre-operative scrub for hand and skin disinfection

---

Phenolics

HEXACHLOROPHENE
(Hexachlorophane)
Indications: see under preparations (below)
Contra-indications: avoid use on badly burned or excoriated skin; pregnancy; children under 2 years except on medical advice
Side-effects: sensitivity; rarely photosensitivity

Ster-Zac DC Skin Cleanser® (SSL) [PoM]
Cream, hexachlorophene 3%. Net price 150 mL = £4.04
Use 3–5 mL instead of soap as pre-operative scrub for hands
Excipients: include chlorocresol, edetic acid (EDTA), propylene glycol, wool fat, fragrance
Ster-Zac Powder® (SSL)
Dusting-powder, hexachlorophene 0.33%, zinc oxide 3%, talc 88.67%, starch 8% (sterile). Net price 30 g = 83p
Excipients: include fragrance
Prevention of neonatal staphylococcal infection, apply to cord immediately after ligature, and to perineum, buttocks, flexures, and axillae; repeat at each nappy change until stump drops away and wound healed
Adjunct for treatment of recurrent furunculosis and for prevention and treatment of pressure sores, apply to affected area (and surrounding skin) daily

TRICLOSAN

Indications: skin disinfection

Cautions: avoid contact with eyes

Aquasept® (SSL)

Skin cleanser, blue, triclosan 2%. Net price
28.5 mL = 33p; 100 mL = 90p; 250 mL = £1.10;
500 mL = £1.68

For disinfection and pre-operative hand preparation

Excipients: include chlorocresol, edetic acid (EDTA), propylene glycol, fragrance

Manusept® (SSL)

Antibacterial hand rub, triclosan 0.5%, isopropyl
alcohol 70%. Net price 100 mL = 59p; 250 mL =
£1.07; 500 mL = £1.56

For disinfection and pre-operative hand preparation

Excipients: none as listed in section 13.1.3

Caution: flammable

Ster-Zac Bath Concentrate® (SSL)

Solution, triclosan 2%. Net price 28.5 mL = 40p;
500 mL = £4.47

For prevention of cross-infection use 28.5 mL/bath

Excipients: include edetic acid (EDTA)

13.11.6 Astringents, oxidisers, and dyes

ALUMINIUM ACETATE

Indications: exudative eczematous reactions and
wounds

Aluminium Acetate Lotion, aluminium acetate
solution 5 mL, purified water, freshly boiled and
cooled, to 100 mL. It should be freshly prepared.
To be used undiluted as a wet dressing

Note. Aluminium acetate solution (13%) for the preparation of aluminium acetate lotion (0.65%) is available
from Martindale (special order)

CRYSTAL VIOLET

(Methylrosanilinium Chloride; Gentian violet)

Indications: see below

Cautions: stains clothes and skin

Side-effects: mucosal ulcerations

Crystal Violet Paint, BP 1980, crystal violet
0.5%, in purified water, freshly boiled and cooled.
To be used undiluted

Note. Licensed for topical application on unbroken skin
only; no longer recommended for application to mucous
membranes or open wounds; restrictions do not apply to
use for skin marking prior to surgery

HYDROGEN PEROXIDE

Indications: skin disinfection, particularly cleansing and deodorising wounds and ulcers

Cautions: large or deep wounds; avoid normal
skin; bleaches fabric

Hydrogen Peroxide Solution, BP

Solution 6% (20 vols). Net price 100 mL = 15p

Solution 3% (10 vols). Net price 100 mL = 25p

Note. The BP directs that when hydrogen peroxide is
prescribed, hydrogen peroxide solution 6% (20 vols)
should be dispensed.

IMPORTANT. Strong solutions of hydrogen peroxide
which contain 27% (90 vols) and 30% (100 vols) are
only for the preparation of weaker solutions

Hioxyl® see section 13.11.7

POTASSIUM PERMANGANATE

Indications: cleansing and deodorising suppurat-
ing eczematous reactions and wounds

Cautions: irritant to mucous membranes; stains
skin and clothing

Administration: wet dressings or baths, approx.
0.01% solution

Potassium Permanganate Solution, potassium permanganate 0.1% (1 in 1000) in water

To be diluted 1 in 10 to provide a 0.01% (1 in 10 000)
solution

Permitabs® (Bioglan)

Solution tablets, for preparation of topical solution, potassium permanganate 400 mg. Net price
30-tab pack = £4.04

1 tablet dissolved in 4 litres of water provides a 0.01% (1
in 10 000) solution

13.11.7 Preparations for promotion of wound healing

Desloughing agents

Desloughing agents for ulcers are second-line treatment and the underlying causes should be treated.
The main beneficial effect is removal of slough and
clot and the ablation of local infection. Preparations
which absorb or help promote the removal of exudate may also help (Appendix 8). It should be noted
that substances applied to an open area are easily
absorbed and perilesional skin is easily sensitised.
Gravitational dermatitis may be complicated by
superimposed contact sensitivity to substances such
as neomycin or lanolin. Enzyme preparations such
as streptokinase-streptodornase or alternatively
dextranomer (Appendix 8) are designed for sloughing ulcers and may help. Sterile larvae (maggots,
Biosurgical Research Unit) [unlicensed] are sometimes used in specialist centres for the management
of sloughing wounds.

Aserbine® (Goldshield)

Cream, benzoic acid 0.025%, malic acid 0.375%,
propylene glycol 1.75%, salicylic acid 0.006%.
Net price 100 g = £2.00

Apply liberally to wound surface (best results with twice
daily wound dressing but more frequent changes may be
needed)

Excipients: include hydroxybenzoates (parabens)

Solution, benzoic acid 0.15%, malic acid 2.25%,
propylene glycol 40%, salicylic acid 0.0375%.
Net price 500 mL = £3.00

Use as wash before each application of cream (or use as
wet dressing)

Excipients: include fragrance

Hioxyl® (Quinoderm Ltd)
Cream, hydrogen peroxide (stabilised) 1.5%. Net price 25 g = £2.16; 100 g = £6.76
For leg ulcers and pressure sores
Excipients: none as listed in section 13.1.3
Apply when necessary and if necessary cover with a dressing

Varidase Topical® (Lederle) [PoM]
Powder, streptokinase 100 000 units, strepto-dornase 25 000 units. For preparing solutions for topical use. Net price per vial = £8.58; with sterile physiological saline 20 mL (combi-pack) = £9.02
Excipients: none as listed in section 13.1.3
Reconstitute with 20 mL sterile physiological saline (or water for injections) and apply as wet dressing 1–2 times daily; cover with semi-occlusive dressing; irrigate lesion thoroughly with physiological saline and remove loosened material before next application; also used to dissolve clots in the bladder or urinary catheters; *contra-indicated:* active haemorrhage; *side-effects:* infrequent allergic reactions (reduced by careful and frequent removal of exudate and thorough irrigation with physiological saline); transient burning reported

Growth factor

A topical preparation of **becaplermin** (recombinant human platelet-derived growth factor) has been introduced recently as an adjunct in the treatment of full-thickness, neuropathic, diabetic ulcers.

Regranex® (Janssen-Cilag) ▼ [PoM]
Gel, becaplermin (recombinant human platelet-derived growth factor) 0.01%, net price 15 g = £275
Excipients: include hydroxybenzoates
Full-thickness, neuropathic, diabetic ulcers (no larger than 5 cm²), apply thin layer daily and cover with gauze dressing moistened with physiological saline; max. duration of treatment 20 weeks (reassess if no healing after first 10 weeks)
Cautions: malignant disease; avoid on sites with infection, malignancy, peripheral arteriopathy, or osteomyelitis
Side-effects: irritation, rarely bullous eruption, oedema

13.12 Antiperspirants

Aluminium chloride is a potent antiperspirant used in the treatment of severe hyperhidrosis. Aluminium salts are also incorporated in preparations used for minor fungal skin infections associated with hyperhidrosis.

ALUMINIUM SALTS

Indications: see under Administration below
Cautions: avoid contact with eyes or mucous membranes; avoid use on broken or irritated skin; do not shave axillae or use depilatories within 12 hours of application; avoid contact with clothing
Side-effects: skin irritation
Administration: hyperhidrosis affecting axillae, hands or feet, apply liquid formulation at night to dry skin, wash off the following morning, initially daily then reduce frequency as condition improves—do not bathe immediately before use;
Hyperhidrosis, bromidrosis, intertrigo, and prevention of tinea pedis and related conditions, apply powder to dry skin

Anhydrol Forte® (Dermal)
Solution (= application), aluminium chloride hexahydrate 20% in an alcoholic basis. Net price 60-mL bottle with roll-on applicator = £2.82. Label: 15
Excipients: none as listed in section 13.1.3

Driclor® (Stiefel)
Application, aluminium chloride hexahydrate 20% in an alcoholic basis. Net price 60-mL bottle with roll-on applicator = £2.82. Label: 15
Note. A 30-mL pack is on sale to the public (*Driclor® Solution*)
Excipients: none as listed in section 13.1.3

ZeaSORB® (Stiefel)
Dusting powder, aldioxa 0.2%, chloroxylenol 0.5%, pulverised maize core 45%. Net price 50 g = £2.15
Excipients: include fragrance

13.13 Wound management products and Elastic Hosiery

Preparations
See Appendix 8

13.14 Topical circulatory preparations

These preparations are used to improve circulation in conditions such as bruising, superficial thrombophlebitis, chilblains and varicose veins but are of little value. Chilblains are best managed by avoidance of exposure to cold; neither systemic nor topical vasodilator therapy is established as being effective. Sclerotherapy of varicose veins is described in section 2.13.

Rubefacients are described in section 10.3.2.

Hirudoid® (Sankyo) 🔲
Cream, heparinoid 0.3% in a vanishing-cream basis. Net price 50 g = £1.35
Excipients: include hydroxybenzoates (parabens)
Gel, heparinoid 0.3%. Net price 50 g = £1.35
Excipients: include propylene glycol, fragrance
Apply up to 4 times daily in superficial soft-tissue injuries and superficial thrombophlebitis

Lasonil® (Bayer Consumer Care) 🔲
Ointment, heparinoid 50 units/g in white soft paraffin, net price 40 g = £1.08
Excipients: include wool fat derivative
Apply 2–3 times daily in superficial soft-tissue injuries

🔲 denotes preparations that are considered to be less suitable for prescribing (see p. vi)

14: Immunological products and vaccines

14.1 Active immunity

Vaccines may consist of:
1. a *live attenuated* form of a virus (e.g. rubella or measles vaccine) or bacteria (e.g. BCG vaccine)
2. *inactivated* preparations of the virus (e.g. influenza vaccine) or bacteria, or
3. *extracts of* or *detoxified exotoxins* produced by a micro-organism (e.g. tetanus vaccine).

They stimulate production of antibodies and other components of the immune mechanism.

For **live attenuated** vaccines, immunisation is generally achieved with a single dose (but 3 doses are required with oral poliomyelitis and oral typhoid vaccines). Live attenuated vaccines usually produce a durable immunity but not always as long as that of the natural infection. When two live virus vaccines are required (and are not available as a combined preparation) they should be given either simultaneously at different sites or with an interval of at least 3 weeks.

Inactivated vaccines may require a primary series of injections of vaccine to produce adequate antibody response and in most cases booster (reinforcing) injections are required; the duration of immunity varies from months to many years.

Extracts of or **detoxified exotoxins** are more immunogenic if adsorbed onto an adjuvant (such as aluminium hydroxide). They require a primary series of injections followed by booster doses.

Guidelines in this chapter reflect those in the handbook *Immunisation against Infectious Disease* (1996), which in turn reflects the advice of the Joint Committee on Vaccination and Immunisation (JCVI). Copies can be obtained from:

The Stationery Office
The Publications Centre
PO Box 276, London SW8 5DT

Telephone orders, 0870 6005522
Fax: 0870 6005533

SIDE-EFFECTS. Some vaccines (e.g. poliomyelitis) produce very few reactions, while others (e.g. measles and rubella) may produce a very mild form of the disease. Some vaccines may produce discomfort at the site of injection and mild fever and malaise. Occasionally there are more serious untoward reactions and these should always be reported to the CSM. Anaphylactic reactions are very rare but can be fatal (see section 3.4.3 for management). For full details of side-effects, the product literature should always be consulted.

CONTRA-INDICATIONS. Most vaccines have some basic contra-indication to their use, and the product literature should always be consulted. In general, vaccination should be postponed if the subject is suffering from an *acute illness*. Minor infections without fever or systemic upset are not contra-indications. A definite severe reaction to a preceding dose is a contra-indication to further doses.

Some viral vaccines contain small quantities of antibiotics such as neomycin or polymyxin B (or both); such vaccines may need to be withheld from individuals who are *sensitive to the antibiotic*. *Hypersensitivity to egg* contra-indicates influenza vaccine (residual egg protein present) and, if evidence of previous anaphylactic reaction, also yellow fever vaccine.

Live vaccines should not be routinely administered to *pregnant women* because of possible harm to the fetus but where there is a significant risk of exposure (e.g. to poliomyelitis or yellow fever), the need for vaccination outweighs any possible risk to the fetus. Live vaccines should not be given to individuals with *impaired immune response*, whether caused by disease (for special reference to *AIDS*, see below) or as a result of radiotherapy or treatment with high doses of corticosteroids or other immunosuppressive drugs[1,2]. They should not be given to those suffering from *malignant conditions* such as leukaemia and tumours of the reticulo-endothelial system[2].

The intramuscular route should not be used in patients with bleeding disorders such as haemophilia or thrombocytopenia.

Note. The Department of Health has advised *against the use of jet guns* for vaccination owing to the risk of transmitting blood-borne infections, such as HIV.

VACCINES AND AIDS. The Department of Health has advised that HIV-positive subjects with or without symptoms can receive the following live vaccines:
measles[2] (or MMR), mumps, poliomyelitis[3], rubella;
and the following inactivated vaccines:
cholera, diphtheria, haemophilus influenzae type b, hepatitis A, hepatitis B, influenza, meningococcal, pertussis, pneumococcal, poliomyelitis[3], rabies, tetanus, typhoid (injection).
HIV-positive subjects should **not** receive:
BCG, yellow fever[4], typhoid (oral)
Note. The above advice differs from that for other immunocompromised patients.

---

1. Live vaccines should be postponed until at least 3 months after stopping corticosteroids and 6 months after stopping chemotherapy.
2. Consideration should be given to use of normal immunoglobulin after exposure to measles (see p. 556) and to varicella-zoster immunoglobulin after exposure to chickenpox or herpes zoster (see p. 557).
3. Virus may be excreted for longer periods than in normal subjects; contacts should be warned of this and of need for washing hands after changing a vaccinated infant's nappies; HIV-positive contacts are at greater risk than normal contacts. For HIV-positive symptomatic subjects inactivated poliomyelitis vaccine may be used at discretion of clinician.
4. Because insufficient evidence of safety.

Immunisation schedule

Vaccines for the childhood immunisation schedule should be obtained **via local Health Authorities** or (in England only) **direct from Farillon**—not for prescribing on FP10 (GP10 in Scotland) since not available to pharmacies.

During first year of life

Adsorbed Diphtheria, Tetanus and Pertussis Vaccine (triple vaccine)

3 doses at intervals of 4 weeks; first dose at 2 months of age

If pertussis component omitted from earlier immunisations 3 doses of Pertussis Vaccine can be given at monthly intervals to provide protection. If basic course against diphtheria and tetanus incomplete, triple vaccine (DTPer/Vac/Ads) may be used to begin or to complete course against pertussis to avoid more injections than necessary

plus

Haemophilus Influenzae type b Vaccine (Hib)

3 doses at intervals of 4 weeks; first dose at 2 months of age

also

Poliomyelitis Vaccine, Live (Oral)

3 doses at intervals of 4 weeks; first dose at 2 months of age

BCG Vaccine (for neonates at risk only)
See section 14.4, BCG Vaccines

During second year of life

Measles, Mumps and Rubella Vaccine, Live (MMR)

Single dose at 12–15 months of age

Haemophilus Influenzae type b Vaccine (Hib) (if not previously immunised)

Single dose at 13 months–4 years of age (over 4 years, see section 14.4, Haemophilus Influenzae type b Vaccine)

Before school or nursery school entry

Adsorbed Diphtheria and Tetanus Vaccine

Single booster dose

Preferably allow interval of at least 3 years after completing basic course; give at same session as MMR Vaccine but use separate syringe and needle, and give after MMR (MMR less painful) in different limb

also

Poliomyelitis Vaccine, Live (Oral)

Single booster dose

Preferably allow interval of at least 3 years after completing basic course

also

Measles, Mumps and Rubella Vaccine, Live (MMR)

Single booster dose

Give at same session as Adsorbed Diphtheria and Tetanus Vaccine but use separate syringe and needle; give MMR first (less painful) and use different limb—alternatively, second appointment can be made

Between 10–14 years of age

BCG Vaccine (for tuberculin-negative children)

Single dose

May be given simultaneously with another live vaccine; otherwise an interval of at least 3 weeks should be allowed between the two

Before leaving school or before employment or further education

Adsorbed Diphtheria and Tetanus Vaccine for Adults and Adolescents

Single booster dose

Adsorbed Diphtheria and Tetanus Vaccine used at school entry **not** to be used for children aged over 10 years and adults

also

Poliomyelitis Vaccine, Live (Oral)

Single booster dose

During adult life

Poliomyelitis Vaccine, Live (Oral) (if not previously immunised)

3 doses at intervals of 4 weeks

No adult should remain unimmunised; health care workers in possible contact with poliomyelitis, and travellers to areas other than Australia, New Zealand, Northern and Western Europe and North America require booster dose if they have not received immunisation within last 10 years

Rubella Vaccine, Live (for susceptible women of child-bearing age)

Single dose

Women of child-bearing age should be tested for rubella antibodies and offered rubella immunisation if sero-negative—exclude pregnancy before immunisation, but see also section 14.4, Rubella Vaccine

Adsorbed Tetanus Vaccine (if not previously immunised)

3 doses at intervals of 4 weeks

Booster dose 10 years after primary course and again 10 years later maintains satisfactory level of protection—if diphtheria cover also needed give Adsorbed Diphtheria and Tetanus Vaccine for Adults and Adolescents

Adsorbed Diphtheria Vaccine for Adults and Adolescents (if not previously immunised)

3 doses at intervals of 4 weeks

Booster dose 10 years after primary course. If tetanus cover also needed give Adsorbed Diphtheria and Tetanus Vaccine for Adults and Adolescents

High-risk groups

For information on high-risk groups, see section 14.4 under individual vaccines

Hepatitis A Vaccine
Hepatitis B Vaccine
Influenza Vaccine
Pneumococcal Vaccine

Post-immunisation pyrexia—Joint Committee on Vaccination and Immunisation recommendation. The doctor should advise the parent that if pyrexia develops after immunisation with triple vaccine the child can be given a dose of paracetamol followed, if necessary, by a second dose 4 to 6 hours later. The dose of paracetamol for post-immunisation pyrexia in an infant aged 2–3 months is 60 mg; an oral syringe can be obtained from any pharmacy to give the small dose-volume required. The doctor should warn the parent that if the pyrexia persists after the second dose medical advice should be sought.

For recommendation relating to advice after MMR vaccine, see p. 550

For full range of paracetamol doses, see p. 205

14.2   Passive immunity

Immunity with immediate protection against certain infective organisms can be obtained by injecting preparations made from the plasma of immune individuals with adequate levels of antibody to the disease for which protection is sought (see under Immunoglobulins, section 14.5). This passive immunity lasts only a few weeks; where necessary passive immunisation can be repeated.

Antibodies of human origin are usually termed *immunoglobulins*. The term *antiserum* is applied to material prepared in animals. Because of serum sickness and other allergic-type reactions that may follow injections of antisera, this therapy has been replaced wherever possible by the use of immunoglobulins. Reactions are theoretically possible after injection of human immunoglobulins but reports of such reactions are very rare.

14.3   Storage and use

Care must be taken to store all vaccines and other immunological products under the conditions recommended in the product literature, otherwise the preparation may become ineffective. **Refrigerated storage** is usually necessary; many vaccines need to be stored at 2–8°C and not allowed to freeze. Vaccines should be protected from light. Unused vaccine in multidose vials without preservative (most live virus vaccines) should be discarded within 1 hour of first use; those containing a preservative (including oral poliomyelitis vaccine) should be discarded within 3 hours or at the end of a session. Unused vaccines should be disposed of by incineration at a registered disposal contractor.

Particular attention must be paid to instructions on the use of diluents. Vaccines which are liquid suspensions or are reconstituted before use should be adequately shaken to ensure uniformity of the material to be injected.

14.4   Vaccines and antisera

AVAILABILITY. Anthrax, rabies, and yellow fever vaccines, botulism antitoxin, and snake and spider venom antitoxins are available from local designated holding centres. Details of names, addresses, and telephone numbers of holding centres are given in:
The Health Service Supply Purchasing Guide, section D pp. 1101–1199

For antivenom, see Emergency Treatment of Poisoning, p. 27

Enquiries for vaccines not available commercially can also be made to
Department of Health
Room 716
133–155 Waterloo Road
London SE1 8UG
Tel (020) 7972 4476/7
In Scotland information about availability of vaccines can be obtained from the Chief Administrative Pharmaceutical Officer of the local Health Board. In Wales enquiries should be directed to the Welsh Office, Cathays Park, Cardiff CF1 3NQ (Tel (029) 2082 5111, extn 4658) and in Northern Ireland the Regional Pharmacist (procurement co-ordination), Eastern Health Social Services Board, 12/22 Linenhall Street, Belfast BT2 8BS (Tel (028) 9055 3795).

For further details of availability, see under individual vaccines.

Anthrax vaccine

Anthrax immunisation is indicated for individuals who handle infected animals, for those exposed to imported infected animal products, and for laboratory staff who work with *Bacillus anthracis*. The vaccine is the alum precipitate of an antigen from *Bacillus anthracis* and, following the primary course of injections, booster doses should be given at about yearly intervals.

Anthrax Vaccine PoM
Dose: initial course 3 doses of 0.5 mL by intramuscular injection at intervals of 3 weeks followed by a 4th dose after an interval of 6 months
Booster doses: 0.5 mL annually
Available from Public Health Laboratory Service

BCG vaccines

BCG (Bacillus Calmette-Guérin) is a live attenuated strain derived from *Mycobacterium bovis* which stimulates the development of hypersensitivity to *M. tuberculosis*. BCG vaccine should be given intradermally by operators skilled in the technique (see below).

Within 2–6 weeks a small swelling appears at the injection site which progresses to a papule or to a benign ulcer about 10 mm in diameter and heals in 6–12 weeks. A dry dressing may be used if the ulcer discharges, but air should **not** be excluded.

The CSM has reported that serious reactions with BCG are uncommon and most often consist of prolonged ulceration or subcutaneous abscess formation due to faulty injection technique.

BCG is recommended for the following groups if BCG immunisation, as evidenced by a characteristic scar, has not previously been carried out and they are negative for tuberculoprotein hypersensitivity:

- contacts of those with active respiratory tuberculosis;

- immigrants (including infants and children) from countries with a high incidence of tuberculosis should be immunised without delay. Their infants born in the UK should also be immunised within a few days of birth, or at two months of age at the same time as the first dose of routine childhood vaccines;

- health service staff (including medical students, hospital medical staff, nurses, physiotherapists, radiographers, technical staff in pathology departments and any others considered to be at special risk because of the likelihood of contact with infective patients or their sputum; particularly important to test staff in contact with the immunocompromised, e.g. in transplant, oncology and HIV units, and staff in maternity and paediatric departments);

- children between 10 and 14 years of age (see schedule, section 14.1);

- veterinary and other staff who handle animal species known to be susceptible to tuberculosis;

- staff working in prisons, in residential homes and in hostels for refugees and the homeless;

- those intending to stay for more than 1 month in countries with a high incidence of tuberculosis (section 14.6)

- newly-born infants, children or adults where the parents or the adults request immunisation;

Apart from infants of up to 3 months, any person being considered for BCG immunisation must first be given a skin test for hypersensitivity to tuberculoprotein (see under Diagnostic agents, below).

BCG vaccine may be given simultaneously with another live vaccine (see also section 14.1), but if they are not given at the same time, an interval of at least 3 weeks should normally be allowed between them. However, when BCG is given to infants, there is no need to delay the primary immunisations, including poliomyelitis.

See section 14.1 for general contra-indications. BCG is also contra-indicated in subjects with generalised septic skin conditions (in the case of eczema, a vaccination site free from lesions should be chosen).

■ Intradermal

Bacillus Calmette-Guérin Vaccine PoM BCG Vaccine, Dried Tub/Vac/BCG. A freeze-dried preparation of live bacteria of a strain derived from the bacillus of Calmette and Guérin.

Dose: 0.1 mL (INFANT under 3 months 0.05 mL) by intradermal injection

Available from Health Authorities or (in England only) direct from Farillon

INTRADERMAL INJECTION TECHNIQUE. After swabbing with spirit and allowing to dry, skin is stretched between thumb and forefinger and needle (size 25G or 26G) inserted (bevel upwards) for about 2 mm into superficial layers of dermis (almost parallel with surface). Needle should be short with short bevel (can usually be seen through epidermis during insertion). Raised blanched bleb showing tips of hair follicles is sign of correct injection; 7 mm bleb ≡ 0.1 mL injection; if considerable resistance not felt, needle is removed and reinserted before giving more vaccine.

Injection site is at insertion of deltoid muscle onto humerus (sites higher on arm more likely to lead to keloid formation); tip of shoulder should be avoided; for cosmetic reasons, upper and lateral surface of thigh may be preferred and this is an acceptable alternative.

Bacillus Calmette-Guérin Vaccine, Isoniazid-Resistant PoM ▬ A freeze-dried preparation of live bacteria of an isoniazid-resistant strain derived from the bacillus of Calmette and Guérin.

Dose: 0.1 mL (INFANT under 3 months 0.05 mL) by intradermal injection; for active immunisation of tuberculosis contacts receiving prophylactic treatment with isoniazid—but **no longer recommended**.

Available from Medeva (special order)

▬ denotes preparations that are considered to be less suitable for prescribing (see p. vi)

■ Percutaneous

The percutaneous multiple puncture technique is an acceptable alternative **only** for young infants in whom the technique of intradermal injection may be difficult (18–20 puncture points are required)

Bacillus Calmette-Guérin Vaccine, Percutaneous Tub/Vac/BCG(Perc) PoM A preparation of live bacteria of a strain derived from the bacillus of Calmette and Guérin (**important:** this preparation must **not** be confused with the intradermal preparation)

Dose: about 0.03 mL by percutaneous administration but only recommended as an alternative for infants, see notes above

Available from Health Authorities or (in England only) direct from Farillon

DIAGNOSTIC AGENTS. In the *Mantoux test,* the diagnostic dose is by intradermal injection of Tuberculin Purified Protein Derivative (PPD):

Routine
10 units PPD i.e. 0.1 mL of 100 units/mL (1 in 1000)

Special (hypersensitive or TB suspected)
1 unit PPD i.e. 0.1 mL of 10 units/mL (1 in 10 000)

Special (low sensitivity)
100 units PPD i.e. 0.1 mL of 1000 units/mL (1 in 100)

In the *Heaf test* (multiple puncture) a solution containing Tuberculin Purified Protein Derivative 100 000 units/mL is used; 1 mL is sufficient for up to about 20 tests.

Note. Tuberculin testing should not be carried out within 4 weeks of receiving a live viral vaccine since response to tuberculin may be inhibited.

Tuberculin PPD PoM Prepared from the heat treated products of growth and lysis of the appropriate species of mycobacterium, and containing 100 000 units/mL, net price 1-mL amp = £5.89. Also available diluted 1 in 100 (1000 units/mL), 1 in 1000 (100 units/mL), and 1 in 10 000 (10 units/mL), net price 1 mL (all) = £2.22

Available from Health Authorities or (in England only) direct from Farillon

Botulism antitoxin

A trivalent botulism antitoxin is available for the post-exposure prophylaxis of botulism and for the treatment of persons thought to be suffering from botulism. It specifically neutralises the toxins produced by *Clostridium botulinum* types A, B, and E. It is not effective against infantile botulism as the toxin (type A) is seldom, if ever, found in the blood in this type of infection.

Hypersensitivity reactions are a problem. It is essential to read the contra-indications, warnings, and details of sensitivity tests on the package insert. Prior to treatment checks should be made regarding previous administration of any antitoxin and history of any allergic condition, e.g. asthma, hay fever, etc. All patients should be tested for sensitivity (diluting the antitoxin if history of allergy).

Botulism Antitoxin. PoM A preparation containing the specific antitoxic globulins that have the power of neutralising the toxins formed by types A, B, and E of *Clostridium botulinum*.

Note. The BP title Botulinum Antitoxin is not used because the preparation currently available has a higher phenol content (0.45% against 0.25%).

Dose: prophylaxis, 20 mL by intramuscular injection as soon as possible after exposure; treatment, 20 mL (diluted to 100 mL with sodium chloride 0.9%) by slow intravenous infusion followed by 10 mL 2–4 hours later if necessary, and further doses at intervals of 12–24 hours.

Available from local designated centres. For supplies outside working hours apply to other designated centres and, as a last resort, to Department of Health Duty Officer (Tel (020) 7210 5371).

Cholera vaccine

Cholera vaccine contains heat-killed Inaba and Ogawa sub-types of *Vibrio cholerae*, Serovar O1. Cholera vaccine provides little protection and cannot control the spread of the disease; it is no longer available in the UK.

Cholera vaccine is no longer required for international travel. The Department of Health has advised that in the rare circumstance where an unofficial demand may be anticipated, confirmation of non-requirement of cholera vaccine may be given on official notepaper signed and stamped by the medical practitioner.

Travellers to a country where cholera exists should be warned that scrupulous attention to food and water and personal hygiene is **essential**.

Diphtheria vaccines

Protection against diphtheria is essentially due to antitoxin, the production of which is stimulated by vaccines prepared from the toxin of *Corynebacterium diphtheriae*. The vaccines are more effective and cause fewer reactions if adsorbed onto a mineral carrier. Adsorbed diphtheria vaccines are recommended for the routine immunisation of babies and are usually given in the form of a triple vaccine, **adsorbed diphtheria, tetanus, and pertussis vaccine** (see schedule, section 14.1). Adsorbed diphtheria and tetanus vaccine is used in place of the triple vaccine when immunisation against pertussis is contra-indicated.

A booster dose of **adsorbed diphtheria and tetanus vaccine** is recommended before school entry (3–5 years of age). This should preferably be given after an interval of at least 3 years from the last dose of the basic course. A further booster dose is now recommended before leaving school; for this purpose **adsorbed diphtheria and tetanus vaccine for adults and adolescents** (a special low-dose version combined in a single injection with tetanus vaccine) is available. For details on booster doses of diphtheria vaccine in a child over 13 years who requires treatment of a tetanus-prone wound, see under Tetanus Vaccines. If there is documented history of a fifth dose of tetanus vaccine having been given when the school-leaving booster dose of adsorbed diphtheria and tetanus vaccine for adults and adolescents is due, then a booster dose of single

antigen adsorbed diphtheria vaccine for adults and adolescents should be given instead.

Other booster doses of adsorbed diphtheria vaccine are not recommended as a routine except for staff in contact with diphtheria patients, or handling clinical specimens which may be pathogenic, or working directly with *Corynebacterium diphtheriae;* they should be considered for a booster or for primary immunisation following a risk assessment. A low-dose vaccine, **adsorbed diphtheria vaccine for adults and adolescents**, is available for this purpose; immunity should be checked by antibody testing at least 3 months after completion of immunisation.

Unimmunised contacts of a diphtheria case require a primary course of 3 doses of adsorbed diphtheria vaccine at monthly intervals. *Immunised* contacts require a single booster dose (**important:** adults and children *over 10 years* must be given a **low-dose** vaccine); those also requiring tetanus cover can be given the appropriate strength of adsorbed diphtheria vaccine combined with tetanus vaccine.

Previously immunised travellers to countries where diphtheria is endemic or epidemic require a booster dose if their primary immunisation was more than 10 years ago. *Unimmunised travellers* require a full course of 3 doses at monthly intervals (**important:** adults and children *over 10 years* requiring either a primary course or a booster should be given a **low-dose** vaccine—those also requiring tetanus cover can be given the special low-dose version combined with tetanus vaccine).

See section 14.1 for general contra-indications.

Diphtheria vaccines for children

IMPORTANT. Not recommended for persons *aged 10 years or over* (use diphtheria vaccines for adults and adolescents instead)

■ With tetanus and pertussis (triple vaccine)

Adsorbed Diphtheria, Tetanus, and Pertussis Vaccine DTPer/Vac/Ads PoM

Injection, suspension of diphtheria formol toxoid, tetanus formol toxoid, and pertussis vaccine adsorbed on a mineral carrier.

Dose: primary immunisation of children, 0.5 mL by intramuscular or deep subcutaneous injection at 2 months followed by second dose after 4 weeks and third dose after another 4 weeks (see schedule, section 14.1)

Available from Health Authorities or (in England only) direct from Farillon as Pasteur Mérieux brand or Wyeth brand (*DTP Vaccine Behring*®)

Note. Adsorbed diphtheria, tetanus and pertussis vaccine is available in combination with Haemophilus influenzae type b vaccine, see under Haemophilus Influenzae type b Vaccine

Infanrix® (SmithKline Beecham) ▼ PoM

Injection, suspension of diphtheria toxoid, tetanus toxoid, and acellular pertussis vaccine components adsorbed on a mineral carrier, net price 0.5-mL prefilled syringe = £11.00

Dose: booster dose for CHILD up to 6 years previously immunised with 3 doses of diphtheria, tetanus, and pertussis (whole cell or acellular) vaccine, by deep intramuscular injection, 0.5 mL

Note. UK immunisation programme does not require booster dose of pertussis vaccine following 3-dose course during first year of life

■ With tetanus

Adsorbed Diphtheria and Tetanus Vaccine
DT/Vac/Ads(Child) PoM

Injection, suspension of diphtheria formol toxoid and tetanus formol toxoid adsorbed on a mineral carrier.

Dose: primary immunisation of children omitting pertussis component, 0.5 mL by intramuscular or deep subcutaneous injection at 2 months followed by second dose after 4 weeks and third dose after another 4 weeks (see schedule, section 14.1); booster at school entry, 0.5 mL (see schedule, section 14.1)

Available from Health Authorities or (in England only) direct from Farillon as Medeva brand or Pasteur Mérieux brand

■ Single antigen

Adsorbed Diphtheria Vaccine Dip/Vac/Ads(Child) PoM

Injection, diphtheria formol toxoid adsorbed on a mineral carrier, net price 0.5-mL amp = £1.12

Note. Used only for contacts of a diphtheria case or carrier; *immunised children under 10 years* are given one dose of 0.5 mL by intramuscular or by deep subcutaneous injection, *unimmunised children under 10 years* are given three doses of 0.5 mL with an interval of 4 weeks between first and second doses and another 4 weeks between second and third; *adults and children over 10 years* must be given adsorbed diphtheria vaccine for adults and adolescents (see below).

Available from Health Authorities or (in England only) direct from Farillon

Diphtheria vaccines for adolescents and adults

IMPORTANT. Also for use in children aged *10 years or over* The small quantity of diphtheria toxoid present in the preparations below is sufficient to recall immunity in individuals previously immunised against diphtheria but whose immunity may have diminished with time; it is insufficient to cause the serious reactions that may occur when diphtheria vaccine of conventional formulation is used in an individual who is already immune. The low dose vaccine must be used when immunising adults and children *over 10 years*; for school leavers a low-dose version combined in a single injection with tetanus vaccine is available (see notes above).

■ With tetanus

Adsorbed Diphtheria and Tetanus Vaccine for Adults and Adolescents DT/Vac/Ads(Adult) PoM

Injection, suspension of diphtheria formol toxoid and tetanus formol toxoid adsorbed on a mineral carrier, net price 0.5-mL prefilled syringe = £2.67

Dose: primary immunisation in *patients over 10 years*, three doses each of 0.5 mL by intramuscular or deep subcutaneous injection separated by intervals of 4 weeks; booster, 0.5 mL after 10 years

Available from Health Authorities or (in England only) direct from Farillon as Pasteur Mérieux (*Diftavax®*) brand

■ Single antigen

Adsorbed Diphtheria Vaccine for Adults and Adolescents Dip/Vac/Ads(Adult) PoM

Injection, diphtheria formol toxoid adsorbed on a mineral carrier.

Dose: primary immunisation in *patients over 10 years*, three doses each of 0.5 mL by intramuscular or deep subcutaneous injection separated by intervals of 1 month; booster, 0.5 mL

Note. Unimmunised adults and children *over 10 years* who are contacts of a diphtheria case or carrier are given the primary immunisation course; immunised adults and children *over 10 years* are given the booster dose.

Available from Health Authorities or (in England only) direct from Farillon

Diphtheria antitoxin

Diphtheria antitoxin is used for passive immunisation; it is prepared in horses therefore reactions are common after administration.

It is now only used in suspected cases of diphtheria (without waiting for bacteriological confirmation); tests for hypersensitivity should be first carried out.

It is no longer used for prophylaxis because of the risk of hypersensitivity; unimmunised contacts should be promptly investigated and given erythromycin prophylaxis (section 5.1, table 2) and vaccine (see notes above).

Diphtheria Antitoxin PoM Dip/Ser.

Dose: prophylactic 500 to 2000 units by intramuscular injection (but **not** used, see notes above); therapeutic 10 000 to 30 000 units increased to 40 000 to 100 000 units in severe cases; doses of up to 30 000 units should be given intramuscularly but for those over 40 000 units a portion is given intramuscularly followed by the bulk of the dose intravenously after an interval of ½–2 hours

Note. Children require the same dose as adults, depending on the severity of the case.

Available from Communicable Disease Surveillance Centre (Tel (020) 8200 6868) or in Northern Ireland from Public Health Laboratory, Belfast City Hospital (Tel (028) 9032 9241).

Haemophilus influenzae type B vaccine

Children under the age of 13 months are at high risk of *Haemophilus influenzae* type b infection. **Haemophilus influenzae type b (Hib) vaccine** is a component of the primary course of childhood immunisation (see schedule, section 14.1). The course consists of 3 doses of haemophilus influenzae type b vaccine with an interval of 1 month between each dose. If primary immunisation against diphtheria, tetanus, pertussis and poliomyelitis has already been commenced or completed, children under the age of 13 months should still receive 3 doses of haemophilus influenzae type b vaccine at monthly intervals. Children over the age of 13 months are at a lower risk of infection and, if not previously immunised, need receive only 1 dose of the vaccine. The risk of infection falls sharply after the age of 4 years therefore the vaccine is not normally required for children over 4 years. However, it may be given to those over 4 years who are considered to be at increased risk of invasive *Haemophilus influenzae* type b disease (such as those with sickle cell disease and those receiving treatment for malignancy). Also, asplenic children and adults, irrespective of age or the interval from splenectomy, should receive a single dose of haemophilus influenzae type b vaccine; those under 1 year should be given three doses. For elective splenectomy, the vaccine should ideally be given at least 2 weeks before the operation. Side-effects reported include fever, headache, malaise, irritability, prolonged crying, loss of appetite, vomiting, diarrhoea, and rash (including urticaria); convulsions, erythema multiforme, and transient cyanosis of the lower limbs have been reported.

See section 14.1 for general contra-indications

■ Single component

Each single component product may be used to complete a course started with any other single component product listed below

HibTITER® (Wyeth) [PoM]

Injection, capsular polysaccharide of *Haemophilus influenzae* type b (conjugated to a protein carrier), net price 0.5-mL vial = £10.20

Dose: by intramuscular injection, 0.5 mL; for primary immunisation, 3 doses are required at intervals of 1 month (see schedule, section 14.1)

Note. If required, haemophilus influenzae type b vaccine is available in combination with adsorbed diphtheria, tetanus and pertussis vaccine (see below)

Available, as part of childhood immunisation schedule, from Health Authorities or (in England only) Farillon

ACT-HIB® (Pasteur Mérieux) [PoM]

Injection, powder for reconstitution, capsular polysaccharide of *Haemophilus influenzae* type b (conjugated to a protein carrier), net price per vial with diluent (0.5 mL) = £8.83

Dose: by intramuscular or deep subcutaneous injection, 0.5 mL; for primary immunisation, 3 doses are required at intervals of 1 month (see schedule, section 14.1)

Note. If required, haemophilus influenzae type b vaccine is available in combination with adsorbed diphtheria, tetanus and pertussis vaccine (see below); alternatively, *ACT-HIB®* may be reconstituted with 0.5 mL of Pasteur Mérieux brand of adsorbed diphtheria, tetanus and pertussis vaccine

Available, as part of childhood immunisation schedule, from Health Authorities or (in England only) Farillon

■ With diphtheria, tetanus and pertussis vaccines

Each combined product may be used to complete a course started with any other combined product listed below; **important** see also under Adsorbed Diphtheria, Tetanus and Pertussis Vaccine (p. 545)

ACT-HIB®DTP dc (Pasteur Mérieux) ▼ [PoM]

Injection, powder for reconstitution, capsular polysaccharide of *Haemophilus influenzae* type b (conjugated to a protein carrier) with diluent containing diphtheria toxoid, tetanus toxoid and *Bordetella pertussis* cells, net price per dual-chamber prefilled syringe = £10.41

Dose: CHILD under 4 years, by intramuscular or deep subcutaneous injection, 0.5 mL; for primary immunisation, 3 doses are required at intervals of 1 month (see schedule, section 14.1)

Available, as part of childhood immunisation schedule, from Health Authorities or (in England only) Farillon

Trivax-HIB® (SmithKline Beecham) [PoM]

Injection, powder for reconstitution, capsular polysaccharide of *Haemophilus influenzae* type b (conjugated to a protein carrier) with diluent containing diphtheria toxoid, tetanus toxoid and *Bordetella pertussis* cells.

Dose: CHILD under 10 years, by intramuscular injection, 0.5 mL; for primary immunisation, 3 doses are required at intervals of 1 month (see schedule, section 14.1)

Available, as part of childhood immunisation schedule, from Health Authorities or (in England only) Farillon

Hepatitis A vaccine

Hepatitis A vaccine is prepared from formaldehyde-inactivated hepatitis A virus grown in human diploid cells.

Immunisation is recommended for:

• laboratory staff who work directly with the virus;
• haemophiliacs treated with Factor VIII or Factor IX concentrates or who have liver disease or who have been infected with hepatitis B or hepatitis C;
• travellers to high-risk areas (see p. 559);
• individuals who are at risk due to their sexual behaviour.

Immunisation should be considered for :

• patients with chronic liver disease;
• staff and residents of homes for those with severe learning difficulties;
• workers at risk of exposure to untreated sewage.

Haemophiliacs and patients with chronic liver disease should be checked for previous exposure before immunisation.

Normal immunoglobulin (section 14.5) provides short-term protection against hepatitis A, but antibody titres after a primary course of hepatitis A vaccine are well in excess of those found after the administration of normal immunoglobulin.

Side-effects of hepatitis A vaccine, usually mild, include transient soreness, erythema, and induration at the injection site. Less common effects include fever, malaise, fatigue, headache, nausea, diarrhoea, and loss of appetite; arthralgia, myalgia, and, generalised rashes are occasionally reported.

See section 14.1 for general contra-indications.

■ Single component

Avaxim® (Pasteur Mérieux) [PoM]

Injection, suspension of formaldehyde-inactivated hepatitis A virus (GBM grown in human diploid cells) 320 antigen units/mL adsorbed onto aluminium hydroxide, net price 0.5-mL prefilled syringe = £20.63

Dose: by intramuscular injection (see note below), 0.5 mL as a single dose; booster dose 0.5 mL 6–12 months following the initial dose; further booster doses, 0.5 mL every 10 years; CHILD under 16 years, not recommended

Note. The deltoid region is the preferred site of injection. The subcutaneous route may be used for patients with haemophilia

Havrix Monodose® (SmithKline Beecham) [PoM]

Injection, suspension of formaldehyde-inactivated hepatitis A virus (HM 175 grown in human diploid cells) 1440 ELISA units/mL adsorbed onto aluminium hydroxide, net price 1-mL (1440 ELISA units) prefilled syringe = £23.81, 0.5-mL (720 ELISA units) prefilled syringe (*Havrix Junior Monodose®*) = £18.03

Dose: by intramuscular injection (see note below), 1 mL as a single dose; booster dose, 1 mL 6–12 months following the initial dose; CHILD 1–15 years 0.5 mL

Note. The deltoid region is the preferred site of injection in adults. The subcutaneous route may be used for patients with haemophilia

Vaqta® Adult (Pasteur Mérieux) ▼ [PoM]

Injection, suspension of formaldehyde-inactivated hepatitis A virus (grown in human diploid cells) 50 antigen units/mL adsorbed onto aluminium hydroxide, net price 1-mL prefilled syringe = £20.63

Dose: by intramuscular injection (see note below), 1 mL as a single dose; booster dose 1 mL 6 months after the initial dose; CHILD and ADOLESCENT under 18 years, not recommended

Note. The deltoid region is the preferred site of injection

Vaqta® Paediatric and Adolescent (Pasteur Mérieux) ▼ PoM

Injection, suspension of formaldehyde-inactivated hepatitis A virus (grown in human diploid cells) 50 antigen units/mL adsorbed onto aluminium hydroxide, net price 0.5-mL prefilled syringe = £15.65

Dose: by intramuscular injection (see note below) CHILD 2–17 years, 0.5 mL as a single dose; booster dose 0.5 mL 6–18 months following the initial dose; under 2 years of age, not recommended

Note. The deltoid region is the preferred site of injection

■ With hepatitis B vaccine
See Hepatitis B Vaccine

■ With typhoid vaccine
Hepatyrix® (SmithKline Beecham) ▼ PoM

Injection, suspension of inactivated hepatitis A virus (grown in human diploid cells) 1440 ELISA units/mL adsorbed onto aluminium hydroxide, combined with typhoid vaccine containing 25 micrograms/mL virulence polysaccharide antigen of *Salmonella typhi*, net price 1-mL prefilled syringe = £34.49

Dose: by intramuscular injection (see note below) ADULT and CHILD 15 years and over, 1-mL as a single dose; booster doses, see under single component hepatitis A vaccine and under polysaccharide typhoid vaccine

Note. The deltoid region is the preferred site of injection. The subcutaneous route may be used for patients with haemophilia

Hepatitis B vaccine

Hepatitis B vaccine contains inactivated hepatitis B virus surface antigen (HBsAg) adsorbed on aluminium hydroxide adjuvant. It is made biosynthetically using recombinant DNA technology. The vaccine is used in individuals at high risk of contracting hepatitis B.

In the UK, high-risk groups include:

- parenteral drug abusers;
- individuals who change sexual partners frequently;
- close family contacts of a case or carrier;
- infants born to mothers who *either* have had hepatitis B during pregnancy, *or* are positive for both hepatitis B surface antigen and hepatitis B e-antigen *or* are surface antigen positive without e markers (or where they have not been determined); active immunisation of the infant is started immediately after delivery and *hepatitis B immunoglobulin* (see p. 557) is given at the same time as the vaccine. Infants born to mothers who are positive for hepatitis B surface antigen and for e-antigen antibody should receive the vaccine but not the immunoglobulin;
- haemophiliacs, those receiving regular blood transfusions or blood products, and carers responsible for the administration of such products;
- patients with chronic renal failure including those on haemodialysis. Haemodialysis patients should be monitored for antibodies annually and re-immunised if necessary;
- health care personnel who have direct contact with blood or blood-stained body fluids or with patients' tissues;
- trainee health care workers;
- other occupational risk groups such as morticians and embalmers;
- staff and patients of day-care or residential accommodation for those with severe learning difficulties;
- inmates of custodial institutions;
- those travelling to areas of high prevalence who are at increased risk or who plan to remain there for lengthy periods (see p. 559);
- families adopting children from countries with a high prevalence of hepatitis B.

Immunisation takes up to 6 months to confer adequate protection; the duration of immunity is not known precisely, but a single booster 5 years after the primary course may be sufficient to maintain immunity for those who continue to be at risk.

More detailed guidance is given in the memorandum *Immunisation against Infectious Disease*. Immunisation does not eliminate the need for commonsense precautions for avoiding the risk of infection from known carriers by the routes of infection which have been clearly established, consult *Guidance for Clinical Health Care Workers: Protection against Infection with HIV and Hepatitis Viruses* and *Protecting Health Care Workers and Patients from Hepatitis B*. Accidental inoculation of hepatitis B virus-infected blood into a wound, incision, needle-prick, or abrasion may lead to infection, whereas it is unlikely that indirect exposure to a carrier will do so.

Specific **hepatitis B immunoglobulin** ('HBIG') is available for use with the vaccine in those accidentally infected and in infants (section 14.5).

A combined hepatitis A and hepatitis B vaccine is also available.

See section 14.1 for general contra-indications.

■ Single component
Engerix B® (SmithKline Beecham) PoM

Injection, suspension of hepatitis B surface antigen (rby, prepared from yeast cells by recombinant DNA technique) 20 micrograms/mL adsorbed onto aluminium hydroxide, net price 0.5 mL (paediatric) vial = £9.85, 1-mL vial = £13.27, 1-mL prefilled syringe = £13.97

Dose: by intramuscular injection (see note below), 3 doses of 1 mL (20 micrograms), the second 1 month and the third 6 months after the first dose; CHILD birth to 12 years 3 doses of 0.5 mL (10 micrograms)

Rapid immunisation, third dose 2 months after first dose and a booster dose at 12 months; exceptionally (e.g. for travellers departing within 1 month), ADULT over 18 years, second dose 7 days after first dose, third dose after a further 14 days and a booster dose at 12 months

INFANTS born to HBsAg-positive mothers (see also above), 3 doses of 0.5 mL (10 micrograms), first dose at birth with hepatitis B immunoglobulin injection (separate site)

Note. Deltoid muscle is preferred site of injection in adults; anterolateral thigh is preferred site in infants and children; not to be injected into the buttock (vaccine efficacy reduced); subcutaneous route used for patients with haemophilia.

HB-Vax® II (Pasteur Mérieux) PoM

Injection, suspension of hepatitis B surface antigen (prepared from yeast cells by recombinant DNA technique) 10 micrograms/mL adsorbed onto aluminium hydroxide, net price 1-mL prefilled syringe = £12.13, 1-mL vial = £11.41, 0.5-mL prefilled syringe (*HB-Vax® II Paediatric*) = £8.99

Dose: ADULT and ADOLESCENT 16 years and over, by intramuscular injection (see note below) 3 doses of 1 mL (10 micrograms), the second 1 month and the third 6 months after the first dose; more rapid (e.g. for travellers), third dose 2 months after first dose with booster at 12 months; CHILD under 15 years, by intramuscular injection (see note below), 3 doses of 0.5 mL (5 micrograms); INFANT born to HBsAg-positive mothers (see also above), 3 doses of 0.5 mL (5 micrograms), first dose at birth with hepatitis B immunoglobulin injection (separate site)

Note. Deltoid muscle is preferred site of injection in adults; anterolateral thigh is preferred site in infants and children; not to be injected into the buttock (vaccine efficacy reduced); subcutaneous route used for patients with haemophilia.

■ Single component for dialysis and predialysis patients

HB-Vax® II 40 (Pasteur Mérieux) PoM

Injection, suspension of hepatitis B surface antigen (prepared from yeast cells by recombinant DNA technique) 40 micrograms/mL adsorbed onto aluminium hydroxide, net price 1-mL vial = £29.37

Dose: by intramuscular injection (see note below) 3 doses of 1 mL (40 micrograms), the second 1 month and the third 6 months after the first dose; booster doses may be required in those with low antibody concentration

Note. Deltoid muscle is preferred site of injection in adults; subcutaneous route used for patients with haemophilia

■ With hepatitis A vaccine

Twinrix® (SmithKline Beecham) ▼ PoM

Injection, inactivated hepatitis A virus 720 ELISA units and recombinant (DNA) hepatitis B surface antigen 20 micrograms/mL adsorbed onto aluminium hydroxide and aluminium phosphate, net price 1-mL prefilled syringe (*Twinrix® Adult*) = £29.85, 0.5-mL prefilled syringe (*Twinrix® Paediatric*) = £22.36

Dose: by intramuscular injection into deltoid muscle (see note below); primary course of 3 doses of 1 mL, the second 1 month and the third 6 months after the first dose; 1 mL booster dose 5 years after the start of primary course for those at continued risk; CHILD 1–15 years 0.5 mL

Note. Primary course should be completed with *Twinrix®* (single component vaccines given at appropriate intervals may be used for booster dose); not to be injected into the buttock (vaccine efficacy reduced); subcutaneous route used for patients with haemophilia (but immune response may be reduced).

IMPORTANT. *Twinrix®* **not** recommended for post-exposure prophylaxis following percutaneous (needle-stick), ocular or mucous membrane exposure to hepatitis B virus.

Influenza vaccines

While most viruses are antigenically stable, the influenza viruses A and B (especially A) are constantly altering their antigenic structure as indicated by changes in the haemagglutinins (H) and neuraminidases (N) on the surface of the viruses. It is essential that influenza vaccines in use contain the H and N components of the prevalent strain or strains. Every year the World Health Organization recommends which strains should be included.

The recommended strains are grown in the allantoic cavity of chick embryos (therefore **contraindicated** in those hypersensitive to eggs).

Since **influenza vaccines** will not control epidemics they are recommended *only for persons at high risk*. Annual immunisation is strongly recommended for those of all ages with any of the following conditions:

- chronic respiratory disease, including asthma;
- chronic heart disease;
- chronic renal failure;
- diabetes mellitus;
- immunosuppression due to disease or treatment, including asplenia or splenic dysfunction.

Influenza immunisation is also recommended for all persons over 75 years of age and for residents of nursing homes, residential homes for the elderly, and other long-stay facilities.

In non-pandemic years routine immunisation of Health Service Staff is not recommended, except for those at high risk (owing to medical disorders).

Interactions: Appendix 1 (influenza vaccine).

See section 14.1 for general contra-indications.

Inactivated Influenza Vaccine (Split Virion) (Pasteur Mérieux) PoM

Injection, suspension of formaldehyde-inactivated influenza virus (split virion) Flu/Vac/Split, net price 0.5-mL prefilled syringe = £5.70

Dose: by deep subcutaneous or by intramuscular injection 0.5 mL; CHILD 6–35 months 0.25 mL (or 0.5 mL) repeated once after 4–6 weeks, 3–12 years, 0.5 mL repeated once after 4–6 weeks; single doses appropriate for children who have already been immunised

Begrivac® (Wyeth) PoM

Injection, suspension of formaldehyde-inactivated influenza virus (split virion) Flu/Vac/Split, net price 0.5-mL prefilled syringe = £5.20

Dose: by deep subcutaneous or by intramuscular injection, 0.5 mL; CHILD 6–35 months 0.25 mL (or 0.5 mL) repeated once after 4–6 weeks, 3–12 years 0.5 mL repeated once after 4–6 weeks; single doses are appropriate for children who have already been immunised

Fluarix® (SmithKline Beecham) PoM

Injection, suspension of formaldehyde-inactivated influenza virus (split virion) Flu/Vac/Split, net price 0.5-mL prefilled syringe = £3.99

Dose: by deep subcutaneous or by intramuscular injection, 0.5 mL; CHILD 6–35 months 0.25 mL (or 0.5 mL) repeated once after 4–6 weeks, 3–12 years 0.5 mL repeated once after 4–6 weeks; single doses are appropriate for children who have already been immunised

Fluvirin® (Medeva) PoM

Injection, suspension of propiolactone-inactivated influenza virus (surface antigen) Flu/Vac/SA, net price 0.5-mL prefilled syringe = £5.69

Dose: by deep subcutaneous or by intramuscular injection, 0.5 mL; CHILD 6–35 months 0.25 mL (or 0.5 mL) repeated once after 4–6 weeks, 3–12 years 0.5 mL repeated once after 4–6 weeks; single doses are appropriate for children who have already been immunised

Influvac Sub-unit® (Solvay) PoM

Injection, suspension of formaldehyde-inactivated influenza virus (surface antigen) Flu/Vac/SA, net price 0.5-mL prefilled syringe = £5.08

Dose: by deep subcutaneous or by intramuscular injection, 0.5 mL; CHILD 6–35 months 0.25 mL (or 0.5 mL) repeated once after 4–6 weeks, 3–12 years 0.5 mL repeated once after 4–6 weeks; single doses are appropriate for children who have already been immunised

Measles vaccine

Measles vaccine has been replaced by a combined measles/mumps/rubella vaccine (MMR vaccine) for all eligible children.

Administration of a measles-containing vaccine to children may be associated with a mild measles-like syndrome with a measles-like rash and pyrexia about a week after injection. Much less commonly, convulsions and, very rarely, encephalitis have been reported. Convulsions in infants are much less frequently associated with measles vaccines than with other conditions leading to febrile episodes.

MMR vaccine may be used in the control of outbreaks of measles (see under MMR Vaccine).

■ Single antigen vaccine
No longer available in the UK

■ Combined vaccines
See MMR vaccine

MMR vaccine

A combined **measles/mumps/rubella vaccine** (MMR vaccine) has been introduced with the aim of eliminating rubella (and congenital rubella syndrome), measles, and mumps. Every child should receive two doses of MMR vaccine by entry to primary school, unless there is a valid contra-indication (see below) or parental refusal.

MMR vaccine has replaced measles vaccine for children of both sexes and should be given irrespective of previous measles, mumps or rubella infection.

The first dose of MMR vaccine is given to children aged 12–15 months. Since October 1996 a second (booster) dose has been given before starting school at 3–5 years of age (see schedule, section 14.1). Children presenting for their pre-school booster who have not received their first dose of MMR vaccine should be given a dose of MMR vaccine followed 3 months later by a second dose. At school-leaving age or at entry into further education, individuals of both sexes who have not received either MR or MMR vaccines should be offered MMR immunisation.

MMR vaccine may also be used in the control of outbreaks of measles and should be offered to susceptible children within 3 days of exposure to infection (**important:** MMR vaccine is not suitable for prophylaxis following exposure to mumps or rubella since the antibody response to the mumps and rubella components is too slow for effective prophylaxis).

Children with partially or totally impaired immune responsiveness should not receive live vaccines (for advice on AIDS see section 14.1). If they have been exposed to measles infection they should be given normal immunoglobulin (section 14.5).

Malaise, fever or a rash may occur following the first dose of MMR vaccine, most commonly about a week after immunisation and lasting about 2 to 3 days. Leaflets are available to provide parents with advice for reducing fever (including the use of paracetamol). Parotid swelling occasionally occurs, usually in the third week. After a second dose of MMR vaccine, adverse reactions are considerably less common than after the first dose. Post-vaccination meningoencephalitis was reported (rarely and with complete recovery) following immunisation with MMR vaccine containing Urabe mumps vaccine, which has now been discontinued; no cases have been confirmed in association with the currently-used Jeryl Lynn mumps vaccine. Children with post-vaccination symptoms are not infectious.

> An expert group of the Medical Research Council has concluded that there is no evidence to indicate any link between MMR vaccination and bowel disease or autism. The Chief Medical Officer has recommended that children should receive MMR vaccine at the appropriate times and should not be given the separate component vaccines since there is no evidence that doing this has any benefit and it may even be harmful.

> The CSM has issued an information leaflet stating that neither the CSM's Working Party on MMR vaccine nor an epidemiological study (*Lancet* 1999; **353**: 2026-9) support an association between MMR (or MR) vaccine and autism or Crohn's disease.

Contra-indications to MMR include:
* children with untreated malignant disease or altered immunity (for advice on vaccines and AIDS see section 14.1), and those receiving immunosuppressive drugs or radiotherapy, or high-dose corticosteroids;
* children who have received another live vaccine by injection within 3 weeks;
* children with allergies to neomycin or kanamycin;
* children with acute febrile illness (vaccination should be deferred);
* if given to women, pregnancy should be avoided for 1 month (as for rubella vaccine);
* should not be given within 3 months of an immuno-globulin injection.

It should be noted that:
children with a personal or close family history of convulsions should be given MMR vaccine, provided the parents understand that there may be a febrile response; doctors should seek specialist paediatric advice rather than withold vaccination; there is increasing evidence that MMR vaccine can be given safely even when the child has had an anaphylactic reaction to food containing egg (dislike of egg or refusal to eat egg is not a contra-indication).

MMR Vaccine PoM
Live measles, mumps, and rubella vaccine
Dose: 0.5 mL by deep subcutaneous or by intramuscular injection
Available from Health Authorities or (in England only) direct from Farillon as *MMR II*® (Pasteur Mérieux) or *Priorix*® ▼ (SmithKline Beecham)

Meningococcal vaccines

Meningococcal Group C conjugate vaccine provides long-term protection against infection by serogroup C of *Neisseria meningitidis* in children from 2 months of age; from autumn 1999 it has become a component of the primary course of childhood immunisation (see schedule, section 14.1). The Department of Health has also announced a 'catch-up' programme targeting the groups at highest risk first; in the initial phase vaccination is recommended for:
* those aged 15–17 years (through programmes based in schools or colleges)
* infants aged 2–4 months (at the same time as routine immunisation against diphteria, tetanus, pertussis poliomyelitis and haemophilus influenzae type B)
* children at around 13 months (at the same time as routine immunisation against measles, mumps and rubella).

As more vaccine becomes available, infants aged 5–12 months will be recalled for immunisation and other high-risk groups will be targeted. The recommended schedule is 3 doses for children aged 2–4 months, 2 doses for children aged over 4 months and a single dose for all individuals aged over 1 year.

Meningoccoal group C conjugate vaccine protects against Group C disease only. Individuals travelling abroad should be immunised with meningococcal polysaccharide A and C vaccine, even if they have already received meningococcal group C conjugate vaccine.

Meningococcal polysaccharide A&C vaccine is effective against serogroup A and C of *N. meningitidis* but infants respond less well than adults. It is indicated for visits of longer than 1 month to areas of the world where the risk of acquiring meningococcal infection is much higher than in the UK, particularly for travellers proposing to travel 'rough' or to live or work with local people. These areas include:

Delhi, Nepal, Bhutan, Pakistan, Mecca (see below), and the meningitis belt of Africa, which encompasses southern sub-Saharan parts of Senegal, Mali, Niger, Chad, and Sudan; all of Gambia, Guinea, Togo, and Benin; Southwest Ethiopia; northern parts of Sierra Leone, Liberia, Ivory Coast, Nigeria, Cameroon, Central African Republic, Uganda, and Kenya.

Saudi Arabia requires vaccination of pilgrims to Mecca during the Haj annual pilgrimage; this may apply to others visiting Saudi Arabia in the months leading up to August.

For advice on the immunisation of *close contacts* of disease cases of Group A and Group C meningococcal meningitis in the UK and on the role of the vaccine in the control of *local outbreaks*, consult the replacement chapter for the memorandum *Immunisation against Infectious Disease*. Meningococcal polysaccharide A and C vaccine should be used until an adequate supply of meningitis conjugate group C vaccine becomes available. See section 5.1 Table 2 for antibiotic prophylaxis to prevent a secondary case of meningococcal meningitis.

The need for immunisation of laboratory staff who work directly with *Neisseria meningitidis* should be determined by assessing the risk.

Side-effects of meningococcal Group C conjugate vaccine include redness and swelling at the site of the injection, mild fever, irritability and headache. Meningococcal polysaccharide A&C vaccine is also associated with injection-site reactions and fever.

See section 14.1 for general contra-indications.

■ Meningococcal Group C conjugate vaccine

Meningitec® (Wyeth) ▼ PoM

Injection, suspension of capsular polysaccharide antigen of *Neisseria meningitidis* (meningococcus) group C (conjugated to *Corynebacterium diphtheriae* protein), net price 0.5-mL vial = £17.95

Dose: by intramuscular injection (see note below)
ADULT and CHILD over 1 year 0.5 mL as a single dose;
INFANT 2–4 months 3 doses of 0.5 mL at intervals of 1 month (see schedule, section 14.1), 5–12 months 2 doses of 0.5 mL at interval of 1 month

Available as part of childhood immunisation schedule from Farillon

Note. Subcutaneous route used for patients with haemophilia

■ Meningococcal groups A and C vaccines

AC Vax® (SmithKline Beecham) PoM

Injection, powder for reconstitution, capsular polysaccharide antigens of *Neisseria meningitidis* (meningococcus) groups A and C, net price single-dose vial (with diluent) = £7.37

Dose: ADULT and CHILD aged 2 months and over, 0.5 mL by deep subcutaneous or intramuscular injection

Mengivac (A+C)® (Pasteur Mérieux) PoM

Injection, powder for reconstitution, capsular polysaccharide antigens of *Neisseria meningitidis* (meningococcus) groups A and C, net price single-dose vial (with syringe containing diluent) = £6.39

Dose: ADULT and CHILD aged over 18 months, 0.5 mL by deep subcutaneous or intramuscular injection

Note. The lower age range for *AC Vax®* and *Mengivac (A+C)®* differ; in the case of *Mengivac (A+C)®* the product literature states that young children and infants respond less well to the vaccine than older children and adults, with little response to the Group C polysaccharide under 18 months of age and a poor response to Group A polysaccharide under 3 months of age. Additionally, protection in infants under 18 months of age is of shorter duration

Mumps vaccine

■ Single antigen vaccine
No longer available in the UK

■ Combined vaccine
See MMR Vaccine

Pertussis vaccine

Pertussis vaccine is usually given combined with diphtheria and tetanus vaccine (in triple vaccine) starting at 2 months of age (see section 14.1).

With some vaccines available in the early 1960s *persistent screaming and collapse* were reported but these reactions are rarely observed with the vaccines now available. *Convulsions and encephalopathy* have been reported as rare complications, but such conditions may arise from other causes and be falsely attributed to the vaccine. Neurological complications *after whooping cough itself* are considerably more common than after the vaccine.

As with any other elective immunisation procedure it is advisable to postpone vaccination if the child is suffering from any acute illness, until fully recovered. Minor infections without fever or systemic upset are not reasons to delay immunisation. Immunisation should not be carried out in children who have a history of severe general reaction to a preceding dose; in these children immunisation should be completed with adsorbed diphtheria and tetanus vaccine. Where there has been a severe local reaction or pyrexia, acellular pertussis vaccine may be used. The following reactions should be regarded as severe:

Local—an extensive area of redness and swelling which becomes indurated and involves most of the antero-lateral surface of the thigh or a major part of the circumference of the upper arm.
General—temperature of 39.5°C or more within 48 hours of vaccine, anaphylaxis, bronchospasm, laryngeal oedema, generalised collapse, prolonged unresponsiveness, prolonged inconsolable screaming, and convulsions occurring within 72 hours.

A personal or family history of allergy is **not** a contra-indication to immunisation against whooping cough; nor are stable neurological conditions such as cerebral palsy or spina bifida.

CHILDREN WITH PROBLEM HISTORIES. When there is a personal or family history of *febrile* convulsions, there is an increased risk of these occurring after pertussis immunisation. In such children, immunisation is *recommended* but advice on the *prevention of fever* (see p. 543) should be given at the time of immunisation.

In a British study, children with a family history of epilepsy were immunised with pertussis vaccine without any significant adverse events. These children's developmental progress has been normal. In children with a close family history (first degree relatives) of *idiopathic epilepsy*, there may be a risk of developing a similar condition, irrespective of vaccine. Immunisation is *recommended* for these children.

Where there is a *still evolving neurological problem*, immunisation should be *deferred* until the condition is stable. Children whose epilepsy is well controlled may receive pertussis vaccine. When there has been a documented history of *cerebral damage in the neonatal period*, immunisation should be *carried out unless there is evidence of an evolving neurological abnormality*. If immunisation is to be deferred, this should be stated on the neonatal discharge summary. Where there is doubt, appropriate advice should be sought from a consultant paediatrician, district immunisation co-ordinator or consultant in communicable disease control *rather than withholding vaccine*.

OLDER CHILDREN. There is no contra-indication to administration of pertussis vaccine to unimmunised older children in order to protect the individuals and siblings under the age of immunisation; there is no upper age limit.

Acellular Pertussis Vaccine, APV (Lederle) ▼ PoM

Unlicensed single-antigen acellular pertussis vaccine (APV) has been made available by the Department of Health under Crown Immunity only for completion of immunisation against pertussis in those children whose course of pertussis vaccine was not given (or not completed) as part of their triple vaccine course
Dose: 0.5 mL by intramuscular or deep subcutaneous injection, 3 doses at intervals of 1 month
Available from Farillon on a named-patient basis
Note. Should be ordered only when required for use
Combined vaccine (*pertussis, tetanus,* and *diphtheria*), see under Diphtheria vaccines

Pneumococcal vaccine

A polyvalent **pneumococcal polysaccharide vaccine** is recommended for the immunisation of persons over the age of 2 years with any of the following conditions:

- Homozygous sickle cell disease;
- Asplenia or severe dysfunction of the spleen;
- Chronic renal disease or nephrotic syndrome;
- Coeliac syndrome;
- Immunodeficiency or immunosuppression due to disease or treatment, including HIV infection;
- Chronic heart disease;
- Chronic lung disease;
- Chronic liver disease including cirrhosis;
- Diabetes mellitus.

Where possible, the vaccine should be given at least 2 weeks before splenectomy and before chemotherapy; patients should be given advice about increased risk of pneumococcal infection (a patient card and information leaflet for patients with asple-

nia are available from the Department of Health). Prophylactic antibiotic therapy against pneumococcal infection should not be stopped after immunisation. The vaccine is effective in a single dose if the types of pneumonia in the community are reflected in the polysaccharides contained in the vaccine. It should not be given in pregnancy, or when breast-feeding, or when there is infection. Hypersensitivity reactions may occur.

REVACCINATION. Revaccination with the previously available 12- or 14-valent vaccines produced severe reactions in some subjects, especially if undertaken less than 3 years after the first injection; the same is likely to apply to revaccination with the currently available 23-valent vaccines. Revaccination is therefore not recommended except, after 5–10 years, in individuals in whom the antibody concentration is likely to decline more rapidly (e.g. asplenia, splenic dysfunction and nephrotic syndrome). If there is doubt about the need for revaccination, this should be discussed with a haematologist and measurement of antibody concentration considered.

IMPORTANT. Not for intradermal injection which may cause severe local reactions
See section 14.1 for general contra-indications.

Pneumovax® II (Pasteur Mérieux) PoM
Polysaccharide from each of 23 capsular types of pneumococcus, net price 0.5-mL vial = £9.49
Dose: 0.5 mL by subcutaneous or intramuscular injection; CHILD under 2 years, not recommended (suboptimal response and also safety and efficacy not established)

Pnu-Imune® (Wyeth) PoM
Polysaccharide from each of 23 capsular types of pneumococcus, net price 0.5-mL vial = £9.94
Dose: 0.5 mL by subcutaneous or intramuscular injection; CHILD under 2 years, not recommended

Poliomyelitis vaccines

There are two types of poliomyelitis vaccine, poliomyelitis vaccine, live (oral) (Sabin) and poliomyelitis vaccine, inactivated (Salk). The oral vaccine, consisting of a mixture of attenuated strains of virus types 1, 2, and 3 is at present generally used in the UK.

A course of primary immunisation consists of 3 doses of **poliomyelitis vaccine, live (oral)**, starting at two months of age with an interval of 1 month between each dose (see schedule, section 14.1). The initial course of 3 doses should also be given to all unimmunised adults; no adult should remain unimmunised against poliomyelitis.

Two booster doses of poliomyelitis vaccine, live (oral), are recommended, the first before school entry and the second before leaving school (see schedule, section 14.1). Booster doses for adults are not necessary except for those at special risk such as travellers to endemic areas, or laboratory staff likely to be exposed to the viruses, or health care workers in possible contact with cases; booster doses should be given to such individuals every 10 years.

Vaccine-associated poliomyelitis and poliomyelitis in contacts of vaccinees are rare. In England and Wales there is an annual average of 1 recipient and 1 contact case for over 2 million doses of oral vaccine. The need for strict personal hygiene must be stressed; the contacts of a recently vaccinated baby should be advised particularly of the need to wash their hands after changing the baby's nappies.

Contra-indications to the use of oral poliomyelitis vaccine include vomiting and diarrhoea, and immunodeficiency disorders (or household contacts of patients with immunodeficiency disorders). See section 14.1 for further contra-indications.

Poliomyelitis vaccine (inactivated) may be used for those in whom poliomyelitis vaccine (oral) is contra-indicated because of immunosuppressive disorders (for advice on AIDS see section 14.1).

Either live (oral) vaccine or inactivated vaccine may be used to complete a course started with the other, except that live (oral) vaccine must **not** be used for immunosuppressed individuals or their household contacts (see also contra-indications).

TRAVELLERS. Travellers to areas other than Australia, New Zealand, Northern and Western Europe, and North America should be given a full course of oral poliomyelitis vaccine if they have not been immunised in the past. Those who have not received immunisation within the last 10 years should be given a booster dose of oral poliomyelitis vaccine.

■ Live (oral) (Sabin)

Poliomyelitis Vaccine, Live (Oral) PoM Pol/ Vac (Oral)[1]. A suspension of suitable live attenuated strains of poliomyelitis virus, types 1, 2, and 3. Available in single-dose and 10-dose containers

Dose: 3 drops from a multidose container or the total contents of a single-dose container; for primary immunisation 3 doses are required (see schedule, section 14.1). May be given on a lump of sugar; not to be given with foods which contain preservatives

Available from Health Authorities or (in England and Scotland only) direct from Farillon
1. BP permits code OPV for vaccine in single doses provided it also appears on pack.
Note. Poliomyelitis vaccine loses potency once the container has been opened, therefore any vaccine remaining at the end of an immunisation session should be discarded; whenever possible sessions should be arranged to avoid undue wastage.

■ Inactivated (Salk)

Poliomyelitis Vaccine, Inactivated PoM Pol/ Vac (Inact). An inactivated suspension of suitable strains of poliomyelitis virus, types 1, 2, and 3.
Dose: 0.5 mL or as stated on the label by subcutaneous injection; for primary immunisation 3 doses are required at intervals of 4 weeks
Available direct from Farillon
Note. Should be ordered one dose at a time (on a named-patient basis) and only when required for use

Rabies vaccine

Pre-exposure, prophylactic immunisation with human diploid cell **rabies vaccine** should be offered to those at high risk—laboratory staff who handle the rabies virus, those working in quarantine stations, animal handlers, veterinary surgeons and field workers who are likely to be exposed to bites of possibly infected wild animals, certain port officials, licensed bat handlers and health workers who are likely to come into close contact with patients with rabies. Pre-exposure immunisation is also recommended for those living or travelling in enzootic areas who may be exposed to unusual risk.

The Department of Health has advised that for *prophylactic use* the vaccine produces a good antibody response when given in a 3-dose schedule on days 0, 7, and 28, with a booster dose every 2–3 years to those at continued risk. For travellers to enzootic areas who are not animal handlers, 2 doses given 4 weeks apart may be acceptable *provided that post-exposure treatment is readily available;* for those who remain at continued risk a booster dose should be given 6–12 months later followed by a booster every 2–3 years.

Post-exposure treatment depends on the level of risk in the country concerned and the individual's immune status. For *post-exposure treatment of fully immunised patients:* countries with no risk, generally no treatment required; countries with low risk and high risk, two booster doses are needed (one on day 0 and one on day 3–7). For *post-exposure treatment of previously unimmunised patients* (or those whose prophylaxis is possibly inadequate): countries with no risk, generally no treatment required; countries with low risk, a course of injections should be started as soon as possible after exposure (days 0, 3, 7, 14 and 30); countries with high risk, as for countries with low risk, **plus** rabies immunoglobulin on day 0 (section 14.5). The course may be discontinued if it is proved that the patient was not at risk.

Staff in attendance on a patient who is highly suspected of, or known to be suffering from, rabies should be offered immunisation. Four intradermal doses of 0.1 mL of human diploid cell vaccine (Pasteur Mérieux) given on the same day at different sites (ensuring correct intradermal technique) has been suggested for this purpose [unlicensed route].

Advice on up-to-date country-by-country information and on post-exposure immunisation and treatment of rabies is available from the Virus Reference Division, Central Public Health Laboratory, Colindale, London NW9 5HT (Tel (020) 8200 4400) or in Scotland from the Scottish Centre for Infection and Environmental Health (Tel 0141-946 7120).

There are no specific contra-indications to this diploid cell vaccine and its use should be considered whenever a patient has been attacked by an animal in a country where rabies is endemic, even if there is no direct evidence of rabies in the attacking animal.

Rabies Vaccine BP Pasteur Mérieux (Pasteur Mérieux) PoM
Freeze-dried inactivated Wistar rabies virus strain PM/WI 38 1503-3M cultivated in human diploid cells. Single-dose vial with syringe containing diluent
IMPORTANT. Studies have shown that when this vaccine is injected into the gluteal region there is a poor response. Concomitant administration of chloroquine may also affect the antibody response. Because of the potential consequences of inadequately treated rabies exposure and because there is no indication that fetal abnormalities have been associated with rabies vaccination, pregnancy is **not** considered a contra-indication to post-exposure prophylaxis. If there is substantial risk of exposure to rabies, pre-exposure prophylaxis may also be indicated during pregnancy
Dose: prophylactic, 1 mL by deep subcutaneous or intramuscular injection in the deltoid region, on days 0, 7, and 28; also booster doses every 2–3 years to those at continued risk; see above for 2-dose schedule
Post-exposure, 1 mL by deep subcutaneous or intramuscular injection in the deltoid region, see notes above
Staff in attendance, see notes above
Also available from local designated centres (special workers and post-exposure treatment)

Rubella vaccine

The selective policy of protecting women of child-bearing age from the risks of rubella (German measles) in pregnancy has been replaced by a policy of eliminating rubella in children; the single-antigen rubella immunisation programme for 10–14 year old girls has been discontinued. All children should be immunised with rubella-containing vaccine (measles, mumps and rubella) at 12–15 months and at 3–5 years (see MMR vaccine, p. 550). Immigrants who enter the UK after the age of school immunisation are particularly likely to require immunisation.

Every effort must be made to identify and immunise with rubella vaccine all *seronegative women of child-bearing age* (see schedule, section 14.1) as well as those who might put pregnant women at risk of infection (e.g. nurses and doctors in obstetric units).

Rubella vaccine may conveniently be offered to previously *unimmunised and seronegative post-partum women.* Immunising susceptible post-partum women a few days after delivery is important as far as the overall reduction of congenital abnormalities in the UK is concerned, for about 60% of these abnormalities occur in the babies of multiparous women.

PREGNANCY. Rubella immunisation should be avoided in early pregnancy, and women of child-bearing age should be advised not to become pregnant within 1 month of immunisation. However, despite active surveillance in the UK, the USA, and Germany, no case of congenital rubella syndrome has been reported following inadvertent immunisation shortly before or during pregnancy. There is thus no evidence that the vaccine is teratogenic, and routine termination of pregnancy following inadvertent immunisation should **not** be recommended; potential parents should be given this information before making a decision about termination.

See section 14.1 for general contra-indications.

Rubella Vaccine, Live PoM Rub/Vac (Live). Prepared from Wistar RA 27/3 strain propagated in human diploid cells

Dose: 0.5 mL by deep subcutaneous or by intramuscular injection (see schedule, section 14.1 and notes above)

Available from Health Authorities or (in England only) direct from Farillon as SmithKline Beecham brand (*Ervevax®*)

■ Combined vaccines
see MMR vaccine

Smallpox vaccine

Smallpox immunisation is no longer required routinely because global eradication has been achieved. Advice on the need for immunisation of workers in laboratories where pox viruses (such as vaccinia) are handled and of others whose work involves an identifiable risk of exposure to pox virus can be obtained from the Virus Reference Laboratory, Central Public Health Laboratory, Colindale (Tel (020) 8200 4400) who will also supply the vaccine.

Tetanus vaccines

Tetanus vaccines stimulate the production of the protective antitoxin. In general, adsorption on aluminium hydroxide, aluminium phosphate, or calcium phosphate improves antigenicity. Adsorbed tetanus vaccine is offered routinely to babies in combination with adsorbed diphtheria vaccine (DT/Vac/Ads(Child)) and more usually also combined with killed *Bordetella pertussis* organisms as a triple vaccine, adsorbed diphtheria, tetanus, and pertussis vaccine (DTPer/Vac/Ads), see schedule, section 14.1.

In children, the triple vaccine not only gives protection against tetanus in childhood but also gives the basic immunity for subsequent booster doses of adsorbed tetanus vaccine at school entry and at school leaving (combined with low-dose adsorbed diphtheria vaccine) and also when a potentially tetanus-contaminated injury has been received. Normally, booster doses of adsorbed tetanus vaccine should not be given unless more than 10 years have elapsed since the last booster dose because of the possibility that hypersensitivity reactions may develop. If a child over the age of 13 years requires a tetanus booster for a wound then, provided more than 10 years have elapsed since the school-entry booster, adsorbed tetanus vaccine combined with low-dose adsorbed diphtheria vaccine can be given; the routine booster at school-leaving age is omitted.

Active immunisation is important for persons in older age groups who may never have had a routine or complete course of immunisation when younger. In these persons a course of adsorbed tetanus vaccine may be given. Very rarely, tetanus has developed after abdominal surgery; patients awaiting elective surgery should be asked about tetanus immunisation and immunised if necessary. All laboratory staff should be offered a primary course if unimmunised.

Any adult who has received 5 doses is likely to have life-long immunity; booster doses on injury should only be required if more than 10 years have elapsed since the last dose.

WOUNDS. Wounds are considered to be tetanus-prone if they are sustained *either* more than 6 hours before surgical treatment *or* at any interval after injury and are puncture-type or show much devitalised tissue or are septic or are contaminated with soil or manure. All wounds should receive thorough surgical toilet.

- For *clean wounds,* a booster dose of adsorbed tetanus vaccine is given if the primary course (or booster dose) was given more than 10 years previously; non-immunised individuals (or whose immunisation status is not known) should be given a full course of the vaccine.
- For *tetanus-prone wounds,* management is as for clean wounds with the addition of a dose of tetanus immunoglobulin (section 14.5); in an immunised individual who has received a dose of adsorbed tetanus vaccine within the previous 10 years, the immunoglobulin may only be needed if the risk of infection is considered to be especially high (e.g. contamination with manure). Antibiotic prophylaxis (with benzylpenicillin, co-amoxiclav, or metronidazole) may also be required for tetanus-prone wounds.

See section 14.1 for general contra-indications

■ Single antigen vaccines

The BP directs that when Tetanus Vaccine is prescribed or demanded and the form is not stated, Adsorbed Tetanus Vaccine may be dispensed or supplied.

Adsorbed Tetanus Vaccine [PoM]

Tet/Vac/Ads.

Injection, suspension of tetanus formol toxoid adsorbed on a mineral carrier

Dose: 0.5 mL or as stated on the label, by intramuscular or deep subcutaneous injection followed after 4 weeks by a second dose and after a further 4 weeks by a third

Available from Medeva (net price 0.5-mL amp = 71p, and as *Clostet*®, net price 0.5-mL single-dose syringe = £1.40) and from Pasteur Mérieux (net price 0.5-mL amp = 55p; 0.5-mL single-dose syringe = £1.20

Combined vaccines, see Diphtheria Vaccines

Typhoid vaccines

Typhoid immunisation is advised for travellers to countries where sanitation standards may be poor, although it is not a substitute for scrupulous personal hygiene (see section 14.6). Immunisation is also advised for laboratory workers handling specimens from suspected cases.

The original **whole cell typhoid vaccine** (no longer available) was normally given in 2 doses at intervals of 4–6 weeks for primary immunisation, with booster doses about every 3 years on continued exposure.

Capsular **polysaccharide typhoid vaccine** is given by *intramuscular or deep subcutaneous injection* with a booster dose every 3 years on continued exposure. Local reactions, including pain, swelling or erythema, may appear 48–72 hours after administration.

An **oral typhoid vaccine** is also available. It is a **live attenuated** vaccine contained in an enteric-coated capsule. It is taken *by mouth* as three doses of one capsule on alternate days, providing protection 7–10 days after the last dose. Protection may persist for up to 3 years in those constantly (or repeatedly) exposed to *Salmonella typhi*, but occasional travellers require a repeat course at intervals of 1 year. Oral typhoid vaccine is **contra-indicated** in individuals who are immunosuppressed (whether due to disease or its treatment) and is inactivated by concomitant administration of *antibiotics* or *sulphonamides*. Oral typhoid vaccine and oral poliomyelitis vaccine should be given at least 3 weeks apart on theoretical grounds. Administration of a dose of oral typhoid vaccine should be coordinated so that *mefloquine* is not taken for at least 12 hours before or after a dose (vaccination with oral typhoid vaccine should preferably be completed at least 3 days before the first dose of mefloquine). Side-effects to oral typhoid vaccine include nausea, vomiting, abdominal cramps, diarrhoea, headache, fever and hypersensitivity reactions including, rarely, anaphylaxis.

For general contra-indications to vaccines, see section 14.1.

■ Whole cell vaccine for injection

Typhoid Vaccine [PoM] Typhoid/Vac. A suspension of killed *Salmonella typhi* organisms.

Note. No longer available.

■ Polysaccharide vaccine for injection

Typherix® (SmithKline Beecham) ▼ [PoM]

Injection, Vi capsular polysaccharide typhoid vaccine, 50 micrograms/mL virulence polysaccharide antigen of *Salmonella typhi*, net price 0.5-mL single-dose prefilled syringe = £10.68

Dose: 0.5 mL by intramuscular injection; CHILD under 2 years may show suboptimal response

Typhim Vi® (Pasteur Mérieux) [PoM]

Injection, Vi capsular polysaccharide typhoid vaccine, 50 micrograms/mL virulence polysaccharide antigen of *Salmonella typhi*, net price 0.5-mL single-dose prefilled syringe = £10.20

Dose: 0.5 mL by deep subcutaneous or intramuscular injection; CHILD under 18 months may show suboptimal response

■ Polysaccharide vaccine with hepatitis A vaccine

See Hepatitis A Vaccine

■ Live oral vaccine

Vivotif® (Medeva) [PoM]

Capsules, e /c, live attenuated *Salmonella typhi* (Ty 21a), net price 3-cap pack = £15.88. Label: 23, 25, C, administration

Dose: ADULT and CHILD over 6 years, 1 capsule on days 1, 3, and 5; under 6 years, not recommended

COUNSELLING. Swallow as soon as possible after placing in mouth with a cold or lukewarm drink; it is important to store capsules in refrigerator

Yellow fever vaccine

Yellow fever vaccine consists of a live attenuated yellow fever virus (17D strain) grown in developing chick embryos. Immunisation is indicated for those travelling or living in areas where infection is endemic (see p. 559) and for laboratory staff who handle the virus or who handle clinical material from suspected cases. Infants under 9 months of age should only be vaccinated if the risk of yellow fever is unavoidable since there is a small risk of encephalitis. The vaccine should not be given to those with impaired immune responsiveness, or who have had an anaphylactic reaction to egg; it should not be given during pregnancy (but where there is a significant risk of exposure the need for immunisation outweighs any risk to the fetus). See section 14.1 for further contra-indications. Reactions are few. The immunity which probably lasts for life is officially accepted for 10 years starting from 10 days after primary immunisation and for a further 10 years immediately after revaccination.

Yellow Fever Vaccine, Live [PoM] Yel/Vac. A suspension of chick embryo proteins containing attenuated 17D strain virus

Dose: 0.5 mL by subcutaneous injection

Available (only to designated Yellow Fever Vaccination centres) as *Arilvax*® (Medeva)

14.5   Immunoglobulins

Human immunoglobulins have replaced immunoglobulins of animal origin (antisera) which were frequently associated with hypersensitivity. Injection of immunoglobulins produces immediate protection lasting for several weeks.

The two types of human immunoglobulin preparation are **normal immunoglobulin** and **specific immunoglobulins**.

Further information about immunoglobulins is included in *Immunisation against Infectious Disease* (see section 14.1).

AVAILABILITY. **Normal immunoglobulin** is now only available from the *Public Health Laboratory Service* laboratories for contacts and the control of outbreaks. It is available commercially for other purposes.

Specific immunoglobulins are available from the *Public Health Laboratory Service* laboratories and *Regional Blood Transfusion Centres* in England and Wales with the exception of **tetanus immunoglobulin** which is distributed through *Regional Blood Transfusion Centres* to hospital pharmacies or blood transfusion departments and is also available to general medical practitioners. **Rabies immunoglobulin** is available from the *Central Public Health Laboratory, London*. The large amounts of **hepatitis B immunoglobulin** required by transplant centres should be obtained commercially.

In Scotland all immunoglobulins are available from the *Blood Transfusion Service*. **Tetanus immunoglobulin** is distributed by the *Blood Transfusion Service* to hospitals and general medical practitioners on demand.

Normal immunoglobulin

Human **normal immunoglobulin** ('HNIG') is prepared from pools of at least 1000 donations of human plasma; it contains antibody to measles, mumps, varicella, hepatitis A, and other viruses that are currently prevalent in the general population.

CAUTIONS AND SIDE-EFFECTS. Side-effects of immunoglobulins include malaise, chills, fever, and rarely anaphylaxis. Normal immunoglobulin is **contra-indicated** in patients with known class specific antibody to immunoglobulin A (IgA).

Normal immunoglobulin may **interfere with the immune response to live virus vaccines** which should therefore only be given **at least 3 weeks before or 3 months after** an injection of normal immunoglobulin (this does not apply to yellow fever vaccine since normal immunoglobulin does not contain antibody to this virus). For travellers, if there is insufficient time, the recommended interval may have to be ignored.

Intramuscular immunoglobulins

Normal immunoglobulin is administered by intramuscular injection for the protection of susceptible contacts against **hepatitis A** virus (infectious hepatitis), **measles** and, to a lesser extent, **rubella**.

HEPATITIS A. Control of hepatitis A depends on good hygiene and many studies have also shown the value of normal immunoglobulin in the prevention and control of outbreaks of this disease. It is recommended for controlling infection in contacts in closed institutions and also, under certain conditions, in school and home contacts, and for occasional or short-term travellers going to areas where the disease is highly endemic (all countries excluding Northern and Western Europe, North America, Australia, and New Zealand). **Hepatitis A vaccine** (see p. 547) is preferred for those visiting such countries frequently or who stay for longer than 3 months.

MEASLES. Normal immunoglobulin may be given for prophylaxis in children with compromised immunity (and in adults with compromised immunity who have no measles antibodies); it should be given as soon as possible after contact with measles. It should also be given to children under 12 months with recent severe illness for whom measles should be avoided; MMR vaccine should then be given (after an interval of **at least** 3 months) at around the usual age.

RUBELLA. Immunoglobulin after exposure does **not** prevent infection in non-immune contacts and is **not** recommended for protection of pregnant women exposed to rubella. It may however reduce the likelihood of a clinical attack which may possibly reduce the risk to the fetus. It should only be used when termination of pregnancy would be unacceptable when it should be given as soon as possible after exposure. Serological follow-up of recipients is essential. For routine prophylaxis, see **Rubella Vaccine** (p. 554).

REPLACEMENT THERAPY. Normal immunoglobulin may also be given intramuscularly for replacement therapy, but intravenous formulations (see below under Intravenous) are normally preferred.

■ For intramuscular use
Normal Immunoglobulin PoM Normal immunoglobulin injection. 250-mg vial; 750-mg vial

Dose: by deep intramuscular injection, Hepatitis A travel prophylaxis (2 months or less abroad), 250 mg; CHILD under 10 years 125 mg; longer travel prophylaxis (3–5 months abroad, but see notes above) and to control outbreaks, 500 mg; CHILD under 10 years 250 mg
Measles prophylaxis, CHILD under 1 year 250 mg, 1–2 years 500 mg, 3 years and over 750 mg; to allow attenuated attack, CHILD under 1 year 100 mg, 1 year and over 250 mg
Rubella in pregnancy, prevention of clinical attack, 750 mg

Available from BPL and Public Health Laboratory Service (for contacts and control of outbreaks only, see above) and from SNBTS

Gammabulin® (Hyland Immuno) PoM
Normal immunoglobulin injection, net price 2-mL vial = £2.98; 10-mL vial = £10.22
Dose: see below

Kabiglobulin® (Pharmacia & Upjohn) PoM
Normal immunoglobulin injection 16%, net price 2-mL amp = £2.78; 5-mL amp = £6.00
Dose: see below

Note. Doses for *Gammabulin*® and *Kabiglobulin*® are expressed in terms of volume:
Dose: by intramuscular injection,
Hepatitis A prophylaxis, ADULT and CHILD 0.02–0.04 mL/kg; greater exposure risk, 0.06–0.12 mL/kg
Measles prophylaxis, 0.2 mL/kg; to allow attenuated attack, 0.04 mL/kg
Rubella in pregnancy, prevention of clinical attack, 20 mL
Antibody deficiency syndromes, consult product literature

Intravenous immunoglobulins

Special formulations for intravenous administration are available for replacement therapy for patients with congenital agammaglobulinaemia and hypogammaglobulinaemia, for the treatment of idiopathic thrombocytopenic purpura and Kawasaki syndrome, and for the prophylaxis of infection following bone marrow transplantation.

Intravenous immunoglobulin is also used in the treatment of Guillain-Barré syndrome and is now preferred to plasma exchange.

■ For intravenous use

Normal Immunoglobulin for Intravenous Use [PoM]

Available as: *Alphaglobin®* (0.5 g, 2.5 g, 5 g, 10 g—Grifols); Human Immunoglobulin (3 g, 5 g, 10 g—SNBTS); *Octagam®* (2.5 g, 5 g, 10 g—Octapharma); *Sandoglobulin®* (1 g, 3 g, 6 g, 12 g—Novartis); *Vigam®S* (2.5 g, 5 g—BPL); *Vigam®Liquid* (2.5 g, 5 g, 10 g—BPL)

Dose: consult product literature

Specific immunoglobulins

Specific immunoglobulins are prepared by pooling the plasma of selected donors with high levels of the specific antibody required.

Although a hepatitis B vaccine is now available for those at high risk of infection, specific **hepatitis B immunoglobulin** ('HBIG') is available for use in association with the vaccine for the prevention of infection in laboratory and other personnel who have been accidentally inoculated with hepatitis B virus, and in infants born to mothers who have become infected with this virus in pregnancy or who are high-risk carriers.

Following exposure of an unimmunised individual to an animal in or from a high-risk country, specific **rabies immunoglobulin** of human origin should be injected at the site of the bite and also given intramuscularly. Rabies vaccine should also be given (for details see Rabies Vaccine, p. 553).

For the management of tetanus-prone wounds, **tetanus immunoglobulin** of human origin ('HTIG') should be used in addition to wound toilet and, where appropriate, antibiotic prophylaxis and adsorbed tetanus vaccine (section 14.4). Tetanus immunoglobulin, together with metronidazole (section 5.1.11) and wound toilet, should also be used for the treatment of established cases of tetanus.

Varicella-zoster immunoglobulin (VZIG) is recommended for individuals who are at increased risk of severe varicella *and* who have no antibodies to varicella-zoster virus *and* who have significant exposure to chickenpox or herpes zoster. Those at increased risk include neonates of women who develop chickenpox 7 days before or 28 days after delivery, women exposed at any stage of pregnancy, and the immunosuppressed including those who have received corticosteroids in the previous 3 months at the following dose equivalents of prednisolone: *children* 2 mg/kg daily for at least 1 week or 1 mg/kg daily for 1 month; *adults* about 40 mg daily for more than 1 week. (**Important:** for full details consult *Immunisation against Infectious Disease*). **Varicella vaccine** is available on a

named-patient basis from SmithKline Beecham or Pasteur Mérieux.

Cytomegalovirus (CMV) immunoglobulin (available on a named-patient basis from SNBTS) is indicated for prophylaxis in patients receiving immunosuppressive treatment. Also batches of normal immunoglobulin with a high CMV titre are available from Grifols for treatment and prophylaxis of CMV infections [unlicensed indication].

■ Hepatitis B

Hepatitis B Immunoglobulin [PoM] See notes above

Dose: by intramuscular injection (as soon as possible after exposure), ADULT 500 units; CHILD under 4 years 200 units, 5–9 years 300 units; NEONATE 200 units as soon as possible after birth; for full details consult *Immunisation against Infectious Disease*

Available from Public Health Laboratory Service (except for Transplant Centres, see p. 556), also available from BPL and SNBTS

Note. Hepatitis B Immunoglobulin for Intravenous Use is available from BPL and SNBTS on a named-patient basis.

■ Rabies

Rabies Immunoglobulin [PoM] (Antirabies Immunoglobulin Injection). See notes above

Dose: 20 units/kg, half by intramuscular injection and half by infiltration around wound

Available from Public Health Laboratory Service (also from BPL and SNBTS)

■ Tetanus

Tetanus Immunoglobulin [PoM] (Antitetanus Immunoglobulin Injection). See notes above

Dose: by intramuscular injection, prophylactic 250 units, increased to 500 units if more than 24 hours have elapsed or there is risk of heavy contamination

Therapeutic, 150 units/kg (multiple sites)

Available from BPL and SNBTS

Tetabulin® (Hyland Immuno) [PoM]

Tetanus immunoglobulin, net price 250-unit pre-filled syringe = £14.80

Dose: by intramuscular injection, prophylactic, 250 units, increased to 500 units if wound older than 12 hours or if risk of heavy contamination or if patient weighs more than 90 kg; second dose of 250 units given after 3–4 weeks if patient immunosuppressed or if active immunisation with vaccine contra-indicated

Therapeutic, 30–300 units/kg

Tetanus Immunoglobulin for Intravenous Use [PoM] Used for proven or suspected clinical tetanus

Dose: by intravenous infusion, 5000–10 000 units

Available from BPL and SNBTS on a named-patient basis

■ Varicella–Zoster

Varicella–Zoster Immunoglobulin [PoM] (Anti-varicella–zoster Immunoglobulin) See notes above

Dose: by deep intramuscular injection, prophylaxis (as soon as possible—not later than 10 days after exposure), CHILD up to 5 years 250 mg, 6–10 years 500 mg, 11–14 years 750 mg, over 15 years 1 g; second dose required if further exposure occurs after 3 weeks

Note. No evidence that effective in treatment of severe disease. Normal immunoglobulin for intravenous use may be used to provide an immediate source of antibody.

Available from Public Health Laboratory Service (also from BPL and SNBTS)

Anti-D (Rh₀) immunoglobulin

Anti-D (Rh₀) immunoglobulin is available to prevent a rhesus-negative mother from forming antibodies to fetal rhesus-positive cells which may pass into the maternal circulation. The objective is to protect any subsequent child from the hazard of haemolytic disease of the newborn.

Anti-D immunoglobulin should be administered following any sensitising episode (e.g. abortion, miscarriage and birth); it should be injected within 72 hours of the episode but even if a longer period has elapsed it may still give protection and should be administered. The dose of anti-D immunoglobulin is determined according to the level of exposure to rhesus-positive blood.

Routine antenatal prophylaxis is also recommended by the Royal College of Obstetricians and Gynaecologists for all rhesus-negative women: two doses of at least 500 units of anti-D immunoglobulin should be given, the first at 28 weeks gestation and the second at 34 weeks.

> Note. Rubella vaccine may be administered in the postpartum period simultaneously with anti-D (Rh₀) immunoglobulin injection providing separate syringes are used and the products are administered into contralateral limbs. If blood is transfused, the antibody response to the vaccine may be inhibited and a test for antibodies should be performed after 8 weeks and the subject revaccinated if necessary.
>
> MMR vaccine should not be given within 3 months of an injection of anti-D (Rh₀) immunoglobulin injection.

Anti-D (Rh₀) Immunoglobulin [PoM]

Dose: by deep intramuscular injection, to rhesus-negative woman for prevention of Rh₀(D) sensitisation:
Following birth of rhesus-positive infant, 500 units immediately or within 72 hours; for transplacental bleed in excess of 4–5 mL fetal red cells, extra 100–125 units per mL fetal red cells
Following any potentially sensitising episode (e.g. still-birth, abortion, amniocentesis) up to 20 weeks' gestation 250 units per episode (after 20 weeks, 500 units) immediately or within 72 hours
Following Rh₀(D) incompatible blood transfusion, 125 units per mL transfused rhesus-positive red cells
Antenatal prophylaxis, 500 units given at weeks 28 and 34 of pregnancy; a further dose is still needed immediately or within 72 hours of delivery
Available from Regional Blood Transfusion Centres and from BPL and SNBTS

Anti-D Immunoglobulin (Hyland Immuno) [PoM]
Anti-D (Rh₀) immunoglobulin 1250 units/mL, net price 1-mL prefilled syringe = £23.90

Dose: by intramuscular injection, to rhesus-negative woman for prevention of Rh₀(D) sensitisation:
Following abortion, miscarriage or birth of rhesus-positive infant, 1250 units immediately or within 72 hours; for transplacental bleed in excess of 25 mL fetal blood (1% of fetal erythrocytes), 5000 units (or 50 units per mL fetal blood)
Following any potentially sensitising episode (e.g. amniocentesis) 1250 units immediately or within 72 hours
Following Rh₀(D) incompatible blood transfusion, at least 50–100 units per mL transfused rhesus-positive blood
Antenatal prophylaxis, 1250 units may be given at weeks 28 and 34 of pregnancy; a further dose is still needed immediately or within 72 hours of delivery
Note. Some UK authorities recommend lower doses for antenatal prophylaxis (see notes above)

WinRho SDF® (Octapharma) [PoM]
Injection, powder for reconstitution, anti-D (Rh₀) immunoglobulin, net price 600-unit vial (with sodium chloride 0.9%) = £30.00; 1500-unit vial (with sodium chloride 0.9%) = £39.00

Dose: to rhesus-negative woman for prevention of Rh₀(D) sensitisation:

Following birth of rhesus-positive infant immediately or within 72 hours, by slow intramuscular injection, 1500 units or by intravenous injection, 600 units; for transplacental bleed in excess of 25 mL fetal blood, by slow intramuscular injection, extra 50 units per mL fetal blood

Following any potentially sensitising episode (e.g mis-carriage, abortion, amniocentesis), by slow intramuscular injection, up to 12 weeks gestation, 600 units (after 12 weeks, 1500 units) immediately or within 72 hours

Following Rh₀(D) incompatible blood transfusion, by slow intramuscular injection, 60 units per mL transfused rhesus-positive blood, in divided doses over several days

Following Rh₀(D) incompatible thrombocyte transfusion, by intravenous injection, 1500 units

Antenatal prophylaxis, by slow intramuscular or intravenous injection, 1500 units at 28 weeks gestation; a further dose should be considered after birth if infant rhesus-positive

Note. For antenatal prophylaxis, some UK authorities recommend a lower dose, which is repeated at 34 weeks gestation (see notes above)

Interferons

Interferon gamma-1b is indicated for chronic granulomatous disease to reduce the frequency of serious infection.

INTERFERON GAMMA-1b

(Immune interferon)

Indications: adjunct to antibiotics to reduce frequency of serious infection in patients with chronic granulomatous disease

Cautions: severe hepatic or renal impairment; seizure disorders or compromised central nervous system function; pre-existing cardiac disease (including ischaemia, congestive heart failure, and arrhythmias); monitor before and during treatment: haematological tests (including full blood count, differential white cell count, and platelet count), blood chemistry tests (including renal and liver function tests) and urinalysis

DRIVING. May impair ability to drive or operate machinery; effects may be enhanced by alcohol

Side-effects: fever, headache, chills, myalgia, fatigue; nausea, vomiting, arthralgia, rashes and injection-site reactions reported

Immukin® (Boehringer Ingelheim) ▼ [PoM]
Injection, recombinant human interferon gamma-1b 200 micrograms/mL, net price 0.5-mL vial = £88.00

Dose: by subcutaneous injection, 50 micrograms/m² 3 times a week; patients with body surface area of 0.5 m² or less, 1.5 micrograms/kg 3 times a week; not yet recommended for children under 6 months

14.6 International travel

Note. For advice on **malaria chemoprophylaxis**, see section 5.4.1.

No particular immunisation is required for travellers to the United States, Europe, Australia, or New Zealand although all travellers should have immunity to tetanus and poliomyelitis (and childhood immunisations should be up to date). In Non-European areas surrounding the Mediterranean, in Africa, the Middle East, Asia, and South America, certain special precautions are required.

Long-term travellers to areas that have a high incidence of **poliomyelitis** or **tuberculosis** should be immunised with the appropriate vaccine; in the case of poliomyelitis previously immunised adults may be given a booster dose of oral poliomyelitis vaccine. BCG immunisation is recommended for travellers proposing to stay for longer than one month (or in close contact with the local population) in Asia, Africa, or Central and South America; it should preferably be given three months or more before departure.

Yellow fever immunisation is recommended for travel to much of Africa and South America. Many countries require an International Certificate of Vaccination from individuals arriving from, or who have been travelling through, endemic areas, whilst other countries require a certificate from all entering travellers (consult the Department of Health Handbook, *Health Information for Overseas Travel*).

Immunisation against **meningococcal meningitis** is recommended for a number of areas of the world (for details, see p. 550).

Protection against **hepatitis A** is recommended for travellers to high-risk areas outside Northern and Western Europe, North America, Australia and New Zealand. Hepatitis A vaccine (see p. 547) is preferred, particularly for frequent travellers or for stays longer than 3 months. Normal immunoglobulin (see p. 556) can be used as an alternative for short or infrequent travel. Those who require immunisation less than 10 days before departure may be given the single-dose vaccine plus normal immunoglobulin at a different injection site. Administration of normal immunoglobulin at the same time as the vaccine, at different injection sites, does not affect rate of seroconversion but the level of antibody may be reduced (see also section 14.5 under Normal Immunoglobulin).

Hepatitis B vaccine (see p. 548) is recommended for those travelling to areas of high prevalence who intend to seek employment as health care workers or who plan to remain there for lengthy periods and who may therefore be at increased risk of acquiring infection as the result of medical or dental procedures carried out in those countries. Short-term tourists or business travellers are not generally at increased risk of infection but may place themselves at risk by their sexual behaviour when abroad.

Prophylactic immunisation against **rabies** (see p. 553) is recommended for travellers to enzootic areas on long journeys to remote areas out of reach of immediate medical attention.

Typhoid vaccine is indicated for travellers to those countries where typhoid is endemic but the vaccine is no substitute for personal precautions. Food should be freshly prepared and hot, and uncooked vegetables (including green salads) should be avoided; only fruits which can be peeled should be eaten. Only suitable bottled water, or tap water that has been boiled, or treated with sterilising tablets should be used for drinking. This advice also applies to cholera and other diarrhoeal diseases (including travellers' diarrhoea).

Cholera vaccine has little value in preventing infections and should **not** be given for international travel (see under Cholera Vaccine). It is no longer available.

Advice on **diphtheria**, on **Japanese encephalitis** (vaccine available on named-patient basis from Pasteur Mérieux) and on **tick-borne encephalitis** (vaccine available on named-patient basis from Hyland Immuno) is included in *Health Information for Overseas Travel*, see below.

Information on health advice for travellers

The Department of Health booklet, *Health Advice For Travellers* (code: T6) includes information on immunisation requirements (or recommendations) around the world. The booklet can be obtained from travel agents, post-offices or by telephoning 0800 555 777 (24-hour service); also available on the Internet at http://www.doh.gov.uk/hat/hatcvr.htm/

The Department of Health handbook, *Health Information for Overseas Travel* (1995), which draws together essential information *for doctors* regarding health advice for travellers, can be obtained from

The Stationery Office
The Publications Centre,
PO Box 276, London SW8 5DT
Telephone orders, 0870 600 5522
Fax: 0870 600 5533

Immunisation requirements change from time to time, and information on the current requirements for any particular country may be obtained from:

Communicable Disease Surveillance Centre Travel Unit, 61 Colindale Avenue, London NW9 5EQ (Tel (020) 8200 6868), (for health care professionals only)

Communicable Diseases (Scotland) Unit, Ruchill Hospital, Bilslend Drive, Glasgow G20 9NB (Tel 0141-946 7120)

Scottish Office Department of Health, Public Health Policy Unit, St. Andrew's House, Edinburgh EH1 3DG (Tel 0131-556 8400)

Welsh Office, Cathays Park, Cardiff CF10 3NQ (Tel (029) 2082 5111)

Department of Health and Social Services, Castle Buildings, Stormont, Belfast BT4 3PP (Tel (028) 9052 0000)

or from the embassy or legation of the appropriate country.

15: Anaesthesia

15.1 General anaesthesia

15.1.1 Intravenous anaesthetics
15.1.2 Inhalational anaesthetics
15.1.3 Antimuscarinic drugs
15.1.4 Sedative and analgesic peri-operative drugs
15.1.5 Muscle relaxants
15.1.6 Anticholinesterases used in anaesthesia
15.1.7 Antagonists for central and respiratory depression
15.1.8 Drugs for malignant hyperthermia

Note. The drugs in section 15.1 should be used only by experienced personnel and where adequate resuscitative equipment is available.

It is now common practice to administer several drugs with different actions to produce a state of surgical anaesthesia with minimal risk of toxic effects. An intravenous anaesthetic is usually used for induction, followed by maintenance with inhalational anaesthetics, perhaps supplemented by other drugs administered intravenously. Specific drugs are often used to produce muscular relaxation. These drugs interfere with spontaneous respiration so intermittent positive pressure ventilation by manual or mechanical means is commonly employed.

For certain procedures controlled hypotension may be required. Labetalol (section 2.4), sodium nitroprusside (section 2.5.1), and glyceryl trinitrate (section 2.6.1) are used.

Beta-blockers (section 2.4), adenosine, amiodarone (section 2.3.2) or verapamil (section 2.6.2) may be used to control arrhythmias during anaesthesia. Esmolol has a very short duration of action and is particularly suited to the peri- and intra-operative management of arrhythmias, including tachycardia, and hypertension (section 2.4).

Glyceryl trinitrate (section 2.6.1) is also used to control hypertension, particularly postoperatively.

SURGERY AND LONG-TERM MEDICATION. The risk of stopping long-term medication before surgery is often greater than the risk of continuing it during surgery; however, surgery itself may alter the need for continued drug therapy of certain conditions. It is vital that the anaesthetist should know of **all** drugs that a patient is (or has been) taking.

Patients with adrenal atrophy due to long-term corticosteroid use (section 6.3.2) may experience a precipitous fall in blood pressure unless corticosteroid cover is provided during anaesthesia and in the immediate postoperative period. Anaesthetists must therefore know whether a patient is, or has been, taking corticosteroids.

Other drugs that should not normally be stopped before surgery include antiepileptics, antipsychotics, bronchodilators, cardiovascular drugs, glaucoma drugs, immunosuppressants, drugs of dependence, and thyroid or antithyroid drugs. For general advice on surgery in diabetic patients see section 6.1.1.

Although it is possible to operate on patients taking oral anticoagulants when the INR is close to 2, many surgeons and anaesthetists prefer to stop oral anticoagulants. Individual circumstances will dictate whether it is appropriate to continue prophylaxis in the peri-operative period with heparin and graduated compression hosiery until oral anticoagulation can be re-established; the haematologist should be consulted for further advice.

Drugs that are stopped before surgery include combined oral contraceptives (see Surgery, section 7.3.1 for details); for advice on hormone replacement therapy, see section 6.4.1.1. If antidepressants need to be stopped, they should be withdrawn gradually to avoid withdrawal symptoms. In view of their hazardous interactions MAOIs should normally be stopped 2 weeks before surgery. Tricyclic antidepressants need not be stopped, but there may be an increased risk of arrhythmias and hypotension (and dangerous interaction with vasopressor drugs); the anaesthetist therefore should be informed if they are not stopped. Lithium should be stopped 24 hours before major surgery but the normal dose can be continued for minor surgery (with careful monitoring of fluids and electrolytes).

ANAESTHESIA AND DRIVING. Patients given sedatives and analgesics during minor outpatient procedures should be very carefully warned about the risk of driving afterwards. For intravenous benzodiazepines and for a short general anaesthetic the risk extends to **at least 24 hours** after administration. Responsible persons should be available to take patients home. The dangers of taking **alcohol** should also be emphasised.

PROPHYLAXIS OF ACID ASPIRATION. Regurgitation and aspiration of gastric contents (Mendelson's syndrome) is an important complication of general anaesthesia, particularly in obstetrics and emergency surgery. The damage to the lung is influenced by the pH, the volume of the gastric contents aspirated, and by the presence of food particles.

H_2-receptor antagonists (section 1.3.1) or omeprazole (section 1.3.5) may be used before surgery to increase the pH and reduce the volume of gastric fluid. They do not affect the pH of fluid already in the stomach and this limits their value in emergency procedures; oral H_2-receptor antagonists can be given 1–2 hours before the procedure but omeprazole must be given at least 12 hours earlier. Antacids are frequently used to neutralise the acidity of the fluid already in the stomach; 'clear' (non-particulate) antacids such as sodium citrate are preferred.

Gas cylinders

Each gas cylinder bears a label with the name of the gas contained in the cylinder. The name or chemical symbol of the gas appears on the shoulder of the cylinder and is also clearly and indelibly stamped on the cylinder valve.

The colours on the valve end of the cylinder extend down to the shoulder; in the case of mixed gases the colours for the individual gases are applied in four segments, two for each colour.

Gas cylinders should be stored in a cool well-ventilated room, free from flammable materials.

No lubricant of any description should be used on the cylinder valves.

15.1.1 Intravenous anaesthetics

Intravenous anaesthetics may be used either to induce anaesthesia or for maintenance of anaesthesia throughout surgery. Intravenous anaesthetics nearly all produce their effect in one arm-brain circulation time and can cause apnoea and hypotension, and so adequate resuscitative facilities **must** be available. They are **contra-indicated** if the anaesthetist is not confident of being able to maintain the airway (e.g. in the presence of a tumour in the pharynx or larynx). Extreme care is required in surgery of the mouth, pharynx, or larynx and in patients with acute circulatory failure (shock) or fixed cardiac output.

Individual requirements vary considerably and the recommended dosage is only a guide. Smaller dosage is indicated in ill, shocked, or debilitated patients, while robust individuals may require more. To facilitate tracheal intubation, induction is followed by a neuromuscular blocking drug (section 15.1.5).

TOTAL INTRAVENOUS ANAESTHESIA. This is a technique in which major surgery is carried out with all anaesthetic drugs given intravenously. Respiration is controlled, the lungs being inflated with oxygen-enriched air. Muscle relaxants are used to provide relaxation and prevent reflex muscle movements. The main problem to be overcome is the assessment of depth of anaesthesia.

ANAESTHESIA AND DRIVING. See section 15.1.

Barbiturates

Thiopental sodium (thiopentone sodium) is a widely used intravenous anaesthetic, but it has no analgesic properties. Induction is generally smooth and rapid, but owing to its narrow therapeutic margin, overdosage with cardiorespiratory depression may occur. The reconstituted solution is highly alkaline and therefore irritant on misplaced injection outside the vein; arterial injection is particularly dangerous.

Awakening from a moderate dose of thiopentone is rapid due to redistribution of the drug in whole body tissues. Metabolism is, however, slow and some sedative effects may persist for 24 hours. Repeated doses have a cumulative effect.

Thiopental is **contra-indicated** in porphyria (section 9.8.2).

THIOPENTAL SODIUM
(Thiopentone Sodium)

Indications: induction of general anaesthesia; anaesthesia of short duration

Cautions: see notes above; reduce induction dose in severe liver disease; **interactions:** Appendix 1 (anaesthetics, general)

Contra-indications: see notes above; porphyria (section 9.8.2)

Side-effects: see notes above

Dose: by intravenous injection as a 2.5% (25 mg/mL) solution, in fit premedicated adults, initially 100–150 mg (reduced in elderly or debilitated) over 10–15 seconds (longer in elderly or debilitated), followed by further quantity if necessary according to response after 30–60 seconds; or up to 4 mg/kg; CHILD induction 2–7 mg/kg

Intraval Sodium® (Rhône-Poulenc Rorer) PoM
Injection 2.5%, powder for reconstitution, thiopental sodium, net price 500-mg amp = £1.75 (with water for injections £2.36)

Other intravenous anaesthetics

Etomidate is an induction agent associated with rapid recovery without hangover effect. It causes less hypotension than other drugs used for induction. There is a high incidence of extraneous muscle movement and of pain on injection; these effects can be minimised by premedication with an opioid analgesic and the use of larger veins. There is evidence that repeated doses of etomidate have an undesirable suppressant effect on adrenocortical function.

Propofol is associated with rapid recovery without hangover effect and is very widely used. There is sometimes pain on intravenous injection, but significant extraneous muscle movements do not occur. The CSM has received reports of convulsions, anaphylaxis, and delayed recovery from anaesthesia after propofol administration; since some of the convulsions are delayed the CSM has advised special caution after day surgery. Propofol has been associated with bradycardia, occasionally profound; intravenous administration of an antimuscarinic may be necessary to prevent this.

Ketamine can be given by the intravenous or the intramuscular route, and has good analgesic properties when used in sub-anaesthetic dosage. The maximum effect occurs after more than one arm-brain circulation time. Muscle tone is increased. There is cardiovascular stimulation and arterial pressure may rise with tachycardia. The main disadvantage is the high incidence of hallucinations and other transient psychotic sequelae, though it is believed that these are much less significant in children. The incidence can be reduced when drugs such as diazepam are also used. Ketamine is **contra-indicated** in patients with hypertension and is best avoided in those prone to hallucinations. It is used mainly for paediatric anaesthesia, particularly when repeated administrations are required. Recovery is relatively slow.

ETOMIDATE

Indications: induction of anaesthesia
Cautions: see notes above; avoid in porphyria (see section 9.8.2); **interactions:** Appendix 1 (anaesthetics, general)
Contra-indications: see notes above
Side-effects: see notes above
Dose: *by slow intravenous injection*, 300 micrograms/kg (ELDERLY 150–200 micrograms/kg); CHILD up to 15 years up to 390 micrograms/kg

Hypnomidate® (Janssen-Cilag) PoM
Injection, etomidate 2 mg/mL in propylene glycol 35%. Net price 10-mL amp = £1.58

KETAMINE

Indications: induction and maintenance of anaesthesia
Cautions: see notes above; **interactions:** Appendix 1 (anaesthetics, general)
Contra-indications: see notes above
Side-effects: see notes above

Dose: *by intramuscular injection,* short procedures, initially 6.5–13 mg/kg (10 mg/kg usually produces 12–25 minutes of surgical anaesthesia)
Diagnostic manoeuvres and procedures not involving intense pain, initially 4 mg/kg
By intravenous injection over at least 60 seconds, short procedures, initially 1–4.5 mg/kg (2 mg/kg usually produces 5–10 minutes of surgical anaesthesia)
By intravenous infusion of a solution containing 1 mg/mL, longer procedures, induction, total dose of 0.5–2 mg/kg; maintenance (using microdrip infusion), 10–45 micrograms/kg/minute, rate adjusted according to response

Ketalar® (Parke-Davis) PoM
Injection, ketamine (as hydrochloride) 10 mg/mL, net price 20-mL vial = £3.52; 50 mg/mL, 10-mL vial = £7.31; 100 mg/mL, 10-mL vial = £13.42

PROPOFOL

Indications: see under preparations below
Cautions: see notes above; monitor blood-lipid concentration if risk of fat overload or if sedation longer than 3 days; **interactions:** Appendix 1 (anaesthetics, general)
Contra-indications: see notes above
Side-effects: see notes above
Dose: see under preparations below

Diprivan® (Zeneca) PoM
1% injection (emulsion), propofol 10 mg/mL, net price 20-mL amp = £3.88, 50-mL vial = £9.70, 50-mL prefilled syringe (for use with *Diprifusor® TCI* system) = £10.67, 100-mL vial = £19.40
Note. Diprifusor® TCI ('target controlled infusion') system is for use **only** for induction and maintenance of general anaesthesia in adults
Dose: induction of anaesthesia, *by intravenous injection or infusion,* 1.5–2.5 mg/kg (less in those over 55 years) at a rate of 20–40 mg every 10 seconds; CHILD over 1 month, administer slowly until response (usual dose in child over 8 years 2.5 mg/kg, may need more in younger child)
Maintenance of anaesthesia, *by intravenous injection,* 25–50 mg repeated according to response *or by intravenous infusion,* 4–12 mg/kg/hour; CHILD over 3 years, *by intravenous injection or infusion,* 9–15 mg/kg/hour
Sedation in intensive care, *by intravenous infusion,* 0.3–4 mg/kg/hour; CHILD under 16 years not recommended
Sedation for surgical and diagnostic procedures, initially *by intravenous injection* over 1–5 minutes, 0.5–1 mg/kg; maintenance, *by intravenous infusion,* 1.5–4.5 mg/kg/hour (additionally, if rapid increase in sedation required, *by intravenous injection,* 10–20 mg); those over 55 years may require lower dose; CHILD not recommended
2% injection (emulsion), propofol 20 mg/mL, net price 50-mL vial = £19.40, 50-mL prefilled syringe (for use with *Diprifusor® TCI* system) = £20.37
Note. Diprifusor® TCI ('target controlled infusion') system is for use **only** for induction and maintenance of general anaesthesia in adults
Dose: induction of anaesthesia, *by intravenous infusion,* 1.5–2.5 mg/kg (less in those over 55 years) at a rate of 20–40 mg every 10 seconds; CHILD over 3 years, administer slowly until response (usual dose in child over 8 years 2.5 mg/kg, may need more in younger child)
Maintenance of anaesthesia, *by intravenous infusion,* 4–12 mg/kg/hour; CHILD over 3 years, *by intravenous infusion,* 9–15 mg/kg/hour
Sedation in intensive care, *by intravenous infusion,* 0.3–4 mg/kg/hour; CHILD under 16 years not recommended

15.1.2   Inhalational anaesthetics

Inhalational anaesthetics may be gases or volatile liquids. They can be used both for induction and maintenance of anaesthesia and may also be used following induction with an intravenous anaesthetic (section 15.1.1).

Gaseous anaesthetics require suitable equipment for storage and administration. They may be supplied via hospital pipelines or from metal cylinders. *Volatile liquid anaesthetics* are administered using calibrated vaporisers, using air, oxygen, or nitrous oxide–oxygen mixtures as the carrier gas. It should be noted that they can all trigger malignant hyperthermia (section 15.1.8).

To prevent hypoxia inhalational anaesthetics must be given with concentrations of oxygen greater than in air.

ANAESTHESIA AND DRIVING. See section 15.1.

Volatile liquid anaesthetics

Halothane is a volatile liquid anaesthetic. Its advantages are that it is potent, induction is smooth, the vapour is non-irritant, pleasant to inhale, and seldom induces coughing or breath-holding. Despite these advantages, however, halothane is much less widely used than previously owing to its association with *severe hepatotoxicity* (**important:** see CSM advice, below).

Halothane causes cardiorespiratory depression. Respiratory depression results in elevation of arterial carbon dioxide tension and perhaps ventricular arrhythmias. Halothane also depresses the cardiac muscle fibres and may cause bradycardia. The result is diminished cardiac output and fall of arterial pressure. Adrenaline (epinephrine) infiltrations should be avoided in patients anaesthetised with halothane as ventricular arrhythmias may result.

Halothane produces moderate muscle relaxation, but this may be inadequate for major abdominal surgery and specific muscle relaxants are then used.

CSM advice (halothane hepatotoxicity). In a publication on findings confirming that *severe hepatotoxicity* can follow halothane anaesthesia the CSM has reported that this occurs more frequently after repeated exposures to halothane and has a high mortality. The risk of severe hepatotoxicity appears to be increased by repeated exposures within a short time interval, but even after a long interval (sometimes of several years) susceptible patients have been reported to develop jaundice. Since there is no reliable way of identifying susceptible patients the CSM recommends the following precautions prior to use of halothane:

1. a careful anaesthetic history should be taken to determine previous exposure and previous reactions to halothane;

2. repeated exposure to halothane within a period of **at least** 3 months should be **avoided** unless there are **overriding** clinical circumstances;

3. a history of unexplained jaundice or pyrexia in a patient following exposure to halothane is an absolute **contra-indication** to its future use in that patient.

Enflurane is a volatile anaesthetic similar to halothane, but less potent, about twice the concentration being necessary for induction and maintenance.

Enflurane is a powerful cardiorespiratory depressant. Shallow respiration is likely to result in a rise of arterial carbon dioxide tension, but ventricular arrhythmias are uncommon and it is probably safe to use adrenaline infiltrations. Myocardial depression may result in a fall in cardiac output and in arterial hypotension. It may cause EEG changes and should be avoided in those liable to epileptic seizures. Enflurane may cause hepatotoxicity in those sensitised to halogenated anaesthetics but the risk is smaller than with halothane.

Isoflurane is an isomer of enflurane. It has a potency intermediate between that of halothane and enflurane, and even less of an inhaled dose is metabolised than with enflurane. Heart rhythm is generally stable during isoflurane anaesthesia, but heart-rate may rise, particularly in younger patients. Systemic arterial pressure may fall, due to a decrease in systemic vascular resistance and with less decrease in cardiac output than occurs with halothane. Respiration is depressed. Muscle relaxation is produced and muscle relaxant drugs potentiated. Isoflurane may also cause hepatotoxicity in those sensitised to halogenated anaesthetics but the risk is appreciably smaller than with halothane.

Desflurane is reported to have about one-fifth the potency of isoflurane. Owing to limited experience it is not recommended in neurosurgical patients. It is not recommended for induction in children because cough, breath-holding, apnoea, laryngospasm and increased secretions can occur. The risk of hepatotoxicity with desflurane in those sensitised to halogenated anaesthetics appears to be remote.

Sevoflurane is a newly introduced rapid acting volatile liquid anaesthetic. Patients may require early postoperative pain relief as emergence and recovery are particularly rapid.

VOLATILE ANAESTHETICS AND CARBOXYHAEMO-GLOBINAEMIA. Carboxyhaemoglobinaemia has been reported during anaesthesia with desflurane, enflurane, or isoflurane used in conjunction with carbon dioxide absorbents in breathing systems in the USA. This phenomenon was very rare and occurred when these absorbents became excessively dried out. The use of barium hydroxide lime produces significantly more carbon monoxide than soda lime particularly at low water content. Barium hydroxide lime is not available in the UK. The CSM has advised that no cases of carboxyhaemoglobinaemia have been reported in the UK and it seems unlikely that this problem will arise with the anaesthetic equipment currently in use in the UK.

DESFLURANE

Indications: see notes above

Cautions: see notes above; **interactions:** Appendix 1 (anaesthetics, general)

Contra-indications: see notes above

Side-effects: see notes above

Dose: using a specifically designed calibrated vaporiser, *induction*, 4–11%; CHILD not recommended for induction

Maintenance, 2–6% in nitrous oxide; 2.5–8.5% in oxygen or oxygen-enriched air; max. 17%

Suprane® (Baxter) [PoM]
Desflurane. Net price 240 mL = £46.50

ENFLURANE

Indications: see notes above

Cautions: see notes above; avoid in porphyria (section 9.8.2); caution is needed in epilepsy; **interactions:** Appendix 1 (anaesthetics, general)

Side-effects: see notes above

Dose: using a specifically calibrated vaporiser, *induction*, increased gradually from 0.4% to max. of 4.5% in air, oxygen, or nitrous oxide–oxygen, according to response

Maintenance, 0.5–3% in nitrous oxide–oxygen

Enflurane (Abbott)
Enflurane. Net price 250 mL = £24.00

HALOTHANE

Indications: see notes above

Cautions: see notes above (**important:** CSM advice, see notes above); avoid in porphyria (section 9.8.2); **interactions:** Appendix 1 (anaesthetics, general)

Contra-indications: see notes above

Side-effects: see notes above

Dose: using a specifically calibrated vaporiser, *induction*, increased gradually to 2–4% in oxygen or nitrous oxide–oxygen; CHILD 1.5–2%
Maintenance, 0.5–2%

Halothane (Concord)
Halothane, net price 250 mL = £16.00

Fluothane® (Zeneca)
Halothane, net price 250 mL = £15.62

ISOFLURANE

Indications: see notes above

Cautions: see notes above; **interactions:** Appendix 1 (anaesthetics, general)

Side-effects: see notes above

Dose: using a specifically calibrated vaporiser, *induction*, increased gradually from 0.5% to 3%, in oxygen or nitrous oxide–oxygen
Maintenance, 1–2.5% in nitrous oxide–oxygen; an additional 0.5–1% may be required when given with oxygen alone; caesarean section, 0.5–0.75% in nitrous oxide–oxygen

Isoflurane (Abbott)
Isoflurane. Net price 250 mL = £47.50

SEVOFLURANE

Indications: see notes above

Cautions: see notes above; **interactions:** Appendix 1 (anaesthetics, general)

IMPORTANT. In low-flow anaesthesia systems with soda lime, sevoflurane forms a vinyl ether ('Compound A') of unknown toxicity. Until further information becomes available, it would be wise to avoid the use of flow rates of less than 2 litres/minute with soda lime in patients with renal disease.

Contra-indications: see notes above

Side-effects: see notes above; also agitation occurs frequently in children

Dose: using a specifically calibrated vaporiser, *induction*, up to 5% in oxygen or nitrous oxide–oxygen; CHILD up to 7%
Maintenance, 0.5–3%

Sevoflurane (Abbott) ▼ PoM
Sevoflurane, net price 250 mL = £123.00

Nitrous oxide

Nitrous oxide is used for maintenance of anaesthesia and, in sub-anaesthetic concentrations, for analgesia. For anaesthesia it is commonly used in a concentration of 50 to 70% in oxygen as part of a balanced technique in association with other inhalational or intravenous agents. Nitrous oxide is unsatisfactory as a sole anaesthetic owing to lack of potency, but is useful as part of a combination of drugs since it allows a significant reduction in dosage.

A mixture of nitrous oxide and oxygen containing 50% of each gas (*Entonox*®, *Equanox*®) is used to produce analgesia without loss of consciousness. Self-administration using a demand valve is popular in obstetric practice, for changing painful dressings, as an aid to postoperative physiotherapy, and in emergency ambulances.

Nitrous oxide may have a deleterious effect if used in patients with an air-containing closed space since nitrous oxide diffuses into such a space with a resulting increase in pressure. This effect may be dangerous in the presence of a pneumothorax which may enlarge to compromise respiration.

Exposure of patients to nitrous oxide for prolonged periods, either by continuous or by intermittent administration, may result in megaloblastic anaemia due to interference with the action of vitamin B_{12}. For the same reason, exposure of theatre staff to nitrous oxide should be minimised. Depression of white cell formation may also occur.

NITROUS OXIDE

Indications: see notes above

Cautions: see notes above; **interactions:** Appendix 1 (anaesthetics, general)

Side-effects: see notes above

Dose: using a suitable anaesthetic apparatus, a mixture with 25–30% oxygen for *maintenance* of light anaesthesia

Analgesic, as a mixture with 50% oxygen, according to the patient's needs

15.1.3   Antimuscarinic drugs

Antimuscarinic drugs are used (less commonly nowadays) as premedicants to dry bronchial and salivary secretions which are increased by intubation, by surgery to the upper airways, and by some inhalational anaesthetics. They are also used before or with neostigmine (section 15.1.6) to prevent bradycardia, excessive salivation, and other muscarinic actions of neostigmine. They are also used to prevent bradycardia and hypotension associated with agents such as halothane, propofol, and suxamethonium.

Atropine is now rarely used for premedication but still has an emergency role in the treatment of vagotonic side-effects. For its role in acute arrhythmias after myocardial infarction, see section 2.3.1; see also cardiopulmonary resuscitation algorithm, section 2.7.3.

Hyoscine effectively reduces secretions and also provides a degree of amnesia, sedation and antiemesis. Unlike atropine it may produce bradycardia rather than tachycardia. In some patients, especially the elderly, hyoscine may cause the central anticholinergic syndrome (excitement, ataxia, hallucinations, behavioural abnormalities, and drowsiness).

Glycopyrronium produces good drying of salivary secretions. When given intravenously it produces less tachycardia than atropine. It is widely used with neostigmine for reversal of non-depolarising muscle relaxants (section 15.1.5).

Phenothiazines have too little drying activity to be effective when used alone.

ATROPINE SULPHATE

Indications: drying secretions, reversal of excessive bradycardia; with neostigmine for reversal of non-depolarising neuromuscular block; antispasmodic (section 1.2); bradycardia (section 2.3.1); eye (section 11.5)

Cautions: cardiovascular disease; see also section 1.2; **interactions:** Appendix 1 (antimuscarinics)

DURATION OF ACTION. Since atropine has a shorter duration of action than neostigmine, late unopposed bradycardia may result; close monitoring of the patient is necessary

Side-effects: tachycardia; see also section 1.2

Dose: premedication, *by intravenous injection*, 300–600 micrograms immediately before induction of anaesthesia, and in incremental doses of 100 micrograms for the treatment of bradycardia

By intramuscular injection, 300–600 micrograms 30–60 minutes before induction; CHILD 20 micrograms/kg

For control of muscarinic side-effects of neostigmine in reversal of competitive neuromuscular block, *by intravenous injection*, 0.6–1.2 mg

Arrhythmias after myocardial infarction, see section 2.3.1; see also cardiopulmonary resuscitation algorithm, section 2.7.3

Atropine (Non-proprietary) PoM
Injection, atropine sulphate 600 micrograms/mL, net price 1-mL amp = 31p
Note. Other strengths also available
Injection, prefilled disposable syringe, atropine sulphate 100 micrograms/mL, net price 5 mL = £3.78, 10 mL = £4.24, 30 mL = £7.75
Available from IMS (*Min-I-Jet®*)
Injection, prefilled disposable syringe, atropine sulphate 200 micrograms/mL, net price 5 mL = £4.24; 300 micrograms/mL, 10 mL = £4.32
Available from Aurum

■ With morphine
See under Morphine Salts (section 4.7.2)

GLYCOPYRRONIUM BROMIDE

Indications: see under Atropine Sulphate
Cautions: see under Atropine Sulphate
Side-effects: see under Atropine Sulphate
Dose: premedication, *by intramuscular or intravenous injection*, 200–400 micrograms, *or* 4–5 micrograms/kg to a max. of 400 micrograms; CHILD, *by intramuscular or* preferably *by intravenous injection*, 4–8 micrograms/kg to a max. of 200 micrograms

Intra-operative use, *by intravenous injection*, as for premedication, repeated if necessary

Control of muscarinic side-effects of neostigmine in reversal of non-depolarising neuromuscular block, *by intravenous injection*, 10–15 micrograms/kg with neostigmine 50 micrograms/kg; CHILD 10 micrograms/kg with neostigmine 50 micrograms/kg

Robinul® (Anpharm) PoM
Injection, glycopyrronium bromide 200 micrograms/mL, net price 1-mL amp = 63p; 3-mL amp = £1.06
Available as a generic from Antigen

■ With neostigmine metilsulphate
Section 15.1.6

HYOSCINE HYDROBROMIDE
(Scopolamine Hydrobromide)
Indications: drying secretions, amnesia; other indications (section 4.6)
Cautions: see under Atropine Sulphate; avoid in the elderly (see notes above)
Contra-indications: porphyria (section 9.8.2)
Side-effects: see under Atropine Sulphate; bradycardia
Dose: premedication, *by subcutaneous or intramuscular injection*, 200–600 micrograms 30–60 minutes before induction of anaesthesia, usually with papaveretum

Hyoscine (Non-proprietary) PoM
Injection, hyoscine hydrobromide 400 micrograms/mL, net price 1-mL amp = £2.67; 600 micrograms/mL, 1-mL amp = £2.73

■ With papaveretum
See under papaveretum (section 4.7.2)

15.1.4 Sedative and analgesic peri-operative drugs

15.1.4.1   Anxiolytics and neuroleptics
15.1.4.2   Non-opioid analgesics
15.1.4.3   Opioid analgesics

These drugs are given to allay the apprehension of the patient in the pre-operative period (including the night before operation), to relieve pain and discomfort when present, and to augment the action of subsequent anaesthetic agents. A number of the drugs used also provide some degree of pre-operative amnesia. The choice will vary with the individual patient, the nature of the operative procedure, the anaesthetic to be used and other prevailing circumstances such as outpatients, obstetrics, recovery facilities etc. The choice would also vary in elective and emergency operations.

PREMEDICATION IN CHILDREN. Oral administration is preferred to injections where possible but is not altogether satisfactory; the rectal route should only be used in exceptional circumstances. Oral alimemazine (trimeprazine) is still used but when given alone it may cause postoperative restlessness when pain is present.

Atropine or hyoscine is often given orally to children, but may be given intravenously immediately before induction.

The use of a suitable local anaesthetic cream (section 15.2) should be considered to avoid pain at injection site.

ANAESTHESIA AND DRIVING. See section 15.1.

Anxiolytics and neuroleptics

Anxiolytic benzodiazepines are widely used whereas neuroleptics such as **chlorpromazine** and **droperidol** (section 4.2.1) are rarely used in the UK for premedication; although chlorpromazine is licensed to prevent shivering in induction of hypothermia, it is no longer in current use for this purpose. **Alimemazine (trimeprazine)** (section 3.4.1) is still occasionally used as a premedicant for children (but see section 15.1.4).

Clomethiazole (chlormethiazole, section 4.1.1) is licensed for use as an intravenous infusion to maintain sleep during surgery carried out under regional anaesthesia, but is no longer in current use for this purpose.

Benzodiazepines

Benzodiazepines possess useful properties for premedication including anxiolysis, sedation, and amnesia; short-acting benzodiazepines taken by mouth are the most common premedicants. They have no analgesic effect so an opioid analgesic may sometimes be required for pain.

Benzodiazepines can alleviate anxiety at doses that do not necessarily cause excessive sedation and they are of particular value during short procedures or during operations under local anaesthesia (including dentistry). Amnesia reduces the likelihood of any unpleasant memories of the procedure (although benzodiazepines, particularly when used for more profound sedation, can sometimes induce sexual fantasies). Benzodiazepines are also used in intensive care units for sedation, particularly in those receiving assisted ventilation.

Benzodiazepines may occasionally cause marked respiratory depression and facilities for its treatment are essential; flumazenil (section 15.1.7) is used to antagonise the effects of benzodiazepines.

Diazepam is used to produce mild sedation with amnesia. It is a long-acting drug with active metabolites and a second period of drowsiness can occur several hours after its administration. Peri-operative use of diazepam in children is not generally recommended; its effect and timing of response are unreliable and paradoxical effects may occur.

Diazepam is relatively insoluble in water and preparations formulated in organic solvents are painful on intravenous injection and give rise to a high incidence of venous thrombosis (which may not be noticed for several days after the injection). Intramuscular injection of diazepam is painful and absorption is erratic. An emulsion preparation for intravenous injection is less irritant and is followed by a negligible incidence of venous thrombosis; it is not suitable for intramuscular injection. Diazepam is also available as a rectal solution.

Temazepam is given by mouth and has a shorter duration of action and a more rapid onset than diazepam given by mouth. It has been used as a premedicant in inpatient and day-case surgery; anxiolytic and sedative effects last about 90 minutes although there may be residual drowsiness.

Lorazepam produces more prolonged sedation than temazepam and it has marked amnesic effects. It is used as a premedicant the night before major surgery; a further, smaller dose may be required the

following morning if any delay in starting surgery is anticipated. Alternatively the first dose may be given early in the morning on the day of operation.

Midazolam is a water-soluble benzodiazepine which is often used in preference to intravenous diazepam; recovery is faster than from diazepam. Midazolam is associated with profound sedation when high doses are given intravenously or when used with certain other drugs.

DIAZEPAM

Indications: premedication; sedation with amnesia, and in conjunction with local anaesthesia; other indications (section 4.1.2, section 4.8.2, and section 10.2.2)

Cautions: see notes above and section 4.1.2 and section 4.8.2

Contra-indications: see notes above and section 4.1.2 and section 4.8.2

Side-effects: see notes above and section 4.1.2 and section 4.8.2

Dose: *by mouth*, 5 mg on night before minor or dental surgery then 5 mg 2 hours before procedure

By intravenous injection, into a large vein 10–20 mg over 2–4 minutes as sedative cover for minor surgical and medical procedures; premedication 100–200 micrograms/kg

By rectum in solution, 10 mg; ELDERLY 5 mg; CHILD not recommended (see notes above)

Note. Diazepam rectal solution doses in the BNF may differ from those in the product literature

Preparations
Section 4.1.2

LORAZEPAM

Indications: sedation with amnesia; premedication; other indications (section 4.1.2 and section 4.8.2)

Cautions: see notes above and under Diazepam (section 4.1.2 and section 4.8.2)

Contra-indications: see notes above and under Diazepam (section 4.1.2 and section 4.8.2)

Side-effects: see notes above and under Diazepam (section 4.1.2 and section 4.8.2)

Dose: *by mouth*, 2–3 mg the night before operation; 2–4 mg 1–2 hours before operation

By slow intravenous injection, preferably diluted with an equal volume of sodium chloride intravenous infusion 0.9% or water for injections, 50 micrograms/kg 30–45 minutes before operation

By intramuscular injection, diluted as above, 50 micrograms/kg 1–1½ hours before operation

Preparations
Section 4.1.2

MIDAZOLAM

Indications: sedation with amnesia, and in conjunction with local anaesthesia; premedication, induction

Cautions: see notes above and under Diazepam (section 4.1.2 and section 4.8.2); **interactions:** Appendix 1 (anxiolytics and hypnotics)

Contra-indications: see notes above and under Diazepam (section 4.1.2 and section 4.8.2)

Side-effects: see notes above and under Diazepam (section 4.1.2 and section 4.8.2); also respiratory depression and respiratory arrest reported, particularly with high doses or on rapid injection

Dose: sedation, *by intravenous injection* over 30 seconds, 2 mg (elderly 1–1.5 mg) followed after 2 minutes by increments of 0.5–1 mg if sedation not adequate; usual range 2.5–7.5 mg (about 70 micrograms/kg), elderly 1–2 mg
Premedication, *by intramuscular injection*, 70–100 micrograms/kg 30–60 minutes before surgery; usual dose 5 mg (2.5 mg in elderly)
Induction, *by slow intravenous injection*, 200–300 micrograms/kg (elderly 100–200 micrograms/kg); CHILD over 7 years, 150 micrograms/kg
Sedation of patients receiving intensive care, *by intravenous infusion*, initially 30–300 micrograms/kg given over 5 minutes, then 30–200 micrograms/kg/hour; reduce dose (or omit initial dose) in hypovolaemia, vasoconstriction, or hypothermia; low doses may be adequate if opioid analgesic also used; avoid abrupt withdrawal after prolonged administration (safety after more than 14 days not established)

Midazolam (Non-proprietary) ▨PoM
Injection, midazolam (as hydrochloride) 1 mg/mL, net price 5 mL-10-mL vial = £6.00
Available from Aurum

Hypnovel® (Roche) ▨PoM
Injection, midazolam (as hydrochloride) 2 mg/mL, net price 5-mL amp = 96p; 5 mg/mL, 2-mL amp = 81p

TEMAZEPAM

Indications: premedication before surgery; anxiety before investigatory procedures; hypnotic (section 4.1.1)
Cautions: see notes above and under Diazepam (section 4.1.2 and section 4.8.2)
Contra-indications: see notes above and under Diazepam (section 4.1.2 and section 4.8.2)
Side-effects: see notes above and under Diazepam (section 4.1.2 and section 4.8.2)
Dose: *by mouth*, premedication, 20–40 mg (elderly, 10–20 mg) 1 hour before operation; CHILD 1 mg/kg (max. 30 mg)

Preparations
Section 4.1.1

15.1.4.2 Non-opioid analgesics

Since non-steroidal anti-inflammatory drugs (NSAIDs) do not depress respiration, do not impair gastro-intestinal motility, and do not cause dependence, they may be useful alternatives (or adjuncts) to the use of opioids for the relief of postoperative pain. NSAIDs may be inadequate for the relief of severe pain.

Diclofenac, flurbiprofen, ketoprofen (section 10.1.1), and **ketorolac** are licensed for postoperative use. Diclofenac, ketoprofen and ketorolac can be given by injection as well as by mouth. Intramuscular injections of diclofenac and ketoprofen are given deep into the gluteal muscle to minimise pain and tissue damage; diclofenac can also be given by intravenous infusion for the treatment or prevention of postoperative pain. Ketorolac is less irritant on intramuscular injection but pain has been reported; it can also be given by intravenous injection.

Suppositories of diclofenac and ketoprofen may be effective alternatives to the parenteral use of these drugs. Flurbiprofen is also available as suppositories.

KETOROLAC TROMETAMOL

Indications: short-term management of moderate to severe acute postoperative pain
Cautions: reduce dose in elderly and in those weighing less than 50 kg; reduce dose and monitor in mild renal impairment (avoid if moderate or severe); heart failure, hepatic impairment and other conditions leading to reduction in blood volume or in renal blood flow (including those taking diuretics); cardiac decompensation, hypertension or similar conditions (fluid retention and oedema reported); **interactions:** Appendix 1 (NSAIDs)
GASTRO-INTESTINAL EFFECTS. Elderly and debilitated more prone to risk of gastro-intestinal effects (risk increases with increased dose and duration; see also under Contra-indications and Side-effects below

Contra-indications: history of hypersensitivity to aspirin or any other NSAID (severe anaphylactic reactions reported), history of asthma, complete or partial syndrome of nasal polyps, angioedema or bronchospasm; history of peptic ulceration or gastro-intestinal bleeding; haemorrhagic diatheses (including coagulation disorders) and operations with high risk of haemorrhage or incomplete haemostasis; confirmed or suspected cerebrovascular bleeding; moderate or severe renal impairment; hypovolaemia or dehydration; pregnancy (including labour and delivery) and breast-feeding

Side-effects: side-effects reported include anaphylaxis (with rash, bronchospasm, laryngeal oedema and hypotension), fluid retention (see Cautions), nausea, dyspepsia, abdominal discomfort, bowel changes, peptic ulceration, gastro-intestinal bleeding (elderly at greater risk, see also above), pancreatitis, drowsiness, dizziness, headache, sweating, dry mouth, excessive thirst, mental and sensory changes, psychotic reactions, convulsions, myalgia, aseptic meningitis, hyponatraemia, hyperkalaemia, raised blood urea and creatinine, urinary symptoms and acute renal failure, flushing or pallor, bradycardia, hypertension, palpitations, chest pain, purpura, thrombocytopenia, prolonged bleeding time, dyspnoea and pulmonary oedema, skin reactions (some severe, including Stevens-Johnson and Lyell's syndromes), postoperative wound haemorrhage, haematoma, epistaxis, oedema, liver function changes (discontinue if clinical symptoms); pain at injection site; for general side-effects of NSAIDs, see section 10.1.1
Dose: *by mouth*, 10 mg every 4–6 hours (ELDERLY every 6–8 hours); max. 40 mg daily; max. duration of treatment 7 days; CHILD under 16 years, not recommended

By intramuscular injection or by intravenous injection over not less than 15 seconds, initially 10 mg, then 10–30 mg every 4–6 hours when required (every 2 hours in initial postoperative period); max. 90 mg daily (ELDERLY and patients weighing less than 50 kg max. 60 mg daily); max. duration of treatment 2 days by either route; CHILD under 16 years, not recommended

Note. Pain relief may not occur for over 30 minutes after intravenous or intramuscular injection. When converting from parenteral to oral administration, total combined dose on the day of converting should not exceed 90 mg (60 mg in the elderly and patients weighing less than 50 kg) of which the oral component should not exceed 40 mg; patients should be converted to oral route as soon as possible

Toradol® (Roche) [PoM]
Tablets, ivory, f/c, ketorolac trometamol 10 mg, net price 20-tab pack = £6.23. Label: 17, 21
Injection, ketorolac trometamol 10 mg/mL, net price 1-mL amp = £1.02; 30 mg/mL, 1-mL amp = £1.22

15.1.4.3   Opioid analgesics

Opioid analgesics are now rarely used as premedicants; they are more likely to be administered at induction. Pre-operative use of opioid analgesics is generally limited to those patients who require control of existing pain. The main side-effects of opioid analgesics are respiratory depression, cardiovascular depression, nausea, and vomiting; for general notes on opioid analgesics and their use in postoperative pain, see section 4.7.2.

For the management of opioid-induced respiratory depression, see section 15.1.7.

INTRA-OPERATIVE ANALGESIA. Opioid analgesics given in small doses before or with induction reduce the dose requirement of some drugs used during anaesthesia. Pethidine, morphine and papaveretum have been used for this purpose, but shorter-acting and more potent drugs such as alfentanil, fentanyl, and remifentanil are now preferred. Nalbuphine is seldom used.

Alfentanil, **fentanyl** and **remifentanil** are particularly useful because they act within 1–2 minutes. The initial doses of alfentanil or fentanyl are followed either by successive intravenous injections or by an intravenous infusion; prolonged infusions increase the duration of effect. Repeated intra-operative doses of alfentanil or fentanyl should be given with care since the respiratory depression can persist into the postoperative period (see below) and occasionally it may become apparent for the first time postoperatively when monitoring of the patient might be less intensive.

In contrast to other opioids which are metabolised in the liver, remifentanil undergoes rapid metabolism by non-specific blood and tissue esterases; its short duration of action allows prolonged administration at high dosage, without accumulation, and with little risk of residual postoperative respiratory depression. Remifentanil should not be given as a bolus injection intra-operatively, but it is well suited to continuous infusion; a supplemental analgesic will often be required after stopping the infusion.

ALFENTANIL

Indications: analgesia especially during short operative procedure and outpatient surgery; enhancement of anaesthesia; analgesia and suppression of respiratory activity in patients receiving intensive care, with assisted ventilation, for up to 4 days
Cautions: see section 4.7.2 and notes above
Contra-indications: see section 4.7.2 and notes above
Side-effects: see section 4.7.2 and notes above

Rapifen® (Janssen-Cilag) [CD]
Injection, alfentanil (as hydrochloride) 500 micrograms/mL. Net price 2-mL amp = 72p; 10-mL amp = £3.31

Intensive care injection, alfentanil (as hydrochloride) 5 mg/mL. To be diluted before use. Net price 1-mL amp = £2.65

FENTANYL

Indications: analgesia during operation, enhancement of anaesthesia; respiratory depressant in assisted respiration; analgesia in other situations (section 4.7.2)
Cautions: see section 4.7.2 and notes above
Contra-indications: see section 4.7.2 and notes above
Side-effects: see section 4.7.2 and notes above
Dose: *by intravenous injection*, with spontaneous respiration,   50–200 micrograms,   then 50 micrograms as required; CHILD 3–5 micrograms/kg, then 1 microgram/kg as required
With assisted ventilation, 0.3–3.5 mg, then 100–200 micrograms as required; CHILD 15 micrograms/kg, then 1–3 micrograms/kg as required

Sublimaze® (Janssen-Cilag) [CD]
Injection, fentanyl (as citrate) 50 micrograms /mL. Net price 2-mL amp = 24p; 10-mL amp = £1.17
Available as a generic from Antigen, Faulding DBL

REMIFENTANIL

Indications: supplementation of general anaesthesia during induction and analgesia during maintenance of anaesthesia
Cautions: see section 4.7.2 and notes above
Contra-indications: see section 4.7.2 and notes above
Side-effects: see section 4.7.2 and notes above
Dose: induction, *by intravenous infusion*, 0.5–1 microgram/kg/minute, *with or without* an initial bolus *by intravenous injection* (of a solution containing 20–250 micrograms/mL) over not less than 30 seconds, 1 microgram/kg
Note. If patient is to be intubated more than 8 minutes after start of intravenous infusion, intial intravenous injection dose is unnecessary
Maintenance in ventilated patients, *by intravenous infusion*, 0.05–2 micrograms/kg/minute according to anaesthetic technique and adjusted according to response; supplemental doses in light anaesthesia, *by intravenous injection* every 2–5 minutes
Maintenance in spontaneous respiration anaesthesia, *by intravenous infusion*, initially 40 nanograms/kg/minute adjusted according to response, usual range 25–100 nanograms/kg/minute
CHILD 2–12 years, limited experience (consult product literature)

Ultiva® (GlaxoWellcome) ▼ [PoM]
Injection, powder for reconstitution, remifentanil (as hydrochloride), net price 1-mg vial = £5.50; 2-mg vial = £11.00; 5-mg vial = £27.50

15.1.5   Muscle relaxants

Muscle relaxants used in anaesthesia are also known as **neuromuscular blocking drugs**. By specific blockade of the neuromuscular junction they enable light levels of anaesthesia to be employed with adequate relaxation of the muscles of the abdomen and diaphragm. They also relax the vocal cords and allow the passage of a tracheal tube.

Their action differs from the muscle relaxants acting on the spinal cord or brain which are used in musculoskeletal disorders (section 10.2.2).

Patients who have received a muscle relaxant should **always** have their respiration assisted or controlled until the drug has been inactivated or antagonised (section 15.1.6).

Non-depolarising muscle relaxants

Non-depolarising muscle relaxants (also known as competitive muscle relaxants) compete with acetylcholine for receptor sites at the neuromuscular junction and their action may be reversed with anticholinesterases such as neostigmine (section 15.1.6). Non-depolarising muscle relaxants may be divided into the **aminosteroid** group which includes pancuronium, rocuronium and vecuronium, and the **benzylisoquinolinium** group which includes atracurium, cisatracurium, gallamine and mivacurium.

Non-depolarising muscle relaxants have a slower onset of action than suxamethonium. These drugs can be classified by their duration of action as short-acting (15–30 minutes), intermediate-acting (30–40 minutes) and long-acting (60–120 minutes), although duration of action is dose-dependent. Drugs with a shorter or intermediate duration of action, such as atracurium and vecuronium, are more widely employed than those with a longer duration of action such as pancuronium.

Non-depolarising muscle relaxants have no sedative or analgesic effects and are not considered to be a triggering factor for malignant hyperthermia.

CAUTIONS. Allergic cross-reactivity between neuromuscular blocking agents has been reported; caution is advised in cases of hypersensitivity to these drugs. Their activity is prolonged in patients with myasthenia gravis and in hypothermia, therefore lower doses are required. Resistance may develop in patients with burns who may require increased doses; low plasma cholinesterase activity in these patients requires dose titration for mivacurium. **Interactions:** Appendix 1 (muscle relaxants)

SIDE-EFFECTS. Benzylisoquinolinium non-depolarising muscle relaxants (except cisatracurium) are associated with histamine release which can cause skin flushing, hypotension, tachycardia, bronchospasm and rarely, anaphylactoid reactions. Aminosteroid muscle relaxants are not associated with histamine release. Drugs possessing vagolytic activity can counteract any bradycardia that occurs during surgery.

Atracurium is a mixture of 10 isomers and is a benzylisoquinolinium muscle relaxant with an intermediate duration of action. It undergoes non-enzymatic metabolism which is independent of liver and kidney function, thus allowing its use in patients with hepatic or renal impairment. Cardiovascular effects are associated with significant histamine release.

Cisatracurium is a single isomer of atracurium. It is more potent and has a slightly longer duration of action than atracurium and provides greater cardiovascular stability because cisatracurium lacks histamine-releasing effects.

Mivacurium, a benzylisoquinolinium muscle relaxant, has a short duration of action. It is metabolised by plasma cholinesterase and muscle paralysis is prolonged in individuals deficient in this enzyme. It is not associated with vagolytic activity or ganglionic blockade although histamine release may occur, particularly with rapid injection.

Pancuronium, an aminosteroid muscle relaxant, has a long duration of action and is often used in patients receiving long-term mechanical ventilation in intensive care units. It lacks a histamine-releasing effect, but vagolytic and sympathomimetic effects can cause tachycardia and hypertension.

Rocuronium exerts an effect within 2 minutes and has the most rapid onset of any of the competitive muscle relaxants. It is an aminosteroid muscle relaxant with an intermediate duration of action. It is reported to have minimal histamine-releasing and cardiovascular effects; high doses produce mild vagolytic activity.

Vecuronium, an aminosteroid muscle relaxant, has an intermediate duration of action. It does not generally produce histamine release and lacks cardiovascular effects.

Gallamine has vagolytic and sympathomimetic properties and frequently increases pulse rate and blood pressure. It is rarely used since the other neuromuscular blocking drugs have a more predictable response and it should be avoided in patients with renal impairment.

ATRACURIUM BESILATE
(Atracurium Besylate)
Indications: muscle relaxation for surgery (short to intermediate duration)
Cautions: see notes above
Side-effects: see notes above
Dose: *by intravenous injection*, ADULT and CHILD over 1 month initially 300–600 micrograms/kg, then 100–200 micrograms/kg as required
By intravenous infusion, 5–10 micrograms/kg/minute (300–600 micrograms/kg/hour)

Tracrium® (GlaxoWellcome) PoM
Injection, atracurium besilate 10 mg/mL. Net price 2.5-mL amp = £1.78; 5-mL amp = £3.23; 25-mL amp = £13.88
Available as a generic from Faulding DBL

CISATRACURIUM
Indications: muscle relaxation for surgery (intermediate duration)
Cautions: see notes above
Side-effects: see notes above
Dose: *by intravenous injection*, intubation, 150 micrograms/kg; maintenance, 30 micrograms/kg approx. every 20 minutes
CHILD over 2 years, initially, 100 micrograms/kg; maintenance, 20 micrograms/kg approx. every 9 minutes
By intravenous infusion, ADULT and CHILD over 2 years, initially, 3 micrograms/kg/minute, *then after stabilisation*, 1–2 micrograms/kg/minute; dose reduced by up to 40% if used with enflurane or isoflurane
CHILD under 2 years not recommended

Nimbex® (GlaxoWellcome) [PoM]
Injection, cisatracurium (as besilate) 2 mg/mL, net price 2.5-mL amp = £2.30, 10-mL amp = £8.50
Forte injection, cisatracurium (as besilate) 5 mg/mL, net price 30-mL vial = £35.00

GALLAMINE TRIETHIODIDE ◣

Indications: muscle relaxation for surgery (intermediate duration)
Cautions: see notes above
Contra-indications: renal impairment
Side-effects: see notes above
Dose: *by intravenous injection*, 80–120 mg, then 20–40 mg as required; NEONATE, 600 micrograms/kg; CHILD, 1.5 mg/kg

Flaxedil® (Concord) [PoM] ◣
Injection, gallamine triethiodide 40 mg/mL. Net price 2-mL amp = £4.97

◣ denotes preparations that are considered to be less suitable for prescribing (see p. vi)

MIVACURIUM

Indications: muscle relaxation for surgery (short duration)
Cautions: see notes above; low plasma cholinesterase activity
Side-effects: see notes above
Dose: *by intravenous injection*, 70–250 micrograms/kg; maintenance 100 micrograms/kg every 15 minutes; CHILD 2–6 months initially 150 micrograms/kg, 7 months–12 years initially 200 micrograms/kg; maintenance (CHILD 2 months–12 years) 100 micrograms/kg every 6–9 minutes
Note. Doses up to 150 micrograms/kg may be given over 5–15 seconds, higher doses should be given over 30 seconds. In patients with asthma, cardiovascular disease or those who are sensitive to falls in arterial blood pressure give over 60 seconds
By intravenous infusion, maintenance of block, 8–10 micrograms/kg/minute, adjusted if necessary every 3 minutes by 1 microgram/kg/minute to usual dose of 6–7 micrograms/kg/minute; CHILD 2 months–12 years, usual dose 11–14 micrograms/kg/minute

Mivacron® (GlaxoWellcome) [PoM]
Injection, mivacurium (as chloride) 2 mg/mL, net price 5-mL amp = £2.73; 10-mL amp = £4.41

PANCURONIUM BROMIDE

Indications: muscle relaxation for surgery (long duration)
Cautions: see notes above; hepatic impairment; reduce dose in renal impairment
Side-effects: see notes above
Dose: *by intravenous injection*, initially for intubation 50–100 micrograms/kg then 10–20 micrograms/kg as required; CHILD initially 60–100 micrograms/kg, then 10–20 micrograms/kg, NEONATE 30–40 micrograms/kg initially then 10–20 micrograms/kg
Intensive care, *by intravenous injection*, 60 micrograms/kg every 60–90 minutes

Pavulon® (Organon-Teknika) [PoM]
Injection, pancuronium bromide 2 mg/mL, net price 2-mL amp = 69p
Available as a generic from Faulding DBL

ROCURONIUM BROMIDE

Indications: muscle relaxation for surgery (intermediate duration)
Cautions: see notes above; hepatic and renal impairment
Side-effects: see notes above
Dose: *by intravenous injection*, intubation, 600 micrograms/kg; maintenance, 150 micrograms/kg
By intravenous infusion, 300–600 micrograms/kg/hour (after initial intravenous injection of 600 micrograms/kg)
CHILD similar sensitivity to adults; NEONATE not recommended

Esmeron® (Organon-Teknika) [PoM]
Injection, rocuronium bromide 10 mg/mL, net price 5-mL vial = £3.38, 10-mL vial = £6.77

VECURONIUM BROMIDE

Indications: muscle relaxation for surgery (intermediate duration)
Cautions: see notes above; reduce dose in renal impairment
Side-effects: see notes above
Dose: *by intravenous injection*, intubation, 80–100 micrograms/kg; maintenance 20–30 micrograms/kg according to response; NEONATE and INFANT up to 4 months, initially 10–20 micrograms/kg then incremental doses to achieve response; CHILD over 5 months, as adult dose (up to 1 year onset more rapid and high intubation dose may not be required)
By intravenous infusion, 0.8–1.4 micrograms/kg/minute (after initial intravenous injection of 40–100 micrograms/kg)

Norcuron® (Organon-Teknika) [PoM]
Injection, powder for reconstitution, vecuronium bromide. Net price 10-mg vial = £4.44 (with water for injections)

Depolarising muscle relaxants

Suxamethonium has the most rapid onset of action of any of the muscle relaxants and is ideal if fast onset and brief duration of action are required e.g. with tracheal intubation. Its duration of action is about 2 to 6 minutes following intravenous doses of about 1 mg/kg; repeated doses can be used for longer procedures.

Suxamethonium acts by mimicking acetylcholine at the neuromuscular junction but hydrolysis is much slower than for acetylcholine; depolarisation is therefore prolonged resulting in neuromuscular blockade. Unlike the non-depolarising muscle relaxants, its action cannot be reversed and recovery is spontaneous; anticholinesterases such as neostigmine potentiate the neuromuscular block.

Suxamethonium should be given after anaesthetic induction because paralysis is usually preceded by painful muscle fasciculations. Bradycardia may occur with repeated doses in adults and with the first dose in children. Premedication with atropine reduces bradycardia as well as the excessive salivation associated with suxamethonium use.

Prolonged paralysis may occur in **dual block**, which occurs with high or repeated doses of suxamethonium and is caused by the development of a non-depolarising block following the initial depolarising block; edrophonium (section 15.1.6) may be used to confirm the diagnosis of dual block. Individuals with myasthenia gravis are resistant to suxamethonium but can develop dual block resulting in delayed recovery. Prolonged paralysis may also occur in those with low or atypical plasma cholinesterase. Assisted ventilation should be continued until muscle function is restored.

SUXAMETHONIUM CHLORIDE

Indications: muscle relaxation (rapid onset, short duration)

Cautions: see notes above; pregnancy (Appendix 4); patients with cardiac, respiratory or neuromuscular disease; raised intra-ocular pressure (avoid in penetrating eye injury); **interactions:** Appendix 1 (muscle relaxants)

Contra-indications: family history of malignant hyperthermia, low plasma cholinesterase activity, hyperkalaemia

Side-effects: see notes above; postoperative muscle pain, myoglobinaemia; tachycardia, arrhythmias, hypertension, hypotension; bronchospasm, apnoea, prolonged respiratory depression; hyperkalaemia; hyperthermia

Dose: *by intravenous injection*, ADULT 1 mg/kg (range 0.3–1.1 mg/kg); usual range 20–100 mg; max. 500 mg/hour; INFANT under 1 year, 2 mg/kg; CHILD 1–12 years, 1–2 mg/kg

By intravenous infusion of a solution containing 1–2 mg/mL (0.1–0.2%), 2–5 mg/minute; max. 500 mg/hour

By intramuscular injection, INFANT up to 4–5 mg/kg; CHILD up to 4 mg/kg; max. 150 mg

Suxamethonium Chloride (Non-proprietary) PoM
Injection, suxamethonium chloride 50 mg/mL, net price 2-mL amp = 70p
Available from Antigen

Anectine® (GlaxoWellcome) PoM
Injection, suxamethonium chloride 50 mg/mL, net price 2-mL amp = 70p

15.1.6 Anticholinesterases used in anaesthesia

Anticholinesterases reverse the effects of the non-depolarising (competitive) muscle relaxant drugs such as pancuronium but they prolong the action of the depolarising muscle relaxant drug suxamethonium.

Edrophonium has a transient action and may be used in the diagnosis of suspected dual block due to suxamethonium.

Neostigmine has a longer duration of action than edrophonium. It is the specific drug for reversal of non-depolarising (competitive) blockade. It acts within one minute of intravenous injection and lasts for 20 to 30 minutes; a second dose may then be necessary. Atropine or preferably glycopyrronium (section 15.1.3) should be given before or with neo-stigmine in order to prevent bradycardia, excessive salivation, and other muscarinic actions of neostigmine.

EDROPHONIUM CHLORIDE

Indications: see under Dose; myasthenia gravis (section 10.2.1)

Cautions: see section 10.2.1 and notes above; atropine should also be given

Contra-indications: see section 10.2.1 and notes above

Side-effects: see section 10.2.1 and notes above

Dose: brief reversal of non-depolarising neuromuscular blockade, *by intravenous injection* over several minutes, 500–700 micrograms/kg (after or with atropine sulphate 600 micrograms)

Diagnosis of dual block, *by intravenous injection*, 10 mg

Edrophonium (Non-proprietary) PoM
Injection, edrophonium chloride 10 mg/mL, net price 1-mL amp = £4.58
Available from Cambridge

NEOSTIGMINE METILSULFATE
(Neostigmine Methylsulphate)

Indications: see under Dose

Cautions: see section 10.2.1 and notes above; atropine should also be given

Contra-indications: see section 10.2.1 and notes above

Side-effects: see section 10.2.1 and notes above

Dose: reversal of non-depolarising neuromuscular blockade, *by intravenous injection* over 1 minute, 50–70 micrograms/kg (max. 5 mg) after or with atropine sulphate 0.6–1.2 mg

Myasthenia gravis, see section 10.2.1

Neostigmine (Non-proprietary) PoM
Injection, neostigmine metilsulfate 2.5 mg/mL, net price 1-mL amp = 54p

■ With glycopyrronium

Robinul-Neostigmine® (Anpharm) PoM
Injection, neostigmine metilsulfate 2.5 mg, glycopyrronium bromide 500 micrograms/mL, net price 1-mL amp = £1.06
Dose: reversal of non-depolarising neuromuscular blockade *by intravenous injection* over 10–30 seconds, 1–2 mL *or* 0.02 mL/kg, dose may be repeated if required (total max. 2 mL); CHILD 0.02 mL/kg (*or* 0.2 mL/kg of a 1 in 10 dilution using water for injections or sodium chloride injection 0.9%), dose may be repeated if required (total max. 2 mL)

15.1.7 Antagonists for central and respiratory depression

Respiratory depression is a major concern with opioid analgesics and it may be treated by artificial ventilation or be reversed by **naloxone**. Naloxone will immediately reverse opioid-induced respiratory depression but the dose may have to be repeated due to the short duration of action of naloxone; however, naloxone will also antagonise the analgesic effect.

Flumazenil is a benzodiazepine antagonist for the reversal of the central sedative effects of benzodiazepines after anaesthetic and similar procedures. Flumazenil has a shorter half-life than that of diazepam and midazolam (and there is a risk that patients may become resedated).

Doxapram is a central and respiratory stimulant but is of limited value.

DOXAPRAM HYDROCHLORIDE

Indications: see under Dose

Cautions: give with oxygen in severe irreversible airways obstruction or severely decreased lung compliance (because of increased work load of breathing); give with beta$_2$-adrenoceptor stimulant in bronchoconstriction; hypertension (avoid if severe), impaired cardiac reserve; hepatic impairment, pregnancy (compelling reasons only); interactions: Appendix 1 (doxapram)

Contra-indications: severe hypertension, status asthmaticus, coronary artery disease, thyrotoxicosis, epilepsy, physical obstruction of respiratory tract

Side-effects: perineal warmth, dizziness, sweating, moderate increase in blood pressure and heart rate; side-effects reported in postoperative period (causal effect not established) include muscle fasciculation, hyperactivity, confusion, hallucinations, cough, dyspnoea, laryngospasm, bronchospasm, sinus tachycardia, bradycardia, extrasystoles, nausea, vomiting and salivation

Dose: postoperative respiratory depression, by intravenous injection over at least 30 seconds, 1–1.5 mg/kg repeated if necessary after intervals of 1 hour or alternatively by intravenous infusion, 2–3 mg/minute adjusted according to response; CHILD not recommended

Acute respiratory failure, by intravenous infusion, 1.5–4 mg/minute adjusted according to response (given concurrently with oxygen and whenever possible monitor with frequent measurement of blood gas tensions); CHILD not recommended

Dopram® (Anpharm) PoM
Injection, doxapram hydrochloride 20 mg/mL. Net price 5-mL amp = £2.14
Intravenous infusion, doxapram hydrochloride 2 mg/mL in glucose 5%. Net price 500-mL bottle = £22.34

FLUMAZENIL

Indications: reversal of sedative effects of benzodiazepines in anaesthetic, intensive care, and diagnostic procedures

Cautions: short-acting (repeat doses may be necessary—benzodiazepine effects may persist for at least 24 hours); benzodiazepine dependence (may precipitate withdrawal symptoms); epileptics who have received prolonged benzodiazepine therapy (risk of convulsions); ensure neuromuscular blockade cleared before giving; avoid rapid injection in high-risk or anxious patients and following major surgery; hepatic impairment; head injury (rapid reversal of benzodiazepine sedation may cause convulsions); elderly, children, pregnancy and breast-feeding

Contra-indications: life-threatening condition (e.g. intracranial pressure, status epilepticus) controlled by benzodiazepines

Side-effects: nausea, vomiting, and flushing; if wakening too rapid, agitation, anxiety, and fear; transient increase in blood pressure and heart-rate in intensive care patients; very rarely convulsions (particularly in epileptics)

Dose: by intravenous injection, 200 micrograms over 15 seconds, then 100 micrograms at 60-second intervals if required; usual dose range, 300–600 micrograms; max. total dose 1 mg (2 mg in intensive care); question aetiology if no response to repeated doses

By intravenous infusion, if drowsiness recurs after injection, 100–400 micrograms/hour, adjusted according to level of arousal

Anexate® (Roche) PoM
Injection, flumazenil 100 micrograms/mL. Net price 5-mL amp = £15.59

NALOXONE HYDROCHLORIDE

Indications: reversal of opioid-induced respiratory depression; overdosage with opioids (Emergency treatment of poisoning)

Cautions: cardiovascular disease or those receiving cardiotoxic drugs (serious adverse cardiovascular effects reported); physical dependence on opioids (precipitates withdrawal); pain (see also under Titration of Dose, below); has short duration of action (repeated doses or infusion may be necessary to reverse effects of opioids with longer duration of action)

TITRATION OF DOSE. In postoperative use, the dose should be titrated for each patient in order to obtain sufficient respiratory response; however, naloxone antagonises analgesia

Side-effects: nausea and vomiting reported; tachycardia and fibrillation also reported

Dose: by intravenous injection, 100–200 micrograms (1.5–3 micrograms/kg); if response inadequate, increments of 100 micrograms every 2 minutes; further doses by intramuscular injection after 1–2 hours if required

CHILD, by intravenous injection, 10 micrograms/kg; subsequent dose of 100 micrograms/kg if no response; if intravenous route not possible, may be given in divided doses by intramuscular or subcutaneous injection

NEONATE, by subcutaneous, intramuscular, or intravenous injection, 10 micrograms/kg, repeated every 2 to 3 minutes or 200 micrograms (60 micrograms/kg) by intramuscular injection as a single dose at birth (onset of action slower)

Naloxone (Non-proprietary) PoM
Injection, naloxone hydrochloride 20 micrograms/mL, net price 2-mL amp = £2.90
Available from Faulding DBL
Injection, naloxone hydrochloride
400 micrograms/mL—see under Emergency Treatment of Poisoning p. 23
Narcan® PoM —see under Emergency Treatment of Poisoning p. 23
Narcan Neonatal® (Du Pont) PoM
Injection, naloxone hydrochloride 20 micrograms/mL. Net price 2-mL amp = £3.32

| 15.1.8 | **Drugs for malignant hyperthermia** |

Dantrolene is used in the treatment of malignant hyperthermia which is a rare but potentially lethal complication of anaesthesia. It is characterised by a rapid rise in temperature, increasing muscle rigidity, tachycardia, and acidosis and can be triggered off by volatile anaesthetics, and suxamethonium. Dantrolene acts on skeletal muscle by interfering with calcium efflux in the muscle cell and stopping the contractile process. Known trigger agents should be avoided during anaesthesia.

DANTROLENE SODIUM
Indications: malignant hyperthermia
Cautions: avoid extravasation; **interactions:** Appendix 1 (muscle relaxants)
Dose: *by rapid intravenous injection*, 1 mg/kg, repeated as required to a cumulative max. of 10 mg/kg

Dantrium Intravenous® (Procter & Gamble Pharm.) PoM
Injection, powder for reconstitution, dantrolene sodium, net price 20-mg vial = £16.67 (hosp. only)

15.2 Local anaesthesia

The use of local anaesthetics by injection or by application to mucous membranes to produce local analgesia is discussed in this section.

See also section 1.7 (colon and rectum), section 11.7 (eye), section 12.3 (oropharynx), and section 13.3 (skin).

USE OF LOCAL ANAESTHETICS. Local anaesthetic drugs act by causing a reversible block to conduction along nerve fibres. The drugs used vary widely in their potency, toxicity, duration of action, stability, solubility in water, and ability to penetrate mucous membranes. These variations determine their suitability for use by various routes, e.g. topical (surface), infiltration, plexus, epidural (extradural) or spinal block.

The cold sensation produced by **ethyl chloride** spray is used to test the onset of regional anaesthesia.

ADMINISTRATION. In estimating the safe dosage of these drugs it is important to take account of the rate at which they are absorbed and excreted as well as their potency. The patient's age, weight, physique, and clinical condition, the degree of vascularity of the area to which the drug is to be applied, and the duration of administration are other factors which must be taken into account.

Local anaesthetics do not rely on the circulation to transport them to their sites of action, but uptake into the systemic circulation is important in terminating their action and producing toxicity. Following most regional anaesthetic procedures, maximum arterial plasma concentrations of anaesthetic develop within about 10 to 25 minutes, so **careful surveillance** for toxic effects is necessary

during the first 30 minutes after injection. Great care must be taken to avoid accidental intravascular injection.

Epidural anaesthesia is commonly used during surgery, often combined with general anaesthesia, because of its protective effect against the stress response of surgery. It is often used when good postoperative pain relief is essential (e.g. aortic aneurysm surgery or major gut surgery).

TOXICITY. Toxic effects associated with local anaesthetics usually result from excessively high plasma concentrations. Effects initially include a feeling of inebriation and lightheadedness followed by sedation, circumoral paraesthesia and twitching; convulsions can occur in severe reactions. On intravenous injection convulsions and cardiovascular collapse may occur very rapidly. Hypersensitivity reactions occur mainly with the ester-type local anaesthetics such as benzocaine, cocaine, procaine, and tetracaine (amethocaine); reactions are less frequent with the amide types such as lidocaine (lignocaine), bupivacaine, prilocaine, and ropivacaine.

When prolonged analgesia is required, a long-acting local anaesthetic is preferred to minimise the likelihood of cumulative systemic toxicity. Toxic effects may also occur if the injection is too rapid. Local anaesthetics should **not** be injected into inflamed or infected tissues nor should they be applied to the traumatised urethra. Under these conditions the drug may be so rapidly absorbed that a systemic rather than a local reaction is produced.

USE OF VASOCONSTRICTORS. Most local anaesthetics, with the exception of cocaine, cause dilation of blood vessels. The addition of a vasoconstrictor such as **adrenaline (epinephrine)** diminishes local blood flow, slows the rate of absorption of the local anaesthetic, and prolongs its local effect. Adrenaline must be used in a low concentration (e.g. 1 in 200 000) for this purpose and it should **not** be given with a local anaesthetic in digits and appendages; it may produce ischaemic necrosis.

When adrenaline is included the final concentration should be 1 in 200 000 (5 micrograms/mL). In dental surgery, up to 1 in 80 000 (12.5 micrograms/mL) of adrenaline is used with local anaesthetics. There is no justification for using higher concentrations.

The total dose of adrenaline should **not** exceed 500 micrograms and it is essential not to exceed a concentration of 1 in 200 000 (5 micrograms/mL) if more than 50 mL of the mixture is to be injected. For general cautions associated with the use of adrenaline, see section 2.7.3. For drug interactions, see Appendix 1 (sympathomimetics).

Lidocaine (Lignocaine)

Lidocaine (lignocaine) is effectively absorbed from mucous membranes and is a useful surface anaesthetic in concentrations of 2 to 4%. Except for surface anaesthesia, solutions should not usually exceed 1% in strength. The duration of the block (with adrenaline) is about 90 minutes.

LIDOCAINE HYDROCHLORIDE/
LIGNOCAINE HYDROCHLORIDE

Indications: see under Dose; also dental anaesthesia (see next page); ventricular arrhythmias (section 2.3.2)

Cautions: epilepsy, hepatic or respiratory impairment, impaired cardiac conduction, bradycardia; porphyria (section 9.8.2); reduce dose in elderly or debilitated; resuscitative equipment should be available; see section 2.3.2 for effects on heart; **interactions:** Appendix 1 (lidocaine)

Contra-indications: hypovolaemia, complete heart block; do not use solutions containing adrenaline for anaesthesia in appendages

Side-effects: CNS effects include confusion, respiratory depression and convulsions; hypotension and bradycardia (may lead to cardiac arrest); hypersensitivity reported; see also notes above

Dose: infiltration anaesthesia, *by injection*, according to patient's weight and nature of procedure, max. 200 mg (or 500 mg if given in solutions containing adrenaline)—see also Administration on p. 573 and see also **important** warning below

Intravenous regional anaesthesia and nerve blocks, seek expert advice

Surface anaesthesia, usual strengths 2–4%, see preparations below

Important: the licensed doses stated above may not be appropriate in some settings and expert advice should be sought

■ Lidocaine hydrochloride injections

Lidocaine/Lignocaine (Non-proprietary) [PoM]
Injection 0.5%, lidocaine hydrochloride 5 mg/mL, net price 10-mL amp = 28p
Injection 1%, lidocaine hydrochloride 10 mg/mL, net price 2-mL amp = 22p; 5-mL amp = 21p; 10-mL amp = 34p; 20-mL amp = 52p
Injection 2%, lidocaine hydrochloride 20 mg/mL, net price 2-mL amp = 27p; 5-mL amp = 23p

Xylocaine® (Astra) [PoM]
Injection 0.5%, anhydrous lidocaine hydrochloride 5 mg/mL. Net price 20-mL vial = 65p
Injection 0.5% with adrenaline 1 in 200 000, anhydrous lidocaine hydrochloride 5 mg/mL, adrenaline 1 in 200 000 (5 micrograms/mL). Net price 20-mL vial = 67p
Injection 1%, anhydrous lidocaine hydrochloride 10 mg/mL. Net price 20-mL vial = 67p
Injection 1% with adrenaline 1 in 200 000, anhydrous lidocaine hydrochloride 10 mg/mL, adrenaline 1 in 200 000 (5 micrograms/mL). Net price 20-mL vial = 69p
Injection 2%, anhydrous lidocaine hydrochloride 20 mg/mL. Net price 20-mL vial = 71p
Injection 2% with adrenaline 1 in 200 000, anhydrous lidocaine hydrochloride 20 mg/mL, adrenaline 1 in 200 000 (5 micrograms/mL). Net price 20-mL vial = 73p

■ Lidocaine injections for dental use
Note. Consult expert dental sources for specific advice in relation to dose of lidocaine for dental anaesthesia
A large variety of lidocaine injections, plain or with adrenaline or noradrenaline, is also available in dental cartridges under the names *Lignospan®*, *Lignostab A®*, *Rexocaine®*, *Xylocaine®*, and *Xylotox®*.

■ Lidocaine for surface anaesthesia
Important. Rapid and extensive absorption may result in systemic side-effects

Emla® (Astra) [PoM]
Drug Tariff cream, lidocaine 2.5%, prilocaine 2.5%, net price 5-g tube = £1.73
Surgical pack cream, lidocaine 2.5%, prilocaine 2.5%, net price 30-g tube = £10.25
Premedication pack cream, lidocaine 2.5%, prilocaine 2.5%, net price 10 × 5-g tube with 25 occlusive dressings = £19.50
Anaesthesia before e.g. venepuncture (not for infants), apply a thick layer under an occlusive dressing 1–5 hours before procedure; split skin grafting, apply a thick layer under an occlusive dressing 2–5 hours before procedure; genital warts (not for children), apply up to 10 g 5–10 minutes before removal
Cautions: not for wounds, mucous membranes (except genital warts in adults) or atopic dermatitis; avoid use near eyes or middle ear; although systemic absorption is low, caution in anaemia, or congenital or acquired methaemoglobinaemia (see also Prilocaine, p. 575); *side-effects* include transient paleness, redness, and oedema; **contra-indicated** in infants under 1 year

Instillagel® (CliniMed)
Gel, lidocaine hydrochloride 2%, chlorhexidine gluconate solution 0.25%, in a sterile lubricant basis in disposable syringe. Net price 6-mL syringe = £1.58; 11-mL syringe = £1.78
Excipients: include hydroxybenzoates (parabens)
Dose: 6–11 mL into urethra

Laryng-O-Jet ® (IMS) [PoM]
Jet spray 4% (disposable kit for laryngotracheal anaesthesia), lidocaine hydrochloride 40 mg/mL. Net price per unit (4-mL vial and disposable sterile cannula with cover and vial injector) = £4.55
Dose: usually 160 mg (4 mL) as a single dose instilled as jet spray into lumen of larynx and trachea (reduce dose according to size, age and condition of patient); max. 200 mg (5 mL)
Caution: may be rapidly and almost completely absorbed from respiratory tract and systemic side-effects may occur; extreme caution if mucosa has been traumatised or if sepsis present

Xylocaine® (Astra)
Antiseptic gel, anhydrous lidocaine hydrochloride 2%, chlorhexidine gluconate solution 0.25% in a sterile lubricant basis. Net price 20 g = £1.06; 20-g single-use syringe (*Accordion®*) = 98p
Dose: into urethra, men 10 mL followed by 3–5 mL; women 5–10 mL
Gel, anhydrous lidocaine hydrochloride 2%, in a sterile lubricant water-miscible basis. Net price 20 g = 76p; 20-g single-use syringe (*Accordion®*) = 98p
Excipients: include hydroxybenzoates (parabens)
Dose:
Into urethra, men 10 mL, followed by further 10 mL (total of up to 40 mL for cystoscopy); women 5–10 mL
Endoscopy, 10–20 mL
Endotracheal intubation, 5 mL applied to surface of tube (avoid introducing gel into lumen)
Ointment, lidocaine 5% in a water-miscible basis. Net price 15 g = 80p
Excipients: include propylene glycol
Dose: max. 20 g in 24 hours
Spray (= pump spray), lidocaine 10% (100 mg/g) supplying 10 mg lidocaine/dose; 500 spray doses per container. Net price 50-mL bottle = £3.13
Dose: dental practice, 1–5 doses; maxillary sinus puncture, 3 doses; during delivery in obstetrics, up to 20 doses; procedures in pharynx, larynx, and trachea, up to 20 doses

Topical 4%, anhydrous lidocaine hydrochloride 40 mg/mL. Net price 30-mL bottle = £1.21
Excipients: include hydroxybenzoates (parabens)
Dose: bronchoscopy, 2–3 mL with suitable spray; biopsy in mouth, 3–4 mL with suitable spray *or* swab (with adrenaline if necessary); max. 7.5 mL

■ Lidocaine for ear, nose, and oropharyngeal use

Lidocaine with Phenylephrine/Lignocaine with Phenylephrine (Non-proprietary)
Topical solution, lidocaine hydrochloride 5%, phenylephrine hydrochloride 0.5%, net price 2.5 mL (with nasal applicator) = £8.00. For cautions, contra-indications and side-effects of phenylephrine, see section 2.7.2
Available from Aurum

Bupivacaine

The advantage of bupivacaine over other local anaesthetics is its longer duration of action. It has a slow onset of action, taking up to 30 minutes for full effect. It is often used in lumbar epidural blockade and is particularly suitable for continuous epidural analgesia in labour. It is the principal drug for spinal anaesthesia in the UK.

BUPIVACAINE HYDROCHLORIDE

Indications: see under Dose
Cautions: see under Lidocaine Hydrochloride and notes above; avoid accidental intravascular injection; myocardial depression may be more severe and more resistant to treatment; **interactions:** Appendix 1 (bupivacaine)
Contra-indications: see under Lidocaine Hydrochloride and notes above; intravenous regional anaesthesia (Bier's block)
Side-effects: see under Lidocaine Hydrochloride and notes above
Dose: adjusted according to patient's weight and nature of procedure—**important**: see also under Administration, above
Local infiltration, 0.25% (up to 60 mL)
Peripheral nerve block, 0.25% (max. 60 mL), 0.375% (max. 40 mL), 0.5% (max. 30 mL)
Epidural block,
   Surgery, *lumbar*, 0.5–0.75% (max. 20 mL of either)
      caudal, 0.5% (max. 30 mL)
   Labour, *lumbar*, 0.25–0.5% (max. 12 mL)
      caudal, but rarely used, 0.25–0.5% (max. 20 mL)
Sympathetic block, 0.25% (max. 50 mL)
Note. 0.75% **contra-indicated** for epidural use in obstetrics.
Important: the licensed doses stated above may not be appropriate in some settings and expert advice should be sought

Marcain® (Astra) PoM
Injection, anhydrous bupivacaine hydrochloride 2.5 mg/mL (*Marcain®* 0.25%), net price 10-mL *Polyamp®* = £1.06; 3.75 mg/mL (*Marcain®* 0.375%), 10-mL *Polyamp®* = £1.16; 5 mg/mL (*Marcain®* 0.5%), 10-mL *Polyamp®* = £1.21; 7.5 mg/mL (*Marcain®* 0.75%), 10-mL *Polyamp®* = £1.82.
Note. Bupivacaine hydrochloride injection 0.25% and 0.5% also available from Antigen, Faulding DBL

Marcain Heavy® (Astra) PoM
Injection, anhydrous bupivacaine hydrochloride 5 mg, glucose 80 mg/mL, net price 4-mL amp = 93p
Dose: spinal anaesthesia, 2–4 mL

Marcain with Adrenaline® (Astra) PoM
Injection 0.25%, bupivacaine hydrochloride 2.5 mg/mL, adrenaline 1 in 200 000 (5 micrograms/mL), net price 10-mL amp = £1.18
Injection 0.5%, bupivacaine hydrochloride 5 mg/mL, adrenaline 1 in 200 000 (5 micrograms/mL), net price 10-mL amp = £1.23

Prilocaine

Prilocaine is a local anaesthetic of low toxicity which is similar to lidocaine (lignocaine). If used in high doses, methaemoglobinaemia may occur which can be treated with intravenous injection of methylthioninium chloride (methylene blue) 1% using a dose of 1 mg/kg. Infants are particularly susceptible to methaemoglobinaemia.

PRILOCAINE HYDROCHLORIDE

Indications: infiltration anaesthesia (higher strengths for dental use only), intravenous regional anaesthesia, nerve block
Cautions: see under Lidocaine Hydrochloride and notes above; renal impairment; **interactions:** Appendix 1 (prilocaine)
Contra-indications: see under Lidocaine Hydrochloride and notes above; anaemia or congenital or acquired methaemoglobinaemia
Side-effects: see under Lidocaine Hydrochloride and notes above; ocular toxicity (including blindness) reported with excessive strengths used for ophthalmic procedures
Dose: adjusted according to site of operation and response of patient, to max. 400 mg used alone, or 300 mg if used with felypressin

Citanest® (Astra) PoM
Injection 0.5%, prilocaine hydrochloride 5 mg/mL, net price 20-mL multidose vial = 71p; 50-mL multidose vial = 99p; 50-mL single dose vial = £1.21
Injection 1%, prilocaine hydrochloride 10 mg/mL, net price 20-mL multidose vial = 73p; 50-mL multidose vial = £1.03
Injection 2%, prilocaine hydrochloride 20 mg/mL, net price 10-mL single dose vial = 70p

■ For dental use

Citanest® (Astra) PoM
Injection 4%, prilocaine hydrochloride 40 mg/mL, net price 2-mL cartridge = 15p

Citanest with Octapressin® (Astra) PoM
Injection 3%, prilocaine hydrochloride 30 mg/mL, felypressin 0.03 unit/mL, net price 2-mL cartridge and self-aspirating cartridge (both) = 15p

Procaine

Procaine is now seldom used. It is as potent as lidocaine (lignocaine) but has a shorter duration of action. It provides less intense analgesia because of reduced spread through the tissues. It is of no value as a surface anaesthetic.

PROCAINE HYDROCHLORIDE ▰▰▰

Indications: local anaesthesia by infiltration and regional routes (but see notes above)
Cautions: see notes above
Side-effects: see notes above
Dose: adjusted according to site of operation and patient's response
By injection, up to 1 g (200 mL of 0.5% solution or 100 mL of 1%) with adrenaline 1 in 200 000

Procaine (Non-proprietary) PoM ▰▰▰
Injection, procaine hydrochloride 2% (20 mg/mL) in sodium chloride intravenous infusion, net price 2-mL amp = 78p; 5-mL amp = £3.49
Available from Martindale

Tetracaine (Amethocaine)

Tetracaine (amethocaine) is an effective local anaesthetic for topical application; a 4% gel is indicated for anaesthesia prior to venepuncture or venous cannulation. It is rapidly absorbed from mucous membranes and should **never** be applied to inflamed, traumatised, or highly vascular surfaces. It should **never** be used to provide anaesthesia for bronchoscopy or cystoscopy, as lidocaine (lignocaine) is a safer alternative. It is used in ophthalmology (section 11.7) and in skin preparations (section 13.3). Hypersensitivity to tetracaine has been reported.

TETRACAINE/AMETHOCAINE

Indications: see under preparation below
Cautions: see notes above
Contra-indications: see notes above
Side-effects: see notes above; also erythema, oedema and pruritus
   Important. Rapid and extensive absorption may result in systemic side-effects (see also notes above)

Ametop® (S&N Hlth.)
Gel, tetracaine 4%, net price 1.5-g tube = £1.15
   Dose: apply contents of tube to site of venepuncture or venous cannulation and cover with occlusive dressing; remove gel and dressing after 30 minutes for venepuncture and after 45 minutes for venous cannulation; PREMATURE INFANT and INFANT under 1 month not recommended

Ropivacaine

Ropivacaine is a recently introduced amide-type local anaesthetic agent.

ROPIVACAINE HYDROCHLORIDE

Indications: see under Dose
Cautions: see Lidocaine Hydrochloride and notes above
Contra-indications: see Lidocaine Hydrochloride and notes above
Side-effects: see Lidocaine Hydrochloride and notes above
Dose: adjust according to patient's physical status and nature of procedure—see also under Administration on p. 573
   Surgical anaesthesia,
      lumbar epidural, 15–20 mL of 10 mg/mL solution *or* 15–25 mL of 7.5 mg/mL solution; caesarean section, 15–20 mL of 7.5 mg/mL solution

   thoracic epidural (to establish block for postoperative pain), 5–15 mL of 7.5 mg/mL solution
   major nerve block (brachial plexus block), 30–40 mL of 7.5 mg/mL solution
   field block, up to 30 mL of 7.5 mg/mL solution
   Acute pain,
      lumbar epidural, 10–20 mL of 2 mg/mL solution followed by 10–15 mL of 2 mg/mL solution at intervals of at least 30 minutes *or* 6–10 mL/hour of 2 mg/mL solution as a continuous epidural infusion for labour pain *or* 6–14 mL/hour of 2 mg/mL solution as a continuous epidural infusion for postoperative pain
      thoracic epidural, 6–14 mL/hour of 2 mg/mL solution as a continuous infusion
      field block, up to 100 mL of 2 mg/mL solution

Naropin® (Astra) PoM
Injection, ropivacaine hydrochloride 2 mg/mL, net price 10-mL *Polyamp®* = £1.37; 7.5 mg/mL, 10-mL *Polyamp®* = £2.65; 10 mg/mL, 10-mL *Polyamp®* = £3.36
Epidural infusion, ropivacaine hydrochloride 2 mg/mL, net price 100-mL *Polybag®* = £8.62, 200-mL *Polybag®* = £14.45

Other local anaesthetics

Benzocaine is a local anaesthetic of low potency and toxicity. It is an ingredient of some proprietary throat lozenges (section 12.3.3).
   Mepivacaine is a local anaesthetic used in dentistry; it is available in dental cartridges with or without adrenaline (epinephrine) as *Scandonest®*. **Articaine (carticaine)** is a newly introduced local anaesthetic for dental use; it is available in cartridges with adrenaline (*Septanest®* ▼).
   Cocaine readily penetrates mucous membranes and is an effective surface anaesthetic with an intense vasoconstrictor action. However, apart from its use in otolaryngology (see below), it has now been replaced by less toxic alternatives. It has marked sympathomimetic activity and should **never** be given by injection because of its toxicity. As a result of its intense stimulant effect it is a drug of addiction. In otolaryngology cocaine is applied to the nasal mucosa in concentrations of 4 to 10% (40–100 mg/mL); an oromucosal solution and nasal spray both containing cocaine hydrochloride 10% are available (Aurum). In order to avoid systemic effects, the maximum dose recommended for application to the nasal mucosa in fit adults is a total of 1.5 mg/kg, which is equivalent to a total topical dose of approximately 100 mg for an adult male; this dose relates to direct application of cocaine (application on gauze may reduce systemic absorption). It should be used only by those skilled in the precautions needed to *minimise absorption* and the *consequent risk of arrhythmias*. Although cocaine interacts with other drugs liable to induce arrhythmias, including adrenaline, some otolaryngologists consider that combined use of topical cocaine with topical adrenaline (in the form of a paste or a solution) improves the operative field and may possibly reduce absorption. Cocaine is a mydriatic as well as a local anaesthetic but owing to corneal toxicity it is now little used in ophthalmology. Cocaine should be avoided in porphyria (section 9.8.2).

Appendix 1: Interactions

Two or more drugs given at the same time may exert their effects independently or may interact. The interaction may be potentiation or antagonism of one drug by another, or occasionally some other effect. Adverse drug interactions should be reported to the CSM as for other adverse drug reactions.

Drug interactions may be **pharmacodynamic** or **pharmacokinetic**.

Pharmacodynamic interactions

These are interactions between drugs which have similar or antagonistic pharmacological effects or side-effects. They may be due to competition at receptor sites, or occur between drugs acting on the same physiological system. They are usually predictable from a knowledge of the pharmacology of the interacting drugs; in general, those demonstrated with one drug are likely to occur with related drugs. They occur to a greater or lesser extent in most patients who receive the interacting drugs.

Pharmacokinetic interactions

These occur when one drug alters the absorption, distribution, metabolism, or excretion of another, thus increasing or reducing the amount of drug available to produce its pharmacological effects. They are not easily predicted and many of them affect only a small proportion of patients taking the combination of drugs. Pharmacokinetic interactions occurring with one drug cannot be assumed to occur with related drugs unless their pharmacokinetic properties are known to be similar.

Pharmacokinetic interactions are of several types:

AFFECTING ABSORPTION. The rate of absorption or the total amount absorbed can both be altered by drug interactions. Delayed absorption is rarely of clinical importance unless high peak plasma concentrations are required (e.g. when giving an analgesic). Reduction in the total amount absorbed, however, may result in ineffective therapy.

DUE TO CHANGES IN PROTEIN BINDING. To a variable extent most drugs are loosely bound to plasma proteins. Protein-binding sites are non-specific and one drug can displace another thereby increasing its proportion free to diffuse from plasma to its site of action. This only produces a detectable increase in effect if it is an extensively bound drug (more than 90%) that is not widely distributed throughout the body. Even so displacement rarely produces more than transient potentiation because this increased concentration of free drug results in an increased rate of elimination.

Displacement from protein binding plays a part in the potentiation of warfarin by phenylbutazone, sulphonamides, and tolbutamide but the importance of these interactions is due mainly to the fact that warfarin metabolism is also inhibited.

AFFECTING METABOLISM. Many drugs are metabolised in the liver. Induction of the hepatic microsomal enzyme system by one drug can gradually increase the rate of metabolism of another, resulting in lower plasma concentrations and a reduced effect. On withdrawal of the inducer plasma concentrations increase and toxicity may occur. Barbiturates, griseofulvin, most antiepileptics, and rifampicin are the most important enzyme inducers in man. Drugs affected include warfarin and the oral contraceptives.

Conversely when one drug inhibits the metabolism of another higher plasma concentrations are produced, rapidly resulting in an increased effect with risk of toxicity. Some drugs which potentiate warfarin and phenytoin do so by this mechanism.

AFFECTING RENAL EXCRETION. Drugs are eliminated through the kidney both by glomerular filtration and by active tubular secretion. Competition occurs between those which share active transport mechanisms in the proximal tubule. Thus probenecid delays the excretion of many drugs including penicillins, some cephalosporins, indometacin, and dapsone; aspirin may increase the toxicity of methotrexate by a similar mechanism.

Relative importance of interactions

Many drug interactions are harmless and many of those which are potentially harmful only occur in a small proportion of patients; moreover, the severity of an interaction varies from one patient to another. Drugs with a small therapeutic ratio (e.g. phenytoin) and those which require careful control of dosage (e.g. anticoagulants, antihypertensives, and antidiabetics) are most often involved.

Patients at increased risk from drug interactions include the elderly and those with impaired renal or liver function.

HAZARDOUS INTERACTIONS. The symbol • has been placed against interactions that are **potentially hazardous** and where combined administration of the drugs involved should be **avoided** (or only undertaken with caution and appropriate monitoring).

Interactions that have no symbol do not usually have serious consequences.

List of drug interactions

The following is an alphabetical list of drugs and their interactions; to avoid excessive cross-referencing each drug or group is listed twice: in the alphabetical list and also under the drug or group with which it interacts; changes in the interactions lists since BNF No. 38 (September 1999) are <u>underlined</u>.

For explanation of symbol • see previous page

Acarbose *see* Antidiabetics
ACE Inhibitors and Angiotensin-II Antagonists
Alcohol: enhanced hypotensive effect
Aldesleukin: enhanced hypotensive effect
Allopurinol: increased risk of toxicity with *captopril*, especially in renal impairment
Alprostadil: enhanced hypotensive effect
• Anaesthetics: enhanced hypotensive effect
• Analgesics: antagonism of hypotensive effect and increased risk of renal impairment with *NSAIDs*; hyperkalaemia with *ketorolac and possibly other NSAIDs*
<u>Antacids</u>: absorption of *captopril, enalapril, fosinopril* and *possibly other ACE inhibitors* reduced
Anti-arrhythmics: *procainamide* increases risk of toxicity with *captopril*, especially in renal impairment
Antibacterials: absorption of *tetracyclines* reduced by *quinapril tablets* (contain magnesium carbonate excipient); *rifampicin* reduces plasma concentration of active metabolite of *imidapril* (reduced antihypertensive effect)
<u>Anticoagulants</u>: increased risk of hyperkalaemia with *heparin*
Antidepressants: possibly enhanced hypotensive effect
Antidiabetics: hypoglycaemic effect possibly enhanced
other Antihypertensives: enhanced hypotensive effect; previous treatment with *clonidine* possibly delays antihypertensive effect of *captopril*
Antipsychotics: severe postural hypotension with *chlorpromazine and possibly other phenothiazines*
Anxiolytics and Hypnotics: enhanced hypotensive effect
Beta-blockers: enhanced hypotensive effect
Calcium-channel Blockers: enhanced hypotensive effect
• <u>Cardiac Glycosides</u>: plasma concentration of *digoxin* increased by *telmisartan* and possibly by *captopril*
• Ciclosporin: increased risk of hyperkalaemia
Corticosteroids: antagonism of hypotensive effect
Cytotoxics: *azathioprine* increases risk of leucopenia with *captopril*
• Diuretics: enhanced hypotensive effect (can be extreme); risk of severe hyperkalaemia with *potassium-sparing diuretics*
Dopaminergics: *levodopa* enhances hypotensive effect
Epoetin: antagonism of hypotensive effect; increased risk of hyperkalaemia
• Lithium: *ACE inhibitors* reduce excretion of *lithium* (increased plasma-lithium concentration)
Moxisylyte: enhanced hypotensive effect
Muscle Relaxants: *baclofen* and *tizanidine* enhance hypotensive effect
Nitrates: enhance hypotensive effect
Oestrogens and Progestogens: *oestrogens* and *combined oral contraceptives* antagonise hypotensive effect
• Potassium Salts: increased risk of hyperkalaemia
Ulcer-healing Drugs: *carbenoxolone* antagonises hypotensive effect
Uricosurics: *probenecid* reduces excretion of *captopril*

Acebutolol *see* Beta-blockers
Aceclofenac *see* NSAIDs
Acemetacin *see* NSAIDs
Acenocoumarol (Nicoumalone) *see* Warfarin and other Coumarins
Acetazolamide *see* Diuretics (carbonic anhydrase inhibitor)
Aciclovir and Famciclovir
Note. Interactions do not apply to topical preparations
Mycophenolate Mofetil: higher plasma concentrations of *aciclovir* and of *mycophenolate mofetil* on concomitant administration
Uricosurics: *probenecid* reduces *aciclovir* and possibly *famciclovir* excretion (increased plasma concentrations)
Acitretin *see* Retinoids
Acrivastine *see* Antihistamines
Adenosine
Note. Possibility of interaction with drugs tending to impair cardiac conduction
• Antiplatelet Drugs: effect enhanced and extended by *dipyridamole* (**important** risk of toxicity)
Theophylline: antagonism of anti-arrhythmic effect
Adrenaline (Epinephrine) *see* Sympathomimetics
Adrenergic Neurone Blockers
Alcohol: enhanced hypotensive effect
Alprostadil: enhanced hypotensive effect
• Anaesthetics: enhanced hypotensive effect
Analgesics: *NSAIDs* antagonise hypotensive effect
Anti-arrhythmics: increased risk of myocardial depression with *bretylium*
Antidepressants: *tricyclics* and *viloxazine* antagonise hypotensive effect
other Antihypertensives: enhanced hypotensive effect
<u>Antipsychotics</u>: *phenothiazines* enhance hypotensive effect (antagonism of hypotensive effect with higher doses of *chlorpromazine*); antagonism of hypotensive effect with *haloperidol*
Anxiolytics and Hypnotics: enhanced hypotensive effect
Beta-blockers: enhanced hypotensive effect
Calcium-channel Blockers: enhanced hypotensive effect
• Cisapride: increased risk of ventricular arrhythmias with *bretylium*—avoid concomitant use
Corticosteroids: antagonism of hypotensive effect
Diuretics: enhanced hypotensive effect
Dopaminergics: *levodopa* enhances hypotensive effect
Moxisylyte: enhanced hypotensive effect
Muscle Relaxants: enhanced hypotensive effect with *tizanidine*
Nitrates: enhance hypotensive effect
Oestrogens and Progestogens: *oestrogens* and *combined oral contraceptives* antagonise hypotensive effect
Pizotifen: antagonism of hypotensive effect
• Sympathomimetics: *some anorectics, some cough and cold remedies (e.g. ephedrine)*, and *methylphenidate* antagonise hypotensive effect
Ulcer-healing Drugs: *carbenoxolone* antagonises hypotensive effect
Alcohol
ACE Inhibitors and Angiotensin-II Antagonists: enhanced hypotensive effect
Analgesics: sedative and hypotensive effect of *opioid analgesics* enhanced
• Antibacterials: disulfiram-like reaction with *cefamandole, metronidazole*, and possibly *tinidazole*; increased risk of seizures with *cycloserine*
• Anticoagulants: *see* Warfarin
• Antidepressants: sedative effect of *tricyclics (and related)* enhanced; *tyramine* (contained in some alcoholic and dealcoholised beverages) interacts with *MAOIs* (hypertensive crisis)—but if no tyramine, enhanced hypotensive effect; effects of alcohol possibly enhanced by *SSRIs*

Alcohol *(continued)*
Antidiabetics: enhanced hypoglycaemic effect;
flushing with *chlorpropamide* (in susceptible
subjects); increased risk of lactic acidosis with
metformin
Antiepileptics: CNS side-effects of *carbamazepine*
possibly enhanced
Antihistamines: enhanced sedative effect
Antihypertensives: enhanced hypotensive effect;
sedative effect of *indoramin* enhanced
Antimuscarinics: sedative effect of *hyoscine*
enhanced
Antipsychotics: enhanced sedative effect
Anxiolytics and Hypnotics: enhanced sedative effect
Barbiturates and Primidone: enhanced sedative effect
Beta-blockers: enhanced hypotensive effect
Calcium-channel Blockers: enhanced hypotensive
effect; plasma-alcohol concentration possibly
increased by *verapamil*
Cisapride: enhanced sedative effect
Cytotoxics: disulfiram-like reaction with *procarbazine*
Dopaminergics: reduced tolerance to *bromocriptine*
Lofexidine: enhanced sedative effect
Muscle Relaxants: *baclofen* and *tizanidine* enhance
sedative effect
Nabilone: enhanced sedative effect
Nitrates: enhanced hypotensive effect
• Paraldehyde: enhanced sedative effect
Retinoids: *etretinate* formed from *acitretin* in
presence of *alcohol*
Aldesleukin
Antihypertensives: enhanced hypotensive effect
Alendronic Acid *see* Bisphosphonates
Alfentanil *see* Opioid Analgesics
Alfuzosin *see* Alpha-blockers (post-synaptic)
Alimemazine (Trimeprazine) *see* Antihistamines
Allopurinol
ACE Inhibitors and Angiotensin-II Antagonists:
increased risk of toxicity with *captopril*, especially
in renal impairment
Anticoagulants: effects of *acenocoumarol* and
warfarin possibly enhanced
Ciclosporin: plasma-ciclosporin concentration
possibly increased (risk of nephrotoxicity)
• Cytotoxics: effects of *azathioprine* and
mercaptopurine enhanced with increased toxicity
(reduce dose when given with allopurinol)
Alpha₂-adrenoceptor Stimulants
Antidepressants: manufacturers of *apraclonidine* and
brimonidine advise avoid concomitant use with
tricyclics or related antidepressants or *MAOIs*
Sympathomimetics: possible risk of hypertension
with *adrenaline* and *noradrenaline*
Alpha-blockers
ACE Inhibitors and Angiotensin-II Antagonists:
enhanced hypotensive effect
Alcohol: enhanced hypotensive effect; sedative effect
of *indoramin* enhanced
Aldesleukin: enhanced hypotensive effect
Alprostadil: enhanced hypotensive effect
• Anaesthetics: enhanced hypotensive effect
Analgesics: *NSAIDs* antagonise hypotensive effect
• Antidepressants: enhanced hypotensive effect;
manufacturer of *indoramin* advises avoid *MAOIs*
other Antihypertensives: additive hypotensive effect
Antipsychotics: enhanced hypotensive effect
Anxiolytics and Hypnotics: enhanced hypotensive
and sedative effect
• Beta-blockers: enhanced hypotensive effect; increased
risk of first-dose hypotensive effect of *post-synaptic
alpha-blockers such as prazosin*
• Calcium-channel Blockers: enhanced hypotensive
effect; increased risk of first-dose hypotensive effect
of *post-synaptic alpha-blockers such as prazosin*
Corticosteroids : antagonism of hypotensive effect
• Diuretics: enhanced hypotensive effect; increased risk
of first-dose hypotensive effect of *post-synaptic
alpha-blockers such as prazosin*

Alpha-blockers *(continued)*
Dopaminergics: *levodopa* enhances hypotensive effect
• Moxisylyte: possible severe postural hypotension
Muscle Relaxants: *baclofen* and *tizanidine* enhance
hypotensive effect
Nitrates: enhanced hypotensive effect
Oestrogens and Progestogens: *oestrogens and
combined oral contraceptives* antagonise
hypotensive effect
Ulcer-healing Drugs: *carbenoxolone* antagonises
hypotensive effect
Alprazolam *see* Anxiolytics and Hypnotics
Alprostadil
Antihypertensives: enhanced hypotensive effect
Altretamine
• Antidepressants: risk of severe postural hypotension
with *MAOIs* and *tricyclics*
• Pyridoxine: reduced response to altretamine
Aluminium Hydroxide *see* Antacids
Amantadine
Antihypertensives: *methyldopa* and *metirosine* have
extrapyramidal side-effects
Antimuscarinics: increased antimuscarinic side-
effects
Antipsychotics: all have extrapyramidal side-effects
Metoclopramide and Domperidone: have
extrapyramidal side-effects
Tetrabenazine: has extrapyramidal side-effects
Amifostine
Note. Limited information available—rapid clearance
from plasma minimises risk of interactions; possibility
of interactions with antihypertensives and other drugs
which potentiate hypotension
Amikacin *see* Aminoglycosides
Amiloride *see* Diuretics (potassium-sparing)
Aminoglutethimide
• Anticoagulants: metabolism of *acenocoumarol* and
warfarin accelerated (reduced anticoagulant effect)
Antidiabetics: manufacturer advises metabolism of
oral antidiabetics possibly accelerated
Cardiac Glycosides: metabolism of *digitoxin*
accelerated (reduced effect)
Corticosteroids: metabolism of *corticosteroids*
accelerated (reduced effect)
Diuretics: increased risk of hyponatraemia
other Hormone Antagonists: plasma concentration of
tamoxifen reduced
Oestrogens and Progestogens: *aminoglutethimide*
reduces plasma concentration of *medroxyprogesterone*
Theophylline: metabolism of *theophylline*
accelerated (reduced effect)
Aminoglycosides
Analgesics: *indometacin* possibly increases plasma
concentration of *gentamicin* and *amikacin* in
neonates
other Antibacterials: increased risk of nephrotoxicity
with *colistin*; increased risk of ototoxicity and
nephrotoxicity with *capreomycin, teicoplanin* and
vancomycin
• Anticoagulants: *see* Phenindione and Warfarin
Antidiabetics: *neomycin* possibly enhances
hypoglycaemic effect of *acarbose* and increases
severity of gastro-intestinal effects
Antifungals: increased risk of nephrotoxicity with
amphotericin
Bisphosphonates: increased risk of hypocalcaemia
• Botulinum Toxin: neuromuscular block enhanced
(risk of toxicity)
• Ciclosporin: increased risk of nephrotoxicity
• Cytotoxics: increased risk of nephrotoxicity and
possibly of ototoxicity with *cisplatin*
• Diuretics: increased risk of ototoxicity with *loop diuretics*
• Muscle Relaxants: effect of *non-depolarising muscle
relaxants* enhanced
• Parasympathomimetics: antagonism of effect of
neostigmine and pyridostigmine
Aminophylline *see* Theophylline

Amiodarone

Note. Amiodarone has a long half-life; there is a potential for drug interactions to occur for several weeks (or even months) after treatment with it has been stopped

* *other* Anti-arrhythmics: additive effect with *disopyramide, flecainide, procainamide, and quinidine* (increased risk of ventricular arrhythmias—avoid concomitant use); increased plasma concentrations of *flecainide, procainamide* and *quinidine*; increased myocardial depression with any anti-arrhythmic
* Antibacterials: increased risk of ventricular arrhythmias with *erythromycin* (parenteral) and *co-trimoxazole* (avoid concomitant use)
* Anticoagulants: metabolism of *acenocoumarol, phenindione* and *warfarin* inhibited (enhanced anticoagulant effect)
* Antidepressants: increased risk of ventricular arrhythmias with *tricyclics* (avoid concomitant use); manufacturer of *reboxetine* advises caution
* Antiepileptics: metabolism of *phenytoin* inhibited (increased plasma concentration)
* Antihistamines: increased risk of ventricular arrhythmias with *mizolastine* and *terfenadine* (avoid concomitant use)
* Antimalarials: increased risk of ventricular arrhythmias with *chloroquine, halofantrine, hydroxychloroquine, mefloquine* and *quinine* (avoid concomitant use)
* Antipsychotics: increased risk of ventricular arrhythmias with *phenothiazines, haloperidol, pimozide* and *sertindole* (avoid concomitant use)
* Antivirals: increased risk of ventricular arrhythmias with *nelfinavir* and *ritonavir* (avoid concomitant use)
* Beta-blockers: increased risk of bradycardia, AV block, and myocardial depression; increased risk of ventricular arrhythmias associated with *sotalol* (avoid concomitant use)
* Calcium-channel Blockers: *diltiazem and verapamil* increase risk of bradycardia, AV block, and myocardial depression
* Cardiac Glycosides: increased plasma concentration of *digoxin* (halve digoxin maintenance dose)

  Ciclosporin: plasma concentration of *ciclosporin* possibly increased
* Cisapride: increased risk of ventricular arrhythmias (avoid concomitant use)

  Diuretics: cardiac toxicity increased if hypokalaemia occurs with *acetazolamide, loop diuretics,* and *thiazides*

  Levothyroxine: for concomitant use see p. 70

  Lithium: increased risk of hypothyroidism
* Pentamidine Isetionate: increased risk of ventricular arrhythmias (avoid concomitant use)

  Tropisetron: risk of ventricular arrhythmias—manufacturer of tropisetron advises caution

  Ulcer-healing Drugs: *cimetidine* increases plasma concentrations of *amiodarone*

Amisulpride *see* Antipsychotics
Amitriptyline *see* Antidepressants, Tricyclic
Amlodipine *see* Calcium-channel Blockers
Amobarbital *see* Barbiturates and Primidone
Amoxapine *see* Antidepressants, Tricyclic
Amoxicillin *see* Penicillins
Amphetamines *see* Sympathomimetics
Amphotericin

Note. Close monitoring required with concomitant administration of nephrotoxic drugs or cytotoxics

  Antibacterials: increased risk of nephrotoxicity with *aminoglycosides*

  other Antifungals: *imidazoles* and *triazoles* possibly antagonise effect of *amphotericin*; renal excretion of *flucytosine* decreased and cellular uptake increased (flucytosine toxicity possibly increased)
* Cardiac Glycosides: increased toxicity if hypokalaemia occurs

Amphotericin *(continued)*

* Ciclosporin: increased risk of nephrotoxicity
* Corticosteroids: increased risk of hypokalaemia (avoid concomitant use unless corticosteroids needed to control reactions)

  Diuretics: increased risk of hypokalaemia with *loop diuretics* and *thiazides*
* Tacrolimus: increased risk of nephrotoxicity

Ampicillin *see* Penicillins
Anabolic Steroids

* Anticoagulants: anticoagulant effect of *acenocoumarol, phenindione, and warfarin* enhanced

  Antidiabetics: hypoglycaemic effect possibly enhanced

Anaesthetics, General *(see also* Surgery and Long-term Medication, section 15.1)

* ACE Inhibitors and Angiotensin-II Antagonists: enhanced hypotensive effect

  Antibacterials: possible potentiation of *isoniazid* hepatotoxicity; effect of *thiopental* enhanced by *sulphonamides*; hypersensitivity-like reactions can occur with concomitant intravenous *vancomycin*

  Antidepressants: risk of arrhythmias and hypotension increased with *tricyclics; MAOIs, see* section 15.1
* Antihypertensives: enhanced hypotensive effect
* Antipsychotics: enhanced hypotensive effect

  Anxiolytics and Hypnotics: enhanced sedative effect
* Beta-blockers: enhanced hypotensive effect
* Calcium-channel Blockers: enhanced hypotensive effect and AV delay with *verapamil*; hypotensive effect of *dihydropyridines* enhanced by *isoflurane*
* Dopaminergics: risk of *volatile liquid anaesthetics such as halothane* given with *levodopa*

  Oxytocin: oxytocic effect possibly reduced by *volatile anaesthetics* (also enhanced hypotensive effect and risk of arrhythmias)
* Sympathomimetics: risk of arrhythmias if *adrenaline or isoprenaline* given with *volatile liquid anaesthetics such as halothane*

  Theophylline: increased risk of arrhythmias with *halothane*; increased risk of convulsions with *ketamine*

Anaesthetics, Local *see* Bupivacaine, Lidocaine, Prilocaine, Ropivacaine
Analgesics *see* Aspirin, Nefopam, NSAIDs, Opioid Analgesics, and Paracetamol
Anion-exchange Resins *see* Colestyramine and Colestipol
Antacids

  ACE Inhibitors and Angiotensin-II Antagonists: reduced absorption of *captopril, enalapril, fosinopril* and *possibly other ACE inhibitors*

  Analgesics: excretion of *aspirin* increased in alkaline urine; absorption of *diflunisal* reduced

  Anti-arrhythmics: excretion of *quinidine* reduced in alkaline urine (may occasionally increase plasma concentrations)

  Antibacterials: reduced absorption of *azithromycin, cefpodoxime, ciprofloxacin, isoniazid, levofloxacin, nitrofurantoin, norfloxacin, ofloxacin, rifampicin, and most tetracyclines*

  Antiepileptics: reduced absorption of *gabapentin* and *phenytoin*

  Antifungals: reduced absorption of *itraconazole* and *ketoconazole*

  Antihistamines: reduced absorption of *fexofenadine*

  Antiplatelet Drugs: *dipyridamole* patient information leaflet advises avoidance of *antacids*

  Antimalarials: reduced absorption of *chloroquine and hydroxychloroquine; magnesium trisilicate* reduces absorption of *proguanil*

  Antipsychotics: reduced absorption of *phenothiazines*

  Antivirals: reduced absorption of *zalcitabine*

  Bile Acids: possibly reduced absorption of *ursodeoxycholic acid*

  Bisphosphonates: reduced absorption

Antacids *(continued)*
Cardiac Glycosides: possibly reduced absorption of *digoxin*
Corticosteroids: reduced absorption of *deflazacort*
Iron: *magnesium trisilicate* reduces absorption of *oral iron*
Lithium: *sodium bicarbonate* increases excretion (reduced plasma-lithium concentration)
Mycophenolate Mofetil: reduced absorption of *mycophenolate mofetil*
Penicillamine: reduced absorption
Ulcer-healing Drugs: possibly reduced absorption of *lansoprazole*

Antazoline *see* Antihistamines
Anti-arrhythmics *see* Adenosine; Amiodarone; Disopyramide; Flecainide; Lidocaine; Mexiletine; Moracizine; Procainamide; Propafenone; Quinidine; Tocainide
Anticholinergics *see* Antimuscarinics
Anticholinesterases *see* Parasympathomimetics
Anticoagulants *see* Heparin, Phenindione, and Warfarin
Antidepressants *see* Antidepressants, SSRI; Antidepressants, Tricyclic; MAOIs; Mianserin; Mirtazapine; Moclobemide; Nefazodone; Reboxetine; Trazodone; Tryptophan; Venlafaxine; Viloxazine
Antidepressants, SSRI
Alcohol: effects possibly enhanced
Anaesthetics: metabolism of *ropivacaine* reduced by *fluvoxamine*—avoid prolonged administration of ropivacaine
Anti-arrhythmics: plasma-flecainide concentration increased by *fluoxetine*
• Anticoagulants: effect of *acenocoumarol* and *warfarin* possibly enhanced
• *other* Antidepressants: CNS effects of *SSRIs* increased by *MAOIs* (risk of serious toxicity), see also p. 191; *moclobemide* see p. 191; plasma concentrations of some *tricyclics* increased; agitation and nausea with *tryptophan*; manufacturer of *reboxetine* advises avoid concomitant use with *fluvoxamine*; *fluvoxamine* increases plasma concentration of *nefazodone*
• Antiepileptics: antagonism (convulsive threshold lowered); plasma concentration of *carbamazepine* increased by *fluoxetine* and *fluvoxamine*; plasma concentration of *phenytoin* increased by *fluoxetine* and *fluvoxamine*; *phenytoin* and possibly other antiepileptics reduce plasma concentration of *paroxetine*
• Antihistamines: *citalopram, fluoxetine,* and *fluvoxamine* increase risk of arrhythmias with *terfenadine*—avoid concomitant use
• Antipsychotics: plasma concentration of *clozapine* possibly increased by *fluoxetine* and *fluvoxamine*; plasma concentration of *haloperidol* and *zotepine* increased by *fluvoxamine*; plasma concentration of *sertindole* increased by *fluoxetine* and *paroxetine*
• Antivirals: plasma concentration possibly increased by *ritonavir*
Anxiolytics and Hypnotics: plasma concentration of some *benzodiazepines* increased by *fluvoxamine*
• Barbiturates and Primidone: *see under* Antiepileptics, above
Beta-blockers: plasma concentration of *propranolol* increased by *fluvoxamine*
• Dopaminergics: hypertension and CNS excitation with *fluoxetine, paroxetine* or *sertraline* and *selegiline* (selegiline should not be started until 5 weeks after discontinuation of fluoxetine, avoid fluoxetine for 2 weeks after stopping selegiline; selegiline should not be started until 2 weeks after stopping sertraline, avoid sertraline for 2 weeks after stopping selegiline)
• 5HT$_1$ Agonists: risk of CNS toxicity increased by *sumatriptan* (avoid concomitant use); *fluvoxamine* possibly inhibits metabolism of *zolmitriptan* (reduce dose of zolmitriptan)

Antidepressants, SSRI *(continued)*
• Lithium: increased risk of CNS effects (lithium toxicity reported)
Opioid Analgesics: *tramadol* possibly increases risk of convulsions
• Theophylline: plasma-theophylline concentration increased by *fluvoxamine* (concomitant use should usually be avoided, but where not possible halve theophylline dose and monitor plasma-theophylline concentration)
Ulcer-healing Drugs: plasma concentration of *sertraline* increased by *cimetidine*
Antidepressants, Tricyclic
• Alcohol: enhanced sedative effect
Alpha$_2$-adrenoceptor Stimulants: manufacturers of *apraclonidine* and *brimonidine* advise avoid concomitant use
• Altretamine: risk of severe postural hypotension
Anaesthetics: risk of arrhythmias and hypotension increased
Analgesics: possibly increased side-effects with *nefopam*; *tramadol* possibly increases risk of convulsions; possibly increased sedation with *opioid analgesics*
• Anti-arrhythmics: increased risk of ventricular arrhythmias with drugs which prolong QT interval, including *amiodarone* (avoid concomitant use), *disopyramide*, *procainamide*, *propafenone* and *quinidine*
Antibacterials: plasma concentrations of some *tricyclics* reduced by *rifampicin* (reduced antidepressant effect)
• *other* Antidepressants: CNS excitation and hypertension with *MAOIs*, see also p. 186; *moclobemide see* p. 191; plasma concentrations of some *tricyclics* increased by *SSRIs*; manufacturer of *reboxetine* advises caution
• Antiepileptics: antagonism (convulsive threshold lowered); plasma concentrations of some *tricyclics* reduced (reduced antidepressant effect)
• Antihistamines: increased antimuscarinic and sedative effects; increased risk of ventricular arrhythmias with *terfenadine* (avoid concomitant use)
• Antihypertensives: in general, hypotensive effect enhanced, but antagonism of effect of *adrenergic neurone blockers* and of *clonidine* (and increased risk of hypertension on clonidine withdrawal)
• Antimalarials: increased risk of ventricular arrhythmias with *halofantrine*
Antimuscarinics: increased antimuscarinic side-effects
• Antipsychotics: increased risk of ventricular arrhythmias—avoid concomitant use with *pimozide* and *sertindole*; increased plasma concentrations of *tricyclic antidepressants* and increased antimuscarinic side-effects with *phenothiazines* and possibly *clozapine*
• Antivirals: plasma concentration possibly increased by *ritonavir*
Anxiolytics and Hypnotics: enhanced sedative effect
• Barbiturates and Primidone: *see under* Antiepileptics, above
• Beta-blockers: risk of ventricular arrhythmias associated with *sotalol* increased
Calcium-channel Blockers: *diltiazem* and *verapamil* increase plasma concentration of *imipramine* and possibly *other tricyclics*
• Cisapride: increased risk of ventricular arrhythmias—avoid concomitant use
Disulfiram: inhibition of metabolism of *tricyclics* (increased plasma concentrations and increased disulfiram reaction reported with *alcohol with amitriptyline*)
Diuretics: increased risk of postural hypotension
• Dopaminergics: manufacturer advises avoid concomitant use with *entacapone*; CNS toxicity reported with *selegiline*

Antidepressants, Tricyclic (continued)

Levothyroxine: manufacturer of *lofepramine* advises avoid *levothyroxine*

Muscle Relaxants: enhanced muscle relaxant effect of *baclofen*

Nitrates: reduced effect of *sublingual nitrates* (owing to dry mouth)

Oestrogens and Progestogens: *oral contraceptives* antagonise antidepressant effect (but side-effects may be increased due to increased plasma concentrations of *tricyclics*)

• Sympathomimetics: hypertension and arrhythmias with *adrenaline* (but local anaesthetics with adrenaline appear to be safe); hypertension with *noradrenaline*; *methylphenidate* may inhibit metabolism of *tricyclics*

Ulcer-healing Drugs: plasma concentrations of *amitriptyline, doxepin, imipramine, nortriptyline, and probably other tricyclics* increased by *cimetidine* (inhibition of metabolism)

Antidiabetics

Note. Includes Acarbose; Insulin; Metformin; Repaglinide, Sulphonylureas

ACE Inhibitors and Angiotensin-II Antagonists: *ACE inhibitors* possibly enhance hypoglycaemic effect

Alcohol: enhanced hypoglycaemic effect; flushing with *chlorpropamide* (in susceptible subjects); risk of lactic acidosis with *metformin*

Anabolic Steroids: possibly enhance hypoglycaemic effect

• Analgesics: *azapropazone, phenylbutazone* and possibly *other NSAIDs* enhance effect of *sulphonylureas*

Anion-exchange Resins: *colestyramine* enhances hypoglycaemic effect of *acarbose*

• Antibacterials: *chloramphenicol, co-trimoxazole,* and *sulphonamides* enhance effect of *sulphonylureas*; *ciprofloxacin* possibly enhances effect of *glibenclamide*; *neomycin* possibly enhances hypoglycaemic effect of *acarbose* and increases severity of gastro-intestinal effects; *rifamycins* reduce effect of *chlorpropamide, tolbutamide* and possibly *other sulphonylureas* (accelerate metabolism); *erythromycin* possibly increases plasma concentration of *repaglinide* (manufacturer advises avoid concomitant use); *rifampicin* possibly reduces plasma concentration of *repaglinide* (manufacturer advises avoid concomitant use)

Anticoagulants: possibly enhanced hypoglycaemic effects of *sulphonylureas* and changes to anticoagulant effects of *warfarin and other coumarins*

Antidepressants: *MAOIs* enhance hypoglycaemic effect

Antiepileptics: *plasma-phenytoin* concentration transiently increased by *tolbutamide* (possibility of toxicity); *phenytoin* possibly reduces plasma concentration of *repaglinide* (manufacturer advises avoid concomitant use)

• Antifungals: *fluconazole* and *miconazole* increase plasma concentrations of *sulphonylureas*—avoid concomitant use of *miconazole* with *glipizide*; *fluconazole, itraconazole,* and *ketoconazole* possibly increase plasma concentration of *repaglinide* (manufacturer advises avoid concomitant use)

Antihistamines: depressed thrombocyte count with concomitant use of *biguanides* and *ketotifen*

Antihypertensives: hypoglycaemic effect antagonised by *diazoxide*

Antipsychotics: *phenothiazines* possibly antagonise hypoglycaemic effect of *sulphonylureas*

Antivirals: *ritonavir* possibly increases plasma concentration of *tolbutamide*

Beta-blockers: enhanced hypoglycaemic effect and masking of warning signs of hypoglycaemia such as tremor

Antidiabetics (continued)

Calcium-channel Blockers: *nifedipine* may occasionally impair glucose tolerance

Corticosteroids: antagonism of hypoglycaemic effect

Diuretics: hypoglycaemic effect antagonised by *loop and thiazide diuretics*; *chlorpropamide* increases risk of hyponatraemia with *thiazides in combination with potassium-sparing diuretics*

Fibrates: may improve glucose tolerance and have an additive effect

Hormone Antagonists: manufacturer advises metabolism of *oral antidiabetics* possibly accelerated by *aminoglutethimide*; *octreotide* possibly reduces *insulin and antidiabetic drug* requirements in diabetes mellitus

Lithium: may occasionally impair glucose tolerance

Oestrogens and Progestogens: *oral contraceptives* antagonise hypoglycaemic effect

Orlistat: manufacturer advises avoid concomitant use with *acarbose* or *metformin*

Pancreatin: hypoglycaemic effect of *acarbose* reduced by *pancreatin*

Testosterone: hypoglycaemic effect possibly enhanced

Ulcer-healing Drugs: *cimetidine* inhibits renal excretion of *metformin* (increased plasma-metformin concentrations); *cimetidine* enhances hypoglycaemic effect of *sulphonylureas*

• Uricosurics: *sulfinpyrazone* enhances effect of *sulphonylureas*; *probenecid* possibly enhances hypoglycaemic effect of *chlorpropamide*

Antiepileptics *see* Carbamazepine; Clomethiazole; Clonazepam; Ethosuximide; Gabapentin; Lamotrigine; Phenytoin; Tiagabine; Topiramate; Valproate; Vigabatrin and p. 222

Antifungals *see* Amphotericin; Antifungals, Imidazole and Triazole; Flucytosine; Griseofulvin; Terbinafine

Antifungals, Imidazole and Triazole

Note. Imidazole antifungals include clotrimazole, ketoconazole and miconazole; triazoles include fluconazole and itraconazole

In general, interactions relate to multiple-dose treatment

Analgesics: metabolism of *alfentanil* inhibited by *ketoconazole* (risk of prolonged or delayed respiratory depression)

Antacids: *antacids* reduce absorption of *itraconazole* and *ketoconazole*

Anti-arrhythmics: plasma concentration of *quinidine* increased by *itraconazole*

• Antibacterials: *rifampicin* accelerates metabolism of *fluconazole, itraconazole* and *ketoconazole* (reduced plasma concentrations); plasma concentration of *rifampicin* may be reduced by *ketoconazole*; plasma concentration of *rifabutin* increased by *fluconazole* and possibly *other triazoles* (risk of uveitis—reduce rifabutin dose); plasma concentration of *ketoconazole* may be reduced by *isoniazid*

• Anticoagulants: effect of *acenocoumarol* and *warfarin* enhanced by *fluconazole, itraconazole, ketoconazole,* and *miconazole* (note: oral gel and possibly vaginal formulations absorbed)

• Antidepressants: manufacturer of *reboxetine* advises avoid concomitant use with *imidazoles* and *triazoles*

• Antidiabetics: plasma concentrations of *sulphonylureas* increased by *fluconazole* and *miconazole*—avoid concomitant use of *miconazole* with *glipizide*; *fluconazole, itraconazole,* and *ketoconazole* possibly increase plasma concentration of *repaglinide* (manufacturer advises avoid concomitant use)

• Antiepileptics: effect of *phenytoin* enhanced by *fluconazole* and *miconazole*; plasma concentrations of *itraconazole* and *ketoconazole* reduced by *phenytoin other* Antifungals: *imidazoles* and *triazoles* possibly antagonise effect of *amphotericin*

Antifungals, Imidazole and Triazole *(continued)*

• Antihistamines: *imidazoles* and *triazoles* inhibit *terfenadine* metabolism (avoid concomitant use of systemic or topical preparations—risk of hazardous arrhythmias); manufacturer advises possibility of increased plasma-loratadine concentration with *ketoconazole*; metabolism of *mizolastine* inhibited by *ketoconazole* and possibly *other imidazoles* (avoid concomitant use)

Antimuscarinics: reduced absorption of *ketoconazole*

• Antipsychotics: *itraconazole* and *ketoconazole* inhibit metabolism of *sertindole* (increased toxicity); risk of ventricular arrhythmias if *imidazoles* or *triazoles* given with *pimozide* (avoid concomitant use)

• Antivirals: *ketoconazole* inhibits metabolism of *indinavir* (reduce dose of indinavir); on theoretical grounds, plasma-indinavir concentration significantly increased by *itraconazole* (avoid concomitant use); plasma concentration of *zidovudine* increased by *fluconazole* (increased risk of toxicity); plasma concentration of *ketoconazole* reduced by *nevirapine* (avoid concomitant use); plasma concentration of *imidazoles* and *triazoles* possibly increased by *ritonavir*; plasma concentration of *saquinavir* increased by *ketoconazole* and possibly by *other imidazoles* and *triazoles*

• Anxiolytics and Hypnotics: plasma concentration of *midazolam* increased by *itraconazole*, *ketoconazole*, and possibly *fluconazole* (prolonged sedative effect)

• Calcium-channel Blockers: *itraconazole* inhibits metabolism of *felodipine* and possibly *other dihydropyridines* (increased plasma concentration)

• Cardiac Glycosides: plasma concentration of *digoxin* increased by *itraconazole*

• Ciclosporin: metabolism inhibited by *itraconazole*, *ketoconazole* and possibly *fluconazole* and *miconazole* (increased plasma-ciclosporin concentration)

• Cisapride: *fluconazole, itraconazole, ketoconazole* and *miconazole* inhibit metabolism (ventricular arrhythmias reported—avoid concomitant use)

Corticosteroids: *ketoconazole* inhibits metabolism of *methylprednisolone* and possibly *other corticosteroids*; *itraconazole* possibly inhibits metabolism of *methylprednisolone*

Cytotoxics: *itraconazole* may inhibit metabolism of *vincristine* (increased risk of neurotoxicity); *in vitro* studies suggest possible interaction between *ketoconazole* and *docetaxel*—consult product literature

Diuretics: plasma concentration of *fluconazole* increased by *hydrochlorothiazide*

• Lipid-regulating Drugs: *itraconazole, ketoconazole*, and possibly *other imidazoles* and *triazoles* increase risk of myopathy with *simvastatin*—avoid concomitant use of *itraconazole* with *simvastatin*; *itraconazole* and possibly *other imidazoles* and *triazoles* may increase risk of myopathy with *atorvastatin*; *itraconazole* increases plasma concentration of *cerivastatin*

Oestrogens and Progestogens: anecdotal reports of contraceptive failure with *fluconazole, itraconazole, ketoconazole* and possibly others

Sildenafil: *ketoconazole* increases plasma-sildenafil concentration (reduce initial dose of sildenafil)

• Tacrolimus: *clotrimazole, fluconazole, ketoconazole* and possibly *other imidazoles* and *triazoles* increase plasma-tacrolimus concentration

• Theophylline: plasma-theophylline concentration increased by *fluconazole* and possibly *ketoconazole*

Ulcer-healing Drugs: *histamine H_2- antagonists* reduce absorption of *itraconazole* and *ketoconazole*; *proton-pump inhibitors* reduce absorption of *ketoconazole* and possibly *itraconazole*; *sucralfate* reduces absorption of *ketoconazole*

Antihistamines

Note. Sedative interactions apply to a lesser extent to the non-sedating antihistamines, and they do not appear to potentiate the effects of alcohol.

Interactions do not generally apply to antihistamines used for topical action (including inhalation)

Grapefruit juice increases plasma concentration of ter-fenadine (avoid)

Alcohol: enhanced sedative effect

Antacids: reduced absorption of *fexofenadine*

• Anti-arrhythmics: increased risk of ventricular arrhythmias with *mizolastine* and *terfenadine* (avoid concomitant use with *amiodarone, disopyramide, procainamide* and *quinidine*)

• Antibacterials: metabolism of *terfenadine* inhibited by *clarithromycin* and *erythromycin* (avoid concomitant use of systemic or topical preparations—risk of hazardous arrhythmias); manufacturer advises possibility of increased plasma-loratadine concentration with *erythromycin*; metabolism of *mizolastine* inhibited by *erythromycin* and possibly *other macrolides* (avoid concomitant use); increased risk of ventricular arrhythmias with *quinupristin/ dalfopristin* (avoid concomitant use)

• Antidepressants: *MAOIs* and *tricyclics* increase antimuscarinic and sedative effects; *tricyclics* increase risk of ventricular arrhythmias with *terfenadine* (avoid concomitant use); *citalopram, fluoxetine, fluvoxamine,* and *nefazodone* increase risk of arrhythmias with *terfenadine*—avoid concomitant use

Antidiabetics: depressed thrombocyte count with concomitant use of *biguanides* and *ketotifen*

• Antifungals: *imidazoles* and *triazoles* inhibit *terfenadine* metabolism (avoid concomitant use of systemic or topical preparations—risk of hazardous arrhythmias); manufacturer advises possibility of increased plasma-loratadine concentration with *ketoconazole*; metabolism of *mizolastine* inhibited by *ketoconazole* and possibly *other imidazoles* (avoid concomitant use)

• Antimalarials: *halofantrine* and *quinine* increase risk of ventricular arrhythmias with *terfenadine* (avoid concomitant use)

Antimuscarinics: increased antimuscarinic side-effects

• Antipsychotics: increased risk of ventricular arrhythmias with *terfenadine*—avoid concomitant use with *pimozide, sertindole* or *thioridazine*

• Antivirals: *efavirenz, indinavir, nelfinavir, ritonavir,* and *saquinavir* increase risk of ventricular arrhythmias with *terfenadine*—avoid concomitant use; plasma concentration of *other non-sedating antihistamines* possibly increased by *ritonavir*

Anxiolytics and Hypnotics: enhanced sedative effect

• Beta-blockers: *sotalol* increases risk of ventricular arrhythmias with *mizolastine* and *terfenadine*

Betahistine: antagonism (theoretical)

• Cisapride: increased risk of ventricular arrhythmias with *terfenadine*—avoid concomitant use

Cytotoxics: *in vitro* studies suggest possible interaction between *docetaxel* and *terfenadine*—consult product literature

• Diuretics: hypokalaemia or other electrolyte imbalance increases risk of ventricular arrhythmias with *terfenadine*

Leukotriene Antagonists: *terfenadine* reduces plasma concentration of *zafirlukast*

• Pentamidine Isetionate: increased risk of ventricular arrhythmias with *terfenadine* (avoid concomitant use)

Ulcer-healing Drugs: manufacturer advises possibility of increased plasma-loratadine concentration with *cimetidine*

Antihypertensives *see* individual drugs or groups

Antimalarials *see* individual drugs

Antimuscarinics

Note. Many drugs have antimuscarinic effects; concomitant use of two or more such drugs can increase side-effects such as dry mouth, urine retention, and constipation; concomitant use can also lead to confusion in the elderly; interactions do not generally apply to antimuscarinics used by inhalation

Alcohol: sedative effect of *hyoscine* enhanced

Analgesics: increased antimuscarinic effects with *nefopam*

Anti-arrhythmics: increased antimuscarinic effects with *disopyramide; atropine* delays absorption of *mexiletine*

Antidepressants: increased antimuscarinic side-effects with *tricyclics* and *MAOIs*

Antifungals: reduced absorption of *ketoconazole*

Antihistamines: increased antimuscarinic side-effects

Antipsychotics: increased antimuscarinic side-effects of *phenothiazines* (but reduced plasma concentrations); increased antimuscarinic side-effects of *clozapine*

Cisapride: antagonism of gastro-intestinal effect

Dopaminergics: increased antimuscarinic side-effects with *amantadine*; absorption of *levodopa* possibly reduced

Metoclopramide and Domperidone: *antimuscarinics* antagonise gastro-intestinal effects

Nitrates: reduced effect of *sublingual nitrates* (failure to dissolve under tongue owing to dry mouth)

Parasympathomimetics: antagonism of effect

Antiplatelet Drugs *see* Aspirin, Clopidogrel, Dipyridamole, and Ticlopidine

Antipsychotics

Note. Increased risk of toxicity with myelosuppressive drugs—clozapine in particular should not be used concurrently with drugs associated with a substantial potential for causing agranulocytosis, such as carbamazepine, co-trimoxazole, chloramphenicol, sulphonamides, pyrazolone analgesics such as azapropazone, penicillamine, or cytotoxics; also avoid clozapine with long-acting depot antipsychotics (have myelosuppressive potential)

ACE Inhibitors and Angiotensin-II Antagonists: severe postural hypotension with *chlorpromazine* and possibly *other phenothiazines*

Alcohol: enhanced sedative effect

• Anaesthetics: enhanced hypotensive effect

Analgesics: enhanced sedative and hypotensive effect with *opioid analgesics*; severe drowsiness possible if *indometacin* given with *haloperidol*

Antacids and Adsorbents: reduced absorption of *phenothiazines* with *antacids* and possibly with *kaolin*

• Anti-arrhythmics: increased risk of ventricular arrhythmias with drugs which prolong QT interval —avoid concomitant use of *pimozide, sertindole* or *thioridazine* with *amiodarone, disopyramide, procainamide* or *quinidine* (also avoid haloperidol with amiodarone)

• Antibacterials: risk of arrhythmias if *clarithromycin* and possibly *erythromycin* given with *pimozide* (avoid concomitant use); *erythromycin* possibly increases plasma concentration of *clozapine* (possible increased risk of convulsions) and *sertindole*; *rifampicin* accelerates metabolism of *haloperidol* (reduced plasma-haloperidol concentration)

• Antidepressants: increased risk of arrhythmias with *tricyclic antidepressants*—avoid concomitant use of *pimozide* or *sertindole* with *tricyclics*; increased plasma concentrations and increased antimuscarinic effects notably on administration of *tricyclics* with *phenothiazines* and possibly *clozapine; fluvoxamine* possibly increase plasma concentration of *clozapine; fluoxetine* increases plasma concentration of *haloperidol* and *zotepine; fluoxetine* and *paroxetine* increase plasma concentration of *sertindole; oxypertine* causes CNS excitation and hypertension with *MAOIs; clozapine* possibly enhances central effects of *MAOIs;* manufacturer of *reboxetine* advises caution with antipsychotics; *nefazodone* increases plasma concentration of *haloperidol*

Antipsychotics *(continued)*

Antidiabetics: hypoglycaemic effect of *sulphonylureas* possibly antagonised by *phenothiazines*

• Antiepileptics: antagonism (convulsive threshold lowered); *carbamazepine* accelerates metabolism of *clozapine, haloperidol, olanzapine,* and *risperidone* (reduced plasma concentrations); *carbamazepine* and *phenytoin* accelerate metabolism of *sertindole* (reduced plasma concentration); *phenytoin* accelerates metabolism of *clozapine* and *quetiapine; phenobarbital* accelerates metabolism of *haloperidol* (reduced plasma concentration)

• Antifungals: *itraconazole* and *ketoconazole* inhibit metabolism of *sertindole* (increased toxicity); risk of ventricular arrhythmias if *imidazoles* or *triazoles* given with *pimozide* (avoid concomitant use)

• Antihistamines: increased risk of ventricular arrhythmias with *terfenadine*—avoid concomitant use with *pimozide, sertindole* or *thioridazine*

Antihypertensives: enhanced hypotensive effect; *haloperidol* and higher doses of *chlorpromazine* antagonise hypotensive effect of *adrenergic neurone blockers*; increased risk of extrapyramidal effects on administration of *methyldopa* and *metirosine*

• Antimalarials: increased risk of ventricular arrhythmias with *halofantrine;* avoid concomitant use of *pimozide* with *mefloquine* and *quinine*

Antimuscarinics: antimuscarinic side-effects of *phenothiazines* increased (but reduced plasma concentrations); antimuscarinic side-effects of *clozapine* increased

• Antivirals: *ritonavir* and possibly other *protease inhibitors* increase plasma concentration of *pimozide* (risk of ventricular arrhythmias—avoid concomitant use); *ritonavir* increases plasma concentration of *clozapine* (risk of toxicity—avoid concomitant use); *ritonavir* possibly increases plasma concentration of *other antipsychotics*

Anxiolytics and Hypnotics: enhanced sedative effect; *diazepam* increases plasma concentration of *zotepine; buspirone* increases plasma concentration of *haloperidol*

Barbiturates and Primidone: *see under* Antiepileptics, above

• Beta-blockers: *phenothiazines* and *pimozide* increase risk of ventricular arrhythmias with *sotalol*; concomitant administration of *propranolol* and *chlorpromazine* may increase plasma concentration of both drugs

Calcium-channel Blockers: enhanced hypotensive effect

• Cisapride: increased risk of ventricular arrhythmias with *haloperidol, phenothiazines, pimozide* and *sertindole*—avoid concomitant use

Desferrioxamine: manufacturer advises avoid *prochlorperazine* (also *levomepromazine* on theoretical grounds)

• Diuretics: hypokalaemia increases risk of ventricular arrhythmias with *pimozide* (avoid concomitant use)

Dopaminergics: antagonism of hypoprolactinaemic and antiparkinsonian effects of *bromocriptine* and *cabergoline*; antagonism of effect of *apomorphine, levodopa, lisuride,* and *pergolide*

Lithium: increased risk of extrapyramidal effects and possibility of neurotoxicity with *clozapine, haloperidol and phenothiazines*

Metoclopramide and Domperidone: increased risk of extrapyramidal effects with *metoclopramide*

Sympathomimetics: antagonise pressor action

Tetrabenazine: increased risk of extrapyramidal effects

Ulcer-healing Drugs: *cimetidine* may enhance effects of *chlorpromazine, clozapine,* and possibly *other antipsychotics*

Antivirals *see* Aciclovir and Famciclovir; Didanosine; Efavirenz; Ganciclovir; Indinavir; Lamivudine; Nelfinavir; Nevirapine; Ritonavir; Saquinavir; Stavudine; Valaciclovir; Zalcitabine; Zidovudine

Anxiolytics and Hypnotics

Alcohol: enhanced sedative effect

Anaesthetics: enhanced sedative effect

Analgesics: *opioid analgesics* enhance sedative effect

• Antibacterials: *erythromycin* and *quinupristin/
dalfopristin* inhibit metabolism of *midazolam*
(increased plasma-midazolam concentration, with
profound sedation) and *zopiclone*; *isoniazid* inhibits
metabolism of *diazepam*; *rifampicin* increases
metabolism of *diazepam* and possibly *other
benzodiazepines*

Anticoagulants: *chloral hydrate* and *triclofos* may
transiently enhance anticoagulant effect of
acenocoumarol and *warfarin*

Antidepressants: enhanced sedative effect;
manufacturer contra-indicates *buspirone* with
MAOIs; plasma concentrations of some
benzodiazepines increased by *fluvoxamine*; plasma
concentration of *alprazolam* increased by
nefazodone (reduce alprazolam dose)

Antiepileptics: metabolism of *clonazepam*
accelerated (reduced effect); plasma-phenytoin
concentrations increased or decreased by *diazepam*
and possibly *other benzodiazepines*

• Antifungals: *itraconazole, ketoconazole*, and possibly
fluconazole increase plasma concentration of
midazolam (prolonged sedative effect)

Antihistamines: enhanced sedative effect

Antihypertensives: enhanced hypotensive effect;
enhanced sedative effect with *alpha-blockers* and
possibly *moxonidine*

Antipsychotics: enhanced sedative effect; *diazepam*
increases plasma concentration of *zotepine*;
buspirone increases plasma concentration of
haloperidol

• Antivirals: *efavirenz, nelfinavir* and *saquinavir*
increase risk of prolonged sedation with *midazolam*
(avoid concomitant use); *indinavir* increases risk of
prolonged sedation with *alprazolam* and
midazolam (avoid concomitant use); *ritonavir*
increases plasma concentration of *alprazolam,
clorazepate, diazepam, flurazepam, midazolam* and
zolpidem (risk of extreme sedation and respiratory
depression—avoid concomitant use); plasma
concentration of *other anxiolytics and hypnotics*
possibly increased by *ritonavir*

Calcium-channel Blockers: *diltiazem* and *verapamil*
inhibit metabolism of *midazolam* (increased
plasma-midazolam concentration, with increased
sedation)

Cisapride: enhanced sedative effect of
benzodiazepines

Disulfiram: metabolism of *benzodiazepines* inhibited,
with enhanced sedative effect (*temazepam* toxicity
reported)

Dopaminergics: *benzodiazepines* occasionally
antagonise effect of *levodopa*

Lofexidine: enhanced sedative effect

Muscle Relaxants: *baclofen* and *tizanidine* enhance
sedative effect

Nabilone: enhanced sedative effect

Ulcer-healing Drugs: *cimetidine* inhibits metabolism
of *benzodiazepines and clomethiazole* (increased
plasma concentrations); *omeprazole* inhibits
metabolism of *diazepam* (increased plasma
concentration)

Apomorphine

Antipsychotics: antagonism of effects

other Dopaminergics: effect possibly enhanced by
entacapone

Apraclonidine *see* Alpha₂-adrenoceptor Stimulants

Aspirin

• *other* Analgesics: avoid concomitant administration
of other *NSAIDs* (increased side-effects)

Antacids and Adsorbents: excretion of *aspirin*
increased in alkaline urine; *kaolin* possibly reduces
absorption

• Anticoagulants: increased risk of bleeding due to
antiplatelet effect

Aspirin *(continued)*

Antiepileptics: enhancement of effect of *phenytoin*
and *valproate*

other Antiplatelet Drugs: increased risk of bleeding
with *clopidogrel* and *ticlopidine*

Corticosteroids: increased risk of gastro-intestinal
bleeding and ulceration; corticosteroids reduce
plasma-salicylate concentration

• Cytotoxics: reduced excretion of *methotrexate*
(increased toxicity)

Diuretics: antagonism of diuretic effect of
spironolactone; reduced excretion of
acetazolamide (risk of toxicity)

Leukotriene Antagonists: aspirin increases plasma
concentration of *zafirlukast*

Metoclopramide and Domperidone: *metoclopramide*
enhances effect of *aspirin* (increased rate of
absorption)

Mifepristone: manufacturer recommends avoid
aspirin until 8–12 days after *mifepristone*

Uricosurics: effect of *probenecid* and *sulfinpyrazone*
reduced

Atenolol *see* Beta-blockers

Atorvastatin *see* Statins

Atovaquone

• Antibacterials: plasma-atovaquone concentration
reduced by *rifampicin* and by *tetracycline* (possible
therapeutic failure of *atovaquone*)

Metoclopramide and Domperidone: plasma-
atovaquone concentration reduced by
metoclopramide

Atracurium *see* Muscle Relaxants (non-depolarising)

Atropine *see* Antimuscarinics

Auranofin *see* Gold

Azapropazone *see* NSAIDs

Azatadine *see* Antihistamines

Azathioprine

ACE Inhibitors and Angiotensin-II Antagonists:
increased risk of leucopenia with *captopril*

• Allopurinol: enhancement of effect with increased
toxicity (reduce dose of azathioprine when given
with allopurinol)

• Antibacterials: manufacturer reports interaction with
rifampicin (transplants possibly rejected);
increased risk of haematological toxicity with *co-
trimoxazole* and *trimethoprim*

• Anticoagulants: anticoagulant effect of warfarin
possibly reduced

Vaccines: see p. 541

Azelastine *see* Antihistamines

Azithromycin *see* Erythromycin and other Macrolides

Aztreonam

• Anticoagulants: anticoagulant effect of
acenocoumarol and *warfarin* possibly enhanced

Baclofen *see* Muscle Relaxants

Bambuterol *see* Sympathomimetics, Beta₂

Barbiturates and Primidone

Alcohol: enhanced sedative effect

Anti-arrhythmics: metabolism of *disopyramide and
quinidine* increased (reduced plasma
concentrations)

Antibacterials: metabolism of *chloramphenicol,
doxycycline, and metronidazole* accelerated
(reduced effect); *sulphonamides* enhance effect of
thiopental

• Anticoagulants: metabolism of *acenocoumarol* and
warfarin accelerated (reduced anticoagulant effect)

• Antidepressants: antagonism of anticonvulsant effect
(convulsive threshold lowered); metabolism of
mianserin and some tricyclics accelerated (reduced
plasma concentrations)

• Antiepileptics: concomitant administration of
phenobarbital or primidone with other
antiepileptics may enhance toxicity without a
corresponding increase in antiepileptic effect;
moreover interactions can complicate monitoring
of treatment; interactions include enhanced effects,
increased sedation, and reductions in plasma
concentrations; for further details see p. 222

Barbiturates and Primidone *(continued)*

Antifungals: *phenobarbital* reduces absorption of *griseofulvin* (reduced effect)

• Antipsychotics: antagonism of anticonvulsant effect (convulsive threshold lowered); *phenobarbital* accelerates metabolism of *haloperidol* (reduced plasma concentration)

• Antivirals: plasma concentration of *indinavir*, *nelfinavir* and *saquinavir* possibly reduced

• Calcium-channel Blockers: effect of *felodipine*, *isradipine* and probably *nicardipine*, *nifedipine* and *other dihydropyridines*, *diltiazem*, and *verapamil* reduced

Cardiac Glycosides: metabolism of *digitoxin only* accelerated (reduced effect)

• Ciclosporin: metabolism of *ciclosporin* accelerated (reduced effect)

• Corticosteroids: metabolism of *corticosteroids* accelerated (reduced effect)

Folic Acid and Folinic Acid: plasma concentration of *phenobarbital* and *primidone* possibly reduced by *folic acid* and *folinic acid*

Hormone Antagonists: metabolism of *toremifene* possibly accelerated

Leukotriene Antagonists: plasma concentration of *montelukast* reduced by *phenobarbital*

Levothyroxine: metabolism of levothyroxine accelerated (may increase levothyroxine requirements in hypothyroidism)

• Oestrogens and Progestogens: metabolism of *gestrinone*, *tibolone*, and *oral contraceptives* accelerated (reduced contraceptive effect, **important:** see p. 368)

Theophylline: metabolism of *theophylline* accelerated (reduced effect)

Tropisetron: *phenobarbitone* reduces plasma concentration of *tropisetron*

Vitamins: *vitamin D* requirements possibly increased

Beclometasone *see* Corticosteroids

Bendrofluazide (Bendroflumethiazide) *see* Diuretics (thiazide)

Bendroflumethiazide (Bendrofluazide) *see* Diuretics (thiazide)

Benorilate *see* Aspirin *and* Paracetamol

Benperidol *see* Antipsychotics

Benzatropine *see* Antimuscarinics

Benzhexol (Trihexyphenidyl) *see* Antimuscarinics

Benzodiazepines *see* Anxiolytics and Hypnotics

Benzthiazide *see* Diuretics (thiazide)

Benzylpenicillin *see* Penicillins

Beta-blockers

Note. Since systemic absorption may follow topical application of beta-blockers to the eye the possibility of interactions, in particular, with drugs such as verapamil should be borne in mind

ACE Inhibitors and Angiotensin-II Antagonists: enhanced hypotensive effect

Alcohol: enhanced hypotensive effect

Aldesleukin: enhanced hypotensive effect

Alprostadil: enhanced hypotensive effect

• Anaesthetics: enhanced hypotensive effect; increased risk of *bupivacaine* toxicity with *propranolol*

Analgesics: *NSAIDs* antagonise hypotensive effect; *morphine* possibly increases plasma concentration of *esmolol*

• Anti-arrhythmics: increased risk of myocardial depression and bradycardia; with *amiodarone* increased risk of bradycardia and AV block; increased risk of *lidocaine* toxicity with *propranolol*; *propafenone* increases plasma concentration of *metoprolol* and *propranolol*; risk of ventricular arrhythmias associated with *sotalol* increased by *amiodarone*, *disopyramide*, *procainamide*, and *quinidine* (avoid concomitant use)

Antibacterials: *rifampicin* accelerates metabolism of *bisoprolol* and *propranolol* (significantly reduced plasma concentration)

Beta-blockers *(continued)*

• Antidepressants: *fluvoxamine* increases plasma concentration of *propranolol*; risk of ventricular arrhythmias associated with *sotalol* increased by *tricyclics*

Antidiabetics: enhanced hypoglycaemic effect and masking of warning signs of hypoglycaemia such as tremor

• Antihistamines: risk of ventricular arrhythmias associated with *sotalol* increased by *mizolastine* and *terfenadine* (avoid concomitant use)

• Antihypertensives: enhanced hypotensive effect; increased risk of withdrawal hypertension with *clonidine* (withdraw beta-blocker several days before slowly withdrawing clonidine); increased risk of first-dose hypotensive effect with *post-synaptic alpha-blockers such as prazosin*

• Antimalarials: risk of ventricular arrhythmias associated with *sotalol* increased by *halofantrine*; increased risk of bradycardia with *mefloquine*

• Antipsychotics: risk of ventricular arrhythmias associated with *sotalol* increased by *phenothiazines* and *pimozide*; concomitant administration of *propranolol* and *chlorpromazine* may increase plasma concentration of both drugs

Anxiolytics and Hypnotics: enhanced hypotensive effect

• Calcium-channel Blockers: increased risk of bradycardia and AV block with *diltiazem*; severe hypotension and heart failure occasionally with *nifedipine* and possibly *other dihydropyridines*; asystole, severe hypotension, and heart failure with *verapamil* (see p. 105); *lercanidipine* may enhance hypotensive effect of *propranolol* and *metoprolol*

Cardiac Glycosides: increased AV block and bradycardia

• Cisapride: increased risk of ventricular arrhythmias with *sotalol* (avoid concomitant use)

Corticosteroids: antagonism of hypotensive effect

Diuretics: enhanced hypotensive effect; risk of ventricular arrhythmias associated with *sotalol* increased by hypokalaemia

Ergotamine: increased peripheral vasconstriction

$5HT_1$ Agonists: *propranolol* may increase plasma concentration of *rizatriptan* (reduce rizatriptan dose)

Levothyroxine: metabolism of *propranolol* accelerated (reduced effect)

• Moxisylyte: possible severe postural hypotension

Muscle Relaxants: *propranolol* enhances effect; possible enhanced hypotensive effect and bradycardia with *tizanidine*

Oestrogens and Progestogens: *oestrogens* and *combined oral contraceptives* antagonise hypotensive effect

Parasympathomimetics: risk of arrhythmias possibly increased by *pilocarpine*; *propranolol* antagonises effect of *neostigmine* and *pyridostigmine*

• Sympathomimetics: severe hypertension with *adrenaline* and *noradrenaline* and possibly with *dobutamine* (especially with *non-selective beta-blockers*)

Theophylline: *beta-blockers* should be avoided on pharmacological grounds (bronchospasm)

Tropisetron: risk of ventricular arrhythmias— manufacturer of tropisetron advises caution

Ulcer-healing Drugs: plasma concentrations of *labetalol*, *metoprolol* and *propranolol* increased by *cimetidine*; hypotensive effect antagonised by *carbenoxolone*

Xamoterol: antagonism of effect of *xamoterol* and reduction in beta-blockade

Betahistine

Antihistamines: antagonism (theoretical)

Betamethasone *see* Corticosteroids

Betaxolol *see* Beta-blockers

Bethanechol *see* Parasympathomimetics

Bezafibrate *see* Fibrates

Bicalutamide
Anticoagulants: effect of *warfarin* possibly enhanced
Bile Acids
Antacids: may reduce absorption of bile acids
Ciclosporin: *ursodeoxycholic acid* increases absorption of *ciclosporin*
Colestyramine and Colestipol: may reduce absorption of bile acids
• Fibrates: *clofibrate* increases elimination of cholesterol in bile
• Oestrogens and Progestogens: *oestrogens* increase elimination of cholesterol in bile
Biperiden *see* Antimuscarinics
Bismuth Chelate *see* Tripotassium Dicitratobismuthate
Bisoprolol *see* Beta-blockers
Bisphosphonates
Analgesics: bioavailability of *tiludronic acid* increased by *indometacin*
Antacids: reduced absorption
Antibacterials: increased risk of hypocalcaemia with *aminoglycosides*
Calcium Salts: reduced absorption
Iron: reduced absorption
Botulinum Toxin
• Antibacterials: effects enhanced by *aminoglycosides* (risk of toxicity)
• Muscle Relaxants: effects enhanced by *non-depolarising muscle relaxants*
Bretylium *see* Adrenergic Neurone Blockers
Brimonidine see Alpha₂-adrenoceptor Stimulants
Bromazepam *see* Anxiolytics and Hypnotics
Bromocriptine and Cabergoline
Alcohol: reduced tolerance to *bromocriptine*
Antibacterials: *erythromycin* and possibly *other macrolides* increase plasma concentration (increased risk of toxicity)
Antipsychotics: antagonism of hypoprolactinaemic and antiparkinsonian effects
Hormone Antagonists: *octreotide* increases concentration of *bromocriptine*
Metoclopramide and Domperidone: antagonise hypoprolactinaemic effect
• Sympathomimetics: increased risk of toxicity with *bromocriptine* and *isometheptene* or *phenylpropanolamine*
Brompheniramine *see* Antihistamines
Buclizine *see* Antihistamines
Budesonide *see* Corticosteroids
Bumetanide *see* Diuretics (loop)
Bupivacaine
Anti-arrhythmics: increased myocardial depression
Beta-blockers: increased risk of *bupivacaine* toxicity with *propranolol*
Buprenorphine *see* Opioid Analgesics
Buspirone *see* Anxiolytics and Hypnotics
Butobarbital *see* Barbiturates and Primidone
Cabergoline *see* Bromocriptine and Cabergoline
Calcium Salts
Antibacterials: reduced absorption of *ciprofloxacin* and *tetracyclines*
Bisphosphonates: reduced absorption
Cardiac Glycosides: large intravenous doses of *calcium* can precipitate arrhythmias
Diuretics: increased risk of hypercalcaemia with *thiazides*
Calcium-channel Blockers
Note. Grapefruit juice increases plasma concentration of dihydropyridine calcium-channel blockers (except amlodipine) and verapamil
Dihydropyridine calcium-channel blockers include amlodipine, felodipine, isradipine, lacidipine, lercanidipine, nicardipine, nifedipine, nimodipine and nisoldipine
ACE Inhibitors and Angiotensin-II Antagonists: enhanced hypotensive effect
Alcohol: enhanced hypotensive effect; plasma-alcohol concentration possibly increased by *verapamil*
Aldesleukin: enhanced hypotensive effect

Calcium-channel Blockers *(continued)*
Alprostadil: enhanced hypotensive effect
• Anaesthetics: *verapamil* increases hypotensive effect of *general anaesthetics* and risk of AV delay; *isoflurane* enhances hypotensive effect of *dihydropyridines*
• Anti-arrhythmics: *amiodarone-induced* risk of bradycardia, AV block, and myocardial depression increased by *diltiazem* and *verapamil*; plasma-concentration of *quinidine* reduced by *nifedipine*; increased risk of myocardial depression and asystole if *verapamil* given with *disopyramide* and *flecainide*; with *verapamil* raised plasma concentration of *quinidine* (extreme hypotension may occur)
• Antibacterials: *erythromycin* possibly inhibits metabolism of *felodipine* (increased plasma concentration); *quinupristin/dalfopristin* increases plasma concentration of *nifedipine*; *rifampicin* increases metabolism of *diltiazem, nifedipine, verapamil* and possibly *isradipine, nicardipine* and *nisoldipine* (plasma concentrations significantly reduced)
Antidepressants: *diltiazem* and *verapamil* increase plasma concentration of *imipramine* and *possibly other tricyclics*
Antidiabetics: *nifedipine* may occasionally impair glucose tolerance
• Antiepileptics: effect of *carbamazepine* enhanced by *diltiazem and verapamil; diltiazem* and *nifedipine* increase plasma concentration of *phenytoin*; effect of *felodipine* and *isradipine* and probably *nicardipine, nifedipine* and *other dihydropyridines* reduced by *carbamazepine, phenobarbital, phenytoin, and primidone*; effect of *diltiazem* and *verapamil* reduced by *phenobarbital* and *phenytoin*; plasma concentration of *nisoldipine* reduced by *phenytoin*
• Antifungals: *itraconazole* inhibits metabolism of *felodipine* and possibly other *dihydropyridines* (increased plasma concentration)
Antihypertensives: enhanced hypotensive effect; increased risk of first-dose hypotensive effect of *post-synaptic alpha-blockers such as prazosin*
Antimalarials: possible increased risk of bradycardia with some *calcium-channel blockers* and *mefloquine*
Antipsychotics: enhanced hypotensive effect
• Antivirals: *ritonavir* possibly increases plasma concentration of calcium-channel blockers
Anxiolytics and Hypnotics: *diltiazem* and *verapamil* inhibit metabolism of *midazolam* (increased plasma-midazolam concentration, with increased sedation)
• Barbiturates and Primidone: *see under* Antiepileptics, above
• Beta-blockers: increased risk of bradycardia and AV block with *diltiazem;* occasionally severe hypotension and heart failure with *nifedipine* and possibly *other dihydropyridines;* asystole, severe hypotension, and heart failure with *verapamil* (see p. 105); *lercanidipine* may enhance hypotensive effect of *propranolol* and *metoprolol*
other Calcium-channel Blockers: clearance of *nifedipine* reduced by *diltiazem* (increased plasma-nifedipine concentration)
• Cardiac Glycosides: plasma concentration of *digoxin* increased by *diltiazem, nicardipine, verapamil* and possibly *nifedipine*; increased AV block and bradycardia with *verapamil*
• Ciclosporin: plasma-ciclosporin concentrations increased by *diltiazem, nicardipine*, and *verapamil*; possibly increases plasma concentration of *nifedipine* (increased risk of side-effects such as gingival hyperplasia)
Diuretics: enhanced hypotensive effect
Lithium: neurotoxicity may occur without increased plasma-lithium concentrations in patients given *diltiazem* and *verapamil*
• Magnesium Salts: profound hypotension reported with *nifedipine* and *intravenous magnesium sulphate* in pre-eclampsia

Calcium-channel Blockers *(continued)*
  Moxisylyte: enhanced hypotensive effect
  Muscle Relaxants: *nifedipine* and *verapamil* enhance
    effect of *non-depolarising muscle relaxants*;
    hypotension, myocardial depression, and
    hyperkalaemia with *verapamil* and intravenous
    dantrolene; risk of arrhythmias with *diltiazem* and
    intravenous *dantrolene*; enhanced hypotensive
    effect with *tizanidine*
• Theophylline: *diltiazem, verapamil* and possibly *other
    calcium-channel blockers* enhance effect (increased
    plasma-theophylline concentration)
  Ulcer-healing Drugs: *cimetidine* inhibits metabolism
    of *some calcium-channel blockers* (increased
    plasma concentrations)
Calcium Levofolinate *see* Folic Acid and Folinic Acid
Candesartan *see* ACE Inhibitors and Angiotensin-II
    Antagonists
Capreomycin
  other Antibacterials: increased risk of nephrotoxicity
    with *colistin*; increased risk of nephrotoxicity and
    ototoxicity with *aminoglycosides and vancomycin*
  Cytotoxics: increased risk of nephrotoxicity and
    ototoxicity with *cisplatin*
Captopril *see* ACE Inhibitors and Angiotensin-II
    Antagonists
Carbachol *see* Parasympathomimetics
Carbamazepine
  Alcohol: CNS side-effects of *carbamazepine*
    possibly enhanced
• Analgesics: *dextropropoxyphene* enhances effect of
    carbamazepine; effect of *methadone* and *tramadol*
    decreased by *carbamazepine*
• Antibacterials: metabolism of *doxycycline* accelerated
    (reduced effect); plasma-carbamazepine
    concentration increased by *clarithromycin,
    erythromycin* and *isoniazid* (also isoniazid
    hepatotoxicity possibly increased); plasma-
    carbamazepine concentration reduced by *rifabutin*
• Anticoagulants: metabolism of *acenocoumarol* and
    warfarin accelerated (reduced anticoagulant effect)
• Antidepressants: antagonism of anticonvulsant effect
    (convulsive threshold lowered); plasma
    concentration of *carbamazepine* increased by
    fluoxetine, fluvoxamine, and *viloxazine*; metabolism
    of *mianserin* and *tricyclics* accelerated (reduced
    plasma concentrations); plasma concentration
    increased by *nefazodone* (also plasma-nefazodone
    concentration reduced); manufacturer advises avoid
    with *MAOIs* or within 2 weeks of *MAOIs*
• *other* Antiepileptics: concomitant administration of
    two or more antiepileptics may enhance toxicity
    without a corresponding increase in antiepileptic
    effect; moreover interactions between individual
    antiepileptics can complicate monitoring of
    treatment; interactions include enhanced effects,
    increased sedation, and reductions in plasma
    concentrations; for further details, see p. 222
• Antimalarials: *chloroquine* and *mefloquine*
    antagonise anticonvulsant effect
• Antipsychotics: antagonism of anticonvulsant effect
    (convulsive threshold lowered); metabolism of
    clozapine, haloperidol, olanzapine, risperidone,
    and *sertindole* accelerated (reduced plasma
    concentrations)
• Antivirals: plasma concentration of *indinavir,
    nelfinavir* and *saquinavir* possibly reduced; plasma
    concentration possibly increased by *ritonavir*
• Calcium-channel Blockers: *diltiazem and verapamil*
    enhance effect of *carbamazepine*; effect of
    felodipine, isradipine and probably *nicardipine,
    nifedipine* and *other dihydropyridines* reduced
  Cardiac Glycosides: metabolism of *digitoxin*
    accelerated (reduced effect)
• Ciclosporin: metabolism accelerated (reduced
    plasma-ciclosporin concentration)
• Corticosteroids: metabolism accelerated (reduced
    effect)

Carbamazepine *(continued)*
• Diuretics: increased risk of hyponatraemia;
    acetazolamide increases plasma-carbamazepine
    concentration
• Hormone Antagonists: *danazol* inhibits metabolism
    of *carbamazepine* (enhanced effect); metabolism of
    gestrinone and possibly *toremifene* accelerated
  Levothyroxine: metabolism accelerated (may
    increase levothyroxine requirements in
    hypothyroidism)
  Lithium: neurotoxicity may occur without increased
    plasma-lithium concentration
  Muscle Relaxants: effect of *non-depolarising muscle
    relaxants* antagonised (recovery from
    neuromuscular blockade accelerated)
• Oestrogens and Progestogens: *carbamazepine*
    accelerates metabolism of *oral contraceptives*
    (reduced contraceptive effect, **important:** see
    p. 368) and of *tibolone*
  Retinoids: plasma concentration possibly reduced by
    isotretinoin
  Theophylline: metabolism of *theophylline*
    accelerated (reduced effect)
• Ulcer-healing Drugs: metabolism inhibited by
    cimetidine (increased plasma-carbamazepine
    concentration)
  Vitamins: *carbamazepine* possibly increases *vitamin
    D* requirements
Carbenoxolone
  Note. Interactions do not apply to small amounts used
    topically on oral mucosa
  Antihypertensives: antagonism of hypotensive effect
  Cardiac Glycosides: toxicity increased if
    hypokalaemia occurs
  Corticosteroids: increased risk of hypokalaemia
  Diuretics: antagonism of diuretic effect; increased
    risk of hypokalaemia with *acetazolamide,
    thiazides,* and *loop diuretics*; inhibition of ulcer
    healing with *amiloride* and *spironolactone*
Carbonic Anhydrase Inhibitors *see* Diuretics
Cardiac Glycosides
• ACE Inhibitors and Angiotensin-II Antagonists:
    telmisartan and possibly *captopril* increase plasma
    concentration of *digoxin*
  Analgesics: *NSAIDs* may exacerbate heart failure,
    reduce GFR and increase plasma-cardiac glycoside
    concentrations
  Anion-exchange Resins: absorption possibly reduced
    by *colestyramine and colestipol*
  Antacids and Adsorbents: *antacids* and kaolin
    possibly reduce absorption of *digoxin*
• Anti-arrhythmics: plasma concentration of *digoxin*
    increased by *amiodarone, propafenone, and
    quinidine* (halve maintenance dose of digoxin)
  Antibacterials: *erythromycin* and possibly *other
    macrolides* enhance effect of *digoxin*; *rifamycins*
    accelerate metabolism of *digoxin* (reduced effect)
  Antidepressants: *nefazodone* increases plasma
    concentration of *digoxin*
  Antiepileptics: metabolism of *digitoxin* accelerated
    (reduced effect)
• Antifungals: increased toxicity if hypokalaemia
    occurs with *amphotericin*; plasma concentration of
    digoxin increased by *itraconazole*
• Antimalarials: *quinine, hydroxychloroquine,* and
    possibly *chloroquine* raise plasma concentration of
    digoxin; possible increased risk of bradycardia with
    mefloquine
  Barbiturates and Primidone: *see under* Antiepileptics,
    above
  Beta-blockers: increased AV block and bradycardia
  Calcium Salts: large intravenous doses of *calcium* can
    precipitate arrhythmias
• Calcium-channel Blockers: plasma concentration of
    digoxin increased by *diltiazem, nicardipine,
    verapamil* and possibly *nifedipine*; increased AV
    block and bradycardia with *verapamil*
  Corticosteroids: increased risk of hypokalaemia

Cardiac Glycosides *(continued)*
- Diuretics: increased toxicity if hypokalaemia occurs with *acetazolamide, loop diuretics, and thiazides*; effects of *digoxin* enhanced by *spironolactone*

  Hormone Antagonists: *aminoglutethimide* accelerates metabolism of *digitoxin only* (reduced effect)

  Lipid-regulating Drugs: plasma concentration of *digoxin* possibly increased by *atorvastatin*

  Muscle Relaxants: arrhythmias with *suxamethonium*; possible bradycardia with *tizanidine*

  Sulfasalazine: absorption of *digoxin* possibly reduced

  Ulcer-healing Drugs: increased toxicity if hypokalaemia occurs with *carbenoxolone*; plasma concentration of *digoxin* possibly increased by *proton pump inhibitors*; absorption possibly reduced by *sucralfate*

Carisoprodol *see* Anxiolytics and Hypnotics
Carteolol *see* Beta-blockers
Carvedilol *see* Beta-blockers
Cefaclor *see* Cephalosporins
Cefadroxil *see* Cephalosporins
Cefalexin *see* Cephalosporins
Cefamandole *see* Cephalosporins
Cefazolin *see* Cephalosporins
Cefixime *see* Cephalosporins
Cefotaxime *see* Cephalosporins
Cefoxitin *see* Cephalosporins
Cefpirome *see* Cephalosporins
Cefpodoxime *see* Cephalosporins
Cefprozil *see* Cephalosporins
Cefradine *see* Cephalosporins
Ceftazidime *see* Cephalosporins
Ceftriaxone *see* Cephalosporins
Cefuroxime *see* Cephalosporins
Celiprolol *see* Beta-blockers
Cephalosporins
  Alcohol: disulfiram-like reaction with *cefamandole*
  Antacids and Adsorbents: *antacids* reduce absorption of *cefpodoxime*
- Anticoagulants: anticoagulant effect of *warfarin and acenocoumarol* enhanced by *cefamandole* and possibly others

  Ulcer-healing Drugs: histamine H_2-antagonists reduce absorption of *cefpodoxime*

  Uricosurics: excretion of *cephalosporins* reduced by *probenecid* (increased plasma concentrations)
Cerivastatin *see* Statins
Certoparin *see* Heparin
Cetirizine *see* Antihistamines
Chloral *see* Anxiolytics and Hypnotics
Chloramphenicol
  other Antibacterials: *rifampicin* accelerates metabolism (reduced chloramphenicol-plasma concentration)
- Anticoagulants: anticoagulant effect of *acenocoumarol* and *warfarin* enhanced
- Antidiabetics: effect of *sulphonylureas* enhanced
- Antiepileptics: metabolism accelerated by *phenobarbital* (reduced chloramphenicol-plasma concentration); increased plasma concentration of *phenytoin* (risk of toxicity)
- Barbiturates and Primidone: *see under* Antiepileptics, above
Chlordiazepoxide *see* Anxiolytics and Hypnotics
Chloroquine and Hydroxychloroquine
  Antacids and Adsorbents: *antacids* reduce absorption of *chloroquine* and *hydroxychloroquine*; *kaolin* reduces absorption of *chloroquine*
- Anti-arrhythmics: *chloroquine* and *hydroxychloroquine* increase risk of ventricular arrhythmias with *amiodarone* (avoid concomitant use)
- Antiepileptics: antagonism of anticonvulsant effect
  other Antimalarials: increased risk of convulsions with *mefloquine*; increased risk of arrhythmias with *halofantrine* (**important:** see also CSM advice under Halofantrine, p. 303)

Chloroquine and Hydroxychloroquine *(continued)*
- Cardiac Glycosides: *hydroxychloroquine* and possibly *chloroquine* increase plasma concentration of *digoxin*
- Ciclosporin: *chloroquine* increases plasma-ciclosporin concentration (increased risk of toxicity)

  Parasympathomimetics: *chloroquine* and *hydroxychloroquine* have potential to increase symptoms of myasthenia gravis and thus diminish effect of *neostigmine* and *pyridostigmine*

  Ulcer-healing Drugs: *cimetidine* inhibits metabolism of *chloroquine* (increased plasma concentration)

  Vaccines: *see* Rabies Vaccine p. 553
Chlorphenamine (Chlorpheniramine) *see* Antihistamines
Chlorpheniramine (Chlorphenamine) *see* Antihistamines
Chlorpromazine *see* Antipsychotics
Chlorpropamide *see* Antidiabetics (sulphonylurea)
Chlortalidone *see* Diuretics (thiazide-related)
Chlortetracycline *see* Tetracyclines
Cholinergics *see* Parasympathomimetics
Ciclosporin
  Note. Grapefruit juice increases plasma-ciclosporin concentration (risk of toxicity)
- ACE Inhibitors and Angiotensin-II Antagonists: increased risk of hyperkalaemia

  Allopurinol: possibly increases plasma-ciclosporin concentration (risk of toxicity)
- Analgesics: increased risk of nephrotoxicity with *NSAIDs*; *ciclosporin* increases plasma concentration of *diclofenac* (halve diclofenac dose)

  Anti-arrhythmics: *amiodarone* and *propafenone* possibly increase plasma-ciclosporin concentration
- Antibacterials: *aminoglycosides, co-trimoxazole* (and *trimethoprim* alone), and *quinolones* increase risk of nephrotoxicity; *doxycycline* possibly increases plasma-ciclosporin concentration; *erythromycin, clarithromycin* and possibly *other macrolides* increase plasma-ciclosporin concentration; *quinupristin/dalfopristin* increases plasma-ciclosporin concentration; *rifampicin, intravenous trimethoprim* (and possibly *sulfadiazine*) reduce plasma-ciclosporin concentration

  Antidepressants: manufacturer of *reboxetine* advises caution
- Antiepileptics: *carbamazepine, phenobarbital, phenytoin, and primidone* accelerate metabolism (reduced plasma-ciclosporin concentration)
- Antifungals: *amphotericin* increases risk of nephrotoxicity; *griseofulvin* possibly reduces plasma-ciclosporin concentration; *itraconazole, ketoconazole,* and possibly *fluconazole* and *miconazole* inhibit metabolism (increased plasma-ciclosporin concentration)
- Antimalarials: *chloroquine* increases plasma-ciclosporin concentration (risk of toxicity)
- Antiplatelet Drugs: *ticlopidine* reduces plasma-ciclosporin concentration
- Antivirals: *ritonavir* possibly increases plasma-ciclosporin concentration
- Barbiturates and Primidone: *see under* Antiepileptics, above
- Bile Acids: *ursodeoxycholic acid* increases absorption of ciclosporin
- Calcium-channel Blockers: *diltiazem, nicardipine,* and *verapamil* increase plasma-ciclosporin concentration; *ciclosporin* possibly increases plasma concentration of *nifedipine* (increased risk of side-effects such as gingival hyperplasia)
- Colchicine: possibly increases risk of nephrotoxicity and myotoxicity (increased plasma-ciclosporin concentration)
- Corticosteroids: *high-dose methylprednisolone* increases plasma-ciclosporin concentration (risk of convulsions); *ciclosporin* increases plasma concentration of *prednisolone*

Ciclosporin *(continued)*
- Cytotoxics: increased risk of neurotoxicity with *doxorubicin*; increased risk of nephrotoxicity with *melphalan*; increased toxicity with *methotrexate*; *in vitro* studies suggest possible interaction with *docetaxel*—consult product literature
- Diuretics: *potassium-sparing diuretics* increase risk of hyperkalaemia
- Hormone Antagonists: *danazol* inhibits metabolism (increased plasma-ciclosporin concentration); *lanreotide* and *octreotide* reduce absorption (reduced plasma-ciclosporin concentration)
- Lipid-regulating Drugs: increased risk of myopathy with *statins*
- Oestrogens and Progestogens: *progestogens* inhibit metabolism (increased plasma-ciclosporin concentration)
- Potassium Salts: increased risk of hyperkalaemia
- Tacrolimus: plasma-ciclosporin half-life prolonged (increased risk of toxicity)
- Ulcer-healing Drugs: *cimetidine* possibly increases plasma-ciclosporin concentration
  Vaccines: *see* p. 541

Cilastatin [ingredient] *see Primaxin*®
Cilazapril *see* ACE Inhibitors and Angiotensin-II Antagonists
Cimetidine *see* Histamine H$_2$-antagonists
Cinnarizine *see* Antihistamines
Cinoxacin *see* Quinolones
Ciprofibrate *see* Fibrates
Ciprofloxacin *see* Quinolones
Cisapride
  Note. Grapefruit juice increases plasma concentration of cisapride (avoid)
  Alcohol: enhanced sedative effect
  Analgesics: *opioid analgesics* possibly antagonise effect on gastro-intestinal motility
- Anti-arrhythmics: increased risk of ventricular arrhythmias with *amiodarone, bretylium, disopyramide, procainamide* and *quinidine*—avoid concomitant use
- Antibacterials: *clarithromycin* and *erythromycin* possibly inhibit metabolism of *cisapride* (risk of ventricular arrhythmias—avoid concomitant use); increased risk of ventricular arrhythmias with *quinupristin/dalfopristin* (avoid concomitant use)
  Anticoagulants: effect of *oral anticoagulants* possibly enhanced
- Antidepressants: increased risk of ventricular arrhythmias with *maprotilene, nefazodone* and *tricyclics* (avoid concomitant use)
- Antifungals: *fluconazole, itraconazole, ketoconazole* and *miconazole* inhibit metabolism of *cisapride* (ventricular arrhythmias reported—avoid concomitant use)
- Antihistamines: increased risk of arrhythmias with *terfenadine*—avoid concomitant use
- Antimalarials: increased risk of ventricular arrhythmias with *halofantrine* and *quinine*—avoid concomitant use
  Antimuscarinics: antagonism of effect on gastro-intestinal motility
- Antipsychotics: increased risk of ventricular arrhythmias with *haloperidol, phenothiazines, pimozide*, and *sertindole*—avoid concomitant use
- Antivirals: increased risk of ventricular arrhythmias with *indinavir, nelfinavir, ritonavir* and possibly *other protease inhibitors* (avoid concomitant use); increased risk of ventricular arrhythmias with *efavirenz* (avoid concomitant use)
  Anxiolytics and Hypnotics: enhanced sedative effect of *benzodiazepines*
- Beta-blockers: increased risk of ventricular arrhythmias with *sotalol*—avoid concomitant use
- Lithium: increased risk of ventricular arrhythmias—avoid concomitant use
- Pentamidine Isetionate: increased risk of ventricular arrhythmias—avoid concomitant use
  Ulcer-healing Drugs: *cimetidine* increases plasma concentration of cisapride

Cisatracurium *see* Muscle Relaxants (non-depolarising)
Cisplatin *see* Platinum Compounds
Citalopram *see* Antidepressants, SSRI
Clarithromycin *see* Erythromycin and other Macrolides
Clemastine *see* Antihistamines
Clindamycin
  Muscle Relaxants: enhancement of effect of *non-depolarising muscle relaxants*
  Parasympathomimetics: antagonism of effect of *neostigmine* and *pyridostigmine*
Clobazam *see* Anxiolytics and Hypnotics
Clodronate Sodium *see* Bisphosphonates
Clofibrate *see* Fibrates
Clomethiazole *see* Anxiolytics and Hypnotics
Clomipramine *see* Antidepressants, Tricyclic
Clonazepam (general sedative interactions *as for* Anxiolytics and Hypnotics)
Clonidine (for general hypotensive interactions *see also* Hydralazine)
  ACE Inhibitors and Angiotensin-II Antagonists: previous treatment with *clonidine* possibly delays antihypertensive effect of *captopril*
- Antidepressants: *tricyclics* antagonise hypotensive effect and also increase risk of rebound hypertension on *clonidine* withdrawal; *viloxazine* possibly antagonises hypotensive effect
- Beta-blockers: increased risk of hypertension on *withdrawal* (withdraw beta-blocker several days before slowly withdrawing clonidine)
Clopamide *see* Diuretics (thiazide)
Clopidogrel
  Analgesics: increased risk of bleeding with *NSAIDs* (including *aspirin*)
- Anticoagulants: enhanced effect due to antiplatelet action of clopidogrel; manufacturer advises avoid concomitant use of *warfarin*
  other Antiplatelet Drugs: increased risk of bleeding
Clorazepate *see* Anxiolytics and Hypnotics
Clotrimazole *see* Antifungals, Imidazole and Triazole
Clozapine *see* Antipsychotics
Co-amoxiclav *see* Penicillins
Co-beneldopa *see* Levodopa
Co-careldopa *see* Levodopa
Codeine *see* Opioid Analgesics
Co-fluampicil *see* Penicillins
Colchicine
- Ciclosporin: possibly increases risk of nephrotoxicity and myotoxicity (increased plasma-ciclosporin concentration)
Cold and Cough Remedies *see* Antihistamines and Sympathomimetics
Colestipol *see* Colestyramine and Colestipol
Colestyramine and Colestipol
  Note. Other drugs should be taken at least 1 hour before or 4–6 hours after colestyramine or colestipol to reduce possible interference with absorption
  Analgesics: absorption of *paracetamol* and *phenylbutazone* reduced by *colestyramine*
  Antibacterials: *colestyramine* antagonises effect of oral *vancomycin*
- Anticoagulants: anticoagulant effect of *acenocoumarol, phenindione,* and *warfarin* enhanced or reduced
  Antidiabetics: hypoglycaemic effect of *acarbose* enhanced by *colestyramine*
  Antiepileptics: absorption of *valproate* possibly reduced
  Bile Acids: absorption of *ursodeoxycholic acid* possibly reduced
  Cardiac Glycosides: possibly reduced absorption
  Diuretics: reduced absorption of *thiazides* (give at least 2 hours apart)
  Levothyroxine: reduced absorption
  Mycophenolate Mofetil: absorption of *mycophenolate mofetil* reduced
  Raloxifene: absorption reduced by *colestyramine* (manufacturer advises avoid concomitant administration)

Colistin (other interactions *as for* Aminoglycosides)
Muscle Relaxants: enhanced muscle relaxant effect

Contraceptives, Oral
Note. Also covers oestrogens taken alone; interactions unlikely with low dose hormone replacement therapy
ACE Inhibitors and Angiotensin-II Antagonists: *oestrogens* and *combined oral contraceptives* antagonise hypotensive effect
• Antibacterials: *rifamycins* accelerate metabolism of both *combined* and *progestogen-only oral contraceptives* (reduced contraceptive effect, **important:** see p. 368); when *broad-spectrum antibiotics such as ampicillin and tetracycline* given with *combined oral contraceptives* possibility of reduced contraceptive effect (risk probably small, but see p. 368)
• Anticoagulants: antagonism of anticoagulant effect of *acenocoumarol, phenindione,* and *warfarin*
Antidepressants: antagonism of antidepressant effect has been reported, but side-effects of *tricyclics* may be increased due to higher plasma concentrations
Antidiabetics: antagonism of hypoglycaemic effect
• Antiepileptics: *carbamazepine, phenobarbital, phenytoin, primidone* and *topiramate* accelerate metabolism (reduced effect of both combined and progestogen-only contraceptives, **important:** see p. 368)
• Antifungals: *griseofulvin* accelerates metabolism (reduced contraceptive effect, **important:** see p. 368); anecdotal reports of contraceptive failure with *fluconazole, itraconazole, ketoconazole* and possibly others
Antihypertensives: *combined oral contraceptives* antagonise hypotensive effect
• Antivirals: *nelfinavir, nevirapine* and *ritonavir* accelerate metabolism of *combined oral contraceptives* (reduced contraceptive effect); *efavirenz* possibly reduces efficacy of *oral contraceptives*
• Barbiturates and Primidone: *see under* Antiepileptics, above
Beta-blockers: *oestrogens* and *combined oral contraceptives* antagonise hypotensive effect
• Bile Acids: *oestrogens* increase elimination of cholesterol in bile
• Ciclosporin: increased plasma-ciclosporin concentration
Corticosteroids: *oral contraceptives* increase plasma concentration of *corticosteroids*
Diuretics: *combined oral contraceptives* antagonise diuretic effect
• Modafinil: accelerates metabolism of *oral contraceptives* (reduced contraceptive effect)
• Retinoids: oral *tretinoin* reduces efficacy of *progestogen-only* and possibly *combined oral contraceptives*
Tacrolimus: efficacy of *oral contraceptives* possibly decreased
Theophylline: *combined oral contraceptives* delay excretion (increased plasma-theophylline concentration)
Ulcer-healing drugs: manufacturer advises *lansoprazole* possibly accelerates metabolism

Corticosteroids
Note. Do not generally apply to corticosteroids used for topical action (including inhalation)
Analgesics: increased risk of gastro-intestinal bleeding and ulceration with *aspirin* and *NSAIDs;* corticosteroids reduce plasma-*salicylate* concentration
Antacids: reduce absorption of *deflazacort*
• Antibacterials: *rifamycins* accelerate metabolism of *corticosteroids* (reduced effect); *erythromycin* inhibits metabolism of *methylprednisolone* and possibly *other corticosteroids*
• Anticoagulants: anticoagulant effect of *acenocoumarol* and *warfarin* possibly altered

Corticosteroids *(continued)*
Antidiabetics: antagonism of hypoglycaemic effect
• Antiepileptics: *carbamazepine, phenobarbital, phenytoin, and primidone* accelerate metabolism of *corticosteroids* (reduced effect)
• Antifungals: increased risk of hypokalaemia with *amphotericin* (avoid concomitant use unless corticosteroids required to control reactions); *ketoconazole* inhibits metabolism of *methylprednisolone* and possibly *other corticosteroids*; *itraconazole* possibly inhibits metabolism of *methylprednisolone*
Antihypertensives: antagonism of hypotensive effect
Antivirals: plasma concentration of *indinavir* and *saquinavir* possibly reduced by *dexamethasone*; *ritonavir* possibly increases plasma concentration of *dexamethasone, prednisolone* and possibly *other corticosteroids*
• Barbiturates and Primidone: *see under* Antiepileptics, above
Cardiac Glycosides: increased toxicity if hypokalaemia occurs with *corticosteroids*
• Ciclosporin: plasma-ciclosporin concentration increased by high-dose *methylprednisolone* (risk of convulsions); *ciclosporin* increases plasma concentration of *prednisolone*
Diuretics: antagonism of diuretic effect; *acetazolamide, loop diuretics, and thiazides* increase risk of hypokalaemia
Hormone Antagonists: *aminoglutethimide* accelerates metabolism of *corticosteroids* (reduced effect)
Oestrogens and Progestogens: *oral contraceptives* increase plasma concentration of *corticosteroids*
Somatropin: growth promoting effect may be inhibited
Sympathomimetics: increased risk of hypokalaemia if high doses of *corticosteroids* given with high doses of *bambuterol, fenoterol, formoterol, reproterol, ritodrine, salbutamol, salmeterol, terbutaline* and *tulobuterol; see also* CSM advice, p. 133; *ephedrine* accelerates metabolism of *dexamethasone*
Ulcer-healing Drugs: *carbenoxolone* increases risk of hypokalaemia
Vaccines: see p. 541

Co-trimoxazole and Sulphonamides
Note. For interactions with co-trimoxazole see also under Trimethoprim
Anaesthetics: effect of *thiopental* enhanced; increased risk of methaemoglobinaemia with *prilocaine*
• Anti-arrhythmics: *co-trimoxazole* increases risk of ventricular arrhythmias with *amiodarone* (avoid concomitant use)
• Anticoagulants: effect of *acenocoumarol* and *warfarin* enhanced
• Antidiabetics: effect of *sulphonylureas* enhanced
• Antiepileptics: antifolate effect and plasma concentration of *phenytoin* increased by *co-trimoxazole* and possibly *other sulphonamides*
• Antimalarials: increased risk of antifolate effect with *pyrimethamine* (includes *Fansidar®* and *Maloprim®*)
• Ciclosporin: increased risk of nephrotoxicity; plasma-ciclosporin concentration possibly reduced by *sulfadiazine*
• Cytotoxics: increased risk of haematological toxicity with *azathioprine* and *mercaptopurine*; antifolate effect of *methotrexate* increased by *co-trimoxazole*; risk of *methotrexate* toxicity increased by *sulphonamides*
Potassium Aminobenzoate: inhibits effect of *sulphonamides*

Cyclizine *see* Antihistamines
Cyclobarbitone *see* Barbiturates
Cyclopenthiazide *see* Diuretics (thiazide)
Cyclopentolate *see* Antimuscarinics

Cyclophosphamide and Ifosfamide
* Anticoagulants: *ifosfamide* possibly enhances effect of *warfarin*
* *other* Cytotoxics: increased toxicity with high-dose cyclophosphamide and *pentostatin* (avoid concomitant use)
   Muscle Relaxants: *cyclophosphamide* enhances effect of *suxamethonium*

Cycloserine
* Alcohol: increased risk of seizures
   other Antibacterials: increased CNS toxicity with *isoniazid*
* Antiepileptics: increased plasma concentration of *phenytoin* (risk of toxicity)

Cyproheptadine *see* Antihistamines
Cytarabine
   Flucytosine: plasma-flucytosine concentration possibly reduced

Cytotoxics *see under* individual drugs
Dalteparin *see* Heparin
Danazol
* Anticoagulants: effect of *acenocoumarol* and *warfarin* enhanced (inhibits metabolism)
* Antiepileptics: inhibits metabolism of *carbamazepine* (increased plasma-carbamazepine concentration)
* Ciclosporin: inhibits metabolism (increased plasma-ciclosporin concentration)
   Tacrolimus: plasma-tacrolimus concentration possibly increased

Dantrolene *see* Muscle Relaxants
Dapsone
   Antibacterials: plasma concentration reduced by *rifamycins*
   Probenecid: *dapsone* excretion reduced (increased risk of side-effects)

Debrisoquine *see* Adrenergic Neurone Blockers
Deflazacort *see* Corticosteroids
Demeclocycline *see* Tetracyclines
Desferrioxamine
   Antipsychotics: manufacturer advises avoid *prochlorperazine* (also *levomepromazine* on theoretical grounds)

Desflurane *see* Anaesthetics, General (volatile liquid)
Desmopressin
   Analgesics: effect of *desmopressin* potentiated by *indometacin*

Desogestrel *see* Progestogens
Dexamethasone *see* Corticosteroids
Dexamfetamine *see* Sympathomimetics
Dexketoprofen *see* NSAIDs
Dextromoramide *see* Opioid Analgesics
Dextropropoxyphene *see* Opioid Analgesics
Diamorphine *see* Opioid Analgesics
Diazepam *see* Anxiolytics and Hypnotics
Diazoxide (general hypotensive interactions *as for* Hydralazine)
   Antidiabetics: antagonism of hypoglycaemic effect

Diclofenac *see* NSAIDs
Dicyclomine (Dicycloverine) *see* Antimuscarinics
Dicycloverine (Dicyclomine) *see* Antimuscarinics
Didanosine
   Note. Antacids in formulation affect absorption of other drugs, *see also* Antacids, p. 580
   other Antivirals: plasma-didanosine concentration possibly increased by *ganciclovir*

Diflunisal *see* NSAIDs
Digitoxin *see* Cardiac Glycosides
Digoxin *see* Cardiac Glycosides
Dihydrocodeine *see* Opioid Analgesics
Dihydroergotamine *see* Ergotamine
Diltiazem *see* Calcium-channel Blockers
Dimenhydrinate *see* Antihistamines
Diphenhydramine *see* Antihistamines
Diphenylpyraline *see* Antihistamines
Diphenoxylate *see* Opioid Analgesics
Dipipanone *see* Opioid Analgesics

Dipivefrine *see* Sympathomimetics (*as for* adrenaline)
Dipyridamole
   Antacids: patient information leaflet advises avoidance of *antacids*
* Anti-arrhythmics: effect of *adenosine* enhanced and extended (**important** risk of toxicity)
* Anticoagulants: enhanced effect due to antiplatelet action of *dipyridamole*
   other Antiplatelet Drugs: increased risk of bleeding with *clopidogrel* and *ticlopidine*
   Cytotoxics: efficacy of *fludarabine* possibly reduced

Disodium Etidronate *see* Bisphosphonates
Disodium Pamidronate *see* Bisphosphonates
Disopyramide
* *other* Anti-arrhythmics: *amiodarone* increases risk of ventricular arrhythmias (avoid concomitant use); increased myocardial depression with any *anti-arrhythmic*
* Antibacterials: plasma concentration of *disopyramide* reduced by *rifampicin* but increased by *erythromycin* and possibly *clarithromycin* (risk of toxicity); increased risk of arrhythmias with *quinupristin/dalfopristin* (avoid concomitant use)
* Antidepressants: increased risk of ventricular arrhythmias with *tricyclics*; manufacturer of *reboxetine* advises caution
   Antiepileptics: plasma concentration of *disopyramide* reduced by *phenobarbital, phenytoin, and primidone*
* Antihistamines: increased risk of ventricular arrhythmias with *mizolastine* and *terfenadine* (avoid concomitant use)
* Antimalarials: increased risk of ventricular arrhythmias with *halofantrine*
   Antimuscarinics: increased antimuscarinic side-effects
* Antipsychotics: increased risk of ventricular arrhythmias—avoid concomitant use with *pimozide, sertindole* or *thioridazine*
* Antivirals: possibly increased risk of arrhythmias with *ritonavir*
   Barbiturates and Primidone: *see under* Antiepileptics, above
* Beta-blockers: increased myocardial depression; increased risk of ventricular arrhythmias associated with *sotalol* (avoid concomitant use)
* Calcium-channel blockers: increased myocardial depression with *verapamil*
* Cisapride: increased risk of ventricular arrhythmias (avoid concomitant use)
* Diuretics: cardiac toxicity of *disopyramide* increased if hypokalaemia occurs with *acetazolamide, loop diuretics,* and *thiazides*
   Nitrates: reduced effect of *sublingual nitrates* (failure to dissolve under tongue owing to dry mouth)
   Tropisetron: risk of arrhythmias—manufacturer of tropisetron advises caution

Distigmine *see* Parasympathomimetics
Disulfiram
   Alcohol: disulfiram reaction (*see* section 4.10)
   Antibacterials: psychotic reaction with *metronidazole* reported
* Anticoagulants: effect of *acenocoumarol* and *warfarin* enhanced
   Antidepressants: inhibition of metabolism of *tricyclic antidepressants* (increased plasma concentrations); increased disulfiram reaction with *alcohol* reported if *amitriptyline* also taken
* Antiepileptics: inhibition of metabolism of *phenytoin* (increased risk of toxicity)
   Anxiolytics and Hypnotics: inhibition of metabolism of *benzodiazepines,* with enhanced sedative effect (*temazepam* toxicity reported)
* Paraldehyde: increased risk of toxicity with *paraldehyde*
   Theophylline: inhibition of metabolism (increased risk of toxicity)

Diuretics

* ACE Inhibitors and Angiotensin-II Antagonists: enhanced hypotensive effect (can be extreme); risk of severe hyperkalaemia with *potassium-sparing diuretics*

Alprostadil: enhanced hypotensive effect

* Analgesics: *diuretics* increase risk of nephrotoxicity of *NSAIDs*; *NSAIDs* notably *indometacin* and *ketorolac* antagonise diuretic effect; *indometacin* and *possibly other NSAIDs* increase risk of hyperkalaemia with *potassium-sparing diuretics*; occasional reports of decreased renal function when *indometacin* given with *triamterene* (avoid concomitant use); diuretic effect of *spironolactone* antagonised by *aspirin; aspirin* reduces excretion of *acetazolamide* (risk of toxicity)

Anion-exchange Resins: *colestyramine and colestipol* reduce absorption of *thiazides* (give at least 2 hours apart)

* Anti-arrhythmics: cardiac toxicity of *amiodarone, disopyramide, flecainide, and quinidine* increased if hypokalaemia occurs; action of *lidocaine* and *mexiletine* antagonised by hypokalaemia; *acetazolamide* reduces excretion of *quinidine* (increased plasma concentration)

* Antibacterials: *loop diuretics* increase ototoxicity of *aminoglycosides, colistin,* and *vancomycin*

Antidepressants: increased risk of postural hypotension with *tricyclics*; possibly increased risk of hypokalaemia if *loop diuretics* or *thiazides* given with *reboxetine*

Antidiabetics: hypoglycaemic effect antagonised by *loop and thiazide diuretics*; *chlorpropamide* increases risk of hyponatraemia associated with *thiazides* in combination with *potassium-sparing diuretics*

* Antiepileptics: increased risk of hyponatraemia with *carbamazepine; acetazolamide* increases plasma concentration of *carbamazepine; carbonic anhydrase inhibitors* possibly increase risk of osteomalacia with *antiepileptics* such as *phenytoin*

Antifungals: increased risk of hypokalaemia if *loop diuretics* and *thiazides* given with *amphotericin; hydrochlorothiazide* increases plasma concentration of *fluconazole*

* Antihistamines: hypokalaemia or other electrolyte imbalance increases risk of ventricular arrhythmias with *terfenadine*

* Antihypertensives: enhanced hypotensive effect; increased risk of first-dose hypotensive effect of post-synaptic *alpha-blockers* such as *prazosin*

* Antimalarials: electrolyte disturbances increase risk of ventricular arrhythmias with *halofantrine*

* Antipsychotics: in hypokalaemia increased risk of ventricular arrhythmias with *pimozide* (avoid concomitant use)

Beta-blockers: enhanced hypotensive effect; in hypokalaemia increased risk of ventricular arrhythmias with *sotalol*

Calcium Salts: increased risk of hypercalcaemia with *thiazides*

Calcium-channel Blockers: enhanced hypotensive effect

* Cardiac Glycosides: increased toxicity if hypokalaemia occurs with *acetazolamide, loop diuretics, and thiazides;* effect enhanced by *spironolactone*

* Ciclosporin: increased risk of hyperkalaemia with *potassium-sparing diuretics*

Corticosteroids: increased risk of hypokalaemia with *acetazolamide, loop diuretics, and thiazides;* antagonism of diuretic effect

Cytotoxics: increased risk of nephrotoxicity and ototoxicity with *cisplatin*

other Diuretics: increased risk of hypokalaemia if *acetazolamide, loop diuretics or thiazides* given together; profound diuresis possible if *metolazone* given with *furosemide*

Diuretics *(continued)*

Hormone Antagonists: increased risk of hyponatraemia with *aminoglutethimide; thiazides* increase risk of hypercalcaemia with *toremifene; trilostane* increases risk of hyperkalaemia with *potassium-sparing diuretics*

* Lithium: *lithium* excretion reduced by *loop diuretics, potassium-sparing diuretics* and *thiazides* (increased plasma-lithium concentration and risk of toxicity—*loop diuretics* safer than *thiazides); lithium* excretion increased by *acetazolamide*

Moxisylyte: enhanced hypotensive effect

Muscle Relaxants: enhanced hypotensive effect with *baclofen* and *tizanidine*

Oestrogens and Progestogens: *oestrogens and combined oral contraceptives* antagonise diuretic effect

* Potassium Salts: hyperkalaemia with *potassium-sparing diuretics*

Sympathomimetics: increased risk of hypokalaemia if *acetazolamide, loop diuretics,* and *thiazides* given with high doses of *bambuterol, fenoterol, formoterol, reproterol, ritodrine, salbutamol, salmeterol, terbutaline,* and *tulobuterol;* see also CSM advice, p. 133

Ulcer-healing Drugs: increased risk of hypokalaemia if *acetazolamide, loop diuretics,* and *thiazides* given with *carbenoxolone; carbenoxolone* antagonises diuretic effect; *amiloride and spironolactone* antagonise ulcer-healing effect of *carbenoxolone*

Vitamins: increased risk of hypercalcaemia if *thiazides* given with *vitamin D*

Dobutamine *see* Sympathomimetics

Docetaxel

Antibacterials: *in-vitro* studies suggest possible interaction with *erythromycin*—consult product literature

Antifungals: *in-vitro* studies suggest possible interaction with *ketoconazole*—consult product literature

Antihistamines: *in-vitro* studies suggest possible interaction with *terfenadine*—consult product literature

Ciclosporin: *in-vitro* studies suggest possible interaction with *ciclosporin*—consult product literature

Domperidone

Analgesics: *opioid analgesics* antagonise effect on gastro-intestinal activity; absorption of *paracetamol* accelerated (enhanced effect)

Antimuscarinics: antagonism of effect on gastro-intestinal activity

Dopaminergics: possible antagonism of hypoprolactinaemic effect of *bromocriptine* and *cabergoline*

Donepezil *see* Parasympathomimetics
Dopamine *see* Sympathomimetics
Dopaminergics *see* Amantadine, Apomorphine, Bromocriptine and Cabergoline, Entacapone, Levodopa, Lisuride, Pramipexole, Quinagolide, Ropinirole
Dopexamine *see* Sympathomimetics
Dorzolamide *see* Diuretics (carbonic anhydrase inhibitor)

Note. Since systemic absorption may follow topical application of dorzolamide to the eye, the possibility of interactions should be borne in mind

Dosulepin (Dothiepin) *see* Antidepressants, Tricyclic
Dothiepin (Dosulepin) *see* Antidepressants, Tricyclic
Doxapram

Antidepressants: *MAOIs* may potentiate *doxapram*

Sympathomimetics: risk of hypertension

Theophylline: increased CNS stimulation

Doxazosin *see* Alpha-blockers (post-synaptic)
Doxepin *see* Antidepressants, Tricyclic
Doxorubicin

Antivirals: may inhibit effect of *stavudine*

* Ciclosporin: increased risk of neurotoxicity

Doxycycline *see* Tetracyclines

Doxylamine *see* Antihistamines
Droperidol *see* Antipsychotics
Dydrogesterone *see* Progestogens
Ecothiopate *see* Parasympathomimetics
Edrophonium *see* Parasympathomimetics
Efavirenz
Antibacterials: increased risk of rash with *clarithromycin*; *rifampicin* reduces plasma concentration of efavirenz (increase efavirenz dose)
• Antihistamines: increased risk of ventricular arrhythmias with *terfenadine* (avoid concomitant use)
other Antivirals: efavirenz reduces plasma concentration of *indinavir* (increase indinavir dose); increased risk of toxicity with efavirenz and *ritonavir* (monitor liver function tests); efavirenz significantly reduces plasma concentration of *saquinavir*
• Anxiolytics and Hypnotics: risk of prolonged sedation with *midazolam* (avoid concomitant use)
• Cisapride: increased risk of ventricular arrhythmias (avoid concomitant use)
Oestrogens and Progestogens: possibly reduced efficacy of *oral contraceptives*
Eformoterol (Formoterol) *see* Sympathomimetics, Beta₂
Enalapril *see* ACE Inhibitors and Angiotensin-II Antagonists
Enflurane *see* Anaesthetics, General (volatile liquid)
Enoxaparin *see* Heparin
Entacapone
Antidepressants: manufacturer advises avoid concomitant use with *MAOIs, tricyclics, maprotiline* or *venlafaxine*
Antihypertensives: effect of *methyldopa* possibly enhanced
other Dopaminergics: effect of *apomorphine* possibly enhanced
Iron: absorption of entacapone reduced
Sympathomimetics: effect of *adrenaline, dobutamine, dopamine, isoprenaline* and *noradrenaline* possibly enhanced
Ephedrine *see* Sympathomimetics
Epinephrine (Adrenaline) *see* Sympathomimetics
Epoetin
ACE Inhibitors and Angiotensin-II Antagonists: antagonism of hypotensive effect; increased risk of hyperkalaemia
Ergotamine
• Antibacterials: risk of ergotism with *azithromycin, clarithromycin* and *erythromycin*—avoid concomitant use
Antidepressants: possibly increased blood pressure with *reboxetine*
• Antivirals: risk of ergotism with *indinavir, nelfinavir, ritonavir* and possibly *saquinavir*—avoid concomitant use
Beta-blockers: increased peripheral vasoconstriction
• 5HT₁ Agonists: increased risk of vasospasm (avoid ergotamine for 6 hours after rizatriptan, sumatriptan or zolmitriptan; avoid rizatriptan or sumatriptan for 24 hours and zolmitriptan for 6 hours after ergotamine)
Erythromycin and other Macrolides
Note. Interactions do not apply to small amounts used topically
Analgesics: plasma concentration of *alfentanil* increased by *erythromycin*
Antacids: *antacids* reduce absorption of *azithromycin*
• Anti-arrhythmics: plasma concentration of *disopyramide* increased by *erythromycin* and possibly *clarithromycin* (risk of toxicity); *erythromycin* (parenteral) increases risk of ventricular arrhythmias with *amiodarone* (avoid concomitant use)
• *other* Antibacterials: *clarithromycin* and possibly *other macrolides* increase plasma concentration of *rifabutin* (risk of uveitis—reduce rifabutin dose)

Erythromycin and other Macrolides *(continued)*
• Anticoagulants: effect of *acenocoumarol* and *warfarin* enhanced by *erythromycin* and possibly enhanced by *clarithromycin* and some *other macrolides*
• Antidepressants: manufacturer of *reboxetine* advises avoid concomitant use
Antidiabetics: *erythromycin* possibly increases plasma concentration of *repaglinide* (manufacturer advises avoid concomitant use)
• Antiepileptics: *clarithromycin* and *erythromycin* inhibit metabolism of *carbamazepine* (increased plasma-carbamazepine concentration); *erythromycin* possibly inhibits metabolism of *valproate* (increased plasma-valproate concentration); *clarithromycin* inhibits metabolism of *phenytoin* (increased plasma-phenytoin concentration)
• Antihistamines: *clarithromycin* and *erythromycin* inhibit metabolism of *terfenadine* (avoid concomitant use of systemic or topical preparations—risk of hazardous arrhythmias, see p. 150); manufacturer advises possibility of increased plasma-loratadine concentration with *erythromycin;* metabolism of *mizolastine* inhibited by *erythromycin* and possibly *other macrolides* (avoid concomitant use)
• Antipsychotics: risk of arrhythmias if *clarithromycin* and possibly *erythromycin* given with *pimozide* (avoid concomitant use); *erythromycin* possibly increases plasma concentration of *clozapine* (possible increased risk of convulsions) and *sertindole*
• Antivirals: *clarithromycin* tablets reduce absorption of *zidovudine; ritonavir* possibly increases plasma concentration of *macrolides*; increased risk of rash when *efavirenz* given with *clarithromycin*
• Anxiolytics and Hypnotics: *erythromycin* inhibits metabolism of *midazolam* (increased plasma-midazolam concentration, with profound sedation) and *zopiclone*
Calcium-channel Blockers: *erythromycin* possibly inhibits metabolism of *felodipine* (increased plasma concentration)
Cardiac Glycosides: effect of *digoxin* enhanced by *erythromycin* and possibly enhanced by *other macrolides*
• Ciclosporin: *erythromycin, clarithromycin* and possibly *other macrolides* inhibit metabolism (increased plasma-ciclosporin concentration)
• Cisapride: *clarithromycin* and *erythromycin* possibly inhibit metabolism of *cisapride* (risk of ventricular arrhythmias—avoid concomitant use)
Corticosteroids: *erythromycin* inhibits metabolism of *methylprednisolone* and possibly *other corticosteroids*
Cytotoxics: *in vitro* studies suggest possible interaction between *erythromycin* and *docetaxel*—consult product literature
Dopaminergics: plasma concentration of *bromocriptine* and *cabergoline* increased by *erythromycin* and possibly *other macrolides*
• Ergotamine: risk of ergotism—avoid concomitant use
Leukotriene Antagonists: *erythromycin* reduces plasma concentration of *zafirlukast*
Lipid-regulating Drugs: *clarithromycin* and *erythromycin* increase risk of myopathy with *simvastatin; erythromycin* possibly increases risk of myopathy with *atorvastatin* and *cerivastatin*
Sildenafil: *erythromycin* increases plasma-sildenafil concentration (reduce initial dose of sildenafil)
• Tacrolimus: *clarithromycin* and *erythromycin* increase plasma-tacrolimus concentration
• Theophylline: *clarithromycin* and *erythromycin* inhibit metabolism (increased plasma-theophylline concentration) (if erythromycin given by mouth, also decreased plasma-erythromycin concentration)
Ulcer-healing Drugs: *cimetidine* increases plasma-erythromycin concentration (increased risk of toxicity, including deafness)

Erythropoietin *see* Epoetin
Esmolol *see* Beta-blockers
Estropipate *see* Contraceptives, Oral
Ethinylestradiol *see* Contraceptives, Oral
Ethosuximide
- Antibacterials: *isoniazid* increases plasma
  concentrations (increased risk of toxicity)
- Antidepressants: antagonism (convulsive threshold
  lowered)
- *other* Antiepileptics: concomitant administration of
  two or more antiepileptics may enhance toxicity
  without a corresponding increase in antiepileptic
  effect; moreover interactions between individual
  antiepileptics can complicate monitoring of
  treatment; interactions include enhanced effects,
  increased sedation, and reductions in plasma
  concentrations; for further details, see p. 222
- Antipsychotics: antagonism (convulsive threshold
  lowered)
Etidronate Disodium *see* Bisphosphonates
Etodolac *see* NSAIDs
Etomidate *see* Anaesthetics, General
Etonogestrel *see* Progestogens
Etynodiol *see* Progestogens
Famciclovir *see* Aciclovir and Famciclovir
Famotidine *see* Histamine H$_2$-antagonists
Fansidar® contains Sulfadoxine and Pyrimethamine
Felodipine *see* Calcium-channel Blockers
Fenbufen *see* NSAIDs
Fenofibrate *see* Fibrates
Fenoprofen *see* NSAIDs
Fenoterol *see* Sympathomimetics, Beta$_2$
Fentanyl *see* Opioid Analgesics
Ferrous Salts *see* Iron
Fexofenadine *see* Antihistamines
Fibrates
- Anticoagulants: enhancement of effect of
  acenocoumarol, phenindione, and *warfarin*
  Antidiabetics: may improve glucose tolerance and
  have additive effect
- Bile Acids: *clofibrate* increases elimination of
  cholesterol in bile
- *other* Lipid-regulating Drugs: increased risk of
  myopathy with *statins*
  Orlistat: manufacturer advises avoid concomitant use
Filgrastim
  Note. Use not recommended in period from 24 hours
  before to 24 hours after chemotherapy—for further
  details consult product literature
  Cytotoxics: possible exacerbation of neutropenia
  with *fluorouracil*
Finasteride
  Note. No clinically important interactions reported
Flavoxate *see* Antimuscarinics
Flecainide
- *other* Anti-arrhythmics: *amiodarone* increases
  plasma-flecainide concentration (and increases risk
  of ventricular arrhythmias—avoid concomitant
  use); increased myocardial depression with any
  anti-arrhythmic
- Antidepressants: *fluoxetine* increases plasma-
  flecainide concentration; increased risk of
  arrhythmias with *tricyclics*; manufacturer of
  reboxetine advises caution
- Antihistamines: increased risk of ventricular
  arrhythmias with *terfenadine*
- Antimalarials: *quinine* increases plasma
  concentration of *flecainide*; increased risk of
  arrhythmias with *halofantrine* (**important:** see
  p. 303)
- Antivirals: plasma concentration increased by
  ritonavir (increased risk of ventricular
  arrhythmias—avoid concomitant use)
- Beta-blockers: increased myocardial depression and
  bradycardia
- Calcium-channel Blockers: increased myocardial
  depression and asystole with *verapamil*

Flecainide *(continued)*
- Diuretics: cardiac toxicity increased if hypokalaemia
  occurs
  Ulcer-healing Drugs: *cimetidine* inhibits metabolism
  of *flecainide* (increased plasma-flecainide
  concentration)
Flucloxacillin *see* Penicillins
Fluconazole *see* Antifungals, Imidazole and Triazole
Flucytosine
  other Antifungals: renal excretion reduced and
  cellular uptake increased by *amphotericin*
  (flucytosine toxicity possibly increased)
  Cytotoxics: *cytarabine* possibly reduces plasma-
  flucytosine concentrations
Fludarabine
  Antiplatelet Drugs: efficacy possibly reduced by
  dipyridamole
- *other* Cytotoxics: increased pulmonary toxicity with
  pentostatin (unacceptably high incidence of
  fatalities)
Fludrocortisone *see* Corticosteroids
Flunisolide *see* Corticosteroids
Flunitrazepam *see* Anxiolytics and Hypnotics
Fluorouracil
  Antibacterials: *metronidazole* inhibits metabolism
  (increased toxicity)
  Filgrastim: possible exacerbation of neutropenia
  Ulcer-healing Drugs: *cimetidine* inhibits metabolism
  (increased plasma-fluorouracil concentration)
Fluoxetine *see* Antidepressants, SSRI
Flupentixol *see* Antipsychotics
Fluphenazine *see* Antipsychotics
Flurazepam *see* Anxiolytics and Hypnotics
Flurbiprofen *see* NSAIDs
Flutamide
- Anticoagulants: effect of *warfarin* enhanced
Fluticasone *see* Corticosteroids
Fluvastatin *see* Statins
Fluvoxamine *see* Antidepressants, SSRI
Folic Acid and Folinic Acid
  Antiepileptics: plasma concentrations of *phenobarbital,
  phenytoin,* and *primidone* possibly reduced
Formoterol (Eformoterol) *see* Sympathomimetics,
  Beta$_2$
Fosinopril *see* ACE Inhibitors
Fosphenytoin *see* Phenytoin
Framycetin *see* Aminoglycosides
Frusemide (Furosemide) *see* Diuretics (loop)
Furosemide (Frusemide) *see* Diuretics (loop)
Gabapentin
  Antacids: reduced gabapentin absorption
  other Antiepileptics: none demonstrated with
  carbamazepine, phenobarbital, phenytoin, or
  valproate
Gallamine *see* Muscle Relaxants (non-depolarising)
Ganciclovir
  Note: Increased risk of myelosuppression with other
  myelosuppressive drugs—consult product literature
- Antibacterials: increased toxicity with *Primaxin*®
  (convulsions reported)
- *other* Antivirals: plasma concentration of *didanosine*
  possibly increased; profound myelosuppression
  with *zidovudine* (if possible avoid concomitant
  administration particularly during initial
  ganciclovir therapy)
  Uricosurics: *probenecid* reduces renal excretion
  (increased plasma half-life)
Gemfibrozil *see* Fibrates
Gentamicin *see* Aminoglycosides
Gestodene *see* Progestogens
Gestonorone *see* Progestogens
Gestrinone
  Antibacterials: *rifampicin* accelerates metabolism
  (reduced plasma concentration)
  Antiepileptics: *carbamazepine, phenobarbital,
  phenytoin, and primidone* accelerate metabolism
  (reduced plasma concentration)
  Barbiturates and Primidone: *see under* Antiepileptics,
  above

Glibenclamide *see* Antidiabetics (sulphonylurea)
Gliclazide *see* Antidiabetics (sulphonylurea)
Glimepiride *see* Antidiabetics (sulphonylurea)
Glipizide *see* Antidiabetics (sulphonylurea)
Gliquidone *see* Antidiabetics (sulphonylurea)
Glyceryl Trinitrate *see* Nitrates
Gold
  Note. Increased risk of toxicity with other nephrotoxic and myelosuppressive drugs
Griseofulvin
• Anticoagulants: metabolism of *acenocoumarol* and *warfarin* accelerated (reduced anticoagulant effect)
  Antiepileptics: absorption reduced by *phenobarbital* (reduced effect)
  Barbiturates and Primidone: *see under* Antiepileptics, above
  Ciclosporin: plasma-ciclosporin concentration possibly reduced
• Oestrogens and Progestogens: metabolism of *oral contraceptives* accelerated (reduced contraceptive effect, **important:** see p. 368)
Guanethidine *see* Adrenergic Neurone Blockers
Guar Gum
  Antibacterials: absorption of *phenoxymethylpenicillin* reduced
Halofantrine
• Anti-arrhythmics: increased risk of ventricular arrhythmias with drugs which prolong QT interval (including amiodarone, disopyramide, flecainide, procainamide and quinidine)
• Antidepressants: increased risk of ventricular arrhythmias with *tricyclics*
• Antihistamines: increased risk of ventricular arrhythmias with *terfenadine* (avoid concomitant use)
• *other* Antimalarials: increased risk of arrhythmias with *chloroquine, mefloquine* and *quinine* (**important:** see also CSM advice under Halofantrine, p. 303)
• Antipsychotics: increased risk of of ventricular arrhythmias with *phenothiazines*
• Beta-blockers: increased risk of ventricular arrhythmias with *sotalol*
• Cisapride: increased risk of ventricular arrhythmias (avoid concomitant use)
• Diuretics: increased risk of ventricular arrhythmias if electrolyte disturbances occur
Haloperidol *see* Antipsychotics
Halothane *see* Anaesthetics, General (volatile liquid)
Heparin
  ACE Inhibitors and Angiotensin-II Antagonists: increased risk of hyperkalaemia
• Analgesics: *aspirin* enhances anticoagulant effect; increased risk of haemorrhage with *intravenous diclofenac* and with *ketorolac* (avoid concomitant use, including low-dose heparin); possibly increased risk of bleeding with NSAIDs
  Antiplatelet Drugs: *aspirin, clopidogrel, dipyridamole* and *ticlopidine* enhance anticoagulant effect
• Nitrates: *glyceryl trinitrate infusion* increases excretion (reduced anticoagulant effect)
Histamine H₁-antagonists *see* Antihistamines
Histamine H₂-antagonists
  Analgesics: *cimetidine* inhibits metabolism of *opioid analgesics* notably *pethidine* (increased plasma concentrations); *cimetidine* possibly increases plasma concentration of *azapropazone*
  Anthelmintics: *cimetidine* possibly inhibits metabolism of *mebendazole* (increased plasma concentration)
• Anti-arrhythmics: *cimetidine* increases plasma concentrations of *amiodarone, flecainide, lidocaine, procainamide, propafenone, quinidine,* and possibly *moracizine*

Histamine H₂-antagonists *(continued)*
  Antibacterials: absorption of *cefpodoxime* reduced; *cimetidine* increases plasma-erythromycin concentration (increased risk of toxicity, including deafness); *rifampicin* accelerates metabolism of *cimetidine* (reduced plasma-cimetidine concentration); *cimetidine* inhibits metabolism of *metronidazole* (increased plasma-metronidazole concentration)
• Anticoagulants: *cimetidine* enhances anticoagulant effect of *acenocoumarol* and *warfarin* (inhibits metabolism)
  Antidepressants: *cimetidine* inhibits metabolism of *amitriptyline, doxepin, imipramine, moclobemide, nortriptyline,* and *sertraline* (increased plasma concentrations)
  Antidiabetics: *cimetidine* inhibits renal excretion of *metformin* (increased plasma concentration); *cimetidine* enhances hypoglycaemic effect of *sulphonylureas*
• Antiepileptics: *cimetidine* inhibits metabolism of *carbamazepine, phenytoin, and valproate* (increased plasma concentrations)
  Antifungals: absorption of *itraconazole and ketoconazole* reduced; plasma concentration of *terbinafine* increased by *cimetidine*
  Antihistamines: manufacturer advises possibility of increased plasma-loratadine concentration with *cimetidine*
  Antimalarials: *cimetidine* inhibits metabolism of *chloroquine* and *quinine* (increased plasma concentrations)
  Antipsychotics: *cimetidine* possibly enhances effect of *chlorpromazine, clozapine, and possibly other antipsychotics*
  Antivirals: plasma concentration of *zalcitabine* possibly increased by *cimetidine*; plasma concentration of *saquinavir* increased by *ranitidine*
  Anxiolytics and Hypnotics: *cimetidine* inhibits metabolism of *benzodiazepines* and *clomethiazole* (increased plasma concentrations)
  Beta-blockers: *cimetidine* inhibits metabolism of *beta-blockers* such as *labetalol, metoprolol* and *propranolol* (increased plasma concentrations)
  Calcium-channel Blockers: *cimetidine* inhibits metabolism of *some calcium-channel blockers* (increased plasma concentrations)
• Ciclosporin: *cimetidine* possibly increases plasma-ciclosporin concentration
  Cisapride: *cimetidine* increases plasma concentration of cisapride
  Cytotoxics: *cimetidine* increases plasma concentration of *fluorouracil*
  Dopaminergics: *cimetidine* inhibits excretion of *pramipexole* (increased plasma-pramipexole concentration)
  Hormone Antagonists: *octreotide* possibly delays absorption of *cimetidine*
  5HT₁ Agonists: *cimetidine* inhibits metabolism of *zolmitriptan* (reduce dose of zolmitriptan)
  Sildenafil: cimetidine increases plasma-sildenafil concentration (reduce initial dose of sildenafil)
• Theophylline: *cimetidine* inhibits metabolism (increased plasma-theophylline concentration)
Homatropine *see* Antimuscarinics
Hormone Antagonists *see* Aminoglutethimide; Bicalutamide; Danazol; Finasteride; Flutamide; Gestrinone; Octeotide; Tamoxifen; Toremifene; Trilostane
5HT₁ Agonists
  Note. There are currently no recognised drug interactions with naratriptan
  Antibacterials: *quinolones* possibly inhibit metabolism of *zolmitriptan* (reduce dose of zolmitriptan)

5HT₁ Agonists *(continued)*
- Antidepressants: risk of CNS toxicity with MAOIs including *moclobemide* (avoid rizatriptan or sumatriptan for 2 weeks after MAOI, reduce dose of zolmitriptan when given with moclobemide); *sumatriptan* increases risk of CNS toxicity with *SSRIs* (avoid concomitant use); *fluvoxamine* possibly inhibits metabolism of *zolmitriptan* (reduce dose of zolmitriptan)

  Beta-blockers: *propranolol* may increase plasma concentration of *rizatriptan* (reduce rizatriptan dose)
- Ergotamine: increased risk of vasospasm (avoid ergotamine for 6 hours after rizatriptan, sumatriptan or zolmitriptan; avoid rizatriptan or sumatriptan for 24 hours and zolmitriptan for 6 hours after ergotamine)

  Ulcer-healing Drugs: *cimetidine* inhibits metabolism of *zolmitriptan* (reduce dose of zolmitriptan)

Hydralazine

ACE Inhibitors and Angiotensin-II Antagonists: enhanced hypotensive effect

Alcohol: enhanced hypotensive effect

Aldesleukin: enhanced hypotensive effect

Alprostadil: enhanced hypotensive effect
- Anaesthetics: enhanced hypotensive effect

Analgesics: *NSAIDs* antagonise hypotensive effect

Antidepressants: enhanced hypotensive effect

other Antihypertensives: additive hypotensive effect

Antipsychotics: enhanced hypotensive effect

Anxiolytics and Hypnotics: enhanced hypotensive effect

Beta-blockers: enhanced hypotensive effect

Calcium-channel Blockers: enhanced hypotensive effect

Corticosteroids: antagonism of hypotensive effect

Diuretics: enhanced hypotensive effect

Dopaminergics: *levodopa* enhances hypotensive effect

Moxisylyte: enhanced hypotensive effect

Muscle Relaxants: *baclofen* and *tizanidine* enhance hypotensive effect

Nitrates: enhanced hypotensive effect

Oestrogens and Progestogens: *oestrogens* and *combined oral contraceptives* antagonise hypotensive effect

Ulcer-healing Drugs: *carbenoxolone* antagonises hypotensive effect

Hydrochlorothiazide *see* Diuretics (thiazide)
Hydrocortisone *see* Corticosteroids
Hydroflumethiazide *see* Diuretics (thiazide)
Hydroxychloroquine *see* Chloroquine and Hydroxychloroquine
Hydroxyprogesterone *see* Progestogens
Hydroxyzine *see* Antihistamines
Hyoscine *see* Antimuscarinics (for general sedative interactions *see also* Antihistamines)
Hypnotics *see* Anxiolytics and Hypnotics
Ibuprofen *see* NSAIDs
Ifosfamide *see* Cyclophosphamide and Ifosfamide
Imipenem *see* Primaxin®
Immunoglobulins
Note. For advice on immunoglobulins and live virus vaccines, see under Normal Immunoglobulin section 14.5
Imidapril *see* ACE Inhibitors and Angiotensin-II Antagonists
Imipramine *see* Antidepressants, Tricyclic
Indapamide *see* Diuretics (thiazide-related)
Indinavir
- Antibacterials: concomitant administration of *indinavir* and *rifabutin* increases plasma-rifabutin concentration and decreases plasma-indinavir concentration (reduce dose of rifabutin and increase dose of indinavir); metabolism enhanced by *rifampicin* (plasma-indinavir concentration significantly reduced—avoid concomitant use)

  Antiepileptics: plasma-indinavir concentration possibly reduced by *carbamazepine, phenobarbital* and *phenytoin*

Indinavir *(continued)*
- Antifungals: metabolism inhibited by *ketoconazole* (reduce dose of indinavir); on theoretical grounds, plasma-indinavir concentration significantly increased by *itraconazole* (avoid concomitant use)
- Antihistamines: increased risk of arrhythmias with *terfenadine*—avoid concomitant use
- Antipsychotics: possibly increased risk of arrhythmias with *pimozide* (avoid concomitant use)

  other Antivirals: combination with *nelfinavir* may lead to increased plasma concentrations of either drug; *indinavir* increases plasma concentration of *saquinavir; ritonavir* increases plasma concentration of *indinavir; efavirenz* reduces plasma concentration of *indinavir* (increase indinavir dose); *nevirapine* reduces plasma concentration of *indinavir*
- Anxiolytics and Hypnotics: increased risk of prolonged sedation with *alprazolam* and *midazolam* (avoid concomitant use)

  Barbiturates and Primidone: *see under* Antiepileptics, above
- Cisapride: increased risk of ventricular arrhythmias (avoid concomitant use)

  Corticosteroids: plasma-indinavir concentration possibly reduced by *dexamethasone*
- Ergotamine: risk of ergotism—avoid concomitant use
- Lipid-regulating Drugs: increased risk of myopathy with *simvastatin*

  Sildenafil: indinavir possibly increases plasma-sildenafil concentration (reduce initial dose of sildenafil)

Indometacin *see* NSAIDs
Indoramin *see* Alpha-blockers
Influenza Vaccine
Anticoagulants: effect of *warfarin* occasionally enhanced

Antiepileptics: effect of *phenytoin* enhanced

Theophylline: effect occasionally enhanced

Insulin *see* Antidiabetics
Interferons
Note. Consult product literature for interactions of interferon beta and gamma

Theophylline: *interferon alfa* inhibits metabolism of *theophylline* (enhanced effect)

Ipratropium *see* Antimuscarinics
Irbesartan *see* ACE Inhibitors and Angiotensin-II Antagonists
Iron
Antacids: *magnesium trisilicate* reduces absorption of *oral iron*

Antibacterials: *tetracyclines* reduce absorption of *oral iron* (and *vice versa*); absorption of *ciprofloxacin, levofloxacin, norfloxacin,* and *ofloxacin* reduced by *oral iron*

Antihypertensives: reduced hypotensive effect of *methyldopa*

Bisphosphonates: reduced absorption

Dopaminergics: absorption of *entacapone* and *levodopa* may be reduced

Penicillamine: reduced absorption of *penicillamine*

Trientine: reduced absorption of *oral iron*

Zinc: reduced absorption of *oral iron* (and *vice versa*)

Isocarboxazid *see* MAOIs
Isoflurane *see* Anaesthetics, General (volatile liquid)
Isometheptene *see* Sympathomimetics
Isoniazid
Anaesthetics: hepatotoxicity possibly potentiated by *isoflurane*

Antacids and Adsorbents: *antacids* reduce absorption

other Antibacterials: increased CNS toxicity with *cycloserine*
- Antiepileptics: metabolism of *carbamazepine, ethosuximide, and phenytoin* inhibited (enhanced effect); also, with *carbamazepine*, isoniazid hepatotoxicity possibly increased

  Antifungals: plasma concentration of *ketoconazole* may be reduced

Isoniazid *(continued)*
  Anxiolytics and Hypnotics: metabolism of *diazepam* inhibited
  Theophylline: *isoniazid* possibly increases plasma *theophylline* concentration
Isoprenaline *see* Sympathomimetics
Isosorbide Dinitrate *see* Nitrates
Isosorbide Mononitrate *see* Nitrates
Isotretinoin *see* Retinoids
Isradipine *see* Calcium-channel Blockers
Itraconazole *see* Antifungals, Imidazole and Triazole
Kanamycin *see* Aminoglycosides
Kaolin
  Analgesics: absorption of *aspirin* possibly reduced
  Anti-arrhythmics: absorption of *quinidine* possibly reduced (possibly reduced plasma concentration)
  Antibacterials: absorption of *tetracyclines* possibly reduced
  Antimalarials: absorption of *chloroquine* reduced
  Antipsychotics: absorption of *phenothiazines* possibly reduced
  Cardiac Glycosides: absorption of *digoxin* possibly reduced
Ketamine *see* Anaesthetics, General
Ketoconazole *see* Antifungals, Imidazole and Triazole
Ketoprofen *see* NSAIDs
Ketorolac *see* NSAIDs
Ketotifen *see* Antihistamines
Labetalol *see* Beta-blockers
Lacidipine *see* Calcium-channel Blockers
Lamivudine
  Antibacterials: *trimethoprim* increases plasma concentration—avoid concomitant use of high-dose *co-trimoxazole*
Lamotrigine
● *other* Antiepileptics: concomitant administration of *two or more antiepileptics* may enhance toxicity without a corresponding increase in antiepileptic effect; moreover interactions between individual antiepileptics can complicate monitoring of treatment; interactions include enhanced effects, increased sedation, and reductions in plasma concentrations; for further details, see p. 222
Lanreotide
  Ciclosporin: absorption of ciclosporin reduced (reduced plasma concentration)
Lansoprazole *see* Proton Pump Inhibitors
Leflunomide
  Vaccines: see p. 541
Lenograstim
  Note. Use not recommended from 24 hours before until 24 hours after chemotherapy—for further details consult product literature
Lercanidipine *see* Calcium-channel Blockers
Leukotriene Antagonists
  Analgesics: *aspirin* increases plasma concentration of *zafirlukast*
  Antibacterials: *erythromycin* reduces plasma concentration of *zafirlukast*
  Anticoagulants: anticoagulant effect of *warfarin* enhanced by *zafirlukast*
  Antihistamines: *terfenadine* reduces plasma concentration of *zafirlukast*
  Barbiturates and Primidone: plasma concentration of *montelukast* reduced by *phenobarbital*
  Theophylline: *zafirlukast* possibly increases plasma-theophylline concentration; plasma-zafirlukast concentration reduced
Levobunolol *see* Beta-blockers
Levocabastine *see* Antihistamines
Levodopa
● Anaesthetics: risk of arrhythmias with *volatile liquid anaesthetics such as* halothane
● Antidepressants: hypertensive crisis with *MAOIs* (including *moclobemide*)—avoid for at least 2 weeks after stopping MAOI

Levodopa *(continued)*
  Antihypertensives: enhanced hypotensive effect
  Antimuscarinics: absorption of levodopa possibly reduced
  Antipsychotics: antagonism of effect
  Anxiolytics and Hypnotics: occasional antagonism of effect by *chlordiazepoxide, diazepam, lorazepam* and possibly *other benzodiazepines*
  Iron: absorption of *levodopa* may be reduced
  Metoclopramide and Domperidone: levodopa-plasma concentrations increased by *metoclopramide*
  Vitamins: effect of *levodopa* antagonised by *pyridoxine* unless a *dopa decarboxylase inhibitor* also given
Levofloxacin *see* Quinolones
Levomepromazine (methotrimeprazine) *see* Antipsychotics
Levonorgestrel *see* Progestogens
Levothyroxine (Thyroxine)
  Analgesics: false low total plasma-thyroxine concentration with *phenylbutazone*
  Anion-exchange Resins: *colestyramine* reduces absorption of *levothyroxine*
  Anti-arrhythmics: for use with *amiodarone*, see p. 70
  Antibacterials: *rifampicin* accelerates metabolism of *levothyroxine* (may increase requirements in hypothyroidism)
● Anticoagulants: effect of *acenocoumarol, phenindione, and warfarin* enhanced
  Antidepressants: manufacturer of *lofepramine* advises avoid *levothyroxine*
  Antiepileptics: *carbamazepine, phenobarbital, phenytoin,* and *primidone* accelerate metabolism of *levothyroxine* (may increase requirements in hypothyroidism)
  Barbiturates and Primidone: *see under* Antiepileptics, above
  Beta-blockers: metabolism of *propranolol* accelerated (reduced effect)
  Ulcer-healing Drugs: *sucralfate* reduces absorption of *levothyroxine*
Lidocaine (lignocaine)
  other Anti-arrhythmics: increased myocardial depression
● Antibacterials: increased risk of ventricular arrhythmias with *quinupristin/dalfopristin* (avoid concomitant use)
  Antidepressants: manufacturer of *reboxetine* advises caution
  Beta-blockers: increased risk of myocardial depression; increased risk of *lidocaine* toxicity with *propranolol*
  Diuretics: effect of *lidocaine* antagonised by hypokalaemia with *acetazolamide, loop diuretics, and thiazides*
  Muscle Relaxants: action of *suxamethonium* prolonged
  Ulcer-healing Drugs: *cimetidine* inhibits metabolism of *lidocaine* (increased risk of toxicity)
Lignocaine *see* Lidocaine
Lipid-regulating Drugs *see* Colestyramine and Colestipol; Fibrates; Nicotinic Acid; Statins
Lisinopril *see* ACE Inhibitors and Angiotensin-II Antagonists
Lisuride
  Antipsychotics: antagonism of effect
Lithium
● ACE Inhibitors and Angiotensin-II Antagonists: *lithium* excretion reduced (increased plasma-lithium concentration)
● Analgesics: excretion of *lithium* reduced by *azapropazone, diclofenac, ibuprofen, indometacin, ketorolac* (avoid concomitant use), *mefenamic acid, naproxen, phenylbutazone, piroxicam,* and probably *other NSAIDs* (risk of toxicity)
  Antacids: *sodium bicarbonate* increases excretion of *lithium* (reduced plasma-lithium concentrations)

Lithium (continued)

Anti-arrhythmics: increased risk of hypothyroidism with *amiodarone*

Antibacterials: *lithium* toxicity reported with *metronidazole*

• Antidepressants: *SSRIs* increase risk of CNS effects (lithium toxicity reported)

Antidiabetics: *lithium* may occasionally impair glucose tolerance

Antiepileptics: neurotoxicity may occur with *carbamazepine* and *phenytoin* without increased plasma-lithium concentration

• Antihypertensives: neurotoxicity may occur with *methyldopa* without increased plasma-lithium concentration

Antipsychotics: increased risk of extrapyramidal effects and possibility of neurotoxicity (notably with *haloperidol*)

Calcium-channel Blockers: neurotoxicity may occur with *diltiazem and verapamil* without increased plasma-lithium concentration

• Cisapride: increased risk of ventricular arrhythmias—avoid concomitant use

• Diuretics: *lithium* excretion reduced by *loop diuretics, potassium-sparing diuretics, and thiazides* (increased plasma-lithium concentration and risk of toxicity—*loop diuretics* safer than *thiazides*); *lithium* excretion increased by *acetazolamide*

Muscle Relaxants: muscle relaxant effect enhanced; *baclofen* possibly aggravates hyperkinesis

Parasympathomimetics: *lithium* antagonises effect of *neostigmine and pyridostigmine*

Theophylline: *lithium* excretion increased (reduced plasma-lithium concentration)

Lofepramine see Antidepressants, Tricyclic

Lofexidine

Alcohol: enhanced sedative effect

Anxiolytics and Hypnotics: enhanced sedative effect

Loprazolam see Anxiolytics and Hypnotics

Loratadine see Antihistamines

Lorazepam see Anxiolytics and Hypnotics

Lormetazepam see Anxiolytics and Hypnotics

Losartan see ACE Inhibitors and Angiotensin-II Antagonists

Loxapine see Antipsychotics

Lymecycline see Tetracyclines

Macrolides see Erythromycin and other Macrolides

Magnesium Salts (see also Antacids and Adsorbents)

• Calcium-channel Blockers: profound hypotension reported with *nifedipine* and *intravenous magnesium sulphate* in pre-eclampsia

Muscle Relaxants: effect of *non-depolarising muscle relaxants* enhanced by *parenteral magnesium salts*

Magnesium Trisilicate see Antacids

Maloprim® contains Dapsone and Pyrimethamine

MAOIs

Note. For interactions of reversible MAO-A inhibitors (RIMAs) see Moclobemide, and for interactions of MAO-B inhibitors see Selegiline

• Alcohol: some *alcoholic* and *dealcoholised beverages* contain *tyramine* which interacts with *MAOIs* (hypertensive crisis)—but if no tyramine, enhanced hypotensive effect; foods, see section 4.3.2

Alpha₂-adrenoceptor Stimulants: manufacturers of *apraclonidine* and *brimonidine* advise avoid concomitant use

• Altretamine: risk of severe postural hypotension

• Analgesics: CNS excitation or depression (hypertension or hypotension) with *pethidine* and possibly *other opioid analgesics*—avoid concomitant use and for 2 weeks after MAOI discontinued; manufacturer advises avoid *nefopam*

Anaesthetics: see section 15.1

• Anorectics: see Sympathomimetics, below

MAOIs (continued)

• *other* Antidepressants: enhancement of CNS effects and toxicity with *other MAOIs* (avoid for at least a week after stopping *previous MAOIs* then start with reduced dose); CNS effects of *SSRIs* increased by *MAOIs* (risk of serious toxicity) , see also p. 191; CNS excitation and hypertension with most *tricyclics and related antidepressants*, see p. 186; CNS excitation and confusion with *tryptophan* (reduce tryptophan dose); enhancement of CNS effects and toxicity possible with *nefazodone*, *reboxetine* and *venlafaxine* (avoid for at least 2 weeks after stopping MAOI, and avoid MAOI for at least 1 week after stopping nefazodone, reboxetine or venlafaxine)

Antidiabetics: effect of *insulin, metformin, and sulphonylureas* enhanced

• Antiepileptics: antagonism of anticonvulsant effect (convulsive threshold lowered); manufacturer advises avoid *carbamazepine* with or within 2 weeks of *MAOIs*

Antihistamines: increased antimuscarinic and sedative effects

• Antihypertensives: hypotensive effect enhanced; manufacturer advises avoidance of *indoramin*; manufacturer advises avoid concomitant use with *methyldopa*

Antimuscarinics: increased side-effects

• Antipsychotics: CNS excitation and hypertension with *oxypertine*; *clozapine* possibly enhances central effects

Anxiolytics and Hypnotics: manufacturer advises avoidance of *buspirone*

• Barbiturates and Primidone: *see under* Antiepileptics, above

• Dopaminergics: hypertensive crisis with *levodopa* (avoid for at least 2 weeks after stopping MAOI); hypotension with *selegiline*; manufacturer advises avoid concomitant use with *entacapone*

Doxapram: potentiated by *MAOIs*

• 5HT₁ Agonists: risk of CNS toxicity (avoid rizatriptan or sumatriptan for 2 weeks after MAOI)

• Sympathomimetics: hypertensive crisis with *sympathomimetics* such as *dexamfetamine and other amfetamines, dopamine, dopexamine, ephedrine, isometheptene, methylphenidate, phentermine, phenylephrine, phenylpropanolamine, and pseudoephedrine*

• Tetrabenazine: CNS excitation and hypertension

Maprotiline see Antidepressants, Tricyclic

Mebendazole

Ulcer-healing Drugs: metabolism possibly inhibited by *cimetidine* (increased plasma-mebendazole concentration)

Medroxyprogesterone see Progestogens

Mefenamic Acid see NSAIDs

Mefloquine

• Anti-arrhythmics: increased risk of ventricular arrhythmias with *amiodarone* (avoid concomitant use) and *quinidine*

• Antiepileptics: antagonism of anticonvulsant effect

other Antimalarials: increased risk of convulsions with *chloroquine* and *quinine*, but should not prevent use of intravenous quinine in severe cases; for full precautions see footnote on p. 299 (also applies to *quinidine*); increased risk of ventricular arrhythmias with *halofantrine* (**important:** see also CSM advice under Halofantrine, p. 303)

• Antipsychotics: increased risk of ventricular arrhythmias—avoid concomitant use with *pimozide*

Beta-blockers: possible increased risk of bradycardia

Calcium-channel Blockers: possible increased risk of bradycardia with some *calcium-channel blockers*

Cardiac Glycosides: possible increased risk of bradycardia with *digoxin*

Vaccines: see Typhoid Vaccine, p. 555

Mefruside *see* Diuretics (thiazide)
Megestrol *see* Progestogens
Meloxicam *see* NSAIDs
Melphalan
  Antibacterials: increased toxicity with *nalidixic acid*
• Ciclosporin: increased risk of nephrotoxicity
Mepacrine
  Antimalarials: increased plasma concentration of
    primaquine (risk of toxicity)
Meprobamate *see* Anxiolytics and Hypnotics
Meptazinol *see* Opioid Analgesics
Mequitazine *see* Antihistamines
Mercaptopurine
• Allopurinol: enhancement of effect (increased
    toxicity—reduce dose of mercaptopurine)
• Antibacterials: increased risk of haematological
    toxicity with *co-trimoxazole* and *trimethoprim*
Mestranol *see* Contraceptives, Oral
Metaraminol *see* Sympathomimetics (*as* noradrenaline)
Metformin *see* Antidiabetics
Methadone *see* Opioid Analgesics
Methenamine
  Potassium Citrate: urine should be acid
Methocarbamol *see* Muscle Relaxants
Methotrexate
• Analgesics: excretion reduced by *aspirin,
    azapropazone* (avoid concomitant use), *diclofenac,
    ibuprofen, indometacin, ketoprofen, meloxicam,
    naproxen, phenylbutazone,* and probably *other
    NSAIDs* (increased risk of toxicity)
• Antibacterials: antifolate effect increased by *co-
    trimoxazole and trimethoprim*; risk of methotrexate
    toxicity increased by *sulphonamides*; excretion
    reduced by *penicillins* (increased risk of toxicity)
  Antiepileptics: *phenytoin* increases antifolate effect
  Antimalarials: antifolate effect increased by
    pyrimethamine (ingredient of *Fansidar®* and
    Maloprim®)
• Ciclosporin: increased toxicity
• Retinoids: plasma concentration of *methotrexate*
    increased by *acitretin* (also increased risk of
    hepatotoxicity)
• Uricosurics: excretion reduced by *probenecid*
    (increased risk of toxicity)
Methotrimeprazine (Levomepromazine) *see*
  Antipsychotics
Methoxamine *see* Sympathomimetics (*as*
  noradrenaline)
Methyldopa
  Alcohol: enhanced hypotensive effect
  Alprostadil: enhanced hypotensive effect
• Anaesthetics: enhanced hypotensive effect
  Analgesics: *NSAIDs* antagonise hypotensive effect
  Antidepressants: enhanced hypotensive effect;
    manufacturer advises avoid concomitant use with
    MAOIs
  other Antihypertensives: enhanced hypotensive effect
  Antipsychotics: increased risk of extrapyramidal
    effects; enhanced hypotensive effect
  Anxiolytics and Hypnotics: enhanced hypotensive
    effect
  Beta-blockers: enhanced hypotensive effect
  Calcium-channel Blockers: enhanced hypotensive
    effect
  Corticosteroids: antagonism of hypotensive effect
  Diuretics: enhanced hypotensive effect
  Dopaminergics: antagonism of antiparkinsonian
    effect; *levodopa* enhances hypotensive effect; effect
    of methydopa possibly enhanced by *entacapone*
  Iron: reduced hypotensive effect
• Lithium: neurotoxicity may occur without increased
    plasma-lithium concentration
  Moxisylyte: enhanced hypotensive effect
  Muscle Relaxants: enhanced hypotensive effect with
    baclofen and *tizanidine*
  Nitrates: enhance hypotensive effect

Methyldopa *(continued)*
  Oestrogens and Progestogens: *oestrogens and
    combined oral contraceptives* antagonise
    hypotensive effect
• Sympathomimetics, Beta$_2$: acute hypotension
    reported with *salbutamol infusion*
  Ulcer-healing Drugs: *carbenoxolone* antagonises
    hypotensive effect
Methylphenidate *see* Sympathomimetics
Methylphenobarbital *see* Barbiturates
Methylprednisolone *see* Corticosteroids
Methysergide *see* Ergotamine
Metipranolol *see* Beta-blockers
Metirosine
  Antipsychotics: increased risk of extrapyramidal
    effects
  Dopaminergics: antagonism
Metoclopramide
  Analgesics: increased absorption of *aspirin and
    paracetamol* (enhanced effect); *opioid analgesics*
    antagonise effect on gastro-intestinal activity
  Antimuscarinics: antagonism of effect on gastro-
    intestinal activity
  Antipsychotics: increased risk of extrapyramidal
    effects
  Atovaquone: plasma concentration reduced by
    metoclopramide
  Dopaminergics: antagonism of hypoprolactinaemic
    effect of *bromocriptine*; increased plasma
    concentration of *levodopa*; antagonism of
    antiparkinsonian effects of *pergolide*
  Tetrabenazine: increased risk of extrapyramidal
    effects
Metolazone *see* Diuretics (thiazide-related)
Metoprolol *see* Beta-blockers
Metronidazole
  Alcohol: disulfiram-like reaction
• Anticoagulants: effect of *acenocoumarol* and
    warfarin enhanced
• Antiepileptics: *metronidazole* inhibits metabolism of
    phenytoin (increased plasma-phenytoin
    concentration); *phenobarbital* accelerates
    metabolism of *metronidazole* (reduced plasma-
    metronidazole concentration)
• Barbiturates and Primidone: *see under* Antiepileptics,
    above
  Cytotoxics: *metronidazole* inhibits metabolism of
    fluorouracil (increased toxicity)
  Disulfiram: psychotic reactions reported
  Lithium: increased toxicity reported
  Ulcer-healing Drugs: *cimetidine* inhibits metabolism
    (increased plasma-metronidazole concentration)
Mexiletine
  Analgesics: *opioid analgesics* delay absorption
• *other* Anti-arrhythmics: increased myocardial
    depression with any combination of *anti-
    arrhythmics*
  Antibacterials: *rifampicin* accelerates metabolism
    (reduced plasma-mexiletine concentration)
  Antidepressants: manufacturer of *reboxetine* advises
    caution
  Antiepileptics: *phenytoin* accelerates metabolism
    (reduced plasma-mexiletine concentration)
  Antimuscarinics: *atropine* delays absorption
• Antivirals: possibly increased risk of arrhythmias with
    ritonavir
  Diuretics: action of *mexiletine* antagonised by
    hypokalaemia due to *acetazolamide, loop diuretics,
    and thiazides*
  Theophylline: plasma-theophylline concentration
    increased
Mianserin
  Alcohol: enhanced effect
  Alpha$_2$-adrenoceptor Stimulants: manufacturers of
    apraclonidine and *brimonidine* advise avoid
    concomitant use
  other Antidepressants: as for Antidepressants,
    Tricyclic

Mianserin *(continued)*
* Antiepileptics: antagonism (convulsive threshold lowered); metabolism accelerated by *carbamazepine, phenobarbital,* and *phenytoin* (reduced plasma-mianserin concentration)
  Anxiolytics and Hypnotics: enhanced effect
* Barbiturates and Primidone: *see under* Antiepileptics, above

Miconazole *see* Antifungals, Imidazole and Triazole

Midazolam *see* Anxiolytics and Hypnotics

Mifepristone
  Analgesics: manufacturer recommends avoid *aspirin* and *NSAIDs* until 8–12 days after *mifepristone* administration

Minocycline *see* Tetracyclines

Minoxidil *see* Hydralazine for general hypotensive interactions

Mirtazapine
  Alcohol: enhanced sedative effect
  Alpha₂-adrenoceptor Stimulants: manufacturers of *apraclonidine* and *brimonidine* advise avoid concomitant use
* *other* Antidepressants: as for Antidepressants, tricyclic
  Anxiolytics and Hypnotics: enhanced sedative effect

Misoprostol
  Analgesics: increased risk of CNS toxicity with *phenylbutazone*

Mivacurium *see* Muscle Relaxants (non-depolarising)

Mizolastine *see* Antihistamines

Moclobemide
  Note. Moclobemide is a reversible MAO-A inhibitor (RIMA), see also p. 191
* Analgesics: CNS excitation or depression (hypertension or hypotension) with *codeine, dextromethorphan, pethidine,* and possibly *fentanyl, morphine,* and *other opioid analgesics*; effects of *ibuprofen* and possibly *other NSAIDs* enhanced
* Anorectics: as for MAOIs (see main list)
* *other* Antidepressants: see p. 191
* Dopaminergics: hypertensive crisis with *levodopa*; avoid concomitant use with *selegiline*
* 5HT₁ Agonists: risk of CNS toxicity (reduce dose of zolmitriptan)
* Sympathomimetics: as for MAOIs (see main list)
  Ulcer-healing Drugs: *cimetidine* inhibits metabolism (increased plasma-moclobemide concentration— halve dose of moclobemide)

Moexipril *see* ACE Inhibitors and Angiotensin-II Antagonists

Modafinil
* Oestrogens and Progestogens: modafinil accelerates metabolism of *oral contraceptives* (reduced contraceptive effect)

Monoamine-oxidase Inhibitors *see* MAOIs, Moclobemide, and Selegiline

Montelukast *see* Leukotriene Antagonists

Moracizine
  other Anti-arrhythmics: increased myocardial depression with any *anti-arrhythmic*
  Antidepressants: manufacturer of *reboxetine* advises caution
  Theophylline: metabolism of *theophylline* accelerated (reduced effect)
  Ulcer-healing Drugs: *cimetidine* possibly increases plasma-moracizine concentration

Morphine *see* Opioid Analgesics

Moxisylyte (Thymoxamine)
* Alpha-blockers: possible severe postural hypotension
  other Antihypertensives: enhanced hypotensive effect
* Beta-blockers: possible severe postural hypotension

Moxonidine
  Alprostadil: enhanced hypotensive effect
  other Antihypertensives: enhanced hypotensive effect
  Anxiolytics and Hypnotics: sedative effect of benzodiazepines possibly enhanced
  Moxisylyte: enhanced hypotensive effect
  Muscle Relaxants: enhanced hypotensive effect with *baclofen* and *tizanidine*

Muscle Relaxants
  ACE Inhibitors and Angiotensin-II Antagonists: enhanced hypotensive effect with *baclofen* and *tizanidine*
  Alcohol: enhanced sedative effect with *baclofen* and *tizanidine*
  Analgesics: *ibuprofen* and *possibly other NSAIDs* reduce excretion of *baclofen* (increased risk of toxicity)
* Anti-arrhythmics: *procainamide* and *quinidine* enhance muscle relaxant effect; *lidocaine* prolongs action of *suxamethonium*
* Antibacterials: effect of *non-depolarising muscle relaxants* enhanced by *aminoglycosides, clindamycin, colistin* and *piperacillin*
  Antidepressants: *tricyclics* enhance muscle relaxant effect of *baclofen*
  Antiepileptics: effect of *non-depolarising muscle relaxants* antagonised by *carbamazepine* and *phenytoin* (recovery from neuromuscular blockade accelerated)
  Antihypertensives: enhanced hypotensive effect with *baclofen* and *tizanidine*
  Anxiolytics and Hypnotics: enhanced sedative effect with *baclofen* and *tizanidine*
  Beta-blockers: *propranolol* enhances muscle relaxant effect; possible enhanced hypotensive effect and bradycardia with *tizanidine*
* Botulinum Toxin: neuromuscular block enhanced by *non-depolarising muscle relaxants* (risk of toxicity)
  Calcium-channel Blockers: *nifedipine* and *verapamil* enhance effect of *non-depolarising muscle relaxants*; hypotension, myocardial depression, and hyperkalaemia reported with intravenous *dantrolene* and *verapamil*; risk of arrhythmias with *diltiazem* and intravenous *dantrolene*
  Cardiac Glycosides: arrhythmias if *suxamethonium* given with *digoxin*; possible bradycardia if *tizanidine* given with *digoxin*
  Cytotoxics: *cyclophosphamide* and *thiotepa* enhance effect of *suxamethonium*
  Diuretics: enhanced hypotensive effect with *baclofen* and *tizanidine*
  Lithium: *lithium* enhances muscle relaxant effect; *baclofen* possibly aggravates hyperkinesis
  Magnesium Salts: *parenteral magnesium* enhances effect of *non-depolarising muscle relaxants*
  Parasympathomimetics: *ecothiopate* eye-drops, *edrophonium, neostigmine, pyridostigmine, rivastigmine* and possibly *donepezil* enhance effect of *suxamethonium* but antagonise effect of *non-depolarising muscle relaxants*
  Sympathomimetics: *bambuterol* enhances effect of *suxamethonium*

Mycophenolate Mofetil
  Anion-exchange Resins: *colestyramine* reduces absorption
  Antacids: reduced absorption of mycophenolate mofetil
  Antivirals: higher plasma concentrations of *mycophenolate mofetil* and of *aciclovir* on concomitant administration

Nabilone
  Alcohol: sedative effect of *nabilone* enhanced
  Anxiolytics and Hypnotics: enhanced sedative effect

Nabumetone *see* NSAIDs

Nadolol *see* Beta-blockers

Nalbuphine *see* Opioid Analgesics

Nalidixic Acid *see* Quinolones

Nandrolone *see* Anabolic Steroids

Naproxen *see* NSAIDs

Naratriptan *see* 5HT₁ Agonists

Nebivolol *see* Beta-blockers

Nefazodone

Note. Although interactions with alcohol, and lithium have not been reported, caution should be observed on concomitant use with nefazodone

- *other* Antidepressants: increased risk of toxicity with *MAOIs* (nefazodone should not be started until 2 weeks after stopping MAOI, and conversely MAOI should not be started until at least 1 week after stopping nefazodone); *fluoxetine* increases plasma concentration of nefazodone

- Antihistamines: increased risk of arrhythmias with *terfenadine*—avoid concomitant use

Antiepileptics: plasma concentration of *carbamazepine* increased and plasma concentration of *nefazodone* reduced

Antihypertensives: hypotensive effect possibly enhanced

Antipsychotics: plasma concentration of *haloperidol* increased

Anxiolytics and Hypnotics: possibly enhanced sedative effect with *benzodiazepines*; plasma concentration of *alprazolam* increased (reduce alprazolam dose)

Cardiac Glycosides: plasma concentration of *digoxin* increased

- Cisapride: increased risk of ventricular arrhythmias (avoid concomitant use)

Lipid-regulating Drugs: increased risk of myopathy with *simvastatin*

Nefopam

- Antidepressants: manufacturer recommends avoid *MAOIs;* possibly increased side-effects with *tricyclics*

Antimuscarinics: increased side-effects

Nelfinavir

- Anti-arrhythmics: increased risk of arrhythmias with *amiodarone* and *quinidine* (avoid concomitant use)

- Antibacterials: *rifampicin* significantly reduces plasma concentration of nelfinavir (avoid concomitant use); nelfinavir increases plasma concentration of *rifabutin* (halve rifabutin dose)

- Antiepileptics: *carbamazepine* and *phenytoin* possibly reduce plasma concentration of nelfinavir

- Antihistamines: increased risk of arrhythmias with *terfenadine* (avoid concomitant use)

- Antipsychotics: possibly increased risk of arrhythmias with *pimozide* (avoid concomitant use) *other* Antivirals: combination of nelfinavir with *indinavir, ritonavir* or *saquinavir* may lead to increased plasma concentrations of either drug (or both)

- Anxiolytics and Hypnotics: risk of prolonged sedation with *midazolam* (avoid concomitant use)

- Barbiturates and Primidone: *phenobarbital* possibly reduces plasma concentration of nelfinavir

- Cisapride: increased risk of arrhythmias (avoid concomitant use)

- Ergotamine: risk of ergotism—avoid concomitant use

- Lipid-regulating Drugs: increased risk of myopathy with *simvastatin*

Oestrogens and Progestogens: possibly reduced efficacy of *oral contraceptives*

Sildenafil: nelfinavir possibly increases plasma-sildenafil concentration (reduce initial dose of sildenafil)

Neomycin *see* Aminoglycosides
Neostigmine *see* Parasympathomimetics
Netilmicin *see* Aminoglycosides
Nevirapine

Antibacterials: *rifabutin* and *rifampicin* reduce plasma concentration of nevirapine

- Antifungals: plasma concentration of *ketoconazole* reduced (avoid concomitant use)

- *other* Antivirals: plasma concentration of *saquinavir* reduced by nevirapine (avoid concomitant use); plasma concentration of *indinavir* reduced by nevirapine

- Oestrogens and Progestogens: accelerated metabolism of *oral contraceptives* and other *hormonal contraceptives* (reduced contraceptive effect)

Nicardipine *see* Calcium-channel Blockers
Nicorandil

Note. Interactions not observed with acenocoumarol, beta-blockers, digoxin, rifampicin, cimetidine, calcium-channel blockers, or furosemide; possibility of hypotensive interaction with vasodilators, tricyclics, or alcohol

- Sildenafil: hypotensive effect significantly enhanced—avoid concomitant use

Nicotine and Tobacco

Theophylline: *tobacco smoking* increases metabolism (reduced plasma-theophylline concentration)

Nicotinic Acid

Note. Interactions apply to lipid-regulating doses of nicotinic acid

- *other* Lipid-regulating Drugs: increased risk of myopathy with *statins*

Nicoumalone (Acenocoumarol) *see* Warfarin and other Coumarins
Nifedipine *see* Calcium-channel Blockers
Nimodipine *see* Calcium-channel Blockers
Nisoldipine *see* Calcium-channel Blockers
Nitrates (general hypotensive interactions *as for* Hydralazine)

Anti-arrhythmics: *disopyramide* may reduce effect of *sublingual nitrates* (owing to dry mouth)

- Anticoagulants: excretion of *heparin* increased by *glyceryl trinitrate infusion* (reduced anticoagulant effect)

Antidepressants: *tricyclics* may reduce effect of *sublingual nitrates* (owing to dry mouth)

Antimuscarinics: *antimuscarinics such as atropine and propantheline* may reduce effect of *sublingual nitrates* (owing to dry mouth)

- Sildenafil: hypotensive effect significantly enhanced—avoid concomitant use

Nitrazepam *see* Anxiolytics and Hypnotics
Nitrofurantoin

Antacids and Adsorbents: *magnesium trisilicate* reduces absorption

Uricosurics: *probenecid* reduces excretion of *nitrofurantoin* (risk of toxicity)

Nitroprusside as for Hydralazine
Nitrous Oxide *see* Anaesthetics, General
Nizatidine *see* Histamine H$_2$-antagonists
Noradrenaline (Norepinephrine) *see* Sympathomimetics
Norepinephrine (Noradrenaline) *see* Sympathomimetics
Norethisterone *see* Progestogens
Norfloxacin *see* Quinolones
Norgestimate *see* Progestogens
Norgestrel *see* Progestogens
Nortriptyline *see* Antidepressants, Tricyclic
NSAIDs (*see also* Aspirin)

Note. Interactions do not generally apply to topical NSAIDs

- ACE Inhibitors and Angiotensin-II Antagonists: antagonism of hypotensive effect; increased risk of renal impairment and increased risk of hyperkalaemia on administration with *ketorolac* and possibly *other NSAIDs*

- *other* Analgesics: avoid concomitant administration of two or more *NSAIDs,* including *aspirin* (increased side-effects)

Anion-exchange Resins: *colestyramine* reduces absorption of *phenylbutazone*

Antacids: absorption of *diflunisal* reduced

- Antibacterials: *NSAIDs* possibly increase risk of convulsions with *quinolones; indometacin* possibly increases plasma concentration of *gentamicin* and *amikacin* in neonates

- Anticoagulants: anticoagulant effect of *acenocoumarol, warfarin* and possibly *phenindione*) seriously enhanced by *azapropazone* and *phenylbutazone* (avoid concomitant use), and possibly enhanced by *diclofenac, diflunisal, flurbiprofen, ibuprofen, mefenamic acid, meloxicam, piroxicam, sulindac,* and *other NSAIDs*; increased risk of haemorrhage with *intravenous diclofenac* and with *ketorolac* and all *anticoagulants,* including *low-dose heparin* (avoid concomitant use); NSAIDs possibly increase risk of bleeding with *heparin*

NSAIDs *(continued)*

Antidepressants: *moclobemide* enhances effect of *ibuprofen* and possibly *other NSAIDs*

• Antidiabetics: effect of *sulphonylureas* enhanced by *azapropazone*, *phenylbutazone* and possibly *other NSAIDs*

• Antiepileptics: effect of *phenytoin* enhanced by *azapropazone* (avoid concomitant use), *phenylbutazone* and possibly *other NSAIDs*

Antihypertensives: antagonism of hypotensive effect

Antiplatelet Drugs: increased risk of bleeding with *clopidogrel* and *ticlopidine*

Antipsychotics: severe drowsiness possible if *indometacin* given with *haloperidol*

• Antivirals: increased risk of haematological toxicity with *zidovudine*; plasma concentration of *piroxicam* increased by *ritonavir* (risk of toxicity—avoid concomitant use); plasma concentration of *other NSAIDs* possibly increased by *ritonavir*

Beta-blockers: antagonism of hypotensive effect

Bisphosphonates: bioavailability of *tiludronic acid* increased by *indometacin*

Cardiac Glycosides: *NSAIDs* may exacerbate heart failure, reduce GFR, and increase plasma-cardiac glycoside concentration

• Ciclosporin: increased risk of nephrotoxicity; *ciclosporin* increases plasma concentration of *diclofenac* (halve diclofenac dose)

Corticosteroids: increased risk of gastro-intestinal bleeding and ulceration

• Cytotoxics: excretion of *methotrexate* reduced by *aspirin*, *azapropazone* (avoid concomitant use), *diclofenac*, *ibuprofen*, *indometacin*, *ketoprofen*, *meloxicam*, *naproxen*, *phenylbutazone* and probably *other NSAIDs* (increased risk of toxicity)

Desmopressin: effect potentiated by *indometacin*

• Diuretics: risk of nephrotoxicity of *NSAIDs* increased; *NSAIDs* notably *indometacin* and *ketorolac* antagonise diuretic effect; *indometacin* and possibly *other NSAIDs* increase risk of hyperkalaemia with *potassium-sparing diuretics*; occasional reports of decreased renal function when *indometacin* given with *triamterene* (avoid concomitant use)

Levothyroxine: false low total plasma-thyroxine concentration with *phenylbutazone*

• Lithium: excretion of *lithium* reduced by *azapropazone*, *diclofenac*, *ibuprofen*, *indometacin*, *ketorolac* (avoid concomitant use), *mefenamic acid*, *naproxen*, *phenylbutazone*, *piroxicam*, and probably *other NSAIDs* (risk of toxicity)

Mifepristone: manufacturer recommends avoid *aspirin* and *NSAIDs* until 8–12 days after *mifepristone* administration

Muscle Relaxants: *ibuprofen* and possibly *other NSAIDs* reduce excretion of *baclofen* (increased risk of toxicity)

• Tacrolimus: *ibuprofen* and possibly other NSAIDs increase risk of nephrotoxicity

Ulcer-healing Drugs: plasma concentration of *azapropazone* possibly increased by *cimetidine*; risk of CNS toxicity with *phenylbutazone* increased by *misoprostol*

• Uricosurics: *probenecid* delays excretion of *indometacin*, *ketoprofen*, *ketorolac* (avoid concomitant use), and *naproxen* and increases plasma-NSAID concentration

• Vasodilators: risk of bleeding associated with *ketorolac* increased by *pentoxifylline* (avoid concomitant use); possibly increased risk of bleeding with *pentoxifylline* and *other NSAIDs*

Octreotide

Antidiabetics: possibly reduces *insulin* and *antidiabetic drug* requirements in diabetes mellitus

Ciclosporin: absorption of *ciclosporin* reduced (reduced plasma concentration)

Dopaminergics: increased concentration of *bromocriptine*

Ulcer-healing Drugs: absorption of *cimetidine* possibly delayed

Oestrogens *see* Contraceptives, Oral
Ofloxacin *see* Quinolones
Olanzapine *see* Antipsychotics
Omeprazole *see* Proton Pump Inhibitors
Opioid Analgesics

Alcohol: enhanced sedative and hypotensive effect

Anti-arrhythmics: delayed absorption of *mexiletine*

Antibacterials: *rifampicin* accelerates metabolism of *methadone* (reduced effect); *erythromycin* increases plasma concentration of *alfentanil*; manufacturer of *ciprofloxacin* advises avoid premedication with *opioid analgesics* (reduced plasma-ciprofloxacin concentration)

• Anticoagulants: *dextropropoxyphene* may enhance effect of *acenocoumarol* and *warfarin*

• Antidepressants: CNS excitation or depression (hypertension or hypotension) if *pethidine* and possibly *other opioid analgesics* given to patients receiving *MAOIs* (including *moclobemide*)—avoid concomitant use and for 2 weeks after *MAOI* discontinued; *tramadol* possibly increases risk of convulsions with *SSRIs* and *tricyclics*; possibly increased sedation with *tricyclics*

• Antiepileptics: *dextropropoxyphene* enhances effect of *carbamazepine*; effect of *methadone* and *tramadol* decreased by *carbamazepine*; *phenytoin* accelerates *methadone* metabolism (reduced effect and risk of withdrawal effects)

Antifungals: metabolism of *alfentanil* inhibited by *ketoconazole* (risk of prolonged or delayed respiratory depression)

Antipsychotics: enhanced sedative and hypotensive effect

• Antivirals: *methadone* possibly increases plasma concentration of *zidovudine*; plasma concentration of *dextropropoxyphene* and *pethidine* increased by *ritonavir* (risk of toxicity—avoid concomitant use); plasma concentration of *other opioid analgesics* (except methadone) possibly increased by *ritonavir*; plasma concentration of *methadone* reduced by *ritonavir*

Anxiolytics and Hypnotics: enhanced sedative effect

• Beta-blockers: *morphine* possibly increases plasma concentration of *esmolol*

Cisapride: possible antagonism of gastro-intestinal effect

• Dopaminergics: hyperpyrexia and CNS toxicity reported if *pethidine* given to patients receiving *selegiline* (avoid concomitant use)

Metoclopramide and Domperidone: antagonism of gastro-intestinal effects

Ulcer-healing Drugs: *cimetidine* inhibits metabolism of opioid analgesics notably *pethidine* (increased plasma concentration)

Orciprenaline *see* Sympathomimetics
Orlistat

Antidiabetics: manufacturer advises avoid concomitant use with *acarbose* or *metformin*

Lipid-regulating Drugs: manufacturer advises avoid concomitant use with *fibrates*

Sympathomimetics: manufacturer advises avoid concomitant use with *phentermine*

Orphenadrine *see* Antimuscarinics
Oxaliplatin *see* Platinum Compounds
Oxazepam *see* Anxiolytics and Hypnotics
Oxitropium *see* Antimuscarinics
Oxpentifylline *see* Pentoxifylline
Oxprenolol *see* Beta-blockers
Oxybutynin *see* Antimuscarinics
Oxymetazoline *see* Sympathomimetics
Oxypertine *see* Antipsychotics
Oxytetracycline *see* Tetracyclines
Oxytocin

Anaesthetics: *inhalational anaesthetics* possibly reduce oxytocic effect (also enhanced hypotensive effect and risk of arrhythmias)

Prostaglandins: uterotonic effect potentiated

Sympathomimetics: enhancement of vasopressor effect of *vasoconstrictor sympathomimetics*

Pamidronate Sodium *see* Bisphosphonates
Pancreatin
  Antidiabetics: hypoglycaemic effect of *acarbose* reduced
Pancuronium *see* Muscle Relaxants (non-depolarising)
Pantoprazole *see* Proton Pump Inhibitors
Papaveretum *see* Opioid Analgesics
Paracetamol
  Anion-exchange Resins: *colestyramine* reduces absorption of *paracetamol*
  Anticoagulants: prolonged regular use of *paracetamol* possibly enhances *warfarin*
  Metoclopramide and Domperidone: *metoclopramide* and *domperidone* accelerate absorption of *paracetamol* (enhanced effect)
Paraldehyde
• Alcohol: enhanced sedative effect
• Disulfiram: increased risk of toxicity with *paraldehyde*
Parasympathomimetics
  Anti-arrhythmics: *procainamide, quinidine* and possibly *propafenone* antagonise effect of *neostigmine* and *pyridostigmine*
• Antibacterials: *aminoglycosides, clindamycin* and *colistin* antagonise effect of *neostigmine* and *pyridostigmine*
  Antimalarials: *chloroquine* and *hydroxychloroquine* have potential to increase symptoms of myasthenia gravis and thus diminish effect of *neostigmine* and *pyridostigmine*
  Antimuscarinics: antagonism of effect
  Beta-blockers: risk of arrhythmias possibly increased by *pilocarpine*; *propranolol* antagonises effect of *neostigmine* and *pyridostigmine*
  Lithium: antagonism of effect of *neostigmine* and *pyridostigmine*
  Muscle Relaxants: *ecothiopate eye-drops, edrophonium, neostigmine, pyridostigmine, rivastigmine* and possibly *donepezil* enhance effect of *suxamethonium*, but antagonise effect of *non-depolarising muscle relaxants*
Paroxetine *see* Antidepressants, SSRI
Penicillamine
  Antacids: reduced absorption of *penicillamine*
  Iron: reduced absorption of *penicillamine*
  Zinc: reduced absorption of *penicillamine*
Penicillins
  Anticoagulants: *see* Phenindione and Warfarin
  Cytotoxics: reduced excretion of *methotrexate* (increased risk of toxicity)
  Guar Gum: reduced absorption of *phenoxymethylpenicillin*
  Muscle Relaxants: effects of *non-depolarising muscle relaxants* enhanced by *piperacillin*
  Oestrogens and Progestogens: *see* Contraceptives, Oral
  Uricosurics: excretion of *penicillins* reduced by *probenecid*
Pentamidine Isetionate
• Anti-arrhythmics: increased risk of ventricular arrhythmias with *amiodarone* (avoid concomitant use)
• Antihistamines: increased risk of ventricular arrhythmias with *terfenadine* (avoid concomitant use)
• Cisapride: increased risk of ventricular arrhythmias (avoid concomitant use)
Pentazocine *see* Opioid Analgesics
Pentostatin
• *other* Cytotoxics: increases pulmonary toxicity of *fludarabine* (unacceptably high incidence of fatalities); increased toxicity with high-dose cyclophosphamide (avoid concomitant use)
Pentoxifylline (Oxpentifylline)
• Analgesics: increased risk of bleeding with *ketorolac* (avoid concomitant use); possibly increased risk of bleeding with *other NSAIDs*
  Theophylline: plasma-*theophylline* concentration increased

Pergolide
  Antipsychotics: antagonism of effect
  Metoclopramide and Domperidone: *metoclopramide* antagonises effect
Pericyazine *see* Antipsychotics
Perindopril *see* ACE Inhibitors and Angiotensin-II Antagonists
Perphenazine *see* Antipsychotics
Pethidine *see* Opioid Analgesics
Phenazocine *see* Opioid Analgesics
Phenelzine *see* MAOIs
Phenindione
  Note. Change in patient's clinical condition, particularly associated with liver disease, intercurrent illness, or drug administration, necessitates more frequent testing. Major changes in diet (especially involving salads and vegetables) and in alcohol consumption may also affect anticoagulant control
• Anabolic Steroids: anticoagulant effect enhanced by *oxymetholone, stanozolol and others*
• Analgesics: anticoagulant effect enhanced by *aspirin* and possibly *other NSAIDs*; increased risk of haemorrhage with *intravenous diclofenac* and with *ketorolac* (avoid concomitant use)
  Anion-exchange Resins: anticoagulant effect enhanced or reduced by *colestyramine*
• Anti-arrhythmics: metabolism inhibited by *amiodarone* (enhanced anticoagulant effect)
  Antibacterials: although studies have failed to demonstrate interaction, common experience in anticoagulant clinics is that INR can be altered by course of *oral broad-spectrum antibiotics* such as *ampicillin* (may also apply to antibiotics given for local action on gut such as *neomycin*)
• Antidepressants: anticoagulant effect possibly enhanced by *viloxazine*
• Antiplatelet Drugs: anticoagulant effect enhanced by *aspirin, clopidogrel, dipyridamole* and ti*clopidine*
• Antivirals: *ritonavir* possibly increases plasma concentration
  Cisapride: anticoagulant effect possibly enhanced
• Fibrates: enhanced anticoagulant effect
• Levothyroxine: enhanced anticoagulant effect
• Oestrogens and Progestogens: anticoagulant effect antagonised by *oral contraceptives*
• Testosterone: anticoagulant effect enhanced
• Vitamins: anticoagulant effect antagonised by *vitamin K* (present in some enteral feeds)
Pheniramine *see* Antihistamines
Phenobarbital *see* Barbiturates
Phenoperidine *see* Opioid Analgesics
Phenothiazines *see* Antipsychotics
Phenoxybenzamine *see* Alpha-blockers
Phenoxymethylpenicillin *see* Penicillins
Phentermine *see* Sympathomimetics
Phentolamine *see* Alpha-blockers
Phenylbutazone *see* NSAIDs
Phenylephrine *see* Sympathomimetics
Phenylpropanolamine *see* Sympathomimetics
Phenytoin
• Analgesics: plasma-phenytoin concentration increased by *aspirin, azapropazone* (avoid concomitant use), *phenylbutazone* and possibly *other NSAIDs*; metabolism of *methadone* accelerated (reduced effect and risk of withdrawal effects)
  Antacids: reduced *phenytoin* absorption
• Anti-arrhythmics: *amiodarone* increases plasma-phenytoin concentration; *phenytoin* reduces plasma concentrations of *disopyramide, mexiletine,* and *quinidine*
• Antibacterials: plasma-phenytoin concentration increased by *chloramphenicol, clarithromycin, cycloserine, isoniazid,* and *metronidazole*; plasma-phenytoin concentration and antifolate effect increased by *co-trimoxazole* and *trimethoprim* and possibly by *other sulphonamides*; plasma-phenytoin concentration reduced by *rifamycins*; plasma concentration of *doxycycline* reduced by *phenytoin*; plasma-phenytoin concentration possibly altered by *ciprofloxacin*

Phenytoin *(continued)*
- Anticoagulants: metabolism of *acenocoumarol* and *warfarin* accelerated (possibility of reduced anticoagulant effect, but enhancement also reported)
- Antidepressants: antagonism of anticonvulsant effect (convulsive threshold lowered); *fluoxetine, fluvoxamine,* and *viloxazine* increase plasma-phenytoin concentration; *phenytoin* reduces plasma concentrations of *mianserin, paroxetine,* and *tricyclics*

  Antidiabetics: plasma-phenytoin concentration transiently increased by *tolbutamide* (possibility of toxicity); phenytoin possibly reduces plasma concentration of *repaglinide* (manufacturer advises avoid concomitant use)
- *other* Antiepileptics: concomitant administration of *two or more antiepileptics* may enhance toxicity without a corresponding increase in antiepileptic effect; moreover interactions between individual antiepileptics can complicate monitoring of treatment; interactions include enhanced effects, increased sedation, and reductions in plasma concentrations; for further details see p. 222
- Antifungals: plasma-phenytoin concentration increased by *fluconazole* and *miconazole*; plasma concentration of *itraconazole* and *ketoconazole* reduced
- Antimalarials: antagonism of anticonvulsant effect; increased risk of antifolate effect with *pyrimethamine* (includes *Fansidar®* and *Maloprim®*)

  Antiplatelet Drugs: plasma-phenytoin concentration increased by *aspirin*
- Antipsychotics: antagonism of anticonvulsant effect (convulsive threshold lowered); *phenytoin* accelerates metabolism of *clozapine, quetiapine* and *sertindole* (reduced plasma concentrations)
- Antivirals: plasma concentration of *indinavir, nelfinavir* and *saquinavir* possibly reduced; plasma-phenytoin concentrations increased or decreased by *zidovudine*

  Anxiolytics and Hypnotics: *diazepam* and possibly *other benzodiazepines* increase or decrease plasma-phenytoin concentration
- Calcium-channel Blockers: *diltiazem* and *nifedipine* increase plasma concentration of *phenytoin*; effect of *felodipine, isradipine, nisoldipine* and probably *nicardipine, nifedipine* and *other dihydropyridines, diltiazam,* and *verapamil* reduced

  Cardiac Glycosides: metabolism of *digitoxin only* accelerated (reduced effect)
- Ciclosporin: metabolism of *ciclosporin* accelerated (reduced plasma concentration)
- Corticosteroids: metabolism of *corticosteroids* accelerated (reduced effect)

  Cytotoxics: reduced absorption of *phenytoin*; increased antifolate effect with *methotrexate*
- Disulfiram: plasma-phenytoin concentration increased

  Diuretics: increased risk of osteomalacia with *carbonic anhydrase inhibitors*

  Folic Acid and Folinic Acid: plasma-phenytoin concentration possibly reduced by *folic acid* and *folinic acid*

  Food: some *enteral foods* may interfere with absorption of *phenytoin*

  Hormone Antagonists: metabolism of *toremifene* possibly accelerated

  Levothyroxine: metabolism of *levothyroxine* accelerated (may increase levothyroxine requirements in hypothyroidism)

  Lithium: neurotoxicity may occur without increased plasma-lithium concentration

  Muscle Relaxants: effect of *non-depolarising muscle relaxants* antagonised (recovery from neuromuscular blockade accelerated)

Phenytoin *(continued)*
- Oestrogens and Progestogens: metabolism of *gestrinone, tibolone, and oral contraceptives* accelerated (reduced contraceptive effect, **important:** see p. 368)

  Sympathomimetics: plasma-phenytoin concentration increased by *methylphenidate*

  Theophylline: metabolism of *theophylline* accelerated (reduced plasma-theophylline concentration)
- Ulcer-healing Drugs: *cimetidine* inhibits metabolism (increased plasma-phenytoin concentration); *sucralfate* reduces absorption; *omeprazole* enhances effect of *phenytoin* (interaction with *lansoprazole* possibly differs)
- Uricosurics: plasma-phenytoin concentration increased by *sulfinpyrazone*

  Vaccines: effect enhanced by *influenza vaccine*

  Vitamins: *vitamin D* requirements possibly increased

Physostigmine *see* Parasympathomimetics
Phytomenadione *see* Vitamins (Vitamin K)
Pilocarpine *see* Parasympathomimetics
Pimozide *see* Antipsychotics
Pindolol *see* Beta-blockers
Piperacillin *see* Penicillins
Pipotiazine *see* Antipsychotics
Piroxicam *see* NSAIDs
Pivmecillinam *see* Penicillins
Pizotifen
  Antihypertensives: hypotensive effect of *adrenergic neurone blockers* antagonised
Platinum Compounds
- Antibacterials: *aminoglycosides* and *capreomycin* increase risk of nephrotoxicity and possibly of ototoxicity

  Diuretics: increased risk of nephrotoxicity and ototoxicity
Polymyxins *see* Colistin
Polythiazide *see* Diuretics (thiazides)
Potassium Aminobenzoate
  Antibacterials: effect of *sulphonamides* inhibited
Potassium Salts (includes Salt Substitutes)
- ACE Inhibitors and Angiotensin-II Antagonists: increased risk of hyperkalaemia
- Ciclosporin: increased risk of hyperkalaemia
- Diuretics: hyperkalaemia with *potassium-sparing diuretics*
Pramipexole
  Ulcer-healing Drugs: *cimetidine* inhibits excretion (increased plasma-pramipexole concentration)
Pravastatin *see* Statins
Prazosin *see* Alpha-blockers (post-synaptic)
Prednisolone *see* Corticosteroids
Prednisone *see* Corticosteroids
Prilocaine
  Antibacterials: increased risk of methaemoglobinaemia with *co-trimoxazole* and *sulphonamides*
Primaquine
  Mepacrine: increased plasma concentration of *primaquine* (risk of toxicity)
Primaxin®
- Antivirals: increased toxicity with *ganciclovir* (convulsions reported)
Primidone *see* Barbiturates and Primidone
Probenecid
  ACE Inhibitors and Angiotensin-II Antagonists: reduced excretion of *captopril*
- Analgesics: *aspirin* antagonises effect; excretion of *indometacin, ketoprofen, ketorolac* (avoid concomitant use), and *naproxen* delayed and increased plasma-NSAID concentrations

  Antibacterials: reduced excretion of *cephalosporins, cinoxacin, ciprofloxacin, dapsone, nalidixic acid, nitrofurantoin, norfloxacin,* and *penicillins* (increased plasma-concentrations); antagonism by *pyrazinamide*

Probenecid (*continued*)
Antidiabetics: hypoglycaemic effect of *chlorpropamide* possibly enhanced
Antivirals: reduced excretion of *aciclovir, ganciclovir, zidovudine*, and possibly *famciclovir* and *zalcitabine* (increased plasma concentrations)
• Cytotoxics: reduced excretion of *methotrexate* (increased risk of toxicity)

Procainamide
ACE Inhibitors and Angiotensin-II Antagonists: increased risk of toxicity with *captopril*, especially in renal impairment
• *other* Anti-arrhythmics: *amiodarone* increases procainamide-plasma concentrations (increased risk of ventricular arrhythmias—avoid concomitant use); increased myocardial depression with *any anti-arrhythmic*
Antibacterials: *trimethoprim* increases plasma concentration of *procainamide*
• Antidepressants: increased risk of ventricular arrhythmias with *tricyclics*; manufacturer of *reboxetine* advises caution
• Antihistamines: increased risk of ventricular arrhythmias with *mizolastine* and *terfenadine* (avoid concomitant use)
• Antimalarials: increased risk of ventricular arrhythmias with *halofantrine*
• Antipsychotics: increased risk of ventricular arrhythmias—avoid concomitant use with *pimozide, sertindole* or *thioridazine*
• Beta-blockers: increased risk of ventricular arrhythmias associated with *sotalol* (avoid concomitant use)
• Cisapride: increased risk of ventricular arrhythmias —avoid concomitant use
• Muscle Relaxants: muscle relaxant effect enhanced
Parasympathomimetics: antagonism of effect of *neostigmine* and *pyridostigmine*
Tropisetron: risk of ventricular arrhythmias—manufacturer of tropisetron advises caution
• Ulcer-healing Drugs: *cimetidine* inhibits excretion (increased plasma-procainamide concentration)

Procarbazine
Alcohol: disulfiram-like reaction

Prochlorperazine *see* Antipsychotics
Procyclidine *see* Antimuscarinics
Progestogens (*see also* Contraceptives, Oral)
Antibacterials: metabolism accelerated by *rifamycins* (reduced effect)
• Antivirals: *nevirapine* accelerates metabolism of *hormonal contraceptives* (reduced contraceptive effect)
• Ciclosporin: increased plasma-ciclosporin concentration (inhibition of metabolism)
Hormone Antagonists: *aminoglutethimide* reduces plasma concentration of *medroxyprogesterone*

Proguanil
• Anticoagulants: effect of *warfarin* possibly enhanced
Antacids: *magnesium trisilicate* reduces absorption of proguanil

Promazine *see* Antipsychotics
Promethazine *see* Antihistamines
Propafenone
other Anti-arrhythmics: *quinidine* increases plasma concentration of *propafenone*; increased myocardial depression with any *anti-arrhythmic*
• Antibacterials: *rifampicin* reduces plasma concentration of *propafenone* (reduced effect)
• Anticoagulants: increased plasma concentration of *acenocoumarol* and *warfarin* (enhanced effect)
• Antidepressants: increased risk of arrhythmias with *tricyclics*; manufacturer of *reboxetine* advises caution
• Antihistamines: increased risk of ventricular arrhythmias with *terfenadine*
• Antivirals: plasma concentration increased by *ritonavir* (increased risk of ventricular arrhythmias—avoid concomitant use)

Propafenone (*continued*)
Beta-blockers: increased plasma concentration of *metoprolol* and *propranolol*
• Cardiac Glycosides: increased plasma concentrations of *digoxin* (halve maintenance dose of digoxin)
Ciclosporin: plasma-ciclosporin concentration possibly increased
Parasympathomimetics: possible antagonism of effect of *neostigmine* and *pyridostigmine*
Theophylline: increased plasma-theophylline concentration
Tropisetron: risk of ventricular arrhythmias—manufacturer of tropisetron advises caution
• Ulcer-healing Drugs: *cimetidine* increases plasma-propafenone concentration

Propantheline *see* Antimuscarinics
Propiverine *see* Antimuscarinics
Propofol *see* Anaesthetics, General
Propranolol *see* Beta-blockers
Prostaglandins
Oxytocin: uterotonic effect enhanced
Protease Inhibitors *see* Indinavir; nelfinavir; Ritonavir; Saquinavir
Proton Pump Inhibitors
Antacids: possibly reduced absorption of *lansoprazole*
• Anticoagulants: effects of *warfarin* enhanced by *omeprazole*; interaction with *lansoprazole* possibly differs
• Antiepileptics: effects of *phenytoin* enhanced by *omeprazole*; interaction with *lansoprazole* possibly differs
Antifungals: absorption of *ketoconazole* and possibly *itraconazole* reduced
Anxiolytics and Hypnotics: metabolism of *diazepam* inhibited by *omeprazole* (increased effect possible)
Cardiac Glycosides: plasma concentration of *digoxin* possibly slightly increased
Oestrogens and Progestogens: manufacturer advises that *lansoprazole* possibly accelerates metabolism of *oral contraceptives*
Tacrolimus: *omeprazole* possibly increases plasma-tacrolimus concentration
Ulcer-healing Drugs: *sucralfate* reduces absorption of lansoprazole

Protriptyline *see* Antidepressants, Tricyclic
Pseudoephedrine *see* Sympathomimetics
Pyrazinamide
Uricosurics: antagonism of effect of *probenecid and sulfinpyrazone*
Pyridostigmine *see* Parasympathomimetics
Pyridoxine *see* Vitamins
Pyrimethamine
• Antibacterials: increased antifolate effect with *co-trimoxazole* and *trimethoprim*
Antiepileptics: increased antifolate effect with *phenytoin*
Cytotoxics: increased antifolate effect with *methotrexate*
Quetiapine *see* Antipsychotics
Quinagolide
Note. No interactions reported; theoretical possibility of reduced effect with dopamine antagonists (eg phenothiazines)
Quinapril *see* ACE Inhibitors and Angiotensin-II Antagonists
Quinidine
Antacids and Adsorbents: reduced excretion in alkaline urine (plasma-quinidine concentration occasionally increased); absorption possibly reduced by *kaolin* (possibly reduced plasma concentration)
• *other* Anti-arrhythmics: *amiodarone* increases plasma-quinidine concentrations (and increases risk of ventricular arrhythmias—avoid concomitant use); plasma concentration of *propafenone* increased; increased myocardial depression with *any anti-arrhythmic*

Quinidine (*continued*)
- Antibacterials: increased risk of arrhythmias with *quinupristin/dalfopristin* (avoid concomitant use); *rifamycins* accelerate metabolism (reduced plasma-quinidine concentration)

  Anticoagulants: effect of *acenocoumarol* and *warfarin* may be enhanced
- Antidepressants: increased risk of ventricular arrhythmias with *tricyclics*; manufacturer of *reboxetine* advises caution

  Antiepileptics: *phenobarbital, phenytoin,* and *primidone* accelerate metabolism (reduced plasma-quinidine concentration)

  Antifungals: plasma concentration increased by *itraconazole*
- Antihistamines: increased risk of ventricular arrhythmias with *mizolastine* and *terfenadine* (avoid concomitant use)
- Antimalarials: increased risk of ventricular arrhythmias with *halofantrine* and *mefloquine*
- Antipsychotics: increased risk of ventricular arrhythmias—avoid concomitant use with *pimozide, sertindole* or *thioridazine*
- Antivirals: increased risk of ventricular arrhythmias with *nelfinavir* and *ritonavir* (avoid concomitant use)

  Barbiturates and Primidone: *see under* Antiepileptics, above
- Beta-blockers: increased risk of ventricular arrhythmias associated with *sotalol* (avoid concomitant use)
- Calcium-channel Blockers: *nifedipine* reduces plasma-quinidine concentration; *verapamil* increases plasma-quinidine concentration (possibility of extreme hypotension)
- Cardiac Glycosides: plasma concentration of *digoxin* increased (halve digoxin maintenance dose)
- Cisapride: increased risk of ventricular arrhythmias (avoid concomitant use)
- Diuretics: *acetazolamide* reduces excretion (plasma-quinidine concentration occasionally increased); quinidine toxicity increased if hypokalaemia occurs with *acetazolamide, loop diuretics,* and *thiazides*
- Muscle Relaxants: muscle relaxant effect enhanced

  Parasympathomimetics: antagonism of effect of *neostigmine and pyridostigmine*

  Tropisetron: risk of ventricular arrhythmias—manufacturer of tropisetron advises caution
- Ulcer-healing Drugs: *cimetidine* inhibits metabolism (increased plasma-quinidine concentration)

Quinine
- Anti-arrhythmics: plasma concentration of *flecainide* increased; increased risk of ventricular arrhythmias with *amiodarone* (avoid concomitant use)
- Antihistamines: increased risk of ventricular arrhythmias with *terfenadine*—avoid concomitant use
- Antipsychotics: increased risk of ventricular arrhythmias—avoid concomitant use with *pimozide*
- *other* Antimalarials: *see* Halofantrine, Mefloquine
- Cardiac Glycosides: plasma concentration of *digoxin* increased
- Cisapride: increased risk of ventricular arrhythmias—avoid concomitant use

  Ulcer-healing Drugs: *cimetidine* inhibits metabolism (increased plasma-quinine concentration)

Quinolones
- Analgesics: possible increased risk of convulsions with *NSAIDs*; manufacturer of *ciprofloxacin* advises avoid premedication with *opioid analgesics* (reduced plasma-ciprofloxacin concentration)

  Antacids and Adsorbents: *antacids* reduce absorption of *ciprofloxacin, levofloxacin, norfloxacin* and *ofloxacin*
- Anticoagulants: anticoagulant effect of *acenocoumarol* and *warfarin* enhanced by *ciprofloxacin, nalidixic acid, norfloxacin* and *ofloxacin*

Quinolones (*continued*)
  Antidiabetics: effect of *glibenclamide* possibly enhanced by *ciprofloxacin*

  Antiepileptics: *ciprofloxacin* possibly alters plasma concentration of *phenytoin*

  Calcium Salts: reduced absorption of *ciprofloxacin*
- Ciclosporin: increased risk of nephrotoxicity

  Cytotoxics: toxicity of *melphalan* increased by *nalidixic acid*

  $5HT_1$ Agonists: quinolones possibly inhibit metabolism of *zolmitriptan* (reduce dose of zolmitriptan)

  Iron: absorption of *ciprofloxacin, levofloxacin, norfloxacin,* and *ofloxacin* reduced by *oral iron*
- Theophylline: possible increased risk of convulsions; *ciprofloxacin* and *norfloxacin* increase plasma-theophylline concentration

  Ulcer-healing Drugs: *sucralfate* reduces absorption of *ciprofloxacin, levofloxacin, norfloxacin,* and *ofloxacin*

  Uricosurics: *probenecid* reduces excretion of *cinoxacin, ciprofloxacin, nalidixic acid* and *norfloxacin*

  Zinc Salts: *zinc* reduces absorption of *ciprofloxacin* and *norfloxacin*

Quinupristin/Dalfopristin
- Anti-arrhythmics: increased risk of ventricular arrhythmias with *disopyramide, lidocaine* and *quinidine*—avoid concomitant use
- Antihistamines: increased risk of ventricular arrhythmias with *terfenadine*—avoid concomitant use
- Anxiolytics and Hypnotics: increased plasma concentration of *midazolam* (risk of profound sedation)
- Calcium-channel Blockers: increased plasma concentration of *nifedipine*
- Cisapride: increased risk of ventricular arrhythmias —avoid concomitant use
- Ciclosporin: increased plasma concentration of ciclosporin
- Tacrolimus: increased plasma concentration of tacrolimus

Rabeprazole *see* Proton Pump Inhibitors
Rabies Vaccine *see* p. 553
Raloxifene
  Anion-exchange Resins: *colestyramine* reduces absorption of raloxifene (manufacturer advises avoid concomitant administration)

  Anticoagulants: antagonism of anticoagulant effect of *warfarin* and *acenocoumarol*
Ramipril *see* ACE Inhibitors and Angiotensin-II Antagonists
Ranitidine *see* Histamine H_2-antagonists
Ranitidine Bismuth Citrate *see* Histamine H_2-antagonists
Reboxetine
  Anti-arrhythmics: manufacturer of reboxetine advises caution
- Antibacterials: manufacturer of reboxetine advises avoid concomitant use with *macrolides*
- *other* Antidepressants: risk of increased toxicity with *MAOIs* (reboxetine should not be started until 2 weeks after stopping MAOI, and conversely MAOI should not be started until at least 1 week after stopping reboxetine); manufacturer of reboxetine advises avoid concomitant use with *fluvoxamine* and caution with *tricyclics*
- Antifungals: manufacturer of reboxetine advises avoid concomitant use with *imidazoles* and *triazoles*

  Antipsychotics: manufacturer of reboxetine advises caution

  Ciclosporin: manufacturer of reboxetine advises caution

  Diuretics: possibly increased risk of hypokalaemia with *loop diuretics* or *thiazides*

  Ergotamine: possibly increased blood pressure
Remifentanil *see* Opioid Analgesics
Repaglinide *see* Antidiabetics
Reproterol *see* Sympathomimetics, Beta$_2$

Retinoids
  Alcohol: etretinate formed from *acitretin* in presence
    of *alcohol*
  Antibacterials: possible increased risk of benign
    intracranial hypertension with *tetracyclines* and
    acitretin, isotretinoin and *tretinoin*
• Anticoagulants: *acitretin* possibly reduces
    anticoagulant effect of *warfarin*
  Antiepileptics: plasma concentration of
    carbamazepine possibly reduced by *isotretinoin*
• Cytotoxics: *acitretin* increases plasma concentration
    of *methotrexate* (also increased risk of
    hepatotoxicity)
• Oestrogens and Progestogens: *tretinoin* reduces
    efficacy of *progestogen-only* and possibly
    combined oral contraceptives
  Vitamins: risk of hypervitaminosis A with *vitamin A*
    and *acitretin, isotretinoin* and *tretinoin*
Rifabutin *see* Rifamycins
Rifampicin *see* Rifamycins
Rifamycins
  ACE Inhibitors and Angiotensin-II Antagonists:
    rifampicin reduces plasma concentration of active
    metabolite of *imidapril* (reduced antihypertensive
    effect)
  Analgesics: metabolism of *methadone* accelerated
    (reduced effect)
  Antacids: reduced absorption of *rifampicin*
• Anti-arrhythmics: metabolism accelerated—reduced
    plasma concentrations of *disopyramide, mexiletine,
    propafenone, quinidine* and *tocainide*
• *other* Antibacterials: metabolism of *chloramphenicol*
    accelerated by *rifampicin* (reduced plasma
    concentration); plasma concentration of *dapsone*
    reduced; plasma concentration of *rifabutin*
    increased by *clarithromycin* and possibly *other
    macrolides* (risk of uveitis—reduce rifabutin dose)
• Anticoagulants: metabolism of *acenocoumarol* and
    warfarin accelerated (reduced anticoagulant effect)
  Antidepressants: metabolism of some *tricyclics*
    accelerated by *rifampicin* (reduced plasma
    concentration)
• Antidiabetics: metabolism of *chlorpropamide,
    tolbutamide and possibly other sulphonylureas*
    accelerated (reduced effect); *rifampicin* possibly
    reduces plasma concentration of *repaglinide*
    (manufacturer advises avoid concomitant use)
• Antiepileptics: metabolism of *phenytoin* accelerated
    (reduced plasma concentration); plasma
    concentration of *carbamazepine* reduced by
    rifabutin
• Antifungals: metabolism of *fluconazole, itraconazole*
    and *ketoconazole* accelerated by *rifampicin* (reduced
    plasma concentrations); plasma concentration of
    rifampicin may be reduced by *ketoconazole*; plasma
    concentration of *terbinafine* reduced by *rifampicin*;
    plasma concentration of *rifabutin* increased by
    fluconazole and possibly *other triazoles* (risk of
    uveitis—reduce rifabutin dose)
  Antipsychotics: metabolism of *haloperidol*
    accelerated by *rifampicin* (reduced plasma
    concentration)
• Antivirals: concomitant administration of *indinavir* and
    rifabutin increases plasma-rifabutin concentration and
    decreases plasma-indinavir concentration (reduce
    dose of rifabutin and increase dose of indinavir);
    metabolism of *indinavir* enhanced by *rifampicin*
    (plasma-indinavir concentration significantly
    reduced—avoid concomitant use); *rifampicin* reduces
    plasma concentration of *efavirenz* (increase efavirenz
    dose); plasma concentration of *nelfinavir* significantly
    reduced by *rifampicin* (avoid concomitant use);
    plasma concentration of *rifabutin* increased by
    nelfinavir (halve rifabutin dose); plasma concentration
    of *rifabutin* increased by *ritonavir* (risk of uveitis—
    avoid concomitant use); plasma concentration of
    saquinavir reduced (avoid concomitant use); plasma
    concentration of *nevirapine* reduced

Rifamycins *(continued)*
  Anxiolytics and Hypnotics: metabolism of *diazepam*
    and possibly *other benzodiazepines* accelerated
    (reduced plasma concentration)
• Atovaquone: plasma concentration reduced by
    rifampicin (possible therapeutic failure of
    atovaquone)
  Beta-blockers: metabolism of *bisoprolol* and
    propranolol accelerated by *rifampicin* (plasma
    concentrations significantly reduced)
• Calcium-channel Blockers: metabolism of *diltiazem,
    nifedipine*, and *verapamil* and possibly *isradipine,
    nicardipine* and *nisoldipine* accelerated by
    rifampicin (plasma concentrations significantly
    reduced)
  Cardiac Glycosides: metabolism of *digitoxin only*
    accelerated (reduced effect)
• Ciclosporin: metabolism accelerated (reduced
    plasma-ciclosporin concentration)
• Corticosteroids: metabolism of *corticosteroids*
    accelerated (reduced effect)
• Cytotoxics: manufacturer reports interaction with
    azathioprine (transplants possibly rejected)
  Levothyroxine: metabolism of *levothyroxine*
    accelerated by *rifampicin* (may increase
    requirements in hypothyroidism)
  Lipid-regulating Drugs: metabolism of *fluvastatin*
    accelerated (reduced effect)
• Oestrogens and Progestogens: metabolism
    accelerated (contraceptive effect of *both combined
    and progestogen-only oral contraceptives* reduced,
    important: see p. 368)
• Tacrolimus: *rifampicin* decreases plasma-tacrolimus
    concentration
  Theophylline: metabolism accelerated by *rifampicin*
    (reduced plasma-theophylline concentration)
  Tropisetron: plasma concentration of *tropisetron*
    reduced by *rifampicin*
  Ulcer-healing Drugs: metabolism of *cimetidine*
    accelerated by *rifampicin* (reduced plasma
    concentration)
Riluzole
  Note. No clinical data available but since riluzole exten-
  sively metabolised by the liver, possibility of interac-
  tions with a number of drugs—consult product literature
  for details
Risperidone *see* Antipsychotics
Ritodrine *see* Sympathomimetics, Sympathomimetics,
  Beta$_2$, and p. 363
Ritonavir
• Analgesics: plasma concentration of
    dextropropoxyphene, pethidine and *piroxicam*
    increased (risk of toxicity—avoid concomitant
    use); plasma concentrations of *other opioid
    analgesics* (except methadone) *and other NSAIDs*
    possibly increased; plasma concentration of
    methadone reduced
• Anti-arrhythmics: increased plasma concentration of
    amiodarone, flecainide, propafenone and *quinidine*
    (increased risk of ventricular arrhythmias—avoid
    concomitant use); possibly increased risk of
    arrhythmias with *disopyramide* and *mexiletine*
• Antibacterials: plasma concentration of *rifabutin*
    increased by *ritonavir* (risk of uveitis—avoid
    concomitant use); plasma concentration of
    macrolides possibly increased
• Anticoagulants: plasma concentration of *warfarin* and
    other anticoagulants possibly increased
• Antidepressants: plasma concentration of *SSRIs* and
    tricyclics possibly increased
  Antidiabetics: plasma concentration of *tolbutamide*
    possibly increased
• Antiepileptics: plasma concentration of
    carbamazepine possibly increased
• Antifungals: plasma concentration of *imidazoles* and
    triazoles possibly increased

Ritonavir *(continued)*
- Antihistamines: increased risk of arrhythmias with *terfenadine*—avoid concomitant use; plasma concentration of *other non-sedating antihistamines* possibly increased
- Antipsychotics: increased plasma concentration of *pimozide* (risk of ventricular arrhythmias—avoid concomitant use); increased plasma concentration of *clozapine* (risk of toxicity—avoid concomitant use); possibly increased plasma concentration of *other antipsychotics*
- *other* Antivirals: combination with *nelfinavir* may lead to increased plasma concentration of either drug; *ritonavir* increases plasma concentration of *indinavir* and *saquinavir*; increased risk of toxicity with *efavirenz* (monitor liver function tests)
- Anxiolytics and Hypnotics: plasma concentration of *alprazolam, clorazepate, diazepam, flurazepam, midazolam* and *zolpidem* increased (risk of extreme sedation and respiratory depression—avoid concomitant use); plasma concentration of *other anxiolytics and hypnotics* possibly increased
- Calcium-channel Blockers: plasma concentration of *calcium-channel blocker* possibly increased
- Ciclosporin: plasma-ciclosporin concentration possibly increased
- Cisapride: plasma-cisapride concentration possibly significantly increased (risk of ventricular arrhythmias—avoid concomitant use)
  Corticosteroids: plasma concentration of *dexamethasone* and *prednisolone* (and possibly other corticosteroids) possibly increased
- Ergotamine: risk of ergotism—avoid concomitant use
- Lipid-regulating Drugs: increased risk of myopathy with simvastatin
- Oestrogens and Progestogens: metabolism accelerated by *ritonavir* (contraceptive effect of combined oral contraceptives reduced)
- Sildenafil: ritonavir significantly increases plasma-*sildenafil* concentration (avoid concomitant use)
- Tacrolimus: plasma-tacrolimus concentration possibly increased
- Theophylline: metabolism accelerated by *ritonavir* (reduced plasma-theophylline concentration)

Rivastigmine *see* Parasympathomimetics
Rizatriptan *see* 5HT$_1$ Agonists
Rocuronium *see* Muscle Relaxants (non-depolarising)
Rofecoxib *see* NSAIDs
Ropinirole
Note. Limited clinical data available, but possibility of interactions—consult product literature for details
Ropivacaine
  Antidepressants: *fluvoxamine* reduces metabolism of ropivacaine—avoid prolonged administration of ropivacaine
Rowachol®
Anticoagulants: effect of *acenocoumarol* and *warfarin* possibly reduced
Salbutamol *see* Sympathomimetics, Beta$_2$
Salmeterol *see* Sympathomimetics, Beta$_2$
Salt Substitutes *see* Potassium Salts
Saquinavir
- Antibacterials: metabolism accelerated by *rifamycins* (reduced plasma concentration—avoid concomitant use)
- Antiepileptics: plasma concentration possibly reduced by *carbamazepine, phenobarbital* and *phenytoin*
  Antifungals: plasma concentration increased by *ketoconazole* and possibly by *other imidazoles* and *triazoles*
- Antihistamines: increased risk of arrhythmias with *terfenadine*—avoid concomitant use
- Antipsychotics: possibly increased risk of arrhythmias with *pimozide* (avoid concomitant use)

Saquinavir *(continued)*
- *other* Antivirals: *nevirapine* reduces plasma concentration of saquinavir (avoid concomitant use); combination with *nelfinavir* may lead to increased plasma concentration of either drug; *indinavir* and *ritonavir* increase plasma concentration of saquinavir; *efavirenz* significantly reduces plasma concentration of saquinavir
- Anxiolytics and Hypnotics: plasma concentration of *midazolam* possibly increased (prolonged sedation—avoid concomitant use)
  Barbiturates and Primidone: *see under* Antiepileptics above
- Cisapride: increased risk of ventricular arrhythmias (avoid concomitant use)
- Corticosteroids: plasma concentration possibly reduced by *dexamethasone*
- Ergotamine: possible risk of ergotism—avoid concomitant use
- Lipid-regulating Drugs: increased risk of myopathy with *simvastatin*
  Sildenafil: saquinavir increases plasma-*sildenafil* concentration (reduce initial dose of sildenafil)
  Ulcer-healing Drugs: plasma concentration increased by *ranitidine*
Secobarbital *see* Barbiturates and Primidone
Selegiline
Note. Selegiline is an MAO-B inhibitor
- Analgesics: hyperpyrexia and CNS toxicity with *pethidine* (avoid concomitant use)
- Antidepressants: hypertension and CNS excitation with *fluoxetine, paroxetine* and *sertraline* (selegiline should not be started until 5 weeks after discontinuation of fluoxetine, avoid fluoxetine for 2 weeks after stopping selegiline; selegiline should not be started until 2 weeks after stopping sertraline, avoid sertraline for 2 weeks after stopping selegiline); hypotension with *MAOIs*; CNS toxicity reported with *tricyclic antidepressants*; avoid concomitant use with *moclobemide*
Sermorelin
Note. Avoid preparations which affect release of growth hormone, see p. 348
Sertindole *see* Antipsychotics
Sertraline *see* Antidepressants, SSRI
Sevoflurane *see* Anaesthetics, General
Sildenafil
Note. Grapefruit juice increases plasma concentration of sildenafil
  Antibacterials: *erythromycin* increases plasma-sildenafil concentration (reduce initial dose of sildenafil)
  Antifungals: *ketoconazole* increases plasma-sildenafil concentration (reduce initial dose of sildenafil)
- Antivirals: *ritonavir* significantly increases plasma-sildenafil concentration (avoid concomitant use); *saquinavir* and possibly *indinavir* and *nelfinavir* increase plasma-sildenafil concentration (reduce initial dose of sildenafil)
- Nicorandil: hypotensive effect significantly enhanced—avoid concomitant use
- Nitrates: hypotensive effect significantly enhanced—avoid concomitant use
  Ulcer-healing Drugs: *cimetidine* increases plasma-sildenafil concentration (reduce initial dose of sildenafil)
Simvastatin *see* Statins
Sodium Aurothiomalate *see* Gold
Sodium Bicarbonate *see* Antacids
Sodium Clodronate *see* Bisphosphonates
Sodium Valproate *see* Valproate
Somatropin
  Corticosteroids: may inhibit growth promoting effect of somatropin

Sotalol see Beta-blockers
Spironolactone see Diuretics (potassium-sparing)
Stanozolol see Anabolic Steroids
Statins
  <u>Antibacterials</u>: metabolism of *fluvastatin* accelerated by *rifampicin* (reduced effect); *clarithromycin* and *erythromycin* increase risk of myopathy with *simvastatin*; *erythromycin* possibly increases risk of myopathy with *atorvastatin* and *cerivastatin*
• Anticoagulants: effect of *acenocoumarol* and *warfarin* enhanced by *simvastatin*
  Antidepressants: *nefazodone* increases risk of myopathy with *simvastatin*
• <u>Antifungals</u>: *itraconazole*, *ketoconazole* and possibly other *imidazoles* and *triazoles* increase risk of myopathy with *simvastatin*—avoid concomitant use of *itraconazole* with *simvastatin*; *itraconazole* and possibly other *imidazoles* and *triazoles* may increase risk of myopathy with *atorvastatin*; *itraconazole* increases plasma concentration of *cerivastatin*
• <u>Antivirals</u>: *protease inhibitors* increase risk of myopathy with *simvastatin*
  Cardiac Glycosides: plasma-digoxin concentration possibly increased by *atorvastatin*
• Ciclosporin: increased risk of myopathy
• *other* Lipid-regulating Drugs: increased risk of myopathy with *fibrates* and *nicotinic acid*
Stavudine
  Cytotoxics: *doxorubicin* may inhibit effect of *stavudine*
Streptomycin see Aminoglycosides
Sucralfate
  Antibacterials: reduced absorption of *ciprofloxacin, levofloxacin, norfloxacin, ofloxacin,* and *tetracycline*
• Anticoagulants: absorption of *warfarin* possibly reduced
• Antiepileptics: reduced absorption of *phenytoin*
  Antifungals: reduced absorption of *ketoconazole*
  Cardiac Glycosides: absorption of *cardiac glycosides* possibly reduced
  Levothyroxine: reduced absorption of *levothyroxine*
  other Ulcer-healing Drugs: reduced absorption of *lansoprazole*
Sulfadiazine see Co-trimoxazole and Sulphonamides
Sulfadoxine see Co-trimoxazole and Sulphonamides
Sulfametopyrazine see Co-trimoxazole and Sulphonamides
Sulfasalazine
  Cardiac Glycosides: absorption of *digoxin* possibly reduced
Sulfinpyrazone
  Analgesics: *aspirin* antagonises uricosuric effect
  Antibacterials: *pyrazinamide* antagonises effect
• Anticoagulants: anticoagulant effect of *acenocoumarol* and *warfarin* enhanced
• Antidiabetics: effect of *sulphonylureas* enhanced
• Antiepileptics: plasma concentration of *phenytoin* increased
  Theophylline: plasma-theophylline concentration reduced
Sulindac see NSAIDs
Sulphonamides see Co-trimoxazole and Sulphonamides
Sulphonylureas see Antidiabetics
Sulpiride see Antipsychotics
Sumatriptan see 5HT$_1$ Agonists
Suxamethonium see Muscle Relaxants
Sympathomimetics (*see below* for Beta$_2$-Sympathomimetics)
  Alpha$_2$-adrenoceptor Stimulants: possible risk of hypertension with *adrenaline* and *noradrenaline*
• Anaesthetics: risk of arrhythmias if *adrenaline and isoprenaline* given with *volatile liquid anaesthetics* such as *halothane*

Sympathomimetics *(continued)*
• Antidepressants: with *tricyclics* administration of *adrenaline* and *noradrenaline* may cause hypertension and arrhythmias (but local anaesthetics with adrenaline appear to be safe); *methylphenidate* may inhibit metabolism of *tricyclics*; with *MAOIs* administration of inotropics such as *dopamine* and *dopexamine* may cause hypertensive crisis; also with *MAOIs* administration of *dexamfetamine and other amfetamines, ephedrine, isometheptene, methylphenidate, phentermine, phenylephrine, phenylpropanolamine,* and *pseudoephedrine* may cause hypertensive crisis (these drugs are contained in anorectics or cold and cough remedies)
  Antiepileptics: *methylphenidate* increases plasma concentration of *phenytoin* and possibly of *phenobarbital* and *primidone*
• Antihypertensives: sympathomimetics in *anorectics and cold and cough remedies (see* above) and *methylphenidate* antagonise hypotensive effect of *adrenergic neurone blockers*
  Barbiturates and Primidone: *see under* Antiepileptics, above
• Beta-blockers: severe hypertension with *adrenaline* and *noradrenaline* and possibly with *dobutamine* (especially with non-selective beta-blockers)
  Corticosteroids: *ephedrine* accelerates metabolism of *dexamethasone*
• Dopaminergics: increased risk of toxicity when *isometheptene* or *phenylpropanolamine* given with *bromocriptine*; effect of *adrenaline, dobutamine, dopamine, isoprenaline* and *noradrenaline* possibly enhanced by *entacapone*
  Orlistat: manufacturer advises avoid concomitant use with *phentermine*
  Doxapram: risk of hypertension
  Oxytocin: hypertension with vasoconstrictor sympathomimetics
• *other* Sympathomimetics: *dopexamine* possibly potentiates effect of *adrenaline* and *noradrenaline*
Sympathomimetics, Beta$_2$
• Antihypertensives: acute hypotension reported with *salbutamol* infusion and *methyldopa*
  Corticosteroids: increased risk of hypokalaemia if high doses of *corticosteroids* given with high doses of *bambuterol, fenoterol, formoterol, reproterol, ritodrine, salbutamol, salmeterol, terbutaline* and *tulobuterol*; *see also* CSM advice, p. 133
  Diuretics: increased risk of hypokalaemia if *acetazolamide, loop diuretics,* and *thiazides* given with high doses of *bambuterol, fenoterol, formoterol, reproterol, ritodrine, salbutamol, salmeterol, terbutaline,* and *tulobuterol*; *see also* CSM advice, p. 133
  Muscle Relaxants: effect of *suxamethonium* enhanced by *bambuterol*
  Theophylline: increased risk of hypokalaemia if given with high doses of *bambuterol, fenoterol, formoterol, reproterol, ritodrine, salbutamol, salmeterol, terbutaline,* and *tulobuterol*; *see also* CSM advice. p. 133
Tacrolimus
• Analgesics: *ibuprofen* and possibly *other NSAIDs* increase risk of nephrotoxicity
• <u>Antibacterials</u>: *clarithromycin* and *erythromycin* increase plasma-tacrolimus concentration; *quinupristin/dalfopristin* increases plasma-tacrolimus concentration; *rifampicin* decreases plasma-tacrolimus concentration
• Antifungals: *amphotericin* increases risk of nephrotoxicity; *clotrimazole, fluconazole, ketoconazole* and possibly *other imidazoles* and *triazoles* increase plasma-tacrolimus concentration
• Antivirals: *ritonavir* possibly increases plasma-tacrolimus concentration
• Ciclosporin: plasma-ciclosporin half-life prolonged (increased risk of toxicity)

Tacrolimus *(continued)*

Hormone Antagonists: *danazol* possibly increases plasma-tacrolimus concentration

Oestrogens and Progestogens: efficacy of *oral contraceptives* possibly decreased

Ulcer-healing Drugs: *omeprazole* possibly increases plasma-tacrolimus concentration

Tamoxifen

• Anticoagulants: anticoagulant effect of *acenocoumarol* and *warfarin* enhanced

other Hormone Antagonists: *aminoglutethimide* reduces plasma-tamoxifen concentration

Tamsulosin *see* Alpha-blockers (post-synaptic)

Teicoplanin

Antibacterials: increased risk of ototoxicity and nephrotoxicity with *aminoglycosides* and *colistin*

Telmisartan *see* ACE Inhibitors and Angiotensin-II Antagonists

Temazepam *see* Anxiolytics and Hypnotics

Temocillin *see* Penicillins

Temozolomide

Antiepileptics: *valproate* increases plasma concentration of temozolomide

Tenoxicam *see* NSAIDs

Terazosin *see* Alpha-blockers (post-synaptic)

Terbinafine

Antibacterials: plasma concentration reduced by *rifampicin*

Ulcer-healing Drugs: plasma concentration increased by *cimetidine*

Terbutaline *see* Sympathomimetics, Beta$_2$

Terfenadine *see* Antihistamines

Testosterone

• Anticoagulants: anticoagulant effect of *warfarin*, *acenocoumarol* and *phenindione* enhanced

Antidiabetics: hypoglycaemic effect possibly enhanced

Tetrabenazine (general extrapyramidal interactions *as for* Antipsychotics)

• Antidepressants: CNS excitation and hypertension with *MAOIs*

Tetracosactide *see* Corticosteroids

Tetracyclines

ACE Inhibitors and Angiotensin-II Antagonists: *quinapril tablets* reduce absorption (contain magnesium carbonate excipient)

Antacids and Adsorbents: reduced absorption with *antacids* and possibly with *kaolin*

Anticoagulants: *see* Phenindione and Warfarin

Antiepileptics: *carbamazepine, phenobarbital, phenytoin,* and *primidone* increase metabolism of *doxycycline* (reduced plasma concentration)

Atovaquone: plasma-atovaquone concentration reduced by *tetracycline*

Barbiturates and Primidone: *see under* Antiepileptics, above

Calcium Salts: reduced absorption of *tetracyclines*

• Ciclosporin: *doxycycline* possibly increases plasma-ciclosporin concentration

Dairy products: reduced absorption (except *doxycycline* and *minocycline*)

Iron: absorption of *oral iron* reduced by *tetracyclines* and *vice versa*

Oestrogens and Progestogens: *see* Contraceptives, Oral (main list)

Retinoids: possible increased risk of benign intracranial hypertension with *tetracyclines* and *acitretin, isotretinoin* and *tretinoin*

Ulcer-healing Drugs: *tripotassium dicitrato-bismuthate* and *sucralfate* reduce absorption

Zinc Salts: reduced absorption (and *vice versa*)

Theophylline

Anaesthetics: increased risk of arrhythmias with *halothane*; increased risk of convulsions with *ketamine*

Anthelmintics: *tiabendazole* may increase plasma-theophylline concentration

Theophylline *(continued)*

Anti-arrhythmics: antagonism of anti-arrhythmic effect of *adenosine*; plasma-theophylline concentration increased by *mexiletine* and *propafenone*; plasma-theophylline concentration reduced by *moracizine*

• Antibacterials: possible increased risk of convulsions with *quinolones*; plasma-theophylline concentration increased by *ciprofloxacin, clarithromycin, erythromycin* (if erythromycin given by mouth, also decreased plasma-erythromycin concentration), and *norfloxacin* and possibly increased by *isoniazid*; plasma-theophylline concentration reduced by *rifampicin*

• Antidepressants: plasma-theophylline concentration increased by *fluvoxamine* (concomitant use should usually be avoided, but where not possible halve theophylline dose and monitor plasma-theophylline concentration) and *viloxazine*

Antiepileptics: plasma-theophylline concentration reduced by *carbamazepine, phenobarbital, phenytoin,* and *primidone*

• Antifungals: plasma-theophylline concentration possibly increased by *fluconazole* and *ketoconazole*

• Antiplatelet Drugs: *ticlopidine* increases plasma-theophylline concentration (risk of toxicity)

• Antivirals: plasma-theophylline concentration reduced by *ritonavir*

Barbiturates and Primidone: *see under* Antiepileptics, above

Beta-blockers: should be avoided on pharmacological grounds (bronchospasm)

• Calcium-channel Blockers: plasma-theophylline concentration increased by *diltiazem, verapamil,* and possibly *other calcium-channel blockers*

Disulfiram: increases plasma-theophylline concentration

Doxapram: increased CNS stimulation

Hormone Antagonists: plasma-theophylline concentration reduced by *aminoglutethimide*

Interferons: plasma-theophylline concentration increased by *interferon alfa*

Leukotriene Antagonists: *zafirlukast* possibly increases plasma-theophylline concentration; plasma-zafirlukast concentration reduced

Lithium: *lithium* excretion accelerated (reduced plasma-lithium concentration)

Nicotine and Tobacco: plasma-theophylline concentration reduced by *tobacco smoking*

Oestrogens and Progestogens: plasma-theophylline concentration increased by *combined oral contraceptives*

Pentoxifylline: plasma-theophylline concentration increased

Sympathomimetics: increased risk of hypokalaemia if *theophylline* given with high doses of *bambuterol, fenoterol, formoterol, reproterol, ritodrine, salbutamol, salmeterol, terbutaline,* and *tulobuterol*; *see also* CSM advice, p. 133

• Ulcer-healing Drugs: plasma-theophylline concentration increased by *cimetidine*

Uricosurics: plasma-theophylline concentration reduced by *sulfinpyrazone*

Vaccines: plasma-theophylline concentration occasionally increased by *influenza vaccine*

Thiopental *see* Anaesthetics, General

Thioridazine *see* Antipsychotics

Thiotepa

Muscle Relaxants: effect of *suxamethonium* enhanced

Thymoxamine *see* Moxisylyte

Thyroxine *see* Levothyroxine

Tiabendazole

Theophylline: plasma concentration may be increased

Tiagabine
- *other* Antiepileptics: concomitant administration of *two or more antiepileptics* may enhance toxicity without a corresponding increase in antiepileptic effect; moreover, interactions between individual antiepileptics can complicate monitoring of treatment; interactions include enhanced effects, increased sedation, and reductions in plasma concentrations; for further details, see p. 222

Tiaprofenic Acid *see* NSAIDs

Tibolone
Antibacterials: *rifampicin* accelerates metabolism (reduced plasma concentration)
Antiepileptics: *carbamazepine, phenobarbital, phenytoin, and primidone* accelerate metabolism (reduced plasma concentration)
Barbiturates and Primidone: *see* Antiepileptics, above

Ticlopidine
Analgesics: increased risk of bleeding with *NSAIDs* (including *aspirin*)
Anticoagulants: increased risk of bleeding
other Antiplatelet Drugs: increased risk of bleeding
- Ciclosporin: reduced plasma concentration of *ciclosporin*
- Theophylline: increased plasma concentration of *theophylline* (risk of toxicity)

Tiludronic Acid *see* Bisphosphonates

Timentin® *see* Penicillins

Timolol *see* Beta-blockers

Tinidazole
Alcohol: possibly disulfiram-like reaction

Tinzaparin *see* Heparin

Tizanidine *see* Muscle Relaxants

Tobramycin *see* Aminoglycosides

Tocainide
Antibacterials: plasma concentration reduced by *rifampicin*
Antidepressants: manufacturer of *reboxetine* advises caution

Tolazamide *see* Antidiabetics (sulphonylurea)

Tolbutamide *see* Antidiabetics (sulphonylurea)

Tolfenamic Acid *see* NSAIDs

Tolterodine *see* Antimuscarinics

Topiramate
- *other* Antiepileptics: concomitant administration of *two or more antiepileptics* may enhance toxicity without a corresponding increase in antiepileptic effect; moreover, interactions between individual antiepileptics can complicate monitoring of treatment; interactions include enhanced effects, increased sedation, and reductions in plasma concentrations; for further details, see p. 222
Oestrogens and Progestogens: metabolism of *oral contraceptives* accelerated (reduced contraceptive effect, **important:** see p. 368)

Torasemide *see* Diuretics (loop)

Toremifene
- Anticoagulants: anticoagulant effect of *acenocoumarol* and *warfarin* possibly enhanced
Antiepileptics: metabolism possibly accelerated by *carbamazepine, phenobarbital* and *phenytoin* (reduced plasma-toremifene concentration)
Diuretics: increased risk of hypercalcaemia with *thiazides*

Tramadol *see* Opioid Analgesics

Trandolapril *see* ACE Inhibitors and Angiotensin-II Antagonists

Tranylcypromine *see* MAOIs

Trazodone
Alcohol: enhanced sedative effect
Alpha$_2$-adrenoceptor Stimulants: manufacturers of *apraclonidine* and *brimonidine* advise avoid concomitant use
- *other* Antidepressants: as for Antidepressants, Tricyclic
- Antiepileptics: antagonism of anticonvulsant effect
Anxiolytics and Hypnotics: enhanced sedative effect

Tretinoin *see* Retinoids

Triamcinolone *see* Corticosteroids

Triamterene *see* Diuretics (potassium-sparing)

Triclofos *see* Anxiolytics and Hypnotics

Trientine
Iron: absorption of *oral iron* reduced

Trifluoperazine *see* Antipsychotics

Trihexyphenidyl (Benzhexol) *see* Antimuscarinics

Trilostane
Diuretics: increased risk of hyperkalaemia with *potassium-sparing diuretics*

Trimeprazine (Alimemazine) *see* Antihistamines

Trimethoprim
Anti-arrhythmics: plasma concentration of *procainamide* increased
Anticoagulants: effect of *acenocoumarol* and *warfarin* possibly enhanced
Antiepileptics: plasma concentration and antifolate effect of *phenytoin* increased
- Antimalarials: increased risk of antifolate effect with *pyrimethamine* (in *Fansidar®* and *Maloprim®*)
Antivirals: plasma concentration of *lamivudine* and possibly *zalcitabine* increased—avoid high-dose co-trimoxazole with *lamivudine*
- Ciclosporin: increased risk of nephrotoxicity; plasma-ciclosporin concentration possibly reduced by *intravenous trimethoprim*
- Cytotoxics: increased risk of haematological toxicity with *azathioprine* and *mercaptopurine*; antifolate effect of *methotrexate* increased

Trimetrexate
Note. Limited clinical data, but potential for serious interactions—consult product literature for details

Trimipramine *see* Antidepressants, Tricyclic

Tripotassium Dicitratobismuthate
Antibacterials: reduced absorption of *tetracyclines*

Triprolidine *see* Antihistamines

Tropicamide *see* Antimuscarinics

Tropisetron
Anti-arrhythmics: risk of ventricular arrhythmias—manufacturer advises caution
Antibacterials: *rifampicin* reduces plasma concentration of tropisetron
Barbiturates and Primidone: *phenobarbitone* reduces plasma concentration of tropisetron
Beta-blockers: risk of ventricular arrhythmias—manufacturer advises caution

Tryptophan
- *other* Antidepressants: CNS excitation and confusion with *MAOIs* (reduce tryptophan dose); agitation and nausea with *fluoxetine, fluvoxamine, paroxetine, and sertraline*

Tulobuterol *see* Sympathomimetics, Beta$_2$

Typhoid Vaccine *see* p. 555

Ulcer-healing Drugs *see* individual drugs

Uricosurics *see* individual drugs

Ursodeoxycholic Acid *see* Bile Acids

Vaccines *see* Influenza Vaccine (p. 597), Rabies Vaccine (p. 553), Typhoid Vaccine (p. 555)
Note. For a general warning on *live vaccines* and *high doses of corticosteroids* or *other immunosuppressive drugs*, see section 14.1; for advice on *live vaccines* and *immunoglobulins*, see under Normal Immunoglobulin, section 14.5

Valaciclovir *see* Aciclovir and Famciclovir
Note. Interactions as for aciclovir

Valproate
Analgesics: *aspirin* enhances effect
Anion-exchange Resins: *colestyramine* possibly reduces absorption
Antibacterials: *erythromycin* possibly inhibits metabolism (increased plasma-valproate concentration)
Anticoagulants: anticoagulant effect of *acenocoumarol* and *warfarin* possibly increased
- Antidepressants: antagonism of anticonvulsant effect (convulsive threshold lowered)

Valproate *(continued)*
- *other* Antiepileptics: concomitant administration of *two or more antiepileptics* may enhance toxicity without a corresponding increase in antiepileptic effect; moreover, interactions between individual antiepileptics can complicate monitoring of treatment; interactions include enhanced effects, increased sedation, and reductions in plasma concentrations; for further details, see p. 222
- Antimalarials: *chloroquine* and *mefloquine* antagonise anticonvulsant effect
- Antipsychotics: antagonism of anticonvulsant effect (convulsive threshold lowered)

  Antivirals: plasma concentration of *zidovudine* possibly increased (risk of toxicity)

  Cytotoxics: plasma concentration of *temozolomide* increased

  Ulcer-healing Drugs: *cimetidine* inhibits metabolism (increased plasma-valproate concentration)

Valsartan *see* ACE Inhibitors and Angiotensin-II Antagonists

Vancomycin

  Anaesthetics: hypersensitivity-like reactions can occur with concomitant vancomycin infusion

  Anion-exchange Resins: antagonism of *oral vancomycin* by *colestyramine*

  other Antibacterials: increased risk of ototoxicity and nephrotoxicity with *aminoglycosides* and *capreomycin*

  Diuretics: increased risk of ototoxicity with *loop diuretics*

Vecuronium *see* Muscle Relaxants (non-depolarising)

Venlafaxine
- *other* Antidepressants: CNS effects of *MAOIs* increased (risk of toxicity); *venlafaxine* should not be started until 2 weeks after stopping *MAOI*; conversely, *MAOI* should not be started until at least 1 week after stopping *venlafaxine*

  Dopaminergics: manufacturer of *entacapone* advises avoid concomitant use

Verapamil *see* Calcium-channel Blockers

Vigabatrin
- *other* Antiepileptics: concomitant administration of *two or more antiepileptics* may enhance toxicity without a corresponding increase in antiepileptic effect; moreover, interactions between individual antiepileptics can complicate monitoring of treatment; interactions include enhanced effects, increased sedation, and reductions in plasma concentrations; for further details, see p. 222

Viloxazine

  Alcohol: enhanced sedative effect

  Alpha$_2$-adrenoceptor Stimulants: manufacturers of *apraclonidine* and *brimonidine* advise avoid concomitant use
- Anticoagulants: anticoagulant effect of *acenocoumarol, warfarin* and *phenindione* possibly enhanced
- *other* Antidepressants: as for Antidepressants, Tricyclic
- Antiepileptics: increased plasma concentrations of *carbamazepine* and *phenytoin*

  Antihypertensives: antagonism of hypotensive effect of *adrenergic neurone blockers* and possibly of *clonidine*

  Theophylline: increased plasma-theophylline concentration

Vincristine

  Antifungals: *itraconazole* may inhibit metabolism (increased risk of neurotoxicity)

Vitamins
- Altretamine: *pyridoxine* reduces response to *altretamine*
- Anticoagulants: anticoagulant effect of *acenocoumarol, phenindione, and warfarin* antagonised by *vitamin K* (present in some enteral feeds)

Vitamins *(continued)*

  Antiepileptics: *vitamin D* requirements possibly increased by *carbamazepine, phenobarbital, phenytoin,* and *primidone*

  Barbiturates and Primidone: *see* Antiepileptics, above

  Diuretics: increased risk of hypercalcaemia if *thiazides* given with *vitamin D*

  Dopaminergics: effect of *levodopa* antagonised by *pyridoxine* (unless a dopa decarboxylase inhibitor also given)

  Retinoids: risk of hypervitaminosis A with *vitamin A* and *acitretin, isotretinoin* and *tretinoin*

Warfarin and other Coumarins

  Note. Change in patient's clinical condition, particularly associated with liver disease, intercurrent illness, or drug administration, necessitates more frequent testing. Major changes in diet (especially involving salads and vegetables) and in alcohol consumption may also affect warfarin control
- Alcohol: enhanced anticoagulant effect with large amounts (see also above)

  Allopurinol: anticoagulant effect possibly enhanced
- Anabolic Steroids: *oxymetholone, stanozolol and others* enhance anticoagulant effect
- Analgesics: *aspirin* increases risk of bleeding due to antiplatelet effect; anticoagulant effect seriously enhanced by *azapropazone* and *phenylbutazone* (avoid concomitant use), and possibly enhanced by *diclofenac, diflunisal, flurbiprofen, ibuprofen, mefenamic acid, meloxicam, piroxicam, sulindac,* and *other NSAIDs*; anticoagulant effect possibly also enhanced by *dextropropoxyphene* and by prolonged regular use of *paracetamol*; increased risk of haemorrhage with *intravenous diclofenac* and with *ketorolac* (avoid concomitant use)
- Anion-exchange Resins: *colestyramine* may enhance or reduce anticoagulant effect
- Anti-arrhythmics: *amiodarone and propafenone* enhance anticoagulant effect; *quinidine* may enhance anticoagulant effect
- Antibacterials: anticoagulant effect reduced by *rifamycins*; anticoagulant effect enhanced by *cefamandole, chloramphenicol, ciprofloxacin, co-trimoxazole, erythromycin, metronidazole, ofloxacin,* and *sulphonamides*; anticoagulant effect possibly also enhanced by *aztreonam, clarithromycin* and some *other macrolides, nalidixic acid, neomycin, norfloxacin, tetracyclines,* and *trimethoprim*; although studies have failed to demonstrate interaction, common experience in anticoagulant clinics is that INR can be altered following doses of oral *broad-spectrum antibiotic, such as ampicillin* (may also apply to antibiotics given for local action on gut such as *neomycin*)
- Antidepressants: *SSRIs* and *viloxazine* possibly enhance anticoagulant effect

  Antidiabetics: possibly enhanced hypoglycaemic effects of *sulphonylureas* and changes to anticoagulant effect
- Antiepileptics: reduced anticoagulant effect with *carbamazepine, phenobarbital, and primidone*; anticoagulant effect possibly increased by *valproate*; both reduced and enhanced effects reported with *phenytoin*
- Antifungals: anticoagulant effect reduced by *griseofulvin*; anticoagulant effect enhanced by *fluconazole, itraconazole, ketoconazole, and miconazole* (note: oral gel and possibly vaginal formulations absorbed)
- Antimalarials: anticoagulant effect possibly enhanced by *proguanil*
- Antiplatelet Drugs: *aspirin, clopidogrel, dipyridamole* and *ticlopidine* increase risk of bleeding due to antiplatelet effect; manufacturer of *clopidogrel* advises avoid concomitant use with *warfarin*
- Antivirals: *ritonavir* possibly increases plasma concentration

Warfarin and other Coumarins *(continued)*

Anxiolytics and Hypnotics: *chloral* and *triclofos* may transiently enhance anticoagulant effect

• Barbiturates and Primidone: anticoagulant effect reduced

Cisapride: effect of *oral anticoagulants* possibly enhanced

• Corticosteroids: anticoagulant effect possibly altered

• <u>Cytotoxics</u>: anticoagulant effect possibly enhanced by *ifosfamide*; anticoagulant effect of *warfarin* possibly reduced by *azathioprine*

• Disulfiram: enhanced anticoagulant effect

• Hormone Antagonists: *aminoglutethimide* reduces anticoagulant effect; *danazol, flutamide, tamoxifen* and possibly *bicalutamide* and *toremifene* enhance anticoagulant effect

Leukotriene Antagonists: *zafirlukast* enhances anticoagulant effect of *warfarin*

• Levothyroxine: enhanced anticoagulant effect

• Lipid-regulating Drugs: *fibrates* and *simvastatin* enhance anticoagulant effect

• Oestrogens and Progestogens: *oral contraceptives* reduce anticoagulant effect

Raloxifene: antagonism of anticoagulant effect

• Retinoids: *acitretin* possibly reduces anticoagulant effect

Rowachol®: possibly reduced anticoagulant effect

• Testosterone: anticoagulant effect of *warfarin* and *acenocoumarol* enhanced

• Ulcer-healing Drugs: *sucralfate* possibly reduces anticoagulant effect (reduced absorption); *cimetidine and omeprazole* enhance anticoagulant effect

• Uricosurics: *sulfinpyrazone* enhances anticoagulant effect

Vaccines: *influenza vaccine* occasionally enhances anticoagulant effect

• Vitamins: *vitamin K* reduces anticoagulant effect; major changes in diet (especially involving vegetables) may affect control; *vitamin K* also present in some enteral feeds

Xamoterol

Beta-blockers: antagonism of effect of *xamoterol* and reduction in beta-blockade

Xipamide *see* Diuretics (thiazide-related)

Xylometazoline *see* Sympathomimetics

Zafirlukast *see* Leukotriene Antagonists

Zalcitabine

Note. Clinical data limited. Avoid use with other drugs which have potential to cause peripheral neuropathy or pancreatitis—for further details consult product literature

Antacids: possibly reduce absorption

Antibacterials: *trimethoprim* possibly increases plasma concentration of zalcitabine

Ulcer-healing Drugs: *cimetidine* possibly increases plasma concentration of zalcitabine

Uricosurics: *probenecid* possibly increases plasma concentration of zalcitabine

Zidovudine

Note. Increased risk of toxicity with nephrotoxic and myelosuppressive drugs—for further details consult product literature

Analgesics: increased risk of haematological toxicity with *NSAIDs*; *methadone* possibly increases plasma-zidovudine concentration

Antibacterials: *clarithromycin tablets* reduce absorption of *zidovudine*

Antiepileptics: plasma-phenytoin concentrations increased or decreased; plasma-zidovudine concentration possibly increased by *valproate* (risk of toxicity)

Antifungals: plasma concentration of *zidovudine* increased by *fluconazole* (increased risk of toxicity)

• *other* Antivirals: profound myelosuppression with *ganciclovir* (if possible avoid concomitant administration, particularly during initial ganciclovir therapy)

Uricosurics: *probenecid* increases plasma-zidovudine concentration and risk of toxicity

Zinc

Antibacterials: reduced absorption of *ciprofloxacin* and *norfloxacin*; *tetracyclines* reduce absorption of *zinc* (and *vice versa*)

Iron: reduced absorption of *oral iron* (and *vice versa*)

Penicillamine: reduced absorption of *penicillamine*

Zolmitriptan *see* 5HT₁ Agonists

Zolpidem *see* Anxiolytics and Hypnotics

Zopiclone *see* Anxiolytics and Hypnotics

Zotepine *see* Antipsychotics

Zuclopenthixol *see* Antipsychotics

Appendix 2: Liver disease

Liver disease may alter the response to drugs in several ways as indicated below, and drug prescribing should be kept to a minimum in all patients with severe liver disease. The main problems occur in patients with jaundice, ascites, or evidence of encephalopathy.

IMPAIRED DRUG METABOLISM. Metabolism by the liver is the main route of elimination for many drugs, but the hepatic reserve appears to be large and liver disease has to be severe before important changes in drug metabolism occur. Routine liver-function tests are a poor guide to the capacity of the liver to metabolise drugs, and in the individual patient it is not possible to predict the extent to which the metabolism of a particular drug may be impaired.

A few drugs, e.g. rifampicin and fusidic acid, are excreted in the bile unchanged and may accumulate in patients with intrahepatic or extrahepatic obstructive jaundice.

HYPOPROTEINAEMIA. The hypoalbuminaemia in severe liver disease is associated with reduced protein binding and increased toxicity of some highly protein-bound drugs such as phenytoin and prednisolone.

REDUCED CLOTTING. Reduced hepatic synthesis of blood-clotting factors, indicated by a prolonged prothrombin time, increases the sensitivity to oral anticoagulants such as warfarin and phenindione.

HEPATIC ENCEPHALOPATHY. In severe liver disease many drugs can further impair cerebral function and may precipitate hepatic encephalopathy. These include all sedative drugs, opioid analgesics, those diuretics that produce hypokalaemia, and drugs that cause constipation.

FLUID OVERLOAD. Oedema and ascites in chronic liver disease may be exacerbated by drugs that give rise to fluid retention, e.g. NSAIDs, corticosteroids, and carbenoxolone.

HEPATOTOXIC DRUGS. Hepatotoxicity is either dose-related or unpredictable (idiosyncratic). Drugs causing dose-related toxicity may do so at lower doses than in patients with normal liver function, and some drugs producing reactions of the idiosyncratic kind do so more frequently in patients with liver disease. These drugs should be avoided.

Table of drugs to be avoided or used with caution in liver disease

The list of drugs given below is not comprehensive and is based on current information concerning the use of these drugs in therapeutic dosage. Products introduced or amended since publication of BNF No. 38 (September 1999) are underlined.

Drug	Comment
Abacavir	No dosage adjustment required in mild hepatic impairment; avoid in moderate or severe hepatic impairment
Abciximab	Avoid in severe liver disease—increased risk of bleeding
Acamprosate	Avoid in severe liver disease
Acarbose	Avoid
ACE Inhibitors	Use of prodrugs such as cilazapril, enalapril, fosinopril, imidapril, moexipril, perindopril, quinapril, ramipril, and trandolapril requires close monitoring in patients with impaired liver function
Aceclofenac	*see* NSAIDs
Acemetacin	*see* NSAIDs
Acenocoumarol (nicoumalone)	*see* Anticoagulants, Oral
Acitretin	Avoid—further impairment of liver function may occur
Aclarubicin	Manufacturer advises caution
Alfentanil	*see* Opioid Analgesics
Alfuzosin	Reduce dose in mild to moderate liver disease; avoid if severe
Alimemazine (trimeprazine)	Avoid—may precipitate coma in severe liver disease; hepatotoxic
Alprazolam	*see* Anxiolytics and Hypnotics
Altretamine	Rare reports of hepatotoxicity
Amifostine	Manufacturer advises avoid
Aminophylline	*see* Theophylline
Amitriptyline	*see* Antidepressants, Tricyclic
Amlodipine	Half-life prolonged—may need dose reduction
Amoxapine	*see* Antidepressants, Tricyclic
Amsacrine	Reduce dose
Anabolic Steroids	Preferably avoid—dose-related toxicity
Analgesics	*see* Aspirin, NSAIDs, Opioid Analgesics and Paracetamol
Anastrozole	Avoid in moderate to severe liver disease
Androgens	Preferably avoid—dose-related toxicity with some, and produce fluid retention

Drug	Comment
Antacids	In patients with fluid retention, avoid those containing large amounts of sodium, e.g. magnesium trisilicate mixture, *Gaviscon*® Avoid those causing constipation—can precipitate coma
Anticoagulants, Oral	Avoid in severe liver disease, especially if prothrombin time already prolonged
Antidepressants, MAOI	*see* MAOIs
Antidepressants, SSRI	Reduce dose or avoid in severe liver disease
Antidepressants, Tricyclic (and related)	Tricyclics preferable to MAOIs but sedative effects increased (avoid in severe liver disease)
Antihistamines	*see* individual entries
Antipsychotics	All can precipitate coma; phenothiazines are hepatotoxic; see also Clozapine, Olanzapine, Quetiapine, Risperidone and Sertindole
Anxiolytics and Hypnotics	All can precipitate coma; small dose of oxazepam or temazepam probably safest; reduce oral dose of clomethiazole; reduce dose of zopiclone (avoid if severe)
Aspirin	Avoid—increased risk of gastro-intestinal bleeding
Atorvastatin	*see* Statins
Atovaquone	Manufacturer advises caution—monitor more closely
Auranofin	*see* Gold
Aurothiomalate	*see* Gold
Azapropazone	*see* NSAIDs
Azatadine	Sedation inappropriate in severe liver disease—avoid
Azathioprine	May need dose reduction
Azithromycin	Avoid; jaundice reported
Bambuterol	Avoid in severe liver disease
Bendrofluazide	*see* Thiazides
Bendroflumethiazide (bendrofluazide)	*see* Thiazides
Benorilate [aspirin-paracetamol ester]	*see* Aspirin
Benperidol	*see* Antipsychotics
Bezafibrate	Avoid in severe liver disease
Bicalutamide	Increased accumulation possible in moderate to severe impairment
Bromazepam	*see* Anxiolytics and Hypnotics
Brompheniramine	Sedation inappropriate in severe liver disease—avoid
Buclizine	Sedation inappropriate in severe liver disease—avoid
Budesonide	Plasma-budesonide concentration may increase on oral administration
Bumetanide	*see* Loop Diuretics
Bupivacaine	*see* Lignocaine
Buprenorphine	*see* Opioid Analgesics
Cabergoline	Reduce dose or avoid in liver disease

Drug	Comment
Candesartan	Halve initial dose in mild or moderate disease; avoid if severe
Carbamazepine	Metabolism impaired in advanced liver disease
Carbenoxolone	Produces sodium and water retention and hypokalaemia
Carvedilol	Avoid
Ceftriaxone	Reduce dose and monitor plasma concentration if both hepatic and severe renal impairment
Cerivastatin	*see* Statins
Certoparin	*see* Heparin
Cetrorelix	Manufacturer advises avoid in moderate liver impairment
Chloral Hydrate	*see* Anxiolytics and Hypnotics
Chloramphenicol	Avoid—increased risk of bone-marrow depression
Chlordiazepoxide	*see* Anxiolytics and Hypnotics
Chlorphenamine (chlorpheniramine)	Sedation inappropriate in severe liver disease—avoid
Chlorpheniramine	*see* Chlorphenamine
Chlorpromazine	*see* Antipsychotics
Chlorpropamide	*see* Sulphonylureas
Chlortetracycline	*see* Tetracyclines
Chlortalidone	*see* Thiazides
Ciclosporin (cyclosporin)	May need dose adjustment
Cilazapril	*see* ACE Inhibitors
Cimetidine	Increased risk of confusion; reduce dose
Cinnarizine	Sedation inappropriate in severe liver disease—avoid
Cinoxacin	*see* Quinolones
Ciprofibrate	Avoid in severe liver disease
Ciprofloxacin	*see* Quinolones
Cisapride	Halve dose initially
Citalopram	Use doses at lower end of range
Cladribine	Regular monitoring recommended
Clarithromycin	Hepatic dysfunction including jaundice reported
Clavulanic Acid [ingredient]	*see* Co-amoxiclav and *Timentin*®
Clemastine	Sedation inappropriate in severe liver disease—avoid
Clindamycin	Reduce dose
Clobazam	*see* Anxiolytics and Hypnotics
Clofibrate	Avoid in severe liver disease
Clomethiazole	*see* Anxiolytics and Hypnotics
Clomifene	Avoid in severe liver disease
Clomipramine	*see* Antidepressants, Tricyclic
Clopamide	*see* Thiazides
Clopidogrel	Manufacturer advises caution (risk of bleeding); avoid in severe liver impairment
Clorazepate	*see* Anxiolytics and Hypnotics
Clozapine	Initial dose 12.5 mg daily increased slowly with regular monitoring of liver function; avoid in symptomatic or progressive liver disease or liver failure

Drug	Comment
Co-amoxiclav	Monitor liver function in liver disease. Cholestatic jaundice, see p. 255
Codeine	*see* Opioid Analgesics
Colestyramine	Interferes with absorption of fat-soluble vitamins and may aggravate malabsorption in primary biliary cirrhosis; likely to be ineffective in complete biliary obstruction
Contraceptives, Oral	Avoid in active liver disease and if history of pruritus or cholestasis during pregnancy
Cyclizine	Sedation inappropriate in severe liver disease—avoid
Cyclofenil	Avoid in severe liver disease
Cyclopenthiazide	*see* Thiazides
Cyclophosphamide	Reduce dose
Cyclosporin	*see* Ciclosporin
Cyproheptadine	Sedation inappropriate in severe liver disease—avoid
Cyproterone Acetate	Dose-related toxicity; *see also* side-effects of cyproterone, section 8.3.4.2
Dacarbazine	Dose reduction may be required in mild to moderate disease; avoid if severe
Dalfopristin [ingredient]	*see Synercid®*
Dalteparin	*see* Heparin
Danaparoid	*see* Heparin
Dantrolene	Avoid—may cause severe liver damage
Daunorubicin	Reduce dose
Debrisoquine	May need dose reduction
Demeclocycline	*see* Tetracyclines
Desflurane	Reduce dose
Desirudin	Monitor activated partial thromboplastin time in mild to moderate impairment; avoid in severe impairment
Desogestrel	*see* Progestogens
Dexfenfluramine	Manufacturer advises avoid
Dexketoprofen	*see* NSAIDs
Dextromethorphan	*see* Opioid Analgesics
Dextromoramide	*see* Opioid Analgesics
Dextropropoxyphene	*see* Opioid Analgesics
Diamorphine	*see* Opioid Analgesics
Diazepam	*see* Anxiolytics and Hypnotics
Diclofenac	*see* NSAIDs
Didanosine	Insufficient information but consider dose reduction
Diethylstilbestrol	*see* Oestrogens
Diflunisal	*see* NSAIDs
Dihydrocodeine	*see* Opioid Analgesics
Diltiazem	Reduce dose
Dimenhydrinate	Caution in mild to moderate liver disease; avoid in severe disease if sedation is inappropriate
Diphenhydramine	Caution in mild to moderate liver disease; avoid in severe disease if sedation is inappropriate
Diphenoxylate	*see* Opioid Analgesics
Diphenylpyraline	Caution in mild to moderate liver disease; avoid in severe disease if sedation is inappropriate
Dipipanone	*see* Opioid Analgesics
Disopyramide	Half-life prolonged—may need dose reduction
Docetaxel	Monitor liver function—reduce dose according to liver enzymes
Dosulepin (dothiepin)	*see* Antidepressants, Tricyclic
Dothiepin	*see* Antidepressants, Tricyclic
Doxazosin	No information—manufacturer advises caution
Doxepin	*see* Antidepressants, Tricyclic
Doxorubicin	Reduce dose according to bilirubin concentration
Doxycycline	*see* Tetracyclines
Doxylamine	Caution in mild to moderate liver disease; avoid in severe disease if sedation is inappropriate
Droperidol	*see* Antipsychotics
Dydrogesterone	*see* Progestogens
Efavirenz	In mild to moderate liver disease, monitor liver function: avoid in severe liver impairment
Eformoterol	*see* Formoterol
Enalapril	*see* ACE Inhibitors
Enoxaparin	*see* Heparin
Entacapone	Avoid
Epirubicin	Reduce dose according to bilirubin concentration
Epoetin	Manufacturers advise caution in chronic liver failure
Eptifibatide	Avoid in severe liver disease—increased risk of bleeding
Ergometrine	Avoid in severe liver disease
Ergotamine	Avoid in severe liver disease—risk of toxicity increased
Erythromycin	May cause idiosyncratic hepatotoxicity
Estradiol	*see* Oestrogens
Estramustine	Manufacturer advises caution and regular liver function tests; avoid in severe liver disease
Estriol	*see* Oestrogens
Estropipate	*see* Oestrogens
Ethinylestradiol	*see* Oestrogens
Etodolac	*see* NSAIDs
Etoposide	Avoid in severe hepatic impairment
Etynodiol Diacetate	*see* Progestogens
Famciclovir	Usual dose in well compensated liver disease (information not available on decompensated)
Felodipine	Reduce dose
Fenbufen	*see* NSAIDs
Fenofibrate	*see* Clofibrate
Fenoprofen	*see* NSAIDs
Fentanyl	*see* Opioid Analgesics

Drug	Comment
Flecainide	Avoid (or reduce dose) in severe liver disease
Flucloxacillin	Cholestatic jaundice, see p. 253
Fluconazole	Toxicity with related drugs
Flunitrazepam	*see* Anxiolytics and Hypnotics
Fluoxetine	*see* Antidepressants, SSRI
Flupentixol	*see* Antipsychotics
Fluphenazine	*see* Antipsychotics
Flurazepam	*see* Anxiolytics and Hypnotics
Flurbiprofen	*see* NSAIDs
Flutamide	Use with caution (hepatotoxic)
Fluvastatin	*see* Statins
Fluvoxamine	*see* Antidepressants, SSRI
Formoterol (eformoterol)	Metabolism possibly reduced in severe cirrhosis
Fosfestrol	*see* Oestrogens
Fosinopril	*see* ACE Inhibitors
Fosphenytoin	Consider 10–25% reduction in dose or infusion rate (except initial dose for status epilepticus)
Frusemide	*see* Loop Diuretics
Furosemide (frusemide)	*see* Loop Diuretics
Fusidic Acid	Impaired biliary excretion; may be increased risk of hepatotoxicity; avoid or reduce dose
Gemcitabine	Manufacturer advises caution
Gemfibrozil	Avoid in liver disease
Gestodene	*see* Progestogens
Gestrinone	Avoid in severe liver disease
Gestronol	*see* Progestogens
Glibenclamide	*see* Sulphonylureas
Gliclazide	*see* Sulphonylureas
Glimepiride	Manufacturer advises avoid in severe liver impairment
Glipizide	*see* Sulphonylureas
Gliquidone	*see* Sulphonylureas
Gold (auranofin, aurothiomalate)	Avoid in severe liver disease—hepatotoxicity may occur
Griseofulvin	Avoid in severe liver disease
Haloperidol	*see* Antipsychotics
Halothane	Avoid if history of unexplained pyrexia or jaundice following previous exposure to halothane
Heparin	Reduce dose in severe disease
Hydralazine	Reduce dose
Hydrochlorothiazide	*see* Thiazides
Hydroflumethiazide	*see* Thiazides
Hydromorphone	*see* Opioid Analgesics
Hydroxyprogesterone Caproate	*see* Progestogens
Hydroxyzine	Sedation inappropriate in severe liver disease—avoid
Hypnotics	*see* Anxiolytics and Hypnotics
Ibuprofen	*see* NSAIDs
Idarubicin	Reduce dose according to bilirubin concentration
Ifosfamide	Avoid
Imidapril	*see* ACE Inhibitors
Imipramine	*see* Antidepressants, Tricyclic
Indapamide	*see* Thiazides

Drug	Comment
Indinavir	Reduce dose to 600 mg every 8 hours in mild to moderate impairment; not studied in severe impairment
Indometacin	*see* NSAIDs
Interferon alfa	Close monitoring in mild to moderate impairment; avoid if severe
Interferon beta	Avoid in decompensated liver disease
Irinotecan	Monitor closely for neutropenia if plasma-bilirubin concentration up to 1.5 times upper limit of normal range; avoid if plasma-bilirubin concentration greater than 1.5 times upper limit of normal range
Isocarboxazid	*see* MAOIs
Isoniazid	Avoid if possible—idiosyncratic hepatotoxicity more common; *see also* p. 276
Isotretinoin	Avoid—further impairment of liver function may occur
Isradipine	Reduce dose
Itraconazole	Half-life prolonged—plasma concentration monitoring advised
Ketoconazole	Avoid
Ketoprofen	*see* NSAIDs
Ketorolac	*see* NSAIDs
Ketotifen	Sedation inappropriate in severe liver disease—avoid
Labetalol	Avoid—severe hepatocellular injury reported
Lacidipine	Antihypertensive effect possibly increased
Lamotrigine	Manufacturer advises avoid
Lansoprazole	In severe liver disease dose should not exceed 30 mg daily
Leflunomide	Avoid—active metabolite may accumulate
Lepirudin	No information—manufacturer advises that cirrhosis may affect renal excretion
Lercanidipine	Avoid in severe liver disease
Levonorgestrel	*see* Progestogens
Levomepromazine (methotrimeprazine)	*see* Antipsychotics
Lidocaine (lignocaine)	Avoid (or reduce dose) in severe liver disease
Lignocaine	*see* Lidocaine
Lofepramine	*see* Antidepressants, Tricyclic
Loop Diuretics	Hypokalaemia may precipitate coma (use potassium-sparing diuretic to prevent this); increased risk of hypomagnesaemia in alcoholic cirrhosis
Loprazolam	*see* Anxiolytics and Hypnotics
Lorazepam	*see* Anxiolytics and Hypnotics
Lormetazepam	*see* Anxiolytics and Hypnotics
Losartan	Consider lower dose
Loxapine	*see* Antipsychotics
Lymecycline	*see* Tetracyclines

Drug	Comment
Magnesium Salts	Avoid in hepatic coma if risk of renal failure
MAOIs	May cause idiosyncratic hepatotoxicity
Maprotiline	*see* Antidepressants, Tricyclic (and related)
Meclozine	Sedation inappropriate in severe liver disease—avoid
Medroxyprogester-one Acetate	*see* Progestogens
Mefenamic Acid	see NSAIDs
Mefloquine	Avoid for prophylaxis in severe liver disease
Mefruside	*see* Thiazides
Megestrol Acetate	*see* Progestogens
Meloxicam	*see* NSAIDs
Meprobamate	*see* Anxiolytics and Hypnotics
Meptazinol	*see* Opioid Analgesics
Mequitazine	Avoid—may precipitate coma in severe liver disease; hepatotoxic
Meropenem	Monitor transaminase and bilirubin concentrations
Mesterolone	*see* Androgens
Mestranol	*see* Oestrogens
Metformin	Avoid—increased risk of lactic acidosis
Methadone	*see* Opioid Analgesics
Methotrexate	Dose-related toxicity—avoid in non-malignant conditions (e.g. psoriasis)
Methotrimeprazine	*see* Antipsychotics
Methoxsalen	Avoid or reduce dose
Methyldopa	Manufacturer advises caution in history of liver disease; avoid in active liver disease
Methysergide	Avoid
Metoclopramide	Reduce dose
Metolazone	*see* Thiazides
Metoprolol	Reduce oral dose
Metronidazole	In severe liver disease reduce total daily dose to one-third, and give once daily
Mexiletine	Avoid (or reduce dose) in severe liver disease
Mianserin	*see* Antidepressants, Tricyclic (and related)
Miconazole	Avoid
Minocycline	*see* Tetracyclines
Mivacurium	Reduce dose
Mizolastine	Manufacturer recommends avoid in significant impairment
Moclobemide	Reduce dose in severe liver disease
Modafinil	Reduce dose by half in severe liver disease
Moexipril	*see* ACE Inhibitors
Monoamine-oxidase Inhibitors	*see* MAOIs
Morphine	*see* Opioid Analgesics
Moxonidine	Avoid in severe liver disease
Nabumetone	*see* NSAIDs
Nalbuphine	*see* Opioid Analgesics
Nalidixic Acid	*see* Quinolones

Drug	Comment
Nandrolone	*see* Anabolic Steroids
Naproxen	*see* NSAIDs
Naratriptan	Max. 2.5 mg in 24 hours in moderate hepatic impairment; avoid if severe
Nebivolol	No information available—manufacturer advises avoid
Nefazodone	Reduce dose
Nelfinavir	No information available—manufacturer advises caution
Neomycin	Absorbed from gastro-intestinal tract in liver disease—increased risk of ototoxicity
Nevirapine	No information available—manufacturer advises avoid
Nicardipine	Reduce dose
Nicoumalone	*see* Anticoagulants, Oral
Nifedipine	Reduce dose
Nisoldipine	Formulation not suitable in hepatic impairment
Nitrazepam	*see* Anxiolytics and Hypnotics
Nitrofurantoin	Cholestatic jaundice and chronic active hepatitis reported
Nitroprusside	Avoid in severe liver disease
Nizatidine	Manufacturer advises caution
Norethisterone	*see* Progestogens
Norfloxacin	*see* Quinolones
Norgestimate	*see* Progestogens
Norgestrel	*see* Progestogens
Nortriptyline	*see* Antidepressants, Tricyclic
NSAIDs	Increased risk of gastro-intestinal bleeding and can cause fluid retention; avoid in severe liver disease; aceclofenac, initially 100 mg daily; rofecoxib max. 12.5 mg daily in mild impairment
Oestrogens	Avoid; *see also* Contraceptives, Oral
Ofloxacin	*see* Quinolones
Olanzapine	Consider initial dose of 5 mg daily
Omeprazole	In liver disease not more than 20 mg daily should be needed
Ondansetron	Reduce dose; not more than 8 mg daily in severe liver disease
Opioid Analgesics	Avoid or reduce dose—may precipitate coma
Oral Contraceptives	*see* Contraceptives, Oral
Oxazepam	*see* Anxiolytics and Hypnotics
Oxprenolol	Reduce dose
Oxypertine	*see* Antipsychotics
Oxytetracycline	*see* Tetracyclines
Paclitaxel	Avoid in severe liver disease
Pantoprazole	Max. 20 mg daily in severe liver impairment and cirrhosis—monitor liver function (discontinue if deterioration)
Papaveretum	*see* Opioid Analgesics
Paracetamol	Dose-related toxicity—avoid large doses
Paroxetine	*see* Antidepressants, SSRI

Drug	Comment
Pentazocine	*see* Opioid Analgesics
Pericyazine	*see* Antipsychotics
Perindopril	*see* ACE Inhibitors
Perphenazine	*see* Antipsychotics
Pethidine	*see* Opioid Analgesics
Phenazocine	*see* Opioid Analgesics
Phenelzine	*see* MAOIs
Phenindione	*see* Anticoagulants, Oral
Pheniramine	Sedation inappropriate in severe liver disease—avoid
Phenobarbital	May precipitate coma
Phenoperidine	*see* Opioid Analgesics
Phenothiazines	*see* Antipsychotics
Phenylbutazone	*see* NSAIDs
Phenytoin	Reduce dose to avoid toxicity
Pholcodine	*see* Opioid Analgesics
Pilocarpine	Reduce oral dose
Pimozide	*see* Antipsychotics
Piperazine	Manufacturer advises avoid
Pipotiazine	*see* Antipsychotics
Piracetam	Avoid
Piroxicam	*see* NSAIDs
Polythiazide	*see* Thiazides
Pravastatin	*see* Statins
Prazosin	Initially 500 micrograms daily; increased with caution
Prednisolone	Side-effects more common
Primidone	Reduce dose; may precipitate coma
Procainamide	Avoid or reduce dose
Prochlorperazine	*see* Antipsychotics
Progesterone	*see* Progestogens
Progestogens	Avoid; *see also* Contraceptives, Oral
Promazine	*see* Antipsychotics
Promethazine	Avoid—may precipitate coma in severe liver disease; hepatotoxic
Propafenone	Reduce dose
Propiverine	Avoid
Propranolol	Reduce oral dose
Propylthiouracil	Reduce dose
Protriptyline	*see* Antidepressants, Tricyclic
Pyrazinamide	Avoid—idiosyncratic hepatotoxicity more common; *see also* p. 276
Quetiapine	Manufacturer advises initial dose of 25 mg daily, increased daily in steps of 25–50 mg
Quinapril	*see* ACE Inhibitors
Quinolones	See section 5.1.12; hepatitis with necrosis reported with *ciprofloxacin*; hepatitis also reported for *norfloxacin; nalidixic acid* partially conjugated in liver; reduce dose of *ofloxacin* in severe liver disease
Quinupristin [ingredient]	*see Synercid®*
Rabeprazole	Manufacturer advises caution in severe hepatic dysfunction
Raloxifene	Manufacturer advises avoid
Raltitrexed	Caution in mild or moderate disease; avoid if severe

Drug	Comment
Ramipril	*see* ACE Inhibitors
Ranitidine	Increased risk of confusion; reduce dose
Reboxetine	Initial dose 2 mg twice daily, increased according to tolerance
Remifentanil	*see* Opioid Analgesics
Repaglinide	Manufacturer advises avoid in severe liver disease
Rifabutin	Reduce dose in severe hepatic impairment
Rifampicin	Impaired elimination; may be increased risk of hepatotoxicity; avoid or do not exceed 8 mg/kg daily; *see also* p. 276
Riluzole	Avoid
Risperidone	Manufacturer advises initial dose of 500 micrograms twice daily increased in steps of 500 micrograms twice daily to 1–2 mg twice daily
Ritonavir	Avoid in severe hepatic impairment
Rivastigmine	No information available—manufacturer advises avoid in severe liver disease
Rizatriptan	Reduce dose to 5 mg in mild to moderate liver disease; avoid in severe liver disease
Rocuronium	Reduce dose
Rofecoxib	*see* NSAIDs
Ropinirole	Avoid in severe hepatic impairment
Saquinavir	Plasma concentration possibly increased; manufacturer advises caution with *Fortovase®* in moderate impairment and with *Invirase®* in severe impairment; avoid *Fortovase®* in severe impairment
Sertindole	Slower titration and lower maintenance dose in mild to moderate impairment; avoid if severe
Sertraline	*see* Antidepressants, SSRI
Sildenafil	Initial dose 25 mg; manufacturer advises avoid in severe impairment
Simvastatin	*see* Statins
Sodium Aurothiomalate	*see* Gold
Sodium Bicarbonate	*see* Antacids
Sodium Fusidate	*see* Fusidic Acid
Sodium Nitroprusside	*see* Nitroprusside
Sodium Valproate	*see* Valproate
Stanozolol	*see* Anabolic Steroids
Statins	Avoid in active liver disease or unexplained persistent elevations in serum transaminases
Sulindac	*see* NSAIDs
Sulphonylureas	Increased risk of hypoglycaemia in severe liver disease; avoid or use small dose; can produce jaundice
Sulpiride	*see* Antipsychotics
Sumatriptan	Manufacturer advises 50 mg oral dose

Drug	Comment
Suxamethonium	Prolonged apnoea may occur in severe liver disease due to reduced hepatic synthesis of pseudocholinesterase
Synercid®	Manufacturer advises caution; dose reduction may be necessary
Tacrolimus	Reduce dose
Telmisartan	Max. 40mg daily in mild or moderate impairment; avoid in severe hepatic impairment or biliary obstruction
Temazepam	*see* Anxiolytics and Hypnotics
Tenoxicam	*see* NSAIDs
Terbinafine	Reduce dose
Terfenadine	Avoid—risk of arrhythmias
Testosterone	*see* Androgens
Tetracyclines	Avoid (or use with caution)
Theophylline	Reduce dose
Thiazides	Avoid in severe liver disease; hypokalaemia may precipitate coma (potassium-sparing diuretic can prevent); increased risk of hypomagnesaemia in alcoholic cirrhosis
Thiopental	Reduce dose for induction in severe liver disease
Thioridazine	*see* Antipsychotics
Tiagabine	Maintenance dose 5–10mg 1–2 times daily initially in mild to moderate impairment; avoid in severe impairment
Tiaprofenic acid	*see* NSAIDs
Tibolone	Avoid in severe liver disease
Ticlopidine	Manufacturer advises caution; discontinue if hepatitis or jaundice develop
Timentin®	Cholestatic jaundice, see p. 257
Tinzaparin	*see* Heparin
Tirofiban	Caution in mild to moderate liver disease; avoid in severe liver disease—increased risk of bleeding
Tizanidine	Avoid in severe liver disease
Tocainide	Reduce initial dose to 400 mg daily in severe liver disease
Tolazamide	*see* Sulphonylureas
Tolbutamide	*see* Sulphonylureas
Tolfenamic Acid	*see* NSAIDs
Tolterodine	Reduce dose to 1 mg twice daily
Topotecan	Avoid in severe hepatic impairment
Torasemide	*see* Loop Diuretics
Toremifene	Elimination decreased in hepatic impairment—avoid if severe
Tramadol	*see* Opioid Analgesics
Trandolapril	*see* ACE Inhibitors
Tranylcypromine	*see* MAOIs
Trazodone	*see* Antidepressants, Tricyclic (and related)
Tretinoin (oral)	Reduce dose

Drug	Comment
Tribavirin	No dosage adjustment required; avoid oral administration in severe hepatic dysfunction or decompensated cirrhosis
Triclofos	*see* Anxiolytics and Hypnotics
Trifluoperazine	*see* Antipsychotics
Trimeprazine	*see* Alimemazine
Trimipramine	*see* Antidepressants, Tricyclic
Triprolidine	Sedation inappropriate in severe liver disease—avoid
Tulobuterol	Avoid
Ursodeoxycholic acid	Avoid in chronic liver disease (but used in primary biliary cirrhosis)
Valproate	Avoid if possible—hepatotoxicity and liver failure may occasionally occur (usually in first 6 months); *see also* p. 228
Valsartan	Halve dose in mild to moderate hepatic impairment; avoid if severe
Venlafaxine	Halve dose in moderate hepatic impairment; avoid if severe
Verapamil	Reduce oral dose
Vinblastine	Dose reduction may be necessary
Vincristine	Dose reduction may be necessary
Vindesine	Dose reduction may be necessary
Vinorelbine	Adjust dosage interval according to degree of hepatic impairment
Warfarin	*see* Anticoagulants, Oral
Xipamide	*see* Thiazides
Zafirlukast	Manufacturer advises avoid
Zalcitabine	Further impairment of liver function may occur
Zidovudine	Accumulation may occur
Zolmitriptan	Max. 5mg in 24 hours in moderate or severe hepatic impairment
Zolpidem	*see* Anxiolytics and Hypnotics
Zopiclone	*see* Anxiolytics and Hypnotics
Zuclopenthixol	*see* Antipsychotics

Appendix 3: Renal impairment

The use of drugs in patients with reduced renal function can give rise to problems for several reasons:

failure to excrete a drug or its metabolites may produce toxicity;

sensitivity to some drugs is increased even if elimination is unimpaired;

many side-effects are tolerated poorly by patients in renal failure;

some drugs cease to be effective when renal function is reduced.

Many of these problems can be avoided by reducing the dose or by using alternative drugs.

Principles of dose adjustment in renal impairment

The level of renal function below which the dose of a drug must be reduced depends on whether the drug is eliminated entirely by renal excretion or is partly metabolised, and on how toxic it is.

For many drugs with only minor or no dose-related side-effects very precise modification of the dose regimen is unnecessary and a simple scheme for dose reduction is sufficient.

For more toxic drugs with a small safety margin dose regimens based on glomerular filtration rate should be used. For those where both efficacy and toxicity are closely related to plasma concentrations recommended regimens should be seen only as a guide to initial treatment; subsequent treatment must be adjusted according to clinical response and plasma concentration.

The total daily maintenance dose of a drug can be reduced either by reducing the size of the individual doses or by increasing the interval between doses. For some drugs, if the size of the maintenance dose is reduced it will be important to give a loading dose if an immediate effect is required. This is because when a patient is given a regular dose of any drug it takes more than five times the half-life to achieve steady-state plasma concentrations. As the plasma half-life of drugs excreted by the kidney is prolonged in renal failure it may take many days for the reduced dosage to achieve a therapeutic plasma concentration. The loading dose should usually be the same size as the initial dose for a patient with normal renal function.

Nephrotoxic drugs should, if possible, be avoided in patients with renal disease because the consequences of nephrotoxicity are likely to be more serious when the renal reserve is already reduced.

Use of dosage table

Dose recommendations are based on the severity of renal impairment. This is expressed in terms of glomerular filtration rate (GFR), usually measured by the **creatinine clearance**. The serum-creatinine concentration can usually be used instead as a measure of renal function but is only a rough guide unless corrected for age, weight, and sex. Nomograms are available for making the correction and should be used where accuracy is important.

For prescribing purposes renal impairment is arbitrarily divided into 3 grades (definitions vary for grades of renal impairment; therefore, where the product literature does not correspond with this grading, values for creatinine clearance or another measure of renal function are included):

Grade	GFR	Serum creatinine (approx.)
Mild	20–50 mL/minute	150–300 µmol/litre
Moderate	10–20 mL/minute	300–700 µmol/litre
Severe	<10 mL/minute	> 700 µmol/litre

Note. Conversion factors are:
Litres/24 hours = mL/minute × 1.44
mL/minute = Litres/24 hours × 0.69

DIALYSIS. **For prescribing in patients on continuous ambulatory peritoneal dialysis (CAPD) or haemodialysis, consult specialist literature.**

Renal function declines with age; many elderly patients have a glomerular filtration rate below 50 mL/minute which, because of reduced muscle mass, may not be indicated by a raised serum creatinine. It is wise to assume at least mild impairment of renal function when prescribing for the elderly.

The following table may be used as a guide to drugs which are known to require a reduction in dose in renal impairment, and to those which are potentially harmful or are ineffective. Drug prescribing should be kept to the minimum in all patients with severe renal disease.

If even mild renal impairment is considered likely on clinical grounds, renal function should be checked before prescribing **any** drug which requires dose modification.

Table of drugs to be avoided or used with caution in renal impairment

Products introduced or amended since publication of BNF No. 38 (September 1999) are <u>underlined</u>.

Drug and degree of impairment	Comment
<u>Abacavir</u>	
Severe	Avoid
Abciximab	
Severe	Avoid—increased risk of bleeding
Acamprosate	
Mild	Avoid; excreted in urine
Acarbose	
Moderate to severe	Manufacturer advises avoid —no information available

Drug and degree of impairment	Comment
ACE Inhibitors	
Mild to moderate	Use with caution and monitor response (see also p. 87). Hyperkalaemia and other side-effects more common. Initial doses: captopril 12.5 mg twice daily, cilazapril 500 micrograms once daily, enalapril 2.5 mg once daily, imidapril 2.5 mg once daily (avoid if creatinine clearance less than 30 mL/minute), moexipril 3.75 mg once daily, perindopril 2 mg once daily (2 mg once daily on alternate days in moderate impairment), quinapril 2.5 mg once daily, ramipril 1.25 mg once daily, trandolapril 500 micrograms once daily
Acebutolol	*see* Beta-blockers
Aceclofenac	*see* NSAIDs
Acemetacin	*see* NSAIDs
Acenocoumarol (nicoumalone)	*see* Anticoagulants, Oral
Acetazolamide	
Mild	Avoid; metabolic acidosis
Aciclovir	
Mild	Reduce intravenous dose
Moderate to severe	Reduce dose
Acipimox	
Mild	Reduce dose; avoid if creatinine clearance less than 30 mL/minute
Acitretin	
Mild	Avoid; increased risk of toxicity
Aclarubicin	Manufacturer advises caution
Acrivastine	
Moderate	Avoid; excreted by kidney
Adrenergic Neurone Blockers	
Moderate to severe	Avoid; increased postural hypotension; decrease in renal blood flow
Alendronic Acid	
Mild	Manufacturer advises avoid if creatinine clearance less than 35 mL/minute
Alfentanil	*see* Opioid Analgesics
Alfuzosin	
Moderate	Reduce dose
Alimemazine (trimeprazine)	
Severe	Avoid
Allopurinol	
Moderate	100mg daily; increased toxicity; rashes
Severe	100mg on alternate days
Alprazolam	*see* Anxiolytics and Hypnotics
Alteplase	
Moderate	Risk of hyperkalaemia

Drug and degree of impairment	Comment
Altretamine	
Mild	Nephrotoxic; if renal function deteriorates reduce dose or discontinue
Aluminium Salts	
Severe	Aluminium is absorbed and may accumulate
	Note. Absorption of aluminium from aluminium salts is increased by citrates, which are contained in many effervescent preparations (such as effervescent analgesics)
Amantadine	
Mild to moderate	Reduce dose; avoid in elderly if creatinine clearance less than 60 mL/minute
Severe	Avoid
Amifostine	Manufacturer advises avoid
Amikacin	*see* Aminoglycosides
Amiloride	*see* Diuretics, Potassium-sparing
Aminoglycosides	
Mild	Reduce dose; monitor plasma concentrations; *see also* section 5.1.4
Amisulpride	
Mild	Manufacturer advises reduce dose by half
Moderate	Manufacturer advises reduce dose by two-thirds
Severe	Manufacturer advises dose reduction and intermittent treatment
Amobarbital	
Severe	Reduce dose; active metabolite accumulates
Amoxicillin	
Severe	Reduce dose; rashes more common
Amphotericin	
Mild	Use only if no alternative; nephrotoxicity may be reduced with use of complexes
Ampicillin	
Severe	Reduce dose; rashes more common
Amsacrine	Reduce dose
Analgesics	*see* Opioid Analgesics and NSAIDs
Anastrozole	
Moderate to severe	Avoid—no information available
Anticoagulants, Oral	
Severe	Avoid
Antipsychotics	
Severe	Start with small doses; increased cerebral sensitivity; *see also* Amisulpride, Clozapine, Olanzapine, Quetiapine, Risperidone and Sulpiride
Anxiolytics and Hypnotics	
Severe	Start with small doses; increased cerebral sensitivity

Drug and degree of impairment	Comment
Aspirin	
Severe	Avoid; sodium and water retention; deterioration in renal function; increased risk of gastro-intestinal bleeding
Atenolol	*see* Beta-blockers
Atovaquone	Manufacturer advises caution—monitor more closely
Auranofin	*see* Gold
Aurothiomalate	*see* Gold
Azapropazone	*see* NSAIDs (excreted by kidney)
Azathioprine	
Severe	Reduce dose
Azithromycin	
Moderate to severe	No information available
Aztreonam	
Moderate	Reduce dose
Baclofen	
Mild	Use smaller doses (e.g. 5 mg daily); excreted by kidney
Balsalazide	
Moderate to severe	Manufacturer advises avoid
Bambuterol	
Mild	Reduce dose
Bendrofluazide	*see* Thiazides
Bendroflumethiazide (bendrofluazide)	*see* Thiazides
Benorilate [aspirin-paracetamol ester]	*see* Aspirin
Benperidol	*see* Antipsychotics
Benzodiazepines	*see* Anxiolytics and Hypnotics
Benzylpenicillin	
Severe	Max. 6 g daily; neurotoxicity—high doses may cause convulsions
Beta-blockers	
Mild	Start with 2.5 mg of nebivolol
Moderate	Start with small dose of acebutolol (active metabolite accumulates); reduce dose of atenolol, nadolol, pindolol, sotalol (all excreted unchanged)
Severe	Start with small dose; higher plasma concentrations after oral administration; may reduce renal blood flow and adversely affect renal function in severe impairment; manufacturer advises avoid celiprolol and sotalol
Betaxolol	*see* Beta-blockers
Bezafibrate	
Mild	Reduce dose
Bicarbonate	*see* Sodium Bicarbonate
Bismuth Chelate	*see* Tripotassium Dicitratobismuthate
Bisoprolol	*see* Beta-blockers
Bleomycin	
Moderate	Reduce dose

Drug and degree of impairment	Comment
Bromazepam	*see* Anxiolytics and Hypnotics
Bumetanide	
Moderate	May need high doses
Buprenorphine	*see* Opioid Analgesics
Candesartan	
Moderate	Halve initial dose
Severe	Avoid
Capreomycin	
Mild	Reduce dose; nephrotoxic; ototoxic
Captopril	*see* ACE Inhibitors
Carbamazepine	Manufacturer advises caution
Carbenoxolone	
Moderate	Avoid; fluid retention
Carboplatin	
Mild	Reduce dose and monitor haematological parameters and renal function
Moderate to severe	Avoid
Cefadroxil	
Moderate	Reduce dose
Cefalexin	
Severe	Max. 500 mg daily
Cefamandole	
Mild	Reduce dose
Cefazolin	
Mild	Reduce dose
Cefixime	
Moderate	Reduce dose
Cefotaxime	
Severe	Use half dose
Cefoxitin	
Mild	Reduce dose
Cefpirome	
Mild	Usual initial dose, then use half dose
Moderate to severe	Usual initial dose, then one-quarter dose
Cefpodoxime	
Moderate	Reduce dose
Cefprozil	Usual initial dose, then use half dose
Cefradine	
Mild	Reduce dose
Ceftazidime	
Mild	Reduce dose
Ceftriaxone	
Severe	Reduce dose; also monitor plasma concentration if both severe renal and hepatic impairment
Cefuroxime	
Moderate to severe	Reduce parenteral dose
Celiprolol	*see* Beta-blockers
Mild	Reduce dose
Certoparin	*see* Heparin
Cetirizine	
Moderate	Use half dose

Drug and degree of impairment	Comment
Cerivastatin	
Moderate to severe	Max. 200 micrograms daily
Cetrorelix	
Moderate	Manufacturer advises avoid
Chloral Hydrate	*see* Anxiolytics and Hypnotics
Chloramphenicol	
Severe	Avoid unless no alternative; dose-related depression of haematopoiesis
Chlordiazepoxide	*see* Anxiolytics and Hypnotics
Chloroquine	
Mild to moderate	Reduce dose (but for malaria prophylaxis see section 5.4.1)
Severe	Avoid (but for malaria prophylaxis see section 5.4.1)
Chlorpromazine	*see* Antipsychotics
Chlorpropamide	Avoid
Chlortetracycline	*see* Tetracyclines
Chlorthalidone	*see* Thiazides
Ciclosporin	*see* p. 399 (*see also* p. 517 if used in atopic dermatitis or psoriasis and p. 461 if used in rheumatoid arthritis)
Cidofovir	
Mild	Avoid; nephrotoxic
Cilastatin [ingredient]	*see* Primaxin®
Cilazapril	*see* ACE Inhibitors
Cimetidine	
Mild to moderate	600–800 mg daily; occasional risk of confusion
Severe	400 mg daily
Cinoxacin	
Mild	Max. 500 mg daily
Moderate	Avoid
Ciprofibrate	
Moderate	100 mg on alternate days
Severe	Avoid
Ciprofloxacin	
Moderate	Use half dose
Cisapride	
Moderate	Start with half dose
Cisplatin	
Mild	Avoid if possible; nephrotoxic and neurotoxic
Citalopram	
Moderate to severe	No information available
Citrates	Absorption of aluminium from aluminium salts is increased by citrates, which are contained in many effervescent preparations (such as effervescent analgesics)
Cladribine	Regular monitoring recommended
Clarithromycin	
Moderate to severe	Use half dose
Clavulanic acid [ingredient]	*see* Co-amoxiclav, *Timentin*®
Clobazam	*see* Anxiolytics and Hypnotics

Drug and degree of impairment	Comment
Clodronate sodium	
Mild to moderate	Use half dose and monitor serum creatinine
Severe	Avoid
Clofibrate	
Mild to moderate	Reduce dose; further deterioration in renal function; myopathy
Severe	Avoid
Clomethiazole	*see* Anxiolytics and Hypnotics
Clopamide	*see* Thiazides
Clopidogrel	Manufacturer advises caution
Clorazepate	*see* Anxiolytics and Hypnotics
Clozapine	
Mild to moderate	Initial dose 12.5 mg daily increased slowly
Severe	Avoid
Co-amoxiclav	
Moderate to severe	Reduce dose
Codeine	*see* Opioid Analgesics
Colchicine	
Severe	Avoid or reduce dose if no alternative
Colistin	
Mild	Reduce dose; nephrotoxic; neurotoxic
Co-trimoxazole	
Moderate	Reduce dose; rashes and blood disorders; may cause further deterioration in renal function
Cyclopenthiazide	*see* Thiazides
Cyclophosphamide	Reduce dose
Cycloserine	
Mild to moderate	Reduce dose
Severe	Avoid
Cyclosporin	*see* Ciclosporin
Dacarbazine	
Mild to moderate	Dose reduction may be required
Severe	Avoid
Dalfopristin [ingredient]	*see* Synercid®
Dalteparin	*see* Heparin
Danaparoid	*see* Heparin
Daunorubicin	
Mild to moderate	Reduce dose
Debrisoquine	*see* Adrenergic Neurone Blockers
Demeclocycline	*see* Tetracyclines
De-Nol®, De-Noltab®	
Severe	Avoid
Desflurane	
Moderate	Reduce dose
Desirudin	
Mild to moderate	Monitor activated partial thromboplastin time if creatinine clearance 31–60 mL/minute; avoid if creatinine clearance less than 30mL/minute
Severe	Avoid
Desmopressin	Antidiuretic effect may be reduced

Drug and degree of impairment	Comment
Dexketoprofen	*see* NSAIDs
Dextromethorphan	*see* Opioid Analgesics
Dextromoramide	*see* Opioid Analgesics
Dextropropoxyphene	*see* Opioid Analgesics
Diamorphine	*see* Opioid Analgesics
Diazepam	*see* Anxiolytics and Hypnotics
Diazoxide	
Severe	75–150 mg i/v; increased sensitivity to hypotensive effect
Diclofenac	*see* NSAIDs
Didanosine	
Mild	Reduce dose; consult product literature
Diflunisal	*see* NSAIDs (excreted by kidney)
Digitoxin	
Severe	Max. 100 micrograms daily
Digoxin	
Mild	Reduce dose; toxicity increased by electrolyte disturbances
Dihydrocodeine	*see* Opioid Analgesics
Diltiazem	Start with smaller dose
Dimenhydrinate	
Severe	Manufacturer advises may accumulate
Diphenoxylate	*see* Opioid Analgesics
Dipipanone	*see* Opioid Analgesics
Disodium Etidronate	*see* Etidronate Disodium
Disodium Pamidronate	*see* Pamidronate Disodium
Disopyramide	
Mild	100 mg every 8 hours *or* 150 mg every 12 hours
Moderate	100 mg every 12 hours
Severe	150 mg every 24 hours

Note. Sustained release preparations may be unsuitable; monitor plasma-disopyramide concentrations

Drug and degree of impairment	Comment
Diuretics, Potassium-sparing	
Mild	Monitor plasma K$^+$; high risk of hyperkalaemia in renal impairment; amiloride excreted by kidney unchanged
Moderate	Avoid
Doxycycline	*see* Tetracyclines
Droperidol	*see* Antipsychotics
Enalapril	*see* ACE Inhibitors
Enflurane	
Severe	Avoid
Enoxaparin	*see* Heparin
Ephedrine	
Severe	Avoid; increased CNS toxicity
Eptifibatide	
Moderate to severe	Avoid if creatinine clearance less than 30 mL/minute
Ergometrine	
Severe	Manufacturer advises avoid
Ergotamine	
Moderate	Avoid; nausea and vomiting; risk of renal vasoconstriction

Drug and degree of impairment	Comment
Erythromycin	
Severe	Max. 1.5 g daily (ototoxicity)
Esmolol	*see* Beta-blockers
Estramustine	Manufacturer advises caution
Ethambutol	
Mild	Reduce dose; optic nerve damage
Etidronate Disodium	
Mild	Max. 5 mg/kg daily; excreted by kidney
Moderate	Avoid
Etodolac	*see* NSAIDs
Famciclovir	
Mild to moderate	Reduce dose
Famotidine	
Severe	Reduce dose
Fenbufen	*see* NSAIDs
Fenofibrate	
Mild	134 mg daily
Moderate	67 mg daily
Severe	Avoid
Fenoprofen	*see* NSAIDs
Fentanyl	*see* Opioid Analgesics
Flecainide	
Mild	Max. initial dose 100 mg daily
Flucloxacillin	
Severe	Reduce dose
Fluconazole	
Mild to moderate	Usual initial dose then halve subsequent doses
Flucytosine	Reduce dose and monitor plasma concentration—consult product literature
Fludarabine	
Mild	Reduce dose; avoid if creatinine clearance less than 30 mL/minute
Flunitrazepam	*see* Anxiolytics and Hypnotics
Fluoxetine	
Mild to moderate	Reduce dose (give on alternate days)
Severe	Avoid
Flupenthixol	*see* Antipsychotics
Fluphenazine	*see* Antipsychotics
Flurazepam	*see* Anxiolytics and Hypnotics
Flurbiprofen	*see* NSAIDs
Fluvastatin	
Severe	Avoid
Fluvoxamine	
Moderate	Start with smaller dose
Foscarnet	
Mild	Reduce dose; consult product literature
Fosinopril	*see* ACE Inhibitors
Fosphenytoin	Consider 10–25% reduction in dose or infusion rate (except initial dose for status epilepticus)
Frusemide	*see* Furosemide

Drug and degree of impairment	Comment
Furosemide (frusemide)	
Moderate	May need high doses; deafness may follow rapid i/v injection
Fybogel Mebeverine®	
Severe	Avoid; contains 7 mmol potassium per sachet
Gabapentin	
Mild	Reduce dose; consult product literature
Gallamine	
Moderate	Avoid; prolonged paralysis
Ganciclovir	
Mild	Reduce dose; consult product literature
Gaviscon®	
Severe	Avoid; high sodium content
Gemcitabine	Manufacturer advises caution
Gemfibrozil	
Severe	Start with 900 mg daily
Gentamicin	*see* Aminoglycosides
Gestrinone	
Severe	Avoid
Glibenclamide	
Severe	Avoid
Gliclazide	
Mild to moderate	Reduce dose
Severe	Avoid if possible; if no alternative reduce dose and monitor closely
Glimepiride	
Severe	Avoid
Glipizide	
Mild to moderate	Increased risk of hypoglycaemia; avoid if hepatic impairment also present
Severe	Avoid
Gliquidone	Avoid in renal failure
Gold (auranofin, aurothiomalate)	
Mild	Avoid; nephrotoxic
Guanethidine	*see* Adrenergic Neurone Blockers
Haloperidol	*see* Antipsychotics
Heparin	
Severe	Risk of bleeding increased
Hetastarch	
Severe	Avoid; excreted by kidney
Hydralazine	Reduce dose if creatinine clearance less than 30 mL/minute
Hydrochlorothiazide	*see* Thiazides
Hydroflumethiazide	*see* Thiazides
Hydromorphone	*see* Opioid Analgesics
Hydroxychloroquine	
Mild to moderate	Reduce dose; only on prolonged use
Severe	Avoid
Hypnotics	*see* Anxiolytics and Hypnotics
Ibuprofen	*see* NSAIDs

Drug and degree of impairment	Comment
Idarubicin	
Mild	Reduce dose
Ifosfamide	
Mild	Avoid if serum creatinine concentration greater than 120 µmol/litre
Imidapril	*see* ACE Inhibitors
Imipenem	*see Primaxin®*
Indapamide	*see* Thiazides
Indometacin	*see* NSAIDs
Inosine Pranobex	
Mild	Avoid; metabolised to uric acid
Insulin	
Severe	May need dose reduction; insulin requirements fall; compensatory response to hypoglycaemia is impaired
Interferon alfa	
Mild to moderate	Close monitoring required
Severe	Avoid
Interferon beta	No information available—monitoring advised
Irinotecan	No information available
Isoniazid	
Severe	Max. 200 mg daily; peripheral neuropathy
Isotretinoin	
Mild	Avoid; increased risk of toxicity
Itraconazole	Bioavailability possibly reduced—plasma concentration monitoring advised
Kanamycin	*see* Aminoglycosides
Ketoprofen	*see* NSAIDs
Ketorolac	*see* NSAIDs
Lamotrigine	
Moderate to severe	Metabolite may accumulate
Lamivudine	
Mild	Reduce dose; consult product literature
Leflunomide	
Moderate to severe	Manufacturer advises avoid—no information available
Lepirudin	
Mild to moderate	Manufacturer advises reducing initial dose by 50% and subsequent doses by 50–85%
Severe	Avoid or stop infusion (unless APTT is below therapeutic levels when alternate day administration may be considered)
Lercanidipine	
Severe	Avoid
Levocabastine	
Severe	Manufacturer advises avoid
Levofloxacin	
Mild	Usual initial dose, then halve dose
Moderate to severe	Reduce dose; consult product literature
Levomepromazine (methotrimeprazine)	*see* Antipsychotics

Drug and degree of impairment	Comment
Lisinopril	*see* ACE Inhibitors
Lithium	
Mild	Avoid if possible or reduce dose and monitor plasma concentration carefully
Moderate	Avoid
Loprazolam	*see* Anxiolytics and Hypnotics
Lorazepam	*see* Anxiolytics and Hypnotics
Lormetazepam	*see* Anxiolytics and Hypnotics
Losartan	
Moderate to severe	Start with 25 mg once daily
Loxapine	*see* Antipsychotics
Lymecycline	*see* Tetracyclines
Magnesium Salts	
Moderate	Avoid or reduce dose; increased risk of toxicity; magnesium carbonate mixture and magnesium trisilicate mixture also have high sodium content
Malarone®	
Severe	Manufacturer advises caution in acute renal failure
Mefenamic Acid	*see* NSAIDs
Mefruside	*see* Thiazides
Meloxicam	*see* NSAIDs
Melphalan	Reduce dose initially; avoid high doses in moderate to severe impairment
Meprobamate	*see* Anxiolytics and Hypnotics
Meptazinol	*see* Opioid Analgesics
Mercaptopurine	
Moderate	Reduce dose
Meropenem	
Mild	Increase dose interval to every 12 hours
Moderate	Half dose every 12 hours
Severe	Half dose every 24 hours
Mesalazine	
Moderate	Use with caution
Severe	Manufacturer advises avoid
Metformin	
Mild	Avoid; increased risk of lactic acidosis
Methadone	*see* Opioid Analgesics
Methenamine	
Mild	Avoid; ineffective
Methocarbamol	
Mild	Avoid; increased plasma urea and acidosis due to solvent in injection
Methotrexate	
Mild	Reduce dose; accumulates; nephrotoxic
Moderate	Avoid
Methotrimeprazine	*see* Antipsychotics
Methyldopa	
Moderate	Start with small dose; increased sensitivity to hypotensive and sedative effect
Methysergide	Avoid

Drug and degree of impairment	Comment
Metoclopramide	
Severe	Avoid or use small dose; increased risk of extrapyramidal reactions
Metolazone	*see* Thiazides
Metoprolol	*see* Beta-blockers
Midazolam	*see* Anxiolytics and Hypnotics
Milrinone	
Mild	Reduce dose and monitor response
Minocycline	*see* Tetracyclines
Mivacurium	
Severe	Reduce dose; prolonged paralysis
Modafinil	
Severe	Reduce dose by half
Moexipril	*see* ACE Inhibitors
Morphine	*see* Opioid Analgesics
Moxonidine	
Mild	Max. single dose 200 micrograms and max. daily dose 400 micrograms
Moderate to severe	Avoid
Nabumetone	*see* NSAIDs
Nadolol	*see* Beta-blockers
Nalbuphine	*see* Opioid Analgesics
Nalidixic Acid	
Moderate to severe	Halve dose; ineffective in renal failure because concentration in urine is inadequate
Naproxen	*see* NSAIDs
Naratriptan	
Moderate	Max. 2.5 mg in 24 hours
Severe	Avoid
Narcotic Analgesics	*see* Opioid Analgesics
Nebivolol	*see* Beta-blockers
Nefazodone	
Severe	Reduce dose
Nelfinavir	No information available—manufacturer advises caution
Neomycin	
Mild	Avoid; ototoxic; nephrotoxic
Neostigmine	
Moderate	May need dose reduction
Netilmicin	*see* Aminoglycosides
Nevirapine	No information available—manufacturer advises avoid
Nicardipine	
Moderate	Start with small dose
Nicotine	
Severe	May affect clearance of nicotine or its metabolites
Nicoumalone	*see* Anticoagulants, Oral
Nitrazepam	*see* Anxiolytics and Hypnotics
Nitrofurantoin	
Mild	Avoid; peripheral neuropathy; ineffective because of inadequate urine concentrations
Nitroprusside	
Moderate	Avoid prolonged use

Drug and degree of impairment	Comment
Nizatidine	
Mild	Use half dose
Moderate	Use one-quarter dose
Norfloxacin	
Mild to moderate	Halve dose if creatinine clearance less than 30 mL/minute
NSAIDs	
Mild	Use lowest effective dose and monitor renal function; sodium and water retention; deterioration in renal function possibly leading to renal failure; deterioration also reported after topical use
Moderate to severe	Avoid if possible
Ofloxacin	
Mild	Usual initial dose, then use half dose
Moderate	Usual initial dose, then 100 mg every 24 hours
Olanzapine	Consider initial dose of 5 mg daily
Olsalazine	
Moderate	Use with caution
Severe	Manufacturer advises avoid
Opioid Analgesics	
Moderate to severe	Reduce doses or avoid; increased and prolonged effect; increased cerebral sensitivity
Oxaliplatin	Manufacturer advises avoid if creatinine clearance less than 30 mL/minute
Oxazepam	*see* Anxiolytics and Hypnotics
Oxpentifylline	*see* Pentoxifylline
Oxprenolol	*see* Beta-blockers
Oxypertine	*see* Antipsychotics
Oxytetracycline	*see* Tetracyclines
Pamidronate Disodium	
Moderate to severe	Max. infusion rate 20 mg/hour
Pancuronium	
Severe	Prolonged duration of block
Pantoprazole	Max. 40 mg daily
Papaveretum	*see* Opioid Analgesics
Paroxetine	
Moderate	Usual initial dose; small increments if necessary
Penicillamine	
Mild	Avoid if possible or reduce dose; nephrotoxic
Pentamidine	
Mild	Reduce dose; consult product literature
Pentazocine	*see* Opioid Analgesics
Pentoxifylline (oxpentifylline)	
Mild	Reduce dose by 30–50% if creatinine clearance less than 30 mL/minute
Pericyazine	*see* Antipsychotics
Perindopril	*see* ACE Inhibitors
Perphenazine	*see* Antipsychotics
Pethidine	*see* Opioid Analgesics

Drug and degree of impairment	Comment
Phenazocine	*see* Opioid Analgesics
Phenindione	*see* Anticoagulants, Oral
Phenobarbital	
Severe	Avoid large doses
Phenoperidine	*see* Opioid Analgesics
Phenothiazines	*see* Antipsychotics
Phenylbutazone	*see* NSAIDs
Pholcodine	*see* Opioid Analgesics
Pimozide	*see* Antipsychotics
Pindolol	*see* Beta-blockers
Piperacillin	
Adult:	
Mild	Max. daily dose 16 g if creatinine clearance is 40–80 mL/minute
Moderate	Max. daily dose 12 g if creatinine clearance is 20–40 mL/minute
Severe	Max. daily dose 8 g if creatinine clearance is less than 20 mL/minute
Child 1 month–12 years:	
Moderate to severe	Reduce dose; consult product literature
Piperazine	
Severe	Reduce dose; neurotoxic
Pipotiazine	*see* Antipsychotics
Piracetam	
Mild	Use half dose
Moderate	Use one-quarter dose
Severe	Avoid
Piroxicam	*see* NSAIDs
Polythiazide	*see* Thiazides
Potassium Salts	
Moderate	Avoid routine use; high risk of hyperkalaemia
Povidone-iodine	
Severe	Avoid regular application to inflamed or broken mucosa
Pramipexole	
Mild	Initially 88 micrograms twice daily; if renal function declines, reduce dose further
Moderate to severe	Initially 88 micrograms daily; if renal function declines, reduce dose further
Pravastatin	
Moderate to severe	Start at lower end of dosage range
Prazosin	
Moderate to severe	Initially 500 micrograms daily; increase with caution
Primaxin®	
Mild	Reduce dose
Primidone	
Severe	Avoid large doses
Probenecid	
Moderate	Avoid; ineffective and toxicity increased
Procainamide	
Mild	Avoid or reduce dose

Drug and degree of impairment	Comment
Procarbazine	
Moderate	Reduce dose
Prochlorperazine	*see* Antipsychotics
Proguanil	
Mild	100 mg once daily
Moderate	50 mg on alternate days
Severe	50 mg once weekly; increased risk of haematological toxicity
Promazine	*see* Antipsychotics
Propiverine	
Severe	Avoid
Propranolol	*see* Beta-blockers
Propylthiouracil	
Mild to moderate	Reduce dose by 25%
Severe	Reduce dose by 50%
Pseudoephedrine	
Severe	Avoid; increased CNS toxicity
Pyridostigmine	
Moderate	Reduce dose; excreted by kidney
Quetiapine	Manufacturer advises initial dose of 25 mg daily; increased daily in steps of 25–50 mg
Quinapril	*see* ACE Inhibitors
<u>Quinupristin</u> [ingredient]	*see Synercid®*
Raloxifene	
Severe	Avoid
Raltitrexed	
Mild	Reduce dose and increase dosing interval
Moderate to severe	Avoid
Ramipril	*see* ACE Inhibitors
Ranitidine	
Severe	Use half normal dose; occasional risk of confusion
Ranitidine Bismuth Citrate	
Severe	Avoid
Reboxetine	Initial dose 2 mg twice daily, increased according to tolerance
Regular®	
Severe	Avoid; contains 6.4 mmol potassium per sachet
Repaglinide	
Mild to moderate	Manufacturer advises caution because insulin sensitivity increased
Severe	Manufacturer advises avoid
<u>Rifabutin</u>	
Mild	Reduce dose by 50% if creatinine clearance less than 30 mL/minute
Riluzole	No information available—manufacturer advises avoid
Risperidone	Manufacturer advises initial dose of 500 micrograms twice daily increased in steps of 500 micrograms twice daily to 1–2 mg twice daily
Rivastigmine	Manufacturer advises caution

Drug and degree of impairment	Comment
Rizatriptan	
Mild to moderate	Reduce dose to 5 mg
Severe	Avoid
Rocuronium	
Moderate	Reduce dose; prolonged paralysis
Rofecoxib	*see* NSAIDs
Ropinirole	
Severe	Avoid
Salicylates	*see* Aspirin
Salt Substitutes	
Moderate	Avoid routine use; high risk of hyperkalaemia
Saquinavir	
Severe	Dose adjustment possibly required
Sertraline	Manufacturer advises caution
Sildenafil	
Mild	Initial dose 25 mg if creatinine clearance less than 30 mL/minute
Simvastatin	
Moderate to severe	Doses above 10 mg daily should be used with caution
Sodium Aurothiomalate	*see* Gold
Sodium Bicarbonate	
Severe	Avoid; specialised role in some forms of renal disease
Sodium Cellulose Phosphate	
Mild to moderate	Reduce dose
Severe	Avoid
Sodium Clodronate	*see* Clodronate Sodium
Sodium Nitroprusside	*see* Nitroprusside
Sodium Salts	
Severe	Avoid
Sodium valproate	*see* Valproate
Solpadeine®	
Severe	Avoid; contains 18.5 mmol sodium per tablet
Solpadol®	
Severe	Avoid; contains 18.6 mmol sodium per tablet
Sotalol	*see* Beta-blockers
Spironolactone	*see* Diuretics, Potassium-sparing
Stavudine	
Mild	20 mg twice daily (15 mg if <60 kg)
Moderate	20 mg once daily (15 mg if <60 kg)
Severe	Information not available
Streptomycin	*see* Aminoglycosides
Sucralfate	
Severe	Avoid; aluminium is absorbed and may accumulate
Sulfadiazine	
Severe	Avoid; high risk of crystalluria
Sulfametopyrazine	*see* Sulphonamides

Drug and degree of impairment	Comment
Sulfasalazine	
Moderate	Risk of toxicity including crystalluria—ensure high fluid intake
Severe	Avoid
Sulfinpyrazone	
Moderate	Avoid; ineffective as uricosuric
Sulindac	*see* NSAIDs
Sulphonamides	
Moderate	Ensure high fluid intake; rashes and blood disorders; crystalluria a risk
Sulphonylureas	*see under* individual drugs
Sulpiride	
Moderate	Avoid if possible, or reduce dose
Synercid®	Manufacturer advises caution
Tazobactam [ingredient]	*see Tazocin*®
Tazocin®	
Adult:	
Moderate	Reduce dose
Child less than 50 kg:	Consult product literature
Teicoplanin	On day 4 reduce dose by half if creatinine clearance is 40–60 mL/minute and by two-thirds if creatinine clearance is less than 40 mL/minute
Telmisartan	
Severe	Avoid
Temazepam	*see* Anxiolytics and Hypnotics
Tenoxicam	*see* NSAIDs
Terbinafine	
Mild	Use half normal dose
Terfenadine	
Mild	Halve dose if creatinine clearance less than 40 mL/minute
Tetracyclines (except doxycycline and minocycline)	
Mild	Avoid—use doxycycline or minocycline if necessary; anti-anabolic effect, increased plasma urea, further deterioration in renal function
Thiazides and Related Diuretics	
Moderate	Avoid; ineffective (metolazone remains effective but risk of excessive diuresis)
Thioridazine	*see* Antipsychotics
Tiaprofenic Acid	*see* NSAIDs
Ticarcillin [ingredient]	*see Timentin*®
Ticlopidine	
Mild	Consider dose reduction; discontinue if haemorrhagic or blood complication occur
Tiludronic Acid	
Moderate to severe	Avoid

Drug and degree of impairment	Comment
Timentin®	
Moderate to severe	Reduce dose
Timolol	*see* Beta-blockers
Tinzaparin	
Severe	May need dose reduction
Tioguanine	
Moderate	Reduce dose
Tirofiban	
Mild	Halve dose if creatinine clearance less than 30 mL/minute
Tizanidine	
Mild	Initially 2 mg once daily; increase once-daily dose gradually before increasing frequency
Tobramycin	*see* Aminoglycosides
Tocainide	
Mild to moderate	Reduce dose to 400 mg twice daily
Severe	Reduce initial dose to 400 mg daily
Tolazamide	Manufacturer advises avoid—no information available
Tolbutamide	
Mild to moderate	Reduce dose
Severe	Avoid if possible; if no alternative reduce dose and monitor closely
Tolfenamic Acid	*see* NSAIDs
Topiramate	
Moderate to severe	Longer time to steady-state plasma concentrations
Topotecan	
Moderate	Reduce dose
Severe	Avoid
Torasemide	
Moderate	May need high doses
Tramadol	*see* Opioid Analgesics
Trandolapril	*see* ACE Inhibitors
Tranexamic acid	
Mild	Reduce dose
Tretinoin (oral)	
Mild	Reduce dose
Triamterene	*see* Diuretics, Potassium-sparing
Tribavirin	
Mild	Avoid oral treatment
Triclofos	*see* Anxiolytics and Hypnotics
Trifluoperazine	*see* Antipsychotics
Trimeprazine	*see* Alimemazine
Trimethoprim	
Moderate	Reduce dose
Tripotassium Dicitrato-bismuthate	
Severe	Avoid
Tulobuterol	
Mild	May need dose reduction; excreted by kidney
Moderate to severe	Avoid

Drug and degree of impairment	Comment
Tylex®	
Moderate to severe	Avoid effervescent tablets; contain 13.6 mmol sodium per tablet
Valaciclovir as for Aciclovir	
Valproate	
Mild to moderate	Reduce dose
Severe	Alter dosage according to free serum valproic acid concentration
Valsartan	
Moderate to severe	Start with 40 mg once daily
Vancomycin	
Mild	Avoid parenteral use if possible; ototoxic; nephrotoxic
Vecuronium	
Severe	Reduce dose; duration of block possibly prolonged
Venlafaxine	
Moderate	Use half dose
Severe	Avoid
Vigabatrin	
Mild	Excreted by kidney—lower maintenance dose may be required
Warfarin	see Anticoagulants, Oral
Xamoterol	
Moderate	Reduce dose; excreted by kidney
Xipamide	*see* Thiazides
Zafirlukast	
Moderate to severe	Manufacturer advises avoid
Zalcitabine	
Mild to moderate	750 micrograms every 12 hours
Severe	750 micrograms daily
Zidovudine	
Severe	Reduce dose; manufacturer advises oral dose of 300–400 mg daily
Zopiclone	*see* Anxiolytics and Hypnotics
Zuclopenthixol	*see* Antipsychotics

Appendix 4: Pregnancy

Drugs can have harmful effects on the fetus at any time during pregnancy. It is important to bear this in mind when prescribing for a woman of *childbearing age*.

During the *first trimester* drugs may produce congenital malformations (teratogenesis), and the period of greatest risk is from the third to the eleventh week of pregnancy.

During the *second* and *third trimesters* drugs may affect the growth and functional development of the fetus or have toxic effects on fetal tissues; and drugs given shortly before term or during labour may have adverse effects on labour or on the neonate after delivery.

The following list includes drugs which may have harmful effects in pregnancy and indicates the trimester of risk. It is based on human data but information on *animal* studies has been included for some newer drugs when its omission might be misleading.

Drugs should be prescribed in pregnancy only if the expected benefit to the mother is thought to be greater than the risk to the fetus, and all drugs should be avoided if possible during the first trimester. Drugs which have been extensively used in pregnancy and appear to be usually safe should be prescribed in preference to new or untried drugs; and the smallest effective dose should be used.

Few drugs have been shown conclusively to be teratogenic in man but no drug is safe beyond all doubt in early pregnancy. Screening procedures are available where there is a known risk of certain defects.

Absence of a drug from the list does not imply safety.

It should be noted that the BNF provides independent advice and may not always agree with the product literature.

Information on drugs and pregnancy is also available from the National Teratology Information Service (telephone: 0191-232 1525).

Table of drugs to be avoided or used with caution in pregnancy

Products introduced or amended since publication of BNF No. 38 (September 1999) are underlined.

Drug (trimester of risk)	Comment
Abacavir	Manufacturer advises avoid (toxicity in *animal* studies)
Abciximab	Manufacturer advises use only if potential benefit outweighs risk—no information available
Acamprosate	Manufacturer advises avoid
Acarbose	Manufacturer advises avoid; insulin is normally substituted in all diabetics

Drug (trimester of risk)	Comment
ACE Inhibitors (1, 2, 3)	Avoid; may adversely affect fetal and neonatal blood pressure control and renal function; also possible skull defects and oligohydramnios; toxicity in *animal* studies
Acebutolol	*see* Beta-blockers
Aceclofenac	*see* NSAIDs
Acemetacin	*see* NSAIDs
Acenocoumarol (nicoumalone)	*see* Anticoagulants, Oral
Acetazolamide	*see* Diuretics
Aciclovir	Experience limited—manufacturers advise use only when potential benefit outweighs risk; limited absorption from topical preparations
Acipimox	Manufacturer advises avoid
Acitretin (1, 2, 3)	Teratogenic; effective contraception must be used for at least 1 month before treatment, during treatment, and for at least 2 years after stopping
Aclarubicin	Avoid (toxicity in *animal* studies); *see also* section 8.1
Acrivastine	*see* Antihistamines
Adapalene	Manufacturer advises teratogenic in *animal* studies and recommends effective contraception during treatment
Albendazole	Manufacturer advises teratogenic in *animal* studies and recommends non-hormonal contraception during and for 1 month after treatment
Alclometasone	*see* Corticosteroids
Alcohol (1, 2)	Regular daily drinking is teratogenic (fetal alcohol syndrome) and may cause growth retardation; occasional single drinks are probably safe
(3)	Withdrawal syndrome may occur in babies of alcoholic mothers
Alendronic Acid	*see* Bisphosphonates
Alfentanil	*see* Opioid Analgesics
Alimemazine (trimeprazine)	Manufacturer advises avoid—no information available
Allopurinol	Toxicity not reported; manufacturer advises avoid; use only if no safer alternative and disease carries risk for mother or child
Alpha-blockers (post-synaptic)	No evidence of teratogenicity; manufacturers advise use only when potential benefit outweighs risk
Alprazolam	*see* Benzodiaepines
Alprostadil (urethral application only)	Manufacturer advises barrier contraception if partner pregnant

Drug (trimester of risk)	Comment
Alteplase	*see* Streptokinase
Altretamine	Avoid (teratogenic and embryo-toxic in *animal* studies); *see also* section 8.1
Amantadine	Avoid; toxicity in *animal* studies
Amifostine	Manufacturer advises avoid—no information available
Amikacin	*see* Aminoglycosides
Amiloride	*see* Diuretics
Aminoglutethimide	Avoid; toxicity in *animal* studies and may affect fetal sexual development
Aminoglycosides (2, 3)	Auditory or vestibular nerve damage; risk greatest with streptomycin; probably very small with gentamicin and tobramycin, but avoid unless essential (if given, monitor plasma concentration)
Aminophylline	*see* Theophylline
Amiodarone (2, 3)	Possible risk of neonatal goitre; use only if no alternative
Amisulpride	Manufacturer advises avoid
Amitriptyline	*see* Antidepressants, Tricyclic
Amlodipine	*see* Calcium-channel Blockers
Amobarbital	*see* Barbiturates
Amorolfine	Systemic absorption very low, but manufacturer advises avoid—no information available
Amoxapine	*see* Antidepressants, Tricyclic
Amphotericin	Not known to be harmful but manufacturers advise avoid unless potential benefit outweighs risk
Amsacrine	Avoid (teratogenic and toxic in *animal* studies); may reduce fertility; *see also* section 8.1
Anabolic Steroids (1, 2, 3)	Masculinisation of female fetus
Anaesthetics, General (3)	Depress neonatal respiration
Anaesthetics, Local (3)	With large doses, neonatal respiratory depression, hypotonia, and bradycardia after paracervical or epidural block; neonatal methaemoglobinaemia with prilocaine and procaine
Analgesics	*see* Opioid Analgesics, Nefopam, NSAIDs and Paracetamol
Androgens (1, 2, 3)	Masculinisation of female fetus
Anistreplase	*see* Streptokinase
Anticoagulants Heparin (1, 2, 3)	Osteoporosis has been reported after prolonged use; multidose vials may contain benzyl alcohol—some manufacturers advise avoid

Drug (trimester of risk)	Comment
Anticoagulants Oral (1, 2, 3)	Congenital malformations; fetal and neonatal haemorrhage *See also* section 2.8.2
Antidepressants	*see* individual drugs (and groups)
Antidepressants, SSRI (1, 2, 3)	Manufacturers advise use only if potential benefit outweighs risk (no evidence of teratogenicity); adverse effects with sertraline in *animals* (manufacturer recommends avoid)
Antidepressants, Tricyclic (and related) (3)	Tachycardia, irritability, and muscle spasms in neonate reported with imipramine
Antiepileptics	Benefit of treatment outweighs risk to fetus; risk of teratogenicity greater if more than one drug used; **important**: *see also* carbamazepine, ethosuximide, phenobarbital, phenytoin, valproate, vigabatrin, and p. 223
Antihistamines	No evidence of teratogenicity; some packs of antihistamines sold to the public carry warning to avoid in pregnancy; embryotoxicity in *animal* studies with high doses of loratadine; manufacturers of mizolastine advise avoid
Antimalarials (1, 3)	Benefit of prophylaxis and treatment in malaria outweighs risk; **important**: *see also* individual drugs and p. 300
Antipsychotics	*See also* amisulpride, clozapine, olanzapine, quetiapine, risperidone, sertindole
(3)	Extrapyramidal effects in neonate occasionally reported
Apomorphine	Avoid
Aspirin (3)	Impaired platelet function and risk of haemorrhage; delayed onset and increased duration of labour with increased blood loss; avoid analgesic doses if possible in last few weeks (low doses probably not harmful); with high doses, closure of fetal ductus arteriosus *in utero* and possibly persistent pulmonary hypertension of newborn; kernicterus in jaundiced neonates
Atenolol	*see* Beta-blockers
Atorvastatin	*see* Statins
Atovaquone	Manufacturer advises avoid unless potential benefit outweighs risk—no information available
Atracurium	Not known to be harmful but manufacturer advises avoid unless benefit outweighs risk
Atropine	Not known to be harmful; manufacturer advises caution
Auranofin	*see* Gold

Drug (trimester of risk)	Comment
Aurothiomalate	*see* Gold
Azapropazone	*see* NSAIDs
Azatadine	*see* Antihistamines
Azathioprine	*see* p. 397
Azelastine	*see* Antihistamines
Azithromycin	Not known to be harmful but manufacturer advises use only if adequate alternatives not available
Aztreonam	Manufacturer advises avoid (but no evidence of teratogenicity)
Baclofen	Manufacturer advises toxicity in *animal* studies
Balsalazide	Manufacturer advises avoid
Bambuterol	*see* section 3.1.1 [text]
Barbiturates (3)	Withdrawal effects in neonate; *see also* Phenobarbital
Basiliximab	Avoid; adequate contraception during and for 8 weeks after last dose
Beclometasone	*see* Corticosteroids
Bendrofluazide	*see* Diuretics
Bendroflumethi- azide (bendrofluazide)	*see* Diuretics
Benorilate [aspirin-paracet- amol ester]	*see* Aspirin
Benperidol	*see* Antipsychotics
Benserazide [ingredient]	*see* Madopar®
Benzodiazepines	Avoid regular use (risk of neonatal withdrawal symptoms); use only if clear indication such as seizure control (high doses during late pregnancy or labour may cause neonatal hypothermia, hypotonia and respiratory depression)
Beta-blockers	May cause intra-uterine growth restriction, neonatal hypoglycaemia, and bradycardia; risk greater in severe hypertension *See also* section 2.5
Betamethasone	*see* Corticosteroids
Betaxolol	*see* Beta-blockers
Bezafibrate	*see* Clofibrate
Bismuth Chelate	Manufacturer advises avoid on theoretical grounds
Bisoprolol	*see* Beta-blockers
Bisphosphonates	Manufacturers advise avoid
Bleomycin	Avoid (teratogenic and carcinogenic in *animal* studies); *see also* section 8.1
Botulinum Toxin	Manufacturers advise avoid
Bromazepam	*see* Benzodiazepines
Brompheniramine	*see* Antihistamines
Buclizine	*see* Antihistamines
Budesonide	*see* Corticosteroids
Bumetanide	*see* Diuretics
Bupivacaine	*see* Anaesthetics, Local

Drug (trimester of risk)	Comment
Buprenorphine	*see* Opioid Analgesics
Buserelin	Avoid
Buspirone	Manufacturer advises avoid (toxicity in *animal* studies)
Busulfan	Avoid (teratogenic in *animals*); manufacturer advises effective contraception during administration to men or women; *see also* section 8.1
Cabergoline	Once regular ovulatory cycles have been achieved manufac- turer advises discontinuation for one month before intended conception (although no evi- dence of teratogenicity)
Calcitonin (salmon) (salcatonin)	Manufacturer advises avoid unless potential benefit outweighs risk (toxicity in *animal* studies)
Calcipotriol	Manufacturer advises avoid if possible
Calcium Folinate	Manufacturer advises use only if potential benefit outweighs risk
Calcium Levofolinate	*see* Calcium Folinate
Calcium-channel Blockers	May inhibit labour and manu- facturers advise that diltiazem and some dihydropyridines are teratogenic in *animals,* but risk to fetus should be balanced against risk of uncontrolled maternal hypertension
Candesartan	As for ACE Inhibitors
Capreomycin	Manufacturer advises teratogenic in *animal* studies
Captopril	*see* ACE Inhibitors
Carbamazepine (1)	Risk of teratogenesis including increased risk of neural tube defects (counselling and screening and adequate folate supplements advised, e.g. 5 mg daily); *see also* Antiepileptics and p. 223
(3)	Because of neonatal bleeding tendency associated with some antiepileptics, manufacturer advises prophylactic vitamin K₁ for mother before delivery (as well as for neonate)
Carbenoxolone (3)	Avoid; causes sodium retention with oedema
Carbimazole (2, 3)	Neonatal goitre and hypo- thyroidism; has been associated with aplasia cutis of the neonate
Carboplatin	Avoid (teratogenic and embryotoxic in *animal* studies); *see also* section 8.1
Carmustine	Avoid (teratogenic and embryotoxic in *animals*); manufacturer advises effective contraception during administration to men or women; *see also* section 8.1
Carvedilol	*see* Beta-blockers
Celiprolol	*see* Beta-blockers

Drug (trimester of risk)	Comment
Cephalosporins	Not known to be harmful
Cerivastatin	*see* Statins
Certoparin	*see* Anticoagulants (Heparin)
Cetirizine	*see* Antihistamines
Chloral hydrate	Avoid
Chlorambucil	Avoid; manufacturer advises effective contraception during administration to men or women; *see also* section 8.1
Chloramphenicol (3)	Neonatal 'grey syndrome'
Chlordiazepoxide	*see* Benzodiazepines
Chlormethine (mustine)	Avoid; *see also* section 8.1
Chloroquine	*see* Antimalarials
Chlorphenamine (chlorphenir-amine)	*see* Antihistamines
Chlorpheniramine	*see* Antihistamines
Chlorpromazine	*see* Antipsychotics
Chlorpropamide	*see* Sulphonylureas
Chlortalidone	*see* Diuretics
Chlortetracycline	*see* Tetracyclines
Ciclosporin	*see* p. 397
Cidofovir	Avoid (toxicity in *animal* studies); effective contraception required during and for 1 month after treatment; also men should avoid fathering a child during and for 3 months after treatment
Cilastatin [ingredient]	*see Primaxin*®
Cilazapril	*see* ACE Inhibitors
Cimetidine	Manufacturer advises avoid unless essential
Cinnarizine	*see* Antihistamines
Cinoxacin	*see* Quinolones
Ciprofibrate	*see* Clofibrate
Ciprofloxacin	*see* Quinolones
Cisapride	Manufacturer advises avoid unless potential benefit outweighs risk
Cisatracurium	Manufacturer advises avoid—no information available
Cisplatin	Avoid (teratogenic and toxic in *animal* studies); *see also* section 8.1
Citalopram	*see* Antidepressants, SSRI
Cladribine	Avoid (teratogenic in *animal* studies); *see also* section 8.1
Clarithromycin	Not known to be harmful but manufacturer advises avoid unless potential benefit outweighs risk
Clemastine	*see* Antihistamines
Clindamycin	Not known to be harmful
Clobazam	*see* Benzodiazepines
Clobetasol	*see* Corticosteroids
Clobetasone	*see* Corticosteroids
Clodronate Sodium	*see* Bisphosphonates

Drug (trimester of risk)	Comment
Clofibrate (1, 2, 3)	Avoid—theoretical possibility of interference with embryonic growth and development due to anticholesterol effect
Clomethiazole	Avoid if possible—especially during first and third trimesters
Clomifene	Possible effects on fetal development
Clomipramine	*see* Antidepressants, Tricyclic
Clomocycline	*see* Tetracyclines
Clonazepam	*see* Antiepileptics
Clopidogrel	Manufacturer advises avoid—no information available
Clorazepate	*see* Benzodiazepines
Clozapine	Manufacturer advises avoid
Co-amoxiclav	No evidence of teratogenicity but manufacturer advises avoid unless essential
Co-cyprindiol (1, 2, 3)	Feminisation of male fetus (due to cyproterone)
Codeine	*see* Opioid Analgesics
Colistin (2, 3)	Avoid—possible risk of fetal toxicity
Contraceptives, Oral	Epidemiological evidence suggests no harmful effects on fetus
Corticosteroids	Benefit of treatment, e.g. in asthma, outweighs risk (see also CSM advice, section 6.3.2); high systemic doses may produce fetal and neonatal adrenal suppression; risk of intra-uterine growth retardation on prolonged or repeated systemic treatment; corticosteroid cover required by mother during labour; monitor closely if fluid retention
Co-trimoxazole (1)	Theoretical teratogenic risk (trimethoprim a folate antagonist)
(3)	Neonatal haemolysis and methaemoglobinaemia; fear of increased risk of kernicterus in neonates appears to be unfounded
Crisantaspase	Avoid; *see also* section 8.1
Cromoglicate	Not known to be harmful; *see also* section 3.1.1 [text]
Cyclizine	*see* Antihistamines
Cyclopenthiazide	*see* Diuretics
Cyclophosphamide	Avoid (manufacturer advises effective contraception during and for at least 3 months after administration to men or women); *see also* section 8.1
Cycloserine	Manufacturer advises use only if potential benefit outweighs risk—crosses the placenta
Cyclosporin	*see* p. 397
Cyproheptadine	*see* Antihistamines
Cyproterone [ingredient]	*see* Co-cyprindiol

Drug (trimester of risk)	Comment
Cytarabine	Avoid (teratogenic in *animal* studies); *see also* section 8.1
Dacarbazine	Avoid (carcinogenic and teratogenic in *animal* studies); ensure effective contraception during and for at least 6 months after administration to men or women; *see also* section 8.1
Daclizumab	Avoid
Dactinomycin	Avoid (teratogenic in *animal* studies); *see also* section 8.1
Dalfopristin [ingredient]	*see Synercid®*
Dalteparin	*see Anticoagulants (Heparin)*
Danaparoid	Insufficient information available
Danazol (1, 2, 3)	Avoid; has weak androgenic effects and virilisation of female fetus reported
Dapsone (3)	Neonatal haemolysis and methaemoglobinaemia; adequate folate supplements should be given to mother
Daunorubicin	Avoid (teratogenic and carcinogenic in *animal* studies); *see also* section 8.1
Debrisoquine	*see Guanethidine*
Deflazacort	*see Corticosteroids*
Demeclocycline	*see Tetracyclines*
Desferrioxamine	Manufacturer advises toxicity in *animal* studies
Desflurane	*see Anaesthetics, General*
Desirudin	Avoid (teratogenic in *animal* studies)
Desmopressin	Small oxytocic effect in third trimester
Desogestrel	*see Contraceptives, Oral*
Desonide	*see Corticosteroids*
Desoximetasone	*see Corticosteroids*
Dexamethasone	*see Corticosteroids*
Dexamfetamine	Manufacturer advises avoid (retrospective evidence of uncertain significance suggesting possible embryotoxicity)
Dexketoprofen	see NSAIDs
Dextromethorphan	*see Opioid Analgesics*
Dextromoramide	*see Opioid Analgesics*
Dextropropoxyphene	*see Opioid Analgesics*
Diamorphine	*see Opioid Analgesics*
Dianette®	*see Co-cyprindiol*
Diazepam	*see Benzodiazepines*
Diazoxide (2, 3)	Prolonged use may produce alopecia and impaired glucose tolerance in neonate; inhibits uterine activity during labour
Diclofenac	*see NSAIDs*
Didanosine	Manufacturer advises use only if potential benefit outweighs risk—no information available
Diethylstilbestrol (1)	High doses associated with vaginal carcinoma, urogenital abnormalities, and reduced fertility in female offspring

Drug (trimester of risk)	Comment
Diflucortolone	*see Corticosteroids*
Diflunisal	*see NSAIDs*
Digoxin	May need dosage adjustment
Dihydrocodeine	*see Opioid Analgesics*
Dihydroergotamine	*see Ergotamine*
Diloxanide	Manufacturer advises avoid— no information available
Diltiazem	*see Calcium-channel Blockers*
Dimenhydrinate	*see Antihistamines*
Diphenhydramine	*see Antihistamines*
Diphenoxylate	*see Opioid Analgesics*
Diphenylpyraline	*see Antihistamines*
Dipipanone	*see Opioid Analgesics*
Disodium Etidronate	*see Bisphosphonates*
Disodium Pamidronate	*see Bisphosphonates*
Disopyramide (3)	May induce labour
Distigmine	Manufacturer advises avoid (may stimulate uterine contractions)
Disulfiram (1)	High concentrations of acetaldehyde which occur in presence of alcohol may be teratogenic
Diuretics	Not used to treat hypertension in pregnancy
(1)	Manufacturers advise avoid acetazolamide and torasemide (toxicity in *animal* studies)
(3)	Thiazides may cause neonatal thrombocytopenia
Docetaxel	Avoid (toxicity and reduced fertility in *animal* studies); manufacturer advises effective contraception during and for at least 3 months after administration; *see also* section 8.1
Domperidone	Manufacturer advises avoid
Dornase alfa	No evidence of teratogenicity; manufacturer advises use only if potential benefit outweighs risk
Dosulepin (dothiepin)	*see Antidepressants, Tricyclic*
Dothiepin	*see Antidepressants, Tricyclic*
Doxazosin	*see Alpha-blockers (post-synaptic)*
Doxepin	*see Antidepressants, Tricyclic*
Doxorubicin	Avoid (teratogenic and toxic in *animal* studies); manufacturer of liposomal product advises effective contraception during and for at least 6 months after administration to men or women; *see also* section 8.1
Doxycycline	*see Tetracyclines*
Doxylamine	*see Antihistamines*
Droperidol	*see Antipsychotics*
Dydrogesterone	*see Progestogens*
Econazole	Not known to be harmful

Drug (trimester of risk)	Comment
Efavirenz	Manufacturer advises use only if potential benefit outweighs risk—no information available
Eformoterol	*see* Formoterol
Enalapril	*see* ACE Inhibitors
Enflurane	*see* Anaesthetics, General
Enoxaparin	Manufacturer advises avoid unless no safer alternative
Entacapone	Manufacturer advises avoid—no information available
Ephedrine	Increased fetal heart rate reported with parenteral ephedrine
Epirubicin	Avoid (carcinogenic in *animal* studies); *see also* section 8.1
Epoetin	Manufacturers advise avoid unless essential—no information available
Eptifibatide	Manufacturer advises use only if potential benefit outweighs risk—no information available
Ergotamine (1, 2, 3)	Oxytocic effects on the pregnant uterus
Erythromycin	Not known to be harmful
Esmolol	*see* Beta-blockers
Ether	*see* Anaesthetics, General
Ethinylestradiol	*see* Contraceptives, Oral
Ethionamide (1)	May be teratogenic
Ethosuximide (1)	May possibly be teratogenic; *see* Antiepileptics
Etidronate Disodium	*see* Bisphosphonates
Etodolac	*see* NSAIDs
Etomidate	*see* Anaesthetics, General
Etoposide	Avoid (teratogenic in *animal* studies); *see also* section 8.1
Etynodiol	*see* Contraceptives, Oral
Famciclovir	*see* Aciclovir
Famotidine	Manufacturer advises avoid unless potential benefit outweighs risk
Fansidar®	
(1)	Possible teratogenic risk (pyrimethamine a folate antagonist)
(3)	Neonatal haemolysis and methaemoglobinaemia; fear of increased risk of kernicterus in neonates appears to be unfounded *see also* Antimalarials
Felodipine	*see* Calcium-channel Blockers
Fenbufen	*see* NSAIDs
Fenofibrate (1, 2, 3)	Manufacturer advises toxicity in *animal* studies; *see also* Clofibrate
Fenoprofen	*see* NSAIDs
Fenoterol	*see* section 3.1.1 [text]
Fentanyl	*see* Opioid Analgesics
Fenticonazole	Manufacturer advises avoid unless essential
Fexofenadine	*see* Antihistamines

Drug (trimester of risk)	Comment
Filgrastim	Toxicity in *animal* studies; manufacturer advises use only if potential benefit outweighs risk
Finasteride (1, 2, 3)	Avoid unprotected intercourse (see section 6.4.2). May cause feminisation of male fetus
Flavoxate	Manufacturer advises avoid unless no safer alternative
Flecainide	Manufacturer advises toxicity in *animal* studies
Fluclorolone	*see* Corticosteroids
Fluconazole	Manufacturer advises avoid
Flucytosine	Teratogenic in *animal* studies; manufacturer advises use only if potential benefit outweighs risk
Fludarabine	Avoid (embryotoxic and teratogenic in *animal* studies); manufacturer advises effective contraception during and for at least 6 months after administration to men or women; *see also* section 8.1
Fludroxycortide (flurandrenolone)	*see* Corticosteroids
Flunisolide	*see* Corticosteroids
Flunitrazepam	*see* Benzodiazepines
Fluocinolone	*see* Corticosteroids
Fluocinonide	*see* Corticosteroids
Fluocortolone	*see* Corticosteroids
Fluorouracil	Avoid (teratogenic); *see also* section 8.1
Fluoxetine	*see* Antidepressants, SSRI
Flupentixol	*see* Antipsychotics
Fluphenazine	*see* Antipsychotics
Flurandrenolone	*see* Corticosteroids
Flurazepam	*see* Benzodiazepines
Flurbiprofen	*see* NSAIDs
Fluticasone	*see* Corticosteroids
Fluvastatin	*see* Statins
Fluvoxamine	*see* Antidepressants, SSRI
Fomepizole	Manufacturer advises use only if potential benefit outweighs risk—no information available
Formoterol (eformoterol)	Manufacturers advise use only if potential benefit outweighs risk; *see also* section 3.1.1.1 [text]
Foscarnet	Manufacturer advises avoid
Fosinopril	*see* ACE Inhibitors
Fosphenytoin	*see* Phenytoin
Framycetin	*see* Aminoglycosides
Frusemide	*see* Diuretics
Furosemide (frusemide)	*see* Diuretics
Gabapentin	*see* Antiepileptics
Gamolenic Acid	Manufacturer advises caution (but no teratogenic effects in *animals*)
Ganciclovir	Avoid—teratogenic risk; *see also* p. 295
Gemcitabine	Avoid (teratogenic in *animal* studies); *see also* section 8.1

Drug (trimester of risk)	Comment
Gemfibrozil	*see* Clofibrate
Gentamicin	*see* Aminoglycosides
Gestodene	*see* Contraceptives, Oral
Gestrinone (1, 2, 3)	Avoid
Glibenclamide	*see* Sulphonylureas
Gliclazide	*see* Sulphonylureas
Glimepiride	*see* Sulphonylureas
Glipizide	*see* Sulphonylureas
Gliquidone	*see* Sulphonylureas
Gold	
Auranofin	Manufacturer advises teratogenicity in *animal* studies; effective contraception should be used during and for at least 6 months after treatment
Aurothiomalate (1, 2, 3)	Manufacturer advises avoid
Goserelin	Manufacturer advises avoid in pregnancy— exclude pregnancy before treatment and use non-hormonal contraceptives during treatment
Granisetron	Manufacturer advises use only when compelling reasons—no information available
Griseofulvin	Avoid (fetotoxicity and teratogenicity in *animals*); effective contraception required during and for at least 1 month after administration (**important:** effectiveness of oral contraceptives reduced, see p. 368); also men should avoid fathering a child during and for at least 6 months after administration
Growth Hormone	*see* Somatropin
Guanethidine (3)	Postural hypotension and reduced uteroplacental perfusion; should not be used to treat hypertension in pregnancy
Haem arginate (human hemin)	Manufacturer advises avoid unless essential
Halcinonide	*see* Corticosteroids
Halofantrine (1)	Manufacturer advises toxicity in *animal* studies
Haloperidol	*see* Antipsychotics
Halothane	*see* Anaesthetics, General
Heparin	*see* Anticoagulants
5HT₁ Agonists	Limited experience—manufacturers advise avoid unless potential benefit outweighs risk
Hydralazine (1, 2)	Manufacturer advises avoid before third trimester; no reports of serious harm following use in third trimester
Hydrochloro-thiazide	*see* Diuretics
Hydrocortisone	*see* Corticosteroids
Hydroflumethiazide	*see* Diuretics
Hydromorphone	*see* Opioid Analgesics

Drug (trimester of risk)	Comment
Hydroxycarbamide (hydroxyurea)	Avoid (teratogenic in *animal* studies); manufacturer advises effective contraception before and during administration; *see also* section 8.1
Hydroxychloro-quine	Avoid for rheumatic disease
Hydroxyprogest-erone	*see* Progestogens
Hydroxyurea	*see* Hydroxycarbamide
Hydroxyzine	*see* Antihistamines
Hyoscine butylbromide	Manufacturer advises use only if potential benefit outweighs risk
Ibuprofen	*see* NSAIDs
Idarubicin	Avoid (teratogenic and toxic in *animal* studies); *see also* section 8.1
Idoxuridine	Manufacturers advise toxicity in *animal* studies
Ifosfamide	Avoid (teratogenic and carcinogenic in *animals*); manufacturer advises adequate contraception during and for at least 6 months after administration to men or women; *see also* section 8.1
Imidapamil	*see* ACE inhibitors
Imiglucerase	Manufacturer advises use only if potential benefit outweighs risk—no information available
Imipenem [ingredient]	*see* Primaxin®
Imipramine	*see* Antidepressants, Tricyclic
Imiquimod	No evidence of teratogenicity or toxicity in *animal* studies; manufacturer advises use only if potential benefit outweighs risk
Immunosuppress-ants	*see* section 8.1
Indapamide	*see* Diuretics
Indinavir	Manufacturer advises use only if potential benefit outweighs risk—no information available
Indometacin	*see* NSAIDs
Infliximab	Avoid; manufacturer advises adequate contraception during and for at least 6 months after last dose
Insulin (1, 2, 3)	Insulin requirements should be assessed frequently by an experienced diabetic physician
Interferons	Manufacturers recommend avoid unless compelling reasons
Iodine and Iodides (2, 3)	Neonatal goitre and hypothyroidism
Radioactive iodine (1, 2, 3)	Permanent hypothyroidism—avoid
Iodoform	*see* Povidone–iodine
Irbesartan	As for ACE Inhibitors

Drug (trimester of risk)	Comment
Irinotecan	Avoid (teratogenic and toxic in *animal* studies); manufacturer advises effective contraception during and for at least 3 months after administration; *see also* section 8.1
Isocarboxazid	*see* MAOIs
Isoflurane	*see* Anaesthetics, General
Isotretinoin (1, 2, 3)	Teratogenic; effective contraception must be used for at least 1 month before oral treatment, during treatment and for at least 1 month after stopping; also avoid topical treatment
Isradipine	*see* Calcium-channel Blockers
Itraconazole	Manufacturer advises use only in life-threatening situations (toxicity at high doses in *animal* studies); ensure effective contraception during and for 1 month after administration
Kanamycin	*see* Aminoglycosides
Ketamine	*see* Anaesthetics, General
Ketoconazole	Manufacturer advises teratogenicity in *animal* studies; packs carry a warning to avoid in pregnancy
Ketoprofen	*see* NSAIDs
Ketorolac	*see* NSAIDs
Ketotifen	*see* Antihistamines
Labetalol	*see* Beta-blockers
Lacidipine	*see* Calcium-channel Blockers
Lamivudine	Manufacturer advises avoid during first trimester—no information available
Lamotrigine	*see* Antiepileptics
Lanreotide	Manufacturer advises avoid—growth retardation in *animal* studies
Lansoprazole	Manufacturer advises avoid
Latanoprost	Manufacturer advises avoid
Leflunomide	Avoid—active metabolite teratogenic in *animal* studies; effective contraception essential during treatment and for at least 2 years after treatment in women and at least 3 months after treatment in men (*see also* Leflunomide section 10.1.3)
Lenograstim	Toxicity in *animal* studies; manufacturer advises use only if potential benefit outweighs risk
Lepirudin	Avoid
Lercanidipine	*see* Calcium-channel blockers
Levocabastine	*see* Antihistamines
Levodopa	Manufacturers advise toxicity in *animal* studies
Levofloxacin	*see* Quinolones
Levomepromazine (methotrimeprazine)	*see* Antipsychotics
Levonorgestrel	*see* Contraceptives, Oral

Drug (trimester of risk)	Comment
Levothyroxine (thyroxine)	Monitor maternal serum-thyrotrophin concentration—dosage adjustment may be necessary
Lidocaine (lignocaine)	*see* Anaesthetics, Local
Lignocaine	*see* Anaesthetics, Local
Lisinopril	*see* ACE Inhibitors
Lithium (1)	Avoid if possible (risk of teratogenicity, including cardiac abnormalities)
(2,3)	Dose requirements increased (but on delivery return to normal abruptly); close monitoring of serum-lithium concentration advised (risk of toxicity in neonate)
Lofepramine	*see* Antidepressants, Tricyclic
Loperamide	Manufacturers advise avoid—no information available
Loprazolam	*see* Benzodiazepines
Loratadine	*see* Antihistamines
Lorazepam	*see* Benzodiazepines
Lormetazepam	*see* Benzodiazepines
Losartan	As for ACE Inhibitors
Lymecycline	*see* Tetracyclines
Madopar®	*see* Levodopa
Malarone®	Manufacturer advises avoid unless essential
Maloprim® (1)	Possible teratogenic risk (pyrimethamine a folate antagonist)
(3)	Neonatal haemolysis and methaemoglobinaemia (due to dapsone); adequate folate supplements should be given to mother; *see also* Antimalarials
MAOIs (including moclobemide) (1, 2, 3)	No evidence of harm but manufacturers advise avoid unless compelling reasons
Maprotiline	*see* Antidepressants, Tricyclic (and related)
Mebendazole	Manufacturer advises toxicity in *animal* studies
Mebeverine	Not known to be harmful; manufacturers advise caution
Mefenamic Acid	*see* NSAIDs
Mefloquine (1)	Manufacturer advises teratogenicity in *animal* studies, but *see* p. 299 and p. 300
Mefruside	*see* Diuretics
Meloxicam	*see* NSAIDs
Melphalan	Avoid (manufacturer advises adequate contraception during administration to men or women); *see also* section 8.1
Menadiol (3)	Neonatal haemolytic anaemia, hyperbilirubinaemia and increased risk of kernicterus in jaundiced infants

Drug (trimester of risk)	Comment
Meprobamate	Manufacturer advises avoid if possible
Meptazinol	*see* Opioid Analgesics
Mercaptamine	Manufacturer advises avoid
Mercaptopurine	Avoid (teratogenic); *see also* section 8.1
Meropenem	Manufacturer advises use only if potential benefit outweighs risk—no information available
Mesalazine	Negligible quantities cross placenta
Mesna	Not known to be harmful; *see also* section 8.1
Mesterolone	*see* Androgens
Mestranol	*see* Contraceptives, Oral
Metaraminol (1, 2, 3)	Avoid—may reduce placental perfusion
Metformin (1, 2, 3)	Avoid; insulin is normally substituted in all diabetics
Methadone	*see* Opioid Analgesics
Methotrexate	Avoid (teratogenic; fertility may be reduced during therapy but this may be reversible); manufacturer advises effective contraception during and for at least 6 months after administration to men or women; *see also* section 8.1
Methotrimeprazine	*see* Antipsychotics
Methyldopa	Not known to be harmful
Methylphenidate	Limited experience; manufacturer advises avoid unless potential benefit outweighs risk
Methylphenobarb-ital	*see* Antiepileptics
Methylprednisolone	*see* Corticosteroids
Methysergide	Manufacturer advises avoid
Metoclopramide	Not known to be harmful but manufacturer advises use only when compelling reasons
Metolazone	*see* Diuretics
Metoprolol	*see* Beta-blockers
Metronidazole	Manufacturer advises avoidance of high-dose regimens
Metyrapone	Avoid (may impair biosynthesis of fetal-placental steroids)
Mianserin	*see* Antidepressants, Tricyclic (and related)
Miconazole	Manufacturer advises avoid unless essential
Mifepristone	Manufacturer advises that if treatment fails, essential that pregnancy be terminated by another method
Minocycline	*see* Tetracyclines
Minoxidil (3)	Neonatal hirsutism reported
Misoprostol (1, 2, 3)	Avoid; increases uterine tone
Mitomycin	Avoid (teratogenic in *animal* studies); *see also* section 8.1

Drug (trimester of risk)	Comment
Mitoxantrone (mitozantrone)	Avoid; manufacturer advises effective contraception during and for at least 6 months after administration to men or women; *see also* section 8.1
Mitozantrone	*see* Mitoxantrone
Mizolastine	*see* Antihistamines
Moclobemide	*see* MAOIs
Modafinil	Manufacturer advises avoid
Moexipril	*see* ACE Inhibitors
Molgramostim	Manufacturer advises toxicity in *animal* studies
Montelukast	Manufacturer advises avoid unless essential
Moracizine	Manufacturer advises use only if potential benefit outweighs risk—no information available
Morphine	*see* Opioid Analgesics
Moxonidine	Manufacturer advises avoid—no information available
Moxisylyte (thymoxamine)	Manufacturer advises avoid
Mustine	*see* Chlormethine
Mycophenolate Mofetil	Manufacturer advises avoid—toxicity in *animal* studies; effective contraception required during and for 6 weeks after discontinuation of treatment
Nabumetone	*see* NSAIDs
Nadolol	*see* Beta-blockers
Nafarelin	Avoid
Nalbuphine	*see* Opioid Analgesics
Nalidixic acid	*see* Quinolones
Naloxone	Manufacturer advises use only if potential benefit outweighs risk
Nandrolone	*see* Anabolic Steroids
Naproxen	*see* NSAIDs
Naratriptan	*see* 5HT$_1$ Agonists
Narcotic Analgesics	*see* Opioid Analgesics
Nebivolol	*see* Beta-blockers
Nedocromil	*see* section 3.1.1 [text]
Nefazodone	No information available—manufacturer advises use only if clearly needed
Nefopam	No information available—manufacturer advises avoid unless no safer treatment
Nelfinavir	No information available—manufacturer advises use only if potential benefit outweighs risk
Neomycin	*see* Aminoglycosides
Neostigmine (3)	Neonatal myasthenia with large doses
Netilmicin	*see* Aminoglycosides
Nevirapine	No information available
Nicardipine	*see* Calcium-channel Blockers
Nicorandil	Manufacturer advises use only if potential benefit outweighs risk—no information available
Nicotine (1,2,3)	Avoid
Nicoumalone	*see* Anticoagulants, Oral

Drug (trimester of risk)	Comment
Nifedipine	*see* Calcium-channel Blockers
Nimodipine	*see* Calcium-channel Blockers
Nisoldipine	*see* Calcium-channel Blockers
Nitrazepam	*see* Benzodiazepines
Nitrofurantoin (3)	May produce neonatal haemolysis if used at term
Nitrous oxide	*see* Anaesthetics, General
Nizatidine	Manufacturer advises avoid unless essential
Noradrenaline (norepinephrine) (1, 2, 3)	Avoid—may reduce placental perfusion
Norethisterone	*see* Contraceptives, Oral
Norfloxacin	*see* Quinolones
Norgestimate	*see* Contraceptives, Oral
Nortriptyline	*see* Antidepressants, Tricyclic
NSAIDs	Most manufacturers advise avoid (or avoid unless potential benefit outweighs risk); ketorolac contra-indicated during pregnancy, labour and delivery
(3)	With regular use closure of fetal ductus arteriosus *in utero* and possibly persistent pulmonary hypertension of the newborn. Delayed onset and increased duration of labour
Nystatin	No information available, but absorption from gastro-intestinal tract negligible
Octreotide (1, 2, 3)	Possible effect on fetal growth; manufacturer advises use only if potential benefit outweighs risk
Oestrogens	*see* Contraceptives, Oral
Ofloxacin	*see* Quinolones
Olanzapine	Manufacturer advises use only if potential benefit outweighs risk
Olsalazine	Manufacturer advises avoid unless potential benefit outweighs risk
Omeprazole	Manufacturer advises toxicity in *animal* studies
Ondansetron	No information available; manufacturer advises avoid unless potential benefit outweighs risk
Opioid Analgesics (3)	Depress neonatal respiration; withdrawal effects in neonates of dependent mothers; gastric stasis and risk of inhalation pneumonia in mother during labour
Orlistat	Manufacturer advises avoid—no information available
Orphenadrine	Manufacturer advises caution
<u>Oxaliplatin</u>	Manufacturer advises avoid—no information available; *see also* section 8.1
Oxazepam	*see* Benzodiazepines
Oxprenolol	*see* Beta-blockers
Oxybutynin	Manufacturer advises toxicity at high doses in *animal* studies

Drug (trimester of risk)	Comment
Oxypertine	*see* Antipsychotics
Oxytetracycline	*see* Tetracyclines
Paclitaxel	Avoid (toxicity in *animal* studies); *see also* section 8.1
Pamidronate Disodium	*see* Bisphosphonates
Pancreatin	Not known to be harmful
Pantoprazole	Manufacturer advises avoid unless potential benefit outweighs risk—fetotoxic in *animals*
Papaveretum	*see* Opioid Analgesics
Paracetamol	Not known to be harmful
Paraldehyde	Manufacturer advises avoid unless essential—crosses the placenta
Paroxetine	*see* Antidepressants, SSRI
Penicillamine (1, 2, 3)	Fetal abnormalities reported rarely; avoid if possible
Penicillins	Not known to be harmful
Pentamidine isetionate	Manufacturer advises avoid unless essential
Pentazocine	*see* Opioid Analgesics
Pentostatin	Avoid (teratogenic in *animal* studies); manufacturer advises that men should not father children during and for 6 months after administration; *see also* section 8.1
Pericyazine	*see* Antipsychotics
Perindopril	*see* ACE Inhibitors
Perphenazine	*see* Antipsychotics
Pethidine	*see* Opioid Analgesics
Phenelzine	*see* MAOIs
Phenindione	*see* Anticoagulants, Oral
Pheniramine	*see* Antihistamines
Phenobarbital (1, 3)	Congenital malformations. Neonatal bleeding tendency—prophylactic vitamin K_1 for mother before delivery (as well as for neonate); *see also* Antiepileptics
Phenothiazines	*see* Antipsychotics
Phentolamine	No information available
Phenytoin (1, 3)	Congenital malformations (screening advised); adequate folate supplements should be given to mother (e.g. folic acid 5 mg daily). Neonatal bleeding tendency—prophylactic vitamin K_1 for mother before delivery (as well as for neonate). Caution in interpreting plasma concentrations—bound may be reduced but free (i.e. effective) unchanged; *see also* Antiepileptics
Pholcodine	*see* Opioid Analgesics
Pilocarpine	Avoid—smooth muscle stimulant
Pimozide	*see* Antipsychotics
Pindolol	*see* Beta-blockers

Drug (trimester of risk)	Comment
Piperazine	No clinical evidence of harm but packs sold to the general public carry a warning to avoid in pregnancy except on medical advice
Piperacillin	*see* Penicillins
Pipotiazine	*see* Antipsychotics
Piracetam	Manufacturer advises avoid
Piroxicam	*see* NSAIDs
Podophyllotoxin	Avoid
Podophyllum resin (1, 2, 3)	Avoid—neonatal death and teratogenesis have been reported
Polythiazide	*see* Diuretics
Povidone–iodine (2, 3)	Sufficient iodine may be absorbed to affect the fetal thyroid
Pramipexole	Manufacturer advises use only if potential benefit outweighs risk—no information available
Pravastatin	*see* Statins
Prazosin	*see* Alpha-blockers (post-synaptic)
Prednisolone	*see* Corticosteroids
Prilocaine (3)	Neonatal methaemoglobinaemia; *see also* Anaesthetics, Local
Primaquine (3)	Neonatal haemolysis and methaemoglobinaemia; *see also* Antimalarials
Primaxin®	Manufacturer advises toxicity in *animal* studies
Primidone	*see* Phenobarbital
Procaine (3)	Neonatal methaemoglobinaemia; *see also* Anaesthetics, Local
Procarbazine	Avoid (teratogenic in *animal* studies and isolated reports in humans); *see also* section 8.1
Prochlorperazine	*see* Antipsychotics
Progestogens (1)	High doses may possibly be teratogenic
Proguanil	Adequate folate supplements should be given to mother; *see also* Antimalarials
Promazine	*see* Antipsychotics
Promethazine	*see* Antihistamines
Propafenone	Manufacturer advises avoid—no information available
Propiverine	Manufacturer advises avoid (retardation of skeletal development in *animals*)
Propofol	*see* Anaesthetics, General
Propranolol	*see* Beta-blockers
Propylthiouracil (2, 3)	Neonatal goitre and hypothyroidism
Protionamide (1)	May be teratogenic
Protriptyline	*see* Antidepressants, Tricyclic
Pseudoephedrine	Not known to be harmful
Pyridostigmine (3)	Neonatal myasthenia with large doses

Drug (trimester of risk)	Comment
Pyrimethamine (1)	Theoretical teratogenic risk (folate antagonist); adequate folate supplements should be given to mother; *see also* Antimalarials
Quetiapine	Manufacturer advises use only if potential benefit outweighs risk
Quinagolide	Manufacturer advises discontinue when pregnancy confirmed unless medical reason for continuing
Quinapril	*see* ACE Inhibitors
Quinine (1)	High doses are teratogenic; but in malaria benefit of treatment outweighs risk
Quinolones (1, 2, 3)	Avoid—arthropathy in *animal* studies; safer alternatives available
Quinupristin [ingredient]	*see Synercid*®
Rabeprazole	Manufacturer advises avoid—no information available
Raltitrexed	Pregnancy must be excluded before treatment; ensure effective contraception during and for at least 6 months after administration to men or women; *see also* section 8.1
Ramipril	*see* ACE Inhibitors
Ranitidine	Manufacturer advises avoid unless essential
Ranitidine bismuth citrate	Safety not established
Razoxane	Avoid (teratogenic in *animal* studies); *see also* section 8.1
Reboxetine	Manufacturer advises avoid (and discontinue if pregnancy occurs)—no information available
Remifentanil	No information available; *see also* Opioid Analgesics
Repaglinide	Manufacturer advises avoid; insulin is normally substituted in all diabetics
Reproterol	*see* section 3.1.1 [text]
Reteplase	*see* Streptokinase
Rifabutin	Manufacturer advises avoid—no information available
Rifampicin (1)	Manufacturers advise very high doses teratogenic in *animal* studies; *see also* p. 274
(3)	Risk of neonatal bleeding may be increased
Riluzole	No information available; manufacturer advises avoid
Risperidone	Manufacturer advises use only if potential benefit outweighs risk
Ritodrine	For use in premature labour see section 7.1.3
Ritonavir	Manufacturer advises use only if potential benefit outweighs risk—no information available;

Drug (trimester of risk)	Comment
Rituximab	Avoid unless potential benefit to mother outweighs risk of B-lymphocyte depletion in fetus—effective contraception required during and for 12 months after treatment
Rivastigmine	Manufacturer advises use only if potential benefit outweighs risk
Rizatriptan	see 5HT₁ Agonists
Rofecoxib	see NSAIDs
Salbutamol	For use in asthma see section 3.1.1 [text]
(3)	For use in premature labour see section 7.1.3
Salcatonin	see Calcitonin (salmon)
Salicylates	see Aspirin
Salmeterol	see section 3.1.1 [text]
Saquinavir	No information available
Sertindole	Manufacturer advises avoid
Sertraline	see Antidepressants, SSRI
Sevoflurane	see Anaesthetics, General
Simvastatin	see Statins
Sodium Aurothiomalate	see Gold
Sodium Clodronate	see Bisphosphonates
Sodium Cromoglicate	see Cromoglicate
Sodium Valproate	see Valproate
Somatropin	Discontinue if pregnancy occurs—no information available but theoretical risk
Sotalol	see Beta-blockers
Spironolactone	Manufacturers advise toxicity in *animal* studies
Stanozolol	see Anabolic Steroids
Statins	Avoid—congenital anomalies reported; decreased synthesis of cholesterol possibly affects fetal development
Stavudine	No information available
Streptokinase (1, 2, 3)	Possibility of premature separation of placenta in first 18 weeks; theoretical possibility of fetal haemorrhage throughout pregnancy; avoid postpartum use—maternal haemorrhage
Streptomycin	see Aminoglycosides
Sulfadiazine	see Sulphonamides
Sulfadoxine	see Sulphonamides
Sulfametopyrazine	see Sulphonamides
Sulfasalazine (3)	Theoretical risk of neonatal haemolysis; adequate folate supplements should be given to mother
Sulindac	see NSAIDs
Sulphonamides (3)	Neonatal haemolysis and methaemoglobinaemia; fear of increased risk of kernicterus in neonates appears to be unfounded

Drug (trimester of risk)	Comment
Sulphonylureas (3)	Neonatal hypoglycaemia; insulin is normally substituted in all diabetics; if oral drugs are used therapy should be stopped at least 2 days before delivery
Sulpiride	see Antipsychotics
Sumatriptan	see 5HT₁ Agonists
Suxamethonium	Mildly prolonged maternal paralysis may occur
Synercid ®	Manufacturer advises avoid unless potential benefit outweighs risk—no information available
Tacalcitol	Manufacturer advises avoid if possible
Tacrolimus	Avoid; manufacturer advises toxicity in *animal* studies
Tamoxifen	Avoid—possible effects on fetal development; effective contraception must be used during treatment and for 2 months after stopping
Tazarotene	Avoid; effective contraception required
Teicoplanin	Manufacturer advises use only if potential benefit outweighs risk
Telmisartan	As for ACE Inhibitors
Temazepam	see Benzodiazepines
Temozolomide	Avoid (teratogenic and embryotoxic in *animal* studies); manufacturer advises adequate contraception during administration; see also section 8.1; also men should avoid fathering a child during and for at least 6 months after treatment
Tenoxicam	see NSAIDS
Terazosin	see Alpha-blockers (post-synaptic)
Terbinafine	Manufacturer advises use only if potential benefit outweighs risk—no information available
Terbutaline	For use in asthma see section 3.1.1 [text]
(3)	For use in premature labour see section 7.1.3
Terfenadine	see Antihistamines
Testosterone	see Androgens
Tetrabenazine	Inadequate information but no evidence of harm
Tetracyclines (1)	Effects on skeletal development in *animal* studies
(2, 3)	Dental discoloration; maternal hepatotoxicity with large parenteral doses
Theophylline (3)	Neonatal irritability and apnoea have been reported
Thiazides (3)	May cause neonatal thrombocytopenia; see also Diuretics
Thiopental	see Anaesthetics, General
Thioridazine	see Antipsychotics

Drug (trimester of risk)	Comment
Thiotepa	Avoid (teratogenic and embryotoxic in *animals*); *see also* section 8.1
Thymoxamine	*see* Moxisylyte
Thyroxine	*see* Levothyroxine
Tiabendazole (1)	Teratogenic in *animal* studies
Tiagabine	Manufacturer advises avoid unless potential benefit outweighs risk
Tiaprofenic Acid	*see* NSAIDs
Ticlodipine	Manufacturer advises avoid unless essential—toxicity in *animal* studies
Tiludronic Acid	*see* Bisphosphonates
Timolol	*see* Beta-blockers
Tinidazole	Manufacturer advises avoid in first trimester
Tinzaparin	Manufacturer advises avoid unless no safer alternative
Tioguanine	Avoid (teratogenicity reported when men receiving thioguanine have fathered children); ensure effective contraception during administration to men or women; *see also* section 8.1
Tirofiban	Manufacturer advises use only if potential benefit outweighs risk—no information available
Tizanidine	Manufacturer advises use only if potential benefit outweighs risk—no information available
Tobramycin	*see* Aminoglycosides
Tocainide	Toxicity in *animal* studies; manufacturer advises use only if potential benefit outweighs risk
Tocopheryl Acetate (1, 2, 3)	No evidence of safety of high doses
Tolbutamide	*see* Sulphonylureas
Tolfenamic Acid	*see* NSAIDs
Tolterodine	Manufacturer advises avoid— no information available
Topiramate	Manufacturer advises avoid unless potential benefit outweighs potential risk; *see also* Antiepileptics
Topotecan	Avoid (teratogenicity and fetal loss in *animal* studies); *see also* section 8.1
Torasemide	*see* Diuretics
Tramadol	No information available; *see also* Opioid Analgesics
Trandolapril	*see* ACE Inhibitors
Tranexamic acid	No evidence of teratogenicity in *animal* studies; manufacturer advises use only if potential benefit outweighs risk
Tranylcypromine	*see* MAOIs
Trazodone	*see* Antidepressants, Tricyclic (and related)
Treosulfan	Avoid; *see also* section 8.1

Drug (trimester of risk)	Comment
Tretinoin (1, 2, 3)	Teratogenic; effective contraception must be used for at least 1 month before oral treatment, during treatment and for at least 1 month after stopping; also avoid topical treatment
Triamcinolone	*see* Corticosteroids
Triamterene	*see* Diuretics
Tribavirin	Avoid; teratogenicity in *animal* studies; ensure effective contraception during oral administration and for 4 months after treatment in women and 7 months after treatment in men; *see also* Tribavirin section 5.3
Triclofos	Avoid
Trifluoperazine	*see* Antipsychotics
Trilostane (1, 2, 3)	Interferes with placental sex hormone production
Trimeprazine	*see* Alimemazine
Trimetaphan (3)	Avoid; risk of paralytic ileus in newborn
Trimethoprim (1)	Theoretical teratogenic risk (folate antagonist)
Trimetrexate	Avoid (fetotoxicity and teratogenicity in *animals*); avoid conception for at least 6 months after administration to woman or man
Trimipramine	*see* Antidepressants, Tricyclic
Tripotassium Dicitratobismuth-ate	*see* Bismuth Chelate
Triprolidine	*see* Antihistamines
Tropisetron	Manufacturer advises toxicity in *animal* studies
Tulobuterol	*see* section 3.1.1 [text]
Ursodeoxycholic acid	No evidence of harm but manufacturer advises avoid
Vaccines (live) (1)	Theoretical risk of congenital malformations, but need for vaccination may outweigh possible risk to fetus (*see also* p. 541); avoid MMR and Rubella vaccines but see p. 554
Valaciclovir	No information available; *see also* Aciclovir
Valproate (1, 3)	Increased risk of neural tube defects (counselling and screening advised— **important**: see also p. 223); neonatal bleeding (related to hypofibrinaemia) and neonatal hepatotoxicity also reported; *see also* Antiepileptics
Valsartan	As for ACE Inhibitors
Vancomycin	Manufacturer advises avoid unless potential benefit outweighs risk—little information available
Vasopressin	Oxytocic effect in third trimester
Venlafaxine	Manufacturer advises avoid— no information available
Verapamil	*see* Calcium-channel Blockers

Drug (trimester of risk)	Comment
Vigabatrin	Congenital anomalies reported—manufacturer advises avoid unless potential benefit outweighs risk; *see also* Antiepileptics
Viloxazine	*see* Antidepressants, Tricyclic (and related)
Vinblastine	Avoid (limited experience suggests fetal harm; teratogenic in *animal* studies); *see also* section 8.1
Vincristine	Avoid (teratogenicity and fetal loss in *animal* studies); *see also* section 8.1
Vindesine	Avoid (teratogenic in *animal* studies); *see also* section 8.1
Vinorelbine	Avoid (teratogenicity and fetal loss in *animal* studies); *see also* section 8.1
Vitamin A (1)	Excessive doses may be teratogenic; *see also* p. 437
Warfarin	*see* Anticoagulants, Oral
Xamoterol	Manufacturer advises toxicity in *animal* studies
Xipamide	*see* Diuretics
Zafirlukast	Manufacturer advises use only if potential benefit outweighs risk
Zalcitabine	Limited information available; use only if potential benefit outweighs risk
Zanamavir	Manufacturer advises use only if potential benefit outweighs risk—no information available
Zidovudine	Limited information available; manufacturer advises use only if clearly indicated; *see also* p. 292
Zolmitriptan	*see* $5HT_1$ Agonists
Zolpidem	*see* Benzodiazepines
Zopiclone	*see* Benzodiazepine
Zuclopenthixol	*see* Antipsychotics

Appendix 5: Breast-feeding

Administration of some drugs (e.g. ergotamine) to nursing mothers may cause toxicity in the infant, whereas administration of others (e.g. digoxin) has little effect on the neonate. Some drugs inhibit lactation (e.g. bromocriptine).

Toxicity to the infant can occur if the drug enters the milk in pharmacologically significant quantities. The concentration in milk of some drugs (e.g. iodides) may exceed those in the maternal plasma so that therapeutic doses in the mother may cause toxicity to the infant. Some drugs inhibit the infant's sucking reflex (e.g. phenobarbital). Drugs in breast milk may, at least theoretically, cause hypersensitivity in the infant even when concentrations are too low for a pharmacological effect.

The following table lists drugs:

- which should be used with caution or which are contra-indicated in breast-feeding for the reasons given above;
- which, on present evidence, may be given to the mother during breast-feeding, because they appear in milk in amounts which are too small to be harmful to the infant;
- which are not known to be harmful to the infant although they are present in milk in significant amounts.

> For many drugs insufficient evidence is available to provide guidance and it is advisable to administer only essential drugs to a mother during breast-feeding. Because of the inadequacy of information on drugs in breast milk the following table should be used only as a guide; absence from the table does not imply safety.

Table of drugs present in breast milk

Products introduced or amended since publication of BNF No. 38 (September 1999) are underlined.

Drug	Comment
Abacavir	Breast-feeding not advised in HIV infection
Abciximab	Manufacturer advises avoid—no information available
Acamprosate	Manufacturer advises avoid
Acarbose	Manufacturer advises avoid
Acebutolol	*see* Beta-blockers
Aceclofenac	Manufacturer advises avoid—no information available
Acemetacin	Manufacturer advises avoid
Acetazolamide	Amount too small to be harmful
Acetohexamide	*see* Sulphonylureas
Aciclovir	Significant amount in milk after systemic administration
Acipimox	Manufacturer advises avoid
Acitretin	Avoid
Aclarubicin	*see* Cytotoxic Drugs
Acrivastine	*see* Antihistamines

Drug	Comment
Adapalene	Manufacturer advises avoid (if used, avoid application to chest)—no information available
Alcohol	Large amounts may affect infant and reduce milk consumption
Alendronic Acid	No information available
Alfacalcidol	*see* Vitamin D
Alimemazine (trimeprazine)	*see* Antihistamines
Allopurinol	Present in milk
Alprazolam	*see* Benzodiazepines
Altretamine	*see* Cytotoxic Drugs
Amantadine	Avoid; present in milk; toxicity in infant reported
Amethocaine	*see* Tetracaine
Amifostine	No information available
Amiloride	Manufacturer advises avoid—no information available
Aminoglutethimide	Avoid
Aminophylline	*see* Theophylline
Amiodarone	Avoid; present in milk in significant amounts; theoretical risk from release of iodine; *see also* Iodine
Amisulpride	Manufacturer advises avoid—no information available
Amitriptyline	*see* Antidepressants, Tricyclic
Amlodipine	Manufacturer advises avoid—no information available
Amobarbital	*see* Barbiturates
Amorolfine	Manufacturer advises avoid—no information available
Amoxapine	*see* Antidepressants, Tricyclic
Amphetamines	Significant amount in milk. Avoid
Amphotericin	No information available
Amsacrine	*see* Cytotoxic Drugs
Androgens	Avoid; may cause masculinisation in the female infant or precocious development in the male infant; high doses suppress lactation
Anthraquinones	Avoid; large doses may cause increased gastric motility and diarrhoea (particularly cascara and dantron)
Anticoagulants, Oral	Risk of haemorrhage; increased by vitamin-K deficiency; warfarin appears safe but phenindione should be avoided; manufacturer of acenocoumarol (nicoumalone) recommends prophylactic vitamin-K for the infant (consult product literature)
Antidepressants, SSRI	*see* individual entries

Drug	Comment
Antidepressants, Tricyclic (and related)	Amount of tricyclic antidepressants (including related drugs such as mianserin and trazodone) too small to be harmful but most manufacturers advise avoid; accumulation of doxepin metabolite may cause sedation and respiratory depression
Antihistamines	Significant amount of some antihistamines; although not known to be harmful some manufacturers advise avoid; drowsiness in infant reported with clemastine
Antipsychotics	Although amount excreted in milk probably too small to be harmful, *animal* studies indicate possible adverse effects of these drugs on developing nervous system therefore avoid unless absolutely necessary; *see also* amisulpride, chlorpromazine, clozapine, olanzapine, quetiapine, risperidone, sertindole, sulpiride
Apomorphine	Manufacturer advises avoid—no information available
Aspirin	Avoid—possible risk of Reye's syndrome; regular use of high doses could impair platelet function and produce hypoprothrombinaemia in infant if neonatal vitamin K stores low
Atenolol	*see* Beta-blockers
Atorvastatin	Manufacturer advises avoid—no information available
Atracurium	No information available
Atropine	Small amount present in milk—manufacturer advises caution
Atovaquone	Manufacturer advises avoid—no information available
Auranofin	*see* Gold
Aurothiomalate	*see* Gold
Azapropazone	Avoid—small amounts in milk
Azatadine	*see* Antihistamines
Azithromycin	Manufacturer advises use only if no suitable alternative—no information available
Baclofen	Amount too small to be harmful
Balsalazide	Manufacturer advises avoid
Barbiturates	Avoid if possible (*see also* phenobarbital); large doses may produce drowsiness
Basiliximab	Avoid
Beclometasone	*see* Corticosteroids
Bendrofluazide	*see* Thiazides
Bendroflumethiazide (bendrofluazide)	*see* Thiazides
Benperidol	*see* Antipsychotics
Benzodiazepines	Present in milk—avoid if possible

Drug	Comment
Beta-blockers and Labetalol	Monitor infant; possible toxicity due to beta-blockade but amount of most beta-blockers excreted in milk too small to affect infant; acebutolol, atenolol, nadolol, and sotalol are present in greater amounts than other beta-blockers; manufacturers advise avoid celiprolol and nebivolol
Betamethasone	*see* Corticosteroids
Betaxolol	*see* Beta-blockers
Bezafibrate	Manufacturer advises avoid
Bisoprolol	*see* Beta-blockers
Bleomycin	*see* Cytotoxic Drugs
Botulinum Toxin	Manufacturers advise avoid
Bromazepam	*see* Benzodiazepines
Bromocriptine	Suppresses lactation
Brompheniramine	*see* Antihistamines
Buclizine	*see* Antihistamines
Budesonide	*see* Corticosteroids
Bumetanide	Manufacturer advises avoid if possible—no information available
Bupivacaine	Amount too small to be harmful
Buprenorphine	Amount too small to be harmful; manufacturer advises contra-indicated in the treatment of opioid dependence
Buserelin	Small amount present in milk—manufacturer advises avoid
Busulfan	*see* Cytotoxic Drugs
Butobarbital	*see* Barbiturates
Cabergoline	Suppresses lactation
Caffeine	Regular intake of large amounts can affect infant
Calciferol	*see* Vitamin D
Calcipotriol	No information available
Calcitonin (salmon) (salcatonin)	Avoid; inhibits lactation in *animals*
Calcitriol	*see* Vitamin D
Calcium Folinate	Manufacturer advises caution—no information available
Calcium Levofolinate	*see* Calcium Folinate
Candesartan	Manufacturer advises avoid—no information available
Captopril	Excreted in milk—manufacturers advise avoid
Carbamazepine	Amount probably too small to be harmful but severe skin reaction reported in 1 infant
Carbimazole	Amounts in milk may be sufficient to affect neonatal thyroid function therefore lowest effective dose should be used (*see also* section 6.2.2)
Carboplatin	*see* Cytotoxic Drugs
Carisoprodol	Concentrated in milk; no adverse effects reported but best avoided
Carmustine	*see* Cytotoxic Drugs
Carvedilol	*see* Beta-blockers
Cascara	*see* Anthraquinones
Celiprolol	*see* Beta-blockers
Cephalosporins	Excreted in low concentrations

Drug	Comment
Cerivastatin	Manufacturer advises avoid
Cetirizine	*see* Antihistamines
Cetrorelix	Manufacturer advises avoid
Chloral Hydrate	Sedation in infant
Chlorambucil	*see* Cytotoxic Drugs
Chloramphenicol	Use another antibiotic; may cause bone-marrow toxicity in infant; concentration in milk usually insufficient to cause 'grey syndrome'
Chlordiazepoxide	*see* Benzodiazepines
Chlormethine (mustine)	*see* Cytotoxic Drugs
Chloroquine	Amount probably too small to be harmful; inadequate for reliable protection against malaria, see section 5.4.1
Chlorphenamine (Chlorpheniramine)	*see* Antihistamines
Chlorpheniramine	*see* Antihistamines
Chlorpromazine	Drowsiness in infant reported; *see* Antipsychotics
Chlorpropamide	*see* Sulphonylureas
Chlortalidone	*see* Thiazides
Chlortetracycline	*see* Tetracyclines
Ciclosporin (cyclosporin)	Present in milk—manufacturer advises avoid
Cidofovir	Manufacturer advises avoid
Cilastatin [ingredient]	*see* Primaxin®
Cilazapril	No information available—manufacturer advises avoid
Cimetidine	Significant amount—not known to be harmful but manufacturer advises avoid
Ciprofibrate	Manufacturer advises avoid—present in milk in *animal* studies
Ciprofloxacin	Avoid—high concentrations in breast milk
Cisapride	Although amount in milk small manufacturer advises avoid
Cisatracurium	No information available
Cisplatin	*see* Cytotoxic Drugs
Citalopram	Present in milk—manufacturer advises caution
Cladribine	*see* Cytotoxic Drugs
Clarithromycin	Excreted in milk
Clavulanic acid (in co-amoxiclav, Timentin®)	Trace amounts in milk
Clemastine	*see* Antihistamines
Clindamycin	Amount probably too small to be harmful but bloody diarrhoea reported in 1 infant
Clobazam	*see* Benzodiazepines
Clodronate Sodium	No information available
Clofibrate	Present in milk—manufacturer advises avoid
Clomethiazole	Amount too small to be harmful
Clomipramine	*see* Antidepressants, Tricyclic
Clomocycline	*see* Tetracyclines
Clopidogrel	Manufacturer advises avoid
Clorazepate	*see* Benzodiazepines
Clozapine	Manufacturer advises avoid

Drug	Comment
Co-amoxiclav	Trace amounts in milk
Codeine	Amount too small to be harmful
Colchicine	Caution because of its cytotoxicity
Colecalciferol	*see* Vitamin D
Contraceptives, Oral	Avoid combined oral contraceptives until weaning or for 6 months after birth (adverse effects on lactation); progestogen-only contraceptives do not affect lactation (start 3 weeks after birth or later)
Corticosteroids	Systemic effects in infant unlikely with maternal dose of prednisolone up to 40 mg daily; monitor infant's adrenal function with higher doses
Cortisone Acetate	*see* Corticosteroids
Co-trimoxazole	Small risk of kernicterus in jaundiced infants and of haemolysis in G6PD-deficient infants (due to sulfamethoxazole)
Cough mixtures containing iodides	Use alternative cough mixtures; *see* Iodine
Crisantaspase	*see* Cytotoxic Drugs
Cromoglicate	Unlikely to be present in milk
Cyclopenthiazide	*see* Thiazides
Cyclophosphamide	Discontinue breast-feeding during and for 36 hours after stopping treatment
Cycloserine	Amount too small to be harmful
Cyclosporin	*see* Ciclosporin
Cyproheptadine	*see* Antihistamines
Cyproterone Acetate	Caution; possibility of anti-androgen effects in neonate
Cytarabine	*see* Cytotoxic Drugs
Cytotoxic Drugs	Discontinue breast-feeding
Daclizumab	Avoid
Dactinomycin	*see* Cytotoxic Drugs
Dalfopristin [ingredient]	*see* Synercid®
Dalteparin	No information available
Danaparoid	No information available
Danazol	No data available but avoid because of possible androgenic effects in infant
Dantron	*see* Anthraquinones
Dapsone	Haemolytic anaemia; although significant amount in milk risk to infant very small
Daunorubicin	*see* Cytotoxic Drugs
Deflazacort	*see* Corticosteroids
Demeclocycline	*see* Tetracyclines
Desirudin	Manufacturer advises avoid—no information available
Desmopressin	Not known to be harmful
Desogestrel	*see* Contraceptives, Oral
Dexamethasone	*see* Corticosteroids
Dexamfetamine	*see* Amphetamines
Dexketoprofen	Manufacturer advises avoid—no information available
Dextropropoxyphene	Amount too small to be harmful

Drug	Comment
Diamorphine	Therapeutic doses unlikely to affect infant; withdrawal symptoms in infants of dependent mothers; breast-feeding no longer considered best method of treating dependence in off-spring of dependent mothers and should be stopped
Diazepam	*see* Benzodiazepines
Diclofenac	Amount too small to be harmful
Didanosine	Breast-feeding not advised in HIV infection
Diflunisal	Manufacturer advises avoid
Digoxin	Amount too small to be harmful
Dihydrotachysterol	*see* Vitamin D
Diloxanide	Manufacturer advises avoid
Diltiazem	Significant amount—manufacturers advise avoid
Diphenhydramine	*see* Antihistamines
Diphenylpyraline	*see* Antihistamines
Disodium Etidronate	No information available
Disodium Pamidronate	Manufacturer advises avoid
Disopyramide	Present in milk—use only if essential and monitor infant for antimuscarinic effects
Docetaxel	*see* Cytotoxic Drugs
Domperidone	Amount probably too small to be harmful
Dosulepin (dothiepin)	*see* Antidepressants, Tricyclic
Dothiepin	*see* Antidepressants, Tricyclic
Doxazosin	Accumulates in milk—manufacturer advises avoid
Doxepin	*see* Antidepressants, Tricyclic
Doxorubicin	*see* Cytotoxic Drugs
Doxycycline	*see* Tetracyclines
Doxylamine	*see* Antihistamines
Droperidol	*see* Antipsychotics
Efavirenz	Breast-feeding not advised in HIV infection
Eformoterol	*see* Formoterol
Enalapril	Amount probably too small to be harmful
Enoxaparin	Manufacturer advises avoid—no information available
Entacapone	Manufacturer advises avoid—no information available
Ephedrine	Irritability and disturbed sleep reported
Epirubicin	*see* Cytotoxic Drugs
Epoetin	Manufacturers advise avoid—no information available
Ergocalciferol	*see* Vitamin D
Ergotamine	Avoid; ergotism may occur in infant; repeated doses may inhibit lactation
Erythromycin	Only small amounts in milk
Esmolol	*see* Beta-blockers
Etamsylate	Significant amount but not known to be harmful
Ethambutol	Amount too small to be harmful
Ethinylestradiol	*see* Contraceptives, Oral

Drug	Comment
Ethosuximide	Avoid—significant amount in milk; hyperexcitability and poor suckling reported
Etodolac	Manufacturer advises avoid
Etoposide	*see* Cytotoxic Drugs
Etynodiol	*see* Contraceptives, Oral
Famciclovir	Manufacturer advises avoid unless potential benefit outweighs risk—present in milk in *animal* studies
Famotidine	Present in milk—not known to be harmful but manufacturer advises avoid
Fansidar®	Small risk of kernicterus in jaundiced infants and of haemolysis in G6PD-deficient infants (due to sulfadoxine)
Felodipine	Appears in milk
Fenbufen	Small amount present in milk—manufacturer advises avoid
Fenofibrate	Manufacturer advises avoid
Fenoprofen	Amount too small to be harmful
Fentanyl	Manufacturer advises avoid
Fenticonazole	Manufacturer advises avoid unless essential—present in milk in *animal* studies
Fexofenadine	*see* Antihistamines
Filgrastim	No information available—manufacturer advises avoid
Flavoxate	Manufacturer advises caution—no information available
Flecainide	Significant amount but not known to be harmful
Fluconazole	Manufacturer advises avoid—present in milk
Flucytosine	Manufacturer advises avoid
Fludarabine	*see* Cytotoxic Drugs
Flunitrazepam	*see* Benzodiazepines
Fluorouracil	*see* Cytotoxic Drugs
Fluoxetine	Significant amounts in milk reported—manufacturer advises avoid
Flupentixol	*see* Antipsychotics
Fluphenazine	*see* Antipsychotics
Flurazepam	*see* Benzodiazepines
Flurbiprofen	Amount too small to be harmful
Fluticasone	*see* Corticosteroids
Fluvastatin	Manufacturer advises avoid
Fluvoxamine	Manufacturer advises avoid
Fomepizole	Manufacturer advises caution—no information available
Formoterol (eformoterol)	Manufacturers advise avoid
Fosinopril	Present in milk—manufacturer advises avoid
Fosphenytoin	*see* Phenytoin
Frusemide	*see* Furosemide
Furosemide (frusemide)	Amount too small to be harmful
Gabapentin	Present in milk—manufacturer advises avoid
Ganciclovir	Avoid; *see also* p. 295
Gemcitabine	*see* Cytotoxic Drugs
Gemfibrozil	Manufacturer advises avoid—no information available

Drug	Comment
Gestodene	see Contraceptives, Oral
Gestrinone	Manufacturer advises avoid
Glibenclamide	see Sulphonylureas
Gliclazide	see Sulphonylureas
Glimepiride	see Sulphonylureas
Glipizide	see Sulphonylureas
Gliquidone	see Sulphonylureas
Glymidine	see Sulphonylureas
Gold (auranofin, aurothiomalate)	Caution—excreted in milk; theoretical possibility of rashes and idiosyncratic reactions
Goserelin	Manufacturer advises avoid
Granisetron	Manufacturer advises avoid—no information available
Growth Hormone	see Somatropin
Haem arginate	Manufacturer advises avoid unless essential—no information available
Halofantrine	Avoid
Haloperidol	see Antipsychotics
Halothane	Excreted in milk
Hepatitis A Vaccine	No information available
Hydralazine	Present in milk but not known to be harmful; monitor infant
Hydrochloro-thiazide	see Thiazides
Hydrocortisone	see Corticosteroids
Hydroflumethiazide	see Thiazides
Hydroxycarbamide (hydroxyurea)	see Cytotoxic Drugs
Hydroxychloro-quine	Avoid—risk of toxicity in infant
Hydroxyurea	see Cytotoxic Drugs
Hydroxyzine	see Antihistamines
Hyoscine	Amount too small to be harmful
Ibuprofen	Amount too small to be harmful but some manufacturers advise avoid (including topical use)
Idarubicin	see Cytotoxic Drugs
Idoxuridine	May possibly make milk taste unpleasant
Ifosfamide	see Cytotoxic Drugs
Imidapril	Manufacturer advises avoid—no information available
Imiglucerase	No information available
Imipenem [ingredient]	see Primaxin®
Imipramine	see Antidepressants, Tricyclic
Imiquimod	Manufacturer advises use only if potential benefit outweighs risk—no information available
Indapamide	No information available—manufacturer advises avoid
Indinavir	Breast-feeding not advised in HIV infection
Indometacin	Amount probably too small to be harmful but convulsions reported in one infant—manufacturers advise avoid
Infliximab	Avoid; manufacturer advises avoid for at least 6 months after last dose
Insulin	Amount too small to be harmful
Interferons	Manufacturers advise avoid—no information available

Drug	Comment
Iodine	Stop breast-feeding; danger of neonatal hypothyroidism or goitre; appears to be concentrated in milk
Radioactive iodine	Breast-feeding contra-indicated after therapeutic doses. With diagnostic doses withhold breast-feeding for at least 24 hours
Irbesartan	Manufacturer advises avoid—no information available
Irinotecan	see Cytotoxic Drugs
Isoniazid	Monitor infant for possible toxicity; theoretical risk of convulsions and neuropathy; prophylactic pyridoxine advisable in mother and infant
Isotretinoin	Avoid
Itraconazole	Small amounts present in milk
Ketoconazole	Manufacturer advises avoid
Ketoprofen	Amount probably too small to be harmful but manufacturer advises avoid unless essential
Ketorolac	Avoid
Ketotifen	see Antihistamines
Labetalol	see Beta-blockers
Lacidipine	Manufacturer advises avoid—no information available
Lamivudine	Present in milk—Manufacturer advises avoid; breast-feeding not advised in HIV infection
Lamotrigine	Present in milk but limited data suggest no harmful effects on infants
Lanreotide	Manufacturer advises avoid—growth retardation in animal studies
Lansoprazole	Manufacturer advises avoid unless essential—present in milk in animal studies
Latanoprost	May be present in milk—manufacturer advises avoid
Leflunomide	Present in milk—manufacturer advises avoid
Lenograstim	Manufacturer advises avoid—no information available
Lepirudin	Avoid
Lercanidipine	Manufacturer advises avoid
Levocabastine	Amount too small to be harmful
Levodopa	No information available
Levofloxacin	Manufacturer advises avoid
Levomepromazine (methotrimeprazine)	see Antipsychotics
Levonorgestrel	see Contraceptives, Oral
Levothyroxine (thyroxine)	Amount too small to affect tests for neonatal hyperthyroidism
Lidocaine (lignocaine)	Amount too small to be harmful
Lignocaine	see Lidocaine
Liothyronine	May interfere with neonatal screening for hypothyroidism
Lisinopril	No information available—manufacturer advises caution
Lisuride	May suppress lactation

Drug	Comment
Lithium salts	Present in milk and risk of toxicity in infant—manufacturers advise avoid
Lofepramine	*see* Antidepressants, Tricyclic
Loperamide	Amount probably too small to be harmful
Loprazolam	*see* Benzodiazepines
Loratadine	Present in milk—manufacturer advises avoid
Lorazepam	*see* Benzodiazepines
Lormetazepam	*see* Benzodiazepines
Losartan	Manufacturer advises avoid—no information available
Lymecycline	*see* Tetracyclines
Malarone®	Manufacturer advises avoid
Maloprim®	Haemolytic anaemia (due to dapsone); risk to infant very small
Maprotiline	*see* Antidepressants, Tricyclic (and related)
Mebendazole	No information available
Mebeverine	Amount too small to be harmful
Medroxyprogesterone Acetate	*see* Progestogens
Mefenamic Acid	Amount too small to be harmful, but manufacturer advises avoid
Mefloquine	Avoid—present in milk
Mefruside	*see* Thiazides
Meloxicam	No information available—manufacturer advises avoid
Melphalan	*see* Cytotoxic Drugs
Meprobamate	Avoid; concentration in milk may exceed maternal plasma concentrations fourfold and may cause drowsiness in infant
Mequitazine	*see* Antihistamines
Mercaptamine	Manufacturer advises avoid
Mercaptopurine	*see* Cytotoxic Drugs
Meropenem	Manufacturer advises avoid unless potential benefit justifies potential risk
Mesalazine	Diarrhoea reported but manufacturers advise negligible amounts detected in breast milk
Mestranol	*see* Contraceptives, Oral
Metformin	Avoid but no information available
Methadone	Withdrawal symptoms in infant; breast-feeding permissible during maintenance but dose should be as low as possible and infant monitored to avoid sedation
Methotrexate	*see* Cytotoxic Drugs
Methotrimeprazine	*see* Antipsychotics
Methyldopa	Amount too small to be harmful
Methylphenidate	No information available—manufacturer advises avoid
Methylprednisolone	*see* Corticosteroids
Methysergide	Manufacturer advises avoid
Metoclopramide	Although amount in milk small, avoid unless essential
Metolazone	*see* Thiazides
Metoprolol	*see* Beta-blockers

Drug	Comment
Metronidazole	Significant amount in milk; manufacturer advises avoid large single doses
Mexiletine	Amount too small to be harmful
Mianserin	*see* Antidepressants, Tricyclic (and related)
Miconazole	Manufacturer advises caution—no information available
Mifepristone	No information available—manufacturer advises stop breast-feeding for 14 days after administration
Minocycline	*see* Tetracyclines
Minoxidil	Significant amount but not known to be harmful
Misoprostol	No information available—manufacturer advises avoid
Mitomycin	*see* Cytotoxic Drugs
Mitoxantrone (mitozantrone)	*see* Cytotoxic Drugs
Mitozantrone	*see* Cytotoxic Drugs
Mizolastine	*see* Antihistamines
Moclobemide	Amount too small to be harmful, but patient leaflet advises avoid
Modafinil	Manufacturer advises avoid—no information available
Moexipril	Manufacturer advises avoid—no information available
Molgramostim	Manufacturer advises avoid (potential for adverse effects in infant)—no information available
Montelukast	Manufacturer advises avoid unless essential
Moracizine	Present in milk—manufacturer advises avoid
Morphine	Therapeutic doses unlikely to affect infant; withdrawal symptoms in infants of dependent mothers; breast-feeding not best method of treating dependence in offspring and should be stopped
Moxonidine	Present in milk— manufacturer advises avoid
Mustine	*see* Cytotoxic Drugs
Mycophenolate Mofetil	No information available—manufacturer advises avoid
Nabumetone	No information available—manufacturer advises avoid
Nadolol	*see* Beta-blockers
Nafarelin	Manufacturer advises avoid—no information available
Nalidixic Acid	Risk to infant very small but one case of haemolytic anaemia reported
Naloxone	No information available
Naproxen	Amount too small to be harmful but manufacturers advise avoid
Naratriptan	Manufacturer advises caution—no information available
Nefazodone	Manufacturer advises avoid—no information available
Nelfinavir	Breast-feeding not advised in HIV infection
Neostigmine	Amount probably too small to be harmful; monitor infant

Drug	Comment
Nevirapine	Breast-feeding not advised in HIV infection
Nicardipine	Manufacturer advises avoid
Nicorandil	No information available—manufacturer advises avoid
Nicotine	Avoid—present in milk
Nicoumalone	see Anticoagulants, Oral
Nifedipine	Amount too small to be harmful but manufacturers advise avoid
Nisoldipine	Manufacturer advises avoid—no information available
Nitrazepam	see Benzodiazepines
Nitrofurantoin	Only small amounts in milk but could be enough to produce haemolysis in G6PD-deficient infants
Nizatidine	Amount too small to be harmful
Norethisterone	see Contraceptives, Oral
Norfloxacin	No information available—manufacturer advises avoid
Norgestimate	see Contraceptives, Oral
Nortriptyline	see Antidepressants, Tricyclic
NSAIDs	see individual entries
Nystatin	No information available, but absorption from gastro-intestinal tract negligible
Octreotide	Manufacturer advises avoid unless essential—no information available
Oestrogens	Avoid; adverse effects on lactation; see also Contraceptives, Oral
Ofloxacin	Manufacturer advises avoid
Olanzapine	Manufacturer advises avoid—no information available
Olsalazine	Manufacturer advises avoid
Omeprazole	Manufacturer advises avoid—no information available
Ondansetron	Manufacturer advises avoid—no information available
Opioid Analgesics	see individual entries
Orlistat	Manufacturer advises avoid—no information available
Orphenadrine	Present in milk—manufacturer advises avoid
Oxaliplatin	see Cytotoxic Drugs
Oxazepam	see Benzodiazepines
Oxitropium	No information available
Oxprenolol	see Beta-blockers
Oxybutynin	Present in milk—manufacturers advise avoid
Oxypertine	see Antipsychotics
Oxytetracycline	see Tetracyclines
Paclitaxel	see Cytotoxic Drugs
Pantoprazole	Manufacturer advises avoid unless potential benefit outweighs risk—small amount present in milk in animal studies
Papaveretum	see Morphine
Paracetamol	Amount too small to be harmful
Paraldehyde	Manufacturer advises avoid unless essential—present in milk

Drug	Comment
Paroxetine	Manufacturer advises avoid unless potential benefit outweighs possible risk
Penicillins	Trace amounts in milk
Pentamidine isetionate	Manufacturer advises avoid unless essential
Pentostatin	see Cytotoxic Drugs
Pergolide	May suppress lactation
Pericyazine	see Antipsychotics
Perindopril	Manufacturer advises avoid—no information available
Perphenazine	see Antipsychotics
Phenindione	see Anticoagulants, Oral
Pheniramine	see Antihistamines
Phenobarbital	Avoid when possible; drowsiness may occur but risk probably small; one report of methaemoglobinaemia with phenobarbital and phenytoin
Phentolamine	No information available
Phenylbutazone	Avoid—small amounts in milk
Phenytoin	Small amount present in milk; manufacturer advises avoid—but see section 4.8.1
Pilocarpine	Manufacturer advises avoid—no information available
Pimozide	see Antipsychotics
Pindolol	see Beta-blockers
Piperacillin	see Penicillins
Piracetam	Manufacturer advises avoid
Piroxicam	Amount too small to be harmful
Pizotifen	Amount probably too small to be harmful, but patient information leaflet advises avoid
Polythiazide	see Thiazides
Povidone-iodine	Avoid; iodine absorbed from vaginal preparations is concentrated in milk
Pramipexole	May suppress lactation; manufacturer advises avoid—present in milk in animal studies
Pravastatin	Small amount excreted in milk—manufacturer advises avoid
Prazosin	Amount probably too small to be harmful
Prednisolone	see Corticosteroids
Primaxin®	Manufacturer advises avoid—no information available
Primidone	see Phenobarbital
Probenecid	No information available
Procarbazine	see Cytotoxic Drugs
Prochlorperazine	see Antipsychotics
Procainamide	Present in milk—manufacturer advises avoid
Progestogens	High doses suppress lactation but see also Contraceptives, Oral
Proguanil	see Chloroquine
Promazine	see Antipsychotics
Promethazine	see Antihistamines
Propafenone	Manufacturer advises avoid—no information available
Propiverine	Manufacturer advises avoid—present in milk in animal studies

Drug	Comment
Propranolol	*see* Beta-blockers
Propylthiouracil	Monitor infant's thyroid status but amounts in milk probably too small to affect infant; high doses might affect neonatal thyroid function
Protirelin	Breast enlargement and leaking of milk reported
Protriptyline	*see* Antidepressants, Tricyclic
Pseudoephedrine	Amount too small to be harmful
Pyrazinamide	Amount too small to be harmful
Pyridostigmine	Amount probably too small to be harmful
Pyrimethamine	Significant amount—avoid administration of other folate antagonists to infant
Quetiapine	Manufacturer advises avoid—no information available
Quinagolide	Suppresses lactation
Quinapril	No information available—manufacturer advises caution
Quinidine	Significant amount but not known to be harmful
Quinupristin [ingredient]	*see Synercid®*
Rabeprazole	Manufacturer advises avoid—no information available
Raltitrexed	*see* Cytotoxic Drugs
Ramipril	Manufacturer advises avoid
Ranitidine	Significant amount but not known to be harmful
Ranitidine Bismuth Citrate	Manufacturer advises avoid—no information available
Razoxane	*see* Cytotoxic Drugs
Reboxetine	Manufacturer advises avoid—no information available
Remifentanil	Manufacturer advises caution—present in milk in *animal* studies
Repaglinide	Manufacturer advises avoid
Rifabutin	Manufacturer advises avoid—no information available
Rifampicin	Amount too small to be harmful
Riluzole	Manufacturer advises avoid—no information available
Risperidone	Manufacturer advises avoid—no information available
Ritonavir	Breast-feeding not advised in HIV infection
Rituximab	Avoid
Rivastigmine	Manufacturer advises avoid—no information available
Rizatriptan	Present in milk in *animal* studies—withhold breast-feeding for 24 hours
Rofecoxib	Manufacturer advises avoid—present in milk in *animal* studies
Salcatonin	*see* Calcitonin (salmon)
Saquinavir	Breast-feeding not advised in HIV infection
Secobarbital	*see* Barbiturates
Senna	*see* Anthraquinones
Sertindole	Manufacturer advises avoid—no information available
Sertraline	Not known to be harmful in short-term use—insufficient data on long-term use

Drug	Comment
Simvastatin	Manufacturer advises avoid—no information available
Sodium Clodronate	No information available
Sodium Cromoglicate	*see* Cromoglicate
Sodium Valproate	*see* Valproate
Somatropin	No information available
Sotalol	*see* Beta-blockers
Stavudine	Breast-feeding not advised in HIV infection
Sulfadiazine	*see* Sulphonamides
Sulfametopyrazine	*see* Sulphonamides
Sulfasalazine	Small amounts in milk (1 report of bloody diarrhoea and rashes); theoretical risk of neonatal haemolysis especially in G6PD-deficient infants
Sulfinpyrazone	No information available
Sulindac	No information available
Sulphonamides	Small risk of kernicterus in jaundiced infants particularly with long-acting sulphonamides, and of haemolysis in G6PD-deficient infants
Sulphonylureas	Theoretical possibility of hypoglycaemia in infant
Sulpiride	Best avoided; significant amounts in milk; *see also* Antipsychotics
Sumatriptan	Present in milk after subcutaneous injection—withhold breast-feeding for 24 hours
Synercid®	Manufacturer advises avoid—no information available
Tacrolimus	Avoid—present in milk
Tamoxifen	Manufacturer advises avoid—no information available
Tazarotene	Manufacturer advises avoid
Teicoplanin	No information available
Telmisartan	Manufacturer advises avoid—no information available
Temazepam	*see* Benzodiazepines
Temozolamide	*see* Cytotoxic Drugs
Tenoxicam	No information available
Terazosin	No information available
Terbinafine	*see* Vasopressin
Terbutaline	Amount too small to be harmful
Terfenadine	*see* Antihistamines
Terlipressin	Not known to be harmful
Tetrabenazine	Manufacturer advises avoid
Tetracaine (amethocaine)	No information available
Tetracyclines	Avoid (although absorption and therefore discoloration of teeth in infant probably usually prevented by chelation with calcium in milk)
Theophylline	Irritability in infant reported; modified-release preparations probably safe
Thiamine	Severely thiamine-deficient mothers should avoid breast-feeding as toxic methylglyoxal excreted in milk

Drug	Comment
Thiazides	Amount too small to be harmful; large doses may suppress lactation
Thioridazine	*see* Antipsychotics
Thiotepa	*see* Cytotoxic Drugs
Thyroxine	*see* Levothyroxine
Tiagabine	Manufacturer advises avoid unless potential benefit outweighs risk
Tiaprofenic Acid	Amount too small to be harmful
Ticlopidine	Manufacturer advises avoid unless essential—present in milk in *animal* studies
Tiludronic Acid	Manufacturer advises avoid—no information available
Timolol	*see* Beta-blockers
Tinidazole	Present in milk—manufacturer advises avoid breast-feeding during and for 3 days after stopping treatment
Tinzaparin	Manufacturer advises avoid—no information available
Tioguanine	*see* Cytotoxic Drugs
Tirofiban	Manufacturer advises avoid—no information available
Tizanidine	Manufacturer advises use only if potential benefit outweighs risk—no information available
Tocainde	No information available
Tolazamide	*see* Sulphonylureas
Tolbutamide	*see* Sulphonylureas
Tolfenamic Acid	Amount too small to be harmful
Tolteridine	Manufacturer advises avoid—no information available
Topiramate	Manufacturer advises avoid
Topotecan	*see* Cytotoxic Drugs
Torasemide	No information available
Tramadol	Amount probably too small to be harmful, but manufacturer advises avoid
Trandolapril	Manufacturers advise avoid
Tranexamic acid	Small amount present in milk—antifibrinolytic effect in infant unlikely
Trazodone	as for Antidepressants, Tricyclic
Treosulfan	*see* Cytotoxic Drugs
Tretinoin	Avoid
Triamcinolone	*see* Corticosteroids
Tribavirin	Avoid—no information available
Trifluoperazine	*see* Antipsychotics
Trimeprazine	*see* Antihistamines
Trimethoprim	Present in milk—short-term use not known to be harmful
Trimetrexate	Manufacturer advises termination of breast-feeding; also breast-feeding not advised in HIV infection
Trimipramine	*see* Antidepressants, Tricyclic
Triprolidine	*see* Antihistamines
Tropisetron	No information available
Tulobuterol	No information available

Drug	Comment
Ursodeoxycholic acid	Not known to be harmful but manufacturer advises avoid
Valaciclovir	No information available; *see also* Aciclovir
Valproate	Amount too small to be harmful
Valsartan	Manufacturer advises avoid—no information available
Vancomycin	Present in milk—manufacturer advises avoid
Vasopressin	Not known to be harmful
Venlafaxine	Manufacturer advises avoid—no information available
Verapamil	Amount too small to be harmful
Vigabatrin	Present in milk—manufacturer advises avoid
Viloxazine	*see* Antidepressants, Tricyclic (and related)
Vinblastine	*see* Cytotoxic Drugs
Vincristine	*see* Cytotoxic Drugs
Vindesine	*see* Cytotoxic Drugs
Vinorelbine	*see* Cytotoxic Drugs
Vitamin A	Theoretical risk of toxicity in infants of mothers taking large doses
Vitamin D (and related compounds)	Caution with high doses; may cause hypercalcaemia in infant
Warfarin	*see* Anticoagulants, Oral
Xipamide	No information available
Zafirlukast	Present in milk—manufacturer advises avoid
Zalcitabine	Breast-feeding not advised in HIV infection
Zanamavir	Manufacturer advises avoid—no information available
Zidovudine	Breast-feeding not advised in HIV infection
Zolmitriptan	No information available—manufacturer advises caution
Zolpidem	Small amounts present in milk—manufacturer advises avoid
Zopiclone	Present in milk—manufacturer advises avoid
Zuclopenthixol	*see* Antipsychotics

Appendix 6: Intravenous Additives

INTRAVENOUS ADDITIVES POLICIES. A local policy on the addition of drugs to intravenous fluids should be drawn up by a multi-disciplinary team in each Health Authority and issued as a document to the members of staff concerned.

Centralised additive services are provided in a number of hospital pharmacy departments and should be used in preference to making additions on wards.

The information that follows should be read in conjunction with local policy documents.

Guidelines

1. Drugs should only be added to infusion containers when constant plasma concentrations are needed or when the administration of a more concentrated solution would be harmful.
2. In general, only one drug should be added to any infusion container and the components should be compatible. Ready-prepared solutions should be used whenever possible. Drugs should not normally be added to blood products, mannitol, or sodium bicarbonate. Only specially formulated additives should be used with fat emulsions or amino-acid solutions (section 9.3).
3. Solutions should be thoroughly mixed by shaking and checked for absence of particulate matter before use.
4. Strict asepsis should be maintained throughout and in general the giving set should not be used for more than 24 hours (for drug admixtures).
5. The infusion container should be labelled with the patient's name, the name and quantity of additives, and the date and time of addition (and the new expiry date or time). Such additional labelling should not interfere with information on the manufacturer's label that is still valid. When possible, containers should be retained for a period after use in case they are needed for investigation.
6. It is good practice to examine intravenous infusions from time to time while they are running. If cloudiness, crystallisation, change of colour, or any other sign of interaction or contamination is observed the infusion should be discontinued.

Problems

MICROBIAL CONTAMINATION. The accidental entry and subsequent growth of micro-organisms converts the infusion fluid pathway into a potential vehicle for infection with micro-organisms, particularly species of Candida, Enterobacter, and Klebsiella. Ready-prepared infusions containing the additional drugs, or infusions prepared by an additive service (when available) should therefore be used in preference to making extemporaneous additions to infusion containers on wards etc. However, when this is necessary strict aseptic procedure should be followed.

INCOMPATIBILITY. Physical and chemical incompatibilities may occur with loss of potency, increase in toxicity, or other adverse effect. The solutions may become opalescent or precipitation may occur, but in many instances there is no visual indication of incompatibility. Interaction may take place at any point in the infusion fluid pathway, and the potential for incompatibility is increased when more than one substance is added to the infusion fluid.

Common incompatibilities. Precipitation reactions are numerous and varied and may occur as a result of pH, concentration changes, 'salting-out' effects, complexation or other chemical changes. Precipitation or other particle formation must be avoided since, apart from lack of control of dosage on administration, it may initiate or exacerbate adverse effects. This is particularly important in the case of drugs which have been implicated in either thrombophlebitis (e.g. diazepam) or in skin sloughing or necrosis caused by extravasation (e.g. sodium bicarbonate and certain cytotoxic drugs). It is also especially important to effect solution of colloidal drugs and to prevent their subsequent precipitation in order to avoid a pyrogenic reaction (e.g. amphotericin).

It is considered undesirable to mix beta-lactam antibiotics, such as semi-synthetic penicillins and cephalosporins, with proteinaceous materials on the grounds that immunogenic and allergenic conjugates could be formed.

A number of preparations undergo significant loss of potency when added singly or in combination to large volume infusions. Examples include ampicillin in infusions that contain glucose or lactates, chlormethine hydrochloride (mustine hydrochloride) in isotonic saline and gentamicin/carbenicillin combinations. The breakdown products of dacarbazine have been implicated in adverse effects.

Blood. Because of the large number of incompatibilities, drugs should not normally be added to blood and blood products for infusion purposes. Examples of incompatibility with blood include hypertonic mannitol solutions (irreversible crenation of red cells), dextrans (rouleaux formation and interference with cross-matching), glucose (clumping of red cells), and oxytocin (inactivated).

If the giving set is not changed after the administration of blood, but used for other infusion fluids, a fibrin clot may form which, apart from blocking the set, increases the likelihood of microbial growth.

Intravenous fat emulsions may break down with coalescence of fat globules and separation of phases when additions such as antibiotics or electrolytes are made, thus increasing the possibility of embolism. Only specially formulated products such as *Vitlipid N®* (section 9.3) may be added to appropriate intravenous fat emulsions.

Other infusions that frequently give rise to incompatibility include amino acids, mannitol, and sodium bicarbonate.

Bactericides such as chlorocresol 0.1% or phenylmercuric nitrate 0.001% are present in some injection solutions. The total volume of such solutions added to a container for infusion on one occasion should not exceed 15 mL.

Method

Ready-prepared infusions should be used whenever available. **Potassium chloride** is usually available in concentrations of 20, 27, and 40 mmol/litre in sodium chloride intravenous infusion (0.9%), glucose intravenous infusion (5%) or sodium chloride and glucose intravenous infusion. **Lidocaine hydrochloride (lignocaine hydrochloride)** is usually available in concentrations of 0.1 or 0.2% in glucose intravenous infusion (5%).

When addition is required to be made extemporaneously, any product reconstitution instructions such as those relating to concentration, vehicle, mixing, and handling precautions should be strictly followed using an aseptic technique throughout. Once the product has been reconstituted, addition to the infusion fluid should be made immediately in order to minimise microbial contamination and, with certain products, to prevent degradation or other formulation change which may occur; e.g. reconstituted ampicillin injection degrades rapidly on standing, and also may form polymers which could cause sensitivity reactions.

It is also important in certain instances that an infusion fluid of specific pH be used (e.g. **furosemide (frusemide)** injection requires dilution in infusions of pH greater than 5.5).

When drug additions are made it is important to mix thoroughly; additions should not be made to an infusion container that has been connected to a giving set, as mixing is hampered. If the solutions are not thoroughly mixed a concentrated layer of the additive may form owing to differences in density. **Potassium chloride** is particularly prone to this 'layering' effect when added without adequate mixing to infusions packed in non-rigid infusion containers; if such a mixture is administered it may have a serious effect on the heart.

A time limit between addition and completion of administration must be imposed for certain admixtures to guarantee satisfactory drug potency and compatibility. For admixtures in which degradation occurs without the formation of toxic substances, an acceptable limit is the time taken for 10% decomposition of the drug. When toxic substances are produced stricter limits may be imposed. Because of the risk of microbial contamination a maximum time limit of 12 hours should be imposed for additions made elsewhere than in hospital pharmacies offering central additive service.

Certain injections must be protected from light during continuous infusion to minimise oxidation, e.g. amphotericin, dacarbazine, and sodium nitroprusside.

Dilution with a small volume of an appropriate vehicle and administration using a motorised infusion pump is advocated for preparations such as heparin where strict control over administration is required. In this case the appropriate dose may be dissolved in a convenient volume (e.g. 24 to 48 mL) of sodium chloride intravenous infusion (0.9%).

Use of table

The table lists preparations given by three methods:
  continuous infusion,
  intermittent infusion, and
  addition via the drip tubing.

Drugs for **continuous infusion** must be diluted in a large volume infusion. Penicillins and cephalosporins are not usually given by continuous infusion because of stability problems and because adequate plasma and tissue concentrations are best obtained by intermittent infusion. Where it is necessary to administer them by continuous infusion, detailed literature should be consulted.

Drugs that are both compatible and clinically suitable may be given by **intermittent infusion** in a relatively small volume of infusion over a short period of time, e.g. 100 mL in 30 minutes. The method is used if the product is incompatible or unstable over the period necessary for continuous infusion; the limited stability of ampicillin or amoxicillin in large volume glucose or lactate infusions may be overcome in this way.

Intermittent infusion is also used if adequate plasma and tissue concentrations are not produced by continuous infusion as in the case of drugs such as carbenicillin, dacarbazine, gentamicin, and ticarcillin.

An in-line burette may be used for intermittent infusion techniques in order to achieve strict control over the time and rate of administration, especially for infants and children and in intensive care units. Intermittent infusion may also make use of the 'piggy-back' technique provided that no additions are made to the primary infusion. In this method the drug is added to a small secondary container connected to a Y-type injection site on the primary infusion giving set; the secondary solution is usually infused within 30 minutes.

Addition *via* the drip tubing is indicated for a number of cytotoxic drugs in order to minimise extravasation. The preparation is added aseptically *via* the rubber septum of the injection site of a fast-running infusion. In general, drug preparations intended for a bolus effect should be given directly into a separate vein where possible. Failing this, administration may be made *via* the drip tubing provided that the preparation is compatible with the infusion fluid when given in this manner.

Table of drugs given by intravenous infusion

Covers addition to *Glucose intravenous infusion* 5 and 10%, *Sodium chloride intravenous infusion* 0.9%, *Compound sodium chloride intravenous infusion* (Ringer's solution), and *Compound sodium lactate intravenous infusion* (Hartmann's solution). Compatibility with glucose 5% and with sodium chloride 0.9% indicates compatibility with *Sodium chloride and glucose intravenous infusion*. Infusion of a large volume of hypotonic solution should be avoided therefore care should be taken if water for injections is used. The information in the Table relates to the proprietary preparations indicated; for other preparations suitability should be checked with the manufacturer

Abciximab (*ReoPro®*)
Continuous *in* Glucose 5% *or* Sodium chloride 0.9%
Withdraw from vial, dilute in infusion fluid and give *via* infusion pump through a non-pyrogenic low protein-binding 0.2 or 0.22 micron filter

Acetylcysteine (*Parvolex®*)
Continuous *in* Glucose 5%
See Emergency Treatment of Poisoning

Aciclovir (as sodium salt) (*Zovirax IV®*; *Aciclovir IV*, Faulding DBL; *Aciclovir Sodium*, Zurich)
Intermittent *in* Sodium chloride 0.9% *or* Sodium chloride and glucose *or* Compound sodium lactate
For *Zovirax IV®* and *Aciclovir Sodium* (Zurich) initially reconstitute to 25 mg/mL in water for injections or sodium chloride 0.9% then dilute to not more than 5 mg/mL with the infusion fluid; to be given over 1 hour; alternatively, may be administered in a concentration of 25 mg/mL using a suitable infusion pump and given over 1 hour; for *Aciclovir IV* (Faulding DBL) dilute to not more than 5 mg/mL with infusion fluid; give over 1 hour

Aclarubicin (as hydrochloride) (*Aclacin®*)
Intermittent *in* Glucose 5% *or* Sodium chloride 0.9%
Dissolve initially in 10 mL water for injections or sodium chloride 0.9% then dilute with 200–500 mL infusion fluid to a concentration of 200–500 micrograms/mL; give over 30–60 minutes and protect from light during administration; pH of glucose infusion should be between 5 and 6

Alfentanil (as hydrochloride) (*Rapifen® preparations*)
Continuous *or* intermittent *in* Glucose 5% *or* Sodium chloride 0.9% *or* Compound sodium lactate

Alprostadil (*Prostin VR®*)
Continuous *in* Glucose 5% *or* Sodium chloride 0.9%
Add directly to the infusion solution avoiding contact with the walls of plastic containers

Alteplase (*Actilyse®*)
Continuous *or* intermittent *in* Sodium chloride 0.9%
Dissolve in water for injections to a concentration of 1 mg/mL and infuse intravenously; alternatively dilute the solution further in the infusion fluid to a concentration of not less than 200 micrograms/mL; not to be infused in glucose solution

Amifostine (*Ethyol®*)
Intermittent *in* Sodium chloride 0.9%

Amikacin sulphate (*Amikin®*)
Intermittent *in* Glucose 5% *or* Sodium chloride 0.9% *or* Compound sodium lactate
To be given over 30 minutes

Aminophylline
Continuous *in* Glucose 5% *or* Sodium chloride 0.9% *or* Compound sodium lactate

Amiodarone hydrochloride (*Cordarone X®*)
Continuous *or* intermittent *in* Glucose 5%
Suggested initial infusion volume 250 mL given over 20–120 minutes; for repeat infusions up to 1.2 g in max. 500 mL; infusion in extreme emergency see section 2.3.2; should not be diluted to less than 600 micrograms/mL; incompatible with sodium chloride infusion

Amoxicillin (as sodium salt) (*Amoxil®*)
Intermittent *in* Glucose 5% *or* Sodium chloride 0.9%
Reconstituted solutions diluted and given without delay; suggested volume 100 mL given over 30–60 minutes
via drip tubing *in* Glucose 5% *or* Sodium chloride 0.9% *or* Ringer's solution *or* Compound sodium lactate
Continuous infusion not usually recommended

Amphotericin (colloidal) (*Amphocil®*)
Intermittent *in* Glucose 5%
Initially reconstitute with water for injections (50 mg in 10 mL, 100 mg in 20 mL), shaking gently to dissolve (fluid may be opalescent) then dilute to a concentration of 625 micrograms/mL (1 volume of reconstituted solution with 7 volumes of infusion fluid); give at a rate of 1–2 mg/kg/hour or slower if not tolerated (initial test dose 2 mg of a 100 microgram/mL solution over 10 minutes); incompatible with sodium chloride or other electrolyte solutions, flush existing intravenous line with glucose 5% or use separate line

Amphotericin (lipid complex) (*Abelcet®*)
Intermittent *in* Glucose 5%
Allow suspension to reach room temperature, shake gently to ensure no yellow settlement, withdraw requisite dose (using 17–19 gauge needle) into one or more 20-mL syringes; replace needle on syringe with a 5-micron filter needle provided (fresh needle for each syringe) and dilute to a concentration of 1 mg/mL (2 mg/mL in fluid restriction); preferably give *via* an infusion pump at a rate of 2.5 mg/kg/hour (initial test dose of 1 mg given over 15 minutes); an in-line filter (pore size no less than 15 micron) may be used; do not use sodium chloride or other electrolyte solutions, flush existing intravenous line with glucose 5% or use separate line

Amphotericin (liposomal) (*AmBisome®*)
Intermittent *in* Glucose 5%
Reconstitute each vial with 12 mL water for injections and shake vigorously to produce a preparation containing 4 mg/mL; withdraw requisite dose from vial and introduce into infusion fluid through the 5 micron filter provided to produce a final concentration of 0.2–2 mg/mL; infuse over 30–60 minutes (initial test dose 1 mg over 10 minutes); incompatible with sodium chloride solutions, flush existing intravenous line with glucose 5% or use separate line

Amphotericin (as sodium deoxycholate complex) (*Fungizone®*)
Intermittent *in* Glucose 5%
Reconstitute each vial with 10 mL water for injections and shake immediately to produce a 5 mg/mL colloidal solution; dilute further in infusion fluid to a concentration of 100 micrograms/mL; pH of the glucose must not be below 4.2 (check each container—see product literature for details of buffer); infuse over 2–4 hours, or longer if not tolerated (initial test dose 1 mg over 20–30

minutes); begin infusion immediately after dilution and protect from light; incompatible with sodium chloride solutions, flush existing intravenous line with glucose 5% or use separate line

Ampicillin sodium (*Penbritin®*)
Intermittent *in* Glucose 5% *or* Sodium chloride 0.9%
Reconstituted solutions diluted and given without delay; suggested volume 100 mL given over 30–60 minutes *via* drip tubing *in* Glucose 5% *or* Sodium chloride 0.9% *or* Ringer's solution *or* Compound sodium lactate
Continuous infusion not usually recommended

Amsacrine (*Amsidine®*)
Intermittent in Glucose 5%
Reconstitute with diluent provided and dilute to suggested volume 500 mL; give over 60–90 minutes; use glass syringes; incompatible with sodium chloride infusion

Atenolol (*Tenormin®*)
Intermittent *in* Glucose 5% *or* Sodium chloride 0.9%
Suggested infusion time 20 minutes

Atracurium besilate (*Tracrium®*)
Continuous *in* Glucose 5% *or* Sodium chloride 0.9% *or* Compound sodium lactate
Stability varies with diluent

Azathioprine (as sodium salt) (*Imuran®*)
Intermittent *in* Sodium chloride 0.9% *or* Sodium chloride and glucose
Reconstitute 50 mg with 5–15 mL water for injections; dilute with 20–200 mL infusion fluid

Azlocillin (as sodium salt) (*Securopen® 5 g*)
Intermittent *in* Glucose 5 and 10% *or* Sodium chloride 0.9% *or* Ringer's solution
Intermittent infusion suggested for doses over 2 g; to be given over 20–30 minutes

Aztreonam (*Azactam®*)
Intermittent *in* Glucose 5% *or* Sodium chloride 0.9% *or* Ringer's solution *or* Compound sodium lactate
Dissolve initially in water for injections (1 g per 3 mL) then dilute to a concentration of less than 20 mg/mL; to be given over 20–60 minutes

Basiliximab (*Simulect®*)
Intermittent *in* Glucose 5% *or* Sodium chloride 0.9%
Reconstitute with water for injections then dilute to at least 50 mL with infusion fluid and give over 20–30 minutes

Benzylpenicillin sodium (*Crystapen®*)
Intermittent *in* Glucose 5% *or* Sodium chloride 0.9%
Suggested volume 100 mL given over 30–60 minutes
Continuous infusion not usually recommended

Betamethasone (as sodium phosphate) (*Betnesol®*)
Continuous *or* intermittent *or via* drip tubing *in* Glucose 5% *or* Sodium chloride 0.9%

Bleomycin sulphate Intermittent *in* Sodium chloride 0.9%
To be given slowly; suggested volume 200 mL

Bumetanide (*Burinex®*)
Intermittent *in* Glucose 5% *or* Sodium chloride 0.9%
Suggested volume 500 mL given over 30–60 minutes

Calcitonin (salmon)/Salcatonin (*Forcaltonin®*, *Miacalcic®*)
Intermittent *in* Sodium chloride 0.9%
Diluted solution given without delay; dilute in 500 mL and give over at least 6 hours; glass or hard plastic containers should not be used; approx. 20% loss of potency on dilution (take into account when calculating dose)

Calcium folinate (*Calcium Leucovorin®*, *Refolinon®*)
Continuous *in* Sodium chloride 0.9%
Calcium Leucovorin® can also be infused in Glucose 5 and 10% or Compound sodium lactate

Calcium gluconate
Continuous *in* Glucose 5% *or* Sodium chloride 0.9%
Avoid bicarbonates, phosphates, or sulphates

Calcium levofolinate (*Isovorin®*)
Intermittent *in* Glucose 5 and 10% *or* Sodium chloride 0.9% *or* Compound sodium lactate
Protect from light

Carboplatin (*Paraplatin®*)
Intermittent *in* Glucose 5% *or* Sodium chloride 0.9%
Final concentration as low as 500 micrograms/mL; give over 15–60 minutes

Carmustine (*BiCNU®*)
Intermittent *in* Glucose 5% *or* Sodium chloride 0.9%
Reconstitute with diluent provided; give over 1–2 hours

Cefamandole (as nafate) (*Kefadol®*)
Intermittent *or via* drip tubing *in* Glucose 5 and 10% *or* Sodium chloride 0.9%
Continuous infusion not usually recommended

Cefazolin (as sodium salt) (*Kefzol®*)
Intermittent *or via* drip tubing *in* Glucose 5 and 10% *or* Sodium chloride 0.9% *or* Compound sodium lactate
Reconstitute initially with water for injections; dilute to 50–100 mL with infusion fluid

Cefodizime sodium (*Timecef®*)
Intermittent *in* Glucose 5% *or* Sodium chloride 0.9% *or* Ringer's solution *or* Compound sodium lactate *or* Water for injections
Dissolve in 40 mL infusion fluid and give over up to 30 minutes

Cefotaxime (as sodium salt) (*Claforan®*)
Intermittent *in* Glucose 5% *or* Sodium chloride 0.9% *or* Compound sodium lactate *or* Water for injections
Suggested volume 40–100 mL given over 20–60 minutes

Cefoxitin (as sodium salt) (*Mefoxin®*)
Intermittent *or via* drip tubing in Glucose 5 and 10% *or* Sodium chloride 0.9%
Continuous infusion not usually recommended

Cefradine (*Velosef®*)
Continuous *or* intermittent *in* Glucose 5 and 10% *or* Sodium chloride 0.9% *or* Ringer's solution *or* Compound sodium lactate

Ceftazidime (as pentahydrate) (*Fortum®, Kefadim®*)
Intermittent *or via* drip tubing *in* Glucose 5 and 10% *or* Sodium chloride 0.9% *or* Compound sodium lactate
Dissolve 2 g initially in 10 mL (3 g in 15 mL) infusion fluid; for *Fortum®* dilute further to a concentration of 40 mg/mL; for *Kefadim®* dilute further to a concentration of 20 mg/mL; give over up to 30 minutes

Ceftriaxone (as sodium salt) (*Rocephin®*)
Intermittent *or via* drip tubing *in* Glucose 5 and 10% *or* Sodium chloride 0.9%
Reconstitute 2-g vial with 40 mL infusion fluid; give intermittent infusion over at least 30 minutes (60 minutes in neonates); not to be given with infusion fluids containing calcium

Cefuroxime (as sodium salt) (*Zinacef®*)
Intermittent *or via* drip tubing *in* Glucose 5% *or* Sodium chloride 0.9% *or* Compound sodium lactate
Dissolve initially in water for injections (at least 2 mL for each 250 mg, 15 mL for 1.5 g); suggested volume 50–100 mL given over 30 minutes

Chloramphenicol (as sodium succinate) (*Kemicetine®*)
Intermittent *or via* drip tubing *in* Glucose 5% *or* Sodium chloride 0.9%

Chlormethine hydrochloride/Mustine hydrochloride (Knoll)
via drip tubing *in* Glucose 5% *or* Sodium chloride 0.9%

Chloroquine sulphate (*Nivaquine®*)
Continuous *in* Sodium chloride 0.9%
See also section 5.4.1

Ciclosporin (*Sandimmun®*)
Continuous *in* Glucose 5% *or* Sodium chloride 0.9%
Dilute to a concentration of 50 mg in 20–100 mL; give over 2–6 hours; not to be used with PVC equipment

Cidofovir (*Vistide®*)
Intermittent *in* Sodium chloride 0.9%
Dilute requisite dose with 100 mL infusion fluid; infuse over 1 hour

Cimetidine (*Tagamet®*)
Continuous *or* intermittent *in* Glucose 5% *or* Sodium chloride 0.9%
For intermittent infusion suggested volume 100 mL given over 30–60 minutes

Cisatracurium (*Nimbex®, Nimbex Forte®*)
Continuous *in* Glucose 5% *or* Sodium chloride 0.9%
Solutions of 2 mg/mL and 5 mg/mL may be infused undiluted; alternatively dilute with infusion fluid to a concentration of 0.1–2 mg/mL

Cisplatin (*Cisplatin*, Lederle; *Cisplatin powder for injection*, Lederle)
Continuous *in* Sodium chloride 0.9% *or* Sodium chloride and glucose
Reconstitute cisplatin powder for injection with water for injections (10 mg in 10 mL, 50 mg in 50 mL); suggested volume 2 litres given over 6–8 hours

Cladribine (*Leustat®*)
Continuous *in* Sodium chloride 0.9%
Dilute with 100–500 mL; glucose solutions are unsuitable

Clarithromycin (*Klaricid® I.V.*)
Intermittent *in* Glucose 5% *or* Sodium chloride 0.9% *or* Ringer's solution *or* Compound sodium lactate
Dissolve initially in water for injections (500 mg in 10 mL) then dilute to a concentration of 2 mg/mL; give over 60 minutes

Clindamycin (as phosphate) (*Dalacin® C Phosphate*)
Continuous *or* intermittent *in* Glucose 5% *or* Sodium chloride 0.9%
Give over at least 10–60 minutes (1.2 g over at least 60 minutes; higher doses by continuous infusion)

Clomipramine hydrochloride (*Anafranil®*)
Intermittent *in* Glucose 5% *or* Sodium chloride 0.9%
See product literature for details of initial dose to test tolerance; suggested volume 125–500 mL given over 45–180 minutes

Clonazepam (*Rivotril®*)
Intermittent *in* Glucose 5 and 10% *or* Sodium chloride 0.9%
Suggested volume 250 mL

Co-amoxiclav (*Augmentin®*)
Intermittent *in* Sodium chloride 0.9% *or* Water for injections; see also package leaflet
Suggested volume 50–100 mL given over 30–40 minutes and completed within 4 hours of reconstitution
via drip tubing *in* Glucose 5% *or* Sodium chloride 0.9%

Co-fluampicil (as sodium salts) (*Magnapen®*)
Intermittent *in* Glucose 5% *or* Sodium chloride 0.9%
Reconstituted solutions diluted and given without delay; suggested volume 100 mL given over 30–60 minutes
via drip tubing *in* Glucose 5% *or* Sodium chloride 0.9% *or* Ringer's solution *or* Compound sodium lactate

Colistimethate sodium (*Colomycin®*)
Continuous *or* intermittent *in* Glucose 5% *or* Sodium chloride 0.9% *or* Ringer's solution
Max. 6 hours between addition and completion of administration

Co-trimoxazole (*Septrin® for infusion*)
Intermittent *in* Glucose 5 and 10% *or* Sodium chloride 0.9% *or* Ringer's solution
Dilute contents of 1 ampoule (5 mL) to 125 mL, 2 ampoules (10 mL) to 250 mL or 3 ampoules (15 mL) to 500 mL; suggested duration of infusion 90 minutes (but may be adjusted according to fluid requirements); if fluid restriction necessary, 1 ampoule may be diluted with 75 mL glucose 5%

Cyclophosphamide (*Endoxana®*)
Intermittent *or via* drip tubing *in* Glucose 5% *or* Sodium chloride 0.9% *or* Water for injections
For intermittent infusion suggested volume 50–100 mL given over 5–15 minutes
via drip tubing in Glucose 5%

Cytarabine (*Cytosar®*)
Continuous *or* intermittent *or via* drip tubing *in* Glucose 5% *or* Sodium chloride 0.9%
Reconstitute *Cytosar®* with water for injections or with infusion fluid; check container for haze or precipitate during administration

Dacarbazine (*DTIC-Dome®*; *Dacarbazine*, Medac)

Intermittent *in* Glucose 5% *or* Sodium chloride 0.9%

Reconstitute initially with water for injections then for *DTIC-Dome®* dilute in 125–250 mL infusion fluid; for *Dacarbazine* (Medac) dilute in 200–300 mL infusion fluid; give over 15–30 minutes; protect infusion from light

Daclizumab (*Zenapax®*)

Intermittent *in* Sodium chloride 0.9%

Dilute requisite dose in 50 mL infusion fluid; infuse over 15 minutes

Dactinomycin (*Cosmegen Lyovac®*)

Intermittent *or via* drip tubing *in* Glucose 5% *or* Sodium chloride 0.9%

Reconstitute with water for injections

Danaparoid sodium (*Orgaran®*)

Continuous *in* Glucose 5% *or* Sodium chloride 0.9%

Daunorubicin (as hydrochloride) (*Cerubidin®*)

via drip tubing *in* Sodium chloride 0.9%

Reconstitute vial with 4 mL water for injections to give 5 mg/mL solution; dilute requisite dose with infusion fluid to a concentration of 1 mg/mL; give over 20 minutes

Daunorubicin (liposomal) (*DaunoXome®*)

Intermittent *in* Glucose 5%

Dilute to a concentration of 0.2–1 mg/mL; give over 30–60 minutes; incompatible with sodium chloride solutions; in-line filter not recommended (if used, pore size should be no less than 5 micron)

Desferrioxamine mesilate (*Desferal®*)

Continuous *or* intermittent *in* Glucose 5% *or* Sodium chloride 0.9%

Dissolve initially in water for injections (500 mg in 5 mL) then dilute with infusion fluid

Desmopressin (*DDAVP®*)

Intermittent *in* Sodium chloride 0.9%

Dilute with 50 mL and give over 20 minutes

Dexamethasone sodium phosphate (*Decadron®*; *Dexamethasone*, Organon)

Continuous *or* intermittent *or via* drip tubing *in* Glucose 5% *or* Sodium chloride 0.9%

Dexamethasone (Organon) can also be infused in Ringer's solution *or* Compound sodium lactate

Diamorphine hydrochloride (*Diamorphine Injection*, CP)

Continuous *in* Glucose 5% *or* Sodium chloride 0.9%

Glucose is preferred as infusion fluid

Diazepam (solution) (*Valium®*)

Continuous *in* Glucose 5% *or* Sodium chloride 0.9%

Dilute to a concentration of not more than 40 mg in 500 mL; max. 6 hours between addition and completion of administration; adsorbed to some extent by the plastics of the infusion set

Diazepam (emulsion) (*Diazemuls®*)

Continuous *in* Glucose 5 and 10%

May be diluted to a max. concentration of 200 mg in 500 mL; max. 6 hours between addition and completion of administration; adsorbed to some extent by the plastics of the infusion set

via drip tubing *in* Glucose 5 and 10% *or* Sodium chloride 0.9%

Adsorbed to some extent by the plastics of the infusion set

Diclofenac sodium (*Voltarol®*)

Continuous *or* intermittent *in* Glucose 5% *or* Sodium chloride 0.9%

Dilute 75 mg with 100–500 mL infusion fluid (previously buffered with 0.5 mL sodium bicarbonate 8.4% solution *or* with 1 mL sodium bicarbonate 4.2% solution); for intermittent infusion give 25–50 mg over 15–60 minutes or 75 mg over 30–120 minutes; for continuous infusion give at a rate of 5 mg/hour

Digoxin (*Lanoxin®*)

Continuous *in* Glucose 5% *or* Sodium chloride 0.9%

To be given slowly; see also section 2.1.1

Digoxin-specific antibody fragments (*Digibind®*)

Intermittent *in* Sodium chloride 0.9%

Dissolve initially in water for injections (4 mL/vial) then dilute with the sodium chloride 0.9% and give through a 0.22 micron sterile, disposable filter over 30 minutes

Dinoprostone (*Prostin E2®*)

Continuous *or* intermittent *in* Glucose 5% *or* Sodium chloride 0.9%

Disodium pamidronate (*Aredia®*)

Continuous *in* Sodium chloride 0.9%

Reconstitute initially with water for injections (15 mg in 5 mL, 30 mg or 90 mg in 10 mL); dilute with infusion fluid to a concentration of not more than 60 mg in 250 mL; give at a rate not exceeding 1 mg/minute; not to be given with infusion fluids containing calcium

Disopyramide (as phosphate) (*Rythmodan®*)

Continuous *or* intermittent *in* Glucose 5% *or* Sodium chloride 0.9% *or* Ringer's solution *or* Compound sodium lactate

Max. rate by continuous infusion 20–30 mg/hour (or 400 micrograms/kg/hour)

Dobutamine (as hydrochloride) (*Dobutrex®*, *Posiject®*)

Continuous *in* Glucose 5% *or* Sodium chloride 0.9%

Dilute to a concentration of 0.5–1 mg/mL and give *via* a controlled infusion device; give higher concentration (max. 5 mg/mL) with infusion pump; incompatible with bicarbonate

Docetaxel (*Taxotere®*)

Intermittent *in* Glucose 5% *or* Sodium chloride 0.9%

Stand docetaxel vials and solvent at room temperature for 5 minutes; add solvent to produce a concentrate containing 10 mg/mL and allow to stand for a further 5 minutes at room temperature; dilute the requisite dose with at least 250 mL infusion fluid to a final concentration not exceeding 740 micrograms/mL; infuse over 1 hour

Dopamine hydrochloride (*Intropin®*)

Continuous *in* Glucose 5% *or* Sodium chloride 0.9% *or* Compound sodium lactate

Dilute to a concentration of 1.6 mg/mL; incompatible with bicarbonate

Dopexamine hydrochloride (*Dopacard®*)

Continuous *in* Glucose 5% *or* Sodium chloride 0.9%

Dilute to a concentration of 400 or 800 micrograms/mL; max. concentration *via* large peripheral vein 1 mg/mL, concentrations up to 4 mg/mL may be infused *via* central vein; give *via* infusion pump or other device which provides accurate control of rate; contact with metal should be minimised; incompatible with bicarbonate

Doxorubicin hydrochloride (*Doxorubicin Rapid Dissolution, Doxorubicin Solution*) (both Pharmacia & Upjohn)

via drip tubing *in* Glucose 5% *or* Sodium chloride 0.9%

Reconstitute *Doxorubicin Rapid Dissolution* with water for injections or sodium chloride 0.9% (10 mg in 5 mL, 50 mg in 25 mL); give over 2–3 minutes

Doxorubicin hydrochloride (liposomal) (*Caelyx®*)

via drip tubing *in* Glucose 5%

Dilute requisite dose in 250 mL infusion fluid; give over 30 minutes

Enoximone (*Perfan®*)

Continuous *or* intermittent *in* Sodium chloride 0.9% *or* Water for injections

Dilute to a concentration of 2.5 mg/mL; incompatible with glucose solutions; use only plastic containers or syringes

Epirubicin hydrochloride (*Pharmorubicin® Rapid Dissolution, Pharmorubicin® Solution*)

via drip tubing *in* Sodium chloride 0.9%

Reconstitute *Pharmorubicin® Rapid Dissolution* with sodium chloride 0.9% or with water for injections (10 mg in 5 mL, 20 mg in 10 mL, 50 mg in 25 mL); give over 3–5 minutes

Epoetin beta (*Recormon®*)

Intermittent *in* Sodium chloride 0.9%

Reconstitute with water for injections provided and dilute in at least 100 mL infusion fluid; complete administration within 2 hours of preparation; avoid glass, use only plastic materials for infusion

Epoprostenol (*Flolan®*)

Continuous *in* Sodium chloride 0.9%

Reconstitute with the diluent provided (pH 10.5) to make a concentrate; use this concentrate within 12 hours and store at 2–8°C; dilute with not more than 6 times the volume of sodium chloride 0.9% before use

Erythromycin (as lactobionate)

Continuous *or* intermittent *in* Glucose 5% (neutralised with sodium bicarbonate) *or* Sodium chloride 0.9%

Dissolve initially in water for injections (1 g in 20 mL) then dilute to a concentration of 1 mg/mL for continuous infusion and 1–5 mg/mL for intermittent infusion; give intermittent infusion over 20–60 minutes

Esmolol hydrochloride (*Brevibloc®*)

Continuous *or* intermittent *in* Glucose 5% *or* Sodium chloride 0.9%

Dilute to a concentration of 10 mg/mL; for continuous infusion use a suitable infusion control device; incompatible with bicarbonate

Ethanol

Continuous *in* Glucose 5% *or* Sodium chloride 0.9% *or* Ringer's solution *or* Compound sodium lactate

Dilute to a concentration of 5–10%

Etoposide (*Eposin®; Vepesid®; Etoposide*, APS)

Intermittent *in* Sodium chloride 0.9%

For *Vepesid®* dilute to a concentration of not more than 250 micrograms/mL and give over not less than 30 minutes; for *Etoposide* (APS) dilute with either sodium chloride 0.9% or glucose 5% to a concentration of 200 micrograms/mL and give over 30–60 minutes; for *Eposin®* dilute with either sodium chloride 0.9% or glucose 5% to a concentration of 200–400 micrograms/mL and give over at least 30 minutes; check container for haze or precipitate during infusion

Etoposide (as phosphate) (*Etopophos®*)

Intermittent *in* Glucose 5% *or* Sodium chloride 0.9%

Reconstitute with 5–10 mL of either water for injections or with infusion fluid then dilute further with infusion fluid to a concentration as low as 100 micrograms/mL and give over 5 minutes to 3.5 hours

Filgrastim (*Neupogen®*)

Continuous *or* intermittent *in* Glucose 5%

For a filgrastim concentration of less than 1 500 000 units/mL (15 micrograms/mL) albumin solution (human serum albumin) is added to produce a final albumin concentration of 2 mg/mL; should not be diluted to a filgrastim concentration of less than 200 000 units/mL (2 micrograms/mL) and should not be diluted with sodium chloride solution

Flecainide acetate (*Tambocor®*)

Continuous *or* intermittent *in* Glucose 5% *or* Sodium chloride 0.9% *or* Compound sodium lactate

Minimum volume in infusion fluids containing chlorides 500 mL

Flucloxacillin (as sodium salt) (*Floxapen®*)

Intermittent *in* Glucose 5% *or* Sodium chloride 0.9%

Suggested volume 100 mL given over 30–60 minutes

via drip tubing *in* Glucose 5% *or* Sodium chloride 0.9% *or* Ringer's solution *or* Compound sodium lactate

Continuous infusion not usually recommended

Fludarabine phosphate (*Fludara®*)

Intermittent *in* Sodium chloride 0.9%

Reconstitute each 50 mg with 2 mL water for injections and dilute requisite dose in 100 mL; give over 30 minutes

Flumazenil (*Anexate®*)

Continuous *in* Glucose 5% *or* Sodium chloride 0.9%

Fluorouracil (as sodium salt)

Continuous *or via* drip tubing *in* Glucose 5%

For continuous infusion suggested volume 500 mL given over 4 hours

Fomepizole (*Antizol®*)

Intermittent *in* Glucose 5% *or* Sodium chloride 0.9%

Dilute requisite dose in at least 100 mL infusion fluid; give over 30 minutes

Foscarnet sodium (*Foscavir®*)

Intermittent *in* Glucose 5% *or* Sodium chloride 0.9%

Dilute to a concentration of 12 mg/mL for infusion into peripheral vein (undiluted solution *via* central venous line only); infuse over at least 1 hour

Fosphenytoin Sodium (*Pro-Epanutin®*)

Intermittent *in* Glucose 5% *or* Sodium chloride 0.9%

Dilute to a concentration of 1.5–25 mg (phenytoin sodium equivalent)/mL

Furosemide/Frusemide (as sodium salt) (*Lasix®*)

Continuous *in* Sodium chloride 0.9% *or* Ringer's solution

Infusion pH must be above 5.5 and rate should not exceed 4 mg/minute; glucose solutions are unsuitable

Fusidic acid (as sodium salt) (*Fucidin*®)

Continuous *in* Glucose 5% (but see below) *or* Sodium chloride 0.9%

Reconstitute with the buffer solution provided and dilute to 500 mL; give through central venous line over 2 hours (or over 6 hours if superficial vein used); incompatible in solution of pH less than 7.4

Ganciclovir (as sodium salt) (*Cymevene*®)

Intermittent *in* Glucose 5% *or* Sodium chloride 0.9% *or* Ringer's solution *or* Compound sodium lactate

Reconstitute initially in water for injections (500 mg/ 10 mL) then dilute to not more than 10 mg/mL with infusion fluid (usually 100 mL); give over 1 hour

Gemcitabine (*Gemzar*®)

Intermittent *in* Sodium chloride 0.9%

Reconstitute initially with sodium chloride 0.9% (200 mg in at least 5 mL, 1 g in at least 25 mL); may be diluted further with infusion fluid; give over 30 minutes

Gentamicin (as sulphate) (*Cidomycin*®)

Intermittent *or via* drip tubing *in* Glucose 5% *or* Sodium chloride 0.9%

Suggested volume for intermittent infusion 50–100 mL given over 20 minutes

Glyceryl trinitrate (*Nitrocine*®, *Nitronal*®, *Tridil*®)

Continuous *in* Glucose 5% *or* Sodium chloride 0.9%

For *Tridil*® dilute to a concentration of not more than 400 micrograms/mL; for *Nitrocine*® suggested infusion concentration 100 micrograms/mL; incompatible with polyvinyl chloride infusion containers such as *Viaflex*® or *Steriflex*®; use glass or polyethylene containers or give *via* a syringe pump

Granisetron (as hydrochloride) (*Kytril*®)

Intermittent *in* Glucose 5% *or* Sodium chloride 0.9% *or* Compound sodium lactate

Dilute 3 mL in 20–50 mL infusion fluid (up to 3 mL in 10–30 mL for children); give over 5 minutes

Haem arginate (*Normosang*®)

Intermittent *in* Sodium chloride 0.9%

Dilute requisite dose in 100 mL infusion fluid in glass bottle and give over at least 30 minutes *via* large antebrachial vein; administer within 1 hour after dilution

Heparin sodium

Continuous *in* Glucose 5% *or* Sodium chloride 0.9%

Administration with a motorised pump advisable

Hydralazine hydrochloride (*Apresoline*®)

Continuous *in* Sodium chloride 0.9% *or* Ringer's solution

Suggested infusion volume 500 mL

Hydrocortisone (as sodium phosphate) (*Efcortesol*®)

Continuous *or* intermittent *or via* drip tubing *in* Glucose 5% *or* Sodium chloride 0.9%

Hydrocortisone (as sodium succinate) (*Efcortelan Soluble*®, *SoluCortef*®)

Continuous *or* intermittent *or via* drip tubing *in* Glucose 5% *or* Sodium chloride 0.9%

Idarubicin hydrochloride (*Zavedos*®)

via drip tubing *in* Sodium chloride 0.9%

Reconstitute with water for injections; give over 5–10 minutes

Ifosfamide (*Mitoxana*®)

Continuous *or* intermittent *or via* drip tubing *in* Glucose 5% *or* Sodium chloride 0.9%

For continuous infusion, suggested volume 3 litres given over 24 hours; for intermittent infusion, give over 30–120 minutes

Imiglucerase (*Cerezyme*®)

Intermittent *in* Sodium chloride 0.9%

Initially reconstitute with 5.1 mL water for injections to give 40 units/mL solution; dilute requisite dose in 100–200 mL infusion fluid and give over 1–2 hours *or* at a rate not exceeding 1 unit/kg/minute; administer within 3 hours after reconstitution

Imipenem with cilastatin (as sodium salt) (*Primaxin*®)

Intermittent *in* Glucose 5% *or* Sodium chloride 0.9%

Dilute to a concentration of 5 mg (as imipenem)/mL; infuse 250–500 mg (as imipenem) over 20–30 minutes, 1 g over 40–60 minutes

Continuous infusion not usually recommended

Infliximab (*Remicade*®)

Intermittent *in* Sodium chloride 0.9%

Reconstitute 100 mg with 10 mL water for injections (swirling gently to dissolve—avoid vigorous agitation) and dilute to 250 mL with infusion fluid; give through an in-line filter (1.2 micron or less) over at least 2 hours at a rate not exceeding 2 mL/minute

Insulin (soluble)

Continuous *in* Sodium chloride 0.9% *or* Compound sodium lactate

Adsorbed to some extent by plastics of infusion set; see also section 6.1.3; ensure insulin is not injected into 'dead space' of injection port of the infusion bag

Interferon alfa-2b (*Intron A*®)

Intermittent *in* Sodium chloride 0.9%

For *Intron A*® solution, dilute requisite dose in 50 mL infusion fluid and administer over 20 minutes; not to be diluted to less than 0.3 million units/mL

For *Intron A*® powder, reconstitute with 1 mL water for injections; dilute requisite dose in 100 mL infusion fluid and administer over 20 minutes

Irinotecan hydrochloride (*Campto*®)

Intermittent *in* Glucose 5% *or* Sodium chloride 0.9%

Dilute requisite dose in 250 mL infusion fluid; give over 30–90 minutes

Isoprenaline hydrochloride (*Saventrine IV*®)

Continuous *in* Glucose 5% *or* Sodium chloride and glucose

Dilute in a large-volume infusion; suggested minimum volume 500 mL; pH of the infusion must be below 5

Isosorbide dinitrate (*Isoket 0.05%*®, *Isoket 0.1%*®)

Continuous *in* Glucose 5% *or* Sodium chloride 0.9%

Adsorbed to some extent by polyvinyl chloride infusion containers; preferably use glass or polyethylene containers or give *via* a syringe pump; *Isoket 0.05%*® can alternatively be administered undiluted using a syringe pump with a glass or rigid plastic syringe

Kanamycin (as acid sulphate) (*Kannasyn*®)

Intermittent *in* Glucose 5% *or* Sodium chloride 0.9%

Dilute to 2.5 mg/mL and give at a rate of 3–4 mL/ minute

Ketamine (as hydrochloride) (*Ketalar®*)

Continuous *in* Glucose 5% *or* Sodium chloride 0.9%

Dilute to 1 mg/mL; microdrip infusion for maintenance of anaesthesia

Labetalol hydrochloride (*Trandate®*)

Intermittent *in* Glucose 5% *or* Sodium chloride and glucose

Dilute to a concentration of 1 mg/mL; suggested volume 200 mL; adjust rate with in-line burette

Lenograstim (*Granocyte®*)

Intermittent *in* Sodium chloride 0.9%

Initially reconstitute with 1 mL water for injection provided (do not shake vigorously) then dilute with up to 50 mL infusion fluid for each vial of *Granocyte-13* or up to 100 mL infusion fluid for *Granocyte-34*; give over 30 minutes

Lepirudin (*Refludan®*)

Continuous *in* Glucose 5% *or* Sodium chloride 0.9%

Reconstitute initially with water for injections *or* sodium chloride 0.9% then dilute to a concentration of 2 mg/mL with infusion fluid

Magnesium sulphate

Continuous *in* Glucose 5% *or* Sodium chloride 0.9%

Suggested concentration up to 200 mg/mL

Melphalan (*Alkeran®*)

Intermittent *or via* drip tubing *in* Sodium chloride 0.9%

Reconstitute with the solvent-diluent provided then dilute with infusion fluid; max. 90 minutes between addition and completion of administration; incompatible with glucose infusion

Meropenem (*Meronem®*)

Intermittent *in* Glucose 5 and 10% *or* Sodium chloride 0.9%

Dilute in 50–200 mL infusion fluid and give over 15–30 minutes

Mesna (*Uromitexan®*)

Continuous *or via* drip tubing *in* Glucose 5% *or* Sodium chloride 0.9%

Metaraminol (as tartrate) (*Aramine®*)

Continuous *or via* drip tubing *in* Glucose 5% *or* Sodium chloride 0.9% *or* Ringer's solution *or* Compound sodium lactate

Suggested infusion volume 500mL

Methocarbamol (*Robaxin®*)

Intermittent *in* Glucose 5% *or* Sodium chloride 0.9%

Dilute to a concentration of not less than 1 g in 250 mL

Methotrexate (as sodium salt) (*Methotrexate*, Lederle)

Continuous *or via* drip tubing *in* Glucose 5% *or* Sodium chloride 0.9% *or* Compound sodium lactate *or* Ringer's solution

Dilute in a large-volume infusion; max. 24 hours between addition and completion of administration

Methyldopa hydrochloride (*Aldomet®*)

Intermittent *in* Glucose 5%

Dilute requisite dose with 100 mL infusion fluid *or* dilute to a concentration of 10 mg/mL; give over 30–60 minutes

Methylprednisolone (as sodium succinate) (*Solu-Medrone®*)

Continuous *or* intermittent *or via* drip tubing *in* Glucose 5% *or* Sodium chloride 0.9%

Reconstitute initially with water for injections; doses up to 250 mg should be given over at least 5 minutes, high doses over at least 30 minutes

Metoclopramide hydrochloride (*Maxolon High Dose®*)

Continuous *or* intermittent *in* Glucose 5% *or* Sodium chloride 0.9% *or* Compound sodium lactate

Continuous infusion recommended; loading dose, dilute with 50–100 mL and give over 15–20 minutes; maintenance dose, dilute with 500 mL and give over 8–12 hours; for intermittent infusion dilute with at least 50 mL and give over at least 15 minutes

Mexiletine hydrochloride (*Mexitil®*)

Continuous *in* Glucose 5% *or* Sodium chloride 0.9%

Milrinone (*Primacor®*)

Continuous *in* Glucose 5% *or* Sodium chloride 0.9%

Dilute to a suggested concentration of 200 micrograms/mL

Mitoxantrone/Mitozantrone (as hydrochloride) (*Novantrone®*)

via drip tubing *in* Glucose 5% *or* Sodium chloride 0.9%

Suggested volume at least 50 mL given over at least 3–5 minutes

Mivacurium (as chloride) (*Mivacron®*)

Continuous *in* Glucose 5% *or* Sodium chloride 0.9%

Dilute to a concentration of 500 micrograms/mL; may also be given undiluted

Molgramostim (*Leucomax®*)

Intermittent *in* Glucose 5% *or* Sodium chloride 0.9%

Reconstitute each vial with 1 mL water for injections; dilute with 25–100 mL infusion fluid to a concentration of not less than 80 000 units/mL; give over 4–6 hours; infusion through low protein binding 0.2 or 0.22 micron filter recommended; some infusion sets (e.g. *Port-A-Cath®*) adsorb molgramostim and should not be used

Mycophenolate mofetil (as hydrochloride) (*CellCept®*)

Intermittent *in* Glucose 5%

Reconstitute each 500-mg vial with 14 mL glucose 5% and dilute the contents of 2 vials in 140 mL infusion fluid; give over 2 hours

Naloxone (*Min-I-Jet® Naloxone Hydrochloride, Narcan®*)

Continuous *in* Glucose 5% *or* Sodium chloride 0.9%

Dilute to a concentration of 4 micrograms/mL

Netilmicin (as sulphate) (*Netillin®*)

Intermittent *or via* drip tubing *in* Glucose 5 and 10% *or* Sodium chloride 0.9%

For intermittent infusion suggested volume 50–200 mL given over 90–120 minutes

Nimodipine (*Nimotop®*)

via drip tubing *in* Glucose 5% *or* Sodium chloride 0.9% *or* Ringer's solution

Not to be added to infusion container; administer *via* an infusion pump through a Y-piece into a central catheter; incompatible with polyvinyl chloride giving sets or containers; protect infusion from light

Nizatidine (*Axid®*)

Continuous *or* intermittent *in* Glucose 5% *or* Sodium chloride 0.9% *or* Compound sodium lactate

For continuous infusion, dilute 300 mg in 150 mL and give at a rate of 10 mg/hour; for intermittent infusion, dilute 100 mg in 50 mL and give over 15 minutes

Noradrenaline acid tartrate/Norepinephrine bitartrate (*Levophed®*)

Continuous *in* Glucose 5% *or* Sodium chloride and glucose

Give *via* controlled infusion device; for administration *via* syringe pump, dilute 4 mg noradrenaline acid tartrate (2 mL solution) with 48 mL; for administration *via* drip counter dilute 40 mg (20 mL solution) with 480 mL; give through a central venous catheter; incompatible with alkalis

Omeprazole (as sodium salt) (*Losec®*)

Intermittent *in* Glucose 5% *or* Sodium chloride 0.9%

Reconstitute with infusion fluid and dilute to 100 mL; give over 20–30 minutes

Ondansetron (as hydrochloride) (*Zofran®*)

Continuous *or* intermittent *in* Glucose 5% *or* Sodium chloride 0.9% *or* Ringer's solution

For intermittent infusion, dilute 32 mg in 50–100 mL and give over at least 15 minutes

Oxaliplatin (*Eloxatin®*)

Continuous *in* Glucose 5%

Reconstitute with water for injections or glucose 5% to a concentration of 5 mg/mL; dilute with 250–500 mL infusion fluid and give over 2–6 hours

Oxytocin (*Syntocinon®*)

Continuous *in* Glucose 5%

Preferably given *via* a variable-speed infusion pump in a concentration appropriate to the pump; if given by drip infusion for *induction or enhancement of labour*, dilute 5 units in 500 mL infusion fluid; for *postpartum uterine haemorrhage* dilute 5–20 units in 500 mL; if high doses given for prolonged period (e.g. for inevitable or missed abortion or for postpartum haemorrhage), use low volume of an electrolyte-containing infusion fluid (not Glucose 5%) given at higher concentration than for induction or enhancement of labour; close attention to patient's fluid and electrolyte status essential

Paclitaxel (*Taxol®*)

Continuous *in* Glucose 5% *or* Sodium chloride 0.9%

Dilute to a concentration of 0.3–1.2 mg/mL and give through a 0.22 micron in-line filter over 3 hours; not to be used with PVC equipment (short PVC inlet or outlet on filter may be acceptable)

Pantoprazole (as sodium sequihydrate) (*Protium®*)

Intermittent *in* Glucose 5 and 10% *or* Sodium chloride 0.9%

Reconstitute 40 mg with 10 mL sodium chloride 0.9% and dilute to 100 mL with infusion fluid

Pentamidine isetionate (*Pentacarinat®*)

Intermittent *in* Glucose 5% *or* Sodium chloride 0.9%

Dissolve initially in water for injections (300 mg in 3–5 mL) then dilute in 50–250 mL; give over at least 60 minutes

Pentostatin (*Nipent®*)

Intermittent *in* Glucose 5% *or* Sodium chloride 0.9%

Reconstitute initially with 5 mL water for injections to produce a 2 mg/mL solution; dilute requisite dose in 25–50 mL infusion fluid and give over 20–30 minutes

Phenoxybenzamine hydrochloride

Intermittent *in* Sodium chloride 0.9%

Dilute in 200–500 mL infusion; give over at least 2 hours; max. 4 hours between dilution and completion of administration

Phentolamine mesilate (*Rogitine®*)

Intermittent *in* Glucose 5% *or* Sodium chloride 0.9%

Phenylephrine hydrochloride

Intermittent *in* Glucose 5% *or* Sodium chloride 0.9%

Dilute 10 mg in 500 mL infusion fluid

Phenytoin sodium (*Epanutin®*)

Intermittent *in* Sodium chloride 0.9%

Flush intravenous line with Sodium chloride 0.9% before and after infusion; dilute in 50–100 mL infusion fluid (final concentration not to exceed 10 mg/mL) and give through an in-line filter (0.22–0.50 micron) at a rate not exceeding 50 mg/minute (neonates, give at a rate of 1–3 mg/kg/minute); complete administration within 1 hour of preparation

Phytomenadione (in mixed micelles vehicle) (*Konakion® MM*)

Intermittent *in* Glucose 5%

Dilute with 55 mL; may be injected into lower part of infusion apparatus

Piperacillin (as sodium salt) (*Pipril®*)

Intermittent *in* Glucose 5% *or* Sodium chloride 0.9% *or* Compound sodium lactate *or* Water for injections

Minimum volume 50 mL given over 20–40 minutes

Piperacillin with tazobactam (as sodium salts) (*Tazocin®*)

Intermittent *in* Glucose 5% *or* Sodium chloride 0.9% *or* Water for injections

Reconstitute initially with water for injections or sodium chloride infusion 0.9% (2.25 g in 10 mL, 4.5 g in 20 mL) then dilute to at least 50 mL with infusion fluid; give over 20–30 minutes

Potassium chloride

Continuous *in* Glucose 5% *or* Sodium chloride 0.9%

Dilute in a large-volume infusion; mix thoroughly to avoid 'layering', especially in non-rigid infusion containers; use ready-prepared solutions when possible

Procainamide hydrochloride (*Pronestyl®*)

Continuous *or* intermittent *in* Glucose 5%

For maintenance, dilute to a concentration of *either* 2 mg/mL and give at a rate of 1–3 mL/minute *or* 4 mg/mL and give at a rate of 0.5–1.5 mL/minute

Propofol (emulsion) (*Diprivan®*)

via drip tubing *in* Glucose 5% *or* Sodium chloride 0.9%

To be administered *via* a Y-piece close to injection site

Continuous *in* Glucose 5%

Dilute to a concentration not less than 2 mg/mL; administer using suitable device to control infusion rate; use glass or PVC containers (if PVC bag used it should be full—withdraw volume of infusion fluid equal to that of propofol to be added); give within 6 hours of preparation; propofol may alternatively be infused undiluted using a suitable infusion pump

Quinine dihydrochloride

Continuous *in* Sodium chloride 0.9%

To be given over 4 hours; see also section 5.4.1

Quinupristin with dalfopristin (*Synercid®*)

Intermittent *in* Glucose 5%

Reconstitute 500 mg with 5 mL water for injections or glucose 5%; gently swirl vial without shaking to dissolve; allow to stand for at least 2 minutes until foam disappears; dilute requisite dose in 250 mL infusion fluid and give over 60 minutes preferably *via* central venous catheter (may be diluted in 100 mL infusion fluid if administered *via* central line only); flush line with glucose 5% before and after infusion; incompatible with sodium chloride solutions

Raltitrexed (*Tomudex®*)

Intermittent *in* Glucose 5% *or* Sodium chloride 0.9%

Reconstitute with water for injections; dilute requisite dose in 50–250 mL infusion fluid and give over 15 minutes

Ranitidine (as hydrochloride) (*Zantac®*)

Intermittent *in* Glucose 5% *or* Sodium chloride 0.9% *or* Compound sodium lactate

Remifentanil (*Ultiva®*)

Intermittent *or via* drip tubing *in* Glucose 5% *or* Sodium chloride 0.9% *or* Water for injections

Reconstitute with infusion fluid to a concentration of 1 mg/mL then dilute further to a concentration of 20–250 micrograms/mL (50 micrograms/mL recommended for general anaesthesia)

Rifampicin (*Rifadin®, Rimactane®*)

Intermittent *in* Glucose 5 and 10% *or* Sodium chloride 0.9% *or* Ringer's solution

Reconstitute with solvent provided then dilute with 250 mL (*Rimactane®*) or 500 mL (*Rifadin®*) infusion fluid; give over 2–3 hours

Ritodrine hydrochloride (*Yutopar®*)

Continuous *in* Glucose 5%

Give *via* controlled infusion device, preferably a syringe pump; if syringe pump available dilute to a concentration of 3 mg/mL; if syringe pump not available dilute to a concentration of 300 micrograms/mL; close attention to patient's fluid and electrolyte status essential

Rituximab (*Mabthera®*)

Intermittent *in* Glucose 5% *or* Sodium chloride 0.9%

Dilute to 1–4 mg/mL and gently invert bag to avoid foaming

Rocuronium bromide (*Esmeron®*)

Continuous *or via* drip tubing *in* Glucose 5% *or* Sodium chloride 0.9%

Salbutamol (as sulphate) (*Ventolin® For Intravenous Infusion*)

Continuous *in* Glucose 5%

For *bronchodilatation* dilute 5 mg with 500 mL glucose 5% or sodium chloride 0.9%; for *premature labour* dilute with glucose 5% to a concentration of 200 micrograms/mL for use in a syringe pump *or* for other infusion methods (preferably *via* controlled infusion device), dilute to a concentration of 20 micrograms/mL; close attention to patient's fluid and electrolyte status essential

Sodium calcium edetate (*Ledclair®*)

Continuous *in* Glucose 5% *or* Sodium chloride 0.9%

Dilute to a concentration of not more than 3%; suggested volume 250–500 mL given over at least 1 hour

Sodium clodronate (*Bonefos® Concentrate, Loron®*)

Continuous *in* Sodium chloride 0.9%

Dilute 300 mg in 500 mL and give over at least 2 hours or 1.5 g in 500 mL and give over at least 4 hours; *Bonefos® Concentrate* can also be diluted in Glucose 5%

Sodium nitroprusside (*Faulding DBL*)

Continuous *in* Glucose 5%

Reconstitute 50 mg with 2–3 mL glucose 5% then dilute immediately with 250–1000 mL infusion fluid; preferably infuse *via* infusion device to allow precise control; protect infusion from light

Sodium valproate (*Epilim®*)

Continuous *or* intermittent *in* Glucose 5% *or* Sodium chloride 0.9%

Reconstitute with solvent provided then dilute with infusion fluid

Sotalol hydrochloride (*Sotacor®*)

Continuous *or* intermittent *in* Glucose 5% *or* Sodium chloride 0.9%

Dilute to a concentration of between 0.01–2 mg/mL

Streptokinase (*Kabikinase®; Streptase®; Streptokinase,* Braun)

Continuous *or* intermittent *in* Glucose 5% *or* Sodium chloride 0.9%

Reconstitute *Kabikinase®* with water for injections, *Streptase®* with sodium chloride 0.9%, and *Streptokinase* (Braun) with either water for injections or sodium chloride 0.9% then dilute further with infusion fluid

Sulfadiazine sodium

Continuous *in* Sodium chloride 0.9%

Suggested volume 500 mL; ampoule solution has a pH of over 10

Suxamethonium chloride (*Anectine®*)

Continuous *in* Glucose 5% *or* Sodium chloride 0.9%

Tacrolimus (*Prograf®*)

Continuous *in* Glucose 5% *or* Sodium chloride 0.9%

Dilute concentrate in infusion fluid to a final concentration of 4–100 micrograms/mL; give over 24 hours; incompatible with PVC

Teicoplanin (*Targocid®*)

Intermittent *in* Glucose 5% *or* Sodium chloride 0.9% *or* Compound sodium lactate

Reconstitute initially with water for injections provided; infuse over 30 minutes

Continuous infusion not usually recommended

Terbutaline sulphate (*Bricanyl®*)

Continuous *in* Glucose 5%

For *bronchodilatation* dilute 1.5–2.5 mg with 500 mL glucose 5% or sodium chloride 0.9% and give over 8–10 hours; for *premature labour* dilute in glucose 5% and give *via* controlled infusion device preferably a syringe pump; if syringe pump available dilute to a concentration of 100 micrograms/mL; if syringe pump not available dilute to a concentration of 10 micrograms/mL; close attention to patient's fluid and electrolyte status essential

Ticarcillin sodium with clavulanic acid
(*Timentin*®)

Intermittent *in* Glucose 5% *or* Water for injections

Suggested volume glucose 5%, 50–150 mL (depending on dose) or water for injections, 25–100 mL; given over 30–40 minutes

Tirofiban (*Aggrastat*®)

Continuous *in* Glucose 5% *or* Sodium chloride 0.9%

Withdraw 50 mL infusion fluid from 250 mL bag and replace with 50 mL tirofiban concentrate (250 micrograms/mL) to give a final concentration of 50 micrograms/mL

Tobramycin (as sulphate) (*Nebcin*®)

Intermittent *or via* drip tubing *in* Glucose 5% *or* Sodium chloride 0.9%

For adult intermittent infusion suggested volume 50–100 mL (children proportionately smaller volume) given over 20–60 minutes

Topotecan (as hydrochloride) (*Hycamtin*®)

Intermittent *in* Glucose 5% *or* Sodium chloride 0.9%

Reconstitute 4 mg with 4 mL water for injections then dilute to a final concentration of 25–50 micrograms/mL; give over 30 minutes

Tramadol hydrochloride (*Zydol*®)

Continuous *or* intermittent *in* Glucose 5% *or* Sodium chloride 0.9% *or* Ringer's solution *or* Compound sodium lactate

Tranexamic acid (*Cyklokapron*®)

Continuous *in* Glucose 5% *or* Sodium chloride 0.9% *or* Ringer's solution

Treosulfan (*Treosulfan*) (Medac)

Intermittent *in* Water for injections

Infusion suggested for doses above 5 g; dilute to a concentration of 5 g in 100 mL

Trimetaphan camsilate (Cambridge)

Intermittent *in* Sodium chloride 0.9% *or* Sodium chloride and glucose

Dilute to a concentration of 0.05–0.1% (0.25% if fluid restriction necessary)

Trimethoprim (as lactate) (*Monotrim*®)

via drip tubing *in* Glucose 5% *or* Sodium chloride 0.9% *or* Compound sodium lactate *or* Ringer's solution

Trimetrexate (*Neutrexin*®)

Intermittent *in* Glucose 5%

Reconstitute each 25 mg with 2 mL glucose 5% or water for injections; dilute further with infusion fluid to a concentration of 0.25–2 mg/mL; infuse over 60–90 minutes; incompatible with solutions containing sodium chloride or other electrolytes, flush intravenous line with glucose 5%

Trisodium edetate (*Limclair*®)

Continuous *in* Glucose 5% *or* Sodium chloride 0.9%

Dilute to a concentration of 10 mg/mL; give over 2–3 hours

Tropisetron (as hydrochloride) (*Navoban*®)

Intermittent *or via* drip tubing *in* Glucose 5% *or* Sodium chloride 0.9% *or* Ringer's solution

Suggested concentration for infusion 50 micrograms/mL

Vancomycin (as hydrochloride) (*Vancocin*®)

Intermittent *in* Glucose 5% *or* Sodium chloride 0.9%

Reconstitute each 500 mg with 10 mL water for injections and dilute with infusion fluid to a concentration of up to 5 mg/mL (10 mg/mL in fluid restriction but increased risk of infusion-related effects); give over at least 60 minutes (rate not to exceed 10 mg/minute for doses over 500 mg); use continuous infusion only if intermittent not feasible

Vasopressin, synthetic (*Pitressin*®)

Intermittent *in* Glucose 5%

Suggested concentration 20 units/100 mL given over 15 minutes

Vecuronium bromide (*Norcuron*®)

Continuous *in* Glucose 5% *or* Sodium chloride 0.9% *or* Ringer's solution

Reconstitute with the solvent provided

Vinblastine sulphate (*Velbe*®)

via drip tubing *in* Sodium chloride 0.9%

Reconstitute with sodium chloride 0.9%; give over approx. 1 minute

Vincristine sulphate (*Oncovin*®)

via drip tubing *in* Glucose 5% *or* Sodium chloride 0.9%

Vindesine sulphate (*Eldisine*®)

via drip tubing *in* Glucose 5% *or* Sodium chloride 0.9%

Reconstitute with sodium chloride 0.9%; give over 1–3 minutes

Vinorelbine (*Navelbine*®)

Intermittent *in* Glucose 5% *or* Sodium chloride 0.9%

Dilute in 125 mL infusion fluid; give over 20–30 minutes

Vitamins B & C (*Pabrinex*® *I/V High potency*)

Intermittent *or via* drip tubing *in* Glucose 5% *or* Sodium chloride 0.9%

Ampoule contents should be mixed, diluted, and administered without delay; give over 10 minutes (see CSM advice, section 9.6.2)

Vitamins, multiple
(*Cernevit*®)

Intermittent *in* Glucose 5% *or* Sodium chloride 0.9%

Dissolve initially in 5 mL water for injections (or infusion fluid)

(*Multibionta*®)

Intermittent *in* Glucose 5% *or* Sodium chloride 0.9%

Dilute 10 mL in not less than 250 mL of infusion fluid (adults); see also section 9.3

(*Solivito N*®)

Intermittent *in* Glucose 5 and 10%

Suggested volume 500–1000 mL given over 2–3 hours; see also section 9.3

Zidovudine (*Retrovir*®)

Intermittent *in* Glucose 5%

Dilute to a concentration of 2 mg/mL or 4 mg/mL and give over 1 hour

Appendix 7: Borderline substances

In certain conditions some foods (and toilet preparations) have characteristics of drugs and the Advisory Committee on Borderline Substances advises as to the circumstances in which such substances may be regarded as drugs. Prescriptions issued in accordance with the Committee's advice and endorsed 'ACBS' will normally not be investigated.

> General Practitioners are reminded that the ACBS recommends products on the basis that they may be regarded as drugs for the management of specified conditions. Doctors should satisfy themselves that the products can safely be prescribed, that patients are adequately monitored and that, where necessary, expert hospital supervision is available.

Foods which may be prescribed on FP10 (GP10 in Scotland)

Note. This is a list of food products which the ACBS has approved. The clinical condition for which the product has approval follows each entry.

Foods included in this Appendix may contain cariogenic sugars and patients should be advised to take appropriate oral hygiene measures.

Advera® (Abbott)
Liquid, providing protein 14.2 g, carbohydrate 48.3 g, fat 5.4 g, energy 1262 kJ (299 kcal)/237 mL, with vitamins and minerals. Gluten-free. Orange and chocolate flavours. Net price 237-mL can = £2.67. For use as a nutritional supplement prescribed on medical grounds for: short-bowel syndrome, intractable malabsorption, preoperative preparation of patients who are undernourished, proven inflammatory bowel disease, following total gastrectomy, bowel fistulas, disease-related malnutrition. Not to be prescribed for any child under 5 years

Aglutella® (Ultrapharm)
Rice, low protein. Net price 500 g = £3.95. For inherited metabolic disorders, renal or liver failure requiring a low-protein diet

AL 110® (Nestlé)
Powder, protein 14 g, fat 25 g, carbohydrate 55.3 g, energy 2100 kJ (502 kcal)/100 g with vitamins and minerals. Net price 400 g = £7.27. For use as lactose intolerance in pre-school children, galactosaemia, and galactokinase deficiency

Alcoholic Beverages *see under* Rectified Spirit
Alembicol D® (Alembic Products)
Fractionated coconut oil. Net price 5 kg = £125.55. For steatorrhoea associated with cystic fibrosis of the pancreas, intestinal lymphangiectasia, surgery of the intestine, chronic liver disease, liver cirrhosis, other proven malabsorption syndromes; in a ketogenic diet in the management of epilepsy; type 1 hyperlipoproteinaemia

Alfare® (Nestlé)
Powder, protein 16.5 g, fat 24 g, carbohydrate 51.7 g, energy 2010 kJ (480 kcal)/100 g with vitamins and minerals. Net price 400 g = £5.49. For disaccharide and/or whole protein intolerance, or where amino acids or peptides are indicated in conjunction with medium chain triglycerides (MCT)

Aminex® (Gluten Free Foods Ltd)
Low-protein. Biscuits, net price 200 g = £3.75. Cookies, 150 g = £3.75. Rusks, 200 g = £3.75. For inherited metabolic disorders, renal or liver failure requiring a low-protein diet

Amino Acid Modules (SHS)
Leucine-Free Amino Acid Mix, powder, essential and non-essential amino acids 93%, except leucine. Net price 200 g = £49.59. For isovaleric acidaemia

Methionine-Free Amino Acid Mix, powder, essential and non-essential amino acids 93%, except methionine. Net price 200 g = £49.59. For homocystinuria or hypermethioninaemia

Methionine, Threonine, Valine-Free and Isoleucine-Low Amino Acid Mix, powder, essential and non-essential amino acids 93%, except methionine, threonine, and valine, with trace amounts of isoleucine. Net price 200 g = £49.59. For methylmalonic acidaemia or propionic acidaemia

Phenylalanine, Tyrosine, and Methionine-Free Amino Acid Mix, powder, essential and non-essential amino acids 93%, except methionine, phenylalanine, and tyrosine. Net price 200 g = £49.59. For tyrosinaemia type I where plasma concentrations are above normal

Tyrosine and Phenylalanine-Free Amino Acid Mix, powder, essential and non-essential amino acids 93%, except phenylalanine and tyrosine. Net price 200 g = £52.07. For tyrosinaemia where plasma methionine concentrations are normal

Aminogran® (UCB Pharma)
Food Supplement, powder, containing all essential amino acids except phenylalanine, for use with mineral mixture (see below), net price 500 g = £42.77. Tablet (≡ 1 g powder), net price 60-tab pack = £9.00. For the dietary management of phenylketonuria. Tablets not to be prescribed for any child under 8 years

Mineral Mixture, powder, containing all appropriate minerals for use with the above food supplement and other synthetic diets. Net price 250 g = £7.24. For phenylketonuria and as a mineral supplement in synthetic diets

Analog® (SHS)
Note. Analog products are generally intended for use in children up to 1 year, see also Flavour Sachets, for use with unflavoured amino acid and peptide products from SHS

LCP Analog, powder, essential and non-essential amino acids except phenylalanine 15.5%, with carbohydrate, fat, vitamins, minerals and trace elements. Gluten- and lactose-free. Net price 400 g = £19.88. For phenylketonuria

MSUD Analog, powder, essential and non-essential amino acids 15.5% except isoleucine, leucine and valine, with carbohydrate, fat, vitamins, minerals, and trace elements. Net price 400 g = £24.00. For maple syrup urine disease

XLeu Analog, powder, essential and non-essential amino acids 15.5% except leucine, with carbohydrate, fat, vitamins, minerals, and trace elements. Net price 400 g = £24.00. For isovaleric acidaemia
Ingredients: include arachis oil (peanut oil)

XLys Analog, powder, essential and non-essential amino acids 15.5% except lysine, with carbohydrate, fat, vitamins, minerals, and trace elements. Net price 400 g = £24.00. For hyperlysinaemia

XLys, Try Low Analog, powder, essential and non-essential amino acids 15.5% except lysine, and low tryptophan, with carbohydrate, fat, vitamins, minerals, and trace elements. Net price 400 g = £24.00. For type 1 glutaric aciduria

XMet Analog, powder, essential and non-essential amino acids 15.5% except methionine, with carbohydrate, fat, vitamins, minerals, and trace elements. Net price 400 g = £24.00. For hypermethioninaemia; homocystinuria

XMet, Thre, Val, Isoleu, Analog, powder, essential and non-essential amino acids 15.5% except methionine, threonine, valine and low isoleucine, with carbohydrate, fat, vitamins, minerals, and trace elements. Net price 400 g = £24.00. For methylmalonic acidaemia or propionic acidaemia

XP Analog, powder, essential and non-essential amino acids 15.5% except phenylalanine, with carbohydrate, fat, vitamins, minerals, and trace elements. Net price 400 g = £17.48. For phenylketonuria

XPhen, Tyr Analog, powder, essential and non-essential amino acids 15.5% except phenylalanine and tyrosine, with carbohydrate, fat, vitamins, minerals and trace elements. Net price 400 g = £24.00. For tyrosinaemia

XPhen, Tyr, Met Analog, powder, essential and non-essential amino acids 15.5% except phenylalanine, tyrosine and methionine, with carbohydrate, fat, vitamins, minerals and trace elements. Net price 400 g = £24.00. For tyrosinaemia

Aproten® (Ultrapharm)

Gluten-free. Flour. Net price 300 g = £1.84. For gluten-sensitive enteropathies including steatorrhoea due to gluten sensitivity, coeliac disease, and dermatitis herpetiformis

Low protein. Low Na+ and K+. Net prices: biscuits 180 g (36) = £2.80; bread mix 250 g = £2.00; cake mix 300 g = £2.10; crispbread 260 g = £3.95; pasta (anellini, ditalini, rigatini, spaghetti) 500 g = £3.95; tagliatelle 250 g = £2.10. For inherited metabolic disorders, renal or liver failure requiring a low-protein diet

L-Arginine (SHS)

Powder, net price 100 g = £7.44. For use as a supplement in urea cycle disorders other than arginase deficiency, such as hyperammonaemia types I and II, citrullaemia, arginosuccinic aciduria, and deficiency of N-acetyl glutamate synthetase

Arnott® (Ultrapharm)

Rice Cookies, gluten-free. Net price 200 g = £1.68. For gluten-sensitive enteropathies including steatorrhoea due to gluten sensitivity, coeliac disease, and dermatitis herpetiformis

Barkat® (Gluten Free Foods Ltd)

Gluten-free. Bread mix, net price 500 g = £4.12. Rice bread (sliced), brown or white, 450 g = £2.79. Rice pizza crust, brown or white, 150 g = £2.21. For gluten-sensitive enteropathies including steatorrhoea due to gluten sensitivity, coeliac disease, and dermatitis herpetiformis

Bi-Aglut® (Ultrapharm)

Gluten-free. Biscuits, net price 180 g = £2.60. Crackers, 150 g = £2.15. Cracker toast, 240 g = £3.60. Pastas (fusilli, macaroni, penne, spaghetti), 500 g = £4.86; Lasagne, 250 g = £2.56. For gluten-sensitive enteropathies including steatorrhoea due to gluten sensitivity, coeliac diseases, and dermatitis herpetiformis

Calogen® (SHS)

Emulsion, arachis oil (peanut oil) 50% in water. Strawberry or natural flavour. Net price 250 mL = £3.67; 1 litre = £14.77. For disease-related malnutrition, malabsorption states or other conditions requiring fortification with a high-fat supplement with or without fluid and electrolyte restrictions

Caloreen® (Nestlé Clinical)

Powder, water-soluble dextrins, with less than 1.8 mmol of Na+ and 0.3 mmol of K+/100 g. Net price 250 g = £1.51. For disease-related malnutrition, malabsorption states or other conditions requiring fortification with a high or readily available carbohydrate supplement

Calsip® (Fresenius)

Liquid, maltodextrin 50%. Flavours: apple, pineapple, neutral. Net price 200-mL carton = 93 p. For disease-related malnutrition, malabsorption states or other conditions requiring fortification with a high or readily available carbohydrate supplement

Caprilon® (SHS)

Powder, protein 11.8%, carbohydrate 55.1%, fat 28.3% (medium chain triglycerides 21.3%). Low in lactose, gluten- and sucrose-free. Used as a 12.7% solution. Net price 420 g = £10.60. For disorders in which a high intake of MCT is beneficial

Carobel, Instant® (Cow & Gate)

Powder, carob seed flour. Net price 45 g = £2.63. For thickening feeds in the treatment of vomiting

Casilan 90® (Heinz)

Powder, whole protein, containing all essential amino acids, 90% with less than 0.1% Na+. Net price 250 g = £5.13. For biochemically proven hypoproteinaemia

Clara's Kitchen® (Gluten Free Foods Ltd)

Gluten-free. Bread mix, net price 500 g = £3.53; hi-fibre bread mix, 500 g = £3.53. For gluten-sensitive enteropathies including steatorrhoea due to gluten-sensitivity, coeliac disease and dermatis herpetiformis.

Clinifeed® (Nestlé Clinical)

Clinifeed Iso, protein 10.5 g, carbohydrate 49.2 g, fat 15.4 g, energy 1575 kJ (375 kcal)/375 mL, with vitamins and minerals, vanilla flavour. Fructose- and sucrose-free, and low sodium. Net price 375-mL can = £1.80. For use as the sole source of nutrition or as a necessary nutritional supplement prescribed on medical grounds for: short-bowel syndrome, intractable malabsorption, pre-operative preparation of patients who are undernourished, proven inflammatory bowel disease, following total gastrectomy, dysphagia, bowel fistulas, disease-related malnutrition. Not to be prescribed for any child under 1 year; use with caution for children under 5 years

Clinutren® (Nestlé Clinical)

Clinutren Dessert, protein 12 g, carbohydrate 19 g, fat 3.3 g, energy 650 kJ (160 kcal)/ 125 g with vitamins and minerals. Gluten-free. Flavours: caramel, chocolate, peach or vanilla. Net price 125-g pot = £1.05. For use as a nutritional supplement prescribed on medical grounds for: short bowel syndrome, intractable malabsorption , pre-operative preparation of undernourished patients, proven inflammatory bowel disease, following total gastrectomy, dysphagia, bowel fistulas, disease-related malnutrition, continuous ambulatory peritoneal dialysis (CAPD), haemodialysis. Not to be prescribed for any child under 1 year; use with caution for children under 5 years.

Clinutren ISO, protein 7.6 g, carbohydrate 28 g, fat 6.6 g, energy 840 kJ (200 kcal)/200 mL with vitamins and minerals. Gluten-free. Flavours: chocolate, coffee, strawberry-raspberry or vanilla. Net price 200-mL pot = £1.18. For use as a nutritional supplement prescribed on medical grounds for: short bowel syndrome, intractable malabsorption, pre-operative preparation of undernourished patients, proven inflammatory bowel disease, following total gastrectomy, dysphagia, bowel fistulas, disease-related malnutrition. Not to be prescribed for any child under 1 year; use with caution for children under 5 years.

Clinutren 1.5, protein 11 g, carbohydrate 42 g, fat 10 g, energy 1260 kJ (300 kcal)/200 mL with vitamins and minerals. Gluten-free; clinically lactose-free. Flavours: apricot, banana, chocolate, strawberry-raspberry or vanilla. Net price 200-mL pot = £1.40. For indications see *Clinutren ISO*

Comminuted Chicken Meat (SHS)

Suspension (aqueous). Net price 150 g = £2.11. For carbohydrate intolerance in association with possible or proven intolerance of milk; glucose and galactose intolerance

Complan® Ready to Drink (Heinz)

Liquid, protein 8.7 g, carbohydrate 35 g, fat 8.3 g, energy 1050 kJ (250 kcal)/230 mL, with vitamins and minerals. Gluten-free. Flavours: chocolate, strawberry, vanilla, net price 230-mL carton = £1.00. For use as a sole source of nutrition or as a nutritional supplement prescribed on medical grounds for: short-bowel syndrome, intractable malabsorption, pre-operative preparation of undernourished patients, proven inflammatory bowel disease, following total gastrectomy, dysphagia, bowel fistulas, disease-related malnutrition. Not to be prescribed for any child under 1 year; use with caution for children under 5 years

Corn flour and corn starch For hypoglycaemia associated with glycogen-storage disease

Dextrose *see* Glucose

Dialamine® (SHS)

Powder, essential amino acids 30%, with carbohydrate 62%, energy 1500 kJ (360 kcal)/100 g, with ascorbic acid, minerals, and trace elements. Flavour: orange. Net price 200 g = £21.14. For oral feeding where essential amino acid supplements are required; e.g. chronic renal failure, hypoproteinaemia, wound fistula leakage with excessive protein loss, conditions requiring a controlled nitrogen intake, and haemodialysis

Dietary Specialities (Nutrition Point)

Gluten-free. Bread mix (brown or white), net price 500 g = £4.20; corn bread mix, 500 g = £4.75; cake mix (white), 750 g = £4.75; white or fibre mix, 500 g = £4.75. For gluten-sensitive enteropathies, coeliac disease, and dermatitis herpetiformis

dp® (SHS)

Cookies, low-protein, butterscotch- or chocolate-flavoured chip cookies. Net price 170 g = £6.16. For inherited metabolic disorders, renal or liver failure requiring a low-protein diet

Duobar® (SHS)

Bar, protein-free (phenylalanine nil added), carbohydrate 49.9 g, fat 49.9 g, energy 2692 kJ (648 kcal)/100 g. Low sodium and potassium. Strawberry or natural flavours. Net price 45-g bar = £1.08. For disease-related malnutrition, malabsorption states or other conditions requiring fortification with fat/carbohydrate supplement

Duocal® (SHS)

Liquid, emulsion providing carbohydrate 23.4 g, fat 7.1 g, energy 661 kJ (158 kcal)/100 mL. Low electrolyte, gluten-, lactose-, and protein-free. Net price 250 mL = £2.27; 1 litre = £8.09

MCT Powder, carbohydrate 74 g, fat 23.2 g (of which MCT 83%), energy 2042 kJ (486 kcal)/100 g. Low electrolyte, gluten-, protein- and lactose-free. Net price 400 g = £13.64

Super Soluble Powder, carbohydrate 72.7 g, fat 22.3 g, energy 2061 kJ (492 kcal)/100 g. Low electrolyte, gluten-, protein-, and lactose-free. Net price 400 g = £11.26
All for disease-related malnutrition, malabsorption states or other conditions requiring fortification with fat/carbohydrate supplement

Elemental 028® (SHS)

Note. see also Flavour Sachets, for use with unflavoured amino acid and peptide products from SHS

028 Powder, amino acids 12%, carbohydrate 70.5–72%, fat 6.64%, energy 1544–1568 kJ (364–370 kcal)/100 g with vitamins and minerals. For preparation with water before use. Net price 100-g box (orange flavoured or plain) = £3.82

028 Extra powder, amino acids 15%, carbohydrate 59%, fat 17.45%, energy 1860 kJ(443 kcal)/100 g, with vitamins, minerals, and trace elements. For preparation with water before use. Net price 100 g (plain) = £4.32; also available orange-flavoured (carbohydrate 55%, energy 1793 kJ (427 kcal)/100 g), 100 g = £4.32

028 Extra liquid, amino acids 7.5 g, carbohydrate 27.5 g, fat 8.7 g, energy 896 kJ (215 kcal)/250 mL, with vitamins, minerals, and trace elements. Flavours: grapefruit, orange and pineapple, summer fruits. Net price 250-mL carton = £2.37

All for use as the sole source of nutrition or as a nutritional supplement prescribed on medical grounds for: short-bowel syndrome, intractable malabsorption, proven inflammatory bowel disease, bowel fistulas. Not to be prescribed for any child under 1 year; use with caution for children up to 5 years

Emsogen® (SHS)

Powder, amino acids 15%, carbohydrate 60%, fat 16.4%, energy 1839 kJ (438 kcal)/100 g, with vitamins, minerals, and trace elements. For preparation with water before use. Net price 100 g = £4.44; also available orange-flavoured (carbohydrate 55%, energy 1754 kJ (418 kcal)/100 g), 100 g = £4.20. For use as the sole source of nutrition or as a nutritional supplement prescribed on medical grounds for short-bowel syndrome, intractable malabsorption, proven inflammatory bowel disease, bowel fistulas. Not to be prescribed for any child under 1 year; use with caution for children up to 5 years

Ener-G® (General Dietary)

Gluten-free. Rice bread (sliced), brown, net price 474 g = £3.75; white, 456 g = £3.75. Rice loaf, 612 g = £3.75. Brown rice and maize bread, 742 g = £3.75. Tapioca bread (sliced), 480 g = £3.75. Rice pasta (macaroni, shells, small shells, and lasagne), 454 g = £3.45; spaghetti, 447 g = £3.45; tagliatelle, 400 g = £3.45; vermicelli, 300 g = £3.45; cannelloni, 284 g = £3.45. Brown rice pasta: lasagne, 454 g = £3.45; macaroni, 454 g = £3.45; spaghetti, 447 g = £3.45. For gluten-sensitive enteropathies including steatorrhoea due to gluten sensitivity, coeliac disease, and dermatitis herpetiformis

Low protein egg replacer, carbohydrate 94 g, energy 1574 kJ (376 kcal)/100 g. Egg-, gluten- and lactose-free. Net price 454 g = £3.00. For phenylketonuria, similar amino acid abnormalities, renal failure, liver failure and liver cirrhosis.

Enfamil® (Mead Johnson)

Lactofree, powder, protein 11.9 g, fat 28 g, carbohydrate 56 g, energy 2176 kJ (520 kcal)/100g with vitamins, minerals and trace elements. Lactose- and sucrose-free. Net price 400 g = £3.22. For proven lactose intolerance

Enlive® (Abbott)

Liquid, protein 9.6 g, carbohydrate 65.4 g, energy 1274 kJ (300 kcal)/240 mL, with vitamins, minerals and trace elements. Fat- and gluten-free; clinically lactose-free. Flavours: apple, fruit punch, grapefruit, lemon and lime, orange, peach, pineapple, strawberry. Net price 240-mL Tetrapak® = £1.60. For use as a nutritional supplement prescribed on medical grounds: for short-bowel syndrome, intractable malabsorption, pre-operative preparation of patients who are undernourished, proven inflammatory bowel disease, following total gastrectomy, dysphagia, bowel fistulas, disease-related malnutrition. Not to be prescribed for any child under 1 year; use with caution for children up to 5 years

Enrich® (Abbott)

Liquid with dietary fibre, providing protein 9.4 g, carbohydrate 34.9 g, fat 8.8 g, fibre 3.4 g, energy 1079 kJ (256 kcal)/250 mL with vitamins and minerals. Lactose- and gluten-free. Vanilla and chocolate flavours. Net price 250-mL can = £2.14. For use as the sole source of nutrition or as a nutritional supplement prescribed on medical grounds for: short-bowel syndrome, intractable malabsorption, pre-operative preparation of patients who are undernourished, proven inflammatory bowel disease, following total gastrectomy, dysphagia, disease-related malnutrition. Not to be prescribed for any child under 1 year; use with caution for children up to 5 years

Ensure® (Abbott)

Liquid, protein 10.0 g, fat 8.4 g, carbohydrate 33.9 g, energy 1057 kJ (251 kcal)/250 mL with minerals and vitamins, lactose- and gluten-free. Vanilla, chocolate, coffee, eggnog, nut, chicken, mushroom, and asparagus flavours. Net price 250-mL can = £1.82

Powder, same composition as Ensure liquid when reconstituted. Vanilla flavour. Net price 400 g = £11.06
Both for use as the sole source of nutrition or as a nutritional supplement prescribed on medical grounds for: short-bowel syndrome, intractable malabsorption, pre-operative preparation of patients who are undernourished, proven inflammatory bowel disease, following total gastrectomy, dysphagia, bowel fistulas, disease-related malnutrition. Neither to be prescribed for any child under 1 year; use with caution for children up to 5 years

Ensure Plus® (Abbott)

Liquid, protein 12.5 g, fat 10.0 g, carbohydrate 40.0 g, with vitamins and minerals, lactose- and gluten-free, energy 1260 kJ (300 kcal)/200 mL. Vanilla flavour. Net price 250-mL can = £1.99; 500-mL ready-to-hang = £3.81; 1-litre ready-to-hang = £7.63; 1.5-litre ready-to-hang = £11.44. Caramel, chocolate, strawberry, banana, fruit of the forest, raspberry, orange, coffee, black currant, peach, vanilla or neutral flavours. Net price 200-mL Tetrapak® = £1.53. As a nutritional supplement prescribed on medical grounds for: short-bowel syndrome, intractable malabsorption, pre-operative preparation of patients who are undernourished, proven inflammatory bowel disease, following total gastrectomy, dysphagia, bowel fistulas, disease-related malnutrition, continuous ambulatory peritoneal dialysis (CAPD), and haemodialysis. Not to be prescribed for any child under 1 year; use with caution for children up to 5 years

Entera® (Fresenius)

Fibre Plus, protein 11.3 g, carbohydrate 37.6 g, fat 11.6 g, fibre 5 g, energy 1260 kJ (300 kcal)/ 200 mL, with vitamins, minerals and trace elements. Gluten-free; clinically lactose-free. Flavours: banana, cappucino, chocolate, lemon, strawberry, vanilla. Net price 200-mL carton = £1.65. For indications see *Entera Liquid*. Not to be prescribed for any child under 1 year; use with caution for children under 5 years.

Liquid, protein 11.3 g, carbohydrate 37.6 g, fat 11.66 g, energy 1260 kJ (300 kcal)/200 mL, with vitamins and minerals. Net price 200-mL carton = £1.50 (flavours: vanilla, strawberry, butterscotch, black currant, banana, orange, pineapple, chocolate-mint, vegetable cream, and neutral): 500-mL bottle = £3.60 (flavour: neutral); 500-mL EasyBag® = £3.65; 1-litre EasyBag® = £7.30. For use as sole source of nutrition or as a nutritional supplement prescribed on medical grounds for: short-bowel syndrome, intractable malabsorption, pre-operative preparation of patients who are undernourished, proven inflammatory bowel disease, following total gastrectomy, dysphagia, bowel fistulas, disease-related malnutrition. Not to be prescribed for any child under 1 year; use with caution for children under 5 years

Farley's Soya Formula (Farley)

Powder, providing protein 2%, carbohydrate 7%, fat 3.8% with vitamins and minerals when reconstituted. Gluten-, sucrose-, and lactose-free. Net price 450 g = £3.79. For proven lactose and associated sucrose intolerance in pre-school children, galactokinase deficiency, galactosaemia, and cow's milk protein intolerance

Flavour Sachets (SHS)

Powder, flavours: cherry-vanilla, grapefruit, lemon-lime, net price 20 x 5-g sachets = £7.15. For use with SHS unflavoured amino acid and peptide products

Formance® (Abbott)

Semi-solid, protein 4 g, carbohydrate 27 g, fat 5 g, energy 711 kJ (170 kcal)/113 g with vitamins and minerals. Gluten-free. Vanilla, chocolate, and butterscotch flavours. Net price 113-g pot = £1.34. As a nutritional supplement prescribed on medical grounds for: short-bowel syndrome, intractable malabsorption, pre-operative preparation of patients who are undernourished, proven inflammatory bowel disease, following total gastrectomy, dysphagia, bowel fistulas, disease-related malnutrition, continuous ambulatory peritoneal dialysis (CAPD), and haemodialysis. Not to be prescribed for any child under 1 year; use with caution for children up to 5 years

Fortifresh® (Nutricia Clinical)

Liquid, protein 13 g, carbohydrate 42.2 g, fat 10 g, energy 1308 kJ (310 kcal)/200 mL with vitamins, minerals and trace elements. Contains porcine gelatin. Gluten-free. Flavours: black currant, mandarin, and raspberry. Net price 200 mL carton = £1.50. For use as a nutritional supplement prescribed on medical grounds for: intractable malabsorption, pre-operative preparation of patients who are undernourished, inflammatory bowel disease, dysphagia, disease-related malnutrition. Not to be prescribed for any child under 1 year; use with caution for children up to 5 years

Fortijuce® (Nutricia Clinical)

Liquid, protein 8 g, carbohydrate 56.8 g, energy 1046 kJ (250 kcal)/200 mL, with vitamins, minerals and trace elements. Fat-free. Flavours: apricot, black currant, dandelion and burdock, lemon and lime, peach and orange, pineapple, summer fruit. Net price 200-mL carton = £1.50. As a nutritional supplement prescribed on medical grounds for: short-bowel syndrome, intractable malabsorption, pre-operative preparation of patients who are undernourished, proven inflammatory bowel disease, following total gastrectomy, dysphagia, bowel fistulas, disease-related malnutrition. Not to be prescribed for any child under 1 year; use with caution for children up to 5 years

Fortimel® (Nutricia Clinical)

Liquid, protein 19.4 g, carbohydrate 20.8 g, fat 4.2 g, energy 840 kJ (200 kcal)/200 mL with vitamins and minerals. Vanilla, strawberry, and forest fruits flavours. Net price 200-mL carton = £1.23. As a nutritional supplement prescribed on medical grounds for: short-bowel syndrome, intractable malabsorption, pre-operative preparation of patients who are undernourished, proven inflammatory bowel disease, following total gastrectomy, dysphagia, bowel fistulas, disease-related malnutrition. Not to be prescribed for any child under 1 year; use with caution for children up to 5 years

Fortipudding® (Nutricia Clinical)

Semi-solid, protein 15.3 g, carbohydrate 24 g, fat 4.5 g, energy 840 kJ (198 kcal)/150 g with vitamins and minerals. Vanilla, chocolate, and coffee flavours. Net price 150-g tub = £1.40. As a nutritional supplement prescribed on medical grounds for: short-bowel syndrome, intractable malabsorption, pre-operative preparation of patients who are undernourished, proven inflammatory bowel disease, following total gastrectomy, dysphagia, bowel fistulas, disease-related malnutrition, continuous ambulatory peritoneal dialysis (CAPD) and haemodialysis. Not to be prescribed for any child under 1 year; use with caution for children up to 5 years

Fortisip® (Nutricia Clinical)

Liquid, protein 10 g, carbohydrate 36 g, fat 13 g, energy 1270 kJ (300 kcal)/200 mL, with vitamins, minerals and trace elements. Gluten-free; clinically lactose-free. Vanilla, banana, chocolate, orange, strawberry, tropical fruits, toffee, chicken, mushroom, and neutral flavours. Net price 200 mL = £1.50. As a nutritional supplement prescribed on medical grounds for: short-bowel syndrome, intractable malabsorption, pre-operative preparation of patients who are undernourished, proven inflammatory bowel disease, following total gastrectomy, dysphagia, bowel fistulas, disease-related malnutrition. Not to be prescribed for any child under 1 year; use with caution for children up to 5 years

Fortisip® Multi Fibre (Nutricia Clinical)

Liquid, protein 10 g, carbohydrate 36 g, fat 13 g, fibre 4.5 g, energy 1260 kJ (300 kcal)/200 mL, with vitamins, minerals and trace elements. Gluten-free, clinically lactose-free. Orange, strawberry, vanilla flavours. Net price 200 mL = £1.55. As a nutritional supplement prescribed on medical grounds for: short-bowel syndrome, intractable malabsorption, pre-operative preparation of undernourished patients, proven inflammatory bowel disease, following total gastrectomy, dysphagia, disease-related malnutrition. Not to be prescribed for any child under 1 year; use with caution for children up to 5 years

Frebini® (Fresenius)

Liquid, protein 5 g, carbohydrate 27 g, fat 8 g, energy 840 kJ (200 kcal)/200 mL, with vitamins, minerals and trace elements. Flavour: neutral. Net price 200-mL bottle = £1.80. For use as the sole source of nutrition or as a nutritional supplement prescribed on medical grounds for short-bowel syndrome, intractable malabsorption, pre-operative preparation of patients who are undernourished, proven inflammatory bowel disease, following total gastrectomy, dysphagia, bowel fistulas, disease-related malnutrition and/or growth failure. Not to be prescribed for any child under 1 year

Fresenius OPD® *see Survimed OPD®*

Fresubin® (Fresenius)

Liquid, protein 7.6 g, carbohydrate 27.6 g, fat 6.8 g, energy 840 kJ (200 kcal)/200 mL with vitamins and minerals. Gluten-free, low lactose and cholesterol. Net price 200-mL carton (nut, peach, black currant, chocolate, mocha, and vanilla flavours) = £1.40; 500-mL bottle (nut, peach and neutral flavours) = £2.85; 500-mL EasyBag® = £2.90; 1-litre EasyBag® = £5.80. For use as the sole source of nutrition or as a nutritional supplement prescribed on medical grounds for: short-bowel syndrome, intractable malabsorption, pre-operative preparation of patients who are undernourished, proven inflammatory bowel disease, following total gastrectomy, dysphagia, bowel fistulas, disease-related malnutrition, and Refsum's disease. Not to be prescribed for any child under 1 year; use with caution for children up to 5 years

Fresubin 750 MCT® (Fresenius)

Liquid, protein 37.5 g, carbohydrate 85 g, fat 30 g, energy 3150 kJ (750 kcal)/500 mL with vitamins, minerals, and trace elements. Gluten-free and low lactose. Vanilla flavour. Net price 500-mL bottle = £3.50; 500-mL EasyBag® = £3.55. As a nutritional supplement prescribed on medical grounds for: short-bowel syndrome, intractable malabsorption, pre-operative preparation of patients who are undernourished, proven inflammatory bowel disease, following total gastrectomy, dysphagia, bowel fistulas, disease-related malnutrition, continuous ambulatory peritoneal dialysis (CAPD), and haemodialysis. Not to be prescribed for any child under 1 year; use with caution for children up to 5 years

Fresubin Isofibre® (Fresenius)

Liquid with dietary fibre, protein 19 g, carbohydrate 69 g, fat 17 g, energy 2100 kJ (500 kcal)/500 mL, with vitamins and minerals. Flavour: neutral. Net price 500-mL bottle = £3.30; 500-mL EasyBag® = £3.35; 1-litre EasyBag® = £6.70. For use as sole source of nutrition or as a nutritional supplement prescribed on medical grounds for: short-bowel syndrome, intractable malabsorption, pre-operative preparation of patients who are undernourished, proven inflammatory bowel disease, following total gastrectomy, dysphagia, disease-related malnutrition. Not to be prescribed for any child under 2 years; use with caution for children up to 5 years

Fructose (laevulose). For proven glucose/galactose intolerance

Galactomin® (SHS)

Formula 17, powder, protein 14.5 g, fat 25.9 g, carbohydrate 56.9 g, mineral salts 3.4 g/100 g. Used as a 13.1% solution with additional vitamins in place of milk. Net price 400 g = £9.76. For proven lactose intolerance in preschool children, galactosaemia and galactokinase deficiency

Formula 19, powder, protein 14.6 g, fat 30.8 g, carbohydrate 49.7 g (fructose as carbohydrate source), mineral salts 2.1 g/100 g, with vitamins. Used as a 12.9% solution in place of milk. Net price 400 g = £25.72. For glucose plus galactose intolerance

Generaid® (SHS)

Powder, whey protein and additional branched-chain amino acids (protein equivalent 81%). Net price 200 g (unflavoured) = £20.39. See also Flavour Sachets. For patients with chronic liver disease and/or porto-hepatic encephalopathy

Plus Powder, whey protein and additional branched-chain amino acids (protein equivalent 11%) carbohydrate 62%, fat 19% with vitamins, minerals and trace elements. Net price 400 g = £14.16. For children over 1 year with hepatic disorders

Glucose (dextrose monohydrate). Net price 100 g = 18p. For glycogen storage disease and sucrose/isomaltose intolerance

Glutafin® (Nutricia Dietary)

Gluten-free. White loaf (sliced or unsliced), net price 400 g = £2.38; part-baked, 400 g = £2.67. Multigrain white loaf (sliced or unsliced), 400 g = £2.67. Fibre loaf (sliced or unsliced), 400 g = £2.38; part-baked, 400 g = £2.67. Fibre rolls (part-baked), 4 = £2.67; long, 2 = £2.67. Multigrain fibre loaf (sliced or unsliced), 400 g = £2.67. White rolls, 4 = £2.67; part-baked, 4 = £2.67; part-baked, long, 2 = £2.67. Multigrain fibre rolls, 4 = £2.67. Mixes (white, multigrain white, fibre and multigrain fibre), 500 g = £4.83. Biscuits, savoury, 125 g = £1.48. Biscuits, digestive, sweet or tea, 150 g = £1.48. Biscuits, 200 g = £3.21. Cake mix, 500 g = £4.83. Crackers, 200 g = £2.41. High fibre crackers, 200 g = £2.02. Pasta (penne, shells, spirals, spaghetti), 500 g = £4.88; (lasagne, tagliatelle), 250 g = £2.56. Pizza bases, 2 × 110 g = £3.34. For gluten-sensitive enteropathies including steatorrhoea due to gluten sensitivity, coeliac disease, and dermatitis herpetiformis

Glutano® (Gluten Free Foods Ltd)

Gluten-free. Biscuits, net price 125 g = £1.58. Crackers, 150 g = £1.58. Flour mix, 750 g = £4.12. Pasta (animal shapes, macaroni, spaghetti, spirals, tagliatelle), 250 g = £1.58. White sliced bread (par-baked), 300 g = £1.86. Wholemeal bread (sliced or par-baked), 500 g = £2.24. Baguette or rolls (par-baked), 200 g = £1.49. For gluten-sensitive enteropathies including steatorrhoea due to gluten sensitivity, coeliac disease, and dermatitis herpetiformis

Hycal® (SmithKline Beecham Healthcare)

Liquid, protein-free, low-electrolyte, glucose syrup solids 49.5%. Flavours: black currant, lemon, orange, and raspberry. Net price 171 mL = 73p. For disease-related malnutrition, malabsorption states or other conditions requiring fortification with high or readily available carbohydrate supplement

InfaSoy® (Cow & Gate)

Powder, carbohydrate 7.1%, fat 3.6%, and protein 1.8% with vitamins and minerals when used as a 12.7% solution. Net price 450 g = £3.77; 900 g = £7.23. For proven lactose and associated sucrose intolerance in preschool children, galactokinase deficiency, galactosaemia, and proven whole cow's milk sensitivity

Infatrini® (Nutricia Clinical)

Liquid, protein 2.6 g, carbohydrate 10.4 g, fat 5.4 g, energy 420 kJ (100 kcal)/100 mL with vitamins, minerals and trace elements. Gluten-free. Net price 100 mL = 85p. For use as a sole source of nutrition or as a nutritional supplement prescribed on medical grounds for: failure to thrive, disease-related malnutrition and malabsorption.

Instant Carobel® see Carobel, Instant®

Isomil® (Abbott)

Powder, protein 1.8%, carbohydrate 6.9%, fat 3.7% with vitamins and minerals when reconstituted. Lactose-free. Net price 400 g = £3.38. For proven lactose intolerance in preschool children, galactokinase deficiency, galactosaemia, and proven whole cow's milk sensitivity

Jevity® (Abbott)

Liquid, protein 4 g, fat 3.5 g, carbohydrate 14.8 g, dietary fibre 1.1 g, energy 441 kJ (106 kcal)/100 mL, with vitamins and minerals. Gluten-, lactose-, and sucrose-free. Net price 500-mL ready-to-hang = £3.31, 1-litre ready-to-hang = £6.62, 1.5-litre ready-to-hang = £9.93. For use as the sole source of nutrition or as a nutritional supplement prescribed on medical grounds for: short-bowel syndrome, intractable malabsorption, pre-operative preparation of patients who are undernourished, proven inflammatory bowel disease, bowel fistulas, following total gastrectomy, dysphagia, disease-related malnutrition. Not to be prescribed for any child under 1 year; use with caution for children up to 5 years

Plus liquid, protein 5.6 g, carbohydrate 16.1 g, fat 3.9 g, dietary fibre 1.2 g, energy 504 kJ (120 kcal)/100 mL, with vitamins and minerals. Gluten- and lactose-free. Net price 500-mL ready-to-hang = £3.88, 1-litre ready-to-hang = £7.94, 1.5-litre ready-to-hang = £11.92. For indications see under *Jevity®*. Not to be prescribed for any child under 10 years

Juvela® (SHS)

Gluten-free. Harvest mix, fibre mix, and flour mix, net price 500 g = £4.83. Bread (whole or sliced), 400-g loaf = £2.34. Fibre bread (sliced and unsliced), 400-g loaf = £2.34. Bread rolls, 6 × 5 = £18.84, fibre bread rolls, 6 × 5 = £18.84, part-baked rolls (with or without fibre), 6 × 5 = £19.68. Crispbread, 210 g = £3.04. Digestive biscuits, 160 g = £1.91. Pizza bases, 2 × 180 g = £5.94. Savoury biscuits, 110 g = £1.79. Tea biscuits, 160 g = £1.91. For gluten-sensitive enteropathies including steatorrhoea due to gluten sensitivity, coeliac disease, and dermatitis herpetiformis

Low Protein. Mix, net price 500 g = £5.00. Bread (whole or sliced), 400-g loaf = £2.32. Bread rolls, 6 × 5 rolls = £17.46. Biscuits, orange and cinnamon flavour, 150 g = £4.66; chocolate chip, 130 g = £4.89. For inherited metabolic disorders, renal or liver failure requiring a low-protein diet

Kindergen PROD® (SHS)

Powder, protein 7.5 g, carbohydrate 60.5 g, fat 26.1 g, energy 2060 kJ (492 kcal)/100 g with vitamins and minerals. Net price 400 g = £16.72. For complete nutritional support or supplementary feeding for infants and children with chronic renal failure who are receiving peritoneal rapid overnight dialysis

Leucine-Free Amino Acid Mix *see* Amino Acid Modules

Lifestyle® (Ultrapharm)

Gluten-free. Brown bread (sliced and unsliced), net price 400 g = £2.28. White bread (sliced and unsliced), 400 g = £2.28. High fibre bread (unsliced), 400 g = £2.38. Bread rolls, 400 g = £2.38. For gluten-sensitive enteropathies including steatorrhoea due to gluten sensitivity, coeliac disease, and dermatitis herpetiformis

Liga® (Jacobs)

Rusks, gluten-free, low sugar. Net price 6 = 88p. For gluten-sensitive enteropathies including steatorrhoea due to gluten sensitivity, coeliac disease, and dermatitis herpetiformis

Liquigen® (SHS)

Emulsion, medium chain triglycerides 52%. Net price 250 mL = £5.75; 1 litre = £23.39. For steatorrhoea associated with cystic fibrosis of the pancreas; intestinal lymphangiectasia, surgery of the intestine; chronic liver disease and liver cirrhosis; other proven malabsorption syndromes; ketogenic diet in the management of epilepsy; type I hyperlipoproteinaemia

Locasol® (SHS)

Powder, protein 14.6 g, carbohydrate 56.5 g, fat 26.1 g, mineral salts 1.9 g, not more than 55 mg of Ca^{2+}/100 g and vitamins. Used as a 13.1% solution in place of milk. Net price 400 g = £13.58. For calcium intolerance

Lofenalac® (Bristol-Myers)

Powder, protein 15%, carbohydrate 60%, fat 18%, phenylalanine not more than 0.1% with vitamins and minerals. Gluten-, sucrose-, and lactose-free. Net price 450 g = £11.61. For phenylketonuria

Loprofin® (SHS)

Low protein. Sweet biscuits, net price 150 g = £1.58; chocolate cream-filled biscuits, 125 g = £1.58; cookies (chocolate chip or cinnamon), 100 g = £4.70; wafers (orange, vanilla, or chocolate), 100 g = £1.52. Breakfast cereal, 375 g = £5.10. Egg replacer, 250 g = £4.55. Bread (sliced or whole), 400-g loaf = £2.34. Bread (white, with or without salt), 227 g = £1.60. Rolls (part-baked) 4 × 65 g = £2.59. Mix, 500 g = £4.98. Crackers, 150 g = £2.14. Pasta (macaroni, pasta spirals, spaghetti), 500 g = £5.44. Pasta (vermicelli), 250 g = £2.59. For inherited metabolic disorders, renal or liver failure requiring a low-protein diet

PKU Drink, protein 0.4 g (phenylalanine 10 mg), lactose 9.4 g, fat 2 g, energy 165 kJ (40 kcal)/100 mL. Net price 200-mL Tetrapak® = 50p. For phenylketonuria

Low protein drink (Milupa)

Powder, protein 0.4%, carbohydrate 5.1%, fat 2% when reconstituted. Net price 400 g = £7.23. For inherited disorders of amino acid metabolism in childhood

Note. Termed *Milupa® lpd* by manufacturer

Maxamaid® (SHS)

Note. Maxamaid products are generally intended for use in children aged 1 to 8 years, see also Flavour Sachets, for use with unflavoured amino acid and peptide products from SHS

MSUD Maxamaid, powder, essential and non-essential amino acids 30% except isoleucine, leucine, and valine, with carbohydrate, fat less than 0.5%, vitamins, minerals, and trace elements. Net price 500 g = £57.06. For maple syrup urine disease

XLeu Maxamaid, powder, essential and non-essential amino acids 28.6% except leucine, with carbohydrate, fat less than 0.5%, vitamins, minerals, and trace elements. Net price 500 g = £57.06. For isovaleric acidaemia

XLys Maxamaid, powder, essential and non-essential amino acids 30% except lysine, with carbohydrate, fat less than 0.5%, vitamins, minerals, and trace elements. Net price 500 g = £57.06. For hyperlysinaemia

XLys, Low Try, Maxamaid, powder, essential and non-essential amino acids 30% except lysine, with carbohydrate, fat less than 0.5%, vitamins, minerals, and trace elements. Net price 500 g = £57.06. For type 1 glutaric aciduria

XMet Maxamaid, powder, essential and non-essential amino acids 30% except methionine, with carbohydrate, fat less than 0.5%, vitamins, minerals, and trace elements. Net price 500 g = £57.06. For hypermethioninaemia, homocystinuria

XMet, Thre, Val, Isoleu Maxamaid, powder, essential and non-essential amino acids 30% except methionine, threonine, valine and low isoleucine, with carbohydrate, fat less than 0.5%, vitamins, minerals, and trace elements. Net price 500 g = £57.06. For methylmalonic acidaemia or propionic acidaemia

XP Maxamaid, essential and non-essential amino acids 30% except phenylalanine, with carbohydrate, vitamins, minerals, and trace elements. Net price powder (unflavoured), 500 g = £35.28; (orange-flavoured), 500 g = £35.28. For phenylketonuria. Not to be prescribed for children under 2 years

XP Maxamaid Concentrate, powder, essential and non-essential amino acids 65% except phenylalanine, with carbohydrate, fat less than 0.5%, vitamins, minerals, and trace elements. Unflavoured. Net price 500 g = £99.15. For phenylketonuria. Not to be prescribed for children under 2 years

XPhen, Tyr Maxamaid, powder, essential and non-essential amino acids 30% except phenylalanine and tyrosine, with carbohydrate, fat less than 0.5%, vitamins, minerals, and trace elements. Unflavoured. Net price 500 g = £57.06. For tyrosinaemia

Maxamum® (SHS)

Note. Maxamum products are generally intended for use in children aged over 8 years

MSUD Maxamum, powder, essential and non-essential amino acids 47% except isoleucine, leucine, and valine, with carbohydrate, fat less than 0.5%, vitamins, minerals, and trace elements. Flavours: orange, unflavoured, see also Flavour Sachets. Net price 500 g = £91.47. For maple syrup urine disease

XMet Maxamum, powder, essential and non-essential amino acids 47% except methionine, with carbohydrate, fat less than 0.5%, vitamins, minerals, and trace elements. Unflavoured, see also Flavour Sachets. Net price 500 g = £91.47. For hypermethioninaemia, homocystinuria

XMet, Thre, Val, Isoleu Maxamum, powder, essential and non-essential amino acids 47% except methionine, threonine, valine and low isoleucine, with carbohydrate, fat less than 0.5%, vitamins, minerals, and trace elements. Unflavoured, see also Flavour Sachets. Net price 500 g = £91.47. For methylmalonic acidaemia or propionic acidaemia

XP Maxamum, powder, essential and non-essential amino acids 47% except phenylalanine, with carbohydrates, vitamins, minerals, and trace elements. Flavours: orange, unflavoured, see also Flavour Sachets. Net price 500 g = £54.52. For phenylketonuria. Not to be prescribed for children under 8 years

Maxijul® (SHS)

Liquid, carbohydrate 50%, with potassium 0.004%, sodium 0.023%. Gluten-, lactose-, and fructose-free. Flavours: black currant, lemon and lime, orange, and natural. Net price 200 mL =90p

LE Powder, modification of *Maxijul®* with lower concentrations of sodium and potassium. Net price 200 g = £3.22, 2 kg = £22.44

Super Soluble Powder, glucose polymer, potassium 0.004%, sodium 0.046%. Gluten-, lactose-, and fructose-free. Net price 4 × 132-g sachet pack = £3.37, 200 g = £1.60, 2.5 kg = £13.71

All for disease-related malnutrition; malabsorption states or other conditions requiring fortification with high or readily available carbohydrate supplement

Maxipro Super Soluble® (SHS)

Powder, whey protein and additional amino acids (protein equivalent 80%). Net price 200 g = £6.89; 1 kg = £27.57. For biochemically proven hypoproteinaemia. Not to be prescribed for any child under 1 year; unsuitable as a sole source of nutrition

Maxisorb® (SHS)

Powder, protein 12 g, carbohydrate 9 g, fat 6 g, energy 579 kJ (138 kcal)/30 g with minerals. Vanilla, strawberry and chocolate flavours. Net price 5 × 30-g sachets = £2.96. For biochemically proven hypoproteinaemia. Not to be prescribed for any child under 1 year; use with caution for children up to 5 years

MCT Oil

Triglycerides from medium chain fatty acids. For steatorrhoea associated with cystic fibrosis of the pancreas; intestinal lymphangiectasia; surgery of the intestine; chronic liver disease and liver cirrhosis; other proven malabsorption syndromes; in a ketogenic diet in the management of epilepsy; in type I hyperlipoproteinaemia

Available from Bristol-Myers (net price 950 mL = £12.18); SHS (net price 500 mL = £8.27)

MCT Pepdite® (SHS)

Powder, essential and non-essential amino acids, peptides, medium chain triglycerides, monoglyceride of sunflower oil, with carbohydrate, fat, vitamins, minerals, and trace elements. Flavour Sachets available.

MCT Pepdite 0–2. Net price 400 g = £12.00

MCT Pepdite 2+. Net price 400 g = £12.00

Both for disorders in which a high intake of medium chain triglyceride is beneficial

Metabolic Mineral Mixture® (SHS)

Powder, essential mineral salts. Net price 100 g = £7.46. For mineral supplementation in synthetic diets

Methionine-Free Amino Acid Mix *see* Amino Acid Modules

Methionine, Threonine, Valine-Free and Isoleucine-Low Amino Acid Mix *see* Amino Acid Modules

Milupa® lpd *see under* Low Protein Drink

Milupa® PKU2 and PKU3 *see under* PKU2 and PKU3

Modulen IBD® (Nestlé)

Powder, protein 18 g, carbohydrate 54 g, fat 23 g, energy 2040 kJ (500 kcal)/100 g with vitamins, minerals and trace elements. Net price 400 g = £9.72. For use as the sole source of nutrition during the active phase of Crohn's disease and for nutritional support during the remission phase in patients who are malnourished. Not to be prescribed for any child under one year; use with caution for young children up to 5 years

Monogen® (SHS)

Powder, protein 11.4 g, carbohydrate 68 g, fat 11.4 g (of which MCT 93%), energy 1772 kJ (420 kcal)/100 g, with vitamins, minerals and trace elements. Net price 400 g = £11.87. For long-chain acyl-CoA dehydrogenase deficiency (LCAD), carnitine palmitoyl transferase deficiency (CPTD), primary and secondary lipoprotin lipase deficiency

MSUD Aid III® (SHS)

Powder, containing full range of amino acids except isoleucine, leucine, and valine, with vitamins, minerals, and trace elements. Net price 500 g = £123.98. For maple syrup urine disease and related conditions where it is necessary to limit the intake of branched chain amino acids

Neocate® (SHS)

Advance, powder, essential and non-essential amino acids, carbohydrate, fat, vitamins, minerals and trace elements. Milk protein-, soy- and lactose-free. Net price 100 g = £3.76. For proven whole protein intolerance, short-bowel syndrome, intractable malabsorption, and other gastrointestinal disorders where an elemental diet is specifically indicated

Powder, essential and non-essential amino acids, maltodextrin, fat, vitamins, minerals, and trace elements. Net price 400 g = £18.28. For proven whole protein intolerance, short-bowel syndrome, intractable malabsorption, and other gastrointestinal disorders where an elemental diet is specifically indicated

Nepro® (Abbott)

Liquid, protein 16.6 g, carbohydrate 60.2 g, fat 26 g, energy 1988 kJ (474 kcal)/237 mL with vitamins and minerals. Net price 237-mL can = £2.28. For patients with chronic renal failure who are on haemodialysis or continuous ambulatory peritoneal dialysis (CAPD), or patients with cirrhosis or other conditions requiring a high energy, low fluid, low electrolyte diet

Nestargel® (Nestlé)

Powder, carob seed flour 96.5%, calcium lactate 3.5%. Net price 125 g = £3.46. For thickening feeds in the treatment of vomiting

Nutilis® (Nutricia Clinical)

Powder, modified maize starch, gluten- and lactose-free. Net price 225 g = £3.40. For thickening of foods in dysphagia. Not to be prescribed for children under 3 years

Nutramigen® (Bristol-Myers)

Powder, protein 13%, carbohydrate 62%, fat 18% with vitamins and minerals. Gluten-, sucrose-, and lactose-free. Net price 425 g = £7.44. For disaccharide and/or whole protein intolerance where additional medium chain triglyceride is not indicated

Nutrini® (Nutricia Clinical)

Extra, liquid, protein 6.8 g, carbohydrate 37.6 g, fat 13.6 g, energy 1260 kJ (300 kcal)/200 mL. Gluten- and sucrose-free; clinically lactose-free. Net price 200-mL bottle = £2.24, 500-mL collapsible pack = £5.70. For use as the sole source of nutrition or as a nutritional supplement prescribed on medical grounds for: disease-related malnutrition and growth failure

Fibre, liquid, protein 5.5 g, carbohydrate 24.4 g, fat 9 g, fibre 1.5 g, energy 840 kJ (200 kcal)/200 mL. Gluten- and sucrose-free; clinically lactose-free. Net price 200-mL bottle = £1.82, 500-mL collapsible pack = £4.55. For indications see *Nutrini Standard*

Standard, liquid, protein 5.5 g, carbohydrate 24.4 g, fat 9 g, energy 840 kJ (200 kcal)/200 mL. Gluten- and sucrose-free; clinically lactose-free. Net price 200-mL bottle = £1.82, 500-mL collapsible pack = £4.55. For use as the sole source of nutrition or as a nutritional supplement prescribed on medical grounds for: short-bowel syndrome, intractable malabsorption, pre-operative preparation of undernourished patients, dysphagia, bowel fistulas, disease-related malnutrition and/or growth failure. Not to be prescribed for any child under 1 year

Nutrison® (Nutricia Clinical)

Energy, liquid, protein 30 g, carbohydrate 92 g, fat 29 g, energy 3200 kJ (750 kcal)/500 mL with vitamins, minerals and trace elements. Gluten- and sucrose-free; clinically lactose-free. Net price 500 mL = £3.25; 1-litre pack = £6.50. As a nutritional supplement prescribed on medical grounds for: short-bowel syndrome, intractable malabsorption, pre-operative preparation of undernourished patients, proven inflammatory bowel disease, following total gastrectomy, dysphagia, bowel fistulas, disease-related malnutrition. Not to be prescribed for any child under 1 year; use with caution for children up to 5 years

Multi Fibre, liquid, protein 20 g, carbohydrate 61.5 g, fibre 7.5 g, energy 2100 kJ (500 kcal)/500 mL with vitamins, minerals and trace elements. Gluten- and sucrose-free; clinically lactose-free. Net price 500-mL bottle = £3.24; 1-litre pack = £6.28. For indications see *Nutrison Standard* excluding bowel fistulas. Not to be prescribed for any child under 1 year; use with caution for children up to 5 years

Soya, liquid, protein 20 g, carbohydrate 61.5 g, fat 19.5 g, energy 2100 kJ (500 kcal)/500 mL, with vitamins, minerals and trace elements. Gluten- and sucrose-free; clinically lactose-free. Net price 500 mL = £3.00; 1-litre pack = £6.68. For indications see *Nutrison Standard*

Standard, liquid, protein 20 g, carbohydrate 61.5 g, fat 19.5 g, energy 2125 kJ (500 kcal)/500 mL, with vitamins, minerals and trace elements. Gluten- and sucrose-free; clinically lactose-free. Net price 500 mL = £2.87; 1-litre pack = £5.74. For use as the sole source of nutrition or as a nutritional supplement prescribed on medical grounds for: short-bowel syndrome, intractable malabsorption, pre-operative preparation of undernourished patients, proven inflammatory bowel disease, following total gastrectomy, dysphagia, bowel fistulas, disease-related malnutrition. Not to be prescribed for any child under 1 year; use with caution for children up to 5 years

Nutrison MCT® (Nutricia Clinical)

Liquid, protein 25 g, carbohydrate 61.5 g, fat 16.5 g, energy 2095 kJ (500 kcal)/500 mL with vitamins, minerals and trace elements. Gluten- and fructose-free, low lactose. Vanilla flavour. Net price 500 mL = £2.94; 1-litre pack = £5.60. For indications see *Nutrison Energy*. Not to be prescribed for any child under 1 year; use with caution for children up to 5 years

Nutrison Pepti® (Nutricia Clinical)

Liquid, protein 20 g, fat 5 g, carbohydrate 94 g, energy 2100 kJ (500 kcal)/500 mL with vitamins, minerals and trace elements. Gluten-free. Net price 500 mL = £4.06; 1-litre pack = £8.61. For use as the sole source of nutrition or as a nutritional supplement prescribed on medical grounds for: short-bowel syndrome, intractable malabsorption, proven inflammatory bowel disease, bowel fistulas. Not to be prescribed for any child under 1 year; use with caution for children up to 5 years

Powder, protein 18 g, fat 5 g, carbohydrate 93 g, energy 2073 kJ (489 kcal)/500 mL when reconstituted, with vitamins and minerals. Net price 126-g sachet = £4.60. For use as a nutritional supplement prescribed on medical grounds for: short bowel syndrome, intractable malabsorption, proven inflammatory bowel disease, bowel fistulas. Not to be prescribed for any child under 1 year; use with caution for children under 5 years

Nutrodrip® (Novartis Consumer Health)

Energy, liquid, protein 28.5 g, carbohydrate 100 g, fat 31 g, energy 3300 kJ (800 kcal)/500 mL with vitamins, minerals and trace elements. Gluten-free; clinically lactose-free. Net price 500-mL bottle = £3.05, 500-mL flexible pouch = £3.05. For indications see *Nutrodrip Standard*

Fibre, liquid, protein 19 g, carbohydrate 68 g, fat 17 g, fibre 7 g, energy 2110 kJ (500 kcal)/500 mL with vitamins, minerals and trace elements. Gluten-free; clinically lactose-free. Net price 500-mL bottle = £2.90, 500-mL flexible pouch = £2.90, 1.5-litre flexible pouch = £8.70. For indications see *Nutrodrip Standard*

Standard, liquid, protein 20.5 g, carbohydrate 71 g, fat 17.5 g, energy 2205 kJ (525 kcal)/500 mL with vitamins minerals and trace elements. Gluten-free; clinically lactose-free. Net price 500-mL bottle = £2.60, 500-mL flexible pouch = £2.60, 1.5-litre flexible pouch = £7.80. For use as a sole source of nutrition or as a nutritional supplement prescribed on medical grounds for: short-bowel syndrome, intractable malabsorption, pre-operative preparation of undernourished patients, proven inflammatory bowel disease, following total gastrectomy, dysphagia, bowel fistulas, disease-related malnutrition. Not to be prescribed for any child under 1 year; use with caution for children up to 5 years

Osmolite® (Abbott)

Liquid, protein 10.0 g, carbohydrate 33.9 g, fat 8.5 g, energy 1060 kJ (252 kcal)/250 mL with vitamins and minerals. Gluten- and lactose-free. Net price 250-mL can = £1.51; 500-mL bottle = £2.91, 1-litre bottle = £5.82, 1.5-litre bottle = £8.73. For use as the sole source of nutrition or as a nutritional supplement prescribed on medical grounds for: short-bowel syndrome, intractable malabsorption, pre-operative preparation of undernourished patients, proven inflammatory bowel disease, following total gastrectomy, bowel fistulas, disease-related malnutrition, dysphagia. Not to be prescribed for any child under 1 year; use with caution for children up to 5 years

Plus, liquid, protein 5.6 g, carbohydrate 15.8 g, fat 3.9 g, energy 508 kJ (121 kcal)/100 mL, with vitamins, minerals and trace elements. Gluten-free and clinically lactose-free. Net price 500-mL ready-to-hang = £3.50, 1-litre ready-to-hang = £6.99, 1.5-litre ready-to-hang = 10.48. For indications see *Osmolite Liquid*.

Paediasure® (Abbott)

Liquid, protein 7 g, carbohydrate 27.9 g, fat 12.5 g, energy 1054 kJ (252 kcal)/250 mL with vitamins and minerals. Gluten-free, clinically lactose-free. Flavours: vanilla (can, ready-to-hang and tetrapaks), strawberry, chocolate and banana (tetrapaks). Net price 250-mL can = £2.26, 500-mL ready-to-hang = £4.52, 200-mL tetrapaks = £1.81. For use as the sole source of nutrition or as a nutritional supplement prescribed on medical grounds for: short-bowel syndrome, intractable malabsorption, pre-operative preparation of undernourished patients, dysphagia, bowel fistulas, and disease-related malnutrition and/or growth failure. Not to be prescribed for any child under 1 year

Liquid with fibre, protein 7 g, carbohydrate 27.9 g, fat 12.5 g, fibre 1.3 g, energy 1054 kJ (252 kcal)/250 mL with vitamins and minerals. Gluten-free, clinically lactose-free. Flavour: vanilla. Net price 250-mL can = £2.57. For indications see *Paediasure Liquid*

Paediatric Seravit® (SHS)

Powder, vitamins, minerals, low sodium and potassium, and trace elements. Net price 200 g (unflavoured) = £10.50; pineapple flavour, 200 g = £11.19. For vitamin and mineral supplementation in restrictive therapeutic diets in infants and children

Pepdite® (SHS)

Powder, peptides, essential and non-essential amino acids, with carbohydrate, fat, vitamins, minerals, and trace elements. Flavour Sachets available.

Pepdite 0–2. Providing 1925 kJ (472 kcal)/100 g. Net price 400 g = £11.80

Pepdite 2+. Providing 1787 kJ (439 kcal)/100 g. Net price 400 g = £11.80

Both for disaccharide and/or whole protein intolerance, or where amino acids or peptides are indicated in conjunction with medium chain triglycerides

Peptamen® (Nestlé Clinical)

Liquid, protein 4 g, carbohydrate 12.7 g, fat 3.7 g, energy 420 kJ (100 kcal)/100 mL, with vitamins, minerals and trace elements. Lactose- and gluten-free. Flavours: unflavoured (can), vanilla (cup, see also *Flavour Sachets*). Net price 375-mL can = £3.69, 200-mL cup = £2.25. For use as the sole source of nutrition or as a nutritional supplement prescribed on medical grounds for: short-bowel syndrome, intractable malabsorption, proven inflammatory bowel disease, bowel fistulas. Not to be prescribed for any child under 1 year; use with caution for children up to 5 years

Flavour Sachets for use with *Peptamen Liquid* 200-mL cup. Flavours: banana, chocolate, coffee, lemon and lime, strawberry. Net price 18-sachet pack = £5.62

Pepti-Junior® (Cow & Gate)

Powder, protein 15.3 g, fat 28.3 g, carbohydrate 55.1 g, energy 2140 kJ (507 kcal)/100 g with vitamins and minerals. Used as a 13.1% solution in place of milk. Net price 450 g = £8.22. For disaccharide and/or whole protein intolerance or where amino acids and peptides are indicated in conjunction with medium chain triglycerides

Perative® (Abbott)

Liquid, providing protein 15.8 g, carbohydrate 42 g, fat 8.8 g, energy 1308 kJ (310 kcal)/237 mL, with vitamins and minerals. Gluten-free, unflavoured. Net price 237-mL can = £2.68, 500-mL ready-to-hang = £5.36, 1-litre ready-to-hang = £10.72. For use as a nutritional supplement prescribed on medical grounds for: short-bowel syndrome, intractable malabsorption, pre-operative preparation of patients who are undernourished, proven inflammatory bowel disease, following total gastrectomy, bowel fistulas, disease-related malnutrition. Not to be prescribed for any child under 5 years

Phenylalanine, Tyrosine and Methionine-Free Amino Acid Mix *see* Amino Acid Modules

Phlexy-10® Exchange System (SHS)

Bar, essential and non-essential amino acids except phenylalanine 8.33 g, carbohydrate 20.5 g, fat 4.5 g/42-g bar. Citrus fruit flavour. Net price per bar = £3.72

Capsules, essential and non-essential amino acids except phenylalanine 500 mg/capsule. Net price 200-cap pack = £25.88

Drink Mix, powder, containing essential and non-essential amino acids except phenylalanine 10 g, carbohydrate 6.8 g/20-g sachet. Blackcurrant and apple flavour. Net price 20-g sachet = £2.59

All for phenylketonuria

PK Aid 4® (SHS)

Powder, containing essential and non-essential amino acids except phenylalanine. Net price 500 g = £86.78. For phenylketonuria

PKU 2® (Milupa)

Granules, containing essential and non-essential amino acids except phenylalanine; with vitamins, minerals, trace elements, 7.1% sucrose. Flavour: vanilla. Net price 500 g = £44.75. For phenylketonuria

PKU 3® (Milupa)

Granules, containing essential and non-essential amino acids except phenylalanine, vitamins, minerals, and trace elements, with 3.4% sucrose. Flavour: vanilla. Net price 500 g = £44.75. For phenylketonuria, not recommended for child under 8 years

Polial® (Ultrapharm)

Biscuits. Gluten- and lactose-free. Net price 200-g pack = £2.85. For gluten-sensitive enteropathies including steatorrhea due to gluten sensitivity, coeliac disease, and dermatitis herpetiformis

Polycal® (Nutricia Clinical)

Powder, glucose, maltose, and polysaccharides, providing 161 kJ (380 kcal)/100 g. Net price 400 g = £2.87

Liquid , glucose polymers providing carbohydrate 61.5 g/100 mL. Low-electrolyte, protein-free. Flavours: apple, black currant, lemon, orange, and neutral. Net price 200 mL = £1.13

Both for disease-related malnutrition; malabsorption states or other conditions requiring fortification with a high or readily available carbohydrate supplement

Polycose® (Abbott)

Powder, glucose polymers, providing carbohydrate 94 g, energy 1598 kJ (376 kcal)/100 g. Net price 350-g can = £3.30. For disease-related malnutrition; malabsorption states or other conditions requiring fortification with a high or readily available carbohydrate supplement

Pregestimil® (Bristol-Myers)

Powder, protein 12.8%, carbohydrate 61.6%, fat 18.3% with vitamins and minerals. Gluten-, sucrose-, and lactose-free. Net price 450 g = £8.49. For disaccharide and/or whole protein intolerance or where amino acids or peptides are indicated in conjunction with medium chain triglycerides

Prejomin® (Milupa)

Granules, protein 13.3 g, carbohydrate 57 g, fat 24.2 g, energy 2090 kJ (499 kcal)/100 g, with vitamins and minerals. Gluten-free. For preparation with water before use. Net price 400 g = £8.11. For disaccharide and/or whole protein intolerance where additional medium chain triglyceride is not indicated

Promin® (Firstplay Dietary)

Low protein. Pasta (alphabets, macaroni, shells, shortcut spaghetti, spirals); Pasta tricolour (alphabets, shells, spirals), net price 250 g = £2.65. Pasta meal, 500 g = £5.30. Pasta imitation rice, 500 g = £5.30. For inherited metabolic disorders, renal or liver failure requiring a low-protein diet

ProMod® (Abbott)

Powder, protein 75 g, carbohydrate 7.5 g, fat 6.9 g/100 g. Gluten-free. Net price 275-g can = £8.82. For biochemically proven hypoproteinaemia

Prosobee® (Bristol-Myers)

Powder, protein 15.6%, carbohydrate 51.4%, fat 27.9% with vitamins and minerals. Gluten-, sucrose-, and lactose-free. Net price 400 g = £3.22

For proven lactose and associated sucrose intolerance in pre-school children, galactokinase deficiency, galactosaemia, and proven whole cow's milk sensitivity

Protein Forte® (Fresenius)

Liquid, protein 20 g, carbohydrate 19 g, fat 5.2 g, energy 840 kJ (200 kcal)/200 mL, with vitamins, minerals, and trace elements. Gluten-free. Vanilla, strawberry, and chocolate flavours. Net price 200-mL carton = £1.25. As a nutritional supplement prescribed on medical grounds for: short-bowel syndrome, intractable malabsorption, pre-operative preparation of patients who are undernourished, proven inflammatory bowel disease, following total gastrectomy, dysphagia, bowel fistulas, disease-related malnutrition, continuous ambulatory peritoneal dialysis (CAPD) and haemodialysis. Not to be prescribed for any child under 1 year; use with caution for young children up to 5 years

Protifar® (Nutricia Clinical)

Powder, protein 88.5%. Low lactose, gluten- and sucrose-free. Net price 225 g = £5.76. For biochemically proven hypoproteinaemia

Provide® (Fresenius)

Xtra Liquid, protein 3.75 g, carbohydrate 27.5 g, energy 525 kJ(125 kcal)/100 mL with vitamins, minerals and trace elements. Gluten-free. Apple, blackcurrant, cherry, citrus cola, lemon & lime, melon, orange & pineapple flavour. Net price 200-mL carton = £1.52.

As a nutritional supplement prescribed on medical grounds for: short-bowel syndrome, intractable malabsorption, pre-operative preparation of patients who are undernourished, proven inflammatory bowel disease, following total gastrectomy, dysphagia, bowel fistulas, disease-related malnutrition. Not to be prescribed for any child under 1 year; use with caution for children up to 5 years

Rectified Spirit. Where the therapeutic qualities of alcohol are required rectified spirit (suitably flavoured and diluted) should be prescribed

Renamil® (Syner-Med)

Powder, protein 4.7 g, carbohydrate 70.2 g, fat 18.7 g, 1984 kJ (468 kcal)/100 g, with vitamins and minerals. Net price 1 kg = £25.40. For chronic renal failure. Not suitable for infants and children under 1 year

Renapro® (Syner-Med)

Powder, whey protein providing protein 92 g, carbohydrate less than 300 mg, fat 500 mg, 1562 kJ (367 kcal)/100 g. Net price 20 g sachet = £2.22. For dialysis and hypoproteinaemia. Not suitable for infants and children under 1 year

Resource® Shake (Novartis Consumer Health)

Liquid, protein 8.9 g, carbohydrate 39.6 g, fat 12.3 g, energy 1280 kJ (305 kcal)/175 mL with vitamins, minerals and trace elements. Gluten-free; low lactose. Flavours: banana, chocolate, strawberry, summer fruits or vanilla. Net price 175-mL carton = £1.46. For use as a nutritional supplement prescribed on medical grounds for: disease-related malnutrition, short-bowel syndrome, intractable malabsorption, proven inflammatory bowel disease, bowel fistulas, dysphagia, pre-operative preparation of undernourished patients, after total gastrectomy. Not to be prescribed for any child under 1 year; use with caution for children up to 5 years

Rite-Diet® Gluten-free (Nutricia Dietary)

Gluten-free. White bread (sliced or unsliced), 400 g = £2.38. White loaf (part-baked), 400 g = £2.67. Fibre bread (sliced or unsliced), 400 g = £2.38. Fibre loaf (part-baked), 400 g = £2.67. White rolls, 4 = £2.42; (part-baked) long, 2 = £2.42. Fibre rolls, 4 = £2.42; (part-baked) long, 2 = £2.67. Flour mix (white or fibre), 500 g = £4.83. For gluten-sensitive enteropathies including steatorrhoea due to gluten sensitivity, coeliac disease, and dermatitis herpetiformis

Rite-Diet® Low-protein (SHS)

Low protein. Baking mix. Net price 500 g = £4.98. Flour mix. 400 g = £4.83. For inherited metabolic disorders, renal or liver failure requiring a low-protein diet

Scandishake® (SHS)

Powder, protein 4 g, carbohydrate 58 g, fat 21 g, energy 1831 kJ (437 kcal)/sachet. For reconstitution with milk. Flavours: chocolate, strawberry, vanilla. Net price 85 g sachet = £1.82. For disease-related malnutrition; malabsorption states or other conditions requiring fortification with a fat/carbohydrate supplement

Schar® (Schär)

Gluten-free. Bread. Net price 250 g = £1.41. Baguette (french bread), 400 g = £2.39. Wholemeal bread, 250 g = £1.41. Bread rolls, 150 g = £1.41. Lunch rolls, 150 g = £1.21. White bread buns, 200 g = £1.41. Bread mix, 1 kg = £4.00. Cake mix, 500 g = £3.95. Flour mix, 1 kg = £3.50. Wholemeal flour, 1 kg = £5.00. Cracker toast, 150 g = £1.72. Crispbread, 250 g = £2.82. Pasta (fusilli, penne, rigati), 500 g = £2.20; (rings, shells, strands) 250 g = £1.40; lasagne, 250 g = £2.80; macaroni pipette, 500 g = £2.20; spaghetti, 500 g = £2.20. Pizza bases, 250 g (2 × 125 g) = £3.78. Biscuits, 175 g = £1.72. Savoy biscuits, 180 g = £1.72. For gluten-sensitive enteropathies including steatorrhoea due to gluten sensitivity, coeliac disease, and dermatitis herpetiformis

SHS Modjul® Flavour System (SHS)

Powder, black currant, orange, pineapple, and savoury tomato flavours. Net price 100 g = £7.15. For use with any unflavoured products based on peptides or amino acids

SMA High Energy® (SMA Nutrition)

Liquid, protein 2 g, carbohydrate 9.8 g, fat 4.9 g, energy 382 kJ (91 kcal)/100mL, with vitamins and minerals. Net price 250 mL = £1.75. For disease-related malnutrition, malabsorption, and growth failure

SMA LF® (SMA Nutrition)

Powder, protein 1.5 g, carbohydrate 7.2 g, fat 3.6 g, energy 282 kJ (67 kcal)/100 mL, with vitamins and minerals. Net price 430 g = £3.99. For proven lactose intolerance

Sno-Pro® (SHS)

Drink, protein 220 mg (phenylalanine 12.5 mg), carbohydrate 8 g, fat 3.8 g, energy 280 kJ (67 kcal)/100 mL. Net price 200 mL = 64p. For phenylketonuria, chronic renal failure, and other inborn errors of metabolism

Sondalis® (Nestlé Clinical)

Sondalis Fibre, protein 3.8 g, carbohydrate 12.5 g, fat 3.9 g, fibre 1.5 g, energy 420 kJ (100 kcal)/100 mL with vitamins, minerals and trace elements. Gluten-free; clinically lactose-free. Flavour: neutral. Net price 500 mL (Dripac-Flex) = £3.20, 1 litre = £6.20. For use as a sole source of nutrition or as a nutritional supplement prescribed on medical grounds for: short bowel syndrome, intractable malabsorption, pre-operative preparation of undernourished patients, proven inflammatory bowel disease, following total gastrectomy, dysphagia, bowel fistulas, disease-related malnutrition. Not to be prescribed for any child under 1 year; use with caution for children under 5 years.

Sondalis ISO, protein 3.8 g, carbohydrate 12.5 g, fat 3.9 g, energy 420 kJ (100 kcal)/100 mL with vitamins, minerals and trace elements. Gluten-free; clinically lactose-free. Flavour: neutral. Net price 500 mL (Dripac-Flex) = £2.60, 1 litre = £5.14. For indications see *Sondalis Fibre*

Sondalis 1.5, protein 5.6 g, carbohydrate 18.8 g, fat 6 g, energy 640 kJ (150 kcal)/100 mL, with vitamins, minerals and trace elements. Gluten-free; clinically lactose-free. Flavour: neutral. Net price 500 mL (Dripac-Flex) = £2.90, 1 litre = £5.70. For indications see *Sondalis Fibre*

Sunnyvale® (Everfresh)

Mixed grain bread, gluten-free. Net price 400 g = £1.39. For gluten-sensitive enteropathies including steatorrhoea due to gluten sensitivity, coeliac disease and dermatitis herpetiformis

Suplena® (Abbott)

Liquid, protein 7.1 g, carbohydrate 60.7 g, fat 22.7 g, energy 1994 kJ (476 kcal)/237 mL. Flavour: vanilla. Net price 237-mL can = £2.28. For patients with chronic or acute renal failure who are not undergoing dialysis; chronic or acute liver disease with fluid restriction; other conditions requiring a high-energy, low-protein, low-electrolyte, low-volume enteral feed

Survimed OPD® (Fresenius)

Liquid, protein 22.5 g, carbohydrate 75 g, fat 13 g, energy 2100 kJ (500 kcal)/500 mL, with vitamins, minerals, and trace elements. Gluten-free, and low lactose. Net price 500-mL bottle = £4.57; 500-mL EasyBag® = £4.62. As a nutritional supplement prescribed on medical grounds for: short-bowel syndrome, intractable malabsorption, pre-operative preparation of patients who are undernourished, proven inflammatory bowel disease, following total gastrectomy, dysphagia, bowel fistulas, disease-related malnutrition. Not to be prescribed for any child under 1 year; use with caution for children up to 5 years

Thick and Easy® (Fresenius)

Powder. Modified maize starch. Net price 225-g can = £3.90; 4.54 kg = £66.94. For thickening of foods in dysphagia. Not to be prescribed for children under 1 year except in cases of failure to thrive

Thickened Juices, liquid, modified food starch. Flavours: apple, cranberry and orange. Net price 1.35-litre bottle = £4.50. For dysphagia. Not suitable for infants and children under 1 year

Thixo-D® (Sutherland)

Powder, modified maize starch, gluten-free. Net price 375-g tub = £5.79. For thickening of foods in dysphagia. Not to be prescribed for children under 1 year except in cases of failure to thrive

Tinkyada® (General Dietary)

Gluten-free. Brown rice pasta (elbows, fettucini, fusilli, penne, shells, spaghetti, spirals). Net price 454 g = £3.00. For gluten-sensitive enteropathies including steatorrhoea due to gluten-sensitivity, coeliac disease and dermatitis herpetiformis

Tritamyl® (Gluten Free Foods Ltd)

Gluten-free. Flour, net price 1 kg = £5.60. Brown bread mix, 1 kg = £5.60. White bread mix, 1 kg = £5.60. For gluten-sensitive enteropathies including steatorrhoea due to gluten sensitivity, coeliac disease and dermatitis herpetiformis

Trufree® (Nutricia Dietary)

Gluten-free, wheat-free flours. For gluten-sensitive enteropathies including steatorrhoea due to gluten sensitivity, coeliac disease, and dermatitis herpetiformis

No. 1, net price 1 kg = £5.59. *No. 4 white*, 1 kg = £5.59. *No. 5 brown*, 1 kg = £5.59. *No. 6 plain*, 1 kg = £5.06. *No. 7 self-raising*, 1 kg = £5.44

L-Tyrosine (SHS)

Powder, net price 100 g = £11.16. For use as a supplement in maternal phenylketonurics who have low plasma tyrosine concentrations

Tyrosine and Phenylalanine-Free Amino Acid Mix

see Amino Acid Modules

Ultra® (Ultrapharm)

Gluten-free. Baguette, net price 400 g = £2.39. Bread, net price 400 g = £2.39. High-fibre bread, 500 g = £3.26. Bread rolls, 400 g = £2.39. Crackerbread, 100 g = £1.72. Pizza base, net price 400 g = £2.57. For gluten-sensitive enteropathies including steatorrhoea due to gluten sensitivity, coeliac disease and dermatitis herpetiformis

Low protein. Brown bread (canned). Net price 500 g = £3.80. White bread (canned), 350 g = £2.75. PKU bread, 400 g = £2.10. PKU flour, 500 g = £2.98. PKU biscuits, 200 g = £2.15. PKU cookies, 250 g = £2.25. PKU pizza base, 400 g = £2.15. PKU savoy biscuits, 150 g = £2.00. For inherited metabolic disorders, renal or liver failure requiring a low-protein diet

Valpiform® (General Dietary)

Gluten-free. Bread mix. Net price 1 kg = £5.18. Country loaf, 400 g = £3.29. Pastry mix, 1 kg = £5.18. Petites baguettes, 2 x 300 g = £2.39. For gluten-sensitive enteropathies including steatorrhoea due to gluten sensitivity, coeliac disease, and dermatitis herpetiformis

Low protein. Shortbread biscuits. Net price 120 g = £3.38. Cookies with chocolate nuggets, 150 g = £4.39. For inherited metabolic disorders, renal or liver failure requiring a low-protein diet

Vitajoule® (Vitaflo)

Powder, glucose polymers, providing carbohydrate 96 g, energy 1610 kJ (380 kcal)/100 g. Net price 125 g = 88p, 200 g = £1.38, 500 g = £2.52, 2.5 kg = £12.55, 25 kg = £84.00. For disease-related malnutrition; malabsorption states or other conditions requiring fortification with a high or readily available carbohydrate supplement

Vitamins and Minerals. Only for use in the management of actual or potential vitamin or mineral deficiency; not to be prescribed as dietary supplements or 'pick-me-ups'

Vitapro® (Vitaflo)

Powder, whole milk proteins, containing all essential amino acids, 75%. Net price 250 g = £5.01, 1 kg = £19.78. For biochemically proven hypoproteinaemia

Vitaquick® (Vitaflo)

Powder. Modified maize starch. Net price 100 g = £2.27, 300 g = £4.77; 1 kg = £12.17; 6 kg = £65.52. For thickening of foods in dysphagia. Not to be prescribed for children under 1 year except in cases of failure to thrive

Wysoy® (Wyeth)

Powder, carbohydrate 6.9%, fat 3.6%, and protein 2.1% with vitamins and minerals when reconstituted. Net price 430 g = £3.98; 860 g = £7.58. For proven lactose and associated sucrose intolerance in preschool children, galactokinase deficiency, galactosaemia and proven whole cow's milk sensitivity

---

Conditions for which foods may be prescribed on FP10 (GP10 in Scotland)

Note. This is a list of clinical conditions for which the ACBS has approved food products. It is essential to check the list of products (above) for availability.

Amino acid metabolic disorders and similar protein disorders: low protein drink (Milupa); see also histidinaemia; homocystinuria; maple syrup urine disease; phenylketonuria; low-protein products; synthetic diets; tyrosinaemia.

Bowel fistulas:

Complete foods: Clinifeed Iso; Complan Ready-to-Drink; Elemental 028 and 028 Extra; Emsogen; Enrich; Ensure; Ensure Powder; Entera Liquid and Fibre Plus; Frebini; Fresubin Liquid and Sip Feeds; Jevity and Plus; Nutrini standard; Nutrison Multi Fibre, Pepti Liquid, Soya and Standard; Nutrodrip Energy, Fibre and Standard; Osmolite Liquid and Plus; Paediasure Liquid and Liquid with fibre; Peptamen; Sondalis Fibres, ISO and 1.5.

Nutritional supplements: Advera; Clinutren Dessert, ISO and 1.5; Enlive; Ensure Plus; Formance; Fortifresh; Fortijuce; Fortimel; Fortipudding; Fortisip; Fortisip Multi Fibre; Fresubin 750 MCT; Nutrison Energy, MCT and Pepti Powder; Perative; Protein Forte; Provide Xtra; Resource Shake; Survimed OPD; Tonexis and 1.5.

Calcium intolerance: Locasol New Formula.

Carbohydrate malabsorption: Duobar. See also synthetic diets; malabsorption states.

(a) Disaccharide intolerance: Alfare; Caloreen; Calsip; Duocal Super Soluble and Duocal Liquid; Maxijul LE, Liquid, Super Soluble; Nutramigen; Pepdite; Pepti-Junior; Polycal; Polycal Liquid; Polycose powder; Pregestimil; Prejomin; Vitajoule. See also lactose intolerance; lactose with associated sucrose intolerance.

(b) Glucose and galactose intolerance: Comminuted Chicken Meat (Cow & Gate); Fructose; Galactomin Formula 19 (fructose formula).

(c) Isomaltose intolerance: Glucose (dextrose).

(d) Lactose intolerance: AL 110; Comminuted chicken meat (Cow & Gate); Enfamil Lactofree; Farley's Soya Formula; Galactomin Formula 17; InfaSoy; Isomil powder; Nutramigen; Pepdite; Pregestimil; Prejomin; Prosobee; SMA LF; Wysoy.

(e) Lactose with associated sucrose intolerance: Comminuted Chicken Meat (Cow & Gate); Farley's Soya For-

mula; Galactomin Formula 17; InfaSoy; Nutramigen; Pepti-Junior; Pregestimil; Prejomin; Prosobee; Wysoy.

(f) Sucrose intolerance: Glucose (dextrose) and see also synthetic diets; malabsorption states; lactose with associated sucrose intolerance.

Note. Lactose or sucrose intolerance is defined as a condition of intolerance to an intake of the relevant disaccharide confirmed by demonstrated clinical benefit of the effectiveness of the disaccharide-free diet, and presence of reducing substances and/or excessive acid in the stools, a low concentration of the corresponding disaccharidase enzyme on intestinal biopsy, or by breath tests or lactose tolerance tests

Carnitine palmitoyl transferase deficiency (CPTD): Monogen

Coeliac disease: see gluten-sensitive enteropathies.

Continuous Ambulatory Peritoneal Dialysis (CAPD): see dialysis.

Cystic fibrosis: see malabsorption states.

Dermatitis Herpetiformis: see gluten-sensitive enteropathies.

Dialysis (nutritional supplements for haemodialysis or continuous ambulatory peritoneal dialysis (CAPD) patients): Clinutren Dessert; Ensure Plus; Formance; Fortipudding; Fresubin 750 MCT; Kindergen PROD; Nepro; Protein Forte; Renapro; Suplena.

Disaccharide intolerance: see carbohydrate malabsorption.

Dysphagia:

Complete foods: Clinifeed Iso; Enrich; Ensure; Ensure Powder; Entera Liquid and Fibre Plus; Frebini; Fresubin Liquid and Sip Feeds, Isofibre; Jevity and Plus; Nutrini Fibre and Standard; Nutrison Multi Fibre, Soya and Standard; Osmolite Liquid and Plus; Paediasure Liquid and Liquid with fibre; Sondalis Fibres, ISO and 1.5.

Nutritional supplements: Advera; Clinutren Dessert, ISO and 1.5; Enlive; Ensure Plus; Formance; Fortifresh; Fortijuce; Fortimel; Fortipudding; Fortisip; Fortisip Multi Fibre; Fresubin 750 MCT; Nutrison Energy and MCT; Protein Forte; Nutrodrip Energy, Fibre and Standard; Provide Xtra; Resource Shake; Survimed OPD.

Thickeners: Nutilis; Thick & Easy powder and thickened juices; Thixo-D; Vitaquick.

Note. Dysphagia is defined as that associated with intrinsic disease of the oesophagus, e.g. oesophagitis; neuromuscular disorders, e.g. multiple sclerosis and motor neurone disease; major surgery and/or radiotherapy for cancer of the upper digestive tract; protracted severe inflammatory disease of the upper digestive tract, e.g. Stevens-Johnson syndrome and epidermolysis bullosa

Epilepsy (ketogenic diet in): Alembicol D; Liquigen; Medium-Chain Triglyceride Oil (MCT).

Flavouring (for use with any unflavoured SHS product based on peptides or amino acids): SHS Flavour Modjul; Flavour Sachets

Galactokinase deficiency and galactosaemia:

AL 110; Farley's Soya Formula; Galactomin Formula 17; InfaSoy; Isomil powder; Prosobee; Wysoy.

Gastrectomy (total):

Complete foods: Clinifeed Iso; Enrich; Ensure; Ensure Powder; Entera Liquid and Fibre Plus; Frebini; Fresubin Liquid and Sip Feeds, Isofibre; Jevity and Plus; Nutrison Multi Fibre, Soya and Standard; Nutrodrip Energy, Fibre and Standard; Osmolite Liquid and Plus; Sondalis Fibres, ISO and 1.5.

Nutritional supplements: Advera; Clinutren Dessert, ISO and 1.5; Enlive; Ensure Plus; Formance; Fortijuce; Fortimel; Fortipudding; Fortisip; Fortisip Multi Fibre; Fresubin 750 MCT; Nutrison Energy and MCT; Perative; Protein Forte; Provide Xtra; Resource Shake; Survimed OPD.

Glucose/galactose intolerance: see carbohydrate malabsorption.

Glutaric aciduria: XLys, Low Try Maxamaid

Gluten-sensitive enteropathies: Aproten flour; Arnott gluten-free rice cookies; Barkat gluten-free bread mix, brown or white rice bread (unsliced), Brown or white rice pizza crust; Bi-Aglut biscuits, crackers, cracker toast, lasagne, pasta (fusilli, macaroni, penne, spaghetti); Clara's Kitchen gluten-free bread mix and hi-fibre bread mix; Dietary Specialities Mixes: brown or white bread, corn bread, white cake, white or fibre; Ener-G brown and white rice bread, brown rice and maize bread, gluten-free tapioca bread, rice loaf, gluten-free rice pasta (cannelloni, lasagna, macaroni, shells, small shells, spaghetti, tagliatelli, vermicelli); brown rice pasta (lasagna, macaroni, spaghetti); Glutafin bread, multigrain white loaf (sliced or unsliced, white or part-baked), rolls (white or part-baked), fibre bread, mixes (white, multigrain white, fibre, multigrain fibre), biscuits (digestive, savoury, sweet (without chocolate or sultanas), tea), crackers, high fibre crackers and pasta (lasagne, penne, spirals, spaghetti), pizza bases; Glutano gluten-free biscuits, crackers, flour mix, pastas (animal shapes, macaroni, spaghetti, spirals, tagliatelle), wholemeal bread (sliced or par-baked), baguette or rolls (par-baked), white sliced bread (par-baked); Juvela gluten-free harvest mix, loaf and high-fibre loaf (sliced and unsliced), bread rolls, fibre bread rolls, part-baked rolls with or without fibre, crispbread, mix and fibre mix; digestive biscuits, savoury biscuits and tea biscuits, pizza bases; Lifestyle gluten-free bread rolls, brown and white bread; Liga gluten-free rusks (Jacobs); Polial gluten-free biscuits; Rite-Diet gluten-free fibre rolls, high-fibre bread (sliced and unsliced), white bread (sliced and unsliced), white rolls; Schar gluten-free bread, bread mix, bread rolls, cake mix, cracker toast, crispbread, flour mix, french bread (baguette), pasta (fusilli, lasagne, macaroni pipette penne, rigati, rings, shells, spaghetti), pizza base, biscuits, savoy biscuits, white bread buns, wholemeal bread, wholemeal flour mix; Sunnyvale gluten-free bread; Tinkyada gluten-free brown rice pasta (elbows, fettucini, fusilli, penne, shells, spaghetti, spirals); Tritamyl flour, brown bread mix and white bread mix; Trufree gluten-free flours No. 1, No. 2 with rice bran, No. 3 for Cantabread, No. 4 white, No. 5 brown, No. 6 plain, No. 7 self-raising, No. 8 special dietary; Ultra gluten-free baguette, high-fibre bread, crackerbread, pizza base; Valpiform bread mix, country loaf, pastry mix, petites baguettes

Glycogen storage disease: Caloreen; Corn Flour or Corn Starch; Glucose (dextrose); Maxijul LE, Liquid (orange flavour), and Super Soluble; Polycal; Polycal Liquid; Polycose; Vitajoule.

Growth Failure (disease related): Frebini; Infatrini; Nutrini Extra, Fibre and Standard; Paediasure Liquid and Liquid with fibre; SMA High Energy; Survimed OPD.

Haemodialysis: see dialysis.

Histidinaemia: see low-protein products; synthetic diets.

Homocystinuria: Analog XMet; Methionine-Free Amino Acid Mix; XMet Maxamaid; XMet Maxamum, and see also low-protein products; synthetic diets.

Hyperlipoproteinaemia type I: Alembicol D; Liquigen; Medium Chain Triglyceride Oil.

Hyperlysinaemia: Analog XLys; XLys Maxamaid

Hypermethioninaemia: Analog XMet; Methionine-Free Amino Acid Mix; XMet Maxamaid; XMet Maxamum.

Hypoglycaemia: Corn Flour or Corn Starch; and see also glycogen storage disease.

Hypoproteinaemia: Casilan 90; Dialamine; Maxipro Super Soluble; Maxisorb; ProMod; Protifar; Renapro; Vitapro.

Inflammatory Bowel Disease:

Complete foods: Clinifeed Iso; Elemental 028; Elemental 028 Extra; Emsogen; Enrich; Ensure; Ensure Powder; Entera Liquid and Fibre Plus; Frebini; Fresubin Liquid, Sip Feeds and Isofibre; Jevity and Plus; Nutrison Multi Fibre, Pepti Liquid, Soya and Standard; Nutrodrip Energy, Fibre and Standard; Osmolite Liquid and Plus; Peptamen, Sondalis Fibres, ISO and 1.5.

Nutritional supplements: Advera; Clinutren Dessert, ISO and 1.5; Enlive; Ensure Plus; Formance; Fortifresh; Fortijuice; Fortimel; Fortipudding; Fortisip; Fortisip Multi Fibre; Fresubin 750 MCT; Nutrison Energy, MCT and Pepti Powder; Perative; Protein Forte; Provide Xtra; Resource Shake; Survimed OPD.

Intestinal lymphangiectasia: see malabsorption states.

Intestinal surgery: see malabsorption states

Isomaltose intolerance: see carbohydrate malabsorption.

Isovaleric acidaemia: Leucine-Free Amino Acid Mix; XLeu Analog; XLeu Maxamaid.

Lactose intolerance: see carbohydrate malabsorption.

Lipoprotein lipase deficiency (primary and secondary): Monogen

Liver failure: Aglutella low-protein rice; Alembicol D; Aminex low-protein biscuits, cookies and rusks; Aproten products (anellini, biscuits, bread mix, cake mix, crispbread, ditalini, rigatini, spaghetti, tagliatelle); dp Low-Protein butterscotch-flavoured or chocolate-flavoured chip cookies; Ener-G low protein egg replacer; Generaid; Generaid Plus; Juvela low-protein (chocolate chip, orange, and cinnamon flavour) cookies, loaf (sliced and unsliced), bread rolls, mix; Liquigen; Loprofin egg replacer; Loprofin low-protein bread (sliced and unsliced), bread (canned, with or without salt), fibre bread (sliced and unsliced), mix, pasta (macaroni, penne, spaghetti long, pasta spirals, vermicelli), sweet biscuits, chocolate cream-filled biscuits, crackers, cookies (chocolate chip, cinnamon), wafers (orange, chocolate, vanilla); Medium Chain Triglyceride Oil; Nepro; Promin low-protein pasta (alphabets, macaroni, shells, shortcut spaghetti, spirals), pasta tricolour (alphabets, shells, spirals), pasta meal, pasta imitation rice; Rite-Diet low-protein baking mix, flour mix; Suplena; Ultra low-protein, canned bread (brown and white); Ultra PKU biscuits, bread, cookies, flour, pizza base and savoy biscuits; Valpiform cookies with chocolate nuggets, shortbread biscuits.

Long chain acyl-CoA dehydrogenase deficiency (LCAD): Monogen

Low-protein products: Aglutella low-protein rice; Aminex low-protein biscuits, cookies and rusks; Aproten products (anellini, biscuits, bread mix, cake mix, crispbread, ditalini, rigatini, spaghetti, tagliatelle); dp Low-Protein butterscotch-flavoured or chocolate-flavoured chip cookies; Ener-G low protein egg replacer; Juvela low-protein (chocolate chip, orange, and cinnamon flavour) cookies, loaf (sliced and unsliced) mix, bread rolls; Loprofin egg replacer; Loprofin low-protein bread (sliced and unsliced), bread (canned, with or without salt), mix, rolls (part-baked) pasta (macaroni, penne, spaghetti long, pasta spirals, vermicelli); sweet biscuits, chocolate cream-filled biscuits, crackers, cookies (chocolate chip, cinnamon), wafers (orange, chocolate, vanilla), breakfast cereal; Promin low-protein pasta (alphabets, macaroni, shells, shortcut spaghetti, spirals), pasta tricolour (alphabets, shells, spirals), pasta meal, pasta imitation rice; Rite-Diet low-protein flour mix, baking mix; Ultra low-protein, canned bread (brown and white); Ultra PKU biscuits, bread, cookies, flour, pizza base and savoy biscuits; Valpiform cookies with chocolate nuggets, shortbread biscuits.

Malabsorption states: (see also gluten-sensitive enteropathies; liver failure; carbohydrate malabsorption; intestinal lymphangiectasia; milk intolerance and synthetic diets).

(a) Protein sources: Caprilon Formula; Comminuted Chicken Meat (Cow & Gate); Duocal Super Soluble and Liquid; Maxipro Super Soluble; MCT Pepdite; Neocate; Neocate Advance; Pepdite.

(b) Fat sources: Alembicol D; Calogen; Caprilon Formula; Liquigen; MCT Pepdite; Medium Chain Triglyceride Oil.

(c) Carbohydrate: Caloreen; Calsip; Hycal; Maxijul LE, Liquid, and Super Soluble; Polycal; Polycal Liquid; Polycose; Vitajoule.

(d) Fat/carbohydrate sources: Duobar; Duocal Liquid and Super Soluble; Scandishake.

(e) Complete Feeds. For use as the sole source of nutrition or as a nutritional supplement prescribed on medical grounds: Caprilon Formula; Clinifeed Iso; Complan Ready-to-Drink; Elemental 028; Elemental 028 Extra; Emsogen; Enrich; Ensure; Ensure Powder; Entera Liquid and Fibre Plus; Frebini; Fresubin Liquid, Sip Feeds and Isofibre; Infatrini; Jevity; MCT Pepdite; Nutrini Standard; Nutrison Multi Fibre, Pepti Liquid, Soya and

Standard; Nutrodrip Energy, Fibre and Standard; Osmolite Liquid and Plus; Paediasure Liquid and Liquid with fibre; Pepdite; Peptamen; Pepti-Junior; Pregestimil; SMA High Energy; Sondalis Fibres, ISO and 1.5.

(f) Nutritional supplements. Nutritional supplements prescribed on medical grounds: Advera; Clinutren Dessert, ISO and 1.5; Enlive; Ensure Plus; Formance; Fortifresh; Fortijuce; Fortimel; Fortipudding; Fortisip; Fortisip Multi Fibre; Fresubin 750 MCT; Nutrison Energy, MCT, and Pepti Powder; Perative; Protein Forte; Provide Xtra; Resource Shake; Survimed OPD.

(g) Minerals: Aminogran Mineral Mixture; Metabolic Mineral Mixture.

(h) Vitamins: As appropriate, and see synthetic diets.

(i) Vitamins and Minerals: Paediatric Seravit

Malnutrition (disease-related):

Complete foods: Calogen; Caloreen; Calsip; Clinifeed Iso; Complan Ready-to-Drink; Duobar; Duocal Liquid and Super Soluble; Enrich; Ensure; Ensure Powder; Entera Liquid and Fibre Plus; Frebini; Fresubin Liquid, Sip Feeds and Isofibre; Hycal; Infatrini; Jevity and Plus; Maxijul LE, Liquid and Super Soluble; Nutrini Extra, Fibre and Standard; Nutrison Multi Fibre, Soya and Standard; Nutrodrip Energy, Fibre and Standard; Osmolite Liquid and Plus; Paediasure Liquid and Liquid with fibre; Polycal Liquid and Powder; Polycose; Scandishake; SMA High Energy; Sondalis Fibres, ISO and 1.5; Vitajoule.

Nutritional supplements: Advera; Clinifeed 400 and Protein Rich; Clinutren Dessert, ISO and 1.5; Enlive; Ensure Plus; Formance; Fortifresh; Fortijuce; Fortimel; Fortipudding; Fortisip; Fortisip Multi Fibre; Fresubin 750 MCT; Nutrison Energy and MCT; Perative; Protein Forte; Provide Xtra; Resource Shake; Survimed OPD.

Maple syrup urine disease: Analog MSUD; MSUD Maxamaid; MSUD Maxamum; MSUD Aid III, and see also low-protein products; synthetic diets.

Methylmalonic acidaemia: Analog XMet, Thre, Val, Isoleu; XMet, Thre, Val, Isoleu Maxamaid; XMet, Thre, Val, Isoleu Maxamum; Methionine, Threonine, Valine-Free and Isoleucine-Low Amino Acid Mix.

Milk protein sensitivity: Comminuted Chicken Meat (Cow & Gate); Farley's Soya Formula; InfaSoy; Isomil powder; Nutramigen; Prosobee; Wysoy, and see also synthetic diets.

Nutritional support for adults

A. **Nutritionally complete feeds.** For use as the sole source of nutrition or as a necessary nutritional supplement prescribed on medical grounds:

(i) Gluten-Free: Clinifeed Iso; Complan Ready-to-Drink; Entera Liquid and Fibre Plus; Fortifresh; Fresubin Liquid and Sip Feeds; Nutrison Multi Fibre and Standard.

(ii) Lactose- and Gluten-Free: Clinifeed 1.0; Enrich; Ensure, Ensure Powder; Fresubin Isofibre; Nutrison Soya; Osmolite Liquid and Plus.

(iii) Containing fibre: Enrich; Fresubin Isofibre; Jevity; Nutrison Multi Fibre; Nutrodrip Fibre.

(iv) Elemental Feeds: Elemental 028; Elemental 028 Extra; Emsogen; Nutrison Pepti; Peptamen.

B. **Nutritional source supplements**: see synthetic diets; malabsorption states.

(a) General supplements. Necessary nutritional supplements prescribed on medical grounds: Advera; Emelis; Enlive; Ensure Plus; Formance; Fortijuce; Fortimel; Fortipudding; Fortisip; Fortisip Multi Fibre; Fresubin 750 MCT; Maxisorb; Nutrison Energy and MCT; Perative; Protein Forte; Provide Xtra; Resource Shake; Survimed OPD.

(b) Carbohydrates; lactose-free and gluten-free: Caloreen*; Calsip*; Hycal*; Maxijul LE*, Liquid, and Super Soluble; Polycal*; Polycal Liquid*; Polycose*; Vitajoule. *Have low electrolyte content.

(c) Fat: Alembicol D; Calogen; Liquigen; MCT Oil.

(d) Fat/carbohydrate sources: Duobar; Duocal Liquid, MCT Powder and Super Soluble (low-electrolyte content); Scandishake.

(e) Nitrogen sources: Casilan 90 (whole protein based, low-sodium); Maxipro Super Soluble (whey protein based, low-sodium); Pro-Mod (whey protein based, low-sodium).

(f) Minerals: Aminogran Mineral Mixture; Metabolic Mineral Mixture.

Phenylketonuria: Aglutella low-protein rice; Aminex low-protein biscuits, cookies and rusks; Aminogran Food Supplement (powder and tablets) and Mineral Mixture; Analog LCP; Analog XP; Aproten products (annellini, biscuits, bread mix, cake mix, crispbread, ditalini, rigatini, spaghetti, tagliatelle); dp Low-Protein butterscotch-flavoured or chocolate-flavoured chip cookies; Ener-G low protein egg replacer; Juvela low-protein loaf (sliced and unsliced), bread rolls, cookies (chocolate chip, orange, and cinnamon flavour), mix; Lofenalac; Loprofin egg replacer; Loprofin low-protein bread (sliced and unsliced), bread (canned, with or without salt), fibre bread (sliced and unsliced), mix and pasta (macaroni, penne, spaghetti long, pasta spirals, vermicelli), sweet biscuits, chocolate cream-filled biscuits, crackers, cookies (chocolate chip, cinnamon), wafers (orange, chocolate, vanilla); Loprofin PKU drink; Metabolic Mineral Mixture; Milupa PKU2 and PKU3; Phlexy-10 exchange system; PK Aid 4; Promin low-protein pasta (alphabets, macaroni, shells, shortcut spaghetti, spirals), pasta tricolour (alphabets, shells, spirals), pasta meal, pasta imitation rice; Rite-Diet low-protein baking mix, flour mix; Sno-Pro; L-Tyrosine supplement; Ultra low-protein, canned white bread; XP PKU biscuits, bread, cookies, flour, pizza base, savoy biscuits; Valpiform shortbread biscuits; XP Maxamaid; XP Bar Maxamaid; XP Concentrate Maxamaid; XP Maxamum; and see low-protein products and synthetic diets

Propionic acidaemia: Analog XMet, Thre, Val, Isoleu; XMet, Thre, Val, Isoleu Maxamaid; XMet Thre, Val, Isoleu Maxamum; Methionine, Threonine, Valine-Free and Isoleucine-Low Amino Acid Mix.

Protein intolerance: *see* amino acid metabolic disorders, low-protein products, milk protein sensitivity, synthetic diets, and whole protein sensitivity.

Refsum's Disease: Fresubin Liquid and Sip Feeds.

Renal dialysis: *see* Dialysis.

Renal failure: Aglutella low-protein rice; Aminex low-protein biscuits, cookies and rusks; Aproten products (annellini, biscuits, bread mix, cake mix, crispbread, ditalini, rigatini, spaghetti, tagliatelle); Dialamine; dp Low-Protein butterscotch-flavoured or chocolate-flavoured chip cookies; Ener-G low protein egg replacer; Juvela low-protein (chocolate chip, orange, and cinnamon flavour) cookies, loaf (sliced and unsliced), bread rolls and flour mix; Kindergen PROD; Loprofin egg replacer; Loprofin low-protein bread (sliced and unsliced), bread (canned, with or without salt), fibre bread (sliced and unsliced), mix and pasta (macaroni, penne, spaghetti long, pasta spirals, vermicelli), sweet biscuits, chocolate cream-filled biscuits, crackers, cookies (chocolate chip, cinnamon), wafers (orange, chocolate, vanilla); Nepro; Promin low-protein pasta (alphabets, macaroni, shells, shortcut spaghetti, spirals), pasta tricolour (alphabets, shells, spirals), pasta meal, pasta imitation rice; Renamil; Rite-Diet low-protein flour mix, baking mix, Sno-Pro Drink; Suplena; Ultra low-protein, canned bread (brown and white); Ultra PKU biscuits, cookies, flour, pizza base and savoy biscuits; Valpiform cookies with chocolate nuggets, shortbread biscuits.

Short bowel syndrome: *see* Malabsorption states.

Sicca Syndrome: Glandosane; Luborant; Oralbalance; Saliva Orthana; Salivace; Saliveze; Salivix.

Sucrose intolerance: *see* Carbohydrate malabsorption.

Synthetic diets:

(a) Fat: Alembicol D; Calogen; Liquigen; Medium Chain Triglyceride Oil.

(b) Carbohydrate: Caloreen; Calsip; Hycal; Maxijul LE, Liquid, Super Soluble; Polycal; Polycal Liquid; Polycose powder; Vitajoule.

(c) Fat/carbohydrate sources: Duobar; Duocal Liquid, MCT Powder and Super Soluble (low-electrolyte content); Scandishake.

(d) Minerals: Aminogran Mineral Mixture; Metabolic Mineral Mixture.

(e) Protein sources: see malabsorption states, complete feeds.

(f) Vitamins: as appropriate and see malabsorption states, nutritional support for adults.

(g) Vitamins and Minerals: Paediatric Seravit.

Tyrosinaemia: Analog XPhen, Tyr; Analog XPhen, Tyr, Met; XPhen, Tyr Maxamaid; Phenylalanine, Tyrosine and Methionine-Free Amino Acid Mix; Tyrosine and Phenylalanine-Free Amino Acid Mix.

Urea cycle disorders: L-Arginine supplement

Vomiting in infancy: Instant Carobel, Nestargel.

Whole protein sensitivity: Alfare; Caprilon Formula; MCT Pepdite; Neocate; Neocate Advance; Nutramigen; Pepdite; Pepti-Junior; Pregestimil; Prejomin.

Note. Defined as intolerance to whole protein, proven by at least two withdrawal and challenge tests, as suggested by an accurate dietary history

Xerostomia: Glandosane; Luborant; Saliva Orthana; Salivace; Saliveze; Salivix.

Conditions for which toilet preparations may be prescribed on FP10 (GP10 in Scotland)

Note. This is a list of clinical conditions for which the ACBS has approved toilet preparations. For details of the preparations see Chapter 13.

Birthmarks: see disfiguring skin lesions.

Dermatitis: Aveeno Bath Oil; Aveeno Cream; Aveeno Bath Additive Sachets Oilated; E45 Emollient Bath Oil; E45 Emollient Wash Oil; E45 Lotion; Vaseline Dermacare Cream and Lotion.

Dermatitis herpetiformis: see gluten-sensitive enteropathies.

Disfiguring skin lesions (birthmarks, mutilating lesions, scars, vitiligo): Boots Covering Cream; Covermark classic foundation and finishing powder; Dermablend Cover Creme, Leg and Body Cover, and Setting Powder; Dermacolor Camouflage cream and fixing powder; Keromask masking cream and finishing powder; Veil Cover cream and Finishing Powder. (Cleansing Creams, Cleansing Milks, and Cleansing Lotions are excluded.)

Eczema: see dermatitis.

Photodermatoses (skin protection in): Ambre Solaire Total Screen for Sun-Sensitive skin SPF 60; Coppertone Ultrashade 23; Piz Buin Sunblock Lotion 20; RoC Total Sunblock Cream SPF 25 (Colourless and tinted); Spectraban 25; Spectraban Ultra 28; Sun E45 Lotion SPF 15, SPF 25, Sunblock SPF 50; Uvistat Babysun Cream 22; Uvistat Lipscreen 15; Uvistat Sun Block Cream 20; Uvistat Tinted Lotion 25; Uvistat Ultrablock Sun Cream 30.

Pruritus: see dermatitis.

Appendix 8: Wound management products and elastic hosiery

A8.1   Wound dressings

An overview of the management of *chronic wounds* (including venous ulcers and pressure sores) and the role of different dressings is given below; the notes do not deal with the management of clean surgical wounds which usually heal very rapidly. The correct dressing for wound management depends not only on the type of wound but also on the stage of the healing process. The principal stages of healing are:

- cleansing, removal of debris;
- granulation, vascularisation;
- epithelialisation.

Greater understanding of the requirements of a surgical dressing, including recognition of the benefits of maintaining a moist environment for wound healing, has improved the management of chronic wounds.

The ideal dressing needs to ensure that the wound remains:

- moist with exudate, but not macerated;
- free of clinical infection and excessive slough;
- free of toxic chemicals, particles or fibres;
- at the optimum temperature for healing;
- undisturbed by the need for frequent changes;
- at the optimum pH value.

As wound healing passes through its different stages, variations in dressing type may be required to satisfy better one or other of these requirements. Depending on the type of wound or the stage of the healing process, the functions of dressings may be summarised as follows:

Type of wound	Role of dressing
Dry, necrotic, black	Moisture retention or rehydration
Yellow, sloughy	If dry, moisture retention or rehydration
	If moist, fluid absorption
	Possibly odour absorption
	Possibly antimicrobial activity
Clean, exuding (granulating)	Fluid absorption
	Thermal insulation
	Possibly odour absorption
	Possibly antimicrobial activity
Dry, low exudate (epithelialising)	Moisture retention or rehydration
	Low adherence
	Thermal insulation

A decrease in pain and reduction in healing time is achieved to a marked extent with **alginate**, **foam**, **hydrogel** and **hydrocolloid** dressings and also to an important extent with **vapour-permeable films** and **membranes**; dressings such as dry gauze have little place. Practices such as the use of irritant cleansers may be harmful and are largely obsolete; removal of debris and dressing remnants should need minimal irrigation.

Alginate, **foam**, **hydrogel** and **hydrocolloid** dressings are designed to absorb wound exudate and thus to control the state of hydration of a wound. All are claimed to be effective, but as yet there have been few trials able to establish a clear advantage for any particular product. The choice between different dressings may therefore often depend not only on the type and stage of the wound, but also on personal experience, availability of the dressing, patient preference or tolerance and site of the wound.

A8.1.1   Alginate dressings

The gelling characteristics of alginate dressings vary according to the product used. Some products only gel to a limited extent to form a partially gelled sheet that can be lifted off; others form an amorphous gel that can be rinsed off with water or physiological saline. A secondary covering is needed. They are highly absorbent and are therefore suitable for moderately or heavily exuding wounds, but not for eschars or for dry wounds.

Algisite® M. Calcium alginate fibre, sterile, flat non-woven dressing, net price 5 cm × 5 cm = 73p, 10 cm × 10 cm = £1.52, 15 cm × 20 cm = £4.07 (S&N Hlth)

Uses: moderately to heavily exuding wounds

Algisite® M Rope, net price 2 cm × 30 cm = £2.70 (S&N Hlth)

Uses: moderately to heavily exuding cavity wounds

Algosteril®. Calcium alginate dressing. Net price 5 cm × 5 cm, 1 = 74p; 10 cm × 10 cm, 1 = £1.69; 10 cm × 20 cm, 1 = £2.86 (Beiersdorf)

Uses: moderately to heavily exuding wounds

Algosteril® Rope, net price 2 g, 30 cm = £3.00 (Beiersdorf)

Uses: moderately to heavily exuding cavity wounds

Kaltogel® (Alginate Dressing, BP 1993, type A). Calcium sodium alginate fibre, highly absorbent, quick gelling dressing, net price 5 cm × 5 cm, each = 72p; 10 cm × 10 cm = £1.51; (NHS) 10 cm × 20 cm = £3.55 (ConvaTec)

Uses: moderately to heavily exuding wounds including leg ulcers, pressure sores, fungating lesions

Kaltostat® (Alginate Dressing, BP 1993, type C). Calcium alginate fibre, flat non-woven pads, 5 cm × 5 cm, net price, each = 74p; 7.5 cm × 12 cm = £1.62; 10 cm × 20 cm = £3.20; 15 cm × 25 cm = £5.50; (NHS) 30 cm × 60 cm, 5 = £123.40 (ConvaTec)

Uses: moderately to heavily exuding wounds

Kaltostat® Wound Packing, net price 2 g = £3.00 (ConvaTec)

Uses: moderately to heavily exuding cavity wounds

Melgisorb®. Calcium sodium alginate fibre, sterile, highly absorbent, gelling dressing, flat non-woven pads, net price 5 cm × 5 cm = 72p, 10 cm × 10 cm = £1.51, 10 cm × 20 cm = £2.83 (Molnlycke)

Uses: moderately to heavily exuding wounds including leg ulcers, dermal lesions and traumatic wounds

Melgisorb® Cavity, calcium sodium alginate fibre, sterile, highly absorbent, gelling filler ribbon, net price 32 cm × 2.2 cm, 3 pieces (2 g) = £2.80 (Molnlycke)

Uses: moderately to heavily exuding cavity wounds, fistulas, sinuses, pressure sores and deep leg ulcers

SeaSorb® (Alginate Dressing, BP 1993), calcium sodium alginate fibre, sterile, highly absorbent, gelling dressing, 4 cm × 6 cm = 73p; 10 cm × 10 cm = £1.53; 15 cm × 15 cm = £3.16 (Coloplast)

Uses: heavily exuding wounds including leg ulcers and pressure sores

SeaSorb® Filler, calcium sodium alginate fibre, highly absorbent, gelling filler, 2 g, 1 = £3.00 (Coloplast)

Uses: moderately to heavily exuding cavity wounds, fistulas, sinus drainage, decubitus and deep leg ulcers

Sorbsan® (Alginate Dressing, BP 1993, type A). Calcium alginate fibre, highly absorbent, flat non-woven pads, 5 cm × 5 cm, net price, each = 93p; 10 cm × 10 cm = £1.63; NHS 10 cm × 20 cm, 5 = £22.75 (Maersk)

Uses: moderately to heavily exuding wounds

Sorbsan® Plus, alginate dressing bonded to a secondary absorbent viscose pad, net price 7.5 cm × 10 cm, 1 = £1.46; 10 cm × 15 cm, 1 = £2.58; 10 cm × 20 cm, 1 = £3.29; 15 cm × 20 cm = £4.65 (Maersk)

Uses: moderately to heavily exuding shallow wounds and ulcers

Sorbsan® Surgical Packing, 2 g, 30 cm = £3.00; *Sorbsan® Ribbon*, 40 cm (with 12.5-cm probe), 1 = £1.75 (Maersk)

Uses: moderately to heavily exuding cavity wounds

NHS *Sorbsan® SA*, calcium alginate fibre, highly absorbent flat non-woven pads for wound contact bonded to adhesive semi-permeable polyurethane foam. Net price 9 cm × 11 cm, 5 = £11.20 (Maersk)

Uses: moderately to lightly exuding shallow wounds

Tegagen® (Alginate Dressing, BP 1993, type B). Net price each 5 cm × 5 cm = 74p; 10 cm × 10 cm = £1.57 (3M)

Uses: for leg ulcers, pressure sores, second degree burns, post-operative wounds, fungating carcinomas

A8.1.2   Foam dressings

Foam dressings vary from products that are suitable for lightly exuding wounds to highly absorbent structures for heavily exuding wounds. They may also be used as secondary dressings. In hypergranulating (or overgranulating) tissue (which may arise from the use of occlusive dressings such as hydrocolloids), changing to a more permeable product such as a foam dressing may be beneficial.

Polyurethane Foam Dressing, BP 1993. Absorbent foam dressing of low adherence; sterile. 7.5 cm × 7.5 cm, net price, each = 90p; 10 cm × 10 cm, each = £1.07; 10 cm × 17.5 cm, each = £1.66; 15 cm × 20 cm, each = £2.24; other sizes (NHS) 10 cm × 25 cm, 35 = £124.15; 25 cm × 30 cm, each = £8.40 (SSL—*Lyofoam®*)

Uses: treatment of burns, decubitus ulcers, donor sites, granulating wounds

Allevyn®. (Drug Tariff title: Polyurethane Foam Film Dressing, Drug Tariff specification 47, type 2) Hydrophilic polyurethane dressing; foam sheets with trilaminate structure, non-adherent would contact layer, foam based central layer, bacteria and waterproof outer layer. 5 cm × 5 cm, each = £1.01; 10 cm × 10 cm, each = £1.99; 10 cm × 20 cm, each = £3.21; 20 cm × 20 cm, each = £5.35; also *Allevyn® Adhesive* (Drug Tariff title: Polyurethane Foam Film Dressing with Adhesive Margin, Drug Tariff specification 47, type 4), 7.5 cm × 7.5 cm = £1.19; 12.5 cm × 12.5 cm = £2.14; 17.5 cm × 17.5 cm = £4.21; 22.5 cm × 22.5 cm = £4.60; *Allevyn® Heel*, net price 10.5 cm × 13.5 cm, 1 = £4.00 (S&N Hlth)

Uses: treatment of light to moderately exuding wounds

Allevyn® Cavity, circular, 5 cm diameter = £3.28, 10 cm = £7.82; tubular, 9 cm × 2.5 cm = £3.18, 12 cm × 4 cm = £5.60 (S&N Hlth)

Uses: moderately to heavily exuding cavity wounds

Askina® Transorbent Sterile, adhesive, polyurethane foam film dressing (with a hydrocolloid layer), net price, 5 cm × 7 cm = 91p, 10 cm × 10 cm = £1.72, 15 cm × 15 cm = £3.16, 20 cm × 20 cm = £5.05 (Braun)

Biatain® Sterile, polyurethane foam film dressing with hydrocolloid adhesive border, net price (each) 12 cm × 12 cm = £2.06; 18 cm × 18 cm = £4.12 (Coloplast)

Uses: moderate to heavily exuding wounds, leg ulcers, pressure sores, diabetic ulcers

Cavi-Care®. [NHS] Soft, conforming cavity wound dressing prepared by mixing thoroughly for 15 seconds immediately before use and allowing to expand its volume within the cavity. Net price 20 g = £16.90 (S&N Hlth)
Uses: in the management of open post-operative granulating cavity wounds (with no underlying tracts or sinuses) such as pilonidal sinus excision, dehisced surgical wounds, hydradenitis suppurativa wounds, perianal wounds, perineal wounds, pressure sores

FlexiPore®. Sterile, semi-permeable, polyurethane foam film adhesive dressing. Net price, 10 cm × 10 cm = £1.73; 20 cm × 20 cm = £5.06; 6 cm × 7 cm = 93p; 10 cm × 30 cm = £3.60; 15 cm × 20 cm = £3.70 (TSL)
Uses: treatment of light to moderately exuding wounds, leg ulcers, pressure sores

Lyofoam Extra®. Extra absorbent polyurethane foam dressing, non-adhesive. Net price 10 cm × 10 cm, 1 = £1.78; 17.5 cm × 10 cm, 1 = £3.02; 20 cm × 15 cm, 1 = £3.91; 25 cm × 10 cm, 1 = £3.65; (with adhesive, 9 cm × 9 cm = £1.12; 15 cm × 15 cm = £2.10; 22 cm × 22 cm = £4.14; 30 cm × 30 cm = £6.02; sacral, 15 cm × 13 cm = £1.72; 22 cm × 26 cm = £3.26 (SSL)
Uses: treatment of light to moderately exuding wounds

Spyrosorb® (Drug Tariff title: Polyurethane Foam Film Dressing, Drug Tariff specification 47, type 1). Sterile, semipermeable, absorbent polyurethane membrane with polyurethane film and hydrophilic adhesive. Net price 10 cm × 10 cm, 10 = £20.20; 20 cm × 20 cm, 5 = £28.75 (S&N Hlth).
Uses: light to moderately exuding wounds

Tielle®. (Drug Tariff title: Polyurethane Foam Film Dressing with Adhesive Margin, Drug Tariff specification 47). Semi-permeable, foamed gel with non-woven wicking layer and polyurethane backing layer. Net price (square) 11 cm × 11 cm = £2.03; 15 cm × 15 cm = £3.31; 18 cm × 18 cm = £4.22; (both rectangular) 7 cm × 9 cm = £1.09; 15 cm × 20 cm = £4.15; *Tielle® Sacrum* 18 cm × 18 cm = £3.07 (J&J)
Uses: light to moderately exuding wounds, leg ulcers
Tielle® Lite (Drug Tariff title: Polyurethane Foam Film Dressing), net price (square) 11 cm × 11 cm = £1.98; (rectangular) 7 cm × 9 cm = £1.05 (J&J)
Uses: light to non-exuding wounds

A8.1.3   Hydrogel dressings

Hydrogel dressings are most commonly supplied as an amorphous, cohesive material that can take up the shape of a wound. These dressings are generally used to donate liquid to dry sloughy wounds and facilitate autolytic debridement but they may also have the ability to absorb limited amounts of exudate. Gel sheets are also available which have a fixed structure; such products have limited fluid handling capacity. Hydrogel sheets are best avoided in the presence of infection.

Aquaform® (Drug Tariff specification 50) Hydrogel containing modified starch copolymer. Net price 15 g = £1.74 (Maersk)
Uses: for dry, sloughy or necrotic wounds, lightly exuding wounds, granulating wounds

Debrisan®
Beads, dextranomer. Net price 60-g castor = £29.01 (Pharmacia & Upjohn)
Uses: for moist wounds, indolent ulcers and small burns, sprinkle onto wound and cover with appropriate dressing, renew before saturation occurs (usually once or twice daily)
Paste, dextranomer in a soft paste basis. Net price 6 × 10-g pouches = £29.93 (Pharmacia & Upjohn)
Uses: for exudative and infected wounds, decubital ulcers, and leg ulcers, apply firmly and cover with appropriate dressing, renew before saturation occurs (usually twice daily to every 2 days)

Geliperm®. [NHS] Gel sheets, wet form and tubed granulated gel. Granulate, 20 g, 6 tubes = £19.92. Wet, 10 cm × 10 cm, net price, 20 sheets = £42.90, 12 cm × 13 cm, 6 sheets = £29.26; 12 cm × 26 cm, 6 sheets = £52.36 (Geistlich)
Uses: wound and ulcer dressing, burns, donor sites

GranuGel® (Drug Tariff Specification 50). Net price 15 g = £1.81 (ConvaTec)
Uses: dry, sloughy or necrotic wounds, lightly exuding wounds, granulating wounds

Intrasite® Gel (formerly Scherisorb®) Drug Tariff specification 50. A ready-mixed hydrogel containing modified carmellose polymer applied directly into the wound. Net price 8-g sachet = £1.41; 15-g sachet = £1.88 (S&N Hlth)
Uses: for dry, sloughy or necrotic wounds; lightly exuding; granulating wounds

Iodoflex®
Paste, iodine 0.9% as cadexomer–iodine in a paste basis with gauze backing, net price 5 × 5-g units = £19.48; 3 × 10-g units = £23.40; 2 × 17-g = £24.68 (S&N Hlth)
Uses: for treatment of chronic leg ulcers, apply to wound surface, remove gauze backing and cover; renew when saturated (usually 2–3 times weekly); max. weekly application 150 g; max. duration up to 3 months in any single course of treatment
Cautions; Contra-indications: avoid in thyroid disorders, in those receiving lithium, and in pregnancy and breast-feeding; caution in patients with history of thyroid disorders; iodine may be absorbed particularly if large wounds treated

Iodosorb®
Ointment, iodine 0.9% as cadexomer–iodine in an ointment basis, net price 4 × 10 g = £17.24; 2 × 20 g = £17.24 (S&N Hlth)
Uses: for treatment of chronic leg ulcers, apply to wound surface to a depth of approx. 3 mm; renew when saturated (usually 3 times weekly); max. weekly application 150 g
Powder, iodine 0.9% as cadexomer–iodine microbeads, net price 3-g sachet = £1.84 (S&N Hlth)
Uses: for treatment of moist wounds, including decubitus ulcers and chronic leg ulcers, apply to wound surface to depth of approx. 3 mm and cover; renew when saturated (usually once daily)
Cautions; Contra-indications: avoid in thyroid disorders, in those receiving lithium, and in pregnancy and breast-feeding; caution in patients with history of thyroid disorders; iodine may be absorbed particularly if large wounds treated

Nu-Gel® (Drug Tariff Specification 50). A ready-mixed hydrogel containing alginate, applied directly into wound and covered with secondary dressing. Net price 15 g = £1.78 (J&J)
Uses: dry, sloughy or necrotic, lightly exuding or granulating wounds

Purilon® Gel (Drug Tariff specification 50). Net price 15 g = £1.82 (Coloplast)
Uses: for dry, sloughy or necrotic wounds; lightly exuding wounds; granulating wounds

Sterigel® (Drug Tariff Specification 50). A ready-mixed hydrogel, applied directly into wound and covered with secondary dressing. Net price 8 g = £1.38; 15 g = £1.81 (SSL)
Uses: dry, sloughy or necrotic, lightly exuding or granulating wounds

Vigilon®. [NHS] Semi-permeable hydrogel sheets on a polyethylene mesh support. Sterile, 3 in × 6 in, net price 10 = £78.30, 4 in × 4 in, 10 = £78.30; non-sterile, 4 in × 4 in, 10 = £54.60, 13 in × 24 in, 2 = £95.05 (SSL)

A8.1.4   Hydrocolloid dressings

Hydrocolloid dressings are usually presented as an absorbent layer on a vapour-permeable film or foam. Owing to the occlusive nature of their backing they are not considered suitable for the treatment of clinically infected or very heavily exuding wounds, but are suitable for softening eschars or for promoting granulation. Recently, fibrous dressings made from modified carmellose fibres have been introduced that resemble alginate dressings (e.g. *Aquacel®*); these are not occlusive.

Aquacel® , soft sterile non-woven pad containing hydrocolloid fibres. Net price 5 cm × 5 cm, 1 = 91p; 10 cm × 10 cm, 1 = £2.16; 15 cm × 15 cm, 1 = £4.06 (ConvaTec)
Uses: moderately to heavily exuding wounds
Aquacel® Ribbon, 2 cm × 45 cm, 1 = £2.20 (ConvaTec)
Uses: moderately to heavily exuding cavity wounds

Askina® Biofilm Transparent Sterile, semi-permeable, polyurethane film dressing with hydrocolloid adhesive, net price, 5 cm × 7 cm = 91p, 10 cm × 10 cm = 95p, 15 cm × 15 cm = £2.15, 20 cm × 20 cm = £3.76 (Braun)

Biofilm S®. ⓃⒽⓈ Hydrocolloid dressing with polyurethane-polyester backing; also in powder form for direct application into wound: 10 cm × 10 cm, net price 10 = £18.04; 20 cm × 20 cm, 5 = £36.24; *Biofilm®* powder, 10 sachets = £23.29 (Braun Biotrol)

CombiDERM®. Dressing with hydrocolloid adhesive border and absorbent wound contact pad. Net price 10 cm × 10 cm, 1 = £1.30; 14 cm × 14 cm, 1 = £1.80; 15 cm × 18 cm (triangular), 1 = £3.11; 20 cm × 20 cm, 1 = £3.46; 20 cm × 23 cm, 1 = £4.17 (ConvaTec)
Uses: chronic exuding wounds such as leg ulcers, pressure sores; postoperative wounds
CombiDERM N®. ⓃⒽⓈ Hydrocolloid absorbent dressing, net price 7.5 cm × 7.5 cm, 1 = £1.03; 14 cm × 14 cm, 1 = £1.84; 15 cm × 25 cm, 1 = £3.75
Uses: chronic wounds (e.g. leg ulcers and diabetic ulcers) and exuding wounds (e.g. biopsies), and surgical wounds

Comfeel®. Soft elastic pad consisting of carmellose sodium particles embedded in adhesive mass; smooth outer layer and polyurethane film backing; available as sheets, powder in plastic blister units and paste for direct application into the wound: Ulcer dressing, 10 cm × 10 cm, net price each = £2.17; 15 cm × 15 cm = £4.35; 20 cm × 20 cm = £6.65; other sizes (ⓃⒽⓈ): 4 cm × 6 cm, 30 = £32.10; powder 6 g, 10 = £35.70; paste 12-g sachet, 10 = £13.70; 50 g, 10 = £52.80 (Coloplast)

Comfeel® Plus. Hydrocolloid dressings containing carmellose sodium and calcium alginate. Contour dressing 6 cm × 8 cm, 1 = £1.73; 9 cm × 11 cm, 1 = £3.00; Ulcer Dressing, 10 cm × 10 cm = £2.23; 15 cm × 15 cm = £4.44; 18 cm × 20 cm = £4.48; 20 cm × 20 cm = £6.66; ⓃⒽⓈ Transparent Dressing, 5 cm × 7 cm, 10 = £12.80; 9 cm × 14 cm, 10 = £37.60; 15 cm × 20 cm, 5 = £42.20; ⓃⒽⓈ Pressure Relieving Dressing, 7 cm × 7 cm, 10 = £37.00; 10 cm × 10 cm, 10 = £37.00; 15 cm × 15 cm, 10 = £76.30 (Coloplast)

Cutinova® Foam. Net price 5 cm × 6 cm = 99p; 10 cm × 10 cm = £2.13; 15 cm × 20 cm = £3.88 (Beiersdorf)
Uses: moderately exuding wounds, burns, decubitus ulcers, and leg ulcers
Cutinova® Cavity. Sterile, highly absorbent polyurethane dressing consisting of a vapour-permeable foam matrix, net price 5 cm × 6 cm = £1.50; 10 cm × 10 cm = £2.50; 15 cm × 20 cm = £5.00 (Beiersdorf)
Uses: heavily exuding deep wounds, including deep leg ulcers, decubitus ulcers, abscesses; management of postoperative wounds including pilonidal sinus excision
Cutinova® Hydro. ⓃⒽⓈ Sterile, highly absorbent semi-transparent two-layered polyurethane dressing with vapour-permeable foam matrix on a semi-permeable film backing, net price 5 cm × 6 cm = £1.28; 10 cm × 10 cm = £5.79; 15 cm × 20 cm = £2.18 (Beiersdorf)
Uses: moderately to heavily exuding wounds including burns and decubitus ulcers
Cutinova® Thin. ⓃⒽⓈ Sterile, highly absorbent, semi-transparent two-layered polyurethane dressing with two-layered vapour-permeable foam matrix on a semi-permeable film backing, net price 5 cm × 6 cm = £1.12;

10 cm × 10 cm = £1.80; 15 cm × 20 cm = £4.93 (Beiersdorf)
Uses: lightly exuding wounds including abrasions, burns, decubitus ulcers, donor sites, skin protection and post-operative wounds

DuoDERM® Extra Thin (formerly Granuflex® ExtraThin), 5 cm × 10 cm, 1 = 60p; 7.5 cm × 7.5 cm, 1 = 62p; 10 cm × 10 cm, 1 = £1.03; 15 cm × 15 cm, 1 = £2.22; ⓃⒽⓈ 5 cm × 20 cm, 1 = £1.38 (ConvaTec)

Granuflex® . Hydrocolloid wound contact layer bonded to plastic foam layer, with outer semipermeable polyurethane film. 10 cm × 10 cm, net price each = £2.18; 15 cm × 15 cm = £4.13; 15 cm × 20 cm = £4.48; 20 cm × 20 cm, 1 = £6.22; ⓃⒽⓈ 20 cm × 30 cm, 5 = £55.75; also *Granuflex® Paste* (ⓃⒽⓈ), net price 30 g = £2.68; also, *Granuflex® Bordered Dressing*, 6 cm × 6 cm, 5 = £6.90; 10 cm × 10 cm, 1 = £2.59; 15 cm × 15 cm, 5 = £24.95; triangular dressing, 10 cm × 13 cm, 1 = £3.06; 15 cm × 18 cm, 1 = £4.77 (ConvaTec)
Uses: chronic ulcers, pressure sores, open wounds, debridement of wounds; powders, gel, and pastes used with sheet dressings to fill deep or heavily exuding wounds

Hydrocoll®. Hydrocolloid dressing with adhesive border and absorbent wound contact pad, net price 5 cm × 5 cm = 88p; 7.5 cm × 7.5 cm = £1.44; 10 cm × 10 cm = £2.08; 15 cm × 15 cm = £4.00; Contour dressing, 6 cm × 14 cm = £1.90; Sacral dressing, 15 cm × 18 cm = £3.20; Basic dressing, 10 cm × 10 cm = £2.15; 15 cm × 20 cm = £4.42; 20 cm × 20 cm = £6.15; Thin film dressing, 7.5 cm × 7.5 cm = 60p; 10 cm × 10 cm = £1.00, 15 cm × 15 cm = £2.20 (Hartmann)
Uses: light to medium exudating wounds

Replicare Ultra® Sterile, adhesive hydrocolloid dressing with outer semipermeable polyurethane film backing, net price 10 cm × 10 cm = £2.06, 15 cm × 15 cm = £4.10, 20 cm × 20 cm = £6.05; Sacral dressing, 15 cm × 18 cm = £3.88 (S&N Hlth)
Uses: lightly to moderately exuding wounds such as leg ulcers, pressure sores; postoperative wounds; superficial burns

Tegasorb®. Hydrocolloid dressing 10 cm × 12 cm (oval), net price each = £2.09; 13 cm × 15 cm (oval), 1 = £3.90; 10 cm × 10 cm, (square) 1= £2.13; 15 cm × 15 cm, (square) 1 = £4.12 (3M)
Uses: chronic wounds such as leg ulcers and pressure sores

■ Keloid dressing
Cica-Care®. ⓃⒽⓈ Soft, self-adhesive, semi-occlusive silicone gel sheet with backing. Net price, 15 cm × 12 cm, 1 sheet = £22.71 (S&N Hlth)
Uses: temporary management of both existing and new hypertrophic and keloid scars; also for temporary prophylaxis of hypertrophic or keloid scarring in closed wounds

■ Hyaluronic acid
Hyalofill®
Hyalofill-F, ⓃⒽⓈ flat, non-woven, absorbent fibrous fleece of *Hyaff* (an ester of hyaluronic acid), net price (each), 5 cm × 5 cm = £9.00, 10 cm × 10 cm = £25.00 (ConvaTec)
Uses: for treatment of chronic or acute wounds, place on surface of lesion and cover with sterile dressing, renew daily or when saturated (at least every 2–3 days)
Hyalofill-R, ⓃⒽⓈ absorbent fibrous rope of *Hyaff* (an ester of hyaluronic acid), net price, 500 mg = £25.00 (ConvaTec)
Uses: for treatment of chronic or acute wounds, position gently inside cavity and cover with sterile dressing, renew daily or when saturated (at least every 2–3 days)

A8.1.5 Vapour-permeable films and membranes

Vapour-permeable films and membranes allow the passage of water vapour and oxygen but not of water or micro-organisms, and are suitable for mildly exuding wounds. They are highly conformable, convenient to use, provide a moist healing environment, and some may permit constant observation of the wound. However, water vapour loss may occur at a slower rate than exudate is generated, so that fluid accumulates under the dressing, which can lead to tissue maceration and to wrinkling at the adhesive contact site (with risk of bacterial entry). Newer versions have increased gaseous permeability; some also contain water-soluble antimicrobials. Despite these advances vapour-permeable films and membranes remain less suitable for large heavily exuding wounds and are probably not suitable for chronic leg ulcers. They are most commonly used as secondary dressings over alginates or gels; they are also sometimes used to protect fragile skin of patients at risk of developing minor skin damage.

Vapour-permeable Adhesive Film Dressing, BP 1993. (Semi-permeable Adhesive Dressing) Sterile, extensible, waterproof, water vapour-permeable polyurethane film coated with synthetic adhesive mass; transparent. Supplied in single-use pieces.
Bioclusive®, net price 10.2 cm × 12.7 cm = £1.31 (J&J); *Cutifilm®*, 5 cm × 7.5 cm = 40p; 7.5 cm × 10 cm = 65p; 10 cm × 14 cm = £1.11 (Beiersdorf); *Epiview®*, 6 cm × 7 cm = 41p; 10 cm × 14 cm = £1.07 (ConvaTec); *Hydrofilm®*, 6 cm × 9 cm = 47p, 10 cm × 15 cm = £1.25, 12 cm × 25 cm = £2.25 (Hartman); *Mefilm®*, 6 cm × 7 cm = 38p, 10 cm × 12.7 cm = £1.01, 10 cm × 25 cm = £1.96, 15 cm × 21.5 cm = £2.49 (Molnlycke); *Opsite® Flexigrid*, 6 cm × 7 cm = 44p; 12 cm × 12 cm = £1.19; 15 cm × 20 cm = £2.95 (S&N Hlth); *Tegaderm®*, 6 cm × 7 cm = 37p; 12 cm × 12 cm = £1.23; 15 cm × 20 cm = £2.30 (3M).
Uses: postoperative dressing, donor sites, i/v sites, superficial decubitus ulcers, amputation stumps, stoma care; protective cover to prevent skin breakdown
Arglaes®. [NHS] Sterile, semi-permeable, self-adhesive, clear, controlled release polyurethane film dressing containing silver. Net price 6 cm × 8 cm, 1 = 99p; 10 cm × 12 cm, 1 = £1.99; 15 cm × 25 cm, 1 = £3.99 (Maersk)
Uses: flat moist wounds including cuts and abrasions; burns and scalds; superficial pressure areas; surgical wounds
Omiderm®. [NHS] Sterile, water-vapour permeable polyurethane film (plain and meshed versions). Net price 5 cm × 7 cm, 20 = £26.09; 8 cm × 10 cm, 20 = £46.12; meshed, 20 = £61.79; 18 cm × 10 cm, 25 = £105.00; meshed, 10 = £61.79; 60 cm × 10 cm, 10 = £154.99; 21 cm × 31 cm, 5 = £79.33; meshed, 5 = £106.30; meshed, 23 cm × 39 cm, 4 = £126.18 (IATRO)
Uses: ulcers; donor sites; superficial and partial thickness burns; meshed: donor sites, skin grafts

A8.1.6 Low adherence dressing and wound contact materials

Perforated film absorbent dressings were developed to overcome the problems of adherence associated with tulle dressings; they are, however, suitable only for wounds with mild to moderate amounts of exudate; they are not, therefore, appropriate for leg ulcers or for other lesions that produce large quantities of viscous exudate.

Knitted viscose primary dressing is an alternative to paraffin gauze for exuding wounds.

Povidone–iodine fabric dressing is a knitted viscose dressing with povidone–iodine incorporated in a hydrophilic polyethylene–glycol basis; this facili-

tates diffusion of the iodine into the wound and permits removal of the dressing by irrigation with water or physiological saline. Although the iodine has a wide spectrum of antimicrobial activity, it is rapidly deactivated by wound exudate and systemic absorption of iodine may occur.

Absorbent Perforated Dressing with Adhesive Border. Low adherence dressing consisting of viscose and rayon absorbent pad with adhesive border.
Mepore®, net price 6 cm × 7 cm = 8p, 9 cm × 10 cm = 18p, 9 cm × 15 cm = 29p, 9 cm × 20 cm = 36p, 9 cm × 25 cm = 49p, 9 cm × 30 cm = 56p, 9 × 35 cm = 61p (Molnlycke)
Primapore®, net price 6 cm × 8.3 cm = 14p, 8 cm × 10 cm = 15p, 8 cm × 15 cm = 26p, 10 cm × 20 cm = 34p, 10 cm × 25 cm = 39p, 10 cm × 30 cm = 49p, 12 cm × 35 cm = 81p (S&N Hlth)
Sterifix®, net price 5 cm × 7 cm = 17p, 7 cm × 10 cm = 28p, 10 cm × 14 cm = 50p (Hartman)
Uses: lightly exuding and post-operative wounds

Absorbent Perforated Plastic Film Faced Dressing (Drug Tariff specification 9). Low-adherence dressing consisting of 3 layers:
Melolin®, 5 cm × 5 cm, net price, each = 13p; 10 cm × 10 cm = 21p; 20 cm × 10 cm = 42p (S&N Hlth)
Release®, 5 cm × 5 cm, net price, each = 12p; 10 cm × 10 cm = 20p; 20 cm × 10 cm = 38p (J&J)
Skintact®, 5 cm × 5 cm, net price, each = 10p; 10 cm × 10 cm = 17p; 20 cm × 10 cm = 33p (Robinson)
Where size not stated, 5 cm size supplied
Uses: dressing for post-operative and low exudate wounds; low adherence property and low absorption capacity

Knitted Viscose Primary Dressing, BP 1993. Warp knitted fabric manufactured from a bright viscose monofilament. Net price 9.5 cm × 9.5 cm = 30p; 9.5 cm × 19 cm = 57p (J&J—*N-A Dressing®*); 9.5 cm × 9.5 cm = 26p (SSL—*Setoprime®*; S&N—*Tricotex®*); silicone-coated, 9.5 cm × 9.5 cm = 29p; 9.5 cm × 19 cm = 54p (J&J—*N-A Ultra®*)
Uses: low adherence wound contact layer for use on ulcerative and other granulating wounds with superimposed absorbent pad

Povidone–iodine Fabric Dressing (Drug Tariff specification 43). Knitted viscose primary dressing impregnated with povidone–iodine ointment 10%, 5 cm × 5 cm, net price, each = 27p; 9.5 cm × 9.5 cm = 41p (J&J—*Inadine®*)
Uses: wound contact layer for abrasions and superficial burns; max. 4 dressings at same time

Ete®. [NHS] Wound pad of rayon wadding with rayon silk wound contact layer stitched in chequered pattern (Molnlycke)
Uses: leg wounds, decubitus ulcers, minor burns, donor sites

Melolite®. [NHS] Absorbent fabric pad covered on both sides by polyethylene net (S&N Hlth)
Uses: primary dressing over clean sutured wounds, lacerations, and abrasions

Mepitel® Non-adherent silicone dressing. Net price 5 cm × 7.5 cm, 1 = £1.44; 7.5 cm × 10 cm, 1 = £2.52; 10 cm × 18 cm = £5.43; 20 cm × 30 cm = £13.73 (Molnlycke)
Uses: leg ulcers, decubitus ulcers, burns, fixation of skin grafts; should be covered with simple absorbent secondary dressing

Mesorb®. Cellulose wadding pad with gauze wound contact layer and non-woven repellent backing, net price 10 cm × 10 cm, 1 = 50p; 10 cm × 15 cm, 1 = 65p; 10 cm × 20 cm, 1 = 80p; 15 cm × 20 cm, 1 = £1.14; 20 cm × 25 cm, 1 = £1.80; 20 cm × 30 cm, 1 = £2.04 (Molnlycke)
Uses: post-operative use for heavily exuding wounds

Perfron®. [NHS] Absorbent pad consisting of alternate layers of absorbent cotton and crepe cellulose tissue, in sleeve of non-woven viscose fabric with coating of polypropylene (J&J)
Uses: low adherence pad for heavily exuding wounds; laminate structure delays strike through

* Surgipad®. DHS Absorbent pad of absorbent cotton and viscose in sleeve of non-woven viscose fabric (J&J)
Uses: for heavily exuding wounds requiring frequent dressing changes
* DHS Except in Sterile Dressing Pack with Non-woven Pads

A8.1.7 Odour absorbent dressings

These dressings have an important role in absorbing the odour of infected wounds. Some dressings may also benefit wound healing by binding bacteria, but this effect awaits confirmation.

Actisorb Plus®. Knitted fabric of activated charcoal, with one-way stretch, with silver residues, within spun-bonded nylon sleeve. Net price (each) 10.5 cm × 10.5 cm = £2.24; 10.5 cm × 19 cm = £4.07 (J&J)

CarboFLEX®. DHS Dressing in 3 layers: wound-facing absorbent layer containing alginate and hydrocolloid; middle layer containing activated charcoal; water-resistant backing layer. Net price 10 cm × 10 cm, each = £2.60; 8 cm × 15 cm, 1 = £4.25; 15 cm × 20 cm, 1 = £6.35 (ConvaTec)

Carbonet®. DHS Activated charcoal dressing. 10 cm × 10 cm, net price, each = £2.47; 10 cm × 20 cm = £4.82 (S&N Hlth)

CliniSorb® Odour Control Dressings. DHS Layer of activated charcoal cloth between viscose rayon with outer polyamide coating. Net price 10 cm × 10 cm, 10 = £15.10; 10 cm × 20 cm, 10 = £20.15; 15 cm × 25 cm, 10 = £32.70 (CliniMed)

Kaltocarb®. DHS Dressing in 3 layers: wound-facing layer of calcium alginate fibre; absorbent middle layer of activated charcoal cloth; backing layer of bonded polyester and viscose non-woven material. Net price 7.5 cm × 12 cm, 25 = £51.48; 15 cm × 15 cm, 15 = £67.80 (ConvaTec)

Lyofoam C®. Lyofoam sheet with layer of activated charcoal cloth and additional outer envelope of polyurethane foam. Net price 10 cm × 10 cm, each = £2.67; 15 cm × 20 cm = £5.91; 25 cm × 10 cm = £4.96 (SSL)

A8.1.8 Dressing packs

The role of dressing packs is very limited. They are used to provide a clean or sterile working surface; packs shown below include cotton wool balls, but they are not recommended for use on wounds.

Sterile Dressing Pack (Drug Tariff specification 10; Scottish, 16). Contains gauze and cotton tissue pad, gauze swabs, absorbent cotton wool balls, absorbent paper towel, water repellent inner wrapper. Net price per pack = 72p

Sterile Dressing Pack with Non-woven Pads (Drug Tariff specification 35). Contains non-woven fabric covered dressing pad, non-woven fabric swabs, absorbent cotton wool balls, absorbent paper towel, water repellent inner wrapper. Net price per pack = 73p (*Vernaid®*)

A8.1.9 Tulle dressings

Tulle dressings are manufactured from cotton or viscose fibres which are impregnated with white or yellow soft paraffin to prevent the fibres from sticking, but this is only partly successful and the paraffin has the disadvantage of reducing absorbency. Versions containing a reduced amount of soft paraffin (i.e. *Paratulle®* and *Unitulle®*) are less liable to interfere with absorption; those containing the traditional amount (such as *Jelonet®*) have been considered more suitable for skin graft transfer.

Paraffin Gauze Dressing, BP 1993 (Tulle Gras). Fabric of leno weave, weft and warp threads of cotton and/or viscose yarn, impregnated with white or yellow soft paraffin; sterile. 10 cm × 10 cm, net price (light loading), each = 25p; (normal loading), each = 32p (most suppliers including SSL—*Paratulle®* (light loading); Hoechst Marion Roussel—*Unitulle®* (light loading); S&N Hlth—*Jelonet®* (normal loading))
Uses: treatment of abrasions, burns, and other injuries of skin, and ulcerative conditions; postoperatively as penile and vaginal dressing and for sinus packing; heavier loading for skin graft transfer

A8.1.10 Medicated tulle dressings

Medicated tulle dressings all have disadvantages; they are not generally recommended for wound care. **Framycetin gauze dressing** is associated with a high incidence of hypersensitivity and exposure to large amounts can lead to absorption of framycetin with the consequent risk of systemic effects such as ototoxicity; its use should be limited to specific indications, on a short-term basis. Hypersensitivity is less of a problem with **sodium fusidate dressing**, but the theoretical possibility of developing bacterial resistance may be of special concern where the antibiotic is likely to be needed for systemic use (e.g. in bone infections and in burns). Although resistance and hypersensitivity are less likely with **chlorhexidine gauze dressing**, its efficacy has been questioned.

Chlorhexidine Gauze Dressing, BP 1993 Fabric of leno weave, weft and warp threads of cotton and/or viscose yarn, impregnated with ointment containing chlorhexidine acetate; sterile. 5 cm × 5 cm, net price each = 23p; 10 cm × 10 cm = 48p (SSL—*Serotulle®*; S&N Hlth—*Bactigras®*)

Framycetin Gauze Dressing, BP 1993. PoM ▰
Fabric of leno weave, weft and warp threads of cotton, impregnated with ointment containing framycetin sulphate 1% in white soft paraffin containing 10% wool fat; sterile. 10 cm × 10 cm, net price each = 24p; DHS 10 cm × 30 cm, 10 = £8.24 (Hoechst Marion Roussel—*Sofra-Tulle®*)
Cautions: large areas (risk of ototoxicity); see also cautions in section 13.10.1
Uses: wide range of infected lesions

Sodium Fusidate Gauze Dressing, BP 1993. PoM
▰ Leno weave cotton gauze impregnated with ointment containing sodium fusidate 2% in white soft paraffin and wool fat. 10 cm × 10 cm, net price = 23p (Leo—*Fucidin Intertulle®*)

▰ denotes preparations that are considered to be less suitable for prescribing (see p. vi)

A8.1.11 Surgical absorbents

Surgical absorbent dressings have many disadvantages, since they adhere to the wound, shed fibres into it, and dehydrate it; they also permit leakage of exudate ('strike through') with an associated risk of infection.

Absorbent Cotton, BP 1988. Carded cotton fibres of not less than 10 mm average staple length, available in rolls and balls. 25 g, net price = 59p; 100 g = £1.34; 500 g = £4.53 (most suppliers). 25-g pack to be supplied when weight not stated
Uses: general purpose cleansing and swabbing, pre-operative skin preparation, application of medicaments; supplementary absorbent pad to absorb excess wound exudate

Absorbent Cotton, Hospital Quality. As for absorbent cotton but lower quality materials, shorter staple length etc. 100 g, net price = 93p; 500 g = £2.95 (most suppliers)

Drug Tariff specifies to be supplied only where specifically ordered

Uses: suitable only as general purpose absorbent, for swabbing, and routine cleansing of incontinent patients; not for wound cleansing

Gauze and Cotton Tissue, BP 1988. Consists of absorbent cotton enclosed in absorbent cotton gauze type 12 or absorbent cotton and viscose gauze type 2. 500 g, net price = £5.74 (most suppliers, including Robinsons—*Gamgee Tissue®* (blue label))

Uses: absorbent and protective pad, as burns dressing on non-adherent layer

Gauze and Cotton Tissue (Drug Tariff specification 14). Similar to above. 500 g, net price = £4.19 (most suppliers, including Robinsons—*Gamgee Tissue®* (pink label))

Drug Tariff specifies to be supplied only where specifically ordered

Uses: absorbent and protective pad, as burns dressing on non-adherent layer

Absorbent Lint, BPC . ▬ Cotton cloth of plain weave with nap raised on one side from warp yarns. 25 g, net price = 73p; 100 g = £2.24; 500 g = £9.43 (most suppliers). 25-g pack supplied where no quantity stated

Note. Not recommended for wound management

Absorbent Cotton Gauze, BP 1988. Cotton fabric of plain weave, in rolls and as swabs (see below), usually Type 13 light, sterile. 90 cm (all) ×1 m, net price = 89p; 3 m = £1.85; 5 m = £2.88; 10 m = £5.61 (most suppliers). 1-m packet supplied when no size stated

Uses: pre-operative preparation, for cleansing and swabbing

Note. Drug Tariff also includes unsterilised absorbent cotton gauze, 25 m roll, net price = £12.63

Cellulose Wadding, BP 1988. Delignified wood pulp bleached white, in multiple laminate form. 500 g, net price = £2.30 (most suppliers)

Uses: absorbing large volumes of fluid

Absorbent Muslin, BP 1988. [NHS] Fabric of plain weave, warp threads of cotton, weft threads of cotton and/or viscose

Uses: wet dressing, soaked in 0.9% sterile sodium chloride solution

Absorbent Cotton Ribbon Gauze, BP. [NHS] Cotton fabric of plain weave in ribbon form with fast selvedge edges

Uses: post-surgery cavity packing for sinus, dental, throat cavities etc.

Absorbent Cotton and Viscose Ribbon Gauze, BP. Woven fabric in ribbon form with fast selvedge edges, warp threads of cotton, weft threads of viscose or combined cotton and viscose yarn, sterile. 5 m (both) × 1.25 cm, net price = 66p; 2.5 m = 74p

Uses: post-surgery cavity packing for sinus, dental, throat cavities etc.

Gauze Swab, BP 1988. Consists of absorbent cotton gauze type 13 light or absorbent cotton and viscose gauze type 1 folded into squares or rectangles of 8-ply with no cut edges exposed. Sterile, 7.5 cm square, net price 5-pad packet = 32p; non-sterile, 10 cm square 100-pad packet = £5.18 (most suppliers)

Filmated Gauze Swab, BP 1988. As for Gauze Swab, but with thin layer of Absorbent Cotton enclosed within. Non-sterile, 10 cm × 10 cm, net price 100-pad packet = £7.11 (Vernon-Carus—*Cotfil®*)

Uses: general swabbing and cleansing

Non-woven Fabric Swab (Drug Tariff specification 28). Consists of non-woven fabric folded 4-ply; alternative to gauze swabs, type 13 light. Sterile, 7.5 cm square, net price 5-pad packet = 21p; non-sterile, 10 cm square, 100-pad packet = £2.43 (J & J—*Topper 8®*); 100-pad pack = £2.43 (CliniMed)

Uses: general purpose swabbing and cleansing; absorbs more quickly than gauze

Filmated Non-woven Fabric Swab (Drug Tariff specification 29). Film of viscose fibres enclosed within non-woven viscose fabric folded 8-ply. Non-sterile, 10 cm square, net price 100-pad packet = £5.26 (J & J—*Regal®*)

Uses: general purpose swabbing and cleansing

▬ denotes preparations that are considered to be less suitable for prescribing (see p. vi)

A8.2 Bandages and adhesives

According to their structure and performance bandages are used for dressing retention, for support, and for compression.

A8.2.1 Non-extensible bandages

Bandages made from non-extensible woven fabrics have generally been replaced by more conformable products therefore their role is now extremely limited. Triangular calico bandage has a role as a sling.

Open-wove Bandage, BP 1988 . Cotton cloth, plain weave, warp of cotton, weft of cotton, viscose, or combination, one continuous length. Type 1, 5 m (all): 2.5 cm, net price = 29p; 5 cm = 48p; 7.5 cm = 67p; 10 cm = 88p (most suppliers) 5 m × 5 cm supplied when size not stated

Uses: protection and retention of absorbent dressings; support for minor strains, sprains; securing splints

Triangular Calico Bandage, BP 1980. Unbleached calico rt. angle triangle. 90 cm × 90 cm × 1.27 m, net price = £1.06 (most suppliers)

Uses: sling

Domette Bandage, BP 1988. [NHS] Fabric, plain weave, cotton warp and wool weft (hospital quality also available, all cotton). 5 m (all): 5 cm, net price = 54p; 7.5 cm = 81p; 10 cm = £1.08; 15 cm = £1.61 (Robert Bailey, Vernon-Carus)

Uses: protection and support where warmth required

Multiple Pack Dressing No. 1 (Drug Tariff). Contains absorbent cotton, absorbent cotton gauze type 13 light (sterile), open-wove bandages (banded). Net price per pack = £3.35

A8.2.2 Light-weight conforming bandages

Lightweight conforming bandages are used for dressing retention, with the aim of keeping the dressing close to the wound without inhibiting movement or restricting blood flow. The elasticity of **conforming-stretch bandages** (also termed contour bandages) is greater than that of **cotton conforming bandages**.

Cotton Conforming Bandage, BP 1988. Cotton fabric, plain weave, treated to impart some elasticity to warp and weft. 3.5 m (all):

type A, 5 cm, net price = 60p; 7.5 cm = 74p; 10 cm = 92p, 15 cm = £1.25 (S&N Hlth—*Crinx®*)

type B, 5 cm = 60p; 7.5 cm = 77p, 10 cm = 94p, 15 cm = £1.23 (J&J—*Kling®*)

Uses: retention of dressings in difficult positions (e.g. over joints)

Knitted Polyamide and Cellulose Contour Bandage, BP 1988. Fabric, knitted warp of polyamide filament, weft of cotton or viscose, fast edges, one continuous length. 4 m stretched (all): 5 cm = 18p, 7 cm = 23p, 10 cm = 25p, 15 cm = 44p (Parema—*K-Band*®); 5 cm = 15p, 7 cm = 20p, 10 cm = 21p, 15 cm = 37p (Boston — *Texband*®)

Polyamide and Cellulose Contour Bandage, BP 1988 (formerly Nylon and Viscose Stretch Bandage). Fabric, plain weave, warp of polyamide filament, weft of cotton or viscose, fast edges, one continuous length. 4 m stretched (all): Robinsons—*Stayform*®(5 cm = 30p, 7.5 cm = 38p, 10 cm = 43p, 15 cm = 73p); SSL—*Slinky*® (net price 5 cm = 38p, 7.5 cm = 55p, 10 cm = 66p, 15 cm = 94p); S&N Hlth—*Easifix* ® (5 cm = 33p, 7.5 cm = 40p, 10 cm = 46p, 15 cm = 78p)
Uses: retention of dressings

A8.2.3 Tubular bandages

Tubular bandages are available in different forms, according to the function required of them. Some are used under orthopaedic casts and some are suitable for protecting areas to which creams or ointments (other than those containing potent corticosteroids) have been applied. The conformability of the elasticated versions makes them particularly suitable for retaining dressings on difficult parts of the body, but their use as the only means of applying pressure to an oedematous limb or to a varicose ulcer is not appropriate, since the pressure they exert is inadequate. Compression hosiery (section A8.3.1) reduces the recurrence of venous leg ulcers and should be considered after wound healing.

Elasticated Tubular Bandage, BP 1993 (formerly Elasticated Surgical Tubular Stockinette). Knitted fabric, elasticated threads of rubber-cored polyamide or polyester with cotton or cotton and viscose yarn, tubular. Lengths 50 cm and 1 m, various widths 6.25 cm–12 cm; B. Braun JLB—*Textube*® (formerly called *Lastogrip*®); Salt—*Rediform*®; S&N Hlth—*Tensogrip*®; SSL—*Tubigrip*®; Sigma—*Sigma ETB*®). Where no brand stated by prescriber, net price of stockinette supplied not to exceed: length 50 cm, 6.25 cm = 57p, 6.75 cm = 60p, 7.5 cm = 60p, 8.75 cm = 68p, 10 cm = 68p, 12 cm = 73p; length 1 m, 6.25 cm = £1.04, 6.75 cm = £1.09, 7.5 cm = £1.09, 8.75 cm = £1.14, 10 cm = £1.14, 12 cm = £1.40
Uses: retention of dressings on limbs, abdomen, trunk

Elasticated Surgical Tubular Stockinette, Foam padded (Drug Tariff specification 25). Fabric as for Elasticated Tubular Bandage with polyurethane foam lining. Heel, elbow, knee, small, net price = £2.45, medium = £2.65, large = £2.83; sacral, small, medium, and large (all) = £12.65 (SSL—*Tubipad*®)
Uses: relief of pressure and elimination of friction in relevant area; porosity of foam lining allows normal water loss from skin surface

Elasticated Viscose Stockinette (Drug Tariff specification 46). Lightweight plain-knitted elasticated tubular bandage, net price 3.5 cm (small limb), length 1 m, 1 = 75p; 5 cm (medium limb), length 1 m, 1 = 81p, 3 m, 1 = £2.31; 5 m, 1 = £3.95; 7.5 cm (large limb), length 1 m, 1 = £1.08, 3 m, 1 = £3.04, 5 m, 1 = £5.30; 10.75 cm (child trunk), length 1 m, 1 = £1.73, 3 m, 1 = £4.95, 5 m, 1 = £8.50; 17.5 cm (adult trunk), length 1 m, 1 = £2.18 (SSL—*Tubifast*®)
Uses: retention of dressings

Elastic Net Surgical Tubular Stockinette (Drug Tariff Specification 26). Lightweight elastic open-work net tubular fabric.
type A : arm/leg, 40 cm × 1.8 cm (size C), net price = 36p; thigh/head, 60 cm × 2.5 cm (size E) = 64p; trunk (adult), 60 cm × 4.5 cm (size F) = 94p; trunk (OS adult) 60 cm × 5.4 cm (size G) = £1.26 (SSL—*Netelast*®)

Cotton Stockinette, Bleached, BP 1988 (formerly Cotton Surgical Tubular Stockinette). Knitted fabric, cotton yarn, tubular. 1 m × 2.5 cm, net price = 28p; 5 cm = 44p; 7.5 cm = 53p; 6 m × 10 cm = £3.60 (J&J, SSL)
Uses: 1 m lengths, basis (with wadding) for Plaster of Paris bandages etc. ; 6 m length, compression bandage

Ribbed Cotton and Viscose Surgical Tubular Stockinette, BP 1988. Knitted fabric of 1:1 ribbed structure, singles yarn spun from blend of two-thirds cotton and one-third viscose fibres, tubular. Length 5 m (all):
type A (lightweight): arm/leg (child), arm (adult) 5 cm, net price = £2.05; arm (OS adult), leg (adult) 7.5 cm = £2.69; leg (OS adult) 10 cm = £3.56; trunk (child) 15 cm = £5.13; trunk (adult) 20 cm = £5.92; trunk (OS adult) 25 cm = £7.08 (SSL)
type B (heavyweight): sizes as for type A, net price £2.01–£6.96 (Sallis—*Eesiban*®)
Drug Tariff specifies various combinations of sizes to provide sufficient material for part or full body coverage
Uses: protective dressings with tar-based and other non-steroid ointments

Tubular Gauze Bandage, Seamless. [NHS]
Unbleached cotton yarn, positioned with applicators. 20 m roll (all): 00, net price = £2.15; 01 = £2.18; 12 = £2.93; 34 = £4.29; 56 = £5.93; 78 = £6.97; T1 = £10.00; T2 = £12.95 (SSL—*Tubegauz*®)
Uses: retention of dressings on limbs, abdomen, trunk

A8.2.4 Support bandages

Light support bandages, which include the various forms of crepe bandage, are used in the prevention of oedema; they are also used to provide support for mild sprains and joints but their effectiveness has not been proven for this purpose. Since they have limited extensibility, they are able to provide light support without exerting undue pressure. For a warning against injudicious compression see section A8.2.5.

Crepe Bandage, BP 1988. Fabric, plain weave, warp of wool threads and crepe-twisted cotton threads, weft of cotton threads; stretch bandage. 4.5 m stretched (all): 5 cm, net price = 84p; 7.5 cm = £1.18; 10 cm = £1.56; 15 cm = £2.25 (most suppliers)
Uses: light support system for strains, sprains, compression over paste bandages for varicose veins

Cotton Crepe Bandage light support bandage, 4.5 m stretched (all): 5 cm, net price = 48p; 7.5 cm = 67p; 10 cm = 87p; 15 cm = £1.27 (Millpledge–*Hospicrepe 239*)

Cotton Crepe Bandage, BP 1988. Fabric, plain weave, warp of crepe-twisted cotton threads, weft of cotton and/or viscose threads; stretch bandage. 4.5 m stretched (both): 7.5 cm, net price = £2.65; 10 cm = £3.40; other sizes [NHS] (most suppliers)
Uses: light support system for strains, sprains, compression over paste bandages for varicose ulcers

Cotton, Polyamide and Elastane Bandage. Fabric, cotton, polyamide, and elastane; light support bandage (Type 2). 4.5 m stretched (all): 5 cm, net price = 62p, 7.5 cm = 89p, 10 cm = £1.14, 15 cm = £1.66 (S&N Hlth —*Soffcrepe*®); 4.5 m stretched, 10 cm = £1.12 (SSL—*Setocrepe*®)
Uses: light support for sprains and strains; retention of dressings

Cotton Stretch Bandage, BP 1988. Fabric, plain weave, warp of crepe-twisted cotton threads, weft of cotton threads; stretch bandage, lighter than cotton crepe. 4.5 m stretched (all): 5 cm, net price = 56p; 7.5 cm = 78p; 10 cm = £1.04; 15 cm = £1.48 (Millpledge—*Hospicrepe 233*)
Uses: light support system for strains, sprains, compression over paste bandages for varicose veins

Cotton Suspensory Bandage (Drug Tariff). Type 1: cotton net bag with draw tapes and webbing waistband; net price small, medium, and large (all) = £1.47, extra large = £1.56. Type 2: cotton net bag with elastic edge and webbing waistband; small = £1.62, medium = £1.67, large = £1.73, extra large = £1.80. Type 3: cotton net bag with elastic edge and webbing waistband with elastic insertion; small, medium, and large (all) = £1.75; extra large = £1.81. Type supplied to be endorsed

Uses: support of scrotum

Knitted Elastomer and Viscose Bandage. Knitted fabric, viscose and elastomer yarn. Type 2: light support bandage, 4.5 m stretched (all): 5 cm, net price = 48p, 7 cm = 68p, 10 cm = 89p, 15 cm = £1.28 (Parema—*K-Lite®*); 5 cm = 38p; 7 cm = 54p; 10 cm = 71p; 15 cm = £1.02 (Boston—*Litetex®*)

Uses: light support for sprains and strains

Type 3a: light compression bandage, 6 m stretched, 10 cm, net price = £2.46; 15 cm = £2.62; 8 m stretched, 10 cm = £3.10 (SSL—*Elset®*); 12 m stretched, 15 cm = £5.20 (SSL—*Elset®S*); 6 m stretched, 10 cm, net price = £1.40; 8.7 m stretched, 10 cm = £1.98 (Parema—*K-Plus®*); 7 m stretched, 10 cm = £3.32 (S&N Hlth—*Litepress®*); 6 m stretched, 10 cm = £1.12; 8.7 m stretched, 10 cm = £1.58 (Boston—*Litetex® Plus*)

Uses: light compression for varicose ulcers

A8.2.5 High compression bandages

High compression products are used to provide the high compression needed for the management of gross varices, post-thrombotic venous insufficiency, venous leg ulcers, and gross oedema in average-sized limbs. Their use calls for an expert knowledge of the elastic properties of the products and experience in the technique of providing careful graduated compression. Inappropriate application can lead to uneven and inadequate pressures or to hazardous levels of pressure. In particular, injudicious use of compression in limbs with arterial disease has been reported to cause severe skin and tissue necrosis (in some instances calling for amputation). Doppler testing is required before treatment with compression.

■ High compression bandages (Drug Tariff specification 52)

PEC High Compression Bandage (Drug Tariff). Polyamide, elastane, and cotton compression (high) extensible bandage, 3.5 m unstretched (both): 7.5 cm, net price = £2.50; 10 cm = £3.23 (SSL—*Setopress®*)

Uses: high compression for varicose ulcers

VEC High Compression Bandage (Drug Tariff). Viscose, elastane, and cotton compression (high) extensible bandage, 3 m unstretched (both); 7.5 cm, net price = £2.43; 10 cm = £3.13 (S&N—*Tensopress®*)

Uses: high compression for varicose ulcers

High Compression Bandage (Drug Tariff). Cotton, viscose, nylon, and Lycra® extensible bandage, 3 m (unstretched), 10 cm = £3.07 (ConvaTec—*SurePress®*)

Uses: high compression for venous leg ulcers

■ Short Stretch Compression Bandage

Short stretch bandages help to reduce oedema and promote healing of venous leg ulcers. They are applied at full stretch over padding (*see* Sub-compression Wadding Bandage below) which protects areas of high pressure and sites at high risk of pressure damage.

Comprilan®. Net price (all 5 m) 8 cm, 1 = £3.08; 10 cm = £3.50; 12 cm = £4.08; ⟨NHS⟩ 6 cm = £4.18 (Beiersdorf)

Uses: venous leg ulcers and lymphoedema

Rosidal K®. Net price (all 5 m) 8 cm, 1 = £3.08; 10 cm = £3.36; 12 cm = £4.08; ⟨NHS⟩ 6 cm = £2.95 (Vernon-Carus)

Uses: venous leg ulcers and lymphoedema

Tensolan K®. Net price (all 5 m) 8 cm, 1 = £3.05; 10 cm = £3.50; 12 cm = £3.85 (S&N Hlth)

Uses: venous leg ulcers and lymphoedema

Varex® short stretch. Net price 5 m x 10 cm, 1 = £3.16 (SSL)

Uses: venous leg ulcers and lymphoedema

■ Sub-compression Wadding Bandage

Cellona® Undercast Padding. Net price 2.75 m unstretched (all): 7.5 cm = 37p; 10 cm = 46p; 15 cm = 59p; ⟨NHS⟩ 5 cm = 33p; 20 cm = 97p (Vernon-Carus)

K-Soft® , net price 3.5 m unstretched, 10 cm = 40p (Parema)

Soffban® Natural , net price 3.5 m unstretched, 10 cm = 60p (S&N Hlth)

Softexe®. Net price 3.5 m unstretched, 10 cm = 59p (SSL)

Sohfast® , soft absorbent bandage, net price 3.5 m unstretched, 10 cm = 42p (Robinsons)

SurePress® , absorbent padding, net price 3 m, 10 cm = 48p (ConvaTec)

A8.2.6 Extra-high performance compression bandages

These bandages are capable of applying pressures even higher than those of high compression bandages, therefore the same stringent warnings apply. Their use is reserved for the largest and most oedematous limbs. Extra-high performance compression bandages are poorly tolerated by patients.

Elastic Web Bandage, BP 1993 (also termed Blue Line Webbing). Characteristic fabric woven ribbon fashion, warp threads of cotton and rubber with mid-line threads coloured blue, weft threads of cotton or combined cotton and viscose; may be dyed skin colour; with or without foot loop. Per m (both) 7.5 cm, net price = 73p; 10 cm = £1.04; with foot loop (Drug Tariff specification 2a) 7.5 cm each = £4.17 (Marlow, SSL)

Uses: provision of support and high compression over large surface

Elastic Web Bandage without Foot Loop (also termed Red Line Webbing) (Drug Tariff specification 2b) (Scott-Curwen). Characteristic fabric woven ribbon fashion, warp threads of cotton and rubber with mid-line threads coloured red, weft threads of cotton or combined cotton and viscose. 7.5 cm × 2.75 m (2.5 m unstretched), net price = £3.30; 7.5 cm × 3.75 m (3.5 m unstretched) = £3.99

Uses: provision of support and high compression over large surfaces

Cotton and Rubber Elastic Bandage, BP 1993. Fabric, plain weave, warp of combined cotton and rubber threads, weft of cotton threads (S&N Hlth)

Uses: provision of high compression and medium support

Heavy Cotton and Rubber Elastic Bandage, BP 1993. Heavy version of above with one end folded as foot loop; fastener also supplied. 1.8 m unstretched × 7.5 cm, net price = £11.20 (Marlow, SSL, S&N Hlth—*Elastoweb®*)

Uses: provision of high even compression over large surface

A8.2.7 Adhesive bandages

Elastic adhesive bandages are used to provide compression in the treatment of varicose veins and for the support of injured joints; they should no longer be used for the support of fractured ribs and clavicles. They have also been used with **zinc paste bandage** in the treatment of venous ulcers, but they can cause skin reactions in susceptible patients and may not produce sufficient pressures for healing (significantly lower than those provided by other compression bandages).

Elastic Adhesive Bandage, BP 1993 Woven fabric, elastic in warp (crepe-twisted cotton threads), weft of cotton and/or viscose threads spread with adhesive mass containing zinc oxide. 4.5 m stretched (all): 5 cm, net price = £3.12; 7.5 cm = £4.51; 10 cm = £6.01 (Robinsons—*Flexoplast*®; S&N Hlth—*Elastoplast*® Bandage). 7.5 cm width supplied when size not stated
Uses: compression for chronic leg ulcers; compression and support for swollen or sprained joints
Half-spread Elastic Adhesive Bandage, BP 1988. [NHS] Fabric as for elastic adhesive bandage but only partially spread with adhesive. (S&N Hlth)
Uses: compression for leg ulcers; compression and support for swollen or sprained joints
Ventilated Elastic Adhesive Bandage, BP 1993. [NHS] Fabric as for elastic adhesive bandage but adhesive spread such that there are regular strips of unspread fabric along length. (S&N Hlth)
Uses: compression for leg ulcers; compression and support for swollen or sprained joints
Extension strapping, BP 1993. [NHS] Woven fabric, elastic in weft, spread with adhesive mass containing zinc oxide, warp threads cotton and/or viscose, weft threads crepe-twisted cotton. (S&N Hlth)
Uses: support of light strains, joints and limbs removed from plaster casts; traction bandaging

A8.2.8 Cohesive bandages

Cohesive bandages adhere to themselves, but not to the skin, and are useful for providing support for sports use where ordinary stretch bandages might become displaced and adhesive bandages are inappropriate. Care is needed in their application, however, since the loss of ability for movement between turns of the bandage to equalise local areas of high tension carries the potential for creating a tourniquet effect. They should not be used if arterial disease is suspected.

■ Cohesive extensible bandages
These elastic bandages adhere to themselves and not to skin; this prevents slipping during use.
Uses: support of sprained joints; outer layer of multilayer compression bandaging
Coban®. Net price 6 m stretched, 10 cm = £2.75; other sizes [NHS] 4.5 m stretched (all): 2.5 cm = £1.05; 5 cm = £1.51; 7.5 cm = £2.26; 10 cm = £3.01; 15 cm = £4.52 (3M)
Cohfast®. Latex-free, net price 6.3 m stretched, 10 cm = £2.77; other sizes [NHS] 4.5 m stretched (both): 5 cm = £1.28; 7.5 cm = £1.98 (Robinson)
Co-Plus®. Net price 6.3 m stretched, 10 cm (flesh, white or mixed) = £2.75; other sizes [NHS] flesh or white, 6.3 m stretched (all): 2.5 cm = £1.07; 3.8 cm = £1.43; 5 cm = £1.65; 7.5 cm (flesh, white, or mixed) = £2.44; 15 cm = £4.87 (S&N Hlth)
Secure® **Forte.** [NHS] Net price 4.5 m stretched, 6 cm = £2.16; 8 cm = £2.90; 10 cm = £3.87 (J&J)

A8.2.9 Medicated bandages

Zinc Paste Bandage remains one of the standard treatments for leg ulcers and can be left on undisturbed for up to a week; it is often used in association with compression for treatment of venous ulcers.

Zinc paste bandages are also used with **coal tar** or **ichthammol** in chronic lichenified skin conditions such as chronic eczema (ichthammol often being preferred since its action is considered to be milder).They are also used with **calamine** in milder eczematous skin conditions (but the inclusion of **clioquinol** may lead to irritation in susceptible subjects).

Zinc Paste Bandage, BP 1993. Cotton fabric, plain weave, impregnated with suitable paste containing zinc oxide; requires additional bandaging. Net price 6 m × 7.5 cm = £3.11 (SSL—*Steripaste*® (15%), excipients: include polysorbate 80); £3.06 (SSL—*Zincaband*® (15%), *excipients: include* hydroxybenzoates); £3.09 (S&N Hlth—*Viscopaste PB7*® (10%), *excipients: include* hydroxybenzoates)
Zinc Paste and Calamine Bandage (Drug Tariff specification 5). Cotton fabric, plain weave, impregnated with suitable paste containing calamine and zinc oxide; requires additional bandaging. Net price 6 m × 7.5 cm = £3.16 (SSL—*Calaband*®)
Zinc Paste, Calamine, and Clioquinol Bandage, BP 1993. Cotton fabric, plain weave, impregnated with suitable paste containing calamine, clioquinol, and zinc oxide; requires additional bandaging. Net price 6 m × 7.5 cm = £3.16 (SSL—*Quinaband*®, *excipients: include* hydroxybenzoates)
Zinc Paste and Coal Tar Bandage, BP 1993. Cotton fabric, plain weave, impregnated with a suitable paste containing coal tar and zinc oxide; requires additional bandaging. Net price 6 m × 7.5 cm = £3.07 (SSL—*Tarband*®, *excipients: include* hydroxybenzoates; S&N Hlth—*Coltapaste*®, *excipients: include* wool fat)
Uses: see section 13.5
Zinc Paste and Ichthammol Bandage, BP 1993. Cotton fabric, plain weave, impregnated with suitable paste containing zinc oxide and ichthammol; requires additional bandaging. Net price 6 m × 7.5 cm = £3.07 (SSL—*Icthaband*®(15/2%), *excipients: include* hydroxybenzoates; S&N Hlth—*Ichthopaste*®(6/2%), *excipients:* none as listed in section 13.1.3)
Uses: see section 13.5

■ Medicated stocking
Zipzoc®. Sterile rayon stocking impregnated with ointment containing zinc oxide 20%. Net price 4-pouch carton = £13.33; 10-pouch carton = £33.33 (S&N Hlth)
Uses: chronic leg ulcers; can be used under appropriate compression bandages or hosiery in chronic venous insufficiency

A8.2.10 Multi-layer compression bandaging

Although multi-layer compression bandaging 'kits' are not prescribable as such on the NHS, individual components of the 'kit' are prescribable; see also Sub-compression Wadding Bandage, section A8.2.5.

K-Four® (Parema)
K-Four # 1 (*K-Soft*®—see Sub-compression Wadding Bandage); *K-Four* # 2 (*K-Lite*®—see Knitted Elastomer and Viscose Bandage); *K-Four* # 3 (*K-Plus*®—see Knitted Elastomer and Viscose Bandage); *K-Four* # 4 (*Ko-Flex*®), net price 10 cm × 6 m (unstretched) = £2.70

Profore® (S&N Hlth.)
Profore® wound contact layer (*Tricotex®*—see Knitted Viscose Primary Dressing); *Profore® #1* (*Soffban® Natural*—see Sub-compression Wadding bandage); *Profore® #2* (*Soffcrepe®*—see Cotton, Polyamide and Elastane Bandage); *Profore® #3* (*Litepress®*—see Knitted Elastomer and Viscose Bandage); *Profore® #4* (*Co-Plus®*—see Cohesive bandages); *Profore® Plus* (*Tensopress®*—see VEC High Compression Bandage)

System 4 (SSL)
System 4 wound contact layer (*Setoprime®*—see Knitted Viscose Primary Dressing); *System 4 #1* (*Softexe®*—see Sub-compression Wadding Bandage); *System 4 #2* (*Setocrepe®*—see Cotton, Polyamide and Elastane Bandage); *System 4 #3* (*Elset®*—see Knitted Elastomer and Viscose Bandage); *System 4 #4* (*Coban®*—see Cohesive bandages)

Ultra Four (Robinsons)
Ultra Four #1 (Robinsons—*Sohfast®*—see Sub-compression Wadding Bandage); *Ultra Four #2* (Parema—*K-Lite®*—see Knitted Elastomer and Viscose Bandage); *Ultra Four #3* (Parema—*K-Plus®*—see Knitted Elastomer and Viscose Bandage); *Ultra Four #4* (Robinsons—*Cohfast®*—see Cohesive bandages)

A8.2.11   Surgical adhesive tapes

Adhesive tapes are useful for retaining dressings on joints or awkward body parts. These tapes, particularly those containing rubber, can cause irritant and allergic reactions in susceptible patients; synthetic adhesives have been developed to overcome this problem, but they, too, may sometimes be associated with reactions. Adhesive tapes that are occlusive may cause skin maceration. Care is needed not to apply these tapes under tension, to avoid creating a tourniquet effect. If applied over joints they need to be orientated so that the area of maximum extensibility of the fabric is in the direction of movement of the limb.

Permeable adhesive tapes

Zinc Oxide Adhesive Tape, BP 1988. (Zinc Oxide Plaster). Fabric, plain weave, warp and weft of cotton and/or viscose, spread with an adhesive containing zinc oxide. 1.25 cm, net price 3 m = 57p, 5 m = 79p; 2.5 cm, 1 m = 37p, 3 m = 84p, 5 m = £1.15; 5 cm × 5 m = £1.94; 7.5 cm × 5 m = £2.92 (most suppliers)
Drug Tariff specifies 1 m × 2.5 cm supplied when size not stated
Uses: securing dressings and immobilising small areas

Permeable Woven Synthetic Adhesive Tape, BP 1988. Non-extensible closely woven fabric, spread with a polymeric adhesive. 5 m (all): 1.25 cm, net price = 65p; 2.5 cm = 95p; 5 cm = £1.66 (Beiersdorf—*Leukosilk®*)
Uses: securing dressings
For patients with skin reaction to other plasters and strapping, requiring use for long periods

Elastic Adhesive Tape, BP 1988 (Elastic Adhesive Plaster). Woven fabric, elastic in warp (crepe-twisted cotton threads), weft of cotton and/or viscose threads, spread with adhesive mass containing zinc oxide. 1.5 m stretched × 2.5 cm, net price = 75p; 4.5 m stretched × 2.5 cm = £1.40 (Robinsons—*Flexoplast®*; S&N—*Elastoplast®*).
Uses: securing dressings
For 5 cm width, see Elastic Adhesive Bandage

Permeable Non-woven Synthetic Adhesive Tape, BP 1988. Backing of paper-based or non-woven textile material spread with a polymeric adhesive mass. 5 m (all): BioDiagnostics—*Scanpor®* (net price 1.25 cm = 39p, 2.5 cm = 63p, 5 cm = £1.09); Beiersdorf—*Leukopor®* (1.25 cm = 44p, 2.5 cm = 69p, 5 cm = £1.21); 3M—*Micropore®* (1.25 cm = 58p, 2.5 cm = 86p, 5 cm = £1.52); S&N Hlth—*Albupore®* (1.25 cm = 44p, 2.5 cm =

69p, 5 cm = £1.20); *Hypal 2®* (1.25 cm = 61p, 2.5 cm = 94p, 5 cm = £1.72). Where no brand stated by prescriber, net price of tape supplied not to exceed 39p (1.25 cm), 63p (2.5 cm), £1.09 (5 cm)
Uses: securing dressings; skin closures for small incisions
For patients with skin reaction to other plasters and strapping, requiring use for long periods

Occlusive adhesive tapes

Impermeable Plastic Adhesive Tape, BP 1988. Extensible water-impermeable plastic film spread with an adhesive mass. 2.5 cm × 3 m, net price = £1.11; 5 m = £1.66; 5 cm × 5 m = £2.11; 7.5 cm × 5 m = £3.06 (Robinsons; SSL; S&N Hlth)
Uses: securing dressings; covering site of infection where exclusion of air, water, and water vapour is required

Impermeable Plastic Synthetic Adhesive Tape, BP 1988. Extensible water-impermeable plastic film spread with a polymeric adhesive mass. 5 m (both): net price, 2.5 cm = £1.58; 5 cm = £3.01 (3M—*Blenderm®*)
Uses: isolating wounds from external environment; covering sites where total exclusion of water and water vapour required; securing dressings and appliances

A8.2.12   Adhesive dressings

Adhesive dressings (also termed 'island dressings') have a limited role for minor wounds only. The inclusion of an antiseptic is not particularly useful and may cause skin irritation in susceptible subjects.

Permeable adhesive dressings

Elastic Adhesive Dressing, BP 1993. [NHS]   Wound dressing or dressing strip, pad attached to piece of extension plaster, leaving suitable adhesive margin; both pad and margin covered with suitable protector; pad may be dyed yellow and may be impregnated with suitable antiseptic (see below); extension plaster may be perforated or ventilated
Uses: general purpose wound dressing
Note. Permitted antiseptics are aminoacridine hydrochloride (aminacrine hydrochloride), chlorhexidine hydrochloride (both 0.07–0.13%), chlorhexidine gluconate (0.11–0.20%); domiphen bromide (0.05–0.25%)

Permeable Plastic Wound Dressing, BP 1993. [NHS]   Consisting of an absorbent pad, which may be dyed and impregnated with a suitable antiseptic (see under Elastic Adhesive Dressing), attached to a piece of permeable plastic surgical adhesive tape, to leave a suitable adhesive margin; both pad and margin covered with suitable protector (most suppliers)
Uses: general purpose wound dressing, permeable to air and water

Vapour permeable adhesive dressings

Vapour-permeable Waterproof Plastic Wound Dressing, BP 1993 (former Drug Tariff title: Semipermeable Waterproof Plastic Wound Dressing). Consists of absorbent pad, may be dyed and impregnated with suitable antiseptic (see under Elastic Adhesive Dressing), attached to piece of semipermeable waterproof surgical adhesive tape, to leave suitable adhesive margin; both pad and margin covered with suitable protector. 8.5 cm × 6 cm, net price = 31p (S&N Hlth—*Elastoplast Airstrip®*)
Uses: general purpose waterproof wound dressing, permeable to air and water vapour

Occlusive adhesive dressings

Impermeable Plastic Wound Dressing, BP

1993. NHS Consists of absorbent pad, may be dyed and impregnated with suitable antiseptic (see under Elastic Adhesive Dressing), attached to piece of impermeable plastic surgical adhesive tape, to leave suitable adhesive margin; both pad and margin covered with suitable protector (most suppliers)

Uses: protective covering for wounds requiring an occlusive dressing

A8.2.13   Skin closure dressings

Skin closure strips are used as an alternative to sutures for minor cuts and lacerations.

Skin closure strips, sterile

Leukostrip®, 6.4 mm × 76 mm, 3 strips per envelope. Net price 10 envelopes = £5.09 (Beiersdorf)

Steri-strip®, 6 mm × 75 mm, 3 strips per envelope. Net price 12 envelopes = £8.23; NHS 3 mm × 75 mm, 12 envelopes = £8.08; 12 mm × 100 mm, 12 envelopes = £10.51 (3M)

Drug Tariff specifies that these are specifically for personal administration by the prescriber

A8.3   Elastic hosiery

Before elastic hosiery can be dispensed, the quantity (single or pair), article (including accessories), and compression class (I, II or III) must be specified by the prescriber; all dispensed articles must state on the packaging that they conform with Drug Tariff technical specification No. 40, for further details see Drug Tariff.

A8.3.1   Graduated compression hosiery

Class I Light Support

Hosiery, compression at ankle 14–17 mm Hg, thigh length or below knee with knitted in heel. Net price per pair, circular knit (standard), thigh length = £6.34, below knee = £5.80; light weight elastic net (made-to-measure), thigh length = £16.98, below knee = £13.26

Uses: superficial or early varices, varicosis during pregnancy

Class 2 Medium Support

Hosiery, compression at ankle 18–24 mm Hg, thigh length or below knee with knitted in heel. Net price per pair, circular knit (standard), thigh length = £9.42, below knee = £8.48, (made-to-measure), thigh length = £31.50, below knee = £19.70; net (made-to-measure), thigh length = £16.98, below knee = £13.26; flat bed (made-to-measure, only with closed heel and open toe), thigh length = £31.50, below knee = £19.70

Uses: varices of medium severity, ulcer treatment and prophylaxis, mild oedema, varicosis during pregnancy

Class 3 Strong Support

Hosiery, compression at ankle 25–35 mm Hg, thigh length or below knee with open or knitted in heel. Net price per pair, circular knit (standard), thigh length = £11.18, below knee = £9.60, (made-to-measure), thigh length = £31.50, below knee = £19.70; flat bed (made-to-measure, only with open heel and open toe), thigh length = £31.50, below knee = £19.70

Uses: gross varices, post thrombotic venous insufficiency, gross oedema, ulcer treatment and prophylaxis

A8.3.2   Accessories

Suspender

Suspender, for thigh stockings, net price = 55p, belt (specification 13), = £4.22, fitted (additional price) = 55p

A8.3.3   Anklets

Class 2 Medium Support

Anklets, compression 18–24 mm Hg, circular knit (standard and made-to-measure), net price per pair = £5.56; flat bed (standard and made-to-measure) = £11.54; net (made-to-measure) = £10.92

Uses: soft tissue support

Class 3 Strong Support

Anklets, compression 25–35 mm Hg, circular knit (standard and made-to-measure), net price per pair = £7.74; flat bed (standard) = £7.74; made-to-measure = £11.54

Uses: soft tissue support

A8.3.4   Knee caps

Class 2 Medium Support

Kneecaps, circular knit (standard and made-to-measure), net price per pair = £5.56; flat bed (standard and made-to-measure) = £11.54; net (standard and made-to-measure) = £9.06

Uses: soft tissue support

Class 3 Strong Support

Kneecaps, circular knit (standard and made-to-measure), net price per pair = £7.40; flat bed (standard) = £7.40; made-to-measure = £11.54

Uses: soft tissue support

Appendix 9: Cautionary and advisory labels for dispensed medicines

Numbers following the preparation entries in the BNF correspond to the codenumbers of the cautionary labels that pharmacists are recommended to add when dispensing. It is also expected that pharmacists will counsel patients when necessary.

Counselling needs to be related to the age, experience, background, and understanding of the individual patient. The pharmacist should ensure that the patient understands how to take or use the medicine and how to follow the correct dosage schedule. Any effects of the medicine on driving or work, any foods or medicines to be avoided, and what to do if a dose is missed should also be explained. Other matters, such as the possibility of staining of the clothes or skin by a medicine should also be mentioned.

For some preparations there is a special need for counselling, such as an unusual method or time of administration or a potential interaction with a common food or domestic remedy, and this is indicated where necessary.

ORIGINAL PACKS. Many preparations are now dispensed in unbroken original packs that bear complete instructions for the patient or provide a leaflet addressed to the patient. These labels or leaflets should not normally be obscured or removed. Where it is known that such instructions are provided with an original pack intended for the patient no label has been listed under the preparation. Label 10 may be used where appropriate. Leaflets are available from various sources advising on the administration of preparations such as eye-drops, eye ointments, inhalers, and suppositories.

SCOPE OF LABELS. In general no label recommendations have been made for injections on the assumption that they will be administered by a health professional or a well-instructed patient. The labelling is not exhaustive and pharmacists are recommended to use their professional discretion in labelling new preparations and those for which no labels are shown.

Individual labelling advice is not given on the administration of the large variety of antacids. In the absence of instructions from the prescriber, and if on enquiry the patient has had no verbal instructions, the directions given under 'Dose' should be used on the label.

It is recognised that there may be occasions when pharmacists will use their knowledge and professional discretion and decide to omit one or more of the recommended labels for a particular patient. In this case counselling is of the utmost importance. There may also be an occasion when a prescriber does not wish additional cautionary labels to be used, in which case the prescription should be endorsed 'NCL' (no cautionary labels). The exact wording that is required instead should then be specified on the prescription.

Pharmacists have traditionally labelled medicines with various wordings in addition to those directions specified on the prescription. Such labels include 'Shake the bottle', 'For external use only', and 'Store in a cool place', as well as 'Discard . . . . days after opening' and 'Do not use after . . . .', which apply particularly to antibiotic mixtures, diluted liquid and topical preparations, and to eye-drops. Although not listed in the BNF these labels should continue to be used when appropriate; indeed, 'For external use only' is a legal requirement on external liquid preparations, while 'Keep out of the reach of children' is a legal requirement on all dispensed medicines.

It is the usual practice for patients to take standard tablets with water or other liquid and for this reason no separate label has been recommended.

The label or labels for each preparation are recommended after careful consideration of the information available. However, it is recognised that in some cases this information may be either incomplete or open to a different interpretation. The Executive Editor will therefore be grateful to receive any constructive comments on the labelling suggested for any preparation.

Recommended label wordings

Wordings which can be given as separate warnings are labels 1–19 and labels 29–33. Wordings which can be incorporated in an appropriate position in the directions for dosage or administration are labels 21–28. A label has been omitted for number 20.

If separate labels are used it is recommended that the wordings be used without modification. If changes are made to suit computer requirements, care should be taken to retain the sense of the original.

1   **Warning. May cause drowsiness**

To be used on *preparations for children* containing antihistamines, or other preparations given to children where the warnings of label 2 on driving or alcohol would not be appropriate.

2   **Warning. May cause drowsiness. If affected do not drive or operate machinery. Avoid alcoholic drink**

To be used on *preparations for adults that can cause drowsiness*, thereby affecting the ability to drive and operate hazardous machinery; label 1 is more appropriate for children. *It is an offence to drive while under the influence of drink or drugs.*

Some of these preparations only cause drowsiness in the first few days of treatment and some only cause drowsiness in higher doses.

In such cases the patient should be told that the advice applies until the effects have worn off. However many of these preparations can produce a slowing of reaction time and a loss of mental concentration that can have the same effects as drowsiness.

Avoidance of alcoholic drink is recommended because the effects of CNS depressants are enhanced by alcohol. Strict prohibition however could lead to some patients not taking the medicine. Pharmacists should therefore explain the risk and encourage compliance, particularly in patients who may think they already tolerate the effects of alcohol (see also label 3). Queries from patients with epilepsy regarding fitness to drive should be referred back to the patient's doctor.

Side-effects unrelated to drowsiness that may affect a patient's ability to drive or operate machinery safely include *blurred vision, dizziness, or nausea*. In general, no label has been recommended to cover these cases, but the patient should be suitably counselled.

3   Warning. May cause drowsiness. If affected do not drive or operate machinery

To be used on *preparations containing monoamine-oxidase inhibitors*; the warning to avoid alcohol and dealcoholised (low alcohol) drink is covered by the patient information leaflet.

Also to be used as for label 2 but where alcohol is not an issue.

4   Warning. Avoid alcoholic drink

To be used on *preparations where a reaction such as flushing may occur if alcohol is taken* (e.g. metronidazole and chlorpropamide). Alcohol may also enhance the hypoglycaemia produced by some oral antidiabetic drugs but routine application of a warning label is not considered necessary.

5   Do not take indigestion remedies at the same time as this medicine

To be used with label 25 on *preparations coated to resist gastric acid* (e.g. enteric-coated tablets). This is to avoid the possibility of premature dissolution of the coating in the presence of an alkaline pH.

Label 5 also applies to drugs such as ketoconazole *where the absorption is significantly affected by antacids*; the usual period of avoidance recommended is 2 to 4 hours.

6   Do not take iron preparations or indigestion remedies at the same time of day as this medicine

To be used on *preparations containing ciprofloxacin, doxycycline, minocycline, and penicillamine*. These drugs chelate iron and calcium ions and are less well absorbed when given with iron or calcium-containing antacids. If necessary these incompatible preparations may be given about two hours apart.

7   Do not take milk, iron preparations or indigestion remedies at the same time of day as this medicine

To be used on *preparations containing tetracyclines that chelate iron, calcium, and magnesium* and are thus less available for absorption; if it is necessary to give milk, iron or antacids, the usual period of avoidance is about 2 hours. Doxycycline and minocycline are less liable to form chelates and therefore only require label 6 (see above).

8   Do not stop taking this medicine except on your doctor's advice

To be used on *preparations that contain a drug which is required to be taken over long periods without the patient necessarily perceiving any benefit* (e.g. antituberculous drugs).

Also to be used on *preparations that contain a drug whose withdrawal is likely to be a particular hazard* (e.g. clonidine for hypertension). Label 10 (see below) is more appropriate for corticosteroids.

9   Take at regular intervals. Complete the prescribed course unless otherwise directed

To be used on *preparations where a course of treatment should be completed* to reduce the incidence of relapse or failure of treatment.

The preparations are antimicrobial drugs given by mouth. Very occasionally, some may have severe side-effects (e.g. diarrhoea in patients receiving clindamycin) and in such cases the patient may need to be advised of reasons for stopping treatment quickly and returning to the doctor.

10   Warning. Follow the printed instructions you have been given with this medicine

To be used particularly on *preparations containing anticoagulants, lithium and oral corticosteroids*. The appropriate treatment card should be given to the patient and any necessary explanations given.

This label may also be used on other preparations to remind the patient of the instructions that have been given.

11   Avoid exposure of skin to direct sunlight or sun lamps

To be used *on preparations that may cause phototoxic or photoallergic reactions* if the patient is exposed to ultraviolet radiation. Many drugs other than those listed (e.g. phenothiazines and sulphonamides) may on rare occasions cause reactions in susceptible patients. Exposure to high intensity ultraviolet radiation from sunray lamps and sunbeds is particularly likely to cause reactions.

12   Do not take anything containing aspirin while taking this medicine

To be used *on preparations containing probenecid and sulfinpyrazone* whose activity is reduced by aspirin.

Label 12 should not be used for anticoagulants since label 10 is more appropriate.

13   Dissolve or mix with water before taking
To be used on *preparations that are intended to be dissolved in water* (e.g. soluble tablets) or *mixed with water* (e.g. powders, granules) before use. In a few cases other liquids such as fruit juice or milk may be used.

14   This medicine may colour the urine
To be used on *preparations that may cause the patient's urine to turn an unusual colour.* These include phenolphthalein (alkaline urine pink), triamterene (blue under some lights), levodopa (dark reddish), and rifampicin (red).

15   Caution flammable: keep away from fire or flames
To be used on *preparations containing sufficient flammable solvent to render them flammable if exposed to a naked flame.*

16   Allow to dissolve under the tongue. Do not transfer from this container. Keep tightly closed. Discard eight weeks after opening
To be used on *glyceryl trinitrate tablets* to remind the patient not to transfer the tablets to plastic or less suitable containers.

17   Do not take more than . . . in 24 hours
To be used on *preparations for the treatment of acute migraine* except those containing ergotamine, for which label 18 is used. The dose form should be specified, e.g. tablets or capsules.
It may also be used on preparations for which no dose has been specified by the prescriber.

18   Do not take more than . . . in 24 hours or
. . . in any one week
To be used on preparations containing ergotamine. The dose form should be specified, e.g. tablets or suppositories.

19   Warning. Causes drowsiness which may continue the next day. If affected do not drive or operate machinery. Avoid alcoholic drink
To be used on *preparations containing hypnotics (or some other drugs with sedative effects) prescribed to be taken at night.* On the rare occasions (e.g. nitrazepam in epilepsy) when hypnotics are prescribed for daytime administration this label would clearly not be appropriate. Also to be used as *an alternative to the label 2 wording* (the choice being at the discretion of the pharmacist) *for anxiolytics prescribed to be taken at night.*
It is hoped that this wording will convey adequately the problem of residual morning sedation after taking 'sleeping tablets'.

21   . . . with or after food
To be used on *preparations that are liable to cause gastric irritation,* or *those that are better absorbed with food.*
Patients should be advised that a *small amount of food is sufficient.*

22   . . . half to one hour before food
To be used on some preparations *whose absorption is thereby improved.* Most oral antibiotics require label 23 instead (see below).

23   . . . an hour before food or on an empty stomach
To be used on *oral antibiotics whose absorption may be reduced by the presence of food and acid in the stomach.*

24   . . . sucked or chewed
To be used on *preparations that should be sucked or chewed.*
The pharmacist should use discretion as to which of these words is appropriate.

25   . . . swallowed whole, not chewed
To be used on *preparations that are enteric-coated or designed for modified-release.*
Also to be used on *preparations that taste very unpleasant or may damage the mouth* if not swallowed whole.

26   . . . dissolved under the tongue
To be used on *preparations designed for sublingual use.* Patients should be advised to hold under the tongue and avoid swallowing until dissolved. The buccal mucosa between the gum and cheek is occasionally specified by the prescriber.

27   . . . with plenty of water
To be used on *preparations that should be well diluted* (e.g. chloral hydrate), *where a high fluid intake is required* (e.g. sulphonamides), or *where water is required to aid the action* (e.g. methylcellulose). The patient should be advised that 'plenty' means at least 150 mL (about a tumblerful). In most cases fruit juice, tea, or coffee may be used.

28   To be spread thinly . . .
To be used on *external preparations* that should be applied sparingly (e.g. corticosteroids, dithranol).

29   Do not take more than 2 at any one time. Do not take more than 8 in 24 hours
To be used on containers of dispensed *solid dose preparations containing paracetamol for adults when the instruction on the label indicates that the dose can be taken on an 'as required' basis.* The dose form should be specified, e.g. tablets or capsules.
This label has been introduced because of the serious consequences of overdosage with paracetamol.

30   Do not take with any other paracetamol products
To be used on all containers of dispensed *preparations containing paracetamol.*

31   Contains aspirin and paracetamol. Do not take with any other paracetamol products
To be used on all containers of dispensed *preparations containing aspirin and paracetamol (e.g. benorilate).*

32 Contains aspirin
  To be used on containers of dispensed *preparations containing aspirin when the name on the label does not include the word 'aspirin'.*

33 Contains an aspirin-like medicine
  To be used on containers of dispensed *preparations containing aspirin derivatives.*

Products and their labels

Products introduced or amended since publication of BNF No. 38 (September 1999) are underlined.
Proprietary names are in *italic.*
C = counselling advised; see BNF = consult product entry in BNF

Acamprosate, 21, 25
Acarbose, C, administration, see BNF
Accolate, 23
Acebutolol, 8
Aceclofenac, 21
Acemetacin, 21, C, driving
Acenocoumarol, 10 anticoagulant card
Acetazolamide, 3
Acetazolamide m/r, 3, 25
Achromycin, 7, 9, 23, C, posture
Aciclovir susp and tabs, 9
Acipimox, 21
Acitretin, 10 patient information leaflet, 7
Acrivastine, C, driving, alcohol, see BNF
Actinac, 28
Acupan, 2, 14 (urine pink)
Adalat LA, 25
Adalat Retard, 25
Adcal-D₃, 24
Adcortyl external preps, 28
Adcortyl with Graneodin, 28
Adipine MR, 21, 25
Adizem preps, 25
AeroBec, 8, C, dose
AeroBec Forte, 8, 10 steroid card, C, dose
Aerocrom, 8
Aerolin Autohaler, C, dose, see BNF
Airomir, C, dose, change to CFC-free inhaler, see BNF
Akineton, 2
Albendazole, 9
Alclometasone external preps, 28
Aldara, 10 patient information leaflet
Aldomet, 3, 8
Alendronic acid, C, administration, see BNF
Alfuzosin, 3, C, dose, see BNF
Alfuzosin m/r, 3, 25, C, dose, see BNF
Alimemazine, 2
Allegron, 2
Allopurinol, 8, 21, 27
Alphosyl HC, 28
Aloxiprin, 12, 21
Alphaderm, 28
Alprazolam, 2
Altretamine, 21
Alupent inhalation, C, dose, see BNF
Alvedon, 30
Alvercol, 25, 27, C, administration, see BNF
Amantadine, C, driving
Aminophylline m/r, see preps
Amiodarone, 11
Amisulpride, 2
Amitriptyline, 2
Amitriptyline m/r, 2, 25

Amobarbital, 19
Amorolfine, 10 patient information leaflet
Amoxapine, 2
Amoxicillin, 9
Amoxicillin chewable tabs, 9, 10 patient information leaflet
Amoxicillin dispersible sachets, 9, 13
Amoxil, 9
Amoxil dispersible sachets, 9, 13
Amoxil paed susp, 9, C, use of pipette
Amphotericin loz, 9, 24, C, after food
Amphotericin mixt (g.i.), 9, C, use of pipette
Amphotericin mixt (mouth), 9, C, use of pipette, hold in mouth, after food
Amphotericin tabs, 9
Ampicillin, 9, 23
Amytal, 19
Anafranil, 2
Anafranil m/r, 2, 25
Androcur, 21
Andropatch, C, administration, see BNF
Angettes-75, 32
Angiopine MR, 25
Angiopine 40 LA, 21, 25
Angitil SR, 25
Angitil XL, 25
Anhydrol Forte, 15
Anquil, 2
Antabuse, 2, C, alcohol reaction, see BNF
Antacids, see BNF dose statements
Antepsin, 5
Anthranol preps, 28
Anticoagulants, oral, 10 anticoagulant card
Antihistamines (see individual preparations)
Antipressan, 8
Anturan, 12, 21
Apsin VK, 9, 23
Arava, 4
Arpimycin, 9
Arpicolin, 9
Artane, C, before or after food, driving, see BNF
Arythmol, 21, 25
Arthrotec, 21, 25
Asacol tabs, 5, 25, C, blood disorder symptoms, see BNF
Asacol enema and supps, 5, C, blood disorder symptoms, see BNF
Asasantin Retard, 21, 25
Ascorbic acid, effervescent, 13
Ascorbic acid tabs (500mg), 24
Asendis, 2

Asmabec preps, 8, 10 steroid card (high-dose preparations only), C, dose
Asmasal, C, dose, see BNF
Aspav, 2, 13, 21, 32
Aspirin and papaveretum dispersible tabs, 2, 13, 21, also 32 (if 'aspirin' not on label)
Aspirin dispersible tabs, 13, 21, also 32 (if 'aspirin' not on label)
Aspirin effervescent, 13, also 32 (if 'aspirin' not on label)
Aspirin e/c, 5, 25, also 32 (if 'aspirin' not on label)
Aspirin m/r, 25, also 32 (if 'aspirin' not on label)
Aspirin supps, 32 (if 'aspirin' not on label)
Aspirin tabs, 21, also 32 (if 'aspirin' not on label)
Aspirin, paracetamol and codeine tabs, 21, 29, also 31 (if 'aspirin' and 'paracetamol' not on label)
Astemizole, C, driving, alcohol, see BNF
Atarax, 2
Atenolol, 8
Ativan, 2 or 19
Atorvastatin, C, muscle effects, see BNF
Atovaquone, 21
Atromid-S, 21
Atrovent inhalations, C, dose, see BNF
Augmentin susp and tabs, 9
Augmentin Duo, 9
Augmentin dispersible tabs, 9, 13
Auranofin, 21, C, blood disorder symptoms, see BNF
Aureocort, 28
Avloclor, 5, C, malaria prophylaxis, see BNF
Avomine, 2
Azapropazone, 11, 21, C, photosensitivity, see BNF
Azatadine, 2
Azathioprine, 21
Azithromycin caps, 5, 9, 23
Azithromycin susp and tabs, 5, 9

> **New British Approved Names (see p. x) used throughout this Appendix**

Baclofen, 2, 8
Balsalazide, 21, 25
Baratol, 2
Baxan, 9
Beclazone, 8, 10 steroid card (250-microgram only), C, dose
Becloforte preps, 8, 10 steroid card, C, dose

Beclometasone external preps, 28
Beclometasone inhalations, 8, 10 steroid card (high-dose preparations only), C, dose
Becodisks, 8, C, dose
Becotide preps, 8, C, dose
Bedranol S.R., 8, 25
Benemid, 12, 21, 27
Benoral susp and tabs, 21, 31
Benoral gran, 13, 21, 31
Benorilate, 21, 31
Benorilate gran, 13, 21, 31
Benperidol, 2
Benzatropine, 2
Benzoin tincture, cpd, 15
Berkolol, 8
Berotec, C, dose, see BNF
Beta-Adalat, 8, 25
Betacap, 15, 28
Beta-Cardone, 8
Betahistine, 21
Betaloc, 8
Betaloc-SA, 8, 25
Betamethasone inj, 10 steroid card
Betamethasone tab, 10 steroid card, 21
Betamethasone external preps, 28
Betamethasone scalp application, 15, 28
Betaxolol tabs, 8
Bethanechol, 22
Betim, 8
Betnelan, 10 steroid card, 21
Betnesol injection, 10 steroid card
Betnesol tabs, 10 steroid card, 13, 21
Betnovate external preps, 28
Betnovate scalp application, 15, 28
Betnovate-RD, 28
Bettamousse, 28
Bezafibrate, 21
Bezalip, 21
Bezalip-Mono, 21, 25
Biorphen, C, driving
Biperiden, 2
Bisacodyl tabs, 5, 25
Bisoprolol, 8
Bonefos caps and tabs, C, food and calcium, see BNF
Brexidol, 21
Bricanyl inhalations, C, dose, see BNF
Bricanyl SA, 25
Britiazim, 25
Britlofex, 2
Broflex, C, before or after food, driving, see BNF
Bromazepam, 2
Bromocriptine, 21, C, hypotensive reactions, see BNF
Brompheniramine, 2
Brufen, 21
Brufen gran, 13, 21
Brufen Retard, 25, 27
Buccastem, 2, C, administration, see BNF
Budenofalk, 5, 10 steroid card, 22, 25
Budesonide inhalations, 8, 10 steroid card (high-dose preparations only), C, dose
Budesonide caps, 5, 10 steroid card, 22, 25
Buprenorphine, 2, 26
Burinex K, 25, 27, C, posture, see BNF
Buserelin nasal spray, C, nasal decongestants, see BNF
Buspar, C, driving

Buspirone, C, driving
Butacote, 5, 21, 25, C, blood disorder symptoms, see BNF
Butobarbital, 19

New British Approved Names (see p. x) used throughout this Appendix

---

Cabaser, 21, C, hypotensive reactions, see BNF
Cabergoline, 21, C, hypotensive reactions, see BNF
Cacit, 13
Cacit D3, 13
Cafergot, 18, C, dosage
Calceos, 24
Calcicard CR, 25
Calcichew preps, 24
Calcidrink, 13
Calcisorb, 13, 21, C, may be sprinkled on food
Calcium-500, 25
Calcium acetate tabs, 25
Calcium carbonate tabs, chewable, 24
Calcium carbonate tabs and gran effervescent, 13
Calcium gluconate tabs, 24
Calcium phosphate sachets, 13
Calcium Resonium, 13
Calcium and ergocalciferol tabs, C, administration, see BNF
Calcort, 5, 10 steroid card
Calmurid HC, 28
Calpol susp, 30
Camcolit 250 tabs, 10 lithium card, C, fluid and salt intake, see BNF
Camcolit 400 tabs, 10 lithium card, 25, C, fluid and salt intake, see BNF
Campral EC, 21, 25
Canesten HC, 28
Canesten spray, 15
Caprin, 5, 25, 32
Carbachol, 22
Carbamazepine chewable, 3, 8, 21, 24, C, blood, hepatic or skin disorder symptoms (see BNF), driving (see BNF, p. 223)
Carbamazepine liq, supps and tabs, 3, 8, C, blood, hepatic or skin disorder symptoms (see BNF), driving (see BNF, p. 223)
Carbamazepine m/r, 3, 8, 25, C, blood, hepatic or skin disorder symptoms (see BNF), driving (see BNF, p. 223)
Carbenoxolone sodium, see preps
Carbimazole, C, blood disorder symptoms, see BNF
Cardene SR, 25
Cardilate MR, 25
Cardinol, 8
Carisoma, 2
Carisoprodol, 2
Carylderm lotion, 15
Catapres, 3, 8
Catapres Perlongets, 3, 8, 25
Caved-S, 24
Cedocard Retard, 25
Cefaclor, 9
Cefaclor m/r, 9, 21, 25
Cefadroxil, 9
Cefalexin, 9
Cefixime, 9
Cefpodoxime, 5, 9, 21
Cefprozil, 9
Cefradine, 9

Cefuroxime susp, 9, 21
Cefuroxime sachets, 9, 13, 21
Cefuroxime tab, 9, 21, 25
Cefzil, 9
Celance, C, hypotensive reactions, see BNF
Celectol, 8, 22
Celevac (constipation or diarrhoea), C, administration, see BNF
Celevac tabs (anorectic), C, administration, see BNF
Celiprolol, 8, 22
CellCept, 23
Centyl K, 25, 27, C, posture, see BNF
Ceporex caps, mixts, and tabs, 9
Cerivastatin, C, muscle effects, see BNF
Cetirizine, C, driving, alcohol, see BNF
Chemydur 60XL, 25
Chloral hydrate, 19, 27
Chloral paed elixir, 1, 27
Chloral mixt, 19, 27
Chlordiazepoxide, 2
Chloroquine, 5, C, malaria prophylaxis, see BNF
Chlorphenamine, 2
Chlorpromazine mixts and supps, 2, 11
Chlorpromazine tabs, 2, 11
Chlorpropamide, 4
Ciclosporin, C, administration, see BNF
Cimetidine chewable tabs, C, administration, see BNF
Cimetidine effervescent tabs, 13
Cinnarizine, 2
Cinobac, 6, 9, C, driving
Cinoxacin, 6, 9, C, driving
Cipramil drops, C, driving, administration
Cipramil tabs, C, driving
Ciprofloxacin, 6, 9, 25, C, driving
Ciproxin susp and tabs, 6, 9, 25, C, driving
Cisapride, C, administration, see BNF
Citalopram drops, C, driving, administration
Citalopram tabs, C, driving
Citramag, 10 patient information leaflet, 13, C, administration
Clarithromycin, 9
Clarithromycin m/r, 9, 21, 25
Clarityn, C, driving, alcohol, see BNF
Clemastine, 2
Clindamycin, 9, 27, C, diarrhoea, see BNF
Clinoril, 21
Clobazam, 2 or 19, 8, C, driving (see BNF, p. 223)
Clobetasol external preps, 28
Clobetasol scalp application, 15, 28
Clofazimine, 8, 14 (urine red), 21
Clofibrate, 21
Clomethiazole, 19
Clomipramine, 2
Clomipramine m/r, 2, 25
Clonazepam, 2, 8, C, driving (see BNF, p. 223)
Clonidine see *Catapres*
Clonidine m/r, 3, 8, 25
Clopixol, 2
Clorazepate, 2 or 19
Clotrimazole spray, 15

Lipostat, C, muscle effects, see BNF

Liquid paraffin, C, administration, see BNF

Liquid paraffin/phenolphthalein mixt, 14 (alkaline urine pink)

Liskonum, 10 lithium card, 25, C, fluid and salt intake, see BNF

Lisuride, 21, C, hypotensive reactions, see BNF

Litarex, 10 lithium card, 25, C, fluid and salt intake, see BNF

Lithium carbonate, 10 lithium card, C, fluid and salt intake, see BNF

Lithium carbonate m/r, 10 lithium card, 25, C, fluid and salt intake, see BNF

Lithium citrate liq, 10 lithium card, C, fluid and salt intake, see BNF

Lithium citrate m/r, 10 lithium card, 25, C, fluid and salt intake, see BNF

Lithonate, 10 lithium card, 25, C, fluid and salt intake, see BNF

Loceryl, 10 patient information leaflet

Locoid cream, oint, and topical emulsion, 28

Locoid scalp lotion, 15, 28

Locoid C, 28

Lofepramine, 2

Lofexidine, 2

Loprazolam, 19

Lopresor, 8

Lopresor SR, 8, 25

Lopresoretic, 8

Loratadine, C, driving, alcohol, see BNF

Lorazepam, 2 *or* 19

Lormetazepam, 19

Loron caps and tabs, 10 patient information leaflet, C, food and calcium, see BNF

Losec, C, administration, see BNF

Lotriderm, 28

Loxapac, 2

Loxapine, 2

Ludiomil, 2

Lugol's solution, 27

Lustral, C, driving, see BNF

Lyclear Dermal cream, 10 patient information leaflet

Lymecycline, 6, 9

Macrobid, 9, 14 (urine yellow or brown), 21, 25

Macrodantin, 9, 14 (urine yellow or brown), 21

Madopar, 14 (urine reddish), 21

Madopar dispersible tabs, 14 (urine reddish), 21, C, administration, see BNF

Madopar CR, 5, 14 (urine reddish), 25

Magnapen, 9, 22

Magnesium citrate effervescent pdr, 10 patient information leaflet, 13, C, administration

Magnesium sulphate, 13, 23

Magnesium trisilicate oral pdr, cpd, 13

Malarone, 21

Maloprim, C, malaria prophylaxis, see BNF

Manerix, 10 patient information leaflet, 21

Manevac, 25, 27

Maprotiline, 2

Marevan, 10 anticoagulant card

Maxalt, 3

Maxalt Melt, 3, C, administration

Maxepa, 21

Maxolon paed liquid, C, use of pipette

Maxolon SR, 25

Maxtrex (methotrexate), C, NSAIDs (see BNF, p. 518)

Mebeverine, C, administration, see BNF

Mecysteine, 5, 22, 25

Medrone tabs, 10 steroid card, 21

Mefenamic acid caps, paed susp, and tabs, 21

Mefloquine, 21, 25, 27, C, driving, malaria prophylaxis, see BNF

Melleril, 2

Meloxicam tabs, 21

Menorest, C, administration, see BNF

Mepacrine, 4, 9, 14, 21

Meprobamate, 2

Meptazinol, 2

Meptid, 2

Mequitazine, 2

Mesalazine e/c, 5, 25, C, blood disorder symptoms, see BNF

Mesalazine m/r, 25, C, administration, blood disorder symptoms, see BNF

Mesalazine enema and supps, C, blood disorder symptoms, see BNF

Metamucil, 13, C, administration, see BNF

Metformin, 21

Methadone, 2

Methadose, 2

Methenamine, 9

Methocarbamol, 2

Methotrexate tabs, C, NSAIDs (see BNF, p. 518)

Methylcellulose (constipation or diarrhoea), C, administration, see BNF

Methylcellulose tabs (anorectic), C, administration, see BNF

Methyldopa, 3, 8

Methylphenobarbital, 2, 8, C, driving (see BNF, p. 223)

Methylprednisolone external preps, 28

Methylprednisolone inj, 10 steroid card

Methylprednisolone tabs, 10 steroid card, 21

Methysergide, 2, 21

Metirosine, 2

Metoclopramide paed liquid, C, use of pipette

Metoclopramide m/r, see preps

Metopirone, 21, C, driving

Metoprolol, 8

Metoprolol m/r, see preps

Metosyn cream and oint, 28

Metosyn scalp lotion, 15, 28

Metrogel, 10 patient information leaflet

Metrolyl supps, 4, 9

Metronidazole gel, see preps

Metronidazole mixt, 4, 9, 23

Metronidazole supps, 4, 9

Metronidazole tabs, 4, 9, 21, 25, 27

Metyrapone, 21, C, driving

Mexiletine m/r, 25

Mexitil PL Perlongets, 25

Mianserin, 2, 25

Micanol, 28

Miconazole denture lacquer, 10 patient information leaflet

Miconazole oral gel, 9, C, hold in mouth, after food

Miconazole tabs, 9, 21

Mictral, 9, 11, 13

Midrid, 30, C, dosage

Mifegyne, 10 patient information leaflet

Mifepristone, 10 patient information leaflet

Migraleve, 2 (pink tablets), 17, 30

Migranal, 18, C, dosage

Migravess, 13, 17, 32

Migravess Forte, 13, 17, 32

Migril, 2, 18, C, dosage

Mildison, 28

Minocin, 6, 9

Minocin MR, 6, 25

Minocycline, 6, 9,

Minocycline m/r, 6, 25

Mintec, 5, 22, 25

Mintezol, 3, 21, 24

Mirapexin, C, hypotensive reactions, driving, see BNF

Miraxid tabs, 9, 21, 27, C, posture, see BNF

Miraxid paed sachets, 9, 13, 21

Mirtazapine, 2, 25

Mistamine, 25, C, driving

Mizolastine, 25, C, driving

Mizollen, 25, C, driving

Mobic tabs, 21

Mobiflex, 21

Moclobemide, 10 patient information leaflet, 21

Modisal XL, 25

Moditen, 2

Modrasone, 28

Modrenal, 21

Moducren, 8

Mogadon, 19

Molipaxin, 2, 21

Molipaxin CR, 2, 21, 25

Mometasone, 28

Monit preps, 25

Mono-Cedocard, 25

Monocor, 8

Monomax SR, 25

Monosorb XL, 25

Monotrim, 9

Monozide-10, 8

Montelukast chewable tabs, 23, 24

Morcap SR, 2, C, administration, see BNF

Morphine preps, 2

Morphine m/r susp, 2, 13

Morphine m/r caps and tabs, see preps

Motens, 21 no longer required

Motifene, 25

Motipress, 2

Motival, 2

Movicol, 13

Moxisylate, 21

Moxonidine, *3*

MST Continus susp, 2, 13

MST Continus tabs, 2, 25

MXL, 2, C, administration, see BNF

Myambutol, 8

Mycobutin, 8, 14 (urine orange-red), C, soft lenses

Mycophenolate mofetil, 23

Mynah, 8, 23

Myocrisin inj, C, blood disorder symptoms, see BNF

Myotonine Chloride, 22

Phentermine m/r, 25, C, driving

Phenylbutazone, e/c, 5, 21, 25, C, blood disorder symptoms, see BNF

Phenytoin caps and tabs, 8, 27, C, administration, blood or skin disorder symptoms (see BNF), driving (see BNF, p. 223)

Phenytoin chewable tabs, 8, 24, C, blood or skin disorder symptoms (see BNF), driving (see BNF, p. 223)

Phenytoin susp, 8, C, administration, blood or skin disorder symptoms (see BNF), driving (see BNF, p. 223)

Phosex, 25

Phosphate-Sandoz, 13

Phyllocontin Continus, 25

Physeptone, 2

Physiotens, 3

Phytomenadione, 24

Picolax, 10 patient information leaflet, 13, C, solution, see BNF

Pilocarpine tabs, 21, 27, C, driving

Pimozide, 2

Pindolol, 8

Piperazine powder, 13

Piracetam, 3

Piriton, 2

Piroxicam caps and tabs, 21

Piroxicam dispersible tabs, 13, 21

<u>Pivmecillinam</u>, 9, 21, 27, C, posture, see BNF

Pizotifen, 2

Plaquenil, 5, 21

Platet, 13, 32

Plendil, 25

Podophyllin paint cpd, 15, C, application, see BNF

Ponstan, 21

Potaba caps and tabs, 21

Potaba Envules, 13, 21

Potassium chloride m/r, see preps

Potassium citrate mixt, 27

Potassium effervescent tabs, 13, 21

Pramipexole, C, hypotensive reactions, driving, see BNF

Pranoxen Continus, 25

Pravastatin, C, muscle effects, see BNF

Praxilene, 25, 27

Prazosin, 3, C, dose, see BNF

Precortisyl, 10 steroid card, 21

Precortisyl Forte, 10 steroid card, 21

Prednesol, 10 steroid card, 13, 21

Prednisolone inj, 10 steroid card

Prednisolone tabs, 10 steroid card, 21

Prednisolone e/c, 5, 10 steroid card, 25

Prefil, 22, 27, C, administration, see BNF

Prepulsid, C, administration, see BNF

Preservex, 21

Prestim, 8

Priadel liq, 10 lithium card, C, fluid and salt intake, see BNF

Priadel tabs, 10 lithium card, 25, C, fluid and salt intake, see BNF

Primalan, 2

Primidone, 2, 8, C, driving (see BNF, p. 223)

Prioderm lotion, 15

Pripsen, 13

Pro-Banthine, 23

Probenecid, 12, 21, 27

Procarbazine, 4

Prochlorperazine, 2

Prochlorperazine buccal tabs, 2, C, administration, see BNF

Prochlorperazine sachets, 2, 13

Procyclidine, C, driving

Prograf, 23, C, driving, see BNF

Proguanil, 21, C, malaria prophylaxis, see BNF

Progynova TS preps, C, administration, see BNF

Promazine, 2

Promethazine, 2

Prominal, 2, 8, C, driving (see BNF, p. 223)

Propaderm, 28

Propafenone, 21, 25

Propantheline, 23

Propiverine hydrochloride, 3

Propranolol, 8

Propranolol m/r, 8, 25

Prothiaden, 2

Protionamide, 8, 21

Protium, 25

Protriptyline, 2, 11

Prozac, C, driving, see BNF

Psorin, 28

Pulmicort, 8, 10 steroid card, C, dose

Pulmicort LS, 8, C, dose

Pulmicort Respules, 8, 10 steroid card, C, dose

Pylorid, C, discoloration (tongue and faeces), see BNF

Pyrazinamide, 8

Pyrogastrone liquid, 21

Pyrogastrone tabs, 21, 24

Questran preps, 13, C, avoid other drugs at same time, see BNF

Quetiapine, 2

Quinagolide, 21, C, hypotensive reactions, see BNF

Quinidine m/r, 25

Quinocort, 28

Quinoderm with Hydrocortisone, 28

Qvar preps, 8, 10 steroid card (high-dose preparations only), C, dose

Rabeprazole, 25

Ranitidine bismuth citrate, C, discoloration (tongue and faeces), see BNF

Ranitidine effervescent tabs, 13

Rebetol, 21

Reboxetine, C, driving

Redoxon effervescent, 13

Redoxon (500mg), 24

Regulan, 13, C, administration, see BNF

Relifex, 21, 25

Relifex susp, 21

Remedeine, 2, 21, 29, 30

Remedeine effervescent tabs, 2, 13, 21, 29, 30

Requip, 21, C, driving, see BNF

Resonium A, 13

Restandol, 21, 25

Retrovir syrup, C, use of oral syringe

Revanil, 21, C, hypotensive reactions, see BNF

Rheumacin SR, 21, 25, C, driving

Rheumox, 11, 21, C, photosensitivity, see BNF

Rhumalgan, 5, 25

Ridaura, 21, C, blood disorder symptoms, see BNF

Rifabutin, 8, 14 (urine orange-red), C, soft lenses

Rifadin, 8, 14 (urine orange-red), 22, C, soft lenses

Rifampicin caps and mixt, 8, 14 (urine orange-red), 22, C, soft lenses

Rifater, 8, 14 (urine orange-red), 22, C, soft lenses

Rifinah, 8, 14 (urine orange-red), 22, C, soft lenses

Rilutek, C, blood disorders, driving

Rimactane, 8, 14 (urine orange-red), 22, C, soft lenses

Rimactazid, 8, 14 (urine orange-red), 22, C, soft lenses

Risperdal, 2

Risperidone, 2

Ritonavir, 21, C, administration, see BNF

Rivastigmine, 21, 25

Rivotril, 2, 8, C, driving (see BNF, p. 223)

Rizatriptan tabs, 3

Rizatriptan wafers, 3, C, administration

Roaccutane, 10 patient information card, 21

Robaxin, 2

Rohypnol, 19

Ronicol Timespan, 25

Ropinirole, 21, C, driving, see BNF

Rowachol, 22

Rowatinex caps, 25

Rozex, 10 patient information leaflet

Rythmodan Retard, 25

Sabril sachets, 3, 8, 13, C, driving (see BNF, p. 223)

Sabril tabs, 3, 8, C, driving (see BNF, p. 223)

Safapryn, 5, 25

Safapryn-Co, 5, 25

Salactol, 15

Salagen, 21, 27, C, driving

Salatac, 15

Salazopyrin, 14 (urine orange-yellow), C, blood disorder symptoms and soft lenses, see BNF

Salazopyrin EN-tabs, 5, 14 (urine orange-yellow), 21, 25, C, blood disorder symptoms and soft lenses, see BNF

Salbulin, C, dose, change to CFC-free inhaler, see BNF

Salbutamol inhalations, C, dose, see BNF

Salbutamol inhalations (CFC-free), C, dose, change to CFC-free inhaler, see BNF

<u>Salbutamol m/r</u>, 25

Salicylic acid collodion, 15

Salicylic acid lotion, 15

Salmeterol, C, dose, see BNF

Salofalk, 5, 25, C, blood disorder symptoms, see BNF

Salsalate, 21, 33

Salts latex adhesive soln, 15

Salts 'SPR' plaster remover, 15

Sandimmun, C, administration, see BNF

Dental Practitioners' Formulary

List of Dental Preparations

The following list has been approved by the appropriate Secretaries of State, and the preparations therein may be prescribed by dental practitioners on form FP10D (GP14 in Scotland).

Sugar-free versions, where available, are preferred.

Aciclovir Cream, BP
Aciclovir Oral Suspension, BP, 200 mg/5 mL
Aciclovir Tablets, BP, 200 mg
Amoxicillin Capsules, BP
Amoxicillin Oral Powder, DPF[1]
Amoxicillin Oral Suspension, BP
Amphotericin Lozenges, BP
Amphotericin Oral Suspension, DPF
Ampicillin Capsules, BP
Ampicillin Oral Suspension, BP
Artificial Saliva, DPF
Ascorbic Acid Tablets, BP
Aspirin Tablets, Dispersible, BP[2]
Benzydamine Mouthwash, DPF[3]
Benzydamine Oral Spray, DPF[3]
Carbamazepine Tablets, BP
Carmellose Gelatin Paste, DPF
Cefalexin Capsules, BP
Cefalexin Oral Suspension, BP
Cefalexin Tablets, BP
Cefradine Capsules, BP
Cefradine Oral Solution, DPF
Chlorhexidine Gluconate 1% Gel, DPF
Chlorhexidine Mouthwash, DPF
Chlorhexidine Oral Spray, DPF
Chlorphenamine Tablets/Chlorpheniramine Tablets, BP
Choline Salicylate Dental Gel, BP
Clindamycin Capsules, BP
Clindamycin Oral Suspension, Paediatric, DPF
Diazepam Oral Solution, BP, 2 mg/5 mL
Diazepam Tablets, BP
Diflunisal Tablets, BP
Dihydrocodeine Tablets, BP, 30 mg
Doxycycline Capsules, BP, 100 mg
Ephedrine Nasal Drops, BP
Erythromycin Ethyl Succinate Oral Suspension, BP
Erythromycin Ethyl Succinate Tablets, BP
Erythromycin Stearate Tablets, BP
Erythromycin Tablets, BP
Fluconazole Capsules, 50 mg, DPF
Fluconazole Oral Suspension, 50 mg/5 mL, DPF
Hydrocortisone Cream, BP, 1%
Hydrocortisone Lozenges, BPC[4]
Hydrocortisone and Miconazole Cream, DPF
Hydrocortisone and Miconazole Ointment, DPF
Hydrogen Peroxide Mouthwash, DPF[3]

Ibuprofen Oral Suspension, BP, sugar-free
Ibuprofen Tablets, BP
Lidocaine 5% Ointment/Lignocaine 5% Ointment, DPF
Menthol and Eucalyptus Inhalation, BP 1980[5]
Metronidazole Oral Suspension, DPF
Metronidazole Tablets, BP
Miconazole Oral Gel, DPF
Mouthwash Solution-tablets, DPF
Nitrazepam Tablets, BP
Nystatin Ointment, BP
Nystatin Oral Suspension, BP
Nystatin Pastilles, DPF
Oxytetracycline Capsules, BP
Oxytetracycline Tablets, BP
Paracetamol Oral Suspension, BP[6]
Paracetamol Tablets, BP
Paracetamol Tablets, Soluble, BP
Penciclovir Cream, DPF
Pethidine Tablets, BP
Phenoxymethylpenicillin Oral Solution, BP
Phenoxymethylpenicillin Tablets, BP
Povidone–iodine Mouthwash, DPF
Probenecid Tablets, BP
Promethazine Hydrochloride Tablets, BP
Promethazine Oral Solution, BP
Sodium Chloride Mouthwash, Compound, BP
Sodium Fluoride Oral Drops, DPF
Sodium Fluoride Tablets, DPF
Sodium Fusidate Ointment, BP
Sodium Perborate Mouthwash, DPF
Temazepam Oral Solution, BP
Temazepam Tablets, DPF
Tetracycline Capsules, BP
Tetracycline Tablets, BP
Thymol Glycerin, Compound, BP 1988[5]
Triamcinolone Dental Paste, BP
Vitamin B Tablets, Compound, Strong, BPC
Zinc Sulphate Mouthwash, DPF

> Preparations in this list which are not included in the BP or BPC are described on next page

1. Amoxicillin Dispersible Tablets are no longer available
2. The BP directs that when soluble aspirin tablets are prescribed, dispersible aspirin tablets should be dispensed
3. Included in the BP
4. Supplies may be difficult to obtain
5. This preparation does not appear in subsequent editions of the BP
6. The BP directs that when Paediatric Paracetamol Oral Suspension or Paediatric Paracetamol Mixture is prescribed and no strength stated Paracetamol Oral Suspension 120 mg/5 mL should be dispensed

Details of DPF preparations

Preparations on the List of Dental Preparations which are specified as DPF are described as follows in the DPF.

Although brand names have sometimes been included for identification purposes preparations on the list should be prescribed by non-proprietary name.

Amoxicillin Oral Powder PoM (proprietary product: *Amoxil Sachets SF*), amoxicillin (as trihydrate) 750 mg[1] and 3 g sachet
  1. 750-mg sachets are no longer available

Amphotericin Oral Suspension PoM (proprietary product: *Fungilin Suspension*), amphotericin 100 mg/mL

Artificial Saliva, (proprietary product: *Luborant*) consists of sorbitol 1.8 g, carmellose sodium (sodium carboxymethylcellulose) 390 mg, dibasic potassium phosphate 48.23 mg, potassium chloride 37.5 mg, monobasic potassium phosphate 21.97 mg, calcium chloride 9.972 mg, magnesium chloride 3.528 mg, sodium fluoride 258 micrograms/60 mL, with preservatives and colouring agents

Benzydamine Mouthwash (proprietary product: *Difflam Oral Rinse*), benzydamine hydrochloride 0.15%

Benzydamine Oral Spray (proprietary product: *Difflam Spray*), benzydamine hydrochloride 0.15%

Carmellose Gelatin Paste (proprietary product: *Orabase Oral Paste*), gelatin, pectin, carmellose sodium, 16.58% of each in a suitable basis

Cefradine Oral Solution PoM (proprietary product: *Velosef Syrup*), cefradine 250 mg/5mL when reconstituted with water

Chlorhexidine Gluconate 1% Gel (proprietary product: *Corsodyl Dental Gel*), chlorhexidine gluconate 1%

Chlorhexidine Mouthwash (proprietary products: *Chlorohex 2000 Mouthwash, Corsodyl Mouthwash*), chlorhexidine gluconate 0.2%

Chlorhexidine Oral Spray (proprietary product: *Corsodyl Oral Spray*), chlorhexidine gluconate 0.2%

Clindamycin Oral Suspension, Paediatric PoM (proprietary product: *Dalacin C Paediatric Suspension*), clindamycin (as palmitate hydrochloride) 75 mg /5mL when reconstituted with purified water (freshly boiled and cooled)

Fluconazole Capsules 50 mg PoM (proprietary product: *Diflucan*), fluconazole 50 mg

Fluconazole Oral Suspension 50 mg/5 mL PoM (proprietary product: *Diflucan*), fluconazole 50 mg/5 mL when reconstituted with water

Hydrocortisone and Miconazole Cream PoM (proprietary product: *Daktacort Cream*), hydrocortisone 1%, miconazole nitrate 2%

Hydrocortisone and Miconazole Ointment PoM (proprietary product: *Daktacort Ointment*), hydrocortisone 1%, miconazole nitrate 2%

Hydrogen Peroxide Mouthwash consists of hydrogen peroxide solution 6% (≡ approx. 20 volume), BP

Lidocaine 5% Ointment/Lignocaine 5% Ointment (proprietary product: *Xylocaine Ointment*), lidocaine 5% in a suitable basis

Metronidazole Oral Suspension PoM (proprietary product: *Flagyl S*), metronidazole (as benzoate) 200 mg /5mL

²Miconazole Oral Gel PoM (proprietary product: *Daktarin Oral Gel*), miconazole 24 mg/mL
  2. For exemption, see p. 496

Mouthwash Solution-tablets consist of tablets which may contain antimicrobial, colouring and flavouring agents in a suitable soluble effervescent basis to make a mouthwash suitable for dental purposes

Nystatin Pastilles PoM (proprietary product: *Nystan Pastilles*), nystatin 100 000 units

Penciclovir Cream ▼ PoM (proprietary product: *Vectavir Cream*), penciclovir 1%

Povidone–iodine Mouthwash (proprietary product: *Betadine Mouthwash*), povidone–iodine 1%

Sodium Fluoride Oral Drops see section 9.5.3

Sodium Fluoride Tablets see section 9.5.3

Sodium Perborate Mouthwash (proprietary product: *Bocasan Mouthwash*), sodium perborate 68.6%

³Temazepam Tablets CD temazepam 10 and 20 mg
  3. See p. 7 for prescribing requirements for temazepam

Zinc Sulphate Mouthwash consists of zinc sulphate lotion, BP. Directions for use: dilute 1 part with 4 parts of warm water
  Note. May be difficult to obtain

Nurse Prescribers' Formulary

Nurse Prescribers' Formulary Appendix
(Appendix NPF). List of preparations approved by
the Secretary of State which may be prescribed on
forms FP10CN and FP10PN (form GP10(N) in
Scotland, form HS21(N) in Northern Ireland) by
Nurses for National Health Service patients

Medicinal preparations

Almond Oil Ear Drops, BP

Arachis Oil Enema, NPF

[1]Aspirin Tablets, Dispersible, 300 mg, BP

Bisacodyl Suppositories, BP (includes 5-mg and 10-mg
strengths)

Bisacodyl Tablets, BP

Cadexomer–Iodine Ointment, NPF

Cadexomer–Iodine Paste, NPF

Cadexomer–Iodine Powder, NPF

Calamine Cream, Aqueous, BP

Calamine Lotion, BP

Calamine Lotion, Oily, BP 1980

Catheter Maintenance Solution, Chlorhexidine, NPF

Catheter Maintenance Solution, Mandelic Acid, NPF

Catheter Maintenance Solution, Sodium Chloride,
NPF

Catheter Maintenance Solution, 'Solution G', NPF

Catheter Maintenance Solution, 'Solution R', NPF

Clotrimazole Cream 1%, BP

Co-danthramer Capsules, NPF

Co-danthramer Capsules, Strong, NPF

Co-danthramer Oral Suspension, NPF

Co-danthramer Oral Suspension, Strong, NPF

Co-danthrusate Capsules, BP

Co-danthrusate Oral Suspension, NPF

Dextranomer Beads, NPF

Dextranomer Paste, NPF

Dimeticone barrier creams containing at least 10%

Docusate Capsules, BP

Docusate Enema, NPF

Docusate Enema, Compound, BP

Docusate Oral Solution, BP

Docusate Oral Solution, Paediatric, BP

Econazole Cream 1%, BP

Emollients as listed below:
  Alcoderm® Cream
  Alcoderm® Lotion
  Aqueous Cream, BP
  Dermamist®
  Diprobase® Cream
  Diprobase® Ointment
  E45® Cream
  Emulsifying Ointment, BP
  Epaderm®
  Humiderm® Cream
  Hydromol® Cream
  Hydrous Ointment, BP
  Keri® Therapeutic Lotion
  LactiCare® Lotion
  Lipobase®
  Neutrogena® Dermatological Cream
  Oilatum® Cream
  Ultrabase®
  Unguentum M®

Emollient Bath Additives as listed below:
  Alpha Keri® Bath Oil
  [2]Balneum®
  Diprobath®
  Emmolate® Bath Oil
  Hydromol® Emollient
  Oilatum® Emollient
  Oilatum® Fragrance Free
  Oilatum® Gel

Folic Acid 400 micrograms/5 mL Oral Solution, NPF

Folic Acid Tablets 400 micrograms, BP

Glycerol Suppositories, BP

Ispaghula Husk Granules, BP

Ispaghula Husk Granules, Effervescent, BP

Ispaghula Husk Oral Powder, BP

Lactitol Powder, NPF

Lactulose Powder, NPF

Lactulose Solution, BP

Lidocaine Gel/Lignocaine Gel, BP

Lidocaine Ointment/Lignocaine Ointment, NPF

Lidocaine and Chlorhexidine Gel/Lignocaine and
Chlorhexidine Gel, BP

Macrogol Oral Powder, Compound, NPF

Magnesium Hydroxide Mixture, BP

Magnesium Sulphate Paste, BP

Malathion alcoholic lotions containing at least 0.5%

Malathion aqueous lotions containing at least 0.5%

Mebendazole Oral Suspension, NPF

Mebendazole Tablets, NPF

Miconazole Cream 2%, BP

Miconazole Oral Gel, NPF

Mouthwash Solution-tablets, NPF

Nystatin Oral Suspension, BP

Nystatin Pastilles, NPF

Olive Oil Ear Drops, BP

Paracetamol Oral Suspension, BP (includes 120 mg/
5 mL and 250 mg/5 mL strengths—both of which are
available as sugar-free formulations)

[1]Paracetamol Tablets, BP

[1]Paracetamol Tablets, Soluble, BP

Permethrin Cream, NPF

Permethrin Cream Rinse, NPF

Phenothrin Alcoholic Lotion, NPF

Phenothrin Aqueous Lotion, NPF

Phenothrin Foam Application, NPF

Phosphates Enema, BP

Piperazine Citrate Elixir, BP

Piperazine and Senna Powder, NPF

Povidone–Iodine Solution, BP

Senna Granules, Standardised, BP

Senna Oral Solution, NPF

Senna Tablets, BP

Senna and Ispaghula Granules, NPF

Sodium Chloride Solution, Sterile, BP

Sodium Citrate Compound Enema, NPF

Sodium Picosulfate Elixir, NPF

Sterculia Granules, NPF

Sterculia and Frangula Granules, NPF

Streptokinase and Streptodornase Topical Powder,
NPF

Thymol Glycerin, Compound, BP 1988

Titanium Ointment, NPF

Zinc and Castor Oil Ointment, BP

Zinc Oxide and Dimeticone Spray, NPF

Zinc Oxide Impregnated Medicated Stocking, NPF

Preparations on this list which are not included in the
BP or BPC are described on p. 711

---

1. Max. 96 tablets; max. pack size 32 tablets
2. Except pack sizes that are not to be prescribed under
   the NHS (see Part XVIIIA of the Drug Tariff, Part XI of
   the Northern Ireland Drug Tariff)

Appliances and Reagents (including Wound Management Products)

Chemical Reagents

The following as listed in Part IXR of the Drug Tariff (Part 9 of the Scottish Drug Tariff, Part II of the Northern Ireland Drug Tariff):

Detection Tablets for Glycosuria

Detection Tablets for Ketonuria

Detection Strips for Glycosuria

Detection Strips for Ketonuria

Detection Strips for Proteinuria

Detection Strips for Blood Glucose

Fertility (Ovulation) Thermometer as listed under Contraceptive Devices in Part IXA of the Drug Tariff (Part 3 of the Scottish Drug Tariff, Part III of the Northern Ireland Drug Tariff)

Film Gloves, Disposable, EMA as listed under Protectives in Part IXA of the Drug Tariff (Part 2 of the Scottish Drug Tariff, Part III of the Northern Ireland Drug Tariff)

Elastic Hosiery including accessories as listed in Part IXA of the Drug Tariff (Part 4 of the Scottish Drug Tariff, Part III of the Northern Ireland Drug Tariff)

Hypodermic Equipment

The following as listed in Part IXA of the Drug Tariff (Part 3 of the Scottish Drug Tariff, Part III of the Northern Ireland Drug Tariff):

Hypodermic Syringes—U100 Insulin

Hypodermic Syringe—Single Use or Single-patient Use, U100 Insulin with Needle

Hypodermic Needles—Sterile, Single-use

Lancets—Sterile, Single-use

Needle Clipping Device

Incontinence Appliances as listed in Part IXB of the Drug Tariff (Part 5 of the Scottish Drug Tariff, Part III of the Northern Ireland Drug Tariff)

Irrigation Fluids as listed in Part IXA of the Drug Tariff (Part 2 of the Scottish Drug Tariff, Part III of the Northern Ireland Drug Tariff)

Pessaries, Ring as listed in Part IXA of the Drug Tariff (Part 3 of the Scottish Drug Tariff, Part III of the Northern Ireland Drug Tariff)

Stoma Appliances and Associated Products as listed in Part IXC of the Drug Tariff (Part 6 of the Scottish Drug Tariff, Part III of the Northern Ireland Drug Tariff)

Urethral Catheters as listed under Catheters in Part IXA of the Drug Tariff (Part 3 of the Scottish Drug Tariff, Part III of the Northern Ireland Drug Tariff)

Urine Sugar Analysis Equipment as listed in Part IXA of the Drug Tariff (Parts 3 and 9 of the Scottish Drug Tariff, Part III of the Northern Ireland Drug Tariff)

Wound Management and Related Products
(including bandages, dressings, gauzes, lint, stockinette, etc)

The following as listed in Part IXA of the Drug Tariff (Part 2 of the Scottish Drug Tariff, Part III of the Northern Ireland Drug Tariff):

Absorbent Cottons

Absorbent Cotton Gauzes

Absorbent Cotton and Viscose Ribbon Gauze, BP 1988

Absorbent Lint, BPC

Absorbent Perforated Plastic Film Faced Dressing

Arm Slings

Cellulose Wadding, BP 1988

Cotton Conforming Bandage, BP 1988

Cotton Crêpe Bandage, BP 1988

Cotton Crêpe Bandage, Hospicrepe 239

Cotton, Polyamide and Elastane Bandage

Cotton Stretch Bandage, BP 1988

Crêpe Bandage, BP 1988

Elastic Adhesive Bandage, BP

Elastic Web Bandages

Elastomer and Viscose Bandage, Knitted

Gauze and Cotton Tissues

Heavy Cotton and Rubber Elastic Bandage, BP

High Compression Bandages (Extensible)

Knitted Polyamide and Cellulose Contour Bandage, BP 1988

Knitted Viscose Primary Dressing, BP, Type 1

Multi-layer Compression Bandaging

Multiple Pack Dressing No. 1

Open-wove Bandage, BP 1988, Type 1

Paraffin Gauze Dressing, BP

Polyamide and Cellulose Contour Bandage, BP 1988

Povidone–Iodine Fabric Dressing, Sterile

Short Stretch Compression Bandage

Skin Closure Strips, Sterile

Sterile Dressing Packs

Stockinettes

Sub-compression Wadding Bandage

Surgical Adhesive Tapes

Suspensory Bandages, Cotton

Swabs

Triangular Calico Bandage, BP 1980

Vapour-permeable Adhesive Film Dressing, BP

Vapour-permeable Waterproof Plastic Wound Dressing, BP, Sterile

Wound Management Dressings (including alginate, cavity, hydrocolloid, hydrogel and foam)

Zinc Paste Bandages (including both plain and with additional ingredients)

In the Drug Tariff Appliances and Reagents which may **not** be prescribed by Nurses are annotated Ⓧ

(**Nx** in the Scottish Drug Tariff and ⋈ in the Northern Ireland Drug Tariff)

Details of NPF preparations

Preparations on the Nurse Prescribers' Formulary which are not included in the BP or BPC are described as follows in the Nurse Prescribers' Formulary.

Although brand names have sometimes been included for identification purposes the non-proprietary names shown on the list should be used for prescribing purposes.

Arachis Oil Enema (proprietary product: *Fletchers' Arachis Oil Retention Enema*), arachis oil

Cadexomer–Iodine Ointment (proprietary product: *Iodosorb Ointment*), cadexomer–iodine containing iodine 0.9% in an ointment basis

Cadexomer–Iodine Paste PoM (proprietary product: *Iodoflex*), cadexomer–iodine containing iodine 0.9% in a paste basis

Cadexomer–Iodine Powder PoM (proprietary product: *Iodosorb Powder*), cadexomer–iodine containing iodine 0.9%

Catheter Maintenance Solution, Chlorhexidine
(proprietary products: *Uro-Tainer Chlorhexidine*; *Uriflex C*), chlorhexidine 0.02%

Catheter Maintenance Solution, Mandelic Acid
(proprietary product: *Uro-Tainer Mandelic Acid*), mandelic acid 1%

Catheter Maintenance Solution, Sodium Chloride
(proprietary products: *Uro-Tainer Sodium Chloride*; *Uriflex-S*), sodium chloride 0.9%

Catheter Maintenance Solution, 'Solution G' (proprietary products: *Uro-Tainer Suby G*, *Uriflex G*), citric acid 3.23%, magnesium oxide 0.38%, sodium bicarbonate 0.7%, disodium edetate 0.01%

Catheter Maintenance Solution, 'Solution R' (proprietary products: *Uro-Tainer Solution R*, *Uriflex R*), citric acid 6%, gluconolactone 0.6%, magnesium carbonate 2.8%, disodium edetate 0.01%

Co-danthramer Capsules PoM co-danthramer 25/200 (dantron 25 mg, poloxamer '188' 200 mg)

Co-danthramer Capsules, Strong PoM co-danthramer 37.5/500 (dantron 37.5 mg, poloxamer '188' 500 mg)

Co-danthramer Oral Suspension PoM (proprietary product: *Codalax*), co-danthramer 25/200 in 5 mL (dantron 25 mg, poloxamer '188' 200 mg/5 mL)

Co-danthramer Oral Suspension, Strong PoM (proprietary product: *Codalax Forte*), co-danthramer 75/1000 in 5 mL (dantron 75 mg, poloxamer '188' 1 g/5 mL)

Co-danthrusate Oral Suspension PoM (proprietary product: *Normax*), co-danthrusate 50/60 (dantron 50 mg, docusate sodium 60 mg/5 mL)

Dextranomer Beads (proprietary product: *Debrisan Beads*), dextranomer

Dextranomer Paste (proprietary product: *Debrisan Paste*), dextranomer in a soft paste basis

Dimeticone barrier creams (proprietary products: *Conotrane Cream*, dimeticone '350' 22%; *Siopel Barrier Cream*, dimeticone '1000' 10%; *Vasogen Barrier Cream*, dimeticone 20%), dimeticone 10–22%

Docusate Enema (proprietary product: *Norgalax Micro-enema*) docusate sodium 120 mg in 10 g

Folic Acid Oral Solution 400 micrograms/5 mL
(proprietary product: *Folicare*), folic acid 400 micrograms/5 mL

Lactitol Powder, lactitol 10 g/sachet

Lactulose Powder (proprietary products: *Lactulose Dry*, *Duphalac Dry*), lactulose 10 g/sachet

Lidocaine Ointment/Lignocaine Ointment (proprietary product: *Xylocaine Ointment*), lidocaine 5%

Macrogol Oral Powder, Compound (proprietary product: *Movicol*), macrogol '3350' 13.125 g, sodium bicarbonate 178.5 mg, sodium chloride 350.7 mg, potassium chloride 46.6 mg/sachet

Malathion alcoholic lotions (proprietary products: *Prioderm Lotion*; *Suleo-M Lotion*), malathion 0.5% in an alcoholic basis

Malathion aqueous lotions (proprietary products: *Derbac-M Liquid; Quellada M Liquid*), malathion 0.5% in an aqueous basis

Mebendazole Oral Suspension PoM (proprietary product: *Vermox*), mebendazole 100 mg/5 mL

[1] **Mebendazole Tablets** PoM (proprietary products: *Ovex, Vermox*), mebendazole 100 mg

1. For PoM exemption, see p. 309

[2] **Miconazole Oral Gel** PoM (proprietary product: *Daktarin Oral Gel*), miconazole 24 mg/mL

2. For PoM exemption, see p. 287

Mouthwash Solution-tablets consist of tablets which may contain antimicrobial, colouring and flavouring agents in a suitable soluble effervescent basis to make a mouthwash

Nystatin Pastilles PoM (proprietary product: *Nystan Pastilles*), nystatin 100 000 units

Permethrin Cream (proprietary product: *Lyclear Dermal Cream*), permethrin 5%

Permethrin Cream Rinse (proprietary product: *Lyclear Cream Rinse*), permethrin 1%

Phenothrin Alcoholic Lotion (proprietary product: *Full Marks Lotion*), phenothrin 0.2% in a basis containing isopropyl alcohol

Phenothrin Aqueous Lotion (proprietary product: *Full Marks Liquid*), phenothrin 0.5% in an aqueous basis

Phenothrin Foam Application (proprietary product: *Full Marks Mousse*), phenothrin 0.5% in an alcoholic basis

Piperazine and Senna Powder (proprietary product: *Pripsen Oral Powder*), piperazine phosphate 4 g, sennosides 15.3 mg/sachet

Senna Oral Solution (proprietary product: *Senokot Syrup*), sennosides 7.5 mg/5 mL

Senna and Ispaghula Granules (proprietary product: *Manevac Granules*), senna fruit 12.4%, ispaghula 54.2%

Sodium Citrate Compound Enema (proprietary products: *Micolette Micro-enema*; *Micralax Micro-enema*; *Relaxit Micro-enema*), sodium citrate 450 mg with glycerol, sorbitol and an anionic surfactant

Sodium Picosulfate Elixir (proprietary products: *Dulcolax Liquid, Laxoberal* NHS), sodium picosulfate 5 mg/5 mL

Sterculia Granules (proprietary product: *Normacol Granules*), sterculia 62%

Sterculia and Frangula Granules (proprietary product: *Normacol Plus Granules*), sterculia 62%, frangula (standardised) 8%

Streptokinase and Streptodornase Topical Powder PoM (proprietary product: *Varidase Topical*), streptokinase 100 000 units, streptodornase 25 000 units

Titanium Ointment (proprietary product: *Metanium Ointment*), titanium dioxide 20%, titanium peroxide 5%, titanium salicylate 3%

Zinc Oxide and Dimeticone Spray (proprietary product: *Sprilon*), dimeticone 1.04%, zinc oxide 12.5% in a pressurised aerosol unit

Zinc Oxide Impregnated Medicated Stocking (proprietary product: *Zipzoc*), sterile rayon stocking impregnated with ointment containing zinc oxide 20%

Index of manufacturers

'Special-order' manufac-
turers—see p. 723

AAH
AAH Specials Laboratory,
Royal Victoria Infirmary,
Newcastle upon Tyne NE1 4LP.
Tel: 0191-261 1709
Fax: 0191-261 1709

Abbott
Abbott Laboratories Ltd,
Abbott House, Norden Rd,
Maidenhead, Berks SL6 4XE.
Tel: (01628) 773355
Fax: (01628) 644185

A&H
Allen & Hanburys Ltd,
see GlaxoWellcome.

Adams
Adams Healthcare Ltd
Lotherton Way,
Garforth, Leeds LS25 2JY.
Tel: (0113) 2320066
Fax: (0113) 2871317

Akita
Akita Pharmaceuticals Ltd,
Manx House,
Spectrum Business Estate,
Maidstone, Kent ME15 9YP.
Tel: (0870) 6071260
Fax: (0870) 6071261

Alcon
Alcon Laboratories (UK) Ltd,
Pentagon Park, Boundary Way,
Hemel Hempstead, Herts
HP2 7UD.
Tel: (01442) 341234
Fax: (01442) 341200

Alembic Products
Alembic Products Ltd,
River Lane, Saltney,
Chester, Cheshire CH4 8RQ.
Tel: (01244) 680147
Fax: (01244) 680155

ALK-Abelló
ALK-Abelló (UK) Ltd,
2 Tealgate, Hungerford
Berks RG17 OYT.
Tel: (01488) 686016
Fax: (01488) 685423

Allerayde
Allerayde,
3 Sanigar Court, Whittle Close,
Newark, Notts NG24 2BW.
Tel: (01636) 613444
Fax: (01636) 611186
Allerayde@aol.com

Allergan
Allergan Ltd,
Coronation Rd, High Wycombe,
Bucks HP12 3SH.
Tel: (01494) 444722
Fax: (01494) 473593

Alliance
Alliance Pharmaceuticals Ltd,
Avonbridge House, Bath Road,
Chippenham, Wilts SN15 2BB.
Tel: (01249) 466966
Fax: (01249) 466977
info@alliancepharma.co.uk

AlphaMed
AlphaMed Ltd,
Bensham House,
340 Bensham Lane,
Thornton Heath,
Surrey CR7 7EQ.
Tel: (020) 8684 0470
Fax: (020) 8665 5397

Amersham
Amersham International plc,
Amersham Place,
Little Chalfont, Bucks
HP7 9NA.
Tel: (01494) 544000
Fax: (01494) 542266

Amgen
Amgen Ltd,
240 Cambridge Science Park,
Milton Rd, Cambridge
CB4 0WD.
Tel: (01223) 436422
Fax: (01223) 426314

Anpharm
see Antigen.
Tel: (01704) 562999

Antigen
Antigen Pharmaceuticals (UK),
Antigen House,
82 Waterloo Rd, Hillside,
Southport PR8 4QW.
Tel: (01704) 562777
Fax: (01704) 562888

APS
Approved Prescription Services
Ltd,
Brampton Rd, Hampden Park,
Eastbourne, East Sussex
BN22 9AG.
Tel: (01323) 501111
Fax: (01323) 520306

Ardern
Ardern Healthcare Ltd,
Pipers Brook Farm, Eastham,
Tenbury Wells, Worcs
WR15 8NP.
Tel: (01584) 781777
Fax: (01584) 781788
info@ardernhealthcare.com

Arun
Arun Pharmaceuticals UK Ltd,
Delta House,
Southwood Crescent,
Southwood, Hants GU14 0NL.
Tel: (01252) 543862
Fax: (01252) 547845

Ashbourne
Ashbourne Pharmaceuticals Ltd,
Victors Barns, Hill Farm,
Brixworth, Northampton
NN6 9DQ.
Tel: (01604) 882190
Fax: (01604) 881640

ASTA Medica
ASTA Medica Ltd,
168 Cowley Rd, Cambridge
CB4 ODL.
Tel: (01223) 423434
Fax: (01223) 420943

Astra
AstraZeneca,
Home Park, Kings Langley,
Herts WD4 8DH.
Tel: (0800) 7830033
Fax: (01923) 260431

Astra Tech
Astra Tech Ltd,
Stroudwater Business Park,
Brunel Way, Stonehouse, Glos
GL10 3SW.
Tel: (01453) 791763
Fax: (01453) 791001

Athena
Athena Neurosciences
(Europe) Ltd,
see Elan.

Aurum
Aurum Pharmaceuticals Ltd,
Bampton Rd, Harold Hill,
Romford,
Essex RM3 8UG.
Tel: (01708) 386660
Fax: (01708) 384032

Bailey, Robert
Robert Bailey & Son plc,
Dysart St, Great Moor,
Stockport, Cheshire
SK2 7PF.
Tel: 0161-483 1133
Fax: 0161-483 5587

Baker Norton
Division of Norton Healthcare
see Norton.

Bard
Bard Ltd,
Forest House, Brighton Rd,
Crawley, West Sussex
RH11 9BP.
Tel: (01293) 527888
Fax: (01293) 552428

Bartholomew Rhodes
Bartholomew Rhodes,
Manor House, Victors Barns,
Northampton Rd, Brixworth,
Northampton NN6 9DQ.
Tel: (01604) 882626
Fax: (01604) 883199

Bausch & Lomb
Bausch & Lomb Surgical,
The Enterprise Centre,
Easthampstead Rd,
Bracknell, Berks RG12 1NF.
Tel: (01344) 300440
Fax: (01344) 454558

Baxter
Baxter Healthcare Ltd,
Caxton Way, Thetford, Norfolk
IP24 3SE.
Tel: (01842) 767189
Fax: (01842) 767134

Baxter Anaesthesia
Baxter Anaesthesia,
Unit 31 Wellington Business
Park, Dukes Ride,
Crowthorne, Berks RG45 6LS.
Tel: (01344) 759300
Fax: (01344) 759330

Bayer
Bayer plc,
Pharmaceutical Division,
Bayer House, Strawberry Hill,
Newbury, Berks RG14 1JA.
Tel: (01635) 563000
Fax: (01635) 563393
medical.affairs@bayer.co.uk

Bayer Consumer Care
see Bayer.

Bayer Diagnostics
Bayer plc,
Diagnostics Division,
Bayer House,
Strawberry Hill,
Newbury, Berks RG14 1JA.
Tel: (01635) 563000
Fax: (01635) 563393

BCM Specials
BCM Specials Manufacturing,
D10 First 114,
Nottingham NG90 2PR.
Tel: (0800) 9521010
Fax: (0115) 9591098

Beambridge
Beambridge Medical,
46 Merrow Lane, Burpham,
Guildford,
Surrey GU4 7LQ.
Tel: (01483) 571928
Fax: (01483) 571928

Becton Dickinson
Becton Dickinson UK Ltd,
Between Towns Rd,
Cowley, Oxford,
Oxon OX4 3LY.
Tel: (01865) 748844
Fax: (01865) 717313

Beiersdorf
Beiersdorf UK Ltd,
Yeomans Drive, Blakelands,
Milton Keynes,
Bucks MK14 5LS.
Tel: (01908) 211444
Fax: (01908) 211555

Bell and Croyden
John Bell and Croyden,
54 Wigmore St, London
W1H 0AU.
Tel: (020) 7935 5555
Fax: (020) 7935 9605

Bencard
see SmithKline Beecham.

Berk
Berk Pharmaceuticals,
see APS.

BHR
BHR Pharmaceuticals Ltd,
41 Centenary Business Centre,
Hammond Close,
Attleborough Fields, Nuneaton,
Warwickshire CV11 6RY.
Tel: (024) 7635 3742
Fax: (024) 7632 7812
inf@bhr.co.uk

Bio Diagnostics
Bio Diagnostics Ltd,
Upton Industrial Estate,
Rectory Rd, Upton-upon-Severn,
Worcs WR8 0XL.
Tel: (01684) 592262
Fax: (01684) 592501

Biocare
Biocare International Inc.
Belvoir House, Chapel St,
Haconby, Lincs
PE10 0UP.
Tel: (01778) 570441
Fax: (01778) 570441

Biogen
Biogen Ltd,
Ocean House,
The Ring, Bracknell,
Berks RG12 1AX.
Tel: (01344) 867033
Fax: (01344) 867416

Bioglan
Bioglan Laboratories Ltd,
5 Hunting Gate, Hitchin,
Herts SG4 0TJ.
Tel: (01462) 438444
Fax: (01462) 421242

Biomatrix
Biomatrix UK Ltd,
Lamb House, Church St,
Chiswick,
London W4 2PD.
Tel: (020) 8987 8830
Fax: (020) 8994 7083

Bio-Medical
Bio-Medical Services,
BMS Laboratories Ltd,
River View Rd, Beverley,
North Humberside HU17 0LD.
Tel: (01482) 860228
Fax: (01482) 872042

Biorex
Biorex Laboratories Ltd,
2 Crossfield Chambers,
Gladbeck Way, Enfield,
Middx EN2 7HT.
Tel: (020) 8366 9301
Fax: (020) 8367 4627

Biosurgical Research
Biosurgical Research Unit,
Surgical Materials Testing
Laboratory,
Princess of Wales Hospital,
Coity Rd, Bridgend,
Mid Glamorgan,
South Wales CF31 1RQ.
Tel: (01656) 752820
Fax: (01656) 752830
maggots@smtl.co.uk

Blackwell
Blackwell Supplies Ltd,
Medcare House,
Centurion Close,
Gillingham Business Park,
Gillingham, Kent ME8 0SB.
Tel: (01634) 877620
Fax: (01634) 877621

Blake
Thomas Blake & Co,
The Byre House, Fearby,
Nr. Masham, North Yorkshire
HG4 4NF.
Tel: (01765) 689042
Fax: (01765) 689042

BOC
BOC Gases,
Priestly Rd, Worsley, Manchester
M28 2UT.
Tel: 0800 111333
Fax: 0800 111555

Boehringer Ingelheim
Boehringer Ingelheim Ltd,
Ellesfield Ave, Bracknell, Berks
RG12 4YS.
Tel: (01344) 424600
Fax: (01344) 741444

Boots
Boots The Chemists,
Medical Services,
D90 East FO8,
Nottingham NG90 1BS.
Tel: (0115) 959 5168
Fax: (0115) 959 2565

Borg
Borg Medicare,
PO Box 99,
Hitchin SG5 2GF.
Tel: (01462) 442993
Fax: (01462) 441293

Boston
Boston Hospital Products,
Unit 1-3 Waymills,
Whitchurch,
Shropshire SY13 1QN.
Tel: (01948) 664487
Fax: (01948) 663099
boston@enterprise.net

BPL
Bio Products Laboratory,
Dagger Lane, Elstree, Herts
WD6 3BX.
Tel: (020) 8905 1818
Fax: (020) 8258 2601

Braun
B. Braun (Medical) Ltd,
Brookdale Rd,
Thorncliffe Park Estate,
Chapeltown,
Sheffield S35 2PW.
Tel: (0114) 225 9000
Fax: (0114) 225 9111
enquiry@bbmuk.demon.co.uk

Braun Biotrol
B. Braun Biotrol,
Parkway Close,
Parkway Industrial Estate,
Sheffield S9 4WJ.
Tel: (0114) 225 9000
Fax: (0114) 225 9111

Bray
Bray Health & Leisure,
1 Regal Way, Faringdon,
Oxon SN7 7BX.
Tel: (01367) 240736
Fax: (01367) 242625
solportltd@btinternet.com

Bristol-Myers Squibb
Bristol-Myers Squibb
Pharmaceuticals Ltd,
141–149 Staines Rd, Hounslow,
Middx TW3 3JA.
Tel: (020) 8572 7422
Fax: (020) 8754 3789

Britannia
Britannia Pharmaceuticals Ltd,
41–51 Brighton Rd, Redhill,
Surrey RH1 6YS.
Tel: (01737) 773741
Fax: (01737) 762672
medicalservices@forumgroup.co.uk

Brodie & Stone

Brodie and Stone plc,
51 Calthorpe St,
London WC1X 0HH.
Tel: (020) 7278 9597
Fax: (020) 7278 2458
mailbox@brodieandstone.com

BSIA

BSIA Ltd,
G4, Middlesex Business Centre,
Bridge Rd, Southall
Middx UB2 4AB.
Tel: (020) 8867 4300
Fax: (020) 8893 6855

Bullen

The Bullen Healthcare Group
Ltd,
3–11 Moss St, Liverpool L6 1EY.
Tel: 0151-207 6995
Fax: 0151-207 0839

Cambridge

Cambridge Laboratories,
Richmond House,
Old Brewery Court,
Sandyford Rd,
Newcastle upon Tyne NE2 1XG.
Tel: 0191-261 5950
Fax: 0191-222 1006

Camp

Camp Ltd,
30–32 Sovereign Rd, Kings
Norton Business Centre,
Birmingham B30 3HN.
Tel: 0121-451 3016
Fax: (01256) 708071

Castlemead

Castlemead Healthcare Ltd,
PO Box 57,
Ware SG10 6LL.
Tel: (07071) 224986
Fax: (07070) 728892

Centeon

Centeon Ltd,
Centeon House,
Market Place,
Haywards Heath,
West Sussex RH16 1DB.
Tel: (01444) 447405
Fax: (01444) 447401
medinfo@uk.centeon.com

Cephalon

Cephalon UK Ltd,
11-13 Frederick Sanger Rd,
Surrey Research Park,
Guildford, Surrey GU2 5YD.
Tel: (0800) 7834869
Fax: (01483) 453324
ukmedinfo@cephalon.com

Ceuta

Ceuta Healthcare Ltd,
Hill House, 41 Richmond Hill,
Bournmouth, Dorset, BH2 6HS.
Tel: (01202) 780558
Fax: (01202) 780559

Chauvin

Chauvin Pharmaceuticals Ltd,
Ashton Rd, Harold Hill,
Romford,
Essex RM3 8SL.
Tel: (01708) 383838
Fax: (01708) 371316

J. Chawner

J. Chawner Surgical Belts Ltd,
Unit 1B Mayfields
Southcrest, Redditch B98 7DU
Tel: (01527) 404353
Fax: (01527) 402157

Chefaro

Chefaro Proprietaries Ltd,
see Organon.

Chiron

Chiron UK Ltd,
Salamander Quay West,
Park Lane, Harefield, Middx
UB9 6NY.
Tel: (01895) 824087
Fax: (01895) 824965

CHS

Cambridge Healthcare Supplies
Ltd,
Contact:
Tudor Health Care Ltd
Martindale House, The Green,
Ruddington,
Nottingham NG11 6HH.
Tel: (0115) 9405393
Fax: (0115) 9405388
tudorhealthcare@compuserve.com

Chugai

Chugai Pharma UK Ltd,
Mulliner House, Flanders Rd
Turnham Green,
London W4 1NN.
Tel: (020) 8987 5680
Fax: (020) 8987 5661

CIBA Vision

CIBA Vision (UK) Ltd,
Flanders Rd, Hedge End,
Southampton SO30 2LG.
Tel: (01489) 785580
Fax: (01489) 798074

Clement Clarke

Clement Clarke International Ltd,
Airmed House, Edinburgh Way,
Harlow, Essex CM20 2ED.
Tel: (01279) 414969
Fax: (01279) 635232

CliniFlex

CliniFlex Ltd,
see CliniMed.

CliniMed

CliniMed Ltd,
Cavell House, Knaves Beech
Way, Loudwater, High
Wycombe, Bucks HP10 9QY.
Tel: (01628) 850100
Fax: (01628) 850331
enquiries@clinimed.demon.co.uk

Codan

Codan Ltd,
308 High Street,
Croydon CR0 1NG.
Tel: (0118) 978 3663
Fax: (0118) 877 6274

Colgate-Palmolive

Colgate-Palmolive Ltd,
Guildford Business Park,
Middleton Rd, Guildford, Surrey
GU2 5LZ.
Tel: (01483) 302222
Fax: (01483) 303003

Coloplast

Coloplast Ltd,
Peterborough Business Park,
Peterborough PE2 6FX.
Tel: (01733) 392000
Fax: (01733) 233348

Concord

Concord Pharmaceuticals Ltd,
Melville House, High Street,
Dunmow, Essex CM6 1AF.
Tel: 0845 602 0137
Fax: (01371) 874883
enquiries@concord-pharma.com

ConvaTec

ConvaTec Ltd,
Harrington House, Milton Rd,
Ickenham, Uxbridge, Middx
UB10 8PU.
Tel: (01895) 628400
Fax: (01895) 628456

Co-Pharma

Co-Pharma Ltd,
Talbot House, Church St,
Rickmansworth, Herts
WD3 1DE.
Tel: (01923) 710934
Fax: (01923) 770199

Cortecs

Cortecs Healthcare Ltd,
Abbey Rd,
Wrexham Industrial Estate,
Wrexham LL13 9PW.
Tel: (01978) 661351
Fax: (01978) 661673

Cover Care

Cover Care,
5 Ancaster Gardens, Wollaton
Park, Nottingham NG8 1FR.
Tel: (0115) 928 7883
Fax: (0115) 928 7883

Cow & Gate

see Nutricia Clinical
Tel: (01225) 768381
Fax: (01225) 768847

Cox

Cox Pharmaceuticals,
A. H. Cox & Co Ltd,
Whiddon Valley, Barnstaple,
Devon EX32 8NS.
Tel: (01271) 311257
Fax: (01271) 311329
med-info-ipd.uk@coxpharma.com

CP

CP Pharmaceuticals Ltd,
Ash Rd North, Wrexham
Industrial Estate, Wrexham,
Clwyd LL13 9UF.
Tel: (01978) 661261
Fax: (01978) 661702
mail@cppharma.co.uk

Crawford

Crawford Pharmaceuticals,
Furtho House,
20 Towcester Rd,
Milton Keynes MK19 6AQ.
Tel: (01908) 262346
Fax: (01908) 567730

Crookes

Crookes Healthcare Ltd,
PO Box 57,
FREEPOST,
Nottingham NG7 1BR.
Tel: (0115) 953 9922
Fax: (0115) 968 8722

Cupal
Cupal Ltd,
See SSL.

Cuxson
Cuxson, Gerrard & Co Ltd,
Oldbury, Warley, West Midlands
B69 4BF.
Tel: 0121-544 7117
Fax: 0121-544 8616

Dansac
Dansac Ltd,
Victory House, Vision Park,
Histon, Cambridge CB4 4ZR.
Tel: (01223) 235100
Fax: (01223) 235146

DDD
DDD Ltd,
94 Rickmansworth Rd, Watford,
Herts WD1 7JJ.
Tel: (01923) 229251
Fax: (01923) 220728

DDSA
DDSA Pharmaceuticals Ltd,
310 Old Brompton Rd, London
SW5 9JQ.
Tel: (020) 7373 7884
Fax: (020) 7370 4321

De Vilbiss
De Vilbiss Health Care UK Ltd,
High St., Wollaston
West Midlands DY8 4PS.
Tel: (01384) 446688
Fax: (01384) 446699

De Witt
E. C. De Witt & Co Ltd,
Tudor Rd, Manor Park, Runcorn,
Cheshire WA7 1SZ.
Tel: (01928) 579029
Fax: (01928) 579712

Dental Health
Dental Health Products Ltd,
60 Boughton Lane,
Maidstone,
Kent ME15 9QS.
Tel: (01622) 749222
Fax: (01622) 744672

Dermal
Dermal Laboratories Ltd,
Penrhyn House,
10 St Mark's Hill,
Surbiton, Surrey KT6 4PW.
Tel: (020) 8399 3040
Fax: (020) 8399 0808
info@dermapharm.co.uk

DermaPharm
DermaPharm Ltd,
Penrhyn House,
10 St Mark's Hill, Surbiton,
Surrey KT6 4PW.
Tel: (020) 8399 3040
Fax: (020) 8399 0808
info@dermapharm.co.uk

Dexcel
Dexcel Pharma Ltd,
Bishop Crewe House,
North St, Daventry,
Northants NN11 5PN.
Tel: (01327) 312266
Fax: (01327) 312262
DexcelPharma@compuserve.com

DF
Duncan, Flockhart & Co Ltd,
see GlaxoWellcome.

Dista
Dista Products Ltd,
see Lilly.

Dominion
Dominion Pharma Ltd,
Dominion House, Lion Lane,
Haslemere, Surrey GU27 1JL.
Tel: (01428) 661078
Fax: (01428) 661075
dominion@dompharm.com

Du Pont
Du Pont Pharmaceuticals Ltd,
Wedgewood Way, Stevenage,
Herts SG1 4QN.
Tel: (0800) 7313339
Fax: (01438) 842533

Dumex
see Cox

Durbin
B & S Durbin Ltd,
240 Northolt Rd, South Harrow,
Middx HA2 8DU.
Tel: (020) 8422 1303
Fax: (020) 8864 6611
durbin@durbin.co.uk

Eastern
Eastern Pharmaceuticals Ltd,
Coomb House, 7 St Johns Rd,
Isleworth, Middx TW7 6NA.
Tel: (020) 8569 8174
Fax: (020) 8569 8175

Eisai
Eisai Ltd,
3 Shortlands, Hammersmith,
London W6 8EE.
Tel: (020) 8600 1400
Fax: (020) 8600 1401
Lmedinfo@eisai.net

Elan
Elan Pharma Ltd,
Elan House, Avenue One,
Letchworth,
Herts SG6 2HU.
Tel: (01462) 707200
Fax: (01462) 707250
medinfo@ElanUK.com

Eldon
Eldon Laboratories,
4 Pooley Close,
Newcastle upon Tyne NE5 2TF.
Tel: 0191-286 0446
Fax: 0191-286 0455
eldon_labsorders@alliance-
unichem.com

Elida Fabergé
Elida Fabergé Ltd,
Coal Rd, Seacroft, Leeds
LS14 2AR.
Tel: (0113) 222 5000
Fax: (0113) 222 5362

Ellis
Ellis, Son & Paramore Ltd,
see Camp

Epiderm
Epiderm Ltd,
52 Main St, Middleton,
Matlock, Derbyshire DE4 4LU.
Tel: (01629) 826833
Fax: (01629) 826844

Everfresh
Everfresh Natural Foods,
Gatehouse Close, Aylesbury,
Bucks HP19 3DE.
Tel: (01296) 425333
Fax: (01296) 422545

Exelgyn
Exelgyn Laboratories,
PO Box 4511,
Henley-on-Thames, Oxon
RG9 1XH.
Tel: (0800) 7316120
Fax: (01491) 577443

Fabre
Pierre Fabre Ltd
Hyde Abbey House
23 Hyde St, Winchester,
Hampshire SO23 7DR
Tel: (01962) 856956
Fax: (01962) 844014
PFabreUK@aol.com

Farillon
Farillon Ltd,
Ashton Rd, Romford,
Essex RM3 8UE.
Tel: (01708) 379000
Fax: (01708) 376554

Farley
Farley Health Products,
Mint Bridge Rd, Kendal,
Cumbria LA9 6NL
Tel: (01539) 723815
Fax: (01539) 730376
Farleys_Heinz@Heinz.co.uk

Faulding DBL
Faulding Pharmaceuticals plc,
Queensway,
Leamington Spa CV31 3RW.
Tel: (01926) 820820
Fax: (01926) 821049

Ferraris
Ferraris Medical Ltd,
Ferraris House, Aden Rd,
Enfield, Middx EN3 7SE.
Tel: (020) 8805 9055
Fax: (020) 8805 9065
ferraris@globalnet.co.uk

Ferring
Ferring Pharmaceuticals UK,
The Courtyard,
Waterside Drive, Langley,
Berks SL3 6EZ.
Tel: (01753) 214800
Fax: (01753) 214801

Firstplay Dietary
Firstplay Dietary Foods Ltd,
338 Turncroft Lane, Offerton,
Stockport, Cheshire SK1 4BP.
Tel: 0161-474 7576
Fax: 0161-474 7576

Florizel
Florizel Ltd,
PO Box 138,
Stevenage SG2 8YN.
Tel: (01462) 436156
Fax: (01462) 457402

Flynn
Flynn Pharma Ltd,
7 Serlby Court, Addison Rd,
London W14 8EE.
Tel: (01462) 458974
Fax: (01462) 450755

Fournier
Fournier Pharmaceuticals Ltd,
22-23 Progress Business Centre,
Whittle Parkway, Slough
SL1 6DG.
Tel: (01753) 740400
Fax: (01753) 740444

Fox

C. H. Fox Ltd,
22 Tavistock St, London
WC2E 7PY
Tel: (020) 7240 3111
Fax: (020) 7379 3410

FP

Family Planning Sales Ltd,
28 Kelburne Rd, Cowley, Oxford
OX4 3SZ.
Tel: (01865) 772486
Fax: (01865) 748746

Fresenius

Fresenius Ltd,
Melbury Park, Birchwood,
Warrington WA3 6FF.
Tel: (01925) 898000
Fax: (01925) 898002

Fresenius Kabi

Fresenius Kabi Ltd,
Parenteral Nutrition Division,
Hampton Court, Tudor Rd
Manor Park, Runcorn,
Cheshire WA7 1UF
Tel: (01928) 594313
Fax: (01928) 594314

Fujisawa

Fujisawa Ltd,
C P House, 8th Floor,
97–107 Uxbridge Rd,
London W5 5TL.
Tel: (020) 8840 9520
Fax: (020) 8840 9521

Futuna

Futuna Ltd,
229 Preston Rd,
Whittle-le-Woods
Preston PR6 7PT.
Tel: (0870) 6012037
Fax: (0870) 6012036

Gainor Medical

Gainor Medical Europe,
Milton Keynes
Distribution Centre, Bradbourne
Drive, Tilbrook,
Milton Keynes MK7 8BN.
Tel: (01908) 365361
Fax: (01908) 365362

Galderma

Galderma (UK) Ltd,
Leywood House,
47 Woodside Rd, Amersham,
Bucks HP6 6AA.
Tel: (01494) 432606
Fax: (01494) 432607

Galen

Galen Ltd,
Seagoe Industrial Estate,
Craigavon, Northern Ireland
BT63 5UA.
Tel: (028) 3833 4974
Fax: (028) 3835 0206

Garnier

Laboratoires Garnier,
Golden Ltd,
PO Box 5, Pontyclun, Glam
CF7 8XW.
Tel: (01443) 233724
Fax: (01443) 233726

GBM

GBM Health Care Ltd,
Beechlawn House,
Hurtmore Rd, Godalming,
Surrey GU7 2RA.
Tel: (01483) 860881
Fax: (01483) 425715
mba_gbm@compuserve.com

Geistlich

Geistlich Pharma,
Newton Bank, Long Lane,
Chester CH2 2PF.
Tel: (01244) 347534
Fax: (01244) 319327

General Dietary

General Dietary Ltd,
PO Box 38,
Kingston upon Thames, Surrey
KT2 7YP.
Tel: (020) 8336 2323
Fax: (020) 8942 8274

Generics

Generics (UK) Ltd,
Albany Gate, Darkes Lane,
Potters Bar,
Herts EN6 1AG.
Tel: (01707) 853000
Fax: (01707) 643148

Genus

Genus Pharmaceuticals,
Benham Valence,
Newbury,
Berks RG20 8LU.
Tel: (01635) 568400
Fax: (01635) 568401

Genzyme

Genzyme Therapeutics,
37 Hollands Rd, Haverhill,
Suffolk CB9 8PU.
Tel: (01440) 703522
Fax: (01440) 714392

GlaxoWellcome

GlaxoWellcome UK,
Stockley Park West, Uxbridge,
Middx UB11 1BT.
Tel: (020) 8990 9000
Fax: (020) 8990 4321

Glenwood

Glenwood Laboratories Ltd,
Jenkins Dale, Chatham,
Kent ME4 5RD.
Tel: (01634) 830535
Fax: (01634) 831345
g.wooduk@virgin.net

Gluten Free Foods Ltd

Gluten Free Foods Ltd,
270 Centennial Park,
Centennial Ave,
Elstree, Borehamwood,
Herts WD6 3SS.
Tel: (020) 8953 4444
Fax: (020) 8953 8285
info@glutenfree-foods.co.uk

Goldshield

Goldshield Pharmaceuticals Ltd,
NLA Tower,
12–16 Addiscombe Rd, Croydon
CR0 0XT.
Tel: (020) 8649 8500
Fax: (020) 8686 0807

Grifols

Grifols UK Ltd,
Howlett Way, Thetford,
Norfolk IP24 1HZ.
Tel: (01842) 761942
Fax: (01842) 766661

Hansam

Hansam Healthcare Ltd,
60 Ondine Rd,
London SE15 4EB.
Tel: 0845 6020137
Fax: (020) 7207 6850

Hartmann

Paul Hartmann Ltd,
Unit P2, Parklands,
Heywood Distribution Park,
Pilsworth Rd, Heywood,
Lancs OL10 2TT.
Tel: (01706) 363200
Fax: (01706) 363201

Hawgreen

Hawgreen Ltd,
PO Box 157,
Hatfield AL10 8ZP.
Tel: (07071) 220777
Fax: (07070) 600678

Heinz

H.J. Heinz Company Ltd,
Stockley Park,
Uxbridge UB11 1HZ
Tel: (020) 8573 7757
Fax: (020) 8482325
Farleys_Heinz@Heinz.co.uk

Helios

Helios Healthcare Ltd,
PO Box 36, Old Warden,
Biggleswade SG18 9UP.
Tel: (07071) 222567
Fax: (07070) 600789

Henleys

Henleys Medical Supplies Ltd,
Brownfields, Welwyn Garden
City, Herts AL7 1AN.
Tel: (01707) 333164
Fax: (01707) 334795

Hillcross

AAH Pharmaceuticals Ltd,
Sapphire Court,
Walsgrave Triangle
Coventry CV2 2TX.
Tel: (024) 7643 2000
Fax: (024) 7643 2001

HK Pharma Ltd

HK Pharma Ltd,
PO Box 105,
Hitchin SG5 2GG.
Tel: (07071) 880292
Fax: (07070) 604101

Hoechst Marion Roussel

Hoechst Marion Roussel Ltd,
Aventis Pharma Ltd,
Aventis House,
50 Kings Hill Avenue,
Kings Hill, West Malling,
Kent ME19 4AH.
Tel: (01732) 584000
Fax: (0870) 5239605

Hollister

Hollister Ltd,
Rectory Court, 42 Broad St,
Wokingham, Berks RG40 1AB.
Tel: (0118) 989 5000
Fax: (0118) 977 5881

Hospital Management & Supplies
Hospital Management and Supplies Ltd,
Brooke House, 4 The Lakes,
Bedford Rd,
Northampton NN4 7YD.
Tel: (01604) 615800
Fax: (01604) 259611

Hutchings
Hutchings Healthcare Ltd,
Rede House, New Barn Lane,
Henfield, West Sussex BN5 9SJ.
Tel: (01273) 495033
Fax: (01273) 495123

Hyland Immuno
Baxter Healthcare Ltd,
Wallingford Rd, Compton,
Nr Newbury,
Berks RG20 7QW.
Tel: (01635) 206000
Fax: (01635) 206115

Hypoguard
Hypoguard Ltd,
Dock Lane, Melton, Woodbridge,
Suffolk IP12 1PE.
Tel: (01394) 387333
Fax: (01394) 380152

IATRO
IATRO Medical Systems,
(Division of SHIVAM Overseas Ltd)
35 Quaggy Walk, Blackheath,
London SE3 9EJ.
Tel: (020) 8297 9081
Fax: (020) 8297 9083
101365.1615@compuserve.com

ICN
ICN Pharmaceuticals Ltd,
1 Elmwood,
Chineham Business Park,
Crockford Lane,
Basingstoke,
Hants RG24 8WG.
Tel: (01256) 707744
Fax: (01256) 707334

IDIS
IDIS Ltd World Medicines,
Millbank House, 171 Ewell Rd,
Surbiton, Surrey.
KT6 6AX.
Tel: (020) 8410 0700
Fax: (020) 8410 0800

Impharm
Impharm Nationwide Ltd,
Valley House,
Britannia Business Park,
Union Rd, Bolton,
Lancs BL2 2HP.
Tel: (01204) 540200
Fax: (01204) 371166

IMS
International Medication Systems
(UK) Ltd,
see Medeva

Incare
see Hollister.

Infai
Infai UK Ltd,
University of York Science Park,
University Rd, Heslington,
York YO1 5DG.
Tel: (01904) 435228
Fax: (01904) 435112
infai@infaiuk.ymn.co.uk

Intrapharm
Intrapharm Laboratories Ltd,
60 Boughton Lane,
Maidstone, Kent ME15 9QS.
Tel: (01622) 749222
Fax: (01622) 744672

Invicta
see Pfizer.

Ipsen
Ipsen Ltd,
1 Bath Rd, Maidenhead,
Berks SL6 4UH
Tel: (01628) 771417
Fax: (01628) 770199

J&J
Johnson & Johnson Ltd,
Foundation Park, Roxborough
Way, Maidenhead,
Berkshire SL6 3UG.
Tel: (01628) 822222
Fax: (01628) 821222

J&J Medical
Johnson & Johnson Medical,
Coronation Rd, Ascot, Berks
SL5 9EY.
Tel: (01344) 871000
Fax: (01344) 872599

J&J MSD
Johnson & Johnson MSD,
Enterprise House, Station Rd,
Loudwater, High Wycombe,
Bucks HP10 9UF.
Tel: (01494) 450778
Fax: (01494) 450487

Jacobs
The Jacobs Bakery Ltd,
PO Box 1, Long Lane,
Liverpool L9 7BQ.
Tel: 0151-525 3661
Fax: 0151-530 3444

Jade-Euro-Med
Jade-Euro-Med
Unit 14, East Hanningfield
Industrial Estate, Oldchurch Rd,
East Hanningfield,
Chelmsford, Essex
CM3 8BG
Tel: (01245) 400413
Fax: (01245) 401415

Janssen-Cilag
Janssen-Cilag Ltd,
PO Box 79, Saunderton,
High Wycombe, Bucks
HP14 4HJ.
Tel: (01494) 567567
Fax: (01494) 567568

JHC
JHC Healthcare Ltd,
The Maltings, Bridge St,
Hitchin, Herts SG5 2DE.
Tel: (01462) 432533
Fax: (01462) 432535

JLB
B. Braun JLB Ltd,
Unit 2A, St Columb Industrial
Estate, St Columb Major,
Cornwall TR9 6SF.
Tel: (01637) 880065
Fax: (01637) 881549

JLJ
JLJ Healthcare Ltd,
Number One, 61 Whitehall Rd,
Halesowen,
West Midlands B63 3JS.
Tel: 0121-602 3943
Fax: 0121-602 3943
jljhealthcare@aol.com

K & K-Greeff
Univar plc,
PO Box 56, Priestley Rd,
Basingstoke,
Hampshire RG24 9QB.
Tel: (01256) 312000
Fax: (01256) 814163

K/L
K/L Pharmaceuticals Ltd,
25 Macadam Place, South
Newmoor Industrial Estate,
Irvine KA11 4HP.
Tel: (01294) 215951
Fax: (01294) 221600

Kendall
The Kendall Co (UK) Ltd,
154 Fareham Rd,
Gosport PO13 OAS
Tel: (01329) 224000
Fax: (01329) 224418

Kendall-Lastonet
see Kendall.

Kent
Kent Pharmaceuticals Ltd,
Wotton Rd, Ashford, Kent
TN23 6LL.
Tel: (01233) 638614
Fax: (01233) 646899

Kestrel
Kestrel Healthcare Ltd,
Network House, Basing View,
Basingstoke RG21 4HG.
Tel: (01256) 307580
Fax: (01256) 307590

Knoll
Knoll Ltd,
9 Castle Quay, Castle Boulevard,
Nottingham NG7 1FW
Tel: (0115) 912 5000
Fax: (0115) 912 5069

Kyowa Hakko
Kyowa Hakko UK Ltd,
258 Bath Rd, Slough,
Berks SL1 4DX.
Tel: (01753) 566020
Fax: (01753) 566030

LAB
Laboratories for Applied Biology
91 Amhurst Park, London
N16 5DR.
Tel: (020) 8800 2252
Fax: (020) 8809 6884

Laclede
Laclede UK Ltd,
20 Cinque Ports St, Rye
East Sussex TN31 7AD.
Tel: (01797) 227570
Fax: (01797) 227571

Lagap
Lagap Pharmaceuticals Ltd,
37 Woolmer Way, Bordon, Hants
GU35 9QE.
Tel: (01420) 478301
Fax: (01420) 474427

Lamberts

Lamberts (Dalston) Ltd,
P O Box 883, Oxford
OX4 3RR.
Tel: (01865) 717300
Fax: (01865) 748746

Lederle

see Wyeth

Leo

Leo Pharmaceuticals,
Longwick Rd, Princes
Risborough, Bucks
HP27 9RR.
Tel: (01844) 347333
Fax: (01844) 342278

LifeScan

LifeScan,
Enterprise House, Station Rd,
Loudwater, High Wycombe,
Bucks HP10 9UF.
Tel: (01494) 450423
Fax: (01494) 463299

Lilly

Eli Lilly & Co Ltd,
Dextra Court, Chapel Hill,
Basingstoke, Hants RG21 5SY.
Tel: (01256) 315000
Fax: (01256) 315858

Link

Link Pharmaceuticals Ltd,
7/8 Sterling Buildings,
Carfax, Horsham, West Sussex
RH12 1DR.
Tel: (01403) 272451
Fax: (01403) 272455

Lipha

see Merck.

LRC

LRC Products Ltd,
London International House,
Turnford Place, Broxbourne,
Herts EN10 6LN.
Tel: (01992) 451111
Fax: (01992) 470133

Lundbeck

Lundbeck Ltd,
Sunningdale House, Caldecotte
Lake Business Park, Caldecotte,
Milton Keynes MK7 8LF.
Tel: (01908) 649966
Fax: (01908) 647888

3M

3M Health Care Ltd,
3M House, Morley St,
Loughborough,
Leics LE11 1EP.
Tel: (01509) 611611
Fax: (01509) 237288

Maersk

Maersk Medical Ltd,
Thornhill Rd,
North Moons Moat, Redditch,
Worcs B98 9NL.
Tel: (01527) 64222
Fax: (01527) 592111

Mandeville

Mandeville Medicines,
Stoke Mandeville Hospital,
Ayelsbury, Bucks HP21 8AL.
Tel: (01296) 394142
Fax: (01296) 397223

Manfred Sauer

Manfred Sauer GMbH,
KG Business Centre,
Kingsfield Way,
Gladstone Industry, Dallington,
Northamptonshire NN5 7QS.
Tel: (01604) 588090
Fax: (01604) 588091

Manx

Manx Pharma,
Unit 2 Spectrum Business Estate,
Parkwood,
Maidstone, Kent ME15 9YP.
Tel: (01622) 766389
Fax: (01622) 761435

Martindale

Martindale Pharmaceuticals Ltd,
Bampton Rd, Harold Hill,
Romford, Essex RM3 8UG.
Tel: (01708) 386660
Fax: (01708) 384032

Mead Johnson

Mead Johnson Nutritional
see Bristol Myers

Medac

Medac (UK),
13 Lynedoch Crescent,
Glasgow G3 6EQ.
Tel: 0141-332 8464
Fax: 0141-332 8619

Medasil

Medasil (Surgical) Ltd,
Medasil House, Hunslet Rd,
Leeds LS10 1AU.
Tel: (0113) 243 3491
Fax: (0113) 242 9276

Medeva

Medeva Pharma Ltd,
Medeva House, Regent Park,
Kingston Rd, Leatherhead,
Surrey KT22 7PQ.
Tel: (01372) 364132
Fax: (01372) 364018

Medic-Aid

Medic-Aid Ltd,
Heath Place, Bognor Regis,
West Sussex PO22 9SL.
Tel: (01243) 840888
Fax: (01243) 846100
info@medic-aid.com

Medigas

Medigas Ltd,
Enterprise Drive, Four Ashes,
Wolverhampton WV10 7DF.
Tel: (01902) 791944
Fax: (01902) 791125

MediSense

MediSense Britain Ltd,
16–17 The Courtyard,
Gorsey Lane, Coleshill,
Birmingham B46 1JA.
Tel: (01675) 467044
Fax: (01675) 467006

Medix

see Clement Clarke.

Menarini

A Menarini Pharmaceuticals UK
Ltd,
Wharfedale Rd, Winnersh,
Wokingham,
Berks RG41 5RA.
Tel: (0118) 944 4128
Fax: (0118) 944 4129

Mepra-pharm

see Co-Pharma.

Merck

E. Merck Pharmaceuticals,
Harrier House, High St,
West Drayton, Middlesex,
UB7 7QG.
Tel: (01895) 452200
Fax: (01895) 452296
info@merck-lipha.co.uk

Merck Consumer Health

see Seven Seas.

Millpledge

Millpledge Healthcare,
Whinleys Estate, Clarborough,
Retford, Notts DN22 9NA.
Tel: (01777) 708440
Fax: (01777) 860020
sales@millpledge.u-net.com

Milupa

Milupa Ltd,
Whitehorse Business Park,
Trowbridge,
Wilts BA14 0XB.
Tel: (01225) 711511
Fax: (01225) 711970

Mölnlycke

Mölnlycke Healthcare Ltd,
Southfields Rd, Dunstable,
Beds LU6 3EJ.
Tel: (01582) 677400
Fax: (01582) 677502

Monmouth

Monmouth Pharmaceuticals,
20 Nugent Rd, The Surrey
Research Park, Guildford, Surrey
GU2 5AF.
Tel: (01483) 565299
Fax: (01483) 563658

MSD

Merck Sharp & Dohme Ltd,
Hertford Rd, Hoddesdon, Herts
EN11 9BU.
Tel: (01992) 467272
Fax: (01992) 451066

Napp

Napp Pharmaceuticals,
Cambridge Science Park,
Milton Rd, Cambridge
CB4 0GW.
Tel: (01223) 424444
Fax: (01223) 424441

Nestlé

Nestlé UK Ltd,
St. George's House, Croydon
CR9 1NR.
Tel: (020) 8686 3333
Fax: (020) 8686 6072

Nestlé Clinical

Nestlé Clinical Nutrition,
St. George's House, Park Lane,
Croydon,
Surrey CR9 1NR.
Tel; (020) 8667 5130
Fax: (020) 8667 6061

Network

Network Health & Beauty,
Network House,
41 Invincible Rd, Farnborough,
Hants GU14 7QU.
Tel: (01252) 533333
Fax: (01252) 533344
networkm@globalnet.co.uk

Neutrogena

see J&J

NeXstar

NeXstar Pharmaceuticals Ltd,
The Quorum, Barnwell Rd,
Cambridge CB5 8RE.
Tel: (01223) 571400
Fax: (01233) 571444
gfox@nexstar.com

Nordic

see Ferring.
Tel: (020) 8898 8665

Norgine

Norgine Ltd,
Chaplin House, Moorhall Rd,
Harefield, Middx UB9 6NS.
Tel: (01895) 826600
Fax: (01895) 825865

North West

North West Medical Supplies
Ltd,
Premier House,
Southgate Way,
Orton Southgate,
Peterborough PE2 6YG.
Tel: (01733) 361336
Fax: (01733) 361336

Norton

Norton Healthcare Ltd,
Albert Basin, Royal Docks,
London E16 2QJ.
Tel: (08705) 020304
Fax: (08705) 323334

Novartis

Novartis Pharmaceuticals UK,
Frimley Business Park,
Frimley, Camberley,
Surrey GU16 5SG.
Tel: (01276) 692255
Fax: (01276) 698449

Novartis Consumer Health

Novartis Consumer Health,
Wimblehurst Rd, Horsham,
West Sussex RH12 5AB.
Tel: (01403) 210211
Fax: (01403) 323939

Novo Nordisk

Novo Nordisk Pharmaceutical
Ltd,
Novo Nordisk House, Broadfield
Park, Brighton Rd, Pease Pottage,
Crawley, West Sussex RH11 9RT.
Tel: (01293) 613555
Fax: (01293) 613535

Nutricia Clinical

Nutricia Clinical Care,
Nutricia Ltd, White Horse
Business Park, Trowbridge,
Wiltshire BA14 0XQ
Tel: (01225) 711677
Fax: (01225) 711798

Nutricia Dietary

Nutricia Dietary Care,
see Nutricia Clinical
Tel: (01225) 711801
Fax: (01225) 711567

Nutrition Point

Nutrition Point Ltd,
13 Taurus Park,
Westbrook, Warrington,
Cheshire WA5 5ZT.
Tel: (07041) 544044
Fax: (07041) 544055
info@nutritionpoint.ltd.uk

Nycomed

Nycomed Amersham plc,
Amersham Laboratories,
White Lion Rd,
Amersham HP7 9LL.
Tel: (01494) 544000
Fax: (01494) 543588
corp.enquiry@nycomed-
amersham.com

Octapharma

Octapharma Ltd,
6 Elm Court, Copse Drive,
Coventry CV5 9RG.
Tel: (01676) 521000
Fax: (01676) 521200
octapharma@octapharma.co.uk

Omex

Omex Medical Ltd,
25 Sea Lane, East Preston,
Littlehampton,
West Sussex BN16 1NH.
Tel: (01903) 738744

Omnicare

The Omnicare Group Ltd,
Enterprise Drive, Four Ashes,
Wolverhampton WV10 7DF.
Tel: 0500 823773
Fax: (01902) 791125

Opus

see Trinity.

Oral B Labs

Oral B Laboratories Ltd,
Gillette Corner,
Great West Rd, Isleworth,
Middx TW7 5NP.
Tel: (020) 8847 7800
Fax: (020) 8847 7828

Organon

Organon Laboratories Ltd,
Cambridge Science Park, Milton
Rd, Cambridge, CB4 0FL.
Tel: (01223) 432700
Fax: (01223) 424368

Organon-Teknika

see Organon
Tel: (01223) 423650

Orion

Orion Pharma (UK) Ltd,
1st Floor, Leat House,
Overbridge Square, Hambridge
Lane, Newbury, Berks
RG14 5UX.
Tel: (01635) 520308
Fax: (01635) 34994

Orphan Europe

Orphan Europe (UK) Ltd,
32 Bell St, Henley-on-Thames,
Oxon RG9 2BH.
Tel: (01491) 414333
Fax: (01491) 414443
info.uk@orphan-europe.com

Orthotic

Orthotic Services Ltd
Heartlands House, 19 Catro St,
The Heartlands,
Birmingham B7 4TS.
Tel: 0121-359 6323
Fax: 0121-359 6324

Owen Mumford

Owen Mumford Ltd,
Brook Hill, Woodstock, Oxford
OX20 1TU.
Tel: (01993) 812021
Fax: (01993) 813466

Oxford

Oxford Pharmaceuticals Ltd,
Masters House, Sandridge Close,
Harrow, Middx HA1 1XD.
Tel: (020) 8861 0788
Fax: (020) 8427 1994

Oxygen Therapy Co Ltd

The Oxygen Therapy Co Ltd,
Dumballs Rd, Cardiff
CF1 6JE.
Tel: 0800 373580

Paines & Byrne

Paines & Byrne Ltd,
Yamanouchi House, Pyrford Rd,
West Byfleet,
Surrey KT14 6RA.
Tel: (01932) 355405
Fax: (01932) 353458

Pantheon

Pantheon Healthcare Ltd,
Studio 8, 48 Tierney Rd,
London SW2 4QS.
Tel: (0845) 6020137

Parema

Parema Ltd,
Sullington Rd, Shepshed,
Loughborough,
Leics LE12 9JJ.
Tel: (01509) 502051
Fax: (01509) 650898

Pari

Pari Medical Ltd,
Enterprise House, Station
Approach, West Byfleet,
Surrey KT14 6NE.
Tel: (01932) 341122
Fax: (01932) 341134

Parkside

Parkside Healthcare
12 Parkside Ave
Salford M7 4HB.
Tel: 0161-795 2792
Fax: 0161-795 4076

Pasteur Mérieux

Pasteur Mérieux MSD Ltd,
Mallards Reach, Bridge Ave,
Maidenhead, Berks SL6 1QP.
Tel: (01628) 785291
Fax: (01628) 671722

PathoGenesis

PathoGenesis Ltd,
PathoGenesis House,
Park Lane, Cranford,
Hounslow TW5 9RR.
Tel: (020) 8580 4000
Fax: (020) 8580 4001

Payne

S G & P Payne,
Percy House, Brook St, Hyde,
Cheshire SK14 2NS.
Tel: 0161-367 8561
Fax: 0161-367 8995

Parke-Davis

Parke-Davis & Co Ltd,
Lambert Court, Chestnut Ave,
Eastleigh, Hants SO53 3ZQ.
Tel: (023) 8062 0500
Fax: (023) 8062 9818

Peckforton

Peckforton Pharmaceuticals Ltd,
Crewe Hall, Crewe,
Cheshire CW1 6UL.
Tel: (01270) 582255
Fax: (01270) 582299

Pelican

Pelican Healthcare Ltd,
Cardiff Business Park,
Cardiff CF4 5WF.
Tel: (029) 2074 7787
Fax: (029) 2074 7001

Penn

Penn Pharmaceuticals Ltd,
Tafarnaubach Industrial Estate,
Tredegar, Gwent, NP2 3AA.
Tel: (01495) 711222
Fax: (01495) 711225

Pennine

Pennine Healthcare,
Pontefract St, Ascot Drive
Industrial Estate,
Derby DE2 8JD.
Tel: (01332) 571111
Fax: (01332) 755324

Perstorp

Perstorp Pharma Ltd,
Intec 2, Wade Rd, Basingstoke,
Hants RG24 8NE.
Tel: (01256) 477868

Pfizer

Pfizer Ltd,
Sandwich, Kent CT13 9NJ.
Tel: (01304) 616161
Fax: (01304) 656221

Pfizer Consumer

Pfizer Consumer Healthcare,
Wilsom Rd, Alton,
Hants GU34 2TJ.
Tel: (01420) 84801
Fax: (01420) 89376

Pharmacia & Upjohn

Pharmacia & Upjohn Ltd,
Davy Ave, Knowlhill,
Milton Keynes, MK5 8PH.
Tel: (01908) 661101
Fax: (01908) 690091

Pharma-Global

Pharma-Global Ltd,
SEQ Ltd, Nerin House,
26 Ridgeway St, Douglas,
Isle of Man IM1 1EL.
Tel: (01624) 613997
Fax: (01624) 613998

Pharmark

Pharmark Ltd,
7 Windermere Rd, West
Wickham, Kent BR4 9AN.
Tel: (020) 8688 5895

Pharmax

Pharmax Ltd,
Bourne Rd, Bexley,
Kent DA5 1NX.
Tel: (01322) 550550
Fax: (01322) 558776

Phoenix

Phoenix Pharmaceuticals Ltd,
Glevum Works, Upton St,
Gloucester GL1 4LA.
Tel: (01452) 522255
Fax: (01452) 306051

Pickles

J. Pickles & Sons,
Beech House, 62 High St,
Knaresborough, N. Yorks
HG5 0EA.
Tel: (01423) 867314
Fax: (01423) 869177

Procter & Gamble

Procter & Gamble UK,
The Heights, Brooklands,
Weybridge, Surrey KT13 0XP.
Tel: (01932) 896000
Fax: (01932) 896200

Procter & Gamble Pharm.

Procter & Gamble
Pharmaceuticals UK Ltd,
Lovett House, Lovett Rd, Staines,
Middx TW18 3AZ.
Tel: (01784) 495000
Fax: (01784) 495253

Quinoderm Ltd

Quinoderm Ltd,
Manchester Rd, Hollinwood,
Oldham, Lancs OL8 4PB.
Tel: 0161-624 9307
Fax: 0161-627 0928

Ranbaxy

Ranbaxy (UK) Ltd,
95 Park Lane,
London W1Y 3TA.
Tel: (020) 7495 5511
Fax: (020) 7491 9504

Rand Rocket

Rand Rocket Ltd,
ABCare House, Hownsgill
Industrial Park, Consett,
County Durham DH8 7NU.
Tel: (01207) 591099
Fax: (01207) 591098

R & C

Reckitt & Colman Products Ltd,
Dansom Lane, Hull HU8 7DS.
Tel: (01482) 326151
Fax: (01482) 582526
miu@eu.reckitt.com

Regent

Regent-GM Laboratories Ltd,
861 Coronation Rd, Park Royal,
London NW10 7PT.
Tel: (020) 8961 6868
Fax: (020) 8961 9311

Respond Plus

Respond Plus Ltd,
Unit 1 The Carlton Business
Centre,
Station Rd, Carlton,
Nottingham NG4 3AT.
Tel: (0115) 900 3001
Fax: (0115) 900 3002

Rhône-Poulenc Rorer

Rhône-Poulenc Rorer Ltd,
Aventis Pharma Ltd,
Aventis House,
50 Kings Hill Ave, Kings Hill
West Malling, Kent ME19 4AH.
Tel: (01732) 584000
Fax: (0870) 5239605

Robinsons

Robinson Healthcare,
Waterside, Walton, Chesterfield,
Derbyshire S40 1YF.
Tel: (01246) 220022
Fax: (01246) 505115

RoC

Laboratoires RoC UK Ltd,
see J & J

Roche

Roche Products Ltd,
40 Broadwater Rd,
Welwyn Garden City,
Herts AL7 3AY.
Tel: (01707) 366000
Fax: (01707) 338297

Roche Consumer Health

see Roche
Tel: (01707) 366000
Fax: (0800) 394353

Roche Diagnostics

Roche Diagnostics Ltd,
Bell Lane, Lewes,
East Sussex BN7 1LG.
Tel: (01273) 480444
Fax: (01273) 480266

Rosemont

Rosemont Pharmaceuticals Ltd,
Rosemont House, Yorkdale
Industrial Park, Braithwaite St,
Leeds LS11 9XE.
Tel: (0113) 244 1999
Fax: (0113) 246 0738

Rowa

Rowa Pharmaceuticals Ltd,
Bantry, Co Cork, Ireland.
Tel: (00 353 27) 50077
Fax: (00 353 27) 50417
rowa@rowa-pharma.ie

Rüsch

Rüsch UK Ltd,
PO Box 138, Halifax Rd,
Cressex Business Park,
High Wycombe,
Bucks HP12 3NB.
Tel: (01494) 532761
Fax: (01494) 524650

Rybar

see Shire

Sallis

E. Sallis Ltd,
Vernon Works, Waterford St,
Basford, Nottingham
NG6 0DH.
Tel: (0115) 978 7841
Fax: (0115) 942 2272

Salts

Salt & Son Ltd,
Lord St,
Birmingham B7 4DS.
Tel: 0121-359 5123
Fax: 0121-359 0830
salt@salts.co.uk

Sangstat

Imtix Sangstat (UK) Ltd,
42 Thames St, Windsor,
Berks SL4 1PR.
Tel: (01753) 625704
Fax: (01753) 625701

Sankyo

Sankyo Pharma UK Ltd,
Sankyo House, Repton Place,
White Lion Rd, Amersham,
Bucks HP7 9LP.
Tel: (01494) 766866
Fax: (01494) 766557

Sanofi-Synthelabo

Sanofi Synthelabo,
One Onslow St, Guildford,
Surrey GU1 4YS.
Tel: (01483) 505515
Fax: (01483) 535432

Schär

Dr Schär,
PO Box 126,
Worcester WR5 2ZN.
Tel: 0808 1000483
Fax: (01905) 357899
info@schaer.com

Schering Health

Schering Health Care Ltd,
The Brow, Burgess Hill,
West Sussex RH15 9NE.
Tel: (01444) 232323
Fax: (01444) 246613
medinfo@schering.co.uk

Schering-Plough

Schering-Plough Ltd,
Shire Park, Welwyn Garden City,
Herts AL7 1TW.
Tel: (01707) 363636
Fax: (01707) 363763

Schwarz

Schwarz Pharma Ltd,
Schwarz House, East St,
Chesham, Bucks HP5 1DG.
Tel: (01494) 797500
Fax: (01494) 773934

Scotia

Scotia Pharmaceuticals Ltd,
Scotia House
Castle Business Park,
Stirling FK9 4TZ.
Tel: (01786) 895100
Fax: (01786) 895450
medenq@scotia-holdings.com

Searle

Searle,
PO Box 53, Lane End Rd, High
Wycombe, Bucks HP12 4HL.
Tel: (01494) 521124
Fax: (01494) 536860

Serono

Serono Pharmaceuticals Ltd,
Bedfont Cross, Stanwell Rd,
Feltham, Middx TW14 8NX.
Tel: (020) 8818 7200
Fax: (020) 8818 7222
serono_uk@serono.com

Servier

Servier Laboratories Ltd,
Fulmer Hall, Windmill Rd,
Fulmer, Slough SL3 6HH.
Tel: (01753) 662744
Fax: (01753) 663456

Seven Seas

Seven Seas Ltd,
Hedon Rd, Marfleet, Hull
HU9 5NJ.
Tel: (01482) 375234
Fax: (01482) 374345

Shannon

T. J. Shannon Ltd,
59 Bradford St, Bolton
BL2 1HT.
Tel: (01204) 521789

Shaw

A. H. Shaw and Partners Ltd,
Manor Rd, Ossett, West
Yorkshire WF5 0LF.
Tel: (01924) 273474

Shire

Shire Pharmaceuticals Ltd,
Fosse House, East Anton Court,
Icknield Way, Andover, Hants
SP10 5RG.
Tel: (01264) 333455
Fax: (01264) 333460
athomson@shiregroup.com

SHS

SHS International Ltd,
100 Wavertree Boulevard,
Liverpool L7 9PT.
Tel: 0151-228 8161
Fax: 0151-280 5447
seve@shsint.co.uk

Sigma

Sigma Pharmaceuticals plc,
PO Box 233, Watford, Herts
WD2 4EW.
Tel: (01923) 250201
Fax: (01923) 241726

SIMS Portex

SIMS Portex Ltd,
Boundary Rd,
Hythe, Kent CT21 6JL.
Tel: (01303) 260551
Fax: (01303) 266761

Sinclair

Sinclair Pharmaceuticals Ltd,
Borough Rd, Godalming, Surrey
GU7 2AB.
Tel: (01483) 426644
Fax: (01483) 860927

S&N Hlth.

Smith & Nephew Healthcare Ltd,
Healthcare House, Goulton St,
Hull HU3 4DJ.
Tel: (01482) 222200
Fax: (01482) 222211
advice@smith-nephew.com

SK&F

see SmithKline Beecham.

SMA Nutrition

see Wyeth

SmithKline Beecham

SmithKline Beecham
Pharmaceuticals,
SmithKline Beecham plc,
Mundells, Welwyn Garden City,
Herts AL7 1EY.
Tel: (0808) 100 2228
Fax: (0808) 100 8802
ukpharma.customer@sb.com

SmithKline Beecham Healthcare

SmithKline Beecham Consumer
Healthcare,
SB House, Brentford,
Middx TW8 9BD.
Tel: (020) 8560 5151

SNBTS

Scottish National Blood
Transfusion Service,
Protein Fractionation Centre,
Ellen's Glen Rd,
Edinburgh EH17 7QT.
Tel: 0131-536 5700
Fax: 0131-536 5781

Solvay

Solvay Healthcare Ltd,
Mansbridge Rd, West End,
Southampton SO18 3JD.
Tel: (023) 8046 7000
Fax: (023) 8046 5350

Sovereign

Sovereign Medical,
Sovereign House, Miles Gray Rd,
Basildon,
Essex SS14 3FR.
Tel: (01268) 535200
Fax: (01268) 535299

Specials Laboratory

The Specials Laboratory Ltd,
Royal Victoria Infirmary,
Queen Victoria Rd,
Newcastle upon Tyne NE1 4LP.
Tel: 0191-261 0555
Fax: 0191-261 0555

Special Products

Special Products Ltd,
Orion House, 49 High St,
Addlestone, Surrey KT15 1TU
Tel: (01932) 820666
Fax: (01932) 850444
JDeanSPL@aol.com

Squibb

see Bristol-Myers.

SSL

SSL International plc,
Tubiton House,
Oldham OL1 3HS.
Tel: 0161-652 2222
Fax: 0161-626 9090

Stafford-Miller

Stafford-Miller Ltd,
Broadwater Rd,
Welwyn Garden City, Herts
AL7 3SP.
Tel: (01707) 331001
Fax: (01707) 373370

STD Pharmaceutical

STD Pharmaceutical Products,
Fields Yard, Plough Lane,
Hereford HR4 0EL.
Tel: (01432) 353684
Fax: (01432) 371314
enquiries@stdpharm.co.uk

Sterling Health

see SmithKline Beecham
Healthcare

Sterwin

see Sanofi-Synthelabo

Stiefel

Stiefel Laboratories (UK) Ltd,
Holtspur Lane, Wooburn Green,
High Wycombe, Bucks
HP10 0AU.
Tel: (01628) 524966
Fax: (01628) 810021
general@stiefel.co.uk

Strakan

Strakan Ltd,
Buckholm Mill,
Buckholm Mill Brae,
Galashiels TD1 2HB.
Tel: (01896) 668060
Fax: (01896) 668061
medinfo@strakan.com

Stuart

see Zeneca

Sussex

Sussex Pharmaceutical Ltd,
Charlwoods Rd,
East Grinstead,
Sussex RH19 2HL.
Tel: (01342) 311311
Fax: (01342) 313078

Sutherland

Sutherland Health Ltd,
Unit 1, Rivermead, Pipers Way,
Thatcham, Berks RG19 4EP.
Tel: (01635) 874488
Fax: (01635) 877622

Syner-Med

Syner-Med (Pharmaceutical
Products) Ltd,
Airport House, Purley Way,
Croydon, Surrey CR0 0XZ.
Tel: (020) 8410 6400
Fax: (020) 8410 6409
synermedpp@aol.com

Takeda

Takeda UK Ltd,
Takeda House,
The Mercury Centre,
Wycombe Lane,
Wooburn Green, High Wycombe,
Bucks HP10 0HH
Tel: (01628) 537900
Fax: (01628) 526615

Thames

see Cortecs

Thornton & Ross

Thornton & Ross Ltd,
Linthwaite Laboratories,
Huddersfield HD7 5QH.
Tel: (01484) 842217
Fax: (01484) 847301
mail@thorntonross.co.uk

Tillomed

Tillomed Laboratories Ltd,
3 Howard Rd,
Eaton Socon, St Neots,
Cambs PE19 3ET.
Tel: (01480) 402400
Fax: (01480) 402402

Timesco

Timesco of London,
Timesco House
1 Knights Rd, London E16 2AT.
Tel: (020) 7511 1234
Fax: (020) 7511 7888

Trinity

Trinity Pharmaceuticals Ltd,
The Old Exchange,
12 Compton Rd, Wimbledon,
London SW19 7QD.
Tel: (020) 8944 9443
Fax: (020) 8947 9325

TSL

Tissue Science Laboratories plc,
Greyholme House,
49 Victoria Rd, Aldershot,
Hants GU11 1SJ.
Tel: (01252) 333002
Fax: (01252) 333010
enquiries@tissuescience.demon.co.uk

Typharm

Typharm Ltd,
Unit 26, Newtown Business Park,
Albion Close, Poole,
Dorset BH12 3LL.
Tel: (01202) 734100
Fax: (01202) 735100

UCB Pharma

UCB Pharma Ltd,
3 George St, Watford,
Herts WD1 8UH.
Tel: (01923) 211811
Fax: (01923) 229002

Ultrapharm

Ultrapharm Ltd,
1,2,3 Centenary Business Park,
Henley-on-Thames,
Oxon RG9 1DS.
Tel: (01491) 578016
Fax: (01491) 570001

Unigreg

Unigreg Ltd,
Enterprise House,
181–189 Garth Rd, Morden,
Surrey SM4 4LL.
Tel: (020) 8330 1421
Fax: (020) 8330 6812
admin@unigreg.co.uk

Universal

Universal Hospital Supplies,
313 Chase Rd,
London N14 6JH.
Tel: (020) 8920 6207
Fax: (020) 8882 6571

Vernon-Carus

Vernon-Carus Ltd,
Penwortham Mills, Preston,
Lancs PR1 9SN.
Tel: (01772) 744493
Fax: (01772) 748754
mail@vernon-carus.co.uk

Vitaflo

Vitaflo Ltd,
11 Century Building,
Brunswick Business Park,
Liverpool L3 4BL.
Tel: 0151-709 9020
Fax: 0151-709 9727
vitaflo@vitaflo.co.uk

Vitaline

Vitaline Pharmaceuticals UK Ltd,
Rx Court, 5 Church St
Aylesbury, Bucks HP20 2QP.
Tel: (01296) 420600
Fax: (01296) 420700

Vitalograph

Vitalograph Ltd,
Maids Moreton House, Maids
Moreton, Buckingham
MK18 1SW.
Tel: (01280) 822811
Fax: (01280) 823302

Wallace Mfg

Wallace Manufacturing Chemists
Ltd,
Randles Rd, Knowsley Industrial
Park, Merseyside
L34 9HX.
Tel: 0151-549 1255
Fax: 0151-549 1064

Wanskerne

Wanskerne Ltd,
31 High Cross St, St. Austell,
Cornwall PL25 4AN.
Tel: (01726) 69500
Fax: (01726) 69135

Ward

Ward Surgical Appliance Co Ltd,
57A Brightwell Ave, Westcliffe-
on-Sea, Essex SS0 9EB.
Tel: (01702) 354064
Fax: (01702) 354064

Warner Lambert

see Parke-Davis

Willis

S. R. Willis & Sons Ltd,
176 Albion Rd,
London N16 9JR.
Tel: (020) 7254 7373

Windsor

see Boehringer Ingelheim.

W-L

Warner Lambert UK Ltd,
see Parke-Davis.

Wyeth

Wyeth Laboratories,
Huntercombe Lane South,
Taplow, Maidenhead,
Berks SL6 0PH.
Tel: (01628) 604377
Fax: (01628) 666368

Wyvern

Wyvern Medical Ltd,
PO Box 17, Ledbury,
Herefordshire HR8 2ES.
Tel: (01531) 631105
Fax: (01531) 634844

Yamanouchi

Yamanouchi Pharma Ltd,
Yamanouchi House, Pyrford Rd,
West Byfleet, Surrey
KT14 6RA.
Tel: (01932) 345535
Fax: (01932) 353458

Zeal

G. H. Zeal Ltd,
8 Lombard Rd, Merton, London
SW19 3UU.
Tel: (020) 8542 2283
Fax: (020) 8543 7840

Zeneca

AstraZeneca,
King's Court, Water Lane,
Wilmslow, Cheshire SK9 5AZ.
Tel: (0800) 200123
Fax: (01625) 712581

Zurich

see Trinity

'Special-order' Manufacturers

The following **companies** manufacture 'special-order' products: AAH Specials, BCM Specials, Eldon Laboratories, Mandeville, Martindale, Oxford Pharmaceuticals, Rosemont, Special Products, The Specials Laboratory.

Hospital manufacturing units also manufacture 'special-order' products, details may be obtained from any of the centres listed below.

It should be noted that when a product has a licence *the Department of Health recommends that the licensed product should be ordered* unless a specific formulation is required.

England

East Anglian and Oxford
Mr G. Hanson,
Production Manager,
Pharmacy Manufacturing Unit,
The Ipswich Hospital NHS Trust,
Heath Rd,
Ipswich IP4 5PD.
Tel: (01473) 703603
Fax: (01473) 703609
con.hanson@ipsh-tr.anglox.nhs.uk

London
Mr M. Lillywhite,
Regional Technical Pharmacist,
St. Bartholomew's Hospital,
West Smithfield, London
EC1A 7BE.
Tel: (020) 7601 7475/7491
Fax: (020) 7601 7486

Mr P. Forsey,
Production Manager,
Guy's and St. Thomas' Hospital
Trust,
St. Thomas' Hospital,
Lambeth Palace Rd
London SE1 7EH.
Tel: (020) 7922 8316
Fax: (020) 7960 5644

Mr C. Evans,
Principal Pharmacist,
Pharmacy Department,
Lanesborough Wing,
St. George's Hospital,
Blackshaw Rd, Tooting,
London SW17 0QT.
Tel: (020) 8725 1770
Fax: (020) 8725 3690

North West
Mr M.D. Booth,
Production & Aseptic Services
Manager,
Stockport Pharmaceuticals,
Stepping Hill Hospital,
Poplar Grove,
Stockport, Cheshire SK2 7JE.
Tel: 0161-419 5657
Fax: 0161-419 5664

Northern
Mr C Adams,
Principal Pharmacist,
Pharmacy Manufacturing Unit,
Newcastle General Hospital,
Westgate Rd,
Newcastle upon Tyne NE4 6BE.
Tel: 0191-273 8811 ext 22689
Fax: 0191-226 0620
adams.fam@virgin.net

South Western
Mr C. W. Lewis,
Principal Pharmacist,
Manorpark Pharmaceuticals,
Blackberry Hill Hospital,
Manor Rd, Bristol BS16 2EW.
Tel: (0117) 975 4852
Fax: (0117) 9586676
chriswlewis@compuserve.com

Trent
Mr R. W. Brookes,
Production Pharmacist,
Royal Hallamshire Hospital,
Glossop Rd,
Sheffield S10 2JF.
Tel: (0114) 271 3104
Fax: (0114) 271 2783
Roger.Brookes@csuh.nhs.uk

Wessex
Dr E. Brierley,
Production Manager
Regional Manufacturing Unit,
Queen Alexandra Hospital,
Cosham, Portsmouth,
Hants PO6 3LY.
Tel: (02392) 286335
Fax: (02392) 378288

West Midlands
Mr P. G. Williams,
Principal Pharmacist,
Pharmacy Manufacturing Unit,
Queens Hospital,
Burton Hospitals NHS Trust,
Belvedere Rd,
Burton-on-Trent DE13 0RB
Tel: (01283) 566333/511511
Extn 5138
Fax: (01283) 593036

Yorkshire
Dr J. Harwood,
Production Manager,
Pharmacy Manufacturing Unit,
Huddersfield Royal Infirmary,
Lindley, Huddersfield,
West Yorks HD3 3EA.
Tel: (01484) 342421
Fax: (01484) 342074
John.Harwood@hudderfd-tr.northy.nhs.uk

Northern Ireland

Mrs S. M. Millership,
Principal Pharmacist,
Central Pharmaceutical
Production Unit,
CSA Distribution Centre,
77 Boucher Cres, Belfast
BT12 6HU.
Tel: (028) 9055 3407

Scotland

Mr J. A. Cook,
Principal Pharmacist—
Production,
Tayside Pharmaceuticals,
Ninewells Hospital,
Dundee DD1 9SY.
Tel: (01382) 632273
Fax: (01382) 632060

Wales

Mr C. Powell
Principal Pharmacist,
Pharmacy Department,
University Hospital of Wales,
Heath Park, Cardiff CF4 4XW.
Tel: (029) 2074 4828
Fax: (029) 2074 3114
colin.powell@UHW-TR.wales.nhs.uk

Index

Where an entry is followed by more than one page reference, the principal reference is printed in **bold** type. Proprietary (trade) names are printed in *italic* type.

Hydrocortisone acetate
  eye, 475
  rheumatic disease, 457
Hydrocortisone butyrate, 508
Hydrocortisone sodium phosphate, 332
  infusion table, 663
Hydrocortisone sodium succinate, 332
  infusion table, 663
Hydrocortistab, 457
Hydrocortone, 332
Hydrofilm, 686
Hydroflumethiazide, 63
Hydrofluoroalkane propellants, 132, 145
Hydromol, 502
Hydromol Emollient, 503
Hydromorphone, 12, **214**
HydroSaluric, 64
Hydrotalcite, 29, **31**
Hydrous ointment, 501
Hydroxocobalamin, 414
Hydroxyapatite *(Ossopan)*, 433
Hydroxycarbamide, 395
Hydroxychloroquine, 458, **461**
Hydroxycholecalciferol, 439
Hydroxyethylcellulose, 483
Hydroxyprogesterone, 340, **341**
Hydroxyquinolone [ingredient], 508
Hydroxyurea *see* Hydroxycarbamide, 395
Hydroxyzine, 152
Hygroton, 64
Hyoscine butylbromide, 33, **34**
Hyoscine hydrobromide
  nausea and vertigo, 198, **203**
  premedication, 564, **565**
Hypal-2, 692
Hyperactive children, 195
Hyperamine-30, 429
Hypercalcaemia, 350–1, 433
Hypercholesterolaemia, 123
Hyperglycaemia, 313
  coma, 322
Hyperhidrosis, 540
Hyperkalaemia, 421, 424–5, 433
Hyperkeratosis, 514
Hyperlipidaemia, 123
Hyperlipoproteinaemia, ACBS, 679
Hyperlysinaemia, ACBS, 679
Hypermethioninaemia, ACBS, 679
Hyperphosphataemia, 435
Hypersensitivity *see* Allergic disorders
Hypersexuality, 343
Hypertension, 63, 75, **82**, 89, 100
  crisis, 83
  diabetes, 83
  elderly, 83
  in renal disease, 83
  malignant, 83
  poisoning and, 19
  pregnancy, 83
  systolic, 83
Hyperthermia
  poisoning and, 20
Hyperthyroidism *see* Thyrotoxicosis, 326
Hyperuricaemia, 385, 463
Hypnomidate, 562
Hypnotics, 164
  poisoning by, 24
  withdrawal, 163
Hypnovel, 567

Hypocalcaemia, 432
Hypochlorhydria, 59
Hypochlorite, 538
Hypodermic equipment, insulin, 318
Hypodermoclysis, 423, 468
Hypogammaglobulinaemia, 557
Hypoglycaemia, 314, 322
  ACBS, 679
  acute, 322
  chronic, 323
Hypogonadism, 342
Hypoguard products, 324
Hypokalaemia, 424
  diuretics and, 63
Hypolar Retard, 104
Hypomagnesaemia, 434
Hypoparathyroidism, 440
Hypophysectomy, 327
Hypopituitarism, 327, 342, 346
Hypoproteinaemia
  ACBS, 679
  liver disease, 615
Hyposensitisation, 153
Hypostop Gel, 322
Hypotears, 484
Hypotension
  controlled, 560
  poisoning and, 19
  sympathomimetics, 109
Hypothalamic hormones, 348
Hypothermia
  antipsychotics and, 172
  poisoning and, 20
Hypothyroidism, 325
  neonatal, 325
Hypovase preparations, 87
  prostatic hyperplasia, 377
Hypovolaemia, 425
Hypoxaemia, 157
Hypromellose, 483
  eye drops, 483
Hypurin Isophane, 316
  biphasic, 317
Hypurin Lente, 316
Hypurin Neutral, 315
Hypurin Protamine Zinc, 317
Hyteneze, 90
Hytrin preparations, 88
  prostatic hyperplasia, 378

Ibrufhalal, 448
IBS Relief, 35
Ibufem, 448
Ibugel, 469
Ibuleve preparations, 470
Ibumousse, 469
Ibuprofen, 448
  pain, 447, 448
  preparations, 448–9, 470
    topical, 469, 470
  rheumatic disease, 447, **448**
Ibuspray, 469
Ibutop, 470
Ichthammol, 513
Ichthopaste, 691
Ichthyosis, 501
Icthaband, 691
Idarubicin, 389, **391**
  infusion table, 663
Idoxuridine, 288
  mouth, 497
  skin, 532, **533**
Ifosfamide, 387, **388**
  infusion table, 663
Ikorel, 106
Ilosone, 268
Ilube, 483
Imazin XL, 99
Imdur, 99

Imidapril, 91
  see also ACE inhibitors
Imidazole antifungal drugs, 283–4
Imiglucerase, 444
  infusion table, 663
Imigran preparations, 220
Imipenem, 262
  infusion table, 663
Imipramine, 185, **188**
Imiquimod, 524
Immukin, 558
Immune interferon *see* Interferons, gamma, 558
Immunisation, 541
  international travel, 559
  schedule, 542
Immunity
  active, 541
  passive, 543
Immunodeficiency, 557
  syndrome, acquired, 289
Immunoglobulins, 543, **555**
  anti-D (Rh$_0$), 558
  cytomegalovirus, 557
  hepatitis B, 557
  normal, 556
  rabies, 557
  tetanus, 557
  varicella-zoster, 557
Immunoprin, 398
Immunostimulants, 401
Immunosuppressants
  malignant disease, 399
  myasthenia gravis, 466
  rheumatic disease, 458, 461
  transplant rejection, 397
Imodium preparations, 45
Impetigo, 250, 528
Implanon, 374
Impotence, 342, **381**
Imunovir, 289
Imuran, 398
Inadine, 686
Incontinence, urinary, 378
Indapamide, **64**, 65
Inderal preparations, 77
Inderetic, 77
Inderex, 77
Indermil, 536
Indian hemp *see* Cannabis regulations, 7
Indinavir, 290, **293**
Indocid preparations, 452
  PDA, 362
Indolar SR, 452
Indomax preparations, 452
Indometacin, 452
  ductus closure, 362
  gout, 463
  premature labour, 363
  preparations, 452
    injection, 362
  rheumatic disease, 447, **452**
Indomethacin *see* Indometacin
Indomod, 452
Indoramin, 87
  cardiovascular, 87
  urinary tract, 377
Indotard, 452
Infacol, 33
Infadrops, 208
Infanrix, 545
Infanrix-Hib, ix
InfaSoy, 672
Infatrini, 672
Infections
  amoebic, 306
  antisera, 543, 555
  bladder, 282
    mycotic, 381

Approximate conversions and units

lb	kg		stones	kg		mL	fl oz
1	0.45		1	6.35		50	1.8
2	0.91		2	12.70		100	3.5
3	1.36		3	19.05		150	5.3
4	1.81		4	25.40		200	7.0
5	2.27		5	31.75		500	17.6
6	2.72		6	38.10		1000	35.2
7	3.18		7	44.45			
8	3.63		8	50.80			
9	4.08		9	57.15			
10	4.54		10	63.50			
11	4.99		11	69.85			
12	5.44		12	76.20			
13	5.90		13	82.55			
14	6.35		14	88.90			
			15	95.25			

Length

1 metre (m)	= 1000 millimetres (mm)
1 centimetre (cm)	= 10 mm
1 inch (in)	= 25.4 mm
1 foot (ft) = 12 inches	= 304.8 mm

Mass

1 kilogram (kg)	= 1000 grams (g)
1 gram (g)	= 1000 milligrams (mg)
1 milligram (mg)	= 1000 micrograms
1 microgram	= 1000 nanograms
1 nanogram	= 1000 picograms

Volume

1 litre	= 1000 millilitres (mL)
1 millilitre (1 mL)	= 1000 microlitres
1 pint	≈ 568 mL

Other units

1 kilocalorie (kcal)	= 4186.8 joules (J)
1000 kilocalories (kcal)	= 4.1868 megajoules (MJ)
1 megajoule (MJ)	= 238.8 kilocalories (kcal)
1 millimetre of mercury (mmHg)	= 133.3 pascals (Pa)
1 kilopascal (kPa)	= 7.5 mmHg (pressure)

Prescribing in children

The **percentage method** below may be used to calculate paediatric doses of commonly prescribed drugs that have a wide margin between the therapeutic and the toxic dose.

	Ideal body-weight		Height		Body-surface	Percentage of adult
Age	kg	lb	cm	inch	m²	dose
Newborn*	3.5	7.7	50	20	0.23	12.5
1 month*	4.2	9	55	22	0.26	14.5
3 months*	5.6	12	59	23	0.32	18
6 months	7.7	17	67	26	0.40	22
1 year	10	22	76	30	0.47	25
3 years	15	33	94	37	0.62	33
5 years	18	40	108	42	0.73	40
7 years	23	51	120	47	0.88	50
12 years	39	86	148	58	1.25	75
Adult						
Male	68	150	173	68	1.80	100
Female	56	123	163	64	1.60	100

* The figures relate to full term and not preterm infants who may need reduced dosage according to their clinical condition.

Plasma-drug concentrations in the BNF are expressed in mass units per litre (e.g. mg/litre). The approximate equivalent in terms of amount of substance units (e.g. micromol/litre) is given in brackets.

Recommended wording of cautionary and advisory labels

For details see Appendix 9

1   Warning. May cause drowsiness
2   Warning. May cause drowsiness. If affected do not drive or operate machinery. Avoid alcoholic drink
3   Warning. May cause drowsiness. If affected do not drive or operate machinery
4   Warning. Avoid alcoholic drink
5   Do not take indigestion remedies at the same time of day as this medicine
6   Do not take iron preparations or indigestion remedies at the same time of day as this medicine
7   Do not take milk, iron preparations or indigestion remedies at the same time of day as this medicine
8   Do not stop taking this medicine except on your doctor's advice
9   Take at regular intervals. Complete the prescribed course unless otherwise directed
10 Warning. Follow the printed instructions you have been given with this medicine
11 Avoid exposure of skin to direct sunlight or sun lamps
12 Do not take anything containing aspirin while taking this medicine
13 Dissolve or mix with water before taking
14 This medicine may colour the urine
15 Caution flammable: keep away from fire or flames
16 Allow to dissolve under the tongue. Do not transfer from this container. Keep tightly closed. Discard 8 weeks after opening
17 Do not take more than ... in 24 hours
18 Do not take more than ... in 24 hours or ... in any one week
19 Warning. Causes drowsiness which may continue the next day. If affected do not drive or operate machinery. Avoid alcoholic drink
21 ... with or after food
22 ... half to one hour before food
23 ... an hour before food or on an empty stomach
24 ... sucked or chewed
25 ... swallowed whole, not chewed
26 ... dissolved under the tongue
27 ... with plenty of water
28 To be spread thinly ...
29 Do not take more than 2 at any one time. Do not take more than 8 in 24 hours
30 Do not take with any other paracetamol products
31 Contains aspirin and paracetamol. Do not take with any other paracetamol products
32 Contains aspirin
33 Contains an aspirin-like medicine